Instructional Course Lectures

Volume 59 2010

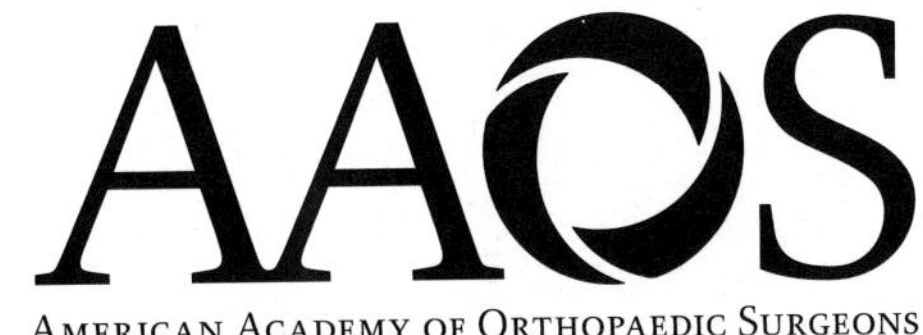

Instructional Course Lectures

Volume 59 2010

Edited by
Mary I. O'Connor, MD
Chair and Associate Professor
Department of Orthopedic Surgery
Mayo Clinic
Jacksonville, Florida

Kenneth A. Egol, MD
Professor and Vice Chairman
Department of Orthopaedic Surgery
Hospital for Joint Diseases
NYU Langone Medical Center
New York, New York

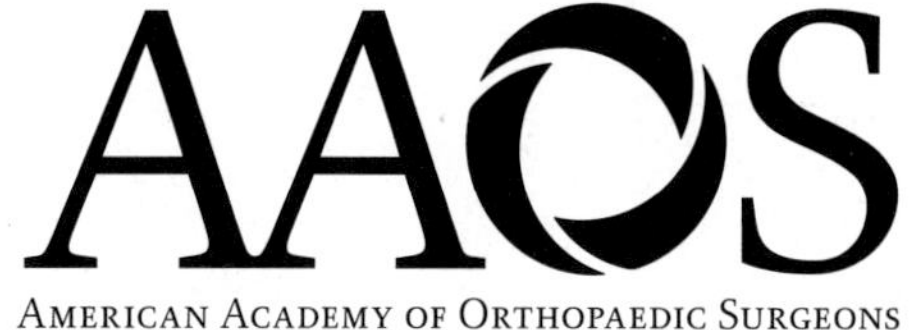

Published 2010 by the

American Academy
of Orthopaedic Surgeons
6300 North River Road
Rosemont, IL 60018

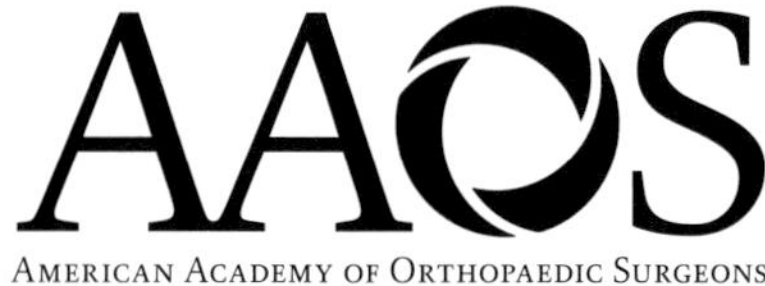

Instructional Course Lectures Volume 59
American Academy of Orthopaedic Surgeons

The material presented in the *Instructional Course Lectures 59* has been made available by the American Academy of Orthopaedic Surgeons for educational purposes only. This material is not intended to present the only, or necessarily best, methods or procedures for the medical situations discussed, but rather is intended to represent an approach, view, statement, or opinion of the author(s) or producer(s), which may be helpful to others who face similar situations.

Some drugs or medical devices demonstrated in Academy courses or described in Academy print or electronic publications have not been cleared by the Food and Drug Administration (FDA) or have been cleared for specific uses only. The FDA has stated that it is the responsibility of the physician to determine the FDA clearance status of each drug or device he or she wishes to use in clinical practice.

Furthermore, any statements about commercial products are solely the opinion(s) of the author(s) and do not represent an Academy endorsement or evaluation of these products. These statements may not be used in advertising or for any commercial purpose.

First Edition

ISBN 978-0-89203-644-8

Printed in the USA

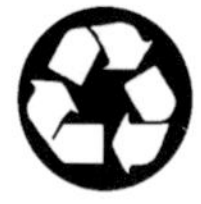

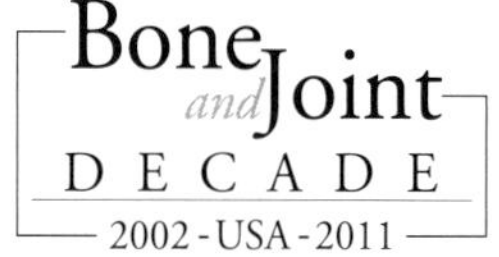

Contributors

Omar Abdul-Hadi, MD, Attending Surgeon, Southern Oregon Orthopedics, Medford, Oregon

Jeffrey S. Abrams, MD, Clinical Associate Professor, Department of Orthopaedic Surgery, Seton Hall University, School of Medical Education, Orange, New Jersey, Associate Director, Princeton Orthopaedic and Rehabilitation Associates, Princeton, New Jersey

Julie E. Adams, MD, Assistant Professor of Orthopaedic Surgery, Department of Orthopaedic Surgery, University of Minnesota, Minneapolis, Minnesota

Behrooz A. Akbarnia, MD, Clinical Professor, Department of Orthopaedics, University of California, San Diego, La Jolla, California

Sahal Altamimi, MD, FRCSC, Fellow, Section of Orthopaedics, University of Manitoba, Pan Am Clinic, Winnipeg, Manitoba, Canada

Annunziato Amendola, MD, Professor, University of Iowa Hospitals and Clinics, Director, University of Iowa Sports Medicine Center, Department of Orthopaedic Surgery and Rehabilitation, University of Iowa Hospitals and Clinics, Iowa City, Iowa

Richard L. Angelo, MD, Clinical Professor of Orthopedics, Department of Orthopedics, University of Washington, Seattle, Washington

Jeffrey O. Anglen, MD, FACS, Professor and Chairman, Department of Orthopaedic Surgery, Indiana University, Indianapolis, Indiana

Robert A. Arciero, MD, Professor of Orthopaedic Surgery, Department of Orthopaedics, University of Connecticut, Farmington, Connecticut

George S. Athwal, MD, FRCSC, Consultant and Assistant Professor, Hand and Upper Limb Centre, University of Western Ontario, London, Ontario, Canada

Matthew S. Austin, MD, Assistant Professor of Orthopaedic Surgery, Department of Orthopaedic Surgery, Thomas Jefferson University Hospital, The Rothman Institute, Philadelphia, Pennsylvania

Michael S. Bahk, MD, Shoulder and Elbow Surgery Fellow, The Rothman Institute, Jefferson Medical College, Philadelphia, Pennsylvania

Craig S. Bartlett III, MD, Assistant Professor of Orthopaedics, Department of Orthopaedics and Rehabilitation, The University of Vermont, Burlington, Vermont

Paul E. Beaulé, MD, FRCSC, Associate Professor, Head, Adult Reconstruction, Division of Orthopaedics, University of Ottawa, Ottawa, Ontario, Canada

Richard A. Berger, MD, Assistant Professor of Orthopedic Surgery, Department of Orthopedic Surgery, Rush Medical College, Chicago, Illinois

Jack M. Bert, MD, Adjunct Clinical Professor, University of Minnesota School of Medicine, Minneapolis, Minnesota, Summit Orthopedics, St. Paul, Minnesota

J. Sybil Biermann, MD, Associate Professor, Department of Orthopaedics/Oncology, University of Michigan, Ann Arbor, Michigan

Laurel C. Blakemore, MD, Chief of Orthopaedic Surgery and Sports Medicine, Children's National Medical Center, Associate Professor, George Washington University, Washington, DC

Pascal Boileau, MD, Professor and Chair, Department of Orthopaedic Surgery and Sports , Traumatology, L'Archet 2 Hospital, University of Nice Sophia Antipolis, Nice, France

Peter M. Bonutti, MD, Director, Bonutti Clinic, Effingham, Illinois

Joseph A. Bosco III, MD, Vice Chair and Associate Professor of Orthopaedic Surgery, New York University Hospital for Joint Diseases, New York, New York

James P. Bradley, MD, Clinical Professor, Department of Orthopaedic Surgery, University of Pittsburgh Medical Center, Burke and Bradley Orthopedics, Pittsburgh, Pennsylvania

William D. Bugbee, MD, Attending Physician, Scripps Clinic, La Jolla, California, Associate Professor, University of California, San Diego, California

Stephen S. Burkhart, MD, Director, Shoulder Fellowship, The San Antonio Orthopaedic Group, San Antonio, Texas

Robert Burks, MD, Professor of Orthopedic Surgery, University of Utah, Salt Lake City, Utah

John J. Callaghan, MD, Lawrence and Marilyn Dorr Chair, Department of Orthopaedics and Rehabilitation, University of Iowa, Iowa City, Iowa

Robert M. Campbell Jr, MD, Attending Physician, Division of Orthopaedic Surgery, The Children's Hospital of Philadelphia, Philadelphia, Pennsylvania

John T. Capo, MD, Associate Professor, Chief, Hand and Microvascular Surgery, Department of Orthopaedics, New Jersey Medical School, Newark, New Jersey

Alessandro Castagna, MD, Department of Orthopaedics, IRCCS Istituto Clinico Humanitas, Milan, Italy

Isabelle Catelas, PhD, Associate Professor and Canada Research Chair (Tier II), Mechanical Engineering, Department of Surgery, University of Ottawa, Ottawa, Ontario, Canada

Sergio L. Checchia, MD, Professor, Department of Orthopaedics, Shoulder and Elbow Service, Santa Casa Hospitals and School of Medicine, Sao Paulo, Brazil

Eli Chen, MD, PhD, Resident, Department of Orthopaedic Surgery, Long Island Jewish Medical Center, New Hyde Park, New York

J. Chris Coetzee, MD, FRCSC, Minnesota Sports Medicine and Twin Cities Orthopedics, Minneapolis, Minnesota

Brian J. Cole, MD, MBA, Professor, Department of Orthopaedic Surgery, Department of Anatomy and Cell Biology, Section Head, Cartilage Restoration Center at Rush, Rush University Medical Center, Chicago, Illinois

Patrick M. Connor, MD, The Shoulder and Elbow Center, The Sports Medicine Center, OrthoCarolina, Charlotte, North Carolina

CAPT Dana C. Covey, MD, MC, USN, Chairman, Department of Orthopaedic Surgery, Naval Medical Center, San Diego, California

Craig J. Della Valle, MD, Associate Professor, Department of Orthopaedic Surgery, Rush University Medical Center, Chicago, Illinois

David G. Dennison, MD, Consultant, Department of Orthopedic Surgery, Mayo Clinic, Rochester, Minnesota

James K. DeOrio, MD, Associate Professor, Department of Orthopedics, Duke University, Durham, North Carolina

Kyle F. Dickson, MD, MBA, Professor, Department of Orthopaedic Surgery, University of Texas Medical School, Houston, Chief of Trauma, Memorial Hermann Hospital, Houston, Texas

David R. Diduch, MD, Professor, Head Orthopaedic Team Physician, Department of Orthopaedic Surgery, University of Virginia, Charlottesville, Virginia

John P. Dormans, MD, FACS, Chief, Division of Orthopaedic Surgery, The Children's Hospital of Philadelphia, Philadelphia, Pennsylvania

Paul J. Dougherty, MD, Associate Professor and Residency Director, Department of Orthopaedic Surgery, University of Michigan, Ann Arbor, Michigan

Clive P. Duncan, MD, MSc, FRCSC, Professor, Division of Lower Limb Reconstruction and Oncology, Department of Orthopaedics, University of British Columbia, Vancouver, British Columbia, Canada

Thomas A. Einhorn, MD, Chairman, Department of Orthopaedic Surgery, Boston University Medical Center, Boston, Massachusetts

Richard D. Ferkel, MD, Director of Sports Medicine and Attending Surgeon, Southern California Orthopaedic Institute, Van Nuys, California, Assistant Clinical Professor of Orthopaedic Surgery, University of California, Los Angeles, California

Diego L. Fernandez, MD, Professor of Orthopedic Surgery, Department of Orthopedic Surgery, University of Bern, Lindenhof Hospital, Bern, Switzerland

Evan L. Flatow, MD, Lasker Professor and Chairman, Department of Orthopaedic Surgery, Mount Sinai School of Medicine, New York, New York

Frank J. Frassica, MD, Robert A. Robinson Professor of Orthopaedics and Oncology, Department of Orthopaedic Surgery, Johns Hopkins University, Baltimore, Maryland

John P. Fulkerson, MD, Orthopedic Associates of Hartford, Clinical Professor, University of Connecticut School of Medicine, Farmington, Connecticut

Leesa M. Galatz, MD, Associate Professor, Shoulder and Elbow Service, Department of Orthopedic Surgery, Washington University, Barnes Jewish Hospital, Saint Louis, Missouri

Rajiv Gandhi, MD, FRCSC, Assistant Professor, Division of Orthopaedic Surgery, University of Toronto, Toronto Western Hospital, University Health Network, Toronto, Ontario, Canada

Donald S. Garbuz, MD, MHSc, FRCSC, Associate Professor, Division of Lower Limb Reconstruction and Oncology, Department of Orthopaedics, University of British Columbia, Vancouver, British Columbia, Canada

Mark Glazebrook, MSc, PhD, MD, FRCSC, Assistant Professor, Division of Orthopaedics, Dalhousie University, Halifax, Nova Scotia, Canada

Robert C. Grumet, MD, Fellow, Sports Medicine, Department of Orthopaedic Surgery, Rush University Medical Center, Chicago, Illinois

Janet P. Haas, DNSc, RN, CIC, Director, Department of Infection Prevention and Control, Westchester Medical Center, Valhalla, New York

George J. Haidukewych, MD, Departments of Orthopaedic Trauma and Adult Reconstruction, Florida Orthopaedic Institute, University of South Florida, Tampa, Florida

Hill Hastings II, MD, Clinical Professor of Orthopaedic Surgery, Indiana University School of Medicine, The Indiana Hand Center, Indianapolis, Indiana

James R. Hebl, MD, Associate Professor, Mayo Clinic College of Medicine, Consultant, Department of Anesthesiology, Mayo Clinic, Rochester, Minnesota

Laurence Higgins, MD, Chief of Sports Medicine and Harvard Shoulder Service, Associate Professor, Harvard Medical School, Department of Orthopaedics, Brigham and Women's Hospital, Boston, Massachusetts

Ginger E. Holt, MD, Assistant Professor of Orthopaedics and Rehabilitation, Vanderbilt Medical Center, Vanderbilt Orthopaedic Institute, Nashville, Tennessee

Terese T. Horlocker, MD, Professor of Anesthesiology and Orthopedics, Mayo College of Medicine, Consultant, Departments of Anesthesiology and Orthopedics, Mayo Clinic, Rochester, Minnesota

Daniel S. Horwitz, MD, Associate Professor, Orthopaedic Trauma, University of Utah Orthopaedic Center, Salt Lake City, Utah

Jerry I. Huang, MD, Assistant Professor, Department of Orthopaedics and Sports Medicine, University of Washington Medical Center, Seattle, Washington

Christopher D. Ingersoll, PhD, ATC, FACSM, Joe H. Gieck Professor of Sports Medicine, Chair, Department of Human Services, University of Virginia, Charlottesville, Virginia

Joshua J. Jacobs, MD, Professor and Chairman, Department of Orthopaedic Surgery, Rush University Medical Center, Chicago, Illinois

Andrew Jawa, MD, Assistant Professor, Department of Orthopaedics, Boston Medical Center, Boston, Massachusetts

Jesse B. Jupiter, MD, Hansjorg Wyss AO Professor of Orthopedic Surgery, Harvard Medical School, Director, Hand and Upper Extremity Service, Massachusetts General Hospital, Boston, Massachusetts

David M. Kalainov, MD, Associate Professor of Clinical Orthopaedic Surgery, Northwestern University, Feinberg School of Medicine, Chicago, Illinois

Brian S. Kern, MD, Sports Medicine Fellow, Department of Sports Medicine, Southern California Orthopaedic Institute, Van Nuys, California

Hanns-Peter Knaebel, MD, MBA, Executive Vice President, Department of Clinical Science, Aesculap, Tuttlingen, Germany

Philip J. Kregor, MD, Jeffrey W. Mast Chair in Orthopaedic Trauma and Hip, Surgery, Associate Professor and Director, Vanderbilt Orthopaedic Institute, Nashville, Tennessee

Aaron J. Krych, MD, Orthopedic Surgery Resident, Department of Orthopedic Surgery, Mayo Clinic College of Medicine, Rochester, Minnesota

Erik N. Kubiak, MD, Assistant Professor, Trauma Orthopaedics, University of Utah Orthopaedic Center, University of Utah, Salt Lake City, Utah

John E. Kuhn, MD, Associate Professor and Chief of Shoulder Surgery, Vanderbilt Sports Medicine, Vanderbilt University Medical Center, Nashville, Tennessee

Amy L. Ladd, MD, Professor of Orthopaedics, Chief of Chase Hand Center, Chase Hand Center Department of Orthopaedics, Stanford University, Stanford, California

Jonathan Lam, MD, PhD, Hand and Upper Extremity Surgeon, Hospital for Special Surgery, New York, New York

Laura W. Lee, MD, MBA, Associate Professor, Department of Physical Medicine and Rehabilitation, University of Virginia School of Medicine, Charlottesville, Virginia

L. Scott Levin, MD, FACS, Professor of Orthopaedic and Plastic Surgery, Chief of Plastic Surgery, Department of Surgery, Duke University Medical Center, Durham, North Carolina

William N. Levine, MD, Vice Chairman and Professor, Department of Orthopaedic Surgery, Columbia University Medical Center, New York, New York

Valerae O. Lewis, MD, Associate Professor and Section Chief, Department of Orthopaedic Oncology, MD Anderson Cancer Center, University of Texas, Houston, Texas

Jess H. Lonner, MD, Director of Knee Replacement Surgery, Booth Bartolozzi Balderston Orthopaedics, Pennsylvania Hospital, Philadelphia, Pennsylvania

Peter B. MacDonald, MD, FRCS, Professor and Head Section of Orthopaedic Surgery, University of Manitoba, Winnipeg, Manitoba, Canada

Nizar N. Mahomed, MD, ScD, FRCSC, Head, Division of Orthopaedic Surgery, Director, Musculoskeletal Health and Arthritis Program, University Health Network, Toronto Western Hospital, Toronto, Ontario, Canada

Bassam A. Masri, MD, FRCSC, Professor and Chairman, Department of Orthopaedics, University of British Columbia, Vancouver, British Columbia, Canada

Wadih Y. Matar, MD, MSc, FRCSC, Department of Orthopaedics, The Rothman Institute of Orthopaedics at Jefferson, Philadelphia, Pennsylvania

CDR Michael T. Mazurek, MD, MC, USN, Residency Program Director, Department of Orthopaedic Surgery, Naval Medical Center, San Diego, California

Mike S. McGrath, MD, Fellow, Rubin Institute for Advanced Orthopedics, Sinai Hospital of Baltimore, Baltimore, Maryland

John B. Medley, PhD, PEng, Professor, Department of Mechanical and Mechatronics Engineering, University of Waterloo, Waterloo, Ontario, Canada

William M. Mihalko, MD, PhD, Associate Professor, Department of Orthopaedic Surgery, Campbell Clinic, University of Tennessee, Memphis, Tennessee

Berton R. Moed, MD, Professor and Chairman Department of Orthopaedic Surgery, Saint Louis University School of Medicine, Saint Louis, Missouri

Michael A. Mont, MD, Director, Center for Joint Preservation and Replacement, Rubin Institute for Advanced Orthopedics, Sinai Hospital of Baltimore, Baltimore, Maryland

Stephen J. Morgan, MD, Associate Director of Orthopaedics, Professor and Orthopaedic Residency Program Director, Department of Orthopaedics, Denver Health Medical Center and University of Colorado Denver School of Medicine, Denver, Colorado

Monica Morman, MD, Shoulder Fellow, Harvard Shoulder Service, Department of Orthopaedics, Brigham and Women's Hospital, Boston, Massachusetts

Michael P. Mott, MD, Associate Professor, Division Head of Musculoskeletal Oncology, Department of Orthopaedic Surgery, Henry Ford Hospital, Detroit, Michigan

Peter M. Murray, MD, Director for Education, Professor of Orthopedic Surgery, Department of Orthopedic Surgery, Mayo Clinic, Jacksonville, Florida

Stephen A. Mussett, MBChB, FRCSC, Fellow, Arthroplasty and Reconstructive Surgery, Department of Orthopaedics, The Ottawa Hospital, Ottawa, Ontario, Canada

Soheil Najibi, MD, PhD, Senior Staff Physician, Department of Orthopaedic Surgery, Henry Ford Health System, Detroit, Michigan

Arvind D. Nana, MD, Associate Professor, Department of Orthopaedic Surgery, University of North Texas Health Science Center, Fort Worth, Texas

Shahryar Noordin, MBBS, FCPS, Clinical Fellow, Division of Lower Limb Reconstruction and Oncology, Department of Orthopaedics, University of British Columbia, Vancouver, British Columbia, Canada

Wendy M. Novicoff, PhD, Manager, Orthopaedic Surgery, Assistant Professor of Public Health Sciences, University of Virginia Health System, Charlottesville, Virginia

A. Lee Osterman, MD, Professor of Orthopedics and Hand Surgery, Department of Orthopedic Surgery, Thomas Jefferson University Hospital, Philadelphia, Pennsylvania

Mark W. Pagnano, MD, Associate Professor of Orthopedic Surgery, Mayo Clinic College of Medicine, Consultant, Department of Orthopedic Surgery, Mayo Clinic, Rochester, Minnesota

Nata Parnes, MD, Fellow, Department of Orthopaedic Surgery, Massachusetts General Hospital, Boston, Massachusetts

Bradford O. Parsons, MD, Assistant Professor, Department of Orthopaedic Surgery, Mount Sinai Medical Center, New York, New York

Theodore W. Parsons III, MD, FACS, Professor and Breech Chair, Department of Orthopaedic Surgery, Henry Ford Hospital, Detroit, Michigan

Javad Parvizi, MD, FRCS, Professor, Department of Orthopedics, The Rothman Institute of Orthopedics, Thomas Jefferson University, Philadelphia, Pennsylvania

Cecilia Pascual-Garrido, MD, Research Fellow, Department of Orthopaedic Surgery, Rush University Medical Center, Chicago, Illinois

Terrance Peabody, MD, Chief, Section of Orthopaedic Surgery and Rehabilitation Medicine, Simon and Kalt Families Professor of Surgery, Department of Orthopaedic Surgery, University of Chicago, Chicago, Illinois

Col Elisha T. Powell IV, MD, MC, USAF (Ret), Department of Orthopaedic Surgery and Sports Medicine, Providence Alaska Medical Center and Alaska Regional Hospital, Anchorage, Alaska

CDR Matthew T. Provencher, MD, MC, USN, Associate Professor of Surgery, Director of Sports Surgery, Naval Medical Center, San Diego, California

Daniel E. Redziniak, MD, Department of Orthopaedic Surgery, Orthopaedic and Sports Medicine Center, Annapolis, Maryland

Mikel L. Reilingh, MD, PhD Candidate, Department of Orthopaedic Surgery, Academic Medical Center, Amsterdam, The Netherlands

Mark C. Reilly, MD, Associate Professor and Co-Chief of Orthopaedic Trauma Service, Department of Orthopaedics, New Jersey Medical School, Newark, New Jersey

Yong Girl Rhee, MD, Professor and Chairman, Chief, Shoulder and Elbow Clinic, Department of Orthopaedic Surgery, Kyung Hee University Hospital, Seoul, Korea

Col Mark W. Richardson, MD, MC, USAF, Chairman Emeritus, Department of Orthopaedic Surgery, Wilford Hall USAF Medical Center, San Antonio, Texas

David C. Ring, MD, PhD, Director of Research, Hand and Upper Extremity Service, Division of Orthopaedic Surgery, Massachusetts General Hospital, Boston, Massachusetts

Andrew W. Ritting, MD, Resident, Department of Orthopaedic Surgery, University of Connecticut Health Center, Farmington, Connecticut

Anthony A. Romeo, MD, Professor, Department of Orthopaedic Surgery, Head, Section of Shoulder and Elbow, Rush University Medical Center, Chicago, Illinois

David S. Ruch, MD, Director of Hand and Upper Extremity Surgery, Division of Orthopaedic Surgery, Duke University Medical Center, Durham, North Carolina

Khaled J. Saleh, MD, MSc, FRCSC, Professor and Chair of Orthopaedic Surgery, Director of Clinical and Translational Research, Southern Illinois University, Springfield, Illinois

Benjamin Sanofsky, BA, Research Assistant, Harvard Shoulder Service, Department of Orthopaedics, Brigham and Women's Hospital, Boston, Massachusetts

Susan A. Scherl, MD, Associate Professor of Orthopaedic Surgery, Department of Orthopaedics, The University of Nebraska, Omaha, Nebraska

Thomas P. Schmalzried, MD, Medical Director, Joint Replacement Institute, Saint Vincent Medical Center, Los Angeles, California

Andrew H. Schmidt, MD, Associate Professor, University of Minnesota, Department of Orthopedic Surgery, Hennepin County Medical Center, Minneapolis, Minnesota

Herbert S. Schwartz, MD, Professor of Orthopaedic Surgery, Vanderbilt University, Vanderbilt Orthopaedic Institute, Nashville, Tennessee

Richard D. Scott, MD, Professor of Orthopaedic Surgery, Harvard Medical School, Department of Orthopaedic Surgery, Brigham and Women's and New England Baptist Hospitals, Boston, Massachusetts

Pierce E. Scranton Jr, MD, Associate Clinical Professor, Department of Orthopaedics, University of Washington, Evergreen Healthcare Center, Kirkland, Washington

Nicholas A. Sgaglione, MD, Associate Clinical Professor of Surgery, Associate Chairman, Department of Orthopaedics, North Shore–Long Island Jewish Medical Center, Manhasset, New York

Shahin Sheibani-Rad, MD, Research Fellow, Orthopaedic Surgery, Department of Orthopaedic Surgery, Maimonides Medical Center, Brooklyn, New York

Alexander Y. Shin, MD, Professor of Orthopedic Surgery, Department of Orthopedic Surgery, Mayo Clinic, Rochester, Minnesota

Craig D. Silverton, DO, Vice Chairman, Department of Orthopaedic Surgery, Henry Ford Hospital, Detroit, Michigan

Anshu Singh, MD, Shoulder and Elbow Surgeon, Kaiser Permanente Medical Center, San Diego, California

James D. Slover, MD, Assistant Professor of Orthopaedic Surgery, Department of Orthopaedics, New York University Hospital for Joint Diseases, New York, New York

David A. Sonnabend, MD, BSc(Med), FRACS, Professor, Department of Orthopaedic and Traumatic Surgery University of Sydney, Sydney, New South Wales, Australia

James W. Stone, MD, Assistant Clinical Professor, Department of Orthopaedic Surgery, Medical College of Wisconsin, Milwaukee, Wisconsin

John S. Taras, MD, Associate Professor, Department of Orthopaedic Surgery, Thomas Jefferson University Hospital and Drexel University, Chief, Division of Hand Surgery, Drexel University, Philadelphia, Pennsylvania

Michael E. Torchia, MD, Consultant, Department of Orthopedic Surgery, Mayo Clinic, Rochester, Minnesota

Alfred J. Tria Jr, MD, Clinical Professor of Orthopaedic Surgery, Robert Wood Johnson Department of Orthopaedics, Robert Wood Johnson Medical School, New Brunswick, New Jersey

Rahul Vaidya, MD, Chief of Orthopaedics, Department of Orthopaedic Surgery, Detroit Receiving Hospital, Detroit, Michigan

Christiaan J.A. van Bergen, MD, PhD Candidate, Department of Orthopaedic Surgery, Academic Medical Center, Amsterdam, The Netherlands

C. Niek van Dijk, MD, PhD, Professor in Orthopaedics, Head, Orthopaedic Department, Academic Medical Center, Amsterdam, The Netherlands

Thomas F. Varecka, MD, Assistant Professor, University of Minnesota, Department of Orthopaedic Surgery, Hennepin County Medical Center, Minneapolis, Minnesota

Eugene R. Viscusi, MD, Director of Acute Pain Management, Department of Anesthesiology, Thomas Jefferson University, Philadelphia, Pennsylvania

Mark S. Vrahas, MD, Partners Chief of Orthopaedic Trauma Services, Department of Orthopaedic Surgery, Brigham and Women's Hospital, Massachusetts General Hospital, Boston, Massachusetts

Xin-Qun Wang, MS, Senior Biostatistician, Department of Public Health Services, University of Virginia, Charlottesville, Virginia

Kristy L. Weber, MD, Associate Professor, Department of Orthopaedic Surgery, Johns Hopkins, Baltimore, Maryland

Gerald R. Williams Jr, MD, Professor of Orthopaedic Surgery, Chief of Shoulder and Elbow Service, The Rothman Institute, Jefferson Medical College, Philadelphia, Pennsylvania

Jennifer Moriatis Wolf, MD, Assistant Professor of Orthopaedic Surgery, Department of Orthopaedic Surgery, University of Colorado, Denver, Colorado

Scott W. Wolfe, MD, Professor of Orthopaedics and Chief of Hand Surgery, Hospital for Special Surgery, Weill Medical College of Cornell University, New York, New York

Robert W. Wysocki, MD, Hand, Upper Extremity, and Microvascular Surgery Fellow, Division of Orthopaedic Surgery, Duke University Medical Center, Durham, North Carolina

Michael J. Yaszemski, MD, PhD, Professor of Orthopedic Surgery and Biomedical Engineering, Director of Tissue Engineering and Biomaterials Laboratory, Department of Orthopedic Surgery, Department of Physiology and Biomedical Engineering, Mayo Clinic, Rochester, Minnesota

Maartje Zengerink, MD, PhD Candidate, Department of Orthopaedic Surgery, Academic Medical Center, Amsterdam, The Netherlands

Michael G. Zywiel, MD, Fellow, Center for Joint Preservation and Replacement, Rubin Institute for Advanced Orthopedics, Sinai Hospital of Baltimore, Baltimore, Maryland

Preface

We became orthopedic surgeons to serve our patients. Our continuing goal is to be highly skilled and compassionate physicians who apply the most effective treatments and achieve optimal results. This objective requires our personal commitment to lifelong learning to stay abreast of the advances in our profession.

Instructional Course Lectures, Volume 59 will assist you in achieving this goal. It represents a collection of lectures from experts in our profession. These lectures focus on the clinical importance of current research and treatments, and the practical applications of these findings. In essence, they translate the "bench" of cutting-edge research to the "bedside" of your practice. The chapters in this volume were written with this same focus on clinical importance and application.

I am grateful to the many individuals who have contributed to this publication. Of greatest importance are the more than 150 authors of the 49 chapters in this volume. These individuals have given of their intellect, experience, and time to create outstanding educational content. Moreover, these chapters were written and published within 1 year of their presentation at the 2009 Annual Meeting of the American Academy of Orthopaedic Surgeons. With the increasing demands of our practices, adhering to such a stringent publication deadline demonstrates the strong professional commitment of these authors.

Volume 59 would not have been possible without the dedicated AAOS staff including Marilyn L. Fox, PhD, director of the AAOS publications department, Lisa Claxton Moore, managing editor for the Instructional Course Lecture series, and Kathleen A. Anderson, senior editor. The material for the DVD, which enhances the educational content of the ICL volume, was organized and edited by Reid L. Stanton, manager, electronic media programs, and his staff. Finally, I want to personally thank Kathie Niesen for the support and guidance given to me as a member and as the Chair of the AAOS Instructional Courses Committee. Kathie is committed to excellence in managing the instructional course lectures program and is a key reason for its success.

It has been my privilege to serve as Chair of the AAOS 2009 Instructional Courses Committee and as the editor of ICL 59. I am grateful to Anthony Rankin, MD, Past President of the AAOS, for these opportunities. I would like to acknowledge the dedication of the Instruction Courses Committee, which included Kenneth A. Egol, MD; Frederick M. Azar, MD; Paul J. Duwelius, MD; Paul Tornetta III, MD; James D. Heckman, MD; and Dempsey S. Springfield, MD. Dr. Egol served as the assistant editor for this volume and has shared in reviewing and editing the chapters. Special thanks go to Drs. Springfield and Heckman for selecting the instructional course lectures for presentation in *The Journal of Bone and Joint Surgery*.

In closing, I dedicate ICL 59 to those in our profession who serve our country and our wounded military heroes. I remain humbled by their sacrifice, dedication, and courage. In particular I would like to acknowledge the late CDR Michael T. Mazurek, MD, MC, USN who contributed to this volume and served with distinction with Bravo Surgical Company in Iraq in 2004. Thank you all for your service.

Mary I. O'Connor, MD
Jacksonville, Florida

Table of Contents

Section 9 Orthopaedic Medicine

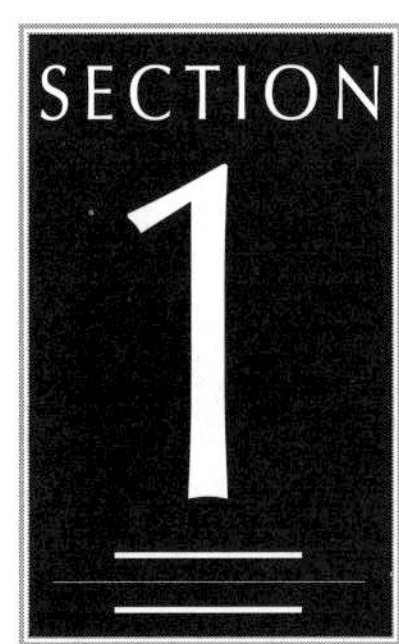

Adult Reconstruction: Hip

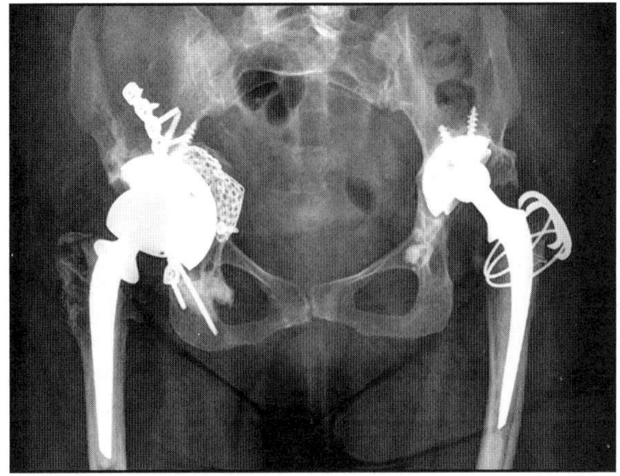

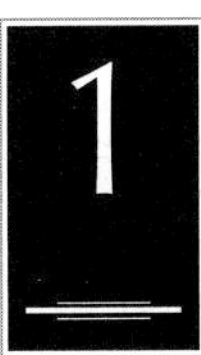

Biologic Activity of Wear Particles

Isabelle Catelas, PhD
Joshua J. Jacobs, MD

Abstract

Aseptic loosening resulting from periprosthetic osteolysis continues to be an important cause of hip implant failure. Wear particles from the bearing surfaces play a major role in initiating periprosthetic osteolysis, which is also potentiated by mechanical factors such as increased synovial fluid pressure. The precise mechanisms by which wear particles induce periprosthetic osteolysis have not been fully elucidated and remain an active subject of research. Particle characteristics such as composition, size, shape, and number (especially for particles in the most biologically active, submicrometer-size range) are recognized to significantly affect the overall cell and tissue response. The production of corrosion products, especially from metal-on-metal implants, also is a clinically significant issue, and individual variability in innate and adaptive immune responses is important but not yet completely defined. Because of the increasing need to implant hip prostheses in younger and more active patients, a better understanding of the biologic activity of wear particles from bearing couples is critical in the attempt to modulate the clinical effects of these particles and to develop materials with improved wear and corrosion resistance.

Instr Course Lect 2010;59:3-16.

Metal-on-polyethylene bearing surfaces have been widely used in total hip replacements for the past 40 years. However, large numbers of polyethylene particles have been detected in the surrounding tissues, and they have been associated with bone resorption and implant failure caused by aseptic loosening.[1-4] The attempts to improve the wear characteristics of polyethylene over the years have included the use of carbon fiber additives, heat pressing, and, most recently, chemical cross-linking. There is strong research and clinical interest in highly cross-linked polyethylene (HXPE), but little is known about the biologic response to wear particles from this new generation of polyethylene. Metal-on-metal and ceramic-on-ceramic bearing surface combinations have been developed based on the concept that the use of harder materials can improve wear resistance.[5] Interest in metal-on-metal implants for total hip replacements has been revived within the past two decades with the introduction of new designs. Although the volumetric wear rate of metal-on-metal bearings is much lower than that of conventional metal-on-polyethylene bearings, the smaller size of the wear particles and the release of corrosion products have raised biologic concerns. Alumina and zirconia (Al_2O_3 and ZrO_2) ceramics are attractive as self-bearing materials because of their low coefficients of friction, high wettability and chemical stability, high hardness and excellent surface finish, and resistance to third-body scratching and wear. However, concerns exist about their extremely high modulus of elasticity compared

Dr. Catelas or an immediate family member is a member of a speakers' bureau or has made paid presentations on behalf of DePuy; and has stock or stock options held in Baxter Healthcare Corporation. Dr. Jacobs or an immediate family member serves as a board member, owner, officer, or committee member of the Bone and Joint Decade, U.S.A., the Hip Society, the Orthopaedic Research and Education Foundation, the Orthopaedic Research Society, InMotion, and NIAMS; serves as a paid consultant to or is an employee of Medtronic Sofamor Danek, the National Institutes of Health (NIAMS & NICHD), Wright Medical Technology, and Zimmer; has received research or institutional support from Arthrex, Biomet, DePuy, DJ Orthopaedics, Johnson & Johnson, Medtronic, Medtronic Sofamor Danek, the National Institutes of Health (NIAMS & NICHD), Nuvasive, Smith & Nephew, Stryker, Wright Medical Technology, Zimmer, Anesiva, Ctr Biom Adv Tech, Don Joy Orthopaedics, Pentax, Pioneer Labs – NUBAC, Spinal Kinetics, Omeros, and Anges; and has received nonincome support (such as equipment or services), commercially derived honoraria, or other non–research-related funding (such as paid travel) from Arthritis and Rheumatism and Taylor and Francis.

with bone, as well as their brittle material properties, which occasionally have caused component fracture.[6-8] This chapter will present a review of the literature that addresses the biologic activity of wear particles from these different types of bearing materials.

Characteristics of Wear Particles

Precise characterization of implant wear particles is important to understand their biologic effects. The composition, size, shape, and number of wear particles are known to play a role in the cell and tissue response.

The size of ultra-high molecular weight polyethylene (UHMWPE) particles isolated from in vitro hip simulators has been reported to be mainly between 0.1 and 1 μm.[9] The in vivo size and morphology of these particles has been demonstrated to be more variable. Most are globular spheroids between 0.1 and 0.4 μm in size, but some are platelet-shaped and are as large as 250 μm; others are fibrils or shreds.[10-13] Richards and associates[14] reported the presence of nanometer-size UHMWPE particles in vivo, but these particles accounted only for a small proportion of the total volume. Laurent and associates[15] studied HXPE particles and found that they were largely spheroidal or oblong and smaller than most UHMWPE particles. However, commercially available HXPE implants differ with respect to type of irradiation, radiation dose, method of thermal stabilization, machining, and final sterilization;[16] therefore, the resulting wear particles may differ in their characteristics.

A direct comparison of the available studies of wear particles from metal-on-metal implants is difficult because of the different implant designs and alloys from different manufacturers, as well as the different particle isolation and characterization techniques used in these studies. Doorn and associates[17] analyzed metal particles following enzymatic digestion of periprosthetic tissues. They found that most particles were round but that a small proportion were shard- or needle-shaped. When comparing different isolation protocols, Catelas and associates[18,19] found that a newly developed enzymatic protocol was less damaging to wear particles than the strong alkaline protocols used by earlier researchers to isolate metal particles. Using this new enzymatic protocol and particle embedding in resin to allow particle dispersion and facilitate morphology and elemental analysis, Catelas and associates[20-22] found that the wear particles produced by metal-on-metal implants in vitro and in vivo were in the nanometer size range and were mostly round or oval, but some were needle-shaped. The quantity of needle-shaped particles depended on the cycling period (for in vitro particles) or the implantation time (for in vivo particles). Most of the particles contained chromium (Cr) and oxygen (O) but no cobalt (Co) and therefore, were most likely chromium oxides. These findings corroborated those of Doorn and associates,[17] but differed to some extent from those reported by Brown and associates[23] who found only round and no needle-shaped cobalt-chromium particles in vitro. These discrepancies in shape and composition may be attributable to differences in the metallurgy of the prosthetic component alloys and the loading parameters; however, all of these researchers agreed that particles from metal-on-metal implants are in the nanometer-size range, have a high specific surface area (surface area/mass), and are subject to corrosion, which leads to the release of metal ions into the surrounding areas. Therefore, the effects of metal ions must be considered when analyzing the biologic response to these wear particles.

Lerouge and associates[24,25] analyzed alumina particles in tissue using scanning electron microscopy. They found uniform round particles with a size of 0.44 μm ($\pm$ 0.25 μm). Yoon and associates[26] reported a similar size of 0.13 μm ($\pm$ 7.21 μm). When using transmission electron microscopy in addition to scanning electron microscopy, some studies revealed a bimodal size range.[27,28] Transmission electron microscopic analysis of particles from tissues revealed the presence of 5- to 90-nm particles (24 nm $\pm$ 19 nm), whereas scanning electron microscopic analysis revealed particles in the size range of 0.05 μm to 3.2 μm.[27] By using microseparation of the prosthesis components with in vitro joint simulations, Tipper and associates[28] also found a bimodal distribution, with nanometer-size particles ranging from 1 to 35 nm and larger micrometer-size particles ranging from 0.021 to 10 μm.

Wear Particle-Induced Periprosthetic Osteolysis

The most common cause of implant failure is aseptic loosening resulting from periprosthetic osteolysis, which is primarily induced by the presence of wear particles and is potentiated by mechanical factors such as synovial fluid pressure. Periprosthetic osteolysis was first described as a cystic erosion of bone by Charnley in 1975.[29] Since then, it has been widely studied using in vitro, animal, and retrieval studies, and has been described as the cumulative result of biologic reactions that lead to increased bone resorption and decreased bone formation.

Many types of cells have been reported to be involved in wear particle-induced periprosthetic osteolysis, including macrophages, giant cells, osteoblasts, and fibroblasts.[30-32] Some studies also have described the recruitment and differentiation of osteoclast progenitors at the bone-implant interface as potentially early events in the pathogenesis of osteolysis.[33-35]

Periprosthetic tissues are characterized by the presence of granulation tissue rich in macrophages, wear particles, as well as inflammatory mediators including interleukin (IL)-1β, tumor necrosis factor (TNF)-α, prostaglandin E_2, and IL-6.[36-39] The cytokine pathways that modulate periprosthetic osteolysis have been extensively studied in recent years, and the importance of the pathway involving the receptor activator of nuclear factor kappa-B (RANK), the receptor activator of nuclear factor kappa-B ligand (RANKL), and osteoprotegerin (OPG) has emerged.[40-42] The RANK-RANKL-OPG pathway has been shown to be fundamental to the process of osteoclastogenesis because osteoclast precursors are unable to differentiate into mature osteoclasts in the absence of RANKL-RANK interaction. RANKL activates key pathways involved in osteoclast differentiation and function. It is a TNF-related cytokine produced by marrow stromal cells and osteoblasts. RANK, a member of the TNF-receptor superfamily, is present on osteoclasts and initiates osteoclastogenesis after binding with RANKL. OPG, a decoy receptor, also can bind to RANKL, thereby preventing its interaction with RANK and limiting its activity in osteoclastogenesis. Mandelin and associates[43] analyzed the particle-initiated inflammatory response in periprosthetic tissues from 11 patients with osteolysis to determine whether the response was associated with the upregulation of the RANK-RANKL-OPG system. They found that RANK and RANKL were upregulated and suggested that RANKL in the interface tissue could stimulate the differentiation of RANK-positive cells into osteoclasts capable of bone resorption.

Other mechanisms that may contribute to wear particle-induced periprosthetic osteolysis include the elevated production of reactive oxygen species by activated macrophages and osteoclasts, impaired periprosthetic bone formation secondary to disrupted osteogenesis, and compromised bone regeneration resulting from increased mesenchymal stem cell mortality caused by the wear particles.[44] The effects of wear particles on bone cells and their progenitors have only recently received attention.[45] Wang and associates[46,47] found that human mesenchymal stem cells exposed to commercially pure titanium (cpTi) particles demonstrated a lower viability and proliferation, reduced collagen type I and bone sialoprotein production, and suppression of bone sialoprotein but not osteocalcin, alkaline phosphatase, or collagen type I gene expression. When cells were exposed to zirconia particles, a decrease in cell proliferation and subsequent mineralization was measured, but there was no significant effect on osteoblastic gene markers. CpTi particles also were found to be more toxic than zirconia particles. These studies show that particle composition influences the viability, proliferation, as well as the gene and protein expression of osteoblast progenitors. Okafor and associates[48] also studied the effects of cpTi on human mesenchymal stem cells and found an increase in apoptosis, a decrease in cell proliferation, and the suppression of osteogenic differentiation after particle endocytosis. The addition of cytochalasin D (an inhibitor of phagocytosis) to the cpTi-stimulated human mesenchymal stem cell cultures inhibited these effects, demonstrating that phagocytosis was key to the adverse effects of cpTi particles on human mesenchymal stem cells. Chiu and associates[49] found that polymethylmethacrylate particles reduced murine bone marrow osteoprogenitor cell proliferation and differentiation when cells were exposed to the particles during the first 5 days of culture in osteogenic medium. Exposure of the bone marrow cells to polymethylmethacrylate particles after the fifth day of differentiation in osteogenic medium resulted in decreased cell proliferation but no reduction of alkaline phosphatase expression or mineralization, thus indicating that the cells were most sensitive to the particles during the first 5 days of differentiation.

In a very recent study, Caicedo and associates[50] examined the potential activation of the inflammasome pathway in human macrophages exposed to soluble metal ions and cobalt-chromium-molybdenum (Co-Cr-Mo) alloy particles. They found that these metal agents stimulate macrophage IL-1β secretion that is inflammasome-mediated. The authors concluded on a potential novel mechanism for implant particle reactivity in which contact with the particles would be sensed and transduced by macrophages into a pro-inflammatory response.

Biologic Response to Polyethylene Particles

Conventional metal-on-polyethylene total hip replacements produce relatively large quantities of polyethylene particles, and these particles have been the most important factor in initiating osteolysis. UHMWPE particles can be observed in histology sections using polarized light microscopy and have been identified in large numbers in tissues surrounding implants associated with bone resorption and failure caused by aseptic loosening.[1-4] These particles have been shown to elicit an inflammatory response due to macrophage and foreign body giant cell interaction and culminating in granuloma formation, osteolysis, and aseptic implant loosening. The influence of particle size and concentration was confirmed by in vivo studies that showed a direct relationship between polyethylene particles, macrophages, and osteolysis.[51-54] Green and associates[55] analyzed the in vitro bone resorption response of C3H murine peritoneal macrophages to grade GUR 1120 polyethylene particles of different sizes (0.24, 0.45, 1.71, and 7.62 μm) and at different doses (particle volume [μm^3] to macrophage ratios of 0.1:1, 1:1, 10:1, and 100:1). The smallest particles were the most active in stimulating bone-resorbing activity, at a ratio of 10 μm^3 per macrophage. Larger doses were necessary for the 0.45 and 1.71 μm particles, and the 7.62 μm particles were inactive at all tested doses. Cytokine amounts followed the same trend. Therefore, the size and dose of UHMWPE particles were important parameters influencing the osteolytic response of macrophages. Yang and associates[56] also analyzed the effects of UHMWPE particle shape, finding that different morphologies could elicit diverse cellular and apoptotic responses in a mouse air pouch model. Using the same model, Ren and associates[41] studied the gene expression of RANK and RANKL during the inflammatory response to globular or elongated UHMWPE particles. Elongated particles generated significantly higher RANK and RANKL gene expression than globular particles in pouch tissue, significantly higher IL-1β and TNF-α gene expression, and a higher cathepsin K gene expression. Histologic analysis revealed clusters of cells that were positive for tartrate-resistant acid phosphatase (TRAP) located in regions in contact with elongated particles. These data suggest that not only the size and dose but also the shape of UHMWPE particles critically influence the biologic response.

In vitro studies of cell response to polyethylene particles demonstrated that UHMWPE particles of different sizes stimulate macrophages to produce cytokines such as IL-1β, IL-6, TNF-α, and prostaglandin E_2.[57-59] However, there are discrepancies in the data, primarily because not all of the studies used the same cell lines, and some used particles that were not endotoxin free (leading to false positive results) or nonphysiologic. When comparing the macrophage response to UHMWPE particles with the macrophage response to other types of particles at similar sizes and concentrations, Petit and associates[60] found that UHMWPE particles induced faster and larger effects on TNF-α release than alumina particles.

The recent development of HXPE raised the question of the influence of cross-linking on the biologic activity of wear particles. Illgen and associates[61] compared the in vitro biologic activity of particles from Longevity HXPE (Zimmer, Warsaw, IN) and grade GUR 1050 conventional polyethylene (Zimmer), isolated from a hip simulator, and found no difference in the secretion of TNF-α and vascular endothelial growth factor (VEGF) at low and intermediate doses (0.1 and 0.75 surface area ratio, respectively). However, at the highest dose tested (2.5 surface area ratio), HXPE was significantly more inflammatory than conventional polyethylene. Both types of particles were predominantly round (granular), but the HXPE particles were somewhat smaller than the conventional polyethylene particles (0.111 μm versus 0.196 μm). Ingram and associates[62] also compared the inflammatory potential of HXPE and conventional polyethylene wear particles (all generated using a multidirectional pin-on-plate wear rig). The authors found that HXPE particles had a greater inflammatory potential than conventional polyethylene particles. Indeed, HXPE particles were able to stimulate cells to produce significantly elevated TNF-α levels at a concentration of only 0.1 μm^3 per cell; in contrast, a concentration of at least 10 μm^3 of the conventional polyethylene particles per cell was required to stimulate the cells. There was also a difference in particle sizes, with a higher percentage of HXPE particles than conventional polyethylene particles in the most biologically active submicrometer-size range. Ingram and associates[62] also reported the influence of the molecular weight and counterface roughness of the polyethylene and showed that higher levels of TNF-α were produced in the presence of particles of higher molecular weight polyethylene or relatively rough surfaces. All these studies show the importance of cross-linking, molecular weight, and

Table 1
Results of Immunohistochemical Staining and In Situ Hybridization Positive Cell Counts in Tissues Surrounding Metal-on-Metal Versus Metal-on-Polyethylene Hip Implants

Patient	CD 3	CD 68	Hybrid	IL-1β	IL-6	PDGF-α	TNF-α	TGF-β
Metal-on-metal								
1	35	36	0	220	1,982	551	1,324	725
2	10	28	0	1,945	3,822	2,900	1,807	662
3	19	33	0	1,627	2,429	2,450	1,719	1,382
4	17	13	0	827	1,064	1,195	889	314
5	7	9	0	1,079	1,301	1,360	632	832
Average	18	24	0	1,140	2,120	1,691	1,274	783
SD	11	12	0	677	1,095	961	511	387
SE	5	5	0	303	490	430	229	173
Metal-on-polyethylene								
1	10	77	0	1,189	2,237	1,206	1,941	1,637
2	5	77	0	2,739	3,572	2,478	3,063	2,284
3	4	36	0	479	798	372	1,239	963
4	5	91	0	2,792	4,284	2,763	3,665	4,003
5	11	97	0	2,125	2,843	1,470	2,623	2,853
Average	7	76	0	1,865	2,747	1,658	2,506	2,348
SD	3	24	0	1,009	1,333	973	948	1,164
SE	1	11	0	451	596	435	424	521
***P*-values**								
t-test	0.07	0.003		0.2	0.4	0.9	0.03	0.02
Mann-Whitney	0.06	0.01		0.2	0.5	0.9	0.05	0.02

CD 3 = CD 3 positive lymphocytes, CD 68 = CD 68 positive macrophages, IL = interleukin, PDGF-α = platelet-derived growth factor-α, TNF-α = tumor necrosis factor-α, TGF-β = transforming growth factor-β, SD = standard deviation, SE = standard error of mean.

(Adapted with permission from Campbell PA, Wang M, Amstutz HC, Goodman SB: Positive cytokine production in failed metal-on-metal total hip replacements. *Acta Orthop Scand* 2002;73:506-512.)

counterface roughness in determining the biologic activity of polyethylene particles. However, it is expected that the increase in particle biologic activity with higher molecular weight or higher cross-linking will probably be mitigated in vivo by lower wear volumes with HXPE.

Biologic Response to Metal Particles

Histiocytic and Specific Immunologic Responses

In a histologic study of periprosthetic tissues from different designs of metal-on-metal total hip replacements, Doorn and associates[17] found that the extent of the inflammatory reaction and the presence of foreign body-type giant cells were much less important in tissues surrounding metal-on-metal implants than in tissues surrounding metal-on-polyethylene implants. The authors postulated that the lower tissue reactivity resulted from the overall smaller size of wear particles from metal-on-metal bearings being an order of magnitude smaller than UHMWPE particles. In a comparison of the tissue response surrounding metal-on-metal and metal-on-polyethylene hip implants, Campbell and associates[63] reported fewer CD 68 positive macrophages and lower levels of transforming growth factor–β and TNF-α in the tissues surrounding metal-on-metal implants, but no difference in the quantities of CD 3 positive lymphocytes, IL-1β, IL-6, or platelet-derived growth factor-α (PDGF-α) (Table 1). Catelas and associates[64] analyzed the relationship between the production of cytokines and the quantity of metal wear particles in tissues and found that tissues surrounding failed metal-on-metal implants with low to moderate quantities of metal particles could induce the production of potentially osteolytic cytokines. However, the number of cells producing these cytokines tended to be lower than the number typically seen in tissues surrounding metal-on-polyethylene implants.

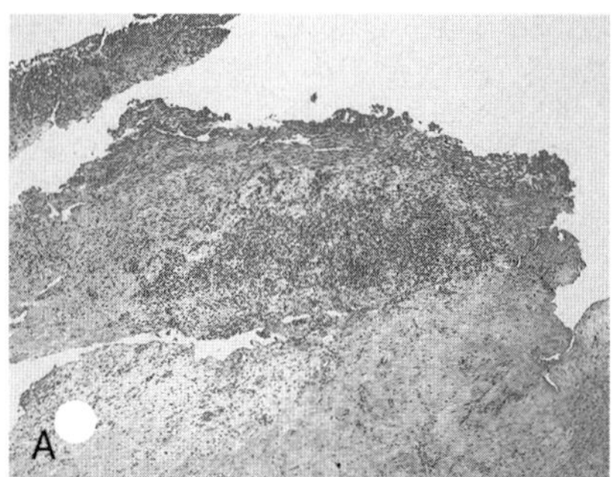

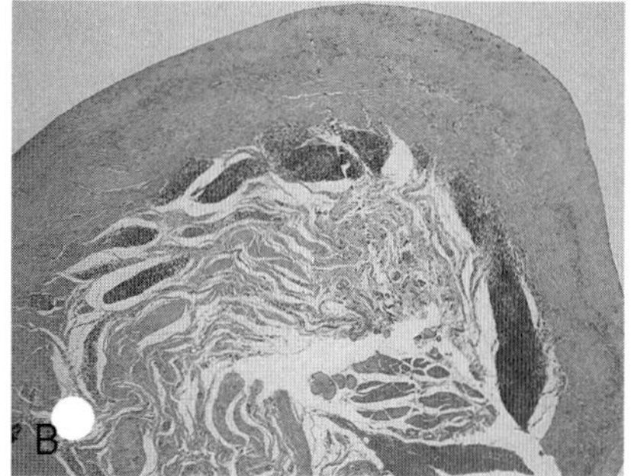

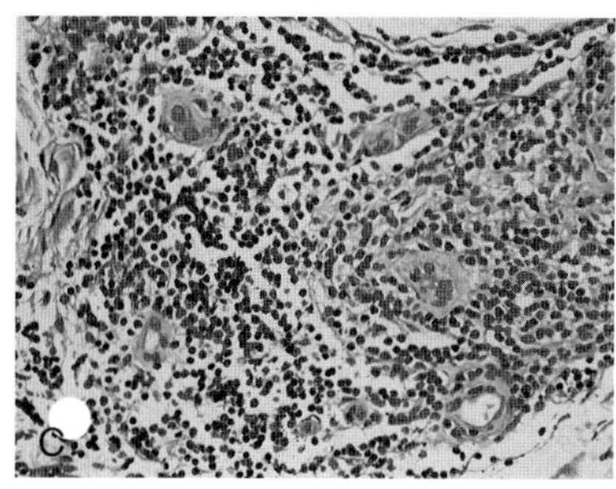

Figure 1 Histologic sections illustrating an ALVAL in tissues surrounding metal-on-metal implants. **A,** Inner capsular layer with infiltrates of diffusely distributed lymphocytes and fibrin exudates at the surface (×4). **B,** Perivascularity agglomerated lymphocytic infiltrates with secondary reaction centers in the intermediate vascular layer of a joint capsule (×20). **C,** High endothelial venules with marrow lumina and dense infiltrates of mononuclear cells in the capsular tissue (×40). (Reproduced with permission from Willert HG, Buchhorn GH, Fayyazi A, et al: Metal-on-metal bearings and hypersensitivity in patients with artificial hip joints: A clinical and histomorphological study. *J Bone Joint Surg Am* 2005;87:28-36.)

In addition to the potential of metal particles to induce osteolysis through macrophage activation, as observed in tissues surrounding conventional metal-on-polyethylene implants, concern has emerged regarding the possibility of specific immunologic responses to metal-on-metal implants. In their comparison study of tissues surrounding metal-on-metal and metal-on-polyethylene implants, Campbell and associates,[63] found a tendency toward more lymphocytes in tissues surrounding metal-on-metal implants. Similarly, Willert and associates[65] reported perivascular lymphocyte accumulations in tissues from 14 failed modern metal-on-metal implants and suggested that this reaction indicated a delayed hypersensitivity response to metal wear products. These immunologic responses could be caused by the release of metal ions that act as antigens and stimulate an allergic (hypersensitivity) reaction when they form an organometallic complex with proteins. However, it is still unclear whether implant loosening can be linked to an increased reactivity of the lymphocytes to metal particles or ions. Hallab and associates[66] investigated the incidence of lymphocyte reactivity to soluble cobalt, chromium, nickel (Ni), and titanium (Ti) using lymphocytes from patients with metal-on-metal implants compared to patients with metal-on-polyethylene implants and to patients with no implants (controls). Patients with metal-on-metal implants had significantly elevated serum cobalt and chromium concentrations (13- and 58-fold, respectively), which were correlated with elevated lymphocyte reactivity to cobalt and nickel, compared to patients having metal-on-polyethylene implants or patients in the control group. However, no etiologic link could be established between this lymphocyte reactivity and the poor performance of the implants. In a more recent study of failed modern metal-on-metal articulations, Willert and associates[67] also reported the presence of lymphocytic infiltrates, plasma cells and sometimes eosinophilic granulocytes, high endothelial venules, localized bleeding, fibrin exudation, necrosis, and macrophages with drop-like inclusions (Figure 1). This response was described as an aseptic, lymphocyte-dominated, vasculitis-associated lesion (ALVAL) or a lymphocyte-dominated immunological answer (LYDIA). Other authors also reported individual cases of lymphocytic infiltration around failed modern metal-on-metal implants.[68-70] In another study, Pandit and associates[71] recently reported the presence of pseudotumors surrounding metal-on-metal surface replacements. These pseudotumors were characterized by an extensive necrosis of dense connective tissue, a focally heavy macrophage and lymphocytic infiltration, and, in some patients, the presence of plasma cells and eosinophils. The observed reaction was somewhat similar to the ALVAL reaction reported by Willert and associates;[67] however, there was a more diffuse lymphocyte infiltrate as well as extensive connective tissue necrosis. The causes of these pseudotumors were not fully elucidated, but the potential effects of wear particles and a possible hypersensitivity reaction were mentioned. All patients in this study were female, and therefore preoperative sensitization to metal might have

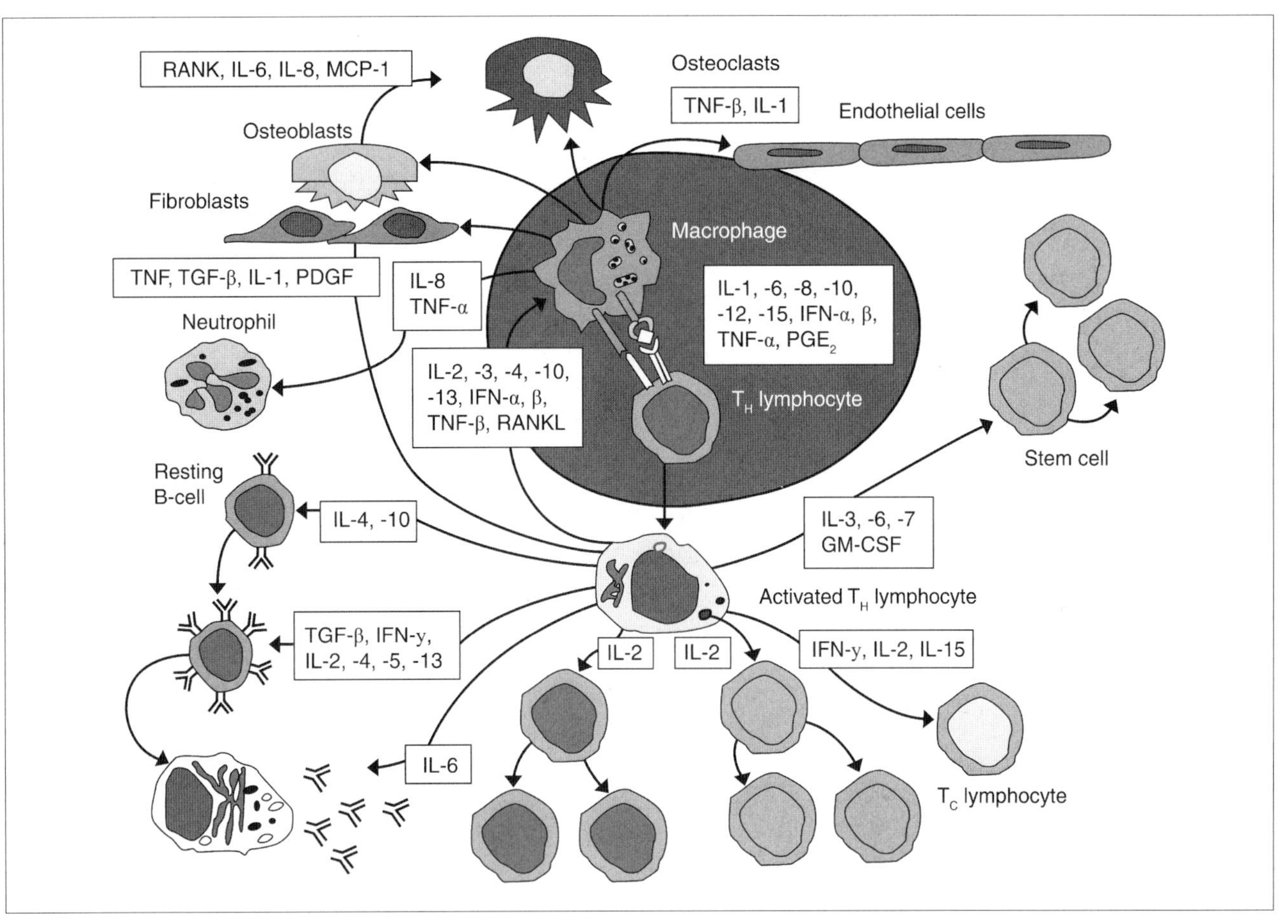

Figure 2 Illustration showing the complex interrelationship between wear products and cells of the innate and adaptive immune systems. GM-CSF = granulocyte monocyte-colony stimulating factor, IFN = interferon, MCP = monocyte chemoattractant protein, PDGF = platelet-derived growth factor, PGE_2 = prostaglandin E_2, T_c = cytotoxic T lymphocyte, TGF = transforming growth factor, T_H = T helper lymphocyte. (Reproduced with permission from Jacobs JJ, Campbell PA, Konttinen YT: Implant Wear Symposium 2007 Biologic Work Group: How has the biologic reaction to wear particles changed with newer bearing surfaces? *J Am Acad Orthop Surg* 2008;16(suppl 1):S49-S55.)

been a factor. Also, all revisions were done within 5 years of implantation (rather short implantation times). Unfortunately, no gold standard test currently exists for the clinical diagnosis of implant-associated metal allergy because cutaneous patch testing to assess metal hypersensitivity may not relate to allergic response in the deep periprosthetic environment.[72] Although the link between aseptic loosening and hypersensitivity reactions remains to be clearly established,[73] there is increasing evidence that hypersensitivity plays a role in the pathogenesis of osteolysis.[74] The incidence of premature failure of metal-on-metal joint arthroplasty caused by a specific immunologic response is probably low but is currently unknown. Figure 2 shows the complex interrelationship between the wear products and cells of the innate and adaptive immune systems.

There are also concerns that the metal wear particles generated by a metal-on-metal hip implants may have cytotoxic effects as they disperse throughout the body. The systemic dissemination of soluble and particulate corrosion products includes the presence of metallic particles in the liver and spleen,[75] raising questions about potential genotoxicity.

Metal Ions and Genotoxic Potential

Ion levels have been measured in whole blood, serum, erythrocytes, and urine. Because of complex issues associated with the analysis of metal ions (including sample collection and statistical methodologies) there has been significant variability in the techniques used by different investigators, and this lack of uniformity makes the comparison of results difficult.[76]

In a randomized clinical trial, MacDonald and associates[77] reported significantly higher levels of metal ions in the urine and erythrocytes of patients with metal-on-metal implants than in patients with metal-on-polyethylene implants. Also, the levels of cobalt, chromium, and titanium ions measured in urine were higher than those measured in erythrocytes. Walter and associates[78] found higher levels of cobalt and chromium ions in serum or plasma than in red blood cells of patients with metal-on-metal implants. Engh and associates[79] also recently found higher levels of chromium and titanium in serum than in erythrocytes. Overall, these studies suggest that serum may better reflect the true ion levels when blood is used to assess systemic ion levels.[78] Brodner and associates[80] specifically studied serum cobalt concentrations in patients during the first 5 years after a total hip arthroplasty with a metal-on-metal articulation and found moderate concentrations of 1 μg/L at 1 year and 0.7 μg/L at 5 years. These results led to the conclusion that the serum cobalt concentrations did not reflect the higher run-in wear of metal-on-metal implants. In a study of modern metal-on-metal surface arthroplasties, Skipor and associates[81] reported that serum chromium levels were 22, 23, and 21 times higher at 3, 6, and 12 months after surgery, respectively, than before surgery; the corresponding serum cobalt levels were eight, seven, and six times higher after surgery. The authors reported that serum chromium and cobalt values found with the current generation of surface arthroplasties were in the same range as those found with conventional metal-on-metal total hip replacements.[81] In contrast, when comparing the levels of serum cobalt and chromium in patients with metal-on-metal resurfacings or metal-on-metal total hip implants, Clarke and associates[82] found median serum levels of 38 nmol/L for cobalt and 53 nmol/L for chromium in patients with metal-on-metal resurfacings compared with 22 nmol/L for cobalt and 19 nmol/L for chromium in patients with metal-on-metal total hip implants. However, this study was a retrospective analysis in which two different metal-on-metal implant designs and shorter follow-up periods were used for patients treated with resurfacing implants compared with patients treated with metal-on-metal total hip implants. In a very recent study, Antoniou and associates[83] compared the blood ion levels of patients after hip resurfacings with the ASR System (DePuy, Warsaw, IN) or metal-on-metal total hip implants using a 28- or 36-mm femoral head. After 1 year, the patients with hip resurfacings had blood metal ion levels similar to those of the patients with total hip implants. Langton and associates[84] analyzed the effects of the femoral head component size and the orientation of the acetabular component and found that both parameters could influence the overall concentration of metal ions in the whole blood of patients with metal-on-metal resurfacings. The authors reported higher ion concentrations in patients with smaller components and when the inclination angle was greater than 45° and the anteversion angle exceeded 20°.[84]

When present in high concentrations, both Co^{2+} and Cr^{3+} ions have been reported to be capable of inducing macrophage necrosis in vitro.[85] However, Co^{2+} appeared to be more toxic than Cr^{3+} considering that 40 to 50 times more Cr^{3+} was needed to induce a similar level of macrophage mortality and TNF-α release.[86,87] In theory, carcinogenic and other biologic risks, including mutagenesis, also can be associated with these metal ions. Although cobalt and chromium ions are most stable as Co^{2+} and Cr^{3+} at neutral pH, soluble Cr^{6+} ions can freely pass through the cell membrane, in comparison with Cr^{3+} ions, which cannot freely move across the lipid membrane and therefore do not easily enter the cells. After Cr^{6+} ions traverse the cell membrane, they are reductively metabolized within the cells, where they can cause a diverse range of genetic lesions. Some of these lesions can present a physical barrier to DNA replication or transcription and can promote apoptosis or terminal growth arrest. Other lesions, such as ternary DNA adducts, may be premutagenic. For example, Cr^{6+} ion exposure has been shown to elicit a classic DNA damage response in cells, including activation of the p53 signaling pathway and cell cycle arrest or apoptosis.[88] Quievryn and associates[89] reported that the reduction of Cr^{6+} led to dose-dependent formation of both mutagenic and replication-blocking DNA lesions in human fibroblasts. Similarly, Papageorgiou and associates[90] found an increase in aneuploidy, chromosome translocations, and DNA damage in human fibroblasts exposed to cobalt-chromium particles. Ladon and associates,[91] investigating changes in metal levels and chromosome aberrations in patients with metal-on-metal Metasul (Zimmer) implants for less than 2 years, showed a statistically significant increase in both chromosome translocations and aneuploidy in peripheral blood lymphocytes at 6, 12, and 24 months after surgery. However, secondary analyses did not show any statistically significant correlations between chromosome translocation indices and cobalt or chromium concentrations in whole blood. Massè and associates[92] also found that the incidence of markers of chromosomal damage in lymphocytes did not correlate with any of the ion levels (cobalt, chromium, nickel, molybdenum) measured in the blood and urine of patients who had received a Metasul component.

Biologic Response to Ceramic Particles

The alumina-on-alumina total hip implants have been in clinical use for more than 30 years, primarily in Europe. Ceramics in bulk form do not undergo oxidative environmental degradation and have been considered inert. However, in particulate form, they have been reported to be capable of eliciting a macrophage response.[93-95] Catelas and associates[95] found an increase in macrophage mortality and TNF-α release with increasing alumina or zirconia particle size and concentration in vitro. There was no significant difference between the cell response to alumina or zirconia but the overall cell response was lower than that observed with high-density polyethylene particles at similar sizes and concentrations. Petit and associates[60] also reported lower levels of TNF-α after macrophage exposure to alumina particles compared with UHMWPE polyethylene particles. Using chemiluminescence assay for reactive oxygen species, Nagase and associates[96] found that the most biologically active size of alumina particles was 1 to 7 μm. Catelas and associates[94] found that both alumina and zirconia induced macrophage apoptotic cell death. The induction of apoptosis was size- and concentration-dependent, and reached a plateau above 150 particles per macrophage with a particle size of 1.3 μm. Hatton and associates[97] compared the effects of two types of ceramic wear particles on TNF-α production by human peripheral blood mononuclear cells (PBMNC) from six donors. When wear particles obtained by microseparation (bimodal size of particles, 5 to 20 nm and 0.2 to 10 μm) were used, a greater volume was required to activate the PBMNC than when alumina powder particles (0.5 μm) were used. PBMNC from all donors produced significantly elevated levels of TNF-α when stimulated with 100 μm³ of alumina powder per cell, but as much as 500 μm³ of the microseparation particles per cell were necessary to have PBMNC from some donors produce similar levels of TNF-α. The authors attributed the differences in cell response to the variations in particle size, as there were fewer particles in the critical size range (0.1 to 1 μm) among the microseparation wear particles. In a comparison of the biologic activity of ceramic particles (both alumina and zirconia) and high-density polyethylene particles on murine calvarial bone, Warashina and associates[98] found that the ceramic particles induced a much lower inflammatory response and much less bone resorption than the polyethylene particles. Considering the high volumetric concentration of ceramic particles needed to generate a significant level of cytokine production, it is unlikely that the concentration threshold would ever be reached in vivo.[97] Overall, these studies suggest that ceramic particles can activate a macrophage response in a fashion similar to the response of the other types of particles, although to a lesser extent.

Lerouge and associates[25] compared the histology of pseudomembranes from ceramic-on-ceramic and metal-on-polyethylene total hip implants in a semiquantitative in vivo study, finding no significant difference in cellular reaction. However, the characterization of the particles from ceramic-on-ceramic hip implants revealed that 76% of these particles consisted of zirconia particles used to opacify the cement used for fixation and only 12% were alumina particles originating from the articulation. The authors concluded that the cellular reaction was caused by the zirconia particles in the cement rather than the alumina particles from the bearing and that the aseptic loosening of the ceramic cups resulted from the cement fragmentation caused by mechanical factors.[25] Nevertheless, osteolysis has been reported in association with ceramic wear particles. Yoon and associates[26] found osteolysis of the femur in 23 hips and osteolysis of the pelvis in 49 hips in a study of 103 noncemented Mittelmeir with a Biolox femoral head (Osteo AG, Selzach, Switzerland) ceramic-on-ceramic total hip implants at a mean 92-month follow-up. Histologic and electron microscopy analysis of the periprosthetic membranes revealed abundant ceramic wear particles with a mean size of 0.71 μm (range, 0.13 to 7.2 μm). The interface tissue consisted of rather vascular fibrous connective tissue rich in macrophages containing electron-dense material within phagosomes. Ten patients had revision surgery for loosening and migration of the acetabular component. The authors concluded that ceramic wear particles could stimulate a foreign body reaction leading to periprosthetic osteolysis.[26] However, Yoo and associates,[99] in a more recent study, reported encouraging results with respect to fracture, osteolysis, and wear at a 5-year minimum follow-up after total hip arthroplasty using a modern cementless-stem, alumina-on-alumina implant. They found radiographic evidence of bone ingrowth, no implant loosening, and no detectable wear. D'Antonio and associates[100] also reported encouraging results at a 62-month follow-up after implantation of a newer alumina-on-alumina cementless design with 99.7% of the cups stable, only 1.4% osteolysis, and no fractures. However, longer follow-up is required before conclusions can be drawn regarding the long-term outcome of using cementless ceramic-on-ceramic implants. A recent study by Yoon and associates[101] analyzed the long-term results of a newer cementless implant design with a tapered, fully porous-coated cobalt-chromium stem (Autophor 900-S; Osteo AG). At an average 17-year follow-up of 127 hip replacements (43 ceramic-on-polyethylene and 84 ceramic-on-ceramic), the femoral component survival rate was 94.5%. In a recent long-term study of ceramic acetabular components with alumina ceramic femoral heads, Hannouche and associates[102] found 85% survival of cemented cups and 61.2% survival of cementless cups in 118 hips after 20 years. Only three hips had osteolysis, and none had detectable wear.

Summary

It is clear that implant wear and corrosion can lead to the production of degradation products, a highly inflammatory biologic response, periprosthetic bone loss, and aseptic loosening. The biologic activity is highly dependent on particle characteristics and the quantity of wear particles in the most biologically active submicrometer-size range. The local and systemic effects of the wear particles and corrosion products also remain clinically significant issues. To minimize the clinical impact of implant wear, efforts should continue to focus not only on developing and studying newer materials with improved wear, corrosion resistance, and less biologic reactivity, but also on elucidating the cellular and molecular mechanisms leading to periprosthetic osteolysis in order to identify new approaches for therapeutic intervention. Several investigations already have been conducted in an attempt to reverse or even suppress the biologic response to wear particles. These approaches include the use of corticosteroids and nonsteroidal anti-inflammatory drugs, antiosteolytic agents (such as bisphosphonates), antioxidants, RANKL inhibitors, gene therapy for the delivery of anti-inflammatory agents (such as anti–TNF-α agents), and osteogenic growth factors to stimulate periprosthetic bone formation. To date, however, there is no approved drug therapy to prevent or inhibit periprosthetic osteolysis.

References

1. Willert HG, Bertram H, Buchhorn GH: Osteolysis in alloarthroplasty of the hip: The role of ultra-high molecular weight polyethylene wear particles. *Clin Orthop Relat Res* 1990;258: 95-107.
2. Amstutz HC, Campbell P, Kossovsky N, Clarke IC: Mechanism and clinical significance of wear debris-induced osteolysis. *Clin Orthop Relat Res* 1992;276:7-18.
3. Cooper RA, McAllister CM, Borden LS, Bauer TW: Polyethylene debris-induced osteolysis and loosening in uncemented total hip arthroplasty: A cause of late failure. *J Arthroplasty* 1992;7:285-290.
4. Schmalzried TP, Jasty M, Harris WH: Periprosthetic bone loss in total hip arthroplasty: Polyethylene wear debris and the concept of the effective joint space. *J Bone Joint Surg Am* 1992; 74:849-863.
5. Schey JA: Systems view of optimizing metal on metal bearings. *Clin Orthop Relat Res* 1996;329:S115-S127.
6. Dorlot JM: Wear patterns of alumina-alumina ceramic hip implants. *Clin Orthop Relat Res* 1991;272:88-93.
7. Nizard RS, Sedel L, Christel P, Meunier A, Soudry M, Witvoet J: Ten-year survivorship of cemented ceramic-ceramic total hip prosthesis. *Clin Orthop Relat Res* 1992;282:53-63.
8. Sedel L: Clinical follow-up of alumina-alumina ceramic bearings in total hip arthroplasty. *Clin Orthop Relat Res* 1994;298:62-69.
9. Endo M, Tipper JL, Barton DC, Stone MH, Ingham E, Fisher J: Comparison of wear, wear debris and functional biological activity of moderately crosslinked and non-crosslinked polyethylene in hip prostheses. *Proc Inst Mech Eng H* 2002;216: 111-122.
10. Campbell P, Ma S, Yeom B, McKellop H, Schmalzried TP, Amstutz HC: Isolation of predominantly submicron sized UHMWPE wear particles from periprosthetic tissues. *J Biomed Mater Res* 1995;29:127-131.
11. Margevicius KJ, Bauer TW, McMahon JT, Brown SA, Merritt K: Isolation and characterization of debris from around total joint prostheses. *J Bone Joint Surg Am* 1994;76: 1664-1675.
12. Shanbhag AS, Jacobs JJ, Glant TT, Gilbert JL, Black J, Galante JO: Composition and morphology of wear debris in failed uncemented total hip replacement. *J Bone Joint Surg Br* 1994; 76:60-67.
13. Visentin M, Stea S, Squarzoni S, Antonietti B, Reggiani M, Toni A: A new

method for isolation of polyethylene wear debris from tissue and synovial fluid. *Biomaterials* 2004;25:5531-5537.

14. Richards L, Brown C, Stone MH, Fisher J, Ingham E, Tipper JL: Identification of nanometre-sized ultra-high molecular weight polyethylene wear particles in samples retrieved in vivo. *J Bone Joint Surg Br* 2008;90: 1106-1113.
15. Laurent MP, Johnson TS, Crowninshield RD, Blanchard CR, Bhambri SK, Yao JQ: Characterization of a highly cross-linked ultrahigh molecular-weight polyethylene in clinical use in total hip arthroplasty. *J Arthroplasty* 2008;23:751-761.
16. Atienza C Jr, Maloney WJ: Highly cross-linked polyethylene bearing surfaces in total hip arthroplasty. *J Surg Orthop Adv* 2008;17:27-33.
17. Doorn PF, Mirra JM, Campbell PA, Amstutz HC: Tissue reaction to metal on metal total hip prostheses. *Clin Orthop Relat Res* 1996;329:S187-S205.
18. Catelas I, Bobyn JD, Medley JB, et al: Effects of digestion protocols on the isolation and characterization of metal-metal wear particles: I. Analysis of particle size and shape. *J Biomed Mater Res* 2001;55:320-329.
19. Catelas I, Bobyn JD, Medley JJ, Zukor DJ, Petit A, Huk OL: Effects of digestion protocols on the isolation and characterization of metal-metal wear particles: Part II. Analysis of ion release and particle composition. *J Biomed Mater Res* 2001;55:330-337.
20. Catelas I, Bobyn JD, Medley JB, Krygier JJ, Zukor DJ, Huk OL: Size, shape, and composition of wear particles from metal-metal hip simulator testing: Effects of alloy and number of loading cycles. *J Biomed Mater Res A* 2003;67:312-327.
21. Catelas I, Medley JB, Campbell PA, Huk OL, Bobyn JD: Comparison of in vitro with in vivo characteristics of wear particles from metal-metal hip implants. *J Biomed Mater Res B Appl Biomater* 2004;70:167-178.
22. Catelas I, Campbell PA, Bobyn JD, Medley JB, Huk OL: Wear particles from metal-on-metal total hip replacements: Effects of implant design and implantation time. *Proc Inst Mech Eng H* 2006;220:195-208.
23. Brown C, Fisher J, Ingham E: Biological effects of clinically relevant wear particles from metal-on-metal hip prostheses. *Proc Inst Mech Eng H* 2006;220:355-369.
24. Lerouge S, Huk O, Yahia LH, Sedel L: Characterization of in vivo wear debris from ceramic-ceramic total hip arthroplasties. *J Biomed Mater Res* 1996;32:627-633.
25. Lerouge S, Huk O, Yahia LH, Witovet J, Sedel L: Ceramic-ceramic and metal-polyethylene total hip replacements: Comparison of pseudomembranes after loosening. *J Bone Joint Surg Br* 1997;79:135-139.
26. Yoon TR, Rowe SM, Jung ST, Seon KJ, Maloney WJ: Osteolysis in association with a total hip arthroplasty with ceramic bearing surfaces. *J Bone Joint Surg Am* 1998;80:1459-1468.
27. Hatton A, Nevelos JE, Nevelos AA, Banks RE, Fisher J, Ingham E: Alumina-alumina artificial hip joints: Part I. A histological analysis and characterization of wear debris by laser capture microdissection of tissues retrieved at revision. *Biomaterials* 2002;23:3429-3440.
28. Tipper JL, Hatton A, Nevelos JE, et al: Alumina-alumina artificial hip joints: Part II. Characterization of the wear debris from in vitro hip joint simulations. *Biomaterials* 2002;23: 3441-3448.
29. Charnley J: Fracture of femoral prostheses in total hip replacement: A clinical study. *Clin Orthop Relat Res* 1975;111:105-120.
30. Rubash HE, Sinha RK, Shanbhag AS, Kim SY: Pathogenesis of bone loss after total hip arthroplasty. *Orthop Clin North Am* 1998;29:173-186.
31. Neale SD, Athanasou NA: Cytokine receptor profile of arthroplasty macrophages, foreign body giant cells and mature osteoclasts. *Acta Orthop Scand* 1999;70:452-458.
32. Jacobs JJ, Roebuck KA, Archibeck M, Hallab NJ, Glant TT: Osteolysis: Basic science. *Clin Orthop Relat Res* 2001; 393:71-77.
33. Neale SD, Fujikawa Y, Sabokbar A, et al: Human bone-derived cells support formation of human osteoclasts from arthroplasty-derived cells in vitro. *J Bone Joint Surg Br* 2000;82: 892-900.
34. Hirashima Y, Ishiguro N, Kondo S, Iwata H: Osteoclast induction from bone marrow cells is due to proinflammatory mediators from macrophages exposed to polyethylene particles: A possible mechanism of osteolysis in failed THA. *J Biomed Mater Res* 2001;56:177-183.
35. Greenfield EM, Bi Y, Ragab AA, Goldberg VM, Van De Motter RR: The role of osteoclast differentiation in aseptic loosening. *J Orthop Res* 2002;20:1-8.
36. Kim KJ, Rubash HE, Wilson SC, D'Antonio JA, McClain EJ: A histologic and biochemical comparison of the interface tissues in cementless and cemented hip prostheses. *Clin Orthop Relat Res* 1993;287:142-152.
37. Xu JW, Konttinen YT, Lassus J, et al: Tumor necrosis factor-alpha (TNF-alpha) in loosening of total hip replacement (THR). *Clin Exp Rheumatol* 1996;14:643-648.
38. Goodman SB, Chin RC, Chiou SS, Schurman DJ, Woolson ST, Masada MP: A clinical-pathologic-biochemical study of the membrane surrounding loosened and non-loosened total hip arthroplasties. *Clin Orthop Relat Res* 1989;244:182-187.
39. Ingham E, Fisher J: The role of macrophages in osteolysis of total joint replacement. *Biomaterials* 2005;26:1271-1286.
40. Haynes DR, Crotti TN, Potter AE, et al: The osteoclastogenic molecules RANKL and RANK are associated with periprosthetic osteolysis. *J Bone Joint Surg Br* 2001;83:902-911.
41. Ren W, Yang SY, Fang HW, Hsu S, Wooley PH: Distinct gene expression of receptor activator of nuclear factor-

kappaB and rank ligand in the inflammatory response to variant morphologies of UHMWPE particles. *Biomaterials* 2003;24:4819-4826.

42. Granchi D, Amato I, Battistelli L, et al: Molecular basis of osteoclastogenesis induced by osteoblasts exposed to wear particles. *Biomaterials* 2005;26: 2371-2379.

43. Mandelin J, Li TF, Liljeström M, et al: Imbalance of RANKL/RANK/ OPG system in interface tissue in loosening of total hip replacement. *J Bone Joint Surg Br* 2003;85:1196-1201.

44. Wang ML, Sharkey PF, Tuan RS: Particle bioreactivity and wear-mediated osteolysis. *J Arthroplasty* 2004;19:1028-1038.

45. Goodman SB, Ma T, Chiu R, Ramachandran R, Smith RL: Effects of orthopaedic wear particles on osteoprogenitor cells. *Biomaterials* 2006;27: 6096-6101.

46. Wang ML, Nesti LJ, Tuli R, et al: Titanium particles suppress expression of osteoblastic phenotype in human mesenchymal stem cells. *J Orthop Res* 2002;20:1175-1184.

47. Wang ML, Tuli R, Manner PA, Sharkey PF, Hall DJ, Tuan RS: Direct and indirect induction of apoptosis in human mesenchymal stem cells in response to titanium particles. *J Orthop Res* 2003;21:697-707.

48. Okafor CC, Haleem-Smith H, Laqueriere P, Manner PA, Tuan RS: Particulate endocytosis mediates biological responses of human mesenchymal stem cells to titanium wear debris. *J Orthop Res* 2006;24:461-473.

49. Chiu R, Ma T, Smith RL, Goodman SB: Polymethylmethacrylate particles inhibit osteoblastic differentiation of bone marrow osteoprogenitor cells. *J Biomed Mater Res A* 2006;77:850-856.

50. Caicedo MS, Desai R, McAllister K, Reddy A, Jacobs JJ, Hallab NJ. Soluble and particulate Co-Cr-Mo alloy implant metals activate the inflammasome danger signaling pathway in human macrophages: A novel mechanism for implant debris reactivity. *J Orthop Res* 2009;27:847-854.

51. Goodman SB, Fornasier VL, Lee J, Kei J: The histological effects of the implantation of different sizes of polyethylene particles in the rabbit tibia. *J Biomed Mater Res* 1990;24:517-524.

52. Goodman S, Aspenberg P, Song Y, et al: Tissue ingrowth and differentiation in the bone-harvest chamber in the presence of cobalt-chromium-alloy and high-density-polyethylene particles. *J Bone Joint Surg Am* 1995; 77:1025-1035.

53. Trindade MC, Song Y, Aspenberg P, Smith RL, Goodman SB: Proinflammatory mediator release in response to particle challenge: Studies using the bone harvest chamber. *J Biomed Mater Res* 1999;48:434-439.

54. Brooks RA, Sharpe JR, Wimhurst JA, Myer BJ, Dawes EN, Rushton N: The effects of the concentration of high density polyethylene particles on the bone implant interface. *J Bone Joint Surg Br* 2000;82:595-600.

55. Green TR, Fisher J, Matthews JB, Stone MH, Ingham E: Effect of size and dose on bone resorption activity of macrophages by in vitro clinically relevant ultra high molecular weight polyethylene particles. *J Biomed Mater Res* 2000;53:490-497.

56. Yang SY, Ren WP, Park YS, et al: Diverse cellular and apoptotic responses to variant shapes of UHMWPE particles in a murine model of inflammation. *Biomaterials* 2002;23:3535-3543.

57. Shanbhag AS, Jacobs JJ, Black J, Galante JO, Glant TT: Human monocyte response to particulate biomaterials generated in vivo and in vitro. *J Orthop Res* 1995;13:792-801.

58. Horowitz SM, Gonzales JB: Effects of polyethylene on macrophages. *J Orthop Res* 1997;15:50-56.

59. Voronov I, Santerre JP, Hinek A, Callahan JW, Sandhu J, Boynton EL: Macrophage phagocytosis of polyethylene particles in vitro. *J Biomed Mater Res* 1998;39:40-51.

60. Petit A, Catelas I, Antoniou J, Zukor DJ, Huk OL: Differential apoptotic response of J774 macrophages to alumina and ultra-high-molecular-weight polyethylene particles. *J Orthop Res* 2002;20:9-15.

61. Illgen RL II , Forsythe TM, Pike JW, Laurent MP, Blanchard CR: Highly crosslinked vs conventional polyethylene particles: An in vitro comparison of biologic activities. *J Arthroplasty* 2008;23:721-731.

62. Ingram JH, Stone M, Fisher J, Ingham E: The influence of molecular weight, crosslinking and counterface roughness on TNF-alpha production by macrophages in response to ultra high molecular weight polyethylene particles. *Biomaterials* 2004;25:3511-3522.

63. Campbell PA, Wang M, Amstutz HC, Goodman SB: Positive cytokine production in failed metal-on-metal total hip replacements. *Acta Orthop Scand* 2002;73:506-512.

64. Catelas I, Campbell PA, Dorey F, Frausto A, Mills BG, Amstutz HC: Semi-quantitative analysis of cytokines in MM THR tissues and their relationship to metal particles. *Biomaterials* 2003;24:4785-4797.

65. Willert H, Buchhorn G, Fayyazi A, Lohmann C: Histopathological changes around metal/metal joints indicate delayed type hypersensitivity: Preliminary results of 14 cases. *Osteologie* 2000;9:2-16.

66. Hallab NJ, Anderson S, Caicedo M, Skipor A, Campbell P, Jacobs JJ: Immune responses correlate with serum-metal in metal-on-metal hip arthroplasty. *J Arthroplasty* 2004;19:88-93.

67. Willert HG, Buchhorn GH, Fayyazi A, et al: Metal-on-metal bearings and hypersensitivity in patients with artificial hip joints: A clinical and histomorphological study. *J Bone Joint Surg Am* 2005;87:28-36.

68. Al-Saffar N: Early clinical failure of total joint replacement in association with follicular proliferation of B-lymphocytes: A report of two cases. *J Bone Joint Surg Am* 2002;84:2270-2273.

69. Böhler M, Kanz F, Schwarz B, et al: Adverse tissue reactions to wear par-

ticles from Co-alloy articulations, increased by alumina-blasting particle contamination from cementless Ti-based total hip implants: A report of seven revisions with early failure. *J Bone Joint Surg Br* 2002;84:128-136.

70. Davies AP, Willert HG, Campbell PA, Learmonth ID, Case CP: An unusual lymphocytic perivascular infiltration in tissues around contemporary metal-on-metal joint replacements. *J Bone Joint Surg Am* 2005;87:18-27.

71. Pandit H, Glyn-Jones S, McLardy-Smith P, et al: Pseudotumours associated with metal-on-metal hip resurfacings. *J Bone Joint Surg Br* 2008;90: 847-851.

72. Jacobs JJ, Campbell PA, T Konttinen YT: How has the biologic reaction to wear particles changed with newer bearing surfaces? *J Am Acad Orthop Surg* 2008;16:S49-S55.

73. Jacobs JJ, Hallab NJ: Loosening and osteolysis associated with metal-on-metal bearings: A local effect of metal hypersensitivity? *J Bone Joint Surg Am* 2006;88:1171-1172.

74. Hallab NJ, Anderson S, Stafford T, Glant T, Jacobs JJ: Lymphocyte responses in patients with total hip arthroplasty. *J Orthop Res* 2005;23:384-391.

75. Urban RM, Tomlinson MJ, Hall DJ, Jacobs JJ: Accumulation in liver and spleen of metal particles generated at nonbearing surfaces in hip arthroplasty. *J Arthroplasty* 2004;19:94-101.

76. MacDonald SJ, Brodner W, Jacobs JJ: A consensus paper on metal ions in metal-on-metal hip arthroplasties. *J Arthroplasty* 2004;19:12-16.

77. MacDonald SJ, McCalden RW, Chess DG, et al: Metal-on-metal versus polyethylene in hip arthroplasty: A randomized clinical trial. *Clin Orthop Relat Res* 2003;406:282-296.

78. Walter LR, Marel E, Harbury R, Wearne J: Distribution of chromium and cobalt ions in various blood fractions after resurfacing hip arthroplasty. *J Arthroplasty* 2008;23:814-821.

79. Engh CA Jr, MacDonald SJ, Sritulanondha S, Thompson A, Naudie D, Engh CA: Metal ion levels after metal-on-metal total hip arthroplasty: A randomized trial [2008 John Charnley Award]. *Clin Orthop Relat Res* 2009;467:101-111.

80. Brodner W, Bitzan P, Meisinger V, Kaider A, Gottsauner-Wolf F, Kotz R: Serum cobalt levels after metal-on-metal total hip arthroplasty. *J Bone Joint Surg Am* 2003;85:2168-2173.

81. Skipor AK, Campbell PA, Patterson LM, Amstutz HC, Schmalzried TP, Jacobs JJ: Serum and urine metal levels in patients with metal-on-metal surface arthroplasty. *J Mater Sci Mater Med* 2002;13:1227-1234.

82. Clarke MT, Lee PT, Arora A, Villar RN: Levels of metal ions after small- and large-diameter metal-on-metal hip arthroplasty. *J Bone Joint Surg Br* 2003;85:913-917.

83. Antoniou J, Zukor DJ, Mwale F, Minarik W, Petit A, Huk OL: Metal ion levels in the blood of patients after hip resurfacing: A comparison between twenty-eight and thirty-six-millimeter-head metal-on-metal prostheses. *J Bone Joint Surg Am* 2008; 90:142-148.

84. Langton DJ, Jameson SS, Joyce TJ, Webb J, Nargol AV: The effect of component size and orientation on the concentrations of metal ions after resurfacing arthroplasty of the hip. *J Bone Joint Surg Br* 2008;90:1143-1151.

85. Catelas I, Petit A, Vali H, et al: Quantitative analysis of macrophage apoptosis vs. necrosis induced by cobalt and chromium ions in vitro. *Biomaterials* 2005;26:2441-2453.

86. Catelas I, Petit A, Zukor DJ, Huk OL: Cytotoxic and apoptotic effects of cobalt and chromium ions on J774 macrophages: Implication of caspase-3 in the apoptotic pathway. *J Mater Sci Mater Med* 2001;12:949-953.

87. Catelas I, Petit A, Zukor DJ, Antoniou J, Huk OL: TNF-alpha secretion and macrophage mortality induced by cobalt and chromium ions in vitro: Qualitative analysis of apoptosis. *Biomaterials* 2003;24:383-391.

88. O'Brien TJ, Ceryak S, Patierno SR: Complexities of chromium carcinogenesis: Role of cellular response, repair and recovery mechanisms. *Mutat Res* 2003;533:3-36.

89. Quievryn G, Peterson E, Messer J, Zhitkovich A: Genotoxicity and mutagenicity of chromium (VI)/ascorbate-generated DNA adducts in human and bacterial cells. *Biochemistry* 2003;42:1062-1070.

90. Papageorgiou I, Yin Z, Ladon D, et al: Genotoxic effects of particles of surgical cobalt chrome alloy on human cells of different age in vitro. *Mutat Res* 2007;619:45-58.

91. Ladon D, Doherty A, Newson R, Turner J, Bhamra M, Case CP: Changes in metal levels and chromosome aberrations in the peripheral blood of patients after metal-on-metal hip arthroplasty. *J Arthroplasty* 2004;19:78-83.

92. Massè A, Bosetti M, Buratti C, Visentin O, Bergadano D, Cannas M: Ion release and chromosomal damage from total hip prostheses with metal-on-metal articulation. *J Biomed Mater Res B Appl Biomater* 2003;67:750-757.

93. Catelas I, Huk OL, Petit A, Zukor DJ, Marchand R, Yahia L: Flow cytometric analysis of macrophage response to ceramic and polyethylene particles: Effects of size, concentration, and composition. *J Biomed Mater Res* 1998; 41:600-607.

94. Catelas I, Petit A, Zukor DJ, Marchand R, Yahia L, Huk OL: Induction of macrophage apoptosis by ceramic and polyethylene particles in vitro. *Biomaterials* 1999;20:625-630.

95. Catelas I, Petit A, Marchand R, Zukor DJ, Yahia L, Huk OL: Cytotoxicity and macrophage cytokine release induced by ceramic and polyethylene particles in vitro. *J Bone Joint Surg Br* 1999;81:516-521.

96. Nagase M, Nishiya H, Takeuchi H: Effect of particle size on alumina-induced production of reactive oxygen metabolites by human leukocytes. *Scand J Rheumatol* 1995;24:102-107.

97. Hatton A, Nevelos JE, Matthews JB, Fisher J, Ingham E: Effects of clinically relevant alumina ceramic wear particles on TNF-alpha production by human peripheral blood mononuclear phagocytes. *Biomaterials* 2003; 24:1193-1204.

98. Warashina H, Sakano S, Kitamura S, et al: Biological reaction to alumina, zirconia, titanium and polyethylene particles implanted onto murine calvaria. *Biomaterials* 2003;24:3655-3661.

99. Yoo JJ, Kim YM, Yoon KS, Koo KH, Song WS, Kim HJ: Alumina-on-alumina total hip arthroplasty: A five-year minimum follow-up study. *J Bone Joint Surg Am* 2005;87:530-535.

100. D'Antonio J, Capello W, Manley M, Naughton M, Sutton K: Alumina ceramic bearings for total hip arthroplasty: Five-year results of a prospective randomized study. *Clin Orthop Relat Res* 2005;436:164-171.

101. Yoon TR, Rowe SM, Kim MS, Cho SG, Seon JK: Fifteen- to 20-year results of uncemented tapered fully porous-coated cobalt-chrome stems. *Int Orthop* 2008;32:317-323.

102. Hannouche D, Hamadouche M, Nizard R, Bizot P, Meunier A, Sedel L: Ceramics in total hip replacement. *Clin Orthop Relat Res* 2005;430:62-71.

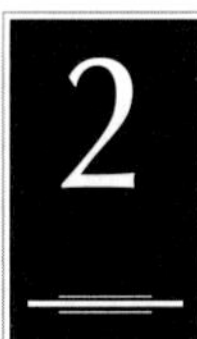

Metal-on-Metal Bearings in Total Hip Arthroplasty

Paul E. Beaulé, MD, FRCSC
Steven A. Mussett, MBChB, FRCSC
John B. Medley, PhD, PEng

Abstract

The demand for total hip arthroplasty is increasing, as are patients' expectations to return to high activity levels. Metal-on-metal bearings are being used in an effort to maximize the longevity of primary hip replacements. Acetabular component inclination has been a recognized aspect of surgical technique for more than 20 years; it now is considered critical, especially in hip resurfacing or implantation of a stem-type device with a larger diameter femoral head and a monoblock acetabular component. It is important to understand the indications for using metal-on-metal bearings as well as the key clinical factors for avoiding early implant failure.

Instr Course Lect 2010;59:17-25.

Metal-on-metal implant articulation bearings were introduced during the 1960s but fell out of favor after poor bearing and implant designs led to disappointing clinical results.[1-4] Metal-on-polyethylene bearings had better clinical results and became the preferred articulation bearing.[5] However, some early metal-on-metal prostheses had satisfactory outcomes, and improved understanding of bearing design eventually led to a renewal of interest in the use of metal-on-metal bearings.[6] A second generation of metal-on-metal bearings with improved design and manufacturing was approved in 1999 for clinical use by the US Food and Drug Administration. The current generation of metal-on-metal bearings has been in use longer than bearings composed of metal on highly cross-linked polyethylene, oxonium on highly cross-linked polyethylene, or delta ceramic on delta ceramic.[7] The advantages of metal on metal compared with other bearing materials include better wear properties and, consequently, potentially greater longevity of the prosthesis; use of a larger femoral head diameter, which permits a greater range of motion and thereby reduces the risk of dislocation after primary or revision surgery; and preservation of acetabular bone stock (when a large-diameter femoral head is used).

Wear Characteristics

Second-generation metal-on-metal bearings have better wear characteristics than first-generation bearings. Decreased wear reduces the risk of wear particle–induced osteolysis[8] or a hypersensitivity reaction.[9,10] Laboratory studies[11-13] comparing different types of cobalt-chromium-molybdenum alloys found that the important factors determining wear resistance are carbon levels, diametral clearance, and surface finish. One study[14] specifically found that the amount of carbon dissolved in the matrix is very important. Cobalt-chromium-molybdenum metal-on-metal bearing alloys are manufactured using either a wrought or cast process. Wrought material has a small grain size with a fine, homogenous distribution of

Dr. Beaulé or an immediate family member is a member of a speakers' bureau or has made paid presentations on behalf of Wright Medical Technology; serves as a paid consultant to or is an employee of Brainlab and Wright Medical Technology; serves as an unpaid consultant to Getinge USA; and has received research or institutional support from Stryker, Wright Medical Technology, and Zimmer. Dr. Medley or an immediate family member has received nonincome support (such as equipment or services), commercially derived honoraria, or other non–research-realted funding (such as paid travel) from Medtronic Spinal & Biologics. Neither Dr. Mussett nor an immediate family member has received anything of value from or owns stock in a commercial company or institution related directly or indirectly to the subject of this chapter.

carbides (a carbide is a compound of carbon with a less electronegative element). Cast material has large grains with blocky carbides; it can be subjected to heat treatment to produce a more uniform distribution of carbides along grain boundaries and in the matrix.[5] Dowson and associates[12] compared wrought and cast cobalt-chromium-molybdenum alloy metal-on-metal hip bearings with a low (less than 0.05%) or high (more than 0.20%) carbon content and found higher wear rates in the bearings with low carbon content. The study did not distinguish between the amount of carbon in carbides compared with the amount dissolved in the alloy matrix. There was no significant difference between the wrought and cast materials in the absence of other factors, and heat treatment did not have a significant effect on wear. This finding was confirmed by other studies.[5]

Rieker and associates[6] found a positive correlation between wear rate and clearance in the laboratory setting. Diametral clearance may be the most important parameter influencing the wear of a metal-on-metal bearing.[9,10] The clearance must be adequate to allow polar (rather than equatorial) articulation of the contact zone that remains polar under the mechanical deformation occurring when the prosthesis is loaded. Polar articulation refers to the femoral head and inner acetabular component surface making contact at the dome, whereas equatorial articulation refers to contact at the widest part of the femoral head. Polar bearing contact patterns result in less wear, probably because fluid ingress optimizes surface-protective, elastohydrodynamic lubrication, which creates beneficial surface deformation in the contact zone, and the subsequent egress of wear-generated particles.[9,10] If the clearance is too small, equatorial bearing occurs and fluid entrainment cannot take place; the resulting high frictional torque leads to seizing and subsequent loosening. McKee[15] recognized inadequate clearance as the mechanism for early failures of the McKee-Farrar prosthesis; as a result, in 1968 the femoral head component was slightly downsized. Seizure also frequently occurred with use of the equatorial-bearing Stanmore metal-on-metal hip implant.[16] Excessive wear also can occur if the diametral clearance is too great; one study reported a wear rate 16 times greater than average.[17] Many manufacturers make metal-on-metal bearings with a diametral clearance of 100 to 200 μm to maximize fluid entrapment and ensure polar bearing.

The influence of diametral clearance recently was considered in more detail. Metal-on-metal implant wear in a hip simulator was found to be related to the film thickness of the lubricant fluid, as determined using Dowson's explanation of elastohydrodynamic theory.[9,10] Efforts were made to relate the thickness of the lubricant fluid film to surface roughness using the λ parameter (the ratio of the thickness of the fluid film to the composite root-mean-square surface roughness). The fluid film thickness and the λ parameter for a specific surface roughness are closely correlated with the effective radius of the bearing.[9,10] The effective radius is a geometric parameter that contains both radial clearance and femoral component head size; it can be expressed by the formula $R = R_H (R_H + C)/C$, where R is the effective radius, R_H is the radius of the head, and C is the radial clearance (the difference between femoral head and acetabular cup radii or, more simply, one half of the diametral clearance). The concept of decreased wear with increasing effective radius was supported by in vitro simulator data and some in vivo clinical data.[18] Effective radius increases with lubricant fluid film thickness and the λ parameter, and wear decreases when the radius of the femoral head is as large as possible and the radial clearance is as small as possible.[9,10] The effective radius can be controlled by the device manufacturer.

A hip bearing with a large effective radius has a larger contact zone and thus a lower contact stress than a bearing with a smaller effective radius. Provided the contact area remains polar and has a small peripheral inlet region, lubricant can be more easily entrained and thus develop into a thicker, more protective fluid film. In addition, a large-diameter head, which often contributes to a large effective radius, has a higher surface velocity during activities and thus creates a higher entrainment velocity for the lubricant, further increasing lubricant film thickness. When activity levels are low, fluid films slowly decrease in thickness and eventually break down; thus, fluid films are not initially available to protect the surface when activity levels subsequently increase. When activity begins, the surfaces are likely to be in direct contact, and other conditions at the surface influence wear.

The manufacturer has some control over the alloy microstructure, particularly over the amount of dissolved carbon. Varano and associates[14] proposed that higher levels of dissolved carbon make the surface microstructure resistant to a strain-induced transformation, which is associated with higher wear. Thus, a higher level of dissolved carbon was considered beneficial. Varano and

Table 1
The Advantages and Disadvantages of Metal-on-Metal Bearings

Advantages
Low wear rate
Reduced risk of osteolysis
Improved longevity
Larger diameter femoral head
Improved range of motion
Reduced risk of dislocation
Preserved acetabular bone stock (compared with a metal-on-polyethylene bearing surface)
Disadvantages
Metal ion release
Risk of carcinogenicity
Risk of chromosomal damage
Pregnancy risk (teratogenic, mutagenic)
Metal hypersensitivity

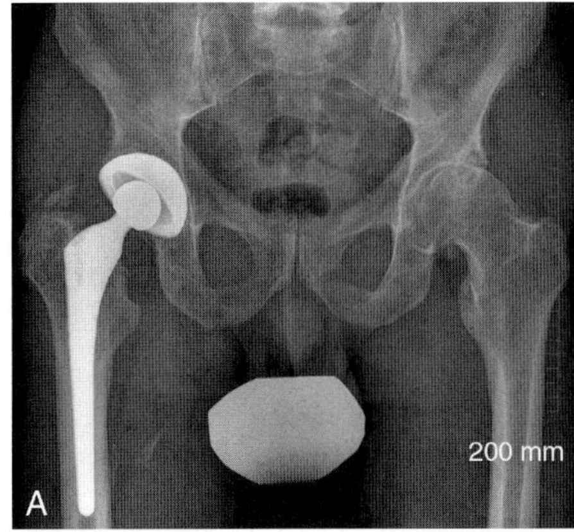

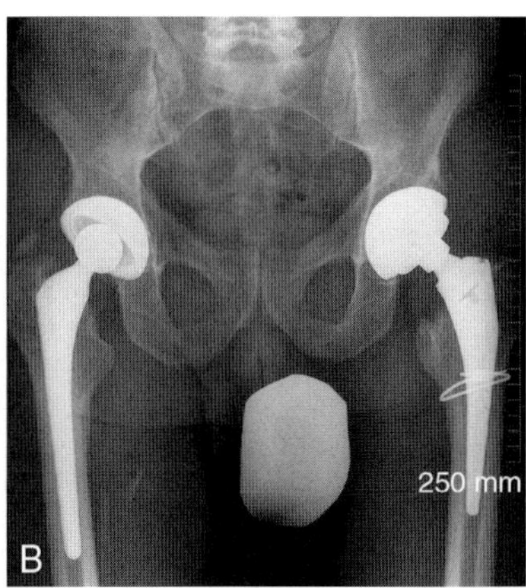

Figure 1 **A,** AP radiograph of the pelvis in a 43-year-old patient showing a right total hip replacement with a cementless metal-on-polyethylene implant and advanced arthritis in the left hip. **B,** AP radiograph of the left total hip replacement using a large metal-on-metal bearing with a modular, large-head femoral component (ProFemur TL Total Hip System, Wright Medical Technology, Memphis, TN).

associates[14] noted that a large effective radius also would reduce contact stress and thus surface strain, thereby reducing strain-induced transformation. Although the effectiveness of higher levels of dissolved carbon in reducing in vivo wear has not been determined, it is interesting to note that a high effective radius might help reduce wear by reducing contact stress during surface contact. A cobalt-chromium-molybdenum alloy with a high level of carbon tends to have a higher level of dissolved carbon; a metal-on-metal hip implant that was made from an alloy with a high carbon content (perhaps having more dissolved carbon) and that has a low clearance and a large diameter (thus, a high effective radius) is likely to have a lower wear rate.

Clinical Indications and Advantages

The use of metal-on-metal implants is associated with several advantages (Table 1). Multiple studies have reported a significant reduction in bearing wear and subsequent osteolysis.[8,19,20] Retrieval analyses of second-generation metal-on-metal implants found a 20-fold reduction in linear wear rate and a more than 60-fold reduction in volumetric wear rate, compared with traditional, not intentionally cross-linked polyethylene implants.[20] This factor may lead to increased implant longevity and a need for fewer revision surgeries, which would be of immense value for young, active patients.

A second advantage of using a metal-on-metal implant is the ability to use a larger diameter femoral head (Figure 1), which has better wear characteristics than a smaller diameter femoral head. In addition, using a larger femoral head component can be important in treating a patient with instability, because increasing the head size reduces the risk of dislocation.[21,22] The increased head size allows for a greater head-to-neck ratio, which increases the primary arc of motion by reducing the risk of the femoral neck impinging on the edge of the cup at opposite ends of the range of motion.[23] Increasing the femoral head size increases the excursion distance from the point the neck impinges to the point the hip dislocates.

The reported incidence of hip instability after revision surgery ranges from 8% to 14%.[24-26] Very large femoral heads (having a diameter greater than 40 mm) with a polyethylene liner have been used with some success in revision procedures necessitated by instability, but the demands on the polyethylene are great.[27,28] The advantage of using a metal-on-metal bearing in revision procedures for instability is that the wall of the acetabular component can be relatively thin (4 mm), permitting the size of the femoral head to be maximized without compromising the acetabular bone stock. A metal-on-metal bearing also can be useful when a liner must be cemented into a well-fixed acetabular shell because the locking mechanism is damaged. Cementing an all-metal liner allows access to a wider range of large femoral heads[29,30] (Figure 2).

Both first- and second-generation metal-on-metal prostheses are associated with good rates of clinical survivorship and low rates of osteol-

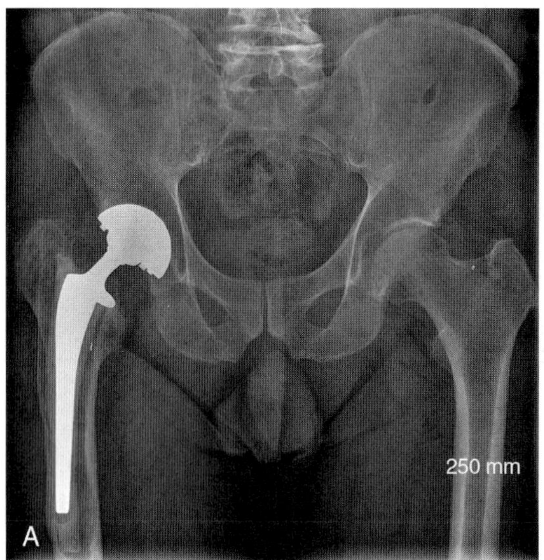

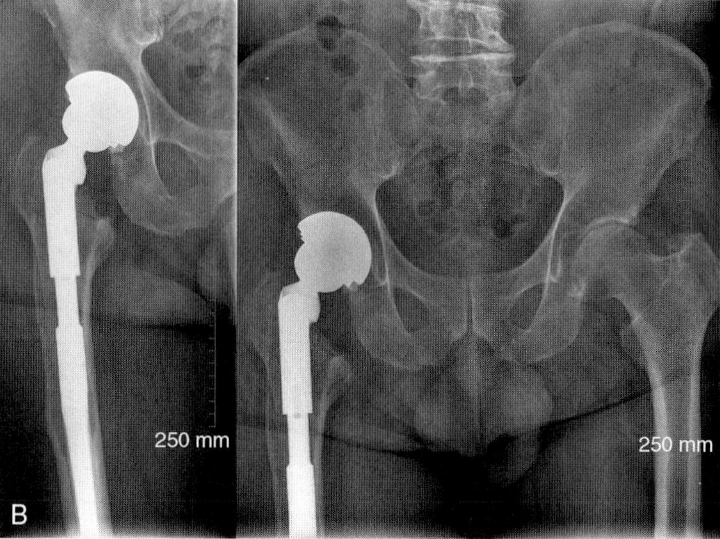

Figure 2 **A,** AP radiograph showing aseptic loosening of a right total hip replacement in a 73-year-old man. **B,** AP hip (left) and AP pelvic (right) radiographs showing revision to a modular femoral stem (Link, Hamburg, Germany) with a large-head metal-on-metal bearing (BFH, Wright Medical Technology), which was achieved by cementing the liner into the well-fixed existing cementless shell.

ysis. Long and associates[31] found good results at 5- to 11-year follow-up after 161 hip replacements using a Metasul hip implant (Zimmer, Warsaw, IN) with a 28-mm femoral head component. Six revision surgeries were needed, including one for aseptic loosening and one for instability. A focal radiolucency, identified as calcar resorption, was identified in nine patients. Saito and associates[32] reported excellent mid-term results at average 6.4-year follow-up after hip replacements using the Metasul implant. The survival rate was 99.1%, and no patients had osteolysis or loosening. Grübl and associates[33] reviewed the 10-year results of 105 hips with a second-generation metal-on-metal total hip replacement. The survival rate was 98.6%, and osteolysis was rarely reported. At a minimum 5-year follow-up, Migaud and associates[34] compared 39 patients treated with a metal-on-metal total hip replacement with a 28-mm femoral head component with 39 matched patients treated with a ceramic-on-polyethylene total hip replacement with a 28-mm femoral head component. The metal-on-metal hip implants fared better than the ceramic-on-polyethylene implants. Nine of the patients with a ceramic-on-polyethylene implant had osteolysis, and seven required revision; neither osteolysis nor revision was found in the patients with a metal-on-metal implant. The 5-year survival rate was 100% for the metal-on-metal implants and 97.2% for the ceramic-on-polyethylene implants.

Cuckler and associates[35] compared the results of using a 28-mm or 38-mm femoral head in metal-on-metal hip replacements. The dislocation rate was 2.5% with the 28-mm head; there were no dislocations with the 38-mm head. Peters and associates[36] found no dislocations in 136 patients with a 38-mm head, compared with a 2.5% rate (four dislocations) in 160 patients with a 28-mm head. The 38-mm heads were inserted using a posterior approach, and the 28-mm heads were inserted using a Hardinge approach. Subsequently, 469 metal-on-metal hip replacements with a 38-mm head were inserted using a posterior approach; only two dislocations occurred.

The use of large-head metal-on-metal hip implants reduces the likelihood of dislocation and therefore leads to fewer postoperative restrictions and a higher postoperative activity level.[35] This factor is especially relevant because returning to recreational activities is an important patient expectation after total hip replacement.[37] Improved activity levels after hip replacement are associated with higher patient satisfaction rates.[38,39] In high-activity patients, a metal-on-metal hip implant has the benefit of being able to withstand impact loading; no implant fractures have been recorded.

The use of metal-on-metal articulations has facilitated the reintroduction of hip resurfacing, with excellent short-term results.[40-42] On the acetabular side, the relatively thin wall of the metal cup and the lack of keyholes means that less bone stock is taken than with the first generation of cemented metal-on-polyethylene hip resurfacing sockets.[43] Although the rate of wear debris–induced failures after hip resurfacing has been significantly reduced with the introduction of metal-on-metal bearings, patient selection and proper surgical technique remain the key determinants of clinical success.[44]

Table 2
The Relationship Between Acetabular Cup Inclination and Metal Ion Concentration in Whole Blood

	Ion Concentration	
Cup Inclination	Cobalt	Chromium
More than 55° (steep)	9.8 μg/L (range, 0.6 to 111.3 μg/L)	9.7 μg/L (range, 0.6 to 94.6 μg/L)
55° or less	2.4 μg/L (range, 0.4 to 31.5 μg/L)	3.6 μg/L (range, 0.2 to 32.2 μg/L)

(Adapted with permission from De Haan R, Pattyn C, Gill HS, Murray DW, Campbell PA, De Smet KA: Correlation between inclination of the acetabular component and metal ion levels in metal-on-metal hip resurfacing replacement. *J Bone Joint Surg Br* 2008;90:1291-1297.)

Clinical Contraindications and Disadvantages

Metal Ion Release

Multiple clinical studies have documented an elevation in patients with a metal-on-metal implant of cobalt and chromium ions in blood, serum, erythrocytes, and urine, as well as an accumulation in the abdominal lymph nodes, liver, and spleen.[45-48] In a randomized, controlled comparison study of metal-on-metal and metal-on-polyethylene total hip replacements, MacDonald and associates[47] reported a 7.9-fold increase in erythrocyte cobalt and a 2.3-fold increase in erythrocyte chromium, as well as a 35-fold increase in urinary cobalt and a 17-fold increase in urinary chromium. Metal-on-metal implants have a biphasic wear pattern. The wear rates are highest during an initial bedding-in phase, with peak levels occurring 6 to 12 months after surgery. The wear rate steadily decreases during the subsequent 12 months to a continuing state of slow, steady wear; however, metal ion levels appear to remain elevated over time.[33] Increased ion concentration has been reported after exercise, but this finding is controversial; the concentration may be related to a decrease in urinary ion excretion rather than an increase in ion production during exercise.[49]

Most metal ions are excreted in the urine and therefore are of most concern in patients with impaired renal function.[50] The value of monitoring metal ion levels is unclear. Jacobs and associates[51] concluded that, although metal ion concentration may be routinely monitored in the future, presently it is primarily useful as a research tool. Nonetheless, assessment of ion levels can be used to identify a malfunctioning or malpositioned total hip replacement.[52] The importance of proper acetabular component orientation (a cup abduction angle of less than 50°) for wear properties and metal ion release was recently discussed[53-55] (Table 2). Langton and associates[53] looked at the influence of acetabular component abduction on metal ion levels, finding that smaller femoral head components (less than 51 mm) were associated with higher levels of metal ion release. It remains unclear how implant design (diametral clearance and inner bearing diameter) influences wear properties in relation to acetabular component position. The inner bearing surface design of monoblock acetabular shells is different from that of modular acetabular metal liners; for example, some monoblock acetabular shells are less than 180° (a hemisphere) and may be only 164°.[56] In addition, some acetabular components have a relatively thick central pole, which lateralizes the hip's center of rotation and decreases the overall surface area for bearing contact. These types of shell designs may have a narrower range of acceptable cup abduction and may be more susceptible to edge-loading wear because of the smaller area of surface contact[54,55] (Table 3). This factor is extremely important because substantial wear of metal-on-metal bearings is associated with significant soft tissue reactions.[57] De Haan and associates[55] recently reported that hip resurfacings with a cup placed at more than 55° of abduction had significantly higher cobalt and chromium ion levels (Table 2) and that smaller femoral component sizes were outliers in terms of ion release. Acetabular component designs with a lower arc of cover (164° compared with an average arc of cover of 170°) had significantly higher concentrations of cobalt and chromium ions when they were placed at more than 55° of abduction (Table 3).

Adverse Tissue Reaction

Metal-on-metal hip replacements may be associated with higher rates of malignancy secondary to metal ion release. However, a review of cancer incidence in all patients on the Finnish registry who underwent

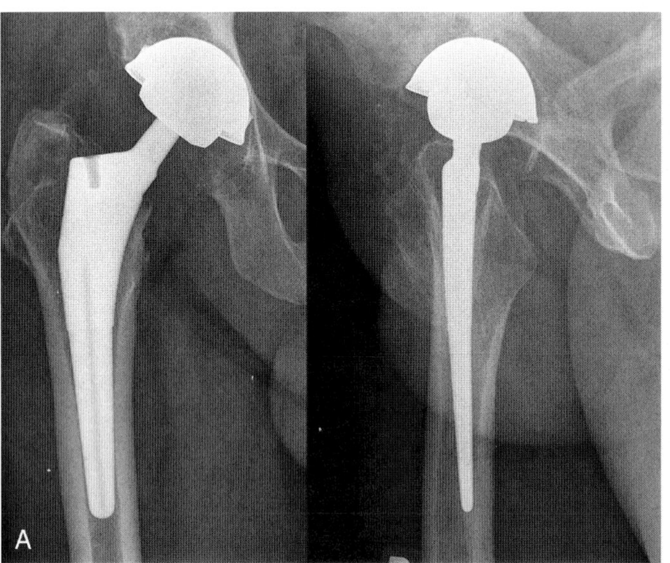

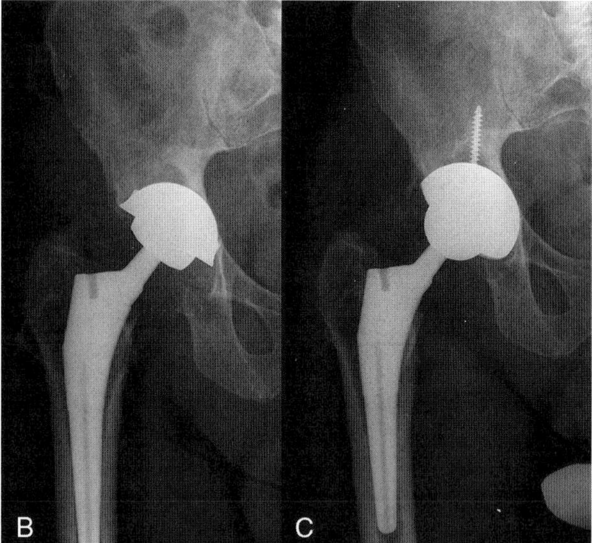

Figure 3 **A,** AP (left) and lateral (right) radiographs of the right hip in a 70-year-old man 14 months after a metal-on-metal total hip replacement and 6 months after the onset of thigh and groin pain. There is evidence of osteolysis at the dome of the acetabular component; the septic workup was negative. **B,** AP radiograph of the right hip (taken 6 months after the radiographs shown in part A) showing migration of the acetabular component. **C,** AP radiograph taken 1 year after isolated revision of the acetabular component with conversion to a metal-on-polyethylene bearing (Trabecular Metal Revision Shell with Longevity liner; Zimmer, Warsaw, IN).

Table 3
The Relationship Between Acetabular Arc of Cover With a Steep Cup Inclination (> 55°) and Metal Ion Concentration in Whole Blood

	Ion Concentration	
Arc of Cover	Cobalt	Chromium
164°	10.2 µg/L (range, 0.8 to 111.3 µg/L)	10.4 µg/L (range, 0.6 to 94.6 µg/L)
170°	2.1 µg/L (range, 0.6 to 6.4 µg/L)	3.0 µg/L (range, 0.9 to 7.6 µg/L)

(Adapted with permission from De Haan R, Pattyn C, Gill HS, Murray DW, Campbell PA, De Smet KA: Correlation between inclination of the acetabular component and metal ion levels in metal-on-metal hip resurfacing replacement. *J Bone Joint Surg Br* 2008;90:1291-1297.)

total hip replacement between 1980 and 1999 found no increased risk among those who had a metal-on-metal implant compared with the general population.[58] Although this study reported an increased incidence of prostate cancer and melanoma after hip arthroplasty, the current evidence does not confirm that the risk is increased. Large epidemiologic studies with longer follow-up periods and an adjustment for comorbidities are necessary to obtain an accurate estimate of the risk.[59]

Chromosomal abnormalities (translocations and aneuploidy) were found to be increased in patients with metal-on-metal or metal-on-polyethylene bearings.[60,61]

Willert and associates[62] described an aseptic, lymphocyte-dominated, vasculitis-associated lesion that appears as persistent hip pain in patients with a metal-on-metal hip implant and in some patients is associated with osteolysis (Figure 3). The incidence of this hypersensitivity reaction was low (less than 0.3%), and it may have been linked to wear of the prosthesis. Although the overall volume of wear particles released from a metal-on-metal implant is less than the volume of polyethylene debris from a metal-on-polyethylene implant, the total number of particles released from a metal-on-metal implant may be greater.[63] Milosev and associates[64] found high levels of osteolysis in low carbon, metal-on-metal alloy articulations, and this clinical experience was confirmed by other studies of low carbon alloy implants.[65] In a retrieval analysis, Reinisch and associates[66] found higher wear rates in low carbon alloy implants, compared with high carbon alloy implants.

Pseudotumors were reported in 17 female patients with metal-on-metal hip resurfacing.[57] These patients had pain or a malfunctioning prosthesis at a mean of 17 months after surgery. A cystic mass was found in

8 of the 13 patients who underwent imaging studies. Fourteen of the 17 patients underwent further surgery; the cup abduction was found to be significantly higher in those with a soft-tissue mass. This study had several limitations—the severity of the soft-tissue reaction was not graded and cystic lesions and masses were not differentiated. Griffiths and associates[67] found that these types of masses, which they called granulomatous pseudotumors, also occurred in female patients with metal-on-polyethylene bearings, with similar destructive processes. Symptoms appeared more rapidly in patients with metal-on-metal bearings than in patients with metal-on-polyethylene bearings, but development of the pseudotumor was related to excessive particulate wear debris in all patients. Additional longitudinal research is required to determine the incidence of pseudotumors and whether they are limited to female patients or to patients with a smaller femoral component.

There has been concern about the use of metal-on-metal bearings in women of childbearing age because the effects of metal ions on a fetus are unknown. Although Brodner and associates[68] did not find that ions cross the placenta, a more recent study by Ziaee and associates,[69] using more sensitive measurement techniques, did find that ions cross the placenta. Because of the theoretic mutagenic and teratogenic risk, women are advised to delay metal-on-metal hip replacement until after childbearing or to delay childbearing for 1 to 2 years after receiving a metal-on-metal hip replacement.

Summary

Improvements in design and manufacturing as well as an improved understanding of in vivo biomechanics and wear have led to renewed interest in the use of metal-on-metal hip bearings. Metal-on-metal bearing surfaces offer several advantages over metal-on-polyethylene, ceramic-on-polyethylene, or ceramic-on-ceramic surfaces. Metal-on-metal bearings have very low wear rates, and osteolysis is infrequent. Metal on metal allows the use of a larger diameter femoral head; the result is a greater range of motion, increased stability, and resistance to fracture. Patients are less restricted and more satisfied. These advantages are important not only for young, high-demand patients but also for patients at risk of dislocation. In revision surgery, the use of a larger femoral head component reduces the risk of dislocation and can successfully treat instability. There are concerns about elevated levels of metal ions and their theoretic consequences, as well as the possibility of metal hypersensitivity; longer term studies are required to resolve the clinical implications of these concerns. With careful patient selection, attention to surgical technique, and vigilant clinical follow-up, metal-on-metal total joint arthroplasty can provide predictable results with excellent long-term survival rates.

References

1. McKee GK, Watson-Farrar J: Replacement of arthritic hips by the McKee-Farrar prosthesis. *J Bone Joint Surg Br* 1966;48:245-259.
2. McKee GK, Chen SC: The statistics of the McKee-Farrar method of total hip replacement. *Clin Orthop Relat Res* 1973;95:26-33.
3. Ring PA: Total replacement of the hip joint: A review of a thousand operations. *J Bone Joint Surg Br* 1974;56: 44-58.
4. Amstutz HC, Grigoris P: Metal on metal bearings in hip arthroplasty. *Clin Orthop Relat Res* 1996;329:S11-S34.
5. Nevelos J, Shelton JC, Fisher J: Metallurgical considerations in the wear of metal-on-metal hip bearings. *Hip Int* 2004;14:1-10.
6. Rieker CB, Schön R, Konrad R, et al: Influence of the clearance on in-vitro tribology of large diameter metal-on-metal articulations pertaining to resurfacing hip implants. *Orthop Clin North Am* 2005;36:135-142.
7. Fisher J, Jin Z, Tipper J, Stone M, Ingham E: Tribology of alternative bearings. *Clin Orthop Relat Res* 2006; 453:25-34.
8. Jacobsson SA, Djerf K, Wahlström O: Twenty-year results of McKee-Farrar versus Charnley prosthesis. *Clin Orthop Relat Res* 1996;139:S60-S68.
9. Dowson D: Tribological principles in metal-on-metal hip joint design. *Proc Inst Mech Eng H* 2006;220:161-171.
10. Rieker CB, Schön R, Köttig P: Development and validation of second-generation metal-on-metal bearing: Laboratory studies and analysis of retrievals. *J Arthroplasty* 2004;19:5-11.
11. Chan FW, Bobyn JD, Medley JB, Krygier JT, Tanzer M: Wear and lubrication of metal-on-metal hip implants. *Clin Orthop Relat Res* 1999;369: 10-24.
12. Dowson D, Hardaker C, Flett M, Isaac GH: A hip joint simulator study of the performance of metal-on-metal joints: Part I. The role of materials. *J Arthroplasty* 2004;19:118-123.
13. Streicher RM, Semlitsch M, Schön R, Weber H, Rieker C: Metal-on-metal articulation for artificial hip joints: Laboratory study and clinical results. *Proc Inst Mech Eng H* 1996;210:223-232.
14. Varano R, Bobyn JD, Medley JB, Yue S: The effect of microstructure on the wear of cobalt-based alloys used in metal-on-metal hip implants. *Proc Inst Mech Eng H* 2006;220:145-159.
15. McKee GK: Development of total prosthetic replacement of the hip. *Clin Orthop Relat Res* 1970;72:85-103.
16. Wilson JN, Scales JT: Loosening of total hip replacements with cement

fixation: Clinical findings and laboratory studies. *Clin Orthop Relat Res* 1970;72:145-160.

17. McKellop H, Park S, Chiesa R, et al: In vivo wear of three types of metal on metal hip prostheses during two decades of use. *Clin Orthop Relat Res* 1996;329:S128-S140.

18. Medley JB: Tribology of bearing materials, in Amstutz HC, ed: *Hip Resurfacing: Principles, Indications, Technique and Results*. Philadelphia, PA, Elsevier, 2008, pp 33-44.

19. Schmalzried TP, Peters PC, Maurer BT, Bragdon CR, Harris WH: Long duration metal-on-metal total hip replacements with low wear of the articulating surfaces. *J Arthroplasty* 1996; 11:322-331.

20. Sieber HP, Rieker CB, Köttig P: Analysis of 118 second-generation metal-on-metal retrieved hip implants. *J Bone and Joint Surg Br* 1999; 81:46-50.

21. Berry DJ, von Knoch M, Schleck CD, Harmsen WS: Effect of femoral head diameter and operative approach on risk of dislocation after primary total hip arthroplasty. *J Bone Joint Surg Am* 2005;87:2456-2463.

22. Amstutz HC, Le Duff MJ, Beaulé PE: Prevention and treatment of dislocation after total hip replacement using large diameter balls. *Clin Orthop Relat Res* 2004;429:108-116.

23. Chandler DR, Glousman R, Hull D, et al: Prosthetic hip range of motion and impingement: The effects of head and neck geometry. *Clin Orthop Relat Res* 1982;166:284-291.

24. Alberton GM, High WA, Morrey BF: Dislocation after revision total hip arthroplasty: An analysis of risk factors and treatment options. *J Bone Joint Surg Am* 2002;84:1788-1792.

25. Phillips CB, Barrett JA, Losina E, et al: Incidence rates of dislocation, pulmonary embolism, and deep infection during the first six months after elective total hip replacement. *J Bone Joint Surg Am* 2003;85:20-26.

26. Mahomed NN, Barrett JA, Katz JN, et al: Rates and outcomes of primary and revision total hip replacement in the United States Medicare population. *J Bone Joint Surg Am* 2003;85: 27-32.

27. Beaulé PE, Schmalzried TP, Udomkiat P, Amstutz HC: Jumbo femoral head for the treatment of recurrent dislocation following total hip replacement. *J Bone Joint Surg Am* 2002;84:256-263.

28. Halley D, Glassman AH, Crowninshield RD: Recurrent dislocation after revision total hip replacement with a large prosthetic femoral head: A case report. *J Bone Joint Surg Am* 2004;86:827-830.

29. Ebramzadeh E, Beaulé PE, Culwell JL, Amstutz HC: Fixation strength of an all-metal acetabular component cemented into an acetabular shell: A biomechanical analysis. *J Arthroplasty* 2004;19:45-49.

30. Beaulé PE, Ebramzadeh E, LeDuff MJ, Prasad R, Amstutz HC: Cementing a liner into a stable cementless acetabular shell in revision hip surgery: The double-socket technique. *J Bone Joint Surg Am* 2004;86:929-934.

31. Long WT, Dorr LD, Gendelman V: An American experience with metal-on-metal total hip arthroplasties: A 7-year follow-up study. *J Arthroplasty* 2004;19:29-34.

32. Saito S, Ryu J, Watanabe T, Ishii K, Saigo K: Midterm results of Metasul metal-on-metal total hip arthroplasty. *J Arthroplasty* 2006;21:1105-1110.

33. Grübl A, Marker M, Brodner W, et al: Long-term follow-up of metal-on-metal total hip replacement. *J Orthop Res* 2007;25:841-848.

34. Migaud H, Jobin A, Chantelot C, Giraud F, Laffargue P, Duquennoy A: Cementless metal-on-metal hip arthroplasty in patients less than 50 years of age: Comparison with a matched control group using ceramic-on-polyethylene after a minimum 5-year follow-up. *J Arthroplasty* 2004;19:23-28.

35. Cuckler JM, Moore KD, Lombardi AV Jr, McPherson E, Emerson R: Large versus small femoral heads in metal-on-metal total hip arthroplasty. *J Arthroplasty* 2004;19:41-44.

36. Peters CL, McPherson E, Jackson JD, Erickson JA: Reduction in early dislocation rate with large-diameter femoral heads in primary total hip arthroplasty. *J Arthroplasty* 2007;22:140-144.

37. Wright JG, Rudicel S, Feinstein AR: Ask patients what they want: Evaluation of individual complaints before total hip replacement. *J Bone Joint Surg Br* 1994;76:229-234.

38. Lieberman JR, Dorey FJ, Shekelle P, et al: Outcome after total hip arthroplasty: Comparison of a traditional disease-specific and a quality-of-life measurement of outcome. *J Arthroplasty* 1997;12:639-645.

39. Beaulé PE, Dorey FJ, Hoke R, Le Duff MJ, Amstutz HC: The value of patient activity level in clinical outcome of total hip arthroplasty. *J Arthroplasty* 2006;21:547-552.

40. Amstutz HC, Beaulé PE, Dorey FJ, Le Duff MJ, Campbell PA, Gruen TA: Metal-on-metal hybrid surface arthroplasty: Two to six-year follow-up. *J Bone Joint Surg Am* 2004;86: 28-39.

41. Daniel J, Pynsent PB, McMinn DJ: Metal-on-metal resurfacing of the hip in patients under the age of 55 years with osteoarthritis. *J Bone Joint Surg Br* 2004;86:177-184.

42. Treacy RB, McBryde CW, Pynsent PB: Birmingham hip resurfacing arthroplasty: A minimum follow-up of five years. *J Bone Joint Surg Br* 2005;87: 167-170.

43. Vendittoli PA, Lavigne M, Girard J, Roy AG: A randomised study comparing resection of acetabular bone at resurfacing and total hip replacement. *J Bone Joint Surg Br* 2006;88:997-1002.

44. Beaulé PE: Surface arthroplasty of the hip: A review and current indications. *Semin Arthroplasty* 2005;16:70-76.

45. Brodner W, Bitzan P, Meisinger V, Kaider A, Gottsauner-Wolf F, Kotz R: Serum cobalt levels after metal-on-metal total hip arthroplasty. *J Bone Joint Surg Am* 2003;85:2168-2173.

46. Schaffer AW, Pilger A, Engelhardt C, Zweymuller K, Ruediger HW: Increased blood cobalt and chromium after total hip replacement. *J Toxicol Clin Toxicol* 1999;37:839-844.

47. MacDonald SJ, McCalden RW, Chess DG, et al: Metal-on-metal versus polyethylene in hip arthroplasty: A randomized clinical trial. *Clin Orthop Relat Res* 2003;406:282-296.

48. Urban RM, Tomlinson MJ, Hall DJ, Jacobs JJ: Accumulation in liver and spleen of metal particles generated at nonbearing surfaces in hip arthroplasty. *J Arthroplasty* 2004;19:94-101.

49. Bitsch RG, Zamorano M, Loidolt T, Heisel C, Jacobs JJ, Schmalzreid TP: Ion production and excretion in a patient with a metal-on-metal bearing hip prosthesis: A case report. *J Bone Joint Surg Am* 2007;89:2758-2763.

50. Brodner W, Grohs JG, Bitzan P, Meisinger V, Kovarik J, Kotz R: Serum cobalt and serum chromium level in 2 patients with chronic renal failure after total hip prosthesis implantation with metal-metal gliding contact. *Z Orthop Ihre Grenzgeb* 2000; 138:425-429.

51. Jacobs JJ, Skipor AK, Campbell PA, Hallab NJ, Urban RM, Amstutz HC: Can metal levels be used to monitor metal-on-metal hip arthroplasties? *J Arthroplasty* 2004;19:59-65.

52. Brodner W, Grübl A, Jankovsky R, Meisinger V, Lehr S, Gottsauner-Wolf F: Cup inclination and serum concentration of cobalt and chromium after metal-on-metal total hip arthroplasty. *J Arthroplasty* 2004;19: 66-70.

53. Langton DJ, Jameson SS, Joyce TJ, Webb J, Nargol AV: The effect of component size and orientation on the concentrations of metal ions after resurfacing arthroplasty of the hip. *J Bone Joint Surg Br* 2008;90:1143-1151.

54. Williams S, Leslie I, Isaac G, Jin Z, Ingham E, Fisher J: Tribology and wear of metal-on-metal hip prostheses: Influence of cup angle and head position. *J Bone Joint Surg Am* 2008;90: 111-117.

55. De Haan R, Pattyn C, Gill HS, Murray DW, Campbell PA, De Smet KA: Correlation between inclination of the acetabular component and metal ion levels in metal-on-metal hip resurfacing replacement. *J Bone Joint Surg Br* 2008;90:1291-1297.

56. Shimmin A, Beaulé PE, Campbell P: Metal-on-metal hip resurfacing arthroplasty. *J Bone Joint Surg Am* 2008; 90:637-654.

57. Pandit H, Glyn-Jones S, McLardy-Smith P, et al: Pseudotumors associated with metal-on-metal hip resurfacings. *J Bone Joint Surg Br* 2008;90: 847-851.

58. Visuri TI, Pukkala E, Pulkkinen P, Paavolainen P: Cancer incidence and causes of death among total hip replacement patients: A review based on Nordic cohorts with a special emphasis on metal-on-metal bearings. *Proc Inst Mech Mech Eng H* 2006;220: 399-407.

59. Tharani R, Dorey FJ, Schmalzreid TP: The risk of cancer following total hip or knee arthroplasty. *J Bone Joint Surg Am* 2001;83:774-780.

60. Ladon D, Doherty A, Newson R, Turner J, Bhamra M, Case CP: Changes in metal levels and chromosome aberrations in the peripheral blood of patients after metal-on-metal hip arthroplasty. *J Arthroplasty* 2004;19:78-83.

61. Daley B, Doherty AT, Fairman B, Case CP: Wear debris from hip or knee replacements causes chromosomal damage in human cells in tissue culture. *J Bone Joint Surg* 2004;86: 598-606.

62. Willert HG, Buchorn G, Fayaayazi A, Lohmann C: Histopathological changes around metal/metal joints indicate delayed type hypersensitivity: Preliminary results of 14 cases. *Osteologie* 2000;9:2.

63. Campbell P, Shen FW, McKellop H: Biologic and tribologic considerations of alternative bearing surfaces. *Clin Orthop Relat Res* 2004;418:98-111.

64. Milosev I, Trebse R, Kovac S, Cör A, Pisot V: Survivorship and retrieval analysis of Sikomet metal-on-metal total hip replacements at a mean of seven years. *J Bone Joint Surg Am* 2006; 88:1173-1182.

65. Park YS, Moon YW, Lim SL, Yang YM, Ahn G, Choi YL: Early osteolysis following second-generation metal-on-metal hip replacement. *J Bone Joint Surg Am* 2005;87:1515-1521.

66. Reinisch G, Judmann KP, Lhotke C, Lintner F, Zweymüller KA: Retrieval study of uncemented metal-metal hip prostheses revised for early loosening. *Biomaterials* 2003;24:1081-1091.

67. Griffiths HJ, Burke J, Bonfiglio TA: Granulomatous pseudotumors in total joint replacement. *Skeletal Radiol* 1987;16:146-152.

68. Brodner W, Grohs JG, Bancher-Todesca D, et al: Does the placenta inhibit the passage of chromium and cobalt after metal-on-metal total hip arthroplasty? *J Arthroplasty* 2004;19: 102-106.

69. Ziaee H, Daniel J, Datta AK, Blunt S, McMinn DJ: Transplacental transfer of cobalt and chromium in patients with metal-on-metal hip arthroplasty: A controlled study. *J Bone Joint Surg Br* 2007;89:301-305.

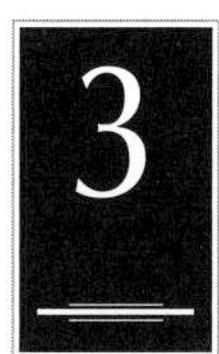

Acetabular Bone Loss in Revision Total Hip Arthroplasty: Principles and Techniques

Shahryar Noordin, MBBS, FCPS
Bassam A. Masri, MD, FRCSC
Clive P. Duncan, MD, MSc, FRCSC
Donald S. Garbuz, MD, MHSc, FRCSC

Abstract

Bone stock deficiency presents the major challenge in acetabular reconstruction during revision hip arthroplasty. The preoperative assessment of acetabular bone stock before revision surgery is critical because the amount and location of pelvic osteolysis can determine the type and success of revision surgery. Traditionally, plain radiographs with AP and lateral views have been used for this purpose; however, Judet views can provide additional information about the integrity of the anterior and posterior columns. CT and MRI scans are indicated in selected patients. A variety of surgical options are available for treating Paprosky type 3 defects. Jumbo cups, the high hip center technique, impaction grafting, bilobed implants, antiprotrusio cages, and structural allografts, in addition to other types of implants, are part of the armamentarium available for revision hip arthroplasty. Segmental bone loss involving more than 50% of the acetabulum is one of the biggest challenges in revision hip replacement. The short-term clinical and radiographic results of treating these large defects with modular, highly porous metal components appear promising. However, potential problems with these components include their unknown long-term durability, potential for debris generation at the shell-augment interface, potential for fatigue failure, and the inability to restore bone stock if future revisions are needed.

Instr Course Lect 2010;59:27-36.

In revision hip arthroplasty, bone stock deficiency is the major challenge in reconstructing the acetabulum. The most common causes of bone deficiency include debris-induced periprosthetic osteolysis (with or without loosening), stress shielding, implant migration, infection, and iatrogenic bone loss during implant extraction. Wear debris-generated osteolysis and loosening of the acetabular cup usually cause proximal and posterior migration of the cup with bone resorption in the posterosuperior wall, giving the acetabular cavity an oblong shape.

With advancing bone loss, reconstructive techniques become more complex. As primary hip arthroplasty is used to treat younger and more active patients, the incidence of revision surgery is likely to further increase, although this factor may be affected by modern wear-resistant bearing surfaces and vigilant follow-up analysis. In patients treated with revision acetabular surgery, the best chance of long-term stable fixation can be achieved with initial stable socket fixation, restoring the center of rotation, and maximizing contact between the host bone and the implant. Limiting the loss of acetabular bone stock is a major factor in achieving these goals.

Diagnosing and Assessing Acetabular Bone Loss

Plain Radiographs and Special Views

Preoperative assessment of acetabular bone stock before revision sur-

Dr. Masri or an immediate family member serves as a board member, owner, officer, or committee member of the Canadian Orthopaedic Association; and has received research or institutional support from Stryker. Dr. Duncan or an immediate family member is a member of a speakers' bureau or has made paid presentations on behalf of Zimmer; and has received research or institutional support from DePuy, Stryker, and Zimmer. Dr. Garbuz or an immediate family member has received research or institutional support from Zimmer. Neither Dr. Noordin nor an immediate family member has received anything of value from or owns stock in a commercial company or institution related directly or indirectly to the subject of this chapter.

gery is critical because the amount and location of pelvic osteolysis can determine the type and success of revision surgery. Plain AP and cross-table lateral radiographs provide important initial information about the size and location of osteolytic lesions involving the acetabulum and the status of cup fixation. Judet oblique views add valuable information, especially about the integrity of the acetabular columns.[1-3] Changes in the location or orientation of the cup on serial radiographs, along with the width and extent of bone-implant radiolucent lines, indicate whether socket fixation is stable or loose. The amount and location of bone stock loss is assessed with the Paprosky classification system.

CT Scans

CT with metal artifact minimization has been shown to be more sensitive than plain radiographs for identifying and quantifying osteolysis around cemented and cementless cups. Because CT scans show the actual extent and location of osteolysis, they are useful adjuncts in planning cup revision in selected patients. Garcia-Cimbrelo and associates[4] preoperatively evaluated 60 hips with CT in addition to routine AP pelvic and lateral hip radiographs. All patients were symptomatic with groin and/or buttock pain. Radiographs showed acetabular lysis in 33 hips, whereas the CT scans showed it in 52 hips. The most frequent locations of osteolysis were the posterior wall and ischium. Puri and associates[5] used the sensitivity of CT to further define the outcome of osteolytic lesions in the pelvis after liner exchange and bone grafting in predominantly asymptomatic patients. They compared preoperative CT scans with postoperative scans done at a minimum of 2 years after liner exchange. Results showed an overall decrease in the size of the lesions from a mean of 6.4 cm² to 2.9 cm², which was highly significant. They also reported that CT scans could be used to more accurately evaluate the quality of graft incorporation.

Magnetic Resonance Imaging

Recent advances in imaging techniques make visualization and quantification of osteolysis feasible with MRI, particularly if titanium alloy prostheses are used.[6] The metal artifact from a prosthesis can make it challenging to assess periacetabular osteolysis, and images are prone to motion artifact, particularly if the patient is uncomfortable lying in a fixed position for a prolonged period. One recent cadaver study comparing the accuracy of radiography, CT, and MRI in assessing periacetabular osteolysis in cadaver models showed a sensitivity of 51.7%, 74.5%, and 95.4% respectively.[7] MRI was most effective in showing small areas of osteolysis, whereas CT was the most accurate modality for calculating lesion volume. Other advantages of MRI include superior soft-tissue contrast, which allows assessment of the surrounding soft-tissue envelope including regional neurovascular structures relative to the pseudocapsule and arthroplasty-bone interface, as well as particle-induced synovitis. Laursen and associates[8] reported dual-energy x-ray absorptiometry can detect bone defects adjacent to cementless cups in human pelvic specimens; however, to the chapter authors' knowledge, this has not yet been confirmed in a clinical study.

The Paprosky Classification System

The Paprosky classification system uses anatomic parameters to classify defects in the acetabulum and guide the selection of reconstructive options.[9] It is important to assess four criteria on preoperative radiographs: superior migration of the hip center, ischial osteolysis, teardrop osteolysis, and the position of the component relative to the Köhler line.

A Paprosky type 1 defect has an undistorted acetabular rim with intact anterior and posterior columns and small focal areas of contained bone loss. The preoperative radiograph shows no migration of the component and no ischial or teardrop osteolysis.[9] In a type 2 defect, adequate host bone remains to support a cementless acetabular component with more than 50% host bone support. Radiographs demonstrate less than 3 cm migration of the hip center from the superior obturator line. Type 2 defects are subdivided into three categories. A type 2A defect is characterized by direct superior migration of the component with an intact rim; a type 2B defect has superior lateral migration of the component with an absent superior rim; and a type 2C defect has medial migration of the component with disruption of the Köhler line. In a type 3A defect, radiographs show more than 3 cm of superior and lateral migration of the component above the superior obturator line, with mild to moderate ischial lysis. In type 3B defects, the radiographs show extensive ischial osteolysis, complete destruction of the teardrop, medial migration to the Köhler line, and more than 3 cm superior migration of the component. This chapter will describe the management of large bone defects (Paprosky types 3A and 3B) (Figure 1). The American Academy of Orthopaedic Surgeons (AAOS) classification of bone defects, described by D'Antonio and associates,[10,11] also identifies the pattern and location of bone loss, which is classified as contained, segmental, combined contained and segmental, pelvic discontinuity, and ankylosis.

Surgical Management Options for Massive Acetabular Bone Loss

Defects, other than Paprosky type 3 defects, can usually be managed with hemispherical shells with or without bone graft or particulate allograft. If massive bone loss is anticipated, an extensile approach is required. This can be achieved with a posterior approach, trochanteric slide, or in some instances, with a direct lateral approach. The authors favor a posterior approach in most cases.

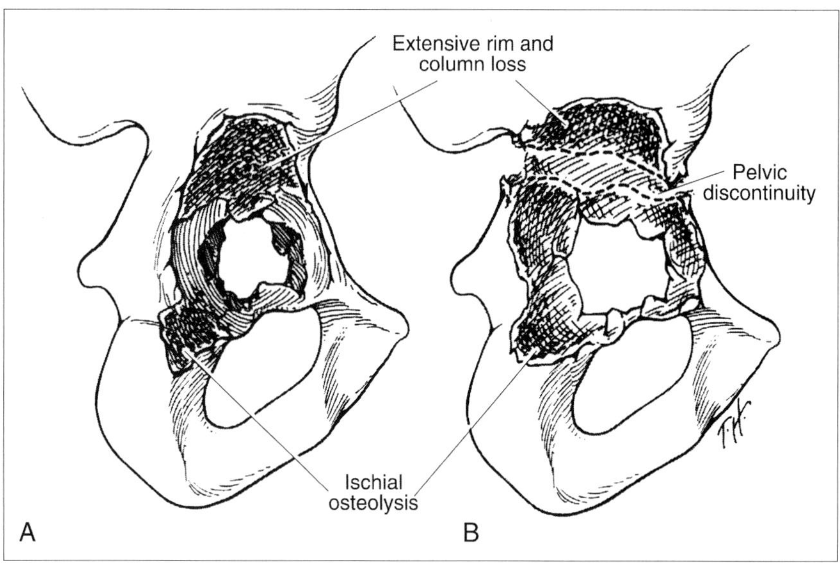

Figure 1 Illustrations of Paprosky acetabular type 3A **(A)** and type 3B **(B)** defects. (Adapted with permission from Buly RL, Nestor BJ: Revision total hip replacement, in Craig EV, ed: *Clinical Orthopaedics*. Philadelphia, PA, Lippincott, Williams & Wilkins, 1999.)

Cementless and Jumbo Cups With Bone Graft

A jumbo acetabular component allows a large surface area for bone ingrowth. Because the center of the hip joint is maintained in a more anatomic position, less bone graft is required and multiple screws can be used for rigid fixation. A jumbo cup also allows the option of using a thicker acetabular liner and a large femoral head.[12]

The definition of a jumbo cup has varied. Dearborn and Harris[13] defined jumbo cups as those with a diameter of more than 65 mm. Other authors suggested a gender-related definition of an extra-large cup as one 66 mm or larger in men and 62 mm or larger in women, a definition that was based on a shell that was more than 10 mm larger than the average size of cups implanted in men and women.[14,15] Ito and associates[16] defined large cups as being "relative to the ratio of the component size to the pelvis and hip joint."

Contraindications to use of a cementless cup for revision include relatively poor host bone quality, less than 50% contact between host bone and the component, the presence of large uncontained defects, and severe damage to the posterior column.[17] The contraindication specifying less than 50% contact between the host bone and the component has been relaxed at the authors' center (the University of British Columbia) since the advent of new technology, such as the Trabecular Metal system (Zimmer, Warsaw, IN). When attempting to convert an oblong defect to a circular defect it is important not to facilitate the conversion by removing an excessive amount of bone, destroying the rim, or damaging the posterior column. Accepting a high hip center is attractive in selected cases, but this has been associated with a higher failure rate.[18]

Della Valle and associates[19] reported their 15- to 19-year postoperative results of 138 total hip arthroplasties in 132 patients using a porous-coated acetabular metal shell (Harris-Galante I [Zimmer]) without cement. The median size of the acetabular components was 62 mm (range, 46 to 78 mm). The 15-year survival rate of the metal shells, with failure defined as revision because of loosening or as radiographic evidence of loosening, was 97%. Hendricks and Harris[12] reported follow-up on an original pool of 24 consecutive patients treated with a jumbo, cementless, hemispheric acetabular component; 12 patients were alive at a minimum follow-up of 12 years (mean, 13.9 years). In patients without infection, no acetabular shell had been revised because of aseptic loosening, and none was radiologically loose.

Geerdink and associates[20] performed acetabular revisions in 72 patients using a hydroxyapatite-coated socket. This treatment was based on the premise that the coating could theoretically compensate for the reduced amount and vitality of host bone in revision surgery. Because fixation by bone ongrowth to the new cup must originate directly from the host bone and is related to the contact area, larger cups were used to enhance this effect. At a mean follow-up of 7.6 years (range, 5 to 13 years) the component survival rate was 90.8% when revision for any reason was the end point (confidence interval, 80.5% to 100%) and 98.1% (confidence interval, 94.5% to 100%) when aseptic loosening of the cup was the end point.

High Hip Center Technique

Insufficient bone stock can prevent reconstruction of the acetabulum at the true anatomic hip center. By placing the component higher in the ilium than the true anatomic hip center, viable host bone can be preserved while maximizing the contact between the host bone and the porous coating. The high hip center technique has been defined as a reconstruction in which the center of rotation of the femoral head is located at least 35 mm proximal to the interteardrop line.[21] Implants with an outer diameter of 40 mm to 44 mm may be required, especially for a very high hip center. The acetabulum should be reamed nearly to the medial wall of the ilium to avoid lateral placement of the component, which has been associated with a higher rate of loosening.[22] The anterior column may be compromised partially during reaming, but it is essential to preserve the posterior column and the proximal medial wall. The socket should be positioned in approximately 45° abduction to achieve maximum contact between the porous-coated implant and the host bone, with at least 70% of the prosthesis in contact with host bone. Bulk and particulate allograft bone should be available if there is insufficient superior acetabular bone stock to place a high hip center.

Superior placement of the acetabulum results in shortening of the leg, decreased abductor muscle tension, and an increased risk of dislocation. These complications can be addressed by using a femoral stem with a longer neck, a calcar replacement, or increased offset. Alternatively, the trochanter can be advanced distally and laterally to restore abductor muscle tension. In addition to inadequate soft-tissue tension, femoral component impingement can result in limited range of motion. The anterior column or the anteroinferior iliac spine can cause the hip to dislocate posteriorly, or impingement of the greater trochanter on the ischium can cause the hip to dislocate anteriorly. These potential complications must be identified at the time of surgery and appropriately treated.

Study results of revision total hip arthroplasty with cemented acetabular components have been generally disappointing, with failure rates as high as 50% reported at relatively short-term follow-ups.[22] Hendricks and Harris[23] reported results (mean follow-up, 16.8 years) for 46 hips treated with porous-coated, cementless, acetabular shells placed at a high hip center at revision because of severe acetabular bone loss. Kaplan-Meier analysis showed a survival rate of 93% with revision of the acetabular shell because of aseptic loosening as the end point, 89% with revision of the shell for any reason as the end point, and 74% with repeat acetabular surgery for any reason as the end point. The authors recommended the use of multiple screws with this technique because of the additional stability provided until bony ingrowth. However, they reported a higher rate of femoral head penetration, suggesting that placement of a high hip center may increase the wear rate of conventional polyethylene. This technique is no longer used at most centers because of potential complications.

Impaction Grafting

Following the pioneering work of groups in The Netherlands and England, impaction allografting of bone has been used successfully as a biologic technique allowing restoration of bone stock in revision hip arthroplasty.[24-26] The procedure involves progressive compaction of morcellized cancellous bone chips into the acetabular cavity, followed by cementing of the prosthesis in place. This technique creates a three-layer composite of implant, cement, and graft. For the acetabular side, it has been shown that large (8-mm to 10-mm) cancellous chips achieve 25% greater stability in a dynamic in vitro acetabular model.[27,28] The better outcomes achieved with cemented impaction grafting are probably the result of the cement producing a solid layer of graft that greatly reduces the potential number of shear planes within the graft, leading to high initial stability and subsequent ingrowth and remodeling.[26] Biologic enhancement of allograft with autologous marrow has shown potential promise.[29] Experimentally, the combination of osteogenic protein and bisphosphonate increase final graft density and bone growth.[30] It is now recognized that bone graft washed before impaction to remove fat and marrow fluid may be preferable for optimal mechanical stability of the acetabular component because of an increase in shear strength of the impacted bone graft.[31,32]

Since its initial description as a treatment, impaction bone grafting in combination with a cemented socket has been used in revision surgery. Favorable outcomes have been reported by Slooff and associates[33] with a follow-up period of 2 years, and by Schreurs and associates[34] at 5.7 years, 11.8 years,[35] and 15 to 20 years.[36] The implant survival rate at 12 years was 85%, with revision of the acetabular component for loosening as the end point. The Kaplan-Meier survivorship for the cup, with revisions for any reason as the end point, was 79% at 15 years. When segmental defects are present, they can be converted to cavitary defects by closure with a metal wire mesh that provides containment for the particulate graft.[37] Radiologic assessment of consolidation of the graft is difficult and perhaps unreliable;[38] however, incorporation does not appear to be a determinant for a successful outcome based on the histologic evidence.[39] Comba and associates[38] reviewed 136 acetabular reconstructions at a minimum 2-year follow-up and a maximum follow-up of 13.1 years. They reported a 95.8% survival rate of the reconstructions, with the need for further revision as the end point. Excluding failure caused by infection, implant survival at a follow-up period of 2 to 13 years rose to 97.9%. However, in a review of 71 acetabular revisions with impaction of bone allograft (mean follow-up, 7.2 years), van Haaren and associates[40] reported the need for 20 rerevisions and an implant survival rate of only 72%. Fourteen of the 20 failed revisions had an AAOS type III or IV (pelvic discontinuity) defect. In the failed revisions, there was a high prevalence of segmental acetabular defects, illustrated by the frequent use of rim meshes (12 of 20 failed revisions) and lack of bony support behind the grafts. The authors hypothesized the underlying mechanism of failure in large defects was primarily micromovement, which led to mechanical instability and graft resorption. For large defects, impaction grafting should be used as an adjunct to other reinforcement techniques.

Bilobed Implants

Eccentric or oblong acetabular implants offer another method of managing large bone deficits. The limited anteroposterior dimension of the pelvis precludes the use of cementless jumbo cups in large segmental defects, particularly in the superolateral region of the acetabulum. The bilobed component has two lobes—the inferior lobe accepts a modular or cemented polyethylene insert, and the other lobe fills the superior defect and allows for additional screw fixation. Bilobed acetabular components maximize host bone implant contact while restoring the normal hip center without a structural bone graft or cement. The design attempts to support the prosthesis entirely on host bone while restoring the anatomic hip center without bulky anterior and posterior projections.[41] These implants can fill large defects with metal, thus avoiding the potential complications of bone graft fracture and resorption.[42] The augmented metallic region increases the area of contact between the porous coating and viable bone, thus enhancing the opportunity for cementless fixation. Reported results for this technique have been mixed and the authors do not recommend this approach.[42-47]

Antiprotrusio Cages

Antiprotrusio cages are indicated in circumstances in which stability cannot be achieved with a cementless, hemispheric, acetabular component and there is so little remaining host bone that biologic fixation of a porous implant is very unlikely.[48] As the name antiprotrusio implies, this cage requires peripheral support on host bone superiorly, posteriorly, and inferiorly. Medial and anterior support is not critical. These cages place the hip center near an anatomic location and restore bone stock, creating the potential for cementless, hemispheric cup placement if rerevision is necessary in the future. The cages also create a stable construct for cementing a polyethylene component, allow local delivery of antibiotics, and permit adjustment of version and abduction independent of the cage position. Cages span the acetabular defect, obtaining support from the ilium superiorly, and the pubis and ischium inferiorly. Acting on the same principle as a snowshoe, it spreads the force across a larger area, decompressing the underlying bone graft and facilitating its integration. Disadvantages of antiprotrusio cages include unacceptable midterm failure if support from allograft or host bone is not adequate.[49] The current designs do not allow for biologic fixation, which compromises the construct's potential for long-term success. In addition, the placement of the flanges requires more dissection, potentially leading to soft-tissue compromise and increasing the likelihood of dislocation.[50]

If the lateral wall of the pelvis above the acetabulum is absent, the cage cannot be used to normalize the hip center. If the posterior column is deficient and does not provide support for the posterior rim of the cage, a bulk allograft should be used to provide support. Inferiorly, the cage is either seated with its inferior rim on bone, or as is most frequently the case, the inferior tab or keel of the cage alone rests against the remaining inferior bone or is inserted into the ischium, which is the preferred technique. Once the cage is securely seated peripherally on host bone and medially on impacted morcellized allograft, it is fixed to the lateral wall of the pelvis with large cancellous screws. The polyethylene cup is then cemented with its orientation independent of the cage orientation to achieve stability.[51]

The results of most studies of antiprotrusio cages show a mechanical failure rate of 0% to approximately 15% at midterm follow-up.[48,52] Undoubtedly the varying results in different studies relate to the varying selection criteria for using antiprotrusio cages and perhaps also to surgical technique.[48] Recently Sembrano and Cheng[52] reviewed 72 cage reconstructions in 68 patients at a mean follow-up of 5.1 years (range, 1.2 to 10.7 years). Five-year, revision-free, cage survivorship was 87.8%. Five-year, loosening-free and acetabular revision-free survivorships were 80.7% and 81.3%, respectively. Interestingly, worsening severity of pelvic deficiency as reflected in any of the three classification systems used (Toronto, D'Antonio, and Paprosky) failed to predict eventual cage failure. In recent years, the use of antiprotrusio cages has diminished because of the availability of more contemporary technologies.

Structural Allograft

Alternatives for providing initial stability for bone ingrowth in Paprosky type 3A defects include the use of implants alone or an implant augmented with a structural allograft. It has been recommended that, in younger patients, restoration of bone stock is preferable if complications such as graft loosening, resorption, and infection can be minimized.[53]

In a study of 48 patients with type 3A defects treated with acetabular reconstruction with a distal femoral allograft and a porous hemispheric shell, Paprosky and associates[54] initially reported a survival rate of 94% (mean follow-up, 6.1 years) with aseptic loosening as the end point. Using the same cohort, continued successful results were published at an average of 10 years postoperatively. At an average of 5.3 years after the index procedure, five components required revision because of aseptic loosening and were converted to a hemispherical shell without the need for additional structural allograft support; thus, a type 3A defect was converted to a type 2 defect.[53] Allograft bone resorption, although difficult to quantitate, was observed around 6 of the 17 stable components and around 2 of the 5 components that failed clinically.

Other authors have reported that the use of structural allograft provides reliable results when more than 50% of host-bone support is present. Woodgate and associates[55] reported an 80.4% survival rate at 10 years postoperatively in a study of 51 hips and concluded that good results can be achieved with the use of structural allograft, especially if there is restoration of nearly normal hip biomechanics.

Total Acetabular Segmental Allograft With a Cage

Segmental bone loss involving more than 50% of the acetabulum is one of the most difficult challenges in revision hip replacement. The bone defect usually involves the dome and posterior column and may be associated with a pelvic discontinuity. The use of a structural allograft has the potential to restore bone stock for possible future surgery and restores the hip to the correct level. These grafts should be protected by a cage that extends from the host ilium to the host ischium. However, a high complication rate is related to the use of allograft and a protective cage.[56] Acetabular allograft bone is usually used in an acetabular revision with a structural allograft protected by a cage, but a male femoral head shaped to fit the defect is acceptable.

In pelvic discontinuity, the superior aspect of the pelvis is separated from the inferior aspect because of bone loss from the anterior and posterior columns combined with a fracture through the acetabulum. Possible reconstruction options include a cementless acetabulum in a high hip center as was previously described, with a major column allograft protected with a pelvic reconstruction plate to span and fix the discontinuity. The graft must be adequately protected to allow osseous integration and prevent mechanical failure.

Garbuz and associates[57] reported on 33 hips (32 patients) with major column grafts at a minimum 5-year follow-up (mean, 7.1 years). Eighteen of 33 hips (55%) in 17 patients had a successful result. In this study, success was defined as an increase in the hip score of at least 20 points; a stable cup with a united, structurally intact allograft; and no additional surgery related to the acetabulum. Six hips required additional surgery for cup loosening, but the grafts were intact and united. One hip required exploration for a sciatic nerve injury. These hips were considered a partial success because no additional grafting was necessary. The overall success rate was 76%. Eight of 33 hips required additional surgical procedures because of graft failure, 7 hips had severe resorption, and 1 hip was infected. The use of structural grafts on the acetabular side is decreasing because of technical difficulties and late biologic failures, which have motivated surgeons to seek alternative treatments.[58]

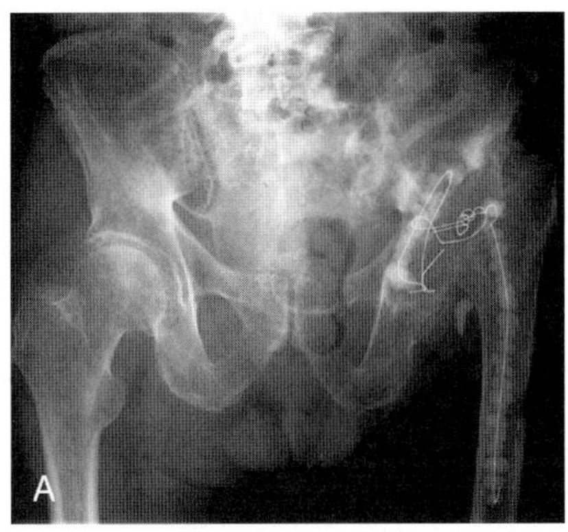

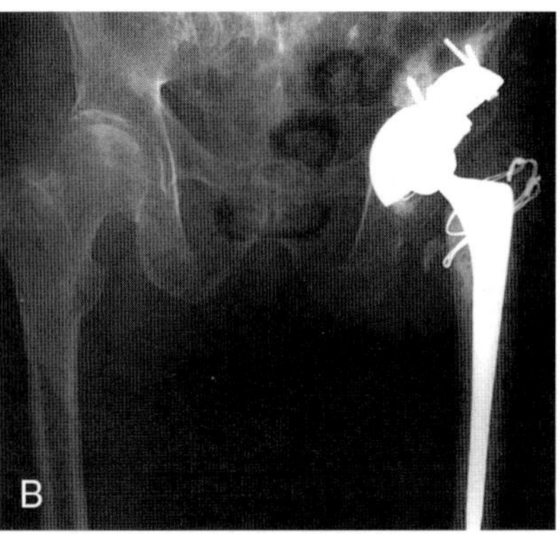

Figure 2 Radiographs of a patient treated with acetabular reconstruction with a Trabecular Metal (tantalum) augment. **A,** AP pelvic view following débridement and insertion of cement beads. **B,** Postoperative AP pelvic view showing the tantalum augment in place.

The Modular Trabecular Metal System and Cup-Cage Construct

Trabecular Metal acetabular implants, because of their porous nature, have the potential to provide a better environment for biologic fixation when limited host bone is available. Tantalum has a high volumetric porosity (ranging from 70% to 80%), a low modulus of elasticity, and a three-dimensional structure composed of a series of interconnected pores that are on average 550 μm in diameter.[59] Tantalum has a very high coefficient of friction, which allows initial component stability. Multiple sizes and shapes of these acetabular augments accommodate a range of acetabular bone defects in addition to the various sizes of the hemispheric acetabular components. The rationale for developing this modular system was to provide an implant that allows the potential for biologic fixation rather than mechanical fixation, to avoid the use of structural allograft, and to obviate the need for custom fabrication of implants.

Siegmeth and associates[60] prospectively reviewed 37 patients treated with acetabular reconstruction with Trabecular Metal augments combined with a Trabecular Metal shell. No patients were lost to follow-up. Three patients died of causes unrelated to their hips before completing the minimum 24-month follow-up; none of those patients had undergone rerevision surgery. The average age of the remaining 34 patients was 64 years at the time of the revision surgery and the minimum follow-up period was 24 months (mean, 34 months; range, 24 to 55 months). Radiographic signs of osseointegration were classified according to Moore and associates.[61] Quality of life was measured with the Medical Outcomes Study 12-Item Short Form, the Western Ontario and McMaster Osteoarthritis Index, and the Oxford Hip Score. At a minimum follow-up of 2 years, 32 of the 34 patients required no further surgery for aseptic loosening and 2 required rerevision surgery. Of the 32 patients who did not require revision surgery, all had radiologically stable cups. All quality-of-life parameters improved. The authors concluded that early results with tantalum augments are promising but longer follow-up periods are required (Figure 2). Similar results have been reported by other researchers.[62-64]

For a massive uncontained or contained defect where contact with the host bone is inadequate to obtain rigid screw fixation of a cementless cup, and bone ingrowth will be a prolonged process, a Trabecular Metal cup-cage construct provides another treatment option (Figure 3). Because of its porosity, Trabecular Metal will provide a better environment for ingrowth of host bone. The cage protects the Trabecular Metal cup until ingrowth has occurred.[65]

Boscainos and associates[66] reviewed 14 patients with Trabecular Metal cup-cage constructs at a mean follow-up of 32 months (range, 6 to 45 months). All patients were walking at the last follow-up. Mean preoperative and postoperative Western Ontario and McMaster Osteoarthritis Index scores were 64 (range, 45 to 82) and 33 (range, 18 to 52), respectively. All implants were stable and none had migrated at the last follow-up. Minor radiolucent lines were observed around the inferior flange of the cage in four patients. Minor graft resorption (less than one third of the graft) occurred in one patient. All but one construct showed graft remodeling. Complications included one thigh seroma; two recurrent dislocations, which were revised to a constrained liner at 2 and 4 months with retention of the cup-

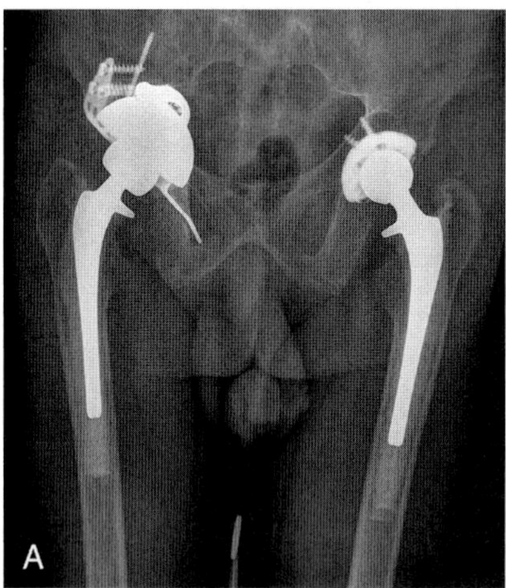

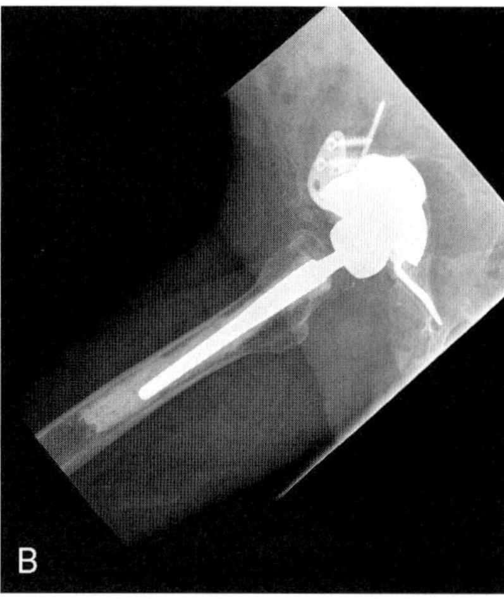

Figure 3 AP **(A)** and lateral **(B)** radiographs of a patient with revision hip arthroplasty managed with a trabecular metal revision shell, a tantalum augment, and a short flange cup-cage construct with an oblique liner.

cage construct; and one death unrelated to surgery.

Potential complications with Trabecular Metal in acetabular reconstruction include unknown long-term durability, potential for debris generation at the shell-augment interface, potential for fatigue failure, and the inability to restore bone stock for future revisions. However, short-term clinical and radiographic results appear promising.[60,64]

Summary

The reconstruction of massive acetabular bone defects remains a challenging issue in revision total hip arthroplasty. The method of acetabular revision must be individualized to meet the mechanical and biologic challenges specific to each reconstruction. No one technique is likely to provide the solution to the full spectrum of acetabular defects. Most revision arthroplasties can be performed using a standard hemispheric component. In a small but increasing subset of patients with considerable acetabular deficiency, the use of a standard cup requires a structural allograft, defect bridging devices with bone graft and/or cement, or placing the component above the anatomic hip center. With the increasing availability of hemispheric cups of larger diameters and improved designs, the use of rings is declining. Antiprotrusio cages are another option in patients with significant acetabular bone loss, but are subject to nonbiologic fixation with the potential for fatigue failure. Modular tantalum or custom-made augments allow for excellent short-term success in complex (type 3) revision arthroplasty. Experience, to date, indicates that this new material provides a more favorable environment for bone ingrowth. Combined with the ability to use modular augments for added support and stability, this technology may change the method for reconstructing major acetabular defects.

References

1. Thomas A, Epstein NJ, Stevens K, Goodman SB: Utility of judet oblique x-rays in preoperative assessment of acetabular periprosthetic osteolysis: A preliminary study. *Am J Orthop* 2007;36:E107-E110.
2. Southwell DG, Bechtold JE, Lew WD, Schmidt AH: Improving the detection of acetabular osteolysis using oblique radiographs. *J Bone Joint Surg Br* 1999;81:289-295.
3. Zimlich RH, Fehring TK: Underestimation of pelvic osteolysis: The value of the iliac oblique radiograph. *J Arthroplasty* 2000;15:796-801.
4. Garcia-Cimbrelo E, Tapia M, Martin-Hervas C: Multislice computed tomography for evaluating acetabular defects in revision THA. *Clin Orthop Relat Res* 2007;463:138-143.
5. Puri L, Lapinski B, Wixson RL, Lynch J, Hendrix R, Stulberg SD: Computed tomographic follow-up evaluation of operative intervention for periacetabular lysis. *J Arthroplasty* 2006; 21:78-82.
6. Weiland DE, Walde TA, Leung SB, et al: Magnetic resonance imaging in the evaluation of periprosthetic acetabular osteolysis: A cadaveric study. *J Orthop Res* 2005;23:713-719.
7. Walde TA, Weiland DE, Leung SB, et al: Comparison of CT, MRI, and radiographs in assessing pelvic osteolysis: A cadaveric study. *Clin Orthop Relat Res* 2005;437:138-144.
8. Laursen MB, Nielsen PT, Søballe K: Detection of bony defects around cementless acetabular components in total hip arthroplasty: A DEXA study on 10 human cadavers. *Acta Orthop* 2006;77:209-217.
9. O'Rourke MR, Paprosky WG, Rosenberg AG: Use of structural allografts in acetabular revision surgery. *Clin Orthop Relat Res* 2004;420:113-121.
10. D'Antonio JA: Periprosthetic bone loss of the acetabulum: Classification and management. *Orthop Clin North Am* 1992;23:279-290.
11. D'Antonio JA, Capello WN, Borden LS, et al: Classification and management of acetabular abnormalities in total hip arthroplasty. *Clin Orthop Relat Res* 1989;243:126-137.
12. Hendricks KJ, Harris WH: Revision of failed acetabular components with use of so-called jumbo noncemented

components: A concise follow-up of a previous report. *J Bone Joint Surg Am* 2006;88:559-563.

13. Dearborn JT, Harris WH: Acetabular revision arthroplasty using so-called jumbo noncemented components: An average 7-year follow-up study. *J Arthroplasty* 2000;15:8-15.
14. Whaley AL, Berry DJ, Harmsen WS: Extra-large uncemented hemispherical acetabular components for revision total hip arthroplasty. *J Bone Joint Surg Am* 2001;83:1352-1357.
15. Patel JV, Masonis JL, Bourne RB, Rorabeck CH: The fate of cementless jumbo cups in revision hip arthroplasty. *J Arthroplasty* 2003;18:129-133.
16. Ito J, Koshino T, Okamoto R, Saito T: 15-year follow-up study of total knee arthroplasty in patients with rheumatoid arthritis. *J Arthroplasty* 2003;18:984-992.
17. Lian YY, Yoo MC, Pei FX, Kim KI, Chun SW, Cheng JQ: Cementless hemispheric acetabular component for acetabular revision arthroplasty: A 5- to 19-year follow-up study. *J Arthroplasty* 2008;23:376-382.
18. Morag G, Zalzal P, Liberman B, Safir O, Flint M, Gross AE: Outcome of revision hip arthroplasty in patients with a previous total hip replacement for developmental dysplasia of the hip. *J Bone Joint Surg Br* 2005;87:1068-1072.
19. Della Valle CJ, Shuaipaj T, Berger RA, et al: Revision of the acetabular component without cement after total hip arthroplasty: A concise follow-up, at fifteen to nineteen years, of a previous report. *J Bone Joint Surg Am* 2005;87:1795-1800.
20. Geerdink CH, Schaafsma J, Meyers WG, Grimm B, Tonino AJ: Cementless hemispheric hydroxyapatite-coated sockets for acetabular revision. *J Arthroplasty* 2007;22:369-376.
21. Russotti GM, Harris WH: Proximal placement of the acetabular component in total hip arthroplasty: A long-term follow-up study. *J Bone Joint Surg Am* 1991;73:587-592.
22. Bozic KJ, Freiberg AA, Harris WH: The high hip center. *Clin Orthop Relat Res* 2004;420:101-105.
23. Hendricks KJ, Harris WH: High placement of noncemented acetabular components in revision total hip arthroplasty: A concise follow-up, at a minimum of fifteen years, of a previous report. *J Bone Joint Surg Am* 2006; 88:2231-2236.
24. Slooff TJ, Huiskes R, van Horn J, Lemmens AJ: Bone grafting in total hip replacement for acetabular protrusion. *Acta Orthop Scand* 1984;55: 593-596.
25. Gie GA, Linder L, Ling RS, Simon JP, Slooff TJ, Timperley AJ: Impacted cancellous allografts and cement for revision total hip arthroplasty. *J Bone Joint Surg Br* 1993;75:14-21.
26. Board TN, Rooney P, Kearney JN, Kay PR: Impaction allografting in revision total hip replacement. *J Bone Joint Surg Br* 2006;88:852-857.
27. Bolder SB, Schreurs BW, Verdonschot N, van Unen JM, Gardeniers JW, Slooff TJ: Particle size of bone graft and method of impaction affect initial stability of cemented cups: Human cadaveric and synthetic pelvic specimen studies. *Acta Orthop Scand* 2003;74:652-657.
28. Ullmark G: Bigger size and defatting of bone chips will increase cup stability. *Arch Orthop Trauma Surg* 2000; 120:445-447.
29. Deakin DE, Bannister GC: Graft incorporation after acetabular and femoral impaction grafting with washed irradiated allograft and autologous marrow. *J Arthroplasty* 2007; 22:89-94.
30. Jeppsson C, Astrand J, Tägil M, Aspenberg P: A combination of bisphosphonate and BMP additives in impacted bone allografts. *Acta Orthop Scand* 2003;74:483-489.
31. Arts JJ, Verdonschot N, Buma P, Schreurs BW: Larger bone graft size and washing of bone grafts prior to impaction enhances the initial stability of cemented cups: Experiments using a synthetic acetabular model. *Acta Orthop* 2006;77:227-233.
32. Dunlop DG, Brewster NT, Madabhushi SP, Usmani AS, Pankaj P, Howie CR: Techniques to improve the shear strength of impacted bone graft: The effect of particle size and washing of the graft. *J Bone Joint Surg Am* 2003;85:639-646.
33. Slooff TJ, Schimmel JW, Buma P: Cemented fixation with bone grafts. *Orthop Clin North Am* 1993;24:667-677.
34. Schreurs BW, Slooff TJ, Buma P, Gardeniers JW, Huiskes R: Acetabular reconstruction with impacted morsellised cancellous bone graft and cement: A 10- to 15-year follow-up of 60 revision arthroplasties. *J Bone Joint Surg Br* 1998;80:391-395.
35. Schreurs BW, Slooff TJ, Gardeniers JW, Buma P: Acetabular reconstruction with bone impaction grafting and a cemented cup: 20 years' experience. *Clin Orthop Relat Res* 2001;393:202-215.
36. Schreurs BW, Bolder SB, Gardeniers JW, Verdonschot N, Slooff TJ, Veth RP: Acetabular revision with impacted morsellised cancellous bone grafting and a cemented cup: A 15- to 20-year follow-up. *J Bone Joint Surg Br* 2004;86:492-497.
37. Oakes DA, Cabanela ME: Impaction bone grafting for revision hip arthroplasty: Biology and clinical applications. *J Am Acad Orthop Surg* 2006;14: 620-628.
38. Comba F, Buttaro M, Pusso R, Piccaluga F: Acetabular reconstruction with impacted bone allografts and cemented acetabular components: A 2- to 13-year follow-up study of 142 aseptic revisions. *J Bone Joint Surg Br* 2006;88:865-869.
39. van der Donk S, Buma P, Slooff TJ, Gardeniers JW, Schreurs BW: Incorporation of morselized bone grafts: A study of 24 acetabular biopsy specimens. *Clin Orthop Relat Res* 2002;396: 131-141.
40. van Haaren EH, Heyligers IC, Alexander FG, Wuisman PI: High rate of failure of impaction grafting in large acetabular defects. *J Bone Joint Surg Br* 2007;89:296-300.

41. Moskal JT, Higgins ME, Shen J: Type III acetabular defect revision with bilobed components: Five-year results. *Clin Orthop Relat Res* 2008; 466:691-695.

42. Abeyta PN, Namba RS, Janku GV, Murray WR, Kim HT: Reconstruction of major segmental acetabular defects with an oblong-shaped cementless prosthesis: A long-term outcomes study. *J Arthroplasty* 2008;23: 247-253.

43. Herrera A, Martínez AA, Cuenca J, Canales V: Management of types III and IV acetabular deficiencies with the longitudinal oblong revision cup. *J Arthroplasty* 2006;21:857-864.

44. DeBoer DK, Christie MJ: Reconstruction of the deficient acetabulum with an oblong prosthesis: Three- to seven-year results. *J Arthroplasty* 1998; 13:674-680.

45. Berry DJ, Sutherland CJ, Trousdale RT, et al: Bilobed oblong porous coated acetabular components in revision total hip arthroplasty. *Clin Orthop Relat Res* 2000;371:154-160.

46. Surace MF, Zatti G, De Pietri M, Cherubino P: Acetabular revision surgery with the LOR cup: Three to 8 years' follow-up. *J Arthroplasty* 2006; 21:114-121.

47. Chen WM, Engh CA Jr , Hopper RH Jr , McAuley JP, Engh CA: Acetabular revision with use of a bilobed component inserted without cement in patients who have acetabular bone-stock deficiency. *J Bone Joint Surg Am* 2000;82:197-206.

48. Berry DJ: Antiprotrusio cages for acetabular revision. *Clin Orthop Relat Res* 2004;420:106-112.

49. Paprosky WG, Sporer SS, Murphy BP: Addressing severe bone deficiency: What a cage will not do. *J Arthroplasty* 2007;22:111-115.

50. Udomkiat P, Dorr LD, Won YY, Longjohn D, Wan Z: Technical factors for success with metal ring acetabular reconstruction. *J Arthroplasty* 2001;16:961-969.

51. Schatzker J, Wong MK: Acetabular revision: The role of rings and cages. *Clin Orthop Relat Res* 1999;369:187-197.

52. Sembrano JN, Cheng EY: Acetabular cage survival and analysis of factors related to failure. *Clin Orthop Relat Res* 2008;466:1657-1665.

53. Sporer SM, O'Rourke M, Chong P, Paprosky WG: The use of structural distal femoral allografts for acetabular reconstruction: Average ten-year follow-up. *J Bone Joint Surg Am* 2005; 87:760-765.

54. Paprosky WG, Bradford MS, Jablonsky WS: Acetabular reconstruction with massive acetabular allografts. *Instr Course Lect* 1996;45:149-159.

55. Woodgate IG, Saleh KJ, Jaroszynski G, Agnidis Z, Woodgate MM, Gross AE: Minor column structural acetabular allografts in revision hip arthroplasty. *Clin Orthop Relat Res* 2000; 371:75-85.

56. Gross AE, Goodman S: The current role of structural grafts and cages in revision arthroplasty of the hip. *Clin Orthop Relat Res* 2004;429:193-200.

57. Garbuz D, Morsi E, Gross AE: Revision of the acetabular component of a total hip arthroplasty with a massive structural allograft: Study with a minimum five-year follow-up. *J Bone Joint Surg Am* 1996;78:693-697.

58. Shinar AA, Harris WH: Bulk structural autogenous grafts and allografts for reconstruction of the acetabulum in total hip arthroplasty: Sixteen-year-average follow-up. *J Bone Joint Surg Am* 1997;79:159-168.

59. Levine B, Della Valle CJ, Jacobs JJ: Applications of porous tantalum in total hip arthroplasty. *J Am Acad Orthop Surg* 2006;14:646-655.

60. Siegmeth A, Duncan CP, Masri BA, Kim WY, Garbuz DS: Modular tantalum augments for acetabular defects in revision hip arthroplasty. *Clin Orthop Relat Res* 2009;467:199-205.

61. Moore MS, McAuley JP, Young AM, Engh CA Sr: Radiographic signs of osseointegration in porous-coated acetabular components. *Clin Orthop Relat Res* 2006;444:176-183.

62. Weeden SH, Schmidt RH: The use of tantalum porous metal implants for Paprosky 3A and 3B defects. *J Arthroplasty* 2007;22:151-155.

63. Nehme A, Lewallen DG, Hanssen AD: Modular porous metal augments for treatment of severe acetabular bone loss during revision hip arthroplasty. *Clin Orthop Relat Res* 2004; 429: 201-208.

64. Sporer SM, Paprosky WG: Acetabular revision using a trabecular metal acetabular component for severe acetabular bone loss associated with a pelvic discontinuity. *J Arthroplasty* 2006;21:87-90.

65. Gross AE, Goodman SB: Rebuilding the skeleton: The intraoperative use of trabecular metal in revision total hip arthroplasty. *J Arthroplasty* 2005; 20:91-93.

66. Boscainos PJ, Kellett CF, Maury AC, Backstein D, Gross AE: Management of periacetabular bone loss in revision hip arthroplasty. *Clin Orthop Relat Res* 2007;465:159-165.

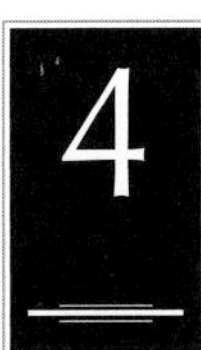

Pelvic Dissociation in Revision Total Hip Arthroplasty: Diagnosis and Treatment

Shahryar Noordin, MBBS, FCPS
Clive P. Duncan, MD, MSc, FRCSC
Bassam A. Masri, MD, FRCSC
Donald S. Garbuz, MD, MHSc, FRCSC

Abstract

Pelvic dissociation is a distinct but uncommon condition, which occurs in association with total hip arthroplasty, in which the superior aspect of the pelvis is separated from the inferior aspect by fracture. Because radiodense implants and cement can obscure pelvic discontinuity on plain radiographs, not all dissociations can be diagnosed preoperatively; therefore, a high index of suspicion for this condition should be maintained. In selected patients, CT angiography may be indicated. Successful treatment requires achieving initial stability of the socket, establishing conditions for long-term stability of the socket, stabilizing the pelvic dissociation, and producing conditions favorable for healing. Applying a posterior pelvic reconstruction plate to the ilium and ischium will achieve stabilization of the dissociation in most patients if sufficient posterior wall and column are present. Occasionally, if there is adequate space, a second plate may be applied. In selected patients, it may be feasible to place anterior column fixation screws using image guidance, which is the preferred technique of the authors rather than the alternate option of using anterior column plating through an anterior exposure. Residual bone loss is then reevaluated and possible options such as a hemispherical socket, a jumbo cup, or a highly porous metal component and augment can be considered. If there is not enough room for a posterior pelvic reconstruction plate, a cup-cage construct with or without an allograft can be used as a reconstruction option.

Instr Course Lect 2010;59:37-43.

Dr. Duncan or an immediate family member is a member of a speakers' bureau or has made paid presentations on behalf of Zimmer; and has received research or institutional support from DePuy, Stryker, and Zimmer. Dr. Masri or an immediate family member serves as a board member, owner, officer, or committee member of the Canadian Orthopaedic Association; and has received research or institutional support from Stryker. Dr. Garbuz or an immediate family member has received research or institutional support from Zimmer. Neither Dr. Noordin nor an immediate family member has received anything of value from or owns stock in a commercial company or institution related directly or indirectly to the subject of this chapter.

Pelvic dissociation is a distinct but uncommon condition that occurs in association with total hip arthroplasty (THA). In pelvic dissociation the superior aspect of the pelvis is separated from the inferior aspect by fracture.[1] Pelvic dissociation may be a result of massive bone loss caused by osteolysis, infection, mechanical abrasion, or fracture. In this setting, revision hip arthroplasty is challenging because of the need to achieve fracture stabilization, to replenish bone stock, to accomplish immediate stabilization of the new socket, and to produce an environment that will permit fracture union, bone regeneration, and long-term implant fixation.

Pelvic osteolysis is a common and well-recognized complication associated with THA.[2-4] It affects cemented and uncemented sockets and has been attributed to the biologic reaction to particulate wear debris, particularly polyethylene debris.[2,5] In instances of massive osteolysis and structural failure, the acetabular rim, quadrilateral plate, and associated columns become

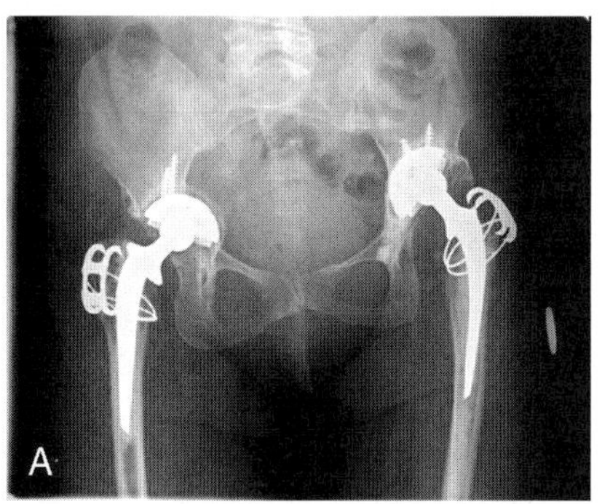

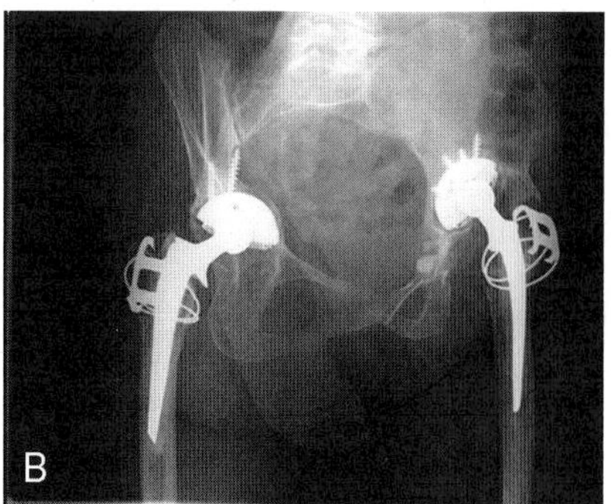

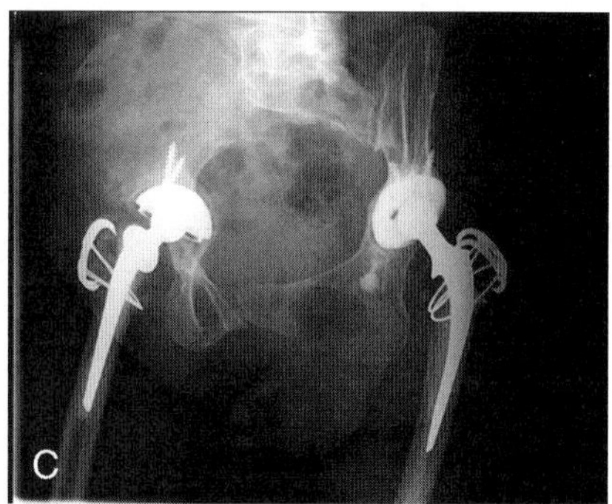

Figure 1 AP **(A)**, obturator oblique **(B)**, and iliac oblique **(C)** views of the pelvis showing pelvic dissociation of the right hip.

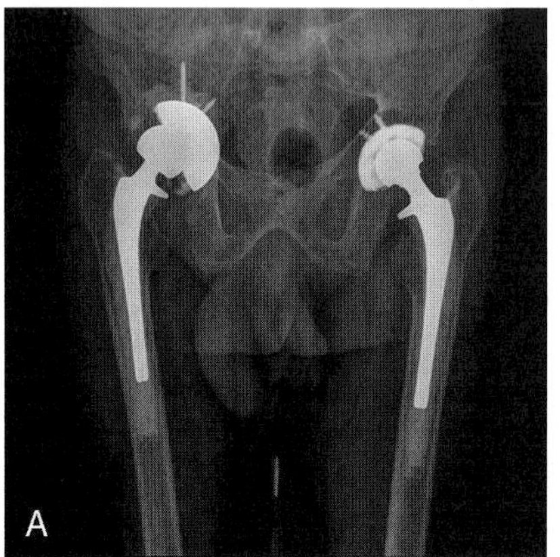

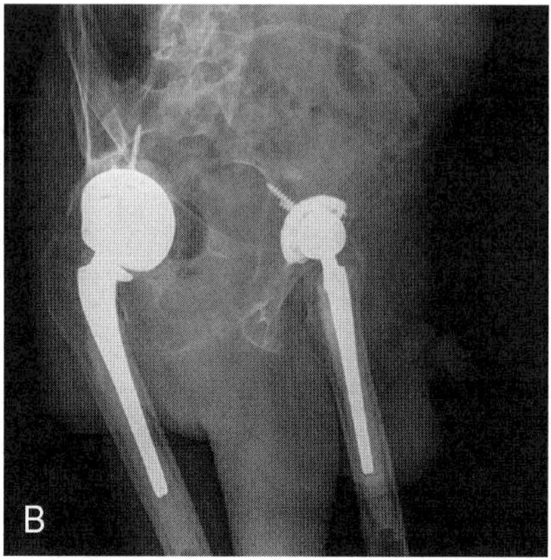

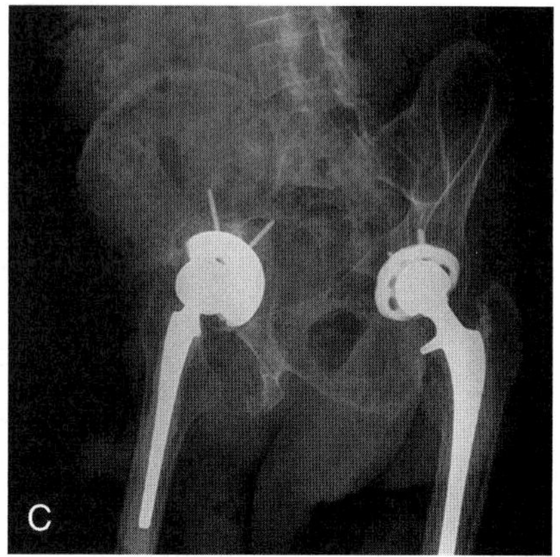

Figure 2 AP **(A)**, obturator oblique **(B)**, and iliac oblique **(C)** views of the pelvis of a patient with pelvic dissociation.

nonsupportive and deficient. In the worst-case scenario, this deficiency occurs in conjunction with pelvic dissociation in which the connection between the ilium and the ischium is disrupted.[6] The incidence of such acetabular destruction is low and most of the literature consists of case reports or small studies. Berry and associates[1] identified this condition in 31 of 3,505 consecutive acetabular revisions. Identified risk factors for pelvic dissociation are female gender, massive pelvic bone loss, and rheumatoid arthritis.

Diagnosis and Radiologic Investigations

Plain Radiographs and Special Views

Because pelvic dissociation is often associated with osteolysis, any investigation for pelvic discontinuity also should have a high predictive value for pelvic osteolysis. In 1999, using computer simulations and cadaver studies, Southwell and associates[7] reported that three radiographic views—the AP view, 45° iliac oblique view, and 60° obturator oblique view—were optimal for accurately assessing pelvic osteolysis. With the AP view alone, linear osteolysis (3 mm or more deep) would be obscured in more than 83% of the cup surface. With two views, 30% to 50% of the cup surface would be obscured. However, with three views, only 7% of the cup surface would be obscured. This assumes that the cup is not severely displaced in a medial direction, which could potentially obscure the posterior column regardless of the radiographic view. Once the degree and location of osteolysis has been determined, signs of pelvic dissociation should be evaluated. These include (1) a visible transverse acetabular fracture on AP, Judet obturator oblique, or iliac oblique pelvic radiographs (Figure 1); (2) medial offset of the inferior pelvis relative to the superior pelvis as seen by a break in the Köhler line (Figure 2); and (3) rotation of the inferior versus superior hemipelvis seen as asymmetry of the obturator rings on a true AP pelvic radiograph.[1] Because radiodense implants and cement can obscure pelvic dissociation on radiographs, not all cases can be diagnosed preoperatively with radiographs, and a high index of suspicion should remain so that such missed cases can be diagnosed intraoperatively. CT scanning is another imaging option to aid in the diagnosis.

CT Scans

The difficulty with observing and underestimating the presence of osteolytic lesions with plain radiographs have led some physicians to advocate CT to evaluate these lesions.[4,8,9] With advances in technology and the development of helical multidetector CT scanners, image quality has greatly improved. The helical CT scanner obtains images in a continuous fashion and has a shorter image acquisition time. Sequential images of the osteolytic lesions can provide volumetric measurements and the shorter scan time decreases the motion artifact. This provides precise information about the lesions located in the ilium, acetabular roof, medial wall, anterior column, posterior column, ischium, or pubic ramus. In patients with significant protrusio, preoperative CT angiography may be required to show the anatomic position of the iliac vessels and other important structures within the pelvis.

Classification and Decision Making

In its classification of acetabular bone loss, the American Academy of Orthopaedic Surgeons (AAOS) defined pelvic dissociation as a type IV deficiency[10] (Table 1). Berry and associates[1] subclassified the degree of bone loss associated with pelvic dissociation as type IVa if the dissociation is associated with cavitary (type II) or mild segmental (type I) bone loss, type IVb if the dissociation is associated with a large segmental (type I) or a combined (type III) defect, and type IVc if the pelvis had been previously irradiated regardless of the presence of cavitary or segmental bone loss.

The treatment of pelvic dissociation requires a full understanding of not only the presence of the fracture but also the degree of bone loss. Preoperatively, the Paprosky classification of bone loss can be used to better plan the equipment and implants required for surgery.[11] This system is based on the severity of bone loss and the ability to support cementless fixation. It is important to assess four radiographic criteria: (1) superior migration of the hip center, (2) ischial osteolysis, (3) teardrop osteolysis, and (4) the position of the implant relative to the Köhler line. Type I and II defects indicate mild to moderate bone loss, and reconstruction is generally straightforward.

With a type IIIa defect, adequate host bone is available and in contact with the ingrowth surface to obtain durable biologic fixation. Preoperative radiographs will show superior and lateral migration of the component more than 3 cm above the obturator line. Ischial lysis will be mild to moderate, extending less than 15 mm inferior to the obturator line. The teardrop will be partially destroyed; however, the medial limb of the teardrop will generally be present. The component will be at or lateral to the Köhler line, and the ilioischial and iliopubic lines will be intact. Pelvic dissociation rarely occurs in type IIIa defects.

In a type IIIb defect, there is less than 40% host bone remaining in contact with the ingrowth surface. The rim defect is greater than 50% of the circumference, usually from the 9 o'clock to 5 o'clock positions. Preoperative radiographs show more extensive ischial osteolysis (> 15 mm below the superior obturator line), complete destruction of the teardrop, migration medial to the Köhler line, and more than 3 cm of superior migration to the obturator line. The failed component migrates superiorly and medially in the type IIIb defect compared with the type IIIa defect in which the migration is superior and lateral. Patients with type IIIb defects are at high risk for occult pelvic dissociation.[11] This condition may be associated with scarring of vital structures, such as the femoral vessels, femoral nerve, ureter, and bowel.

Table 1
Classification of Acetabular Deficiencies

Type I	Segmental deficiencies Peripheral Superior Anterior Posterior Central (medial wall absent)
Type II	Cavitary deficiencies Peripheral Superior Anterior Posterior Central (medial wall intact)
Type III	Combined deficiencies
Type IV	Pelvic discontinuity
Type V	Arthrodesis

(Reproduced with permission from D'Antonio JA, Capello WN, Borden LS, et al: Classification and management of acetabular abnormalities in total hip arthroplasty. *Clin Orthop Relat Res* 1989;243:123-137.)

Intraoperatively, once the acetabulum is fully exposed, the anterior and posterior columns are compressed with a Cobb elevator and motion between the superior and inferior hemipelvis is assessed. Important intraoperative findings include the amount of host bone present, the location of structural defects, and the location of the dissociation.

Surgical Treatment

Goals

Surgical goals include pain relief and restoration of ambulatory status in patients who are suitable candidates for surgery. Successful treatment achieves initial stability of the socket, establishes conditions for long-term stability of the socket, stabilizes the pelvic dissociation, and produces conditions favorable for healing.[1]

Treatment Algorithm

If a trial component has partial inherent stability, there is generally enough contact with host bone to support ingrowth and the defect is type IIIa.[12] Options for reconstruction include a structural distal femoral graft with a cementless hemispherical cup, a modular highly porous metal component (such as the Trabecular Metal cup [Zimmer, Warsaw, IN]) augment with a hemispherical cup, or a high hip center hemispherical cup. When there is no inherent stability of the hemispherical trial component, the defect is type IIIb. Treatment options for these defects include augments and pelvic reconstruction plates (posterior and/or anterior). If there is not enough room for a posterior reconstruction plate, a cup-cage construct with or without an allograft can be used.

Principles of Treatment

Guiding principles for the treatment of pelvic dissociation include identifying the condition, stabilizing or effectively bypassing the dissociation, bone grafting at the site of the discontinuity, treating any associated bone loss, and placing a stable acetabular implant.[1] Once pelvic dissociation is detected, the posterior column and wall should be evaluated first. If there is sufficient wall and column, a posterior pelvic reconstruction plate into the ilium and ischium will stabilize the dissociation in most patients. Occasionally, if there is adequate space, a second plate may be applied. In selected cases, under image guidance, the use of an anterior column fixation screw may be feasible. Alternatively, plating of the anterior column can be used. The residual bone loss is then reevaluated; possible treatment options include a hemispherical socket or highly porous metal socket and augment. If there is not enough room for a posterior pelvic reconstruction plate, then a cup-cage construct with or without an allograft can be used as a reconstruction option.[13] Osseointegration of the implant provides secondary stability to the pelvic dissociation and effectively eliminates the instability, protecting the hardware from fracture. To achieve stability of the dissociated fragments, it may be necessary to intentionally distract them, placing the highly porous metal socket to act as a biointegrative bridge.

Results

Cementless Sockets

Reliable and durable fixation of cementless acetabular components requires an environment with adequate biologic potential and mechanical stability to allow bone ingrowth.[12] Sporer and Paprosky[12] reported on a 6-year follow-up study of 13 patients (13 hips) with type IIIb acetabular defects and an associated pelvic dissociation. A highly porous metal socket acetabular component with or without an augment was used to obtain fixation proximal and distal to the dissociation. At a mean follow-up of 2.6 years, two patients required the use of a walker, two required the use of a cane, and nine walked without support for more than six blocks. Eleven patients had no pain or mild pain, whereas two had moderate pain. Clinically, the modified Postel-Merle d'Aubigné score improved from 6.1 preoperatively to 10.3 postoperatively ($P < 0.05$). Radiographically, one patient had possible acetabular loosening secondary to screw breakage, despite being clinically asymptomatic. None of the remaining patients required any repeat surgery.

Acetabular Cages and Ring

When bone loss and instability preclude the use of a hemispherical cementless socket, another approach involves the use of reconstruction metal cages that distribute forces to a larger area to bypass areas of bone loss into which a cup is cemented (Figure 3).

Paprosky and associates[14] reported on 15 patients with 16 acetabular cage reconstructions at a mean follow-up of 5 years (range, 2 to 8 years). The presence of pelvic dissociation was based on intraoperative findings after removing any pseudomembrane and exposing the remaining host bone. There were two Paprosky type IIc defects, six type IIIa defects, and eight type IIIb defects. Posterior column plate fixation was used in 11 of 16 patients and structural allograft was used in 7 patients. Revision or resection occurred in 5 of 16 hips (31%) at intermediate-term follow-up. Four hips were revised for aseptic loosening including three fractured cages. The cage type did not correlate with the revision. More type IIIb defects (3 of 8) were associated with rerevision compared with type IIIa defects (1 of 6). Use of a plate and the type of allograft used did not seem to affect rerevision rates. Complications included one infection, four nerve palsies, and one dislocation. Study limitations included missing data, heterogeneity of the underlying diagnoses, the heterogeneity of the implants and/or allografts used, and the small number of patients studied. Despite these limitations, with a 31% revision rate and 44% rate of overall loosening, the authors concluded that acetabular cages in the setting of pelvic dissociation did not provide encouraging results at intermediate term follow-up.

Eggli and associates[15] reported the clinical outcome of seven patients with pelvic dissociation following revision THA after a mean follow-up of 96 months. Surgical treatment consisted of three consecutive steps beginning with mechanical stabilization of the two acetabular columns, followed by bony acetabular reconstruction (filling the osteolytic defect with allograft chips covered with autologous bone to achieve a contained defect after healing of the autograft), and anchorage of the cup using an acetabular reinforcement ring (five with a hook and two without a hook). A high complication rate was reported, including a partial ischial nerve lesion, one intraoperative femoral shaft fracture, and one recurrent dislocation. One patient had revision surgery after 12 months because of aseptic loosening; another patient required removal of two prominent screws.

Goodman and associates[13] reported the results of 61 acetabular revisions with ilioischial cages at 1 to 7 years showing an overall successful result in 76%; however, in patients with pelvic dissociation only 5 of 10 revisions (50%) were considered successful and 8 of 10 (80%) had complications.

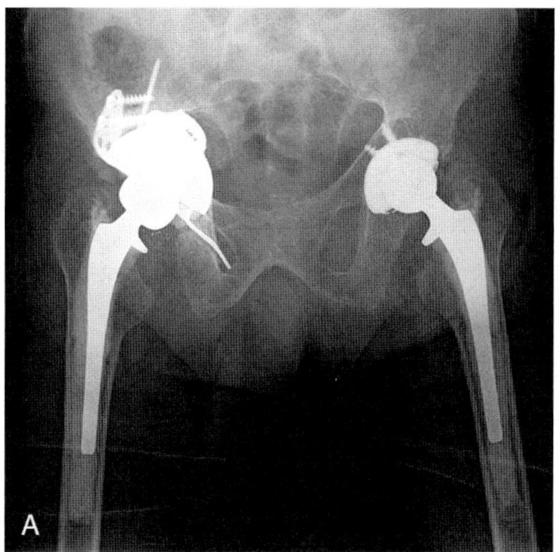

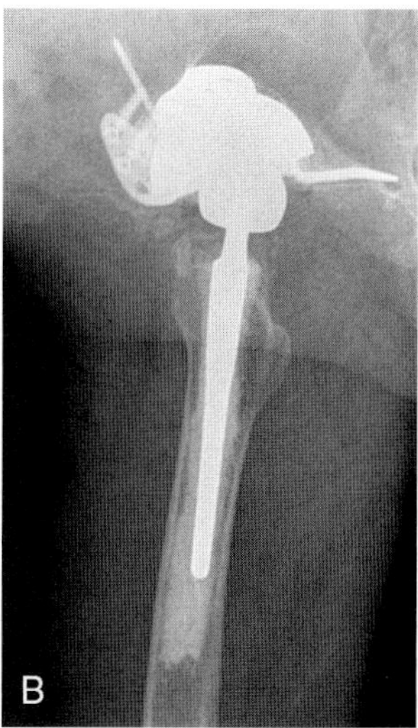

Figure 3 AP (**A**) and lateral (**B**) views showing 1-year postoperative radiographs of a pelvic dissociation treated with a cup-cage construct.

Custom Triflange Acetabular Prosthesis

A triflange cup provides another option for difficult acetabular reconstruction in a patient with pelvic dissociation and massive bone loss. It achieves stable implant fixation on host bone, reapproximates anatomic load bearing, and provides the potential for biologic fixation. DeBoer and associates[16] reported the results of 28 patients (30 hips) with failed THA and pelvic dissociation (most were type IVb). The prosthesis was custom manufactured on the basis of a three-dimensional model of the hemipelvis created with CT. The locations of the three flanges were identified by the surgeon on the ilium, ischium, and pubis; the center of rotation of the femoral head and orientation of the cup were then determined. Initial stability of the implant was provided with screw fixation, which was first placed in the ischial flange. The iliac flange was then fixed with screws that pulled the flange into intimate contact with bone, often reduced the dissociation, and rotated the caudad half of the hemipelvis into correct orientation relative to the cephalad aspect of the hemipelvis. Twenty hips in 18 patients were followed for a mean of 10 years (range, 7.4 to 13 years). Definite healing of the pelvic dissociation was indicated by the presence of bridging callus in 18 of the 20 hips. There were no broken screws and no implant migration, even when the discontinuity persisted. Small nonprogressive radiolucent lines were observed in six hips. Complications included one partial sciatic nerve palsy that resolved completely and one instance of loose ischial screws in a radiographically stable implant in the same patient. Five patients had one or more dislocations postoperatively. The mean Harris hip score improved from 41 points preoperatively to 80 points at the time of the latest follow-up (range, 7.4 to 13 years). Eleven patients required ambulatory aids postoperatively. No component was revised.

Structural Allografts

Bulk acetabular bone grafting has been used with bulk femoral heads with limited screw fixation as well as with whole acetabular allografts. Acetabular reamers are used to size the acetabular cavity and identify the location of the remaining bone to support the allograft. A pelvic recon-

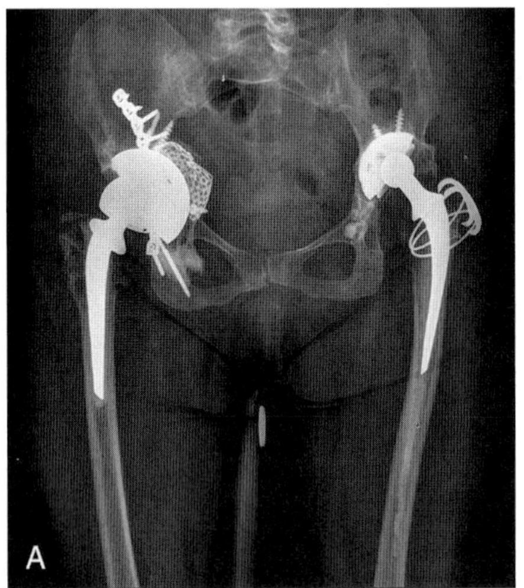

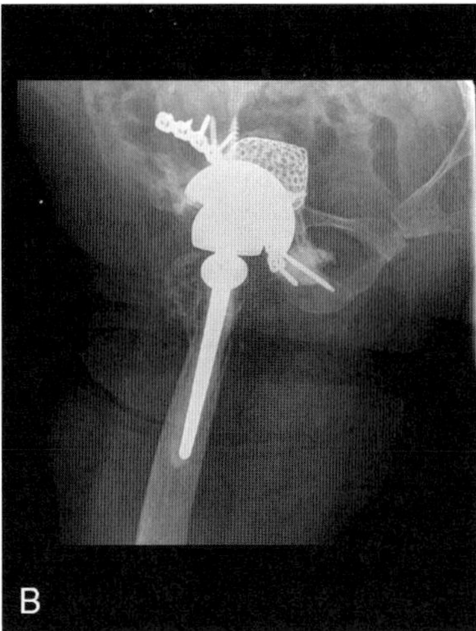

Figure 4 Two-year postoperative AP **(A)** and lateral **(B)** radiographs of a pelvic dissociation reconstructed with porous tantalum implant and posterior plating.

struction plate may be required to stabilize the posterior column as previously mentioned. A cage is recommended to protect allografts. Cage-host bone screws and cage-allograft bone screws achieve fixation. The inferior flange of the cage should be inserted into a slot in the ischium for fixation. Some cages have an inferior flange designed for screw fixation into ischium; however, because of complications associated with screws in the ischium, this technique is not preferred. A metal shell or a polyethylene liner is then cemented into the cage or allograft composite, avoiding the tendency to place the component in a vertical and retroverted position.

Type IIIb acetabular defects treated with an acetabular allograft and a cemented acetabular component have shown poor clinical results. Sporer and associates[11] reported on 16 patients at a minimum 8-year follow-up (mean follow-up, 10 years). Six hips were functioning without loosening, six were revised for aseptic loosening at an average of 2.9 years, and four hips showed radiographic loosening.

Stiehl and associates[6] reported on 17 patients with massive acetabular bone loss. Ten of these patients had a type IV pelvic dissociation, with nine having a type IVb deficiency and one having a type IVc deficiency. Bulk structural allograft was used in combination with posterior and/or anterior column plates. At follow-up (mean, 7 years postoperatively), 6 of 10 patients (60%) required re-revision surgery. Cementless cups that rested on a bulk allograft had high failure rates.

Highly Porous Metal Modular Implants With or Without Plating

Porous coated acetabular components provide effective long-term stability in the revision setting through biologic fixation to the host bone in addition to plating (Figure 4). Porous tantalum, with a high volumetric porosity (ranging from 70% to 80%) and low modulus of elasticity, has a propensity for bony ingrowth and biologic fixation.[17,18]

The acetabular defect is sized with acetabular reamers in the desired location to find the dimension of the cavity until two points of fixation are achieved (anterior to posterior, anteroinferior to posteroinferior, posterosuperior to anteroinferior). Augments are used to decrease acetabular volume and restore a rim to support a revision cup. The location and orientation of the augments are highly variable depending on the bone-loss pattern. Augments are often placed on the medial aspect of the ilium, or they may be stacked. It is more common to use the augments with the wide base placed laterally and the apex medially. The augments are initially secured to the host bone with the use of multiple screws. Portions of the augments may need to be removed with a burr to optimize the surface area contact between the revision shell and the augments. Multiple screw fixation is then used through the revision shell.[11]

Potential Complications

In addition to the risk of mechanical and biologic failure of the construct, serious complications related to these large-scale, difficult reconstructions include intraoperative fractures, recurrent dislocations, deep infections, injuries to the sciatic nerve, nonunions, and fixation failures. Delayed sciatic neuropathy following complex acetabular reconstruction for pelvic dissociation has been reported by Stiehl and Stewart.[19] Sciatic nerve exploration at 12 months postoperatively showed dense scar tissue directly over the plate as the nerve crossed the ischium. One pelvic plate screw had worked out approximately 3 mm and was directly pressing on the nerve. Substantial improvement in clinical symptoms resulted from screw removal and nerve release. Palmer and associates[20] reported a hip-vagina fistula in a 46-year-old woman who had multiple revision procedures complicated by infection after a primary THA that failed because of recurrent dislocation. The patient presented with a hip-vagina fistula 18 months after reconstruction of pelvic dissociation using an antiprotrusio cage. Radiographs showed a fracture of the cage with superomedial migration into the pelvis. The fistula was possibly formed by pressure necrosis from the failed acetabular cage against the intrapelvic vaginal wall. The patient was treated with a salvage procedure that included primary closure of the fistula with rotational muscle flaps, the use of an oversized bipolar acetabular component to avoid Girdlestone resection, and chronic bacterial suppression with antibiotics.

Summary

Pelvic dissociation following THA is a challenging condition requiring complex reconstructive procedures. Despite the technical feasibility of such revisions and the good clinical results, the main goal should be early recognition of acetabular loosening to minimize osteolytic loss of bone stock. Modular highly porous metal component revision systems have not been used long enough to provide definitive recommendations; however, early results from various centers are encouraging. For large defects in patients with pelvic dissociation, highly porous metal cups should be supported with either augments or a cage, when indicated, to improve initial mechanical stability and long-term biologic fixation.

References

1. Berry DJ, Lewallen DG, Hanssen AD, Cabanela ME: Pelvic discontinuity in revision total hip arthroplasty. *J Bone Joint Surg Am* 1999;81:1692-1702.
2. Harris WH: Wear and periprosthetic osteolysis: The problem. *Clin Orthop Relat Res* 2001;393:66-70.
3. Hozack WJ, Mesa JJ, Carey C, Rothman RH: Relationship between polyethylene wear, pelvic osteolysis, and clinical symptomatology in patients with cementless acetabular components: A framework for decision making. *J Arthroplasty* 1996;11: 769-772.
4. Chiang PP, Burke DW, Freiberg AA, Rubash HE: Osteolysis of the pelvis: Evaluation and treatment. *Clin Orthop Relat Res* 2003;417:164-174.
5. Jacobs JJ, Roebuck KA, Archibeck M, Hallab NJ, Glant TT: Osteolysis: Basic science. *Clin Orthop Relat Res* 2001; 393:71-77.
6. Stiehl JB, Saluja R, Diener T: Reconstruction of major column defects and pelvic discontinuity in revision total hip arthroplasty. *J Arthroplasty* 2000;15:849-857.
7. Southwell DG, Bechtold JE, Lew WD, Schmidt AH: Improving the detection of acetabular osteolysis using oblique radiographs. *J Bone Joint Surg Br* 1999;81:289-295.
8. Puri L, Wixson RL, Stern SH, Kohli J, Hendrix RW, Stulberg SD: Use of helical computed tomography for the assessment of acetabular osteolysis after total hip arthroplasty. *J Bone Joint Surg Am* 2002;84:609-614.
9. Stulberg SD, Wixson RL, Adams AD, Hendrix RW, Bernfield JB: Monitoring pelvic osteolysis following total hip replacement surgery: An algorithm for surveillance. *J Bone Joint Surg Am* 2002;84:116-122.
10. D'Antonio JA, Capello WN, Borden LS, et al: Classification and management of acetabular abnormalities in total hip arthroplasty. *Clin Orthop Relat Res* 1989;243 :126-137.
11. Sporer SM, O'Rourke M, Paprosky WG: The treatment of pelvic discontinuity during acetabular revision. *J Arthroplasty* 2005;20:79-84.
12. Sporer SM, Paprosky WG: Acetabular revision using a trabecular metal acetabular component for severe acetabular bone loss associated with a pelvic discontinuity. *J Arthroplasty* 2006;21:87-90.
13. Goodman S, Saastamoinen H, Shasha N, Gross A: Complications of ilioischial reconstruction rings in revision total hip arthroplasty. *J Arthroplasty* 2004;19:436-446.
14. Paprosky W, Sporer S, O'Rourke MR: The treatment of pelvic discontinuity with acetabular cages. *Clin Orthop Relat Res* 2006;453:183-187.
15. Eggli S, Müller C, Ganz R: Revision surgery in pelvic discontinuity: An analysis of seven patients. *Clin Orthop Relat Res* 2002;398:136-145.
16. DeBoer DK, Christie MJ, Brinson MF, Morrison JC: Revision total hip arthroplasty for pelvic discontinuity. *J Bone Joint Surg Am* 2007;89:835-840.
17. Levine B, Della Valle CJ, Jacobs JJ: Applications of porous tantalum in total hip arthroplasty. *J Am Acad Orthop Surg* 2006;14:646-655.
18. Weeden SH, Schmidt RH: The use of tantalum porous metal implants for Paprosky 3A and 3B defects. *J Arthroplasty* 2007;22:151-155.
19. Stiehl JB, Stewart WA: Late sciatic nerve entrapment following pelvic plate reconstruction in total hip arthroplasty. *J Arthroplasty* 1998;13:586-588.
20. Palmer SW, Luu HH, Finn HA: Hip-vagina fistula after acetabular revision. *J Arthroplasty* 2003;18:533-536.

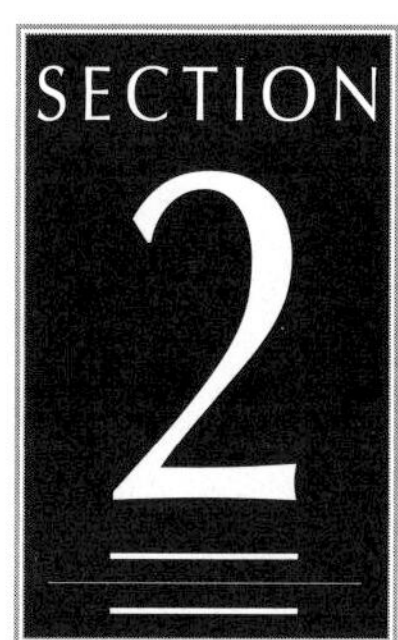

Adult Reconstruction: Knee

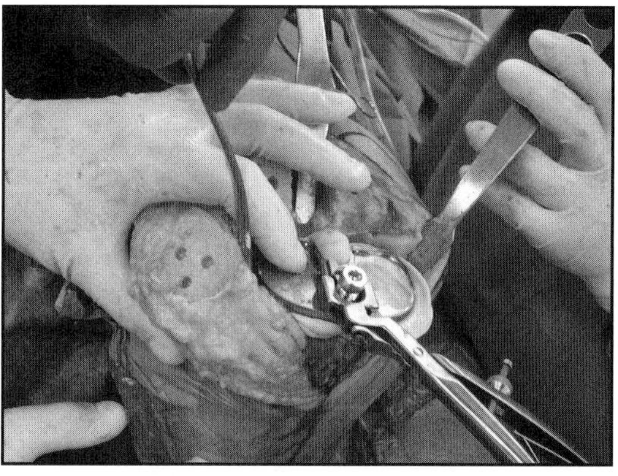

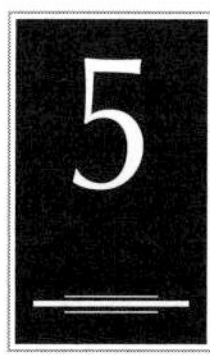

Unicompartmental Knee Arthroplasty: Indications, Techniques, and Results

Richard A. Berger, MD
Craig J. Della Valle, MD

Abstract

Unicompartmental knee arthroplasty (UKA) was introduced in the early 1970s but did not receive substantial support because total knee arthroplasty was flourishing. In the early 1990s, interest in UKA increased with the introduction of a minimally invasive surgical approach. It is important that the indications for this demanding but achievable surgical technique be strictly observed. The extension and flexion gaps for UKA can be addressed in a similar fashion to total knee arthroplasty and should be equalized. The femoral and tibial components must be properly sized so that the surfaces are well covered without overhang or impingement. UKA results at 10- to 15-year follow-ups are encouraging and are similar to many reported results of total knee arthroplasty.

Instr Course Lect 2010;59:47-59.

Initially introduced in the early 1970s, unicompartmental knee arthroplasty (UKA) gained popularity secondary to the relative ease of prosthetic implantation, the requirement for minimal bone sacrifice, and the potential ease of future revision to a total knee arthroplasty (TKA) if required. However, the combination of poor prosthetic design and instrumentation and an inadequate understanding of appropriate patient selection criteria resulted in an unacceptably high rate of failure. UKA was nearly abandoned in the United States by the late 1980s.

More than any other surgeon, Repicci was responsible for reintroducing UKA in the United States in the 1990s.[1,2] He developed a minimally invasive technique for UKA that was appealing to orthopaedic surgeons who were increasingly aware of the potential benefits that minimally invasive approaches had offered in other areas of surgery for reducing tissue trauma.

UKA has enjoyed a resurgence in popularity because of a combination of studies that have reported implant survivorship (in appropriately selected patients) that rivals that of TKA and the development of improved minimally invasive surgical techniques, which facilitate implantation with reduced disruption of the soft-tissue envelope.[1-8] The benefits of minimally invasive techniques include less discomfort, a shorter hospital stay, and a more rapid return of range of motion and function.

Indications

General

Because the outcomes of UKA seem to be highly dependent on patient selection criteria, a thorough understanding of the appropriate indications for the procedure is critical to both short- and long-term success. The ideal candidate for UKA has noninflammatory arthritis that has

Dr. Berger or an immediate family member has received royalties from Zimmer; is a member of a speakers' bureau or has made paid presentations on behalf of Biomet and Zimmer; serves as a paid consultant to or is an employee of TissueLink and Zimmer; and has received research or institutional support from Wright Medical Technology, Zimmer, and Smith & Nephew. Dr. Della Valle or an immediate family member is a member of a speakers' bureau or has made paid presentations on behalf of Angiotech; serves as a paid consultant to or is an employee of Zimmer; serves as an unpaid consultant to Biomet and Kinamed; has received research or institutional support from Zimmer; and has received nonincome support (such as equipment or services), commercially derived honoraria, or other non–research-related funding (such as paid travel) from Smith & Nephew and Stryker.

been unresponsive to nonsurgical treatment, clinical symptoms confined to the medial or lateral joint line, and radiographic evidence of isolated tibiofemoral arthritis in a single compartment. Optimal results have been reported in nonobese patients without patellofemoral symptoms who have functioning cruciate ligaments and knee range of motion greater than 90°. Minimal varus or valgus deformity (less than 15°) and a flexion contracture of less than 10° are additional prerequisites for optimal results.

Patient History and Pain Pattern

The single most important factor in selecting the proper candidate for UKA is the patient's pain pattern; pain should be localized to the involved compartment without patellofemoral or contralateral compartment symptoms. More diffuse pain, particularly in the patellofemoral region, during activities such as stair climbing, is a relative contraindication, as is the presence of pain at rest or at night. It is also important to differentiate between anterior patellofemoral pain (indicating a poor candidate for UKA) and anteromedial pain, which is more inferior and medial to the patella (indicating a good candidate for UKA).

Physical Examination

A physical examination of the potential UKA candidate should show good range of motion, stable ligaments, and only minimal angular deformity. The varus or valgus deformity should be less than 15°. In general, a flexion contracture of 10° or less can be corrected at the time of UKA. A flexion contracture of more than 10° cannot be corrected by UKA and residual flexion will remain. The residual flexion is not well tolerated by most patients and leads to quadriceps fatigue. It is also important to identify clinically relevant patellofemoral disease; a patellofemoral grind test is helpful in this regard. Patients also should report more pain in the suspected compartment than the front of the knee when they rise from a squatting position. Excessive retropatellar crepitus may also indicate clinically relevant patellofemoral disease.

Because UKA relies on normal ligament kinematics to stabilize the joint, both cruciate ligaments should be competent. However, some patients with anterior cruciate ligament (ACL) deficiency but without instability are well suited for a fixed-bearing UKA. Mobile-bearing implants cannot be used in patients with an ACL-deficient knee, as bearing dislocation is more likely in this subset of patients. A significant effusion is usually a sign of a diffuse inflammatory response and indicates a patient with more pervasive arthritis who is not well suited for UKA.

Varus or valgus correction of the knee to stress or overcorrection of the knee to stress is another important consideration. This test can be done either clinically by visually assessing alignment while applying stress or radiographically with a stress view. In either instance, a knee that does not correct to a neutral alignment during stress is better suited for UKA because the knee will remain slightly deformed and spare the opposite noninvolved compartment increased weight-bearing forces when the replacement compartment is stressed; stress is well tolerated by the UKA. Conversely, a knee that fully corrects or overcorrects to varus or valgus stress is a poor candidate for UKA. Full correction or overcorrection increases the force in the normal contralateral compartment; with time this force will lead to deterioration and pain in the normal compartment. Overcorrection of the knee during stress indicates a loss of joint space in the contralateral compartment. Overcorrection offers the worst prognosis for a UKA. The overcorrected knee places more of the weight-bearing forces through the already diseased opposite compartment. Rapid deterioration of the contralateral compartment is likely.

Radiographic Evaluation

Radiographically, degenerative disease should be limited to the involved compartment. An AP standing radiograph, a PA flexion view (skier's view), and a Merchant view are mandatory for proper evaluation. Although the presence of small osteophytes in the noninvolved compartments is acceptable, they should not be clinically painful. Similarly, a small area of notch impingement of the tibial spine into the contralateral femoral condyle is sometimes seen and is not a contraindication, as this area will be unloaded with correction of the knee into a more neutral alignment with UKA. Loss of joint space, however, in the contralateral compartment is a contraindication because it indicates disease that may be subclinical; stress radiographs can be particularly helpful in identifying such patients. Excessive tibial subluxation also is a worrisome sign because it indicates either instability or contralateral compartment disease. Moderate degenerative disease is preferred over more severe disease because more severe radiographic changes are suggestive of contralateral or patellofemoral disease as well as ACL insufficiency. Inflammatory arthritis is a strict contraindication because of the risk of arthritis progression.

Other Considerations

In some instances, patient age, physical demand level, and personality may play a role in the decision between UKA and TKA. When considering a patient for UKA, it is important to educate the patient regarding the known differences between UKA and TKA so that they may assist in the decision-making process.

If it is assumed that many younger patients (younger than 60 years) will likely need another knee arthroplasty at some point during their lifetime and that elderly patients (older than 75 years) probably will not, then UKA should be the first knee procedure for a young patient and the last knee procedure for an older patient. Patients 60 years of age or older and those 75 years or younger may be better served with a TKA, given that their risk for resurgery may be higher with UKA than TKA.

Patient Demand Level and Personality

One of the advantages of UKA is that it retains the cruciate ligaments, the contralateral compartment, and the patella, resulting in more normal kinematics. This may help explain why patients treated with UKA feel more normal than those treated with TKA. Following UKA, patients usually report a more stable knee with greater strength and endurance. Because a large portion of the knee is unresurfaced with UKA, there are more potential sources for persistent discomfort postoperatively.

A patient who has fewer physical demands, is more sensitive to discomfort, and who does not want to worry about the development of knee arthritis in the remainder of the knee may be better suited for TKA. Conversely, a patient with greater physical demands who is more tolerant of discomfort is a better UKA candidate.

Although the typical decision is between TKA and UKA for a given patient, UKA is an alternative to high tibial osteotomy (HTO) for the treatment of isolated medial compartment arthritis in the younger patient. UKA usually offers better pain relief, a faster recovery, a lower risk of complications, improved function, and a decreased rate of conversion to TKA than does HTO. A well-performed UKA is typically easier to convert to a TKA than is an HTO, and outcomes following conversion are better.

Contraindications

Contraindications to UKA include inflammatory and contralateral compartment arthritis as well as symptomatic patellofemoral disease. Long-term studies have reported that progression of arthritis in the other compartments (particularly the patellofemoral joint) is the most common reason for a UKA failure requiring conversion to TKA.[3,4,9,10] Therefore, preoperative symptoms or full-thickness cartilage loss seen in the patellofemoral or contralateral compartment at the time of surgery is considered a contraindication to UKA. Another contraindication is radiographic evidence of tibiofemoral subluxation, which is a sign of contralateral compartment joint space loss and instability and is difficult to correct surgically with a UKA. Persistent subluxation in a UKA can lead to edge loading of the polyethylene and accelerated failure. Absence of the ACL has been considered a relative contraindication because patients may have symptoms of instability; however, in patients without symptomatic instability, a fixed-bearing UKA has been shown to work well.[3,9] A mobile-bearing UKA is contraindicated in patients without an ACL because the polyethylene bearing may dislocate.

Surgical Technique for Minimally Invasive Medial Compartment UKAs

A minimally invasive approach is most easily accomplished in thin, elderly women and is most difficult in young, heavy, muscular men. Both intramedullary and extramedullary guides have been developed for femoral component preparation. Although the extramedullary technique is faster and usually preferred by a surgeon who performs a larger volume of UKAs, the use of intramedullary alignment for the femoral component is familiar to most knee surgeons and allows placement of a fixed retractor that keeps the patella laterally subluxated.

Exposure of the Medial Compartment

After the knee is prepped and draped, a tourniquet is applied. The tibial tubercle, patella, and joint line are outlined and an incision is made extending from the proximal medial border of the patella superiorly to a point 1 cm distal to the joint line along the medial aspect of the tibial tubercle. Subcutaneous dissection proximal and distal to the skin incision aids in exposure by creating a mobile window. An arthrotomy is performed from the superior pole of the patella to just distal to the joint line (Figure 1).

The synovium and a portion of the patellar fat pad are resected to aid in visualization. Although additional exposure is rarely required, if needed, the capsular arthrotomy can be extended proximally into the quadriceps tendon or into the vastus medialis, or the capsule can be fur-

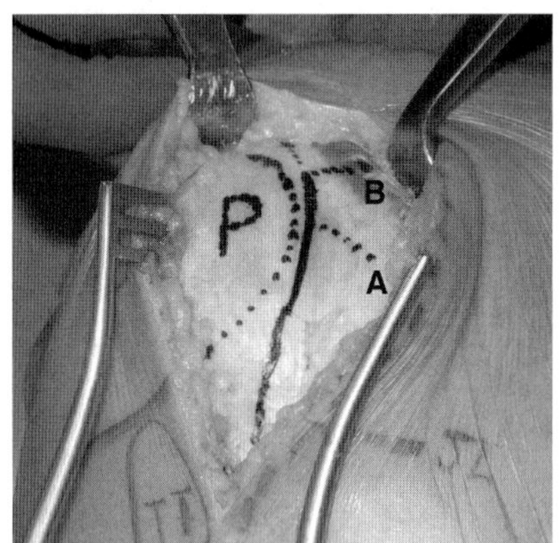

Figure 1 Intraoperative photograph of an arthrotomy from the superior pole of the patella to approximately 1 cm distal to the joint line. P = patella, B = arthrotomy for a midvastus approach, A = the arthrotomy for a subvastus approach.

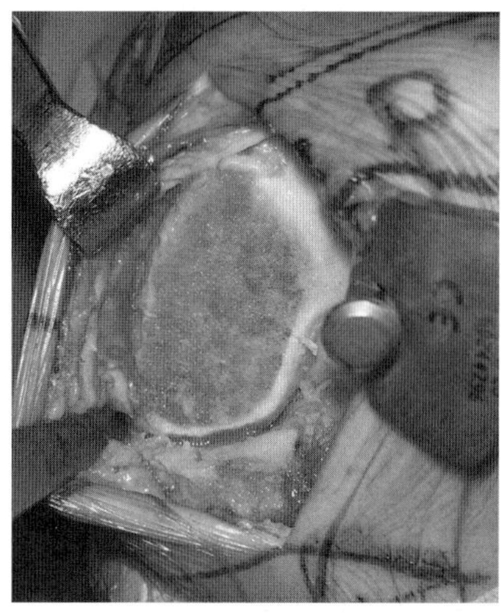

Figure 2 A patellar retractor aids visualization. Intraoperative photograph of the cut surface of the distal femur.

ther opened by incising it perpendicular to the longitudinal arthrotomy below the vastus medialis. The proximal medial tibia is exposed with an electric cautery or curved osteotome to the posteromedial corner and is extended approximately 1 cm distal to the joint line. The patellofemoral and lateral compartment are then inspected; extension of the knee often aids in visualization.

Distal Femoral and Proximal Tibial Preparation With Intramedullary Alignment

The knee is flexed approximately 30°. The patella is displaced laterally with a single point retractor and a pilot hole is drilled on the medial side of the intercondylar notch just anterior to the insertion of the posterior cruciate ligament. This starting point is just medial to the typical starting point used in TKA.

The intramedullary alignment guide is then set for the distal femoral cut, which is typically 4° or 6°. This angle determines the position that the round femoral component will contact the flat tibial component. In TKA, the angle of the distal femoral cut determines the overall alignment of the knee because only one condyle is resected and the space is made up by the thickness of the polyethylene liner. The distal femoral cutting guide is then placed into the pilot hole and seated flush with the femoral condyle. The distal femur is cut with an oscillating saw. The amount of bone resected should equal the thickness of the femoral component to be inserted, usually 6 mm. A patellar retractor is then inserted into the intramedullary hole to keep the patella laterally subluxated, which aids with exposure for subsequent steps (Figure 2).

Tibial Preparation

Although the femur can be finished prior to the tibia, balancing a UKA is much easier if the tibia is resected first. An extramedullary alignment guide is placed onto the anterior tibia, as it would be in a TKA. The guide is set for a resection that is perpendicular to the mechanical axis of the tibia, with a posterior slope that matches the native slope of the tibia (approximately 7°), although some variation is sometimes helpful. Because the proximal portion of the guide is aligned with the medial portion of the tibial tubercle, the guide distally usually needs to be aligned approximately 5 to 10 mm medial to the center of the ankle. The guide also should be parallel to the tibial shaft, when viewed from the side, to re-create the native tibial slope. The depth of the tibial cut is then set to resect 2 to 4 mm of bone from the medial tibial plateau.

With the guide pinned in place, a thin metal wedge can be inserted through the cutting slot in the tibial guide to ensure both an appropriate level of resection and slope. A retractor is placed to protect the medial collateral ligament, and the proximal tibia is cut, taking care not to undermine the cruciate ligament insertions. The sagittal cut in the tibia is then made at the apex of the medial tibial spine, corresponding to the medial border of the cruciate ligaments (Figure 3). The piece is removed and the medial meniscus is resected.

Balancing a UKA

Basic Techniques

Balancing a UKA is similar to balancing a TKA—the goal is to create nearly equal flexion and extension spaces to allow for proper knee kinematics. However, unlike those treated with TKA, patients treated with UKA usually have minimal deformity and excellent range of motion. The preoperative flexion and extension spaces are nearly equal in size, and if a measured resection technique is used, the flexion and extension spaces should remain symmetric.

The flexion space should be 1 mm larger than the extension

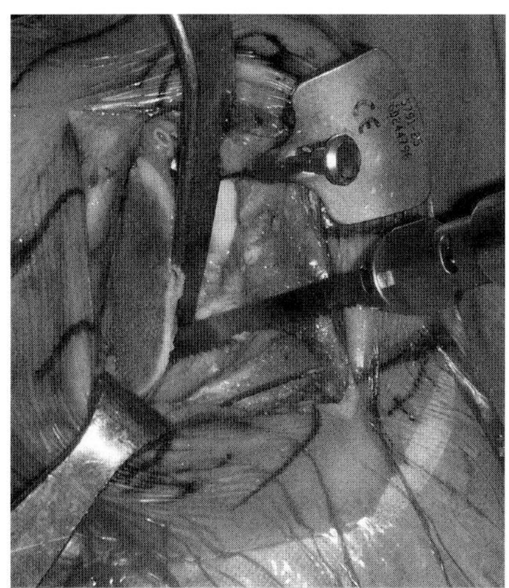

Figure 3 Intraoperative photograph showing a sagittal tibial cut made at the apex of the medial tibial spine, corresponding to the medial border of the cruciate ligaments.

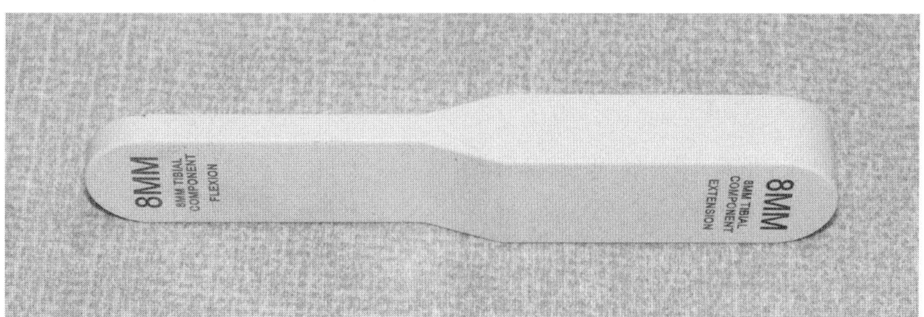

Figure 4 Photograph of an 8-mm spacer with a thinner end for judging the flexion gap before femoral resection and a thicker end for measuring the extension space after both sides of the joint have been resected.

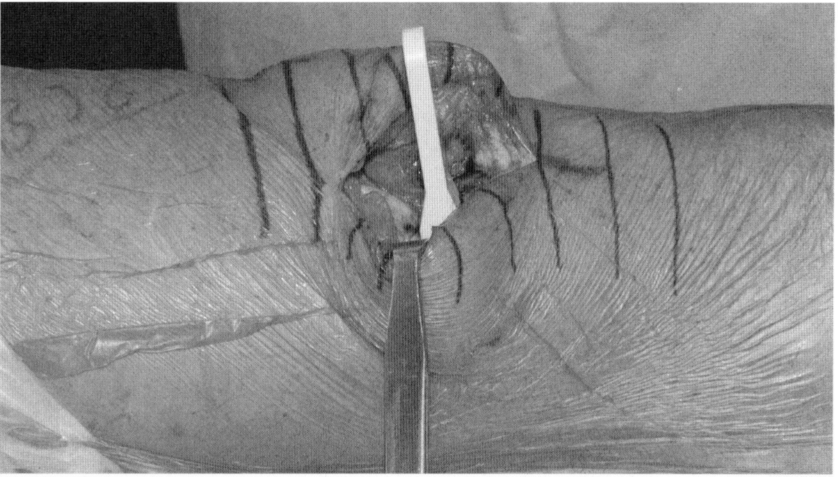

Figure 5 The thicker side of the spacer block is inserted in full extension with both the distal femoral and proximal tibial resections completed.

space for a medial unicompartmental replacement and 1 to 2 mm larger for a lateral unicompartmental replacement. After the components are in place, the overall laxity remaining in the replaced compartment should be 2 mm in full extension and 3 mm in 90° of flexion for a medial unicompartmental replacement (4 mm for a lateral unicompartmental replacement).

Initial Balancing

Spacer blocks have been designed for UKAs that measure 8, 10, 12, and 14 mm in thickness (Figure 4). These spacers typically have two ends, a thicker end for checking the extension space after the distal femur and the proximal tibia have been resected (Figure 5) and a thinner end for checking the size of the flexion space once the tibia has been cut prior to resecting the posterior femoral condyle (Figure 6).

The technique for a fixed-bearing UKA includes resection of the same amount of distal femur as is replaced by the femoral component. Preoperative assessment of the knee's flexion and extension can aid in adjusting the slope of the tibial resection, which assists in creating appropriate flexion and extension gaps. In a knee with both full extension and good flexion, the slope of the tibial resection should match the slope of the native tibia. In some knees, altering the slope of the tibial resection can assist the surgeon in creating symmetric flexion and extension gaps.

The most common situation is a patient with a small flexion contracture and good flexion (the extension space is slightly smaller than the flexion space). In this situation, it is helpful to decrease the posterior slope of the tibial cut, resulting in an asymmetric resection of the tibia (more bone is removed anteriorly than posteriorly) that selectively increases the extension space compared with the flexion space. In rare instances, the patient has full extension and poor flexion. In this situation, the tibial slope can be increased slightly by resecting more tibia posteriorly than anteriorly; this increases the flexion space compared with the extension space. If this algorithm is routinely followed, many of the commonly encountered UKA discrepancies can be accommodated.

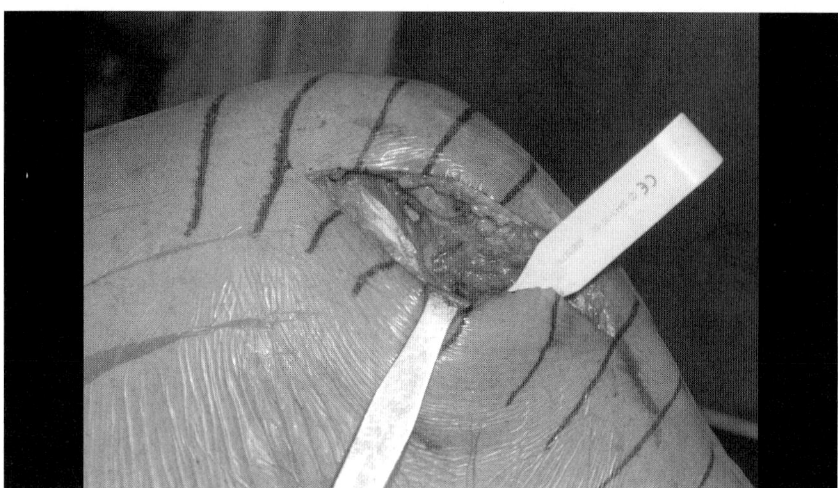

Figure 6 The thinner side of the spacer block is inserted in flexion with only the proximal tibial resection completed.

Using the Extension and Flexion Spacer Blocks

With the leg in extension, and after the distal femur and proximal tibia have been resected, the extension side of the spacer is inserted (Figure 5). The thicker extension side of the spacer simulates the thickness of the distal femoral component combined with the tibial component and polyethylene liner. At a minimum, the 10-mm block should fit into that space. This process will simulate the thickness of the femoral component with the thickness of the smallest tibial polyethylene liner (8 mm) and allow 2 mm of laxity in extension the appropriate amount of residual laxity for a UKA. Once the extension space is appropriately measured, the knee is flexed up to 90°.

In 90° of flexion, the flexion side of the spacer (the thin side) is inserted into the flexion gap (Figure 6). This spacer simulates the thickness of the tibial component and the polyethylene liner, without resection of the posterior femoral condyle. At a minimum, a 10-mm spacer block should be able to fit into this space. Usually, the flexion and extension spaces will be similar or equal at this point; however, because of variations in the patient's preoperative ligament balance or bony anatomy (or if the bony resections have not been performed accurately) a mismatch between the flexion and extension spaces may be present.

Equalizing the Flexion and Extension Spaces

The goal is to have the flexion space approximately 1 mm larger than the extension space for a properly balanced medial UKA (2 mm larger for a lateral UKA).The most common problem is an extension space that is tighter than the flexion space, which may be a residual complication of a preoperative flexion contracture. Several steps can fix these mismatched spaces.

As is done routinely in TKA, removal of posterior condylar osteophytes and the posterior capsule with a curved osteotome can increase the size of the extension gap. If this maneuver does not remedy the problem, the tibia can be recut with slightly less slope as was previously described. The distal femur can be recut by 1 or 2 mm, which will selectively increase the size of the extension space; this is typically required only in instances in which the initial distal femoral resection was inadequate (less than 6 mm of distal femur was resected). The final alternative is to move the femoral cutting block posteriorly, reducing the amount of posterior femoral condyle resected and thus reducing the size of the flexion space; balance is subsequently achieved by using a smaller polyethylene spacer, but only if enough tibia has been resected to accommodate the 10-mm block.

A less common scenario is the occurrence of a flexion space that is smaller than the extension space. In this instance, the tibia can be recut with slightly more posterior slope as was previously described. If this does not remedy the problem, the posterior femoral condyle can be shaved by 1 or 2 mm with a saw prior to fitting and sizing the femoral component. This additional resection of the posterior femoral condyle will move the femoral component anteriorly, enlarging the flexion space. The process of balancing the flexion and extension spaces can be an iterative process in which slight corrections are made until the flexion and extension spaces are equal and appropriately sized (at least 10 mm) to allow for proper knee kinematics (Table 1).

Femoral Component Sizing and Final Distal Femoral Preparation

The femoral component size is selected by placing the foot of the femoral finishing guide underneath the posterior femoral condyle and selecting the largest size that will not overhang the junction between the remaining articular cartilage and the cut end of the distal femur (Figure 7, *A*). If the component overhangs and extends beyond this point, the native patella can impinge on the femoral component (Figure 7, *B*). In general, if the surgeon is choosing between sizes, the smaller size is selected.[10] It is important to recognize that this is a posterior referencing system; therefore, femoral component size does not affect balancing of the flexion and extension gap. The amount of bone removed from the posterior femoral condyle is the same regardless of the femoral component size selected with a resection that is equivalent to the thickness of the posterior condyle of the component.

When placing the femoral finishing guide on the cut end of the distal femur, care should be taken to ensure it is rotated appropriately so that the final femoral component will track centrally on the tibial tray. The best way to achieve this goal is to place the flexion side (the thin end) of the 8-mm balancing block under the femoral guide; this derotates the femur and aligns the guide perpendicular to the cut end of the upper tibia. The removal of osteophytes from the intercondylar notch also can assist the surgeon in appropriately rotating this guide. The guide is then affixed to the femur with multiple pins, and the lug holes for the femoral component are drilled. The femoral chamfer and posterior femoral cuts are then made with an oscillating saw.

Table 1
Flexion and Extension Space Balancing in UKA

Following distal femoral and proximal tibial resection:
Extension space is smaller than the flexion space:
Remove posterior condylar osteophytes and release posterior capsule
Decrease tibial slope
Translate femoral component posteriorly (reduce size of flexion gap)
Resect more distal femur
Flexion space is smaller than extension space:
Shave posterior femoral condyle prior to finishing the femoral component
Increase tibial slope

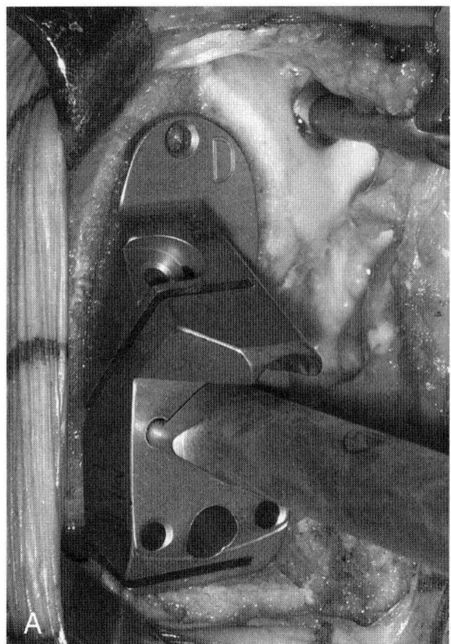

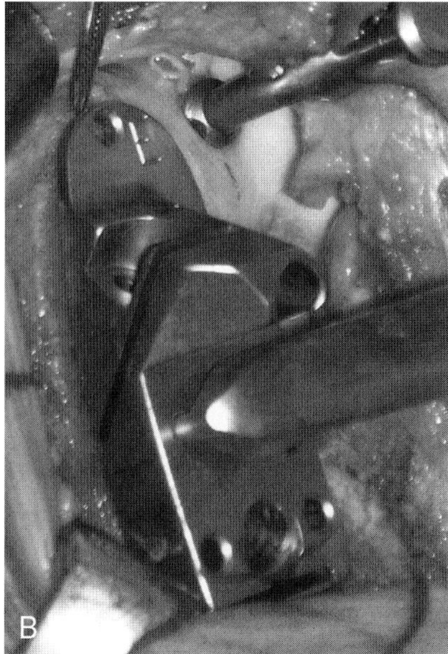

Figure 7 **A,** Intraoperative photograph showing an appropriately sized femoral component in place approximately 2 mm below the remaining trochlear cartilage. **B,** This component is too large and will impinge on the remaining trochlear cartilage.

Tibial Component Sizing

The remainder of the posterior horn of the medial meniscus and any other remaining soft tissues are removed from the posterior aspect of the joint. The largest size tibial component that will not overhang the cut surface of the tibia is selected using the sizing guides; if the tibial cut was removed as a single piece, this can aid in tibial sizing. The trial tibial component is then impacted into place.

Trial Reduction

The trial femoral component is inserted along with the trial polyethylene insert. The knee is brought through a range of motion to ensure that the femoral component tracks centrally on the tibial component throughout a range of motion and that the femur does not impinge against the patella (Figure 8).

At this point, the knee is extended fully; there should be 2 mm of laxity in this position. In the system used by the authors, the laxity is assessed using a plastic spacer that measures 2 mm on one side and 3 mm on the opposite side (Figure 9). With the knee in extension, the 2 mm side of the spacer should be insertable into the extension space. The knee is then flexed to 90° and the 3 mm side of the plastic spacer should be placeable between the trial femoral component and polyethylene spacer.

If the flexion and extension spaces are unequal with the trial components in place, modification of the tibial slope is usually the easiest way to balance the knee. Once

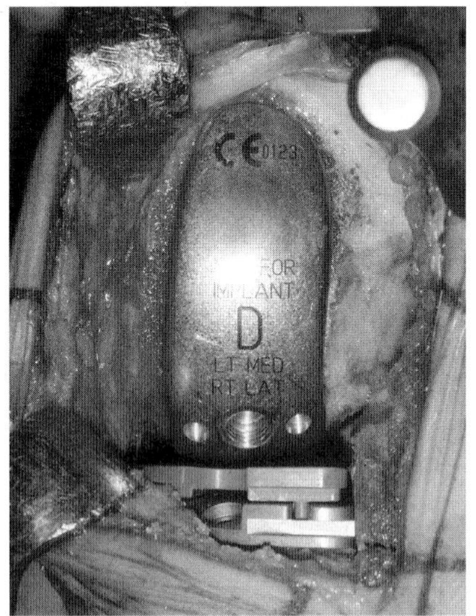

Figure 8 Intraoperative photograph showing the trial components in place with central placement of the femur on the tibia without overhang.

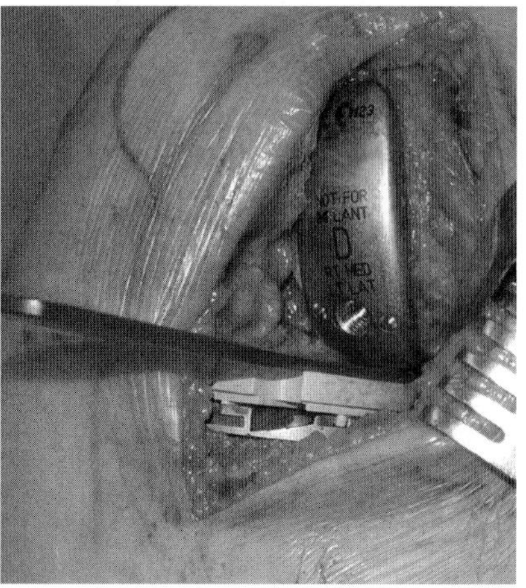

Figure 9 Intraoperative photograph showing the 2-mm end of the plastic spacer inserted between the components in 90° of flexion.

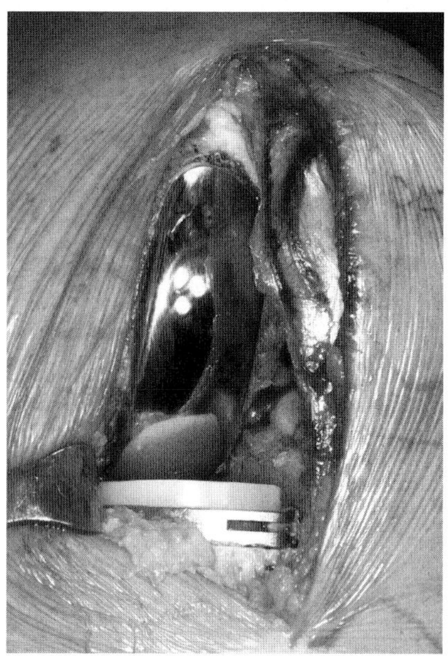

Figure 10 Intraoperative photograph of the final components in place.

component position is determined to be acceptable, lug holes for the tibial component are drilled and the trial components are then removed.

Cementing the Components

Areas of sclerotic bone can be drilled with a small drill bit to improve cement intrusion. The bony surfaces are cleansed using pulsatile lavage and thoroughly dried. A sponge is placed around the medial and posterior aspects of the tibial plateau to allow easy removal of extruded, excess cement. The tibia is cemented first and cement is inserted onto the bony surfaces with a gun and pressurized; an angled tip is helpful in this process. The posterior edge is forced down first, followed by the anterior edge to allow the excess cement to be extruded anteriorly for easy removal. The sponge that was previously placed around the tibia is now removed, withdrawing excess cement from the posterior aspect of the knee. The knee is then placed into approximately 110° of flexion and a valgus stress is applied, which allows the femur to be easily inserted. A trial polyethylene liner of the appropriate thickness is placed and the knee is flexed approximately 90° until the cement hardens. The previously described 2-mm spacer can be inserted to maintain pressure on the tibiofemoral articulation while the cement is hardening. Once the appropriate polyethylene spacer is selected, the surgeon should carefully search for any remaining cement because retained cement fragments can cause pain and damage to the bearing surface.[11] The final polyethylene insert is then engaged into the locking mechanism of the tibial tray (Figure 10). A drain can be inserted exiting laterally and the arthrotomy closed with the knee flexed. The subcutaneous tissues and skin are then closed in a routine fashion.

Video 5.1: Medial Unicompartmental Knee Arthroplasty Utilizing an Intramedullary Guide. Craig J. Della Valle, MD (30 min)

Surgical Technique for Minimally Invasive Lateral Compartment UKAs

The surgical steps and principles for a lateral compartment UKA are similar to those of a medial compartment UKA; however, some subtle differences are important to recognize.

Exposure of the Lateral Compartment

Although a medial approach for a lateral UKA has been described, the authors prefer a lateral approach to minimize the size of the incision and the soft-tissue dissection required. The incision should extend from the proximal lateral border of the patella to 1 cm distal to the joint line on the lateral side of the tibial tubercle; if additional exposure is required, the arthrotomy can be extended proximally. It is important to recognize that even in obese patients there is minimal soft tissue between the skin and the lateral retinaculum. Subcutaneous dissection proximal and distal to the skin incision may aid exposure. An arthrotomy is performed from the superior pole of the patella to the lateral side of the tibial tubercle without incising the patellar tendon. Because there is minimal synovium in the lateral compartment, this should be preserved to enhance soft-tissue coverage at the time of closure. After removal of the anterior horn of the lateral meniscus, a retractor is placed into the intercondylar notch to allow inspection of the patellofemoral and lateral compartments; slight extension of the knee aids visualization. If the surgeon is uncomfortable with the potential for performing a TKA through a laterally based incision (in the event that more diffuse arthritis is identified), then arthroscopy can be considered to inspect the remainder of the knee prior to the arthrotomy.

Given the relative tendency for lateral tracking of the patella, exposure can be more difficult for a lateral UKA. When preparing the hole for the intramedullary alignment guide, the hole is placed slightly more laterally, and thus less travel of the patella will be required.

Osseous Preparation

There are several critical differences between the bony preparations of a lateral UKA and a medial UKA. The lateral tibial plateau often has more bone loss than is found on the medial side and thus a minimal tibial resection is critical to prevent the use of a large polyethylene spacer or the necessity for intraoperative conversion to a TKA if an overly thick spacer is required. Given the relative tendency for lateral tracking of the patella, the risk of impingement of the patella against the femoral component is greater in the lateral compartment.[10] Therefore, the femoral component must be sized so that the most anterior border of the component is at least 2 mm below the junction of the cut distal end of the femur and the remaining articular cartilage, resulting in a component that is typically one size smaller than would be expected for a medial UKA.

Soft-Tissue Balancing

Because there is normally more laxity and translation of the femur on the lateral as opposed to the medial side of the knee, there should be slightly more laxity of the knee in flexion when performing a lateral UKA.

Component Insertion

The femoral component is often more difficult to introduce on the lateral side because of the relative lateral position of the patella. This difficulty can be overcome by flexing the knee to only 60° or 70° and applying a varus stress to the knee, which opens up the lateral compartment to facilitate insertion of both the trial and the final components.

Results

Several studies have reported excellent long-term results of fixed-bearing UKAs performed with a standard arthrotomy, with survivorship that rivals that of TKA in appropriately selected patients.[3-7,9] Berger and associates[3,9] reported a 10-year survivorship of 98% and a 15-year survivorship of 96% using a standard open arthrotomy in a cohort of patients who had a mean age of 68 years at the time of surgery. In a report of UKA in patients older than age 60 years, Swienckowski and Pennington[12] reported an 11-year survivorship of 92%. Similarly, Squire and associates[13] reported a revision rate of 10% in an average 18-year follow-up of 140 cemented UKAs.

Mobile-bearing UKA also has shown excellent results when performed via a standard medial parapatellar arthrotomy. Murray and associates[14] reported the results of 143 Oxford medial UKAs with a 10-year survivorship of 98%. Another study of 124 mobile-bearing UKAs reported a 10-year survivorship of 95%.[15] However, both studies involving mobile-bearing UKAs reported revisions resulting from dislocation of the mobile polyethylene bearing.

In early reports of the minimally invasive UKA surgical technique, 136 fixed-bearing UKAs were followed for 8 years. A 7% failure rate was reported with 10 revision surgeries.[1] Price and associates[16] compared 40 Oxford UKAs using a minimally invasive incision with 20 Oxford UKAs performed with a standard incision. They found that the average rate of recovery of the minimally invasive UKAs was twice as fast without compromising the final result. Gesell and Tria[8] reported on 47 minimally invasive UKAs with 2- to 4-year follow-up. Clinically, the patients did well with Knee Society pain scores that improved from 45 to 80, functional scores that improved from 47 to 78, and revision surgery in 1 of 47 patients (2%).

Although some studies support the safety of the minimally invasive approach,[17,18] one study demonstrated that results can be compromised if proper instrumentation and training is not ensured.[19] Robertsson and Lidgren[19] studied 13,299 knees that were implanted with three commonly used prosthetic designs over a 20-year period and assessed whether the introduction of minimally invasive techniques affected revision rates. The outcomes for one type of implant, which had good results prior to the introduction of a minimally invasive approach, showed deteriorated results following the use of a more limited exposure. Conversely, outcomes for another design, which was associated with poorer results initially, improved when a minimally invasive approach was introduced along with improved instrumentation and training. In the third prosthetic design, which was associated with excellent results, there was no change in results with the introduction of specialized instruments and proper training in minimally invasive techniques. It was concluded that proper instrumentation and training is crucial to maintaining good results.

Summary

UKA has seen a resurgence in popularity because of studies that have reported survivorship rates that rival those of TKA in appropriately selected patients along with the development of minimally invasive surgical techniques that facilitate implantation with minimal disruption of the soft-tissue envelope. The benefits of this minimally invasive UKA include less discomfort, a shorter hospital stay, and a more rapid return of range of motion and function. Although several recent studies show that a less invasive approach can result in acceptable implant alignment and excellent early clinical results when meticulous surgical technique is used, other studies show that proper instrumentation and training are necessary to maintain low failure rate for these procedures.

References

1. Repicci JA, Eberle RW: Minimally invasive surgical technique for unicondylar knee arthroplasty. *J South Orthop Assoc* 1999;8:20-27.
2. Romanowski MR, Repicci JA: Minimally invasive unicondylar arthroplasty: Eight year follow-up. *J Knee Surg* 2002;15:17-22.
3. Berger RA, Meneghini RM, Jacobs JJ, et al: Results of unicompartmental knee arthroplasty at a minimum of ten years of follow-up. *J Bone Joint Surg Am* 2005;87:999-1006.
4. Argenson JN, Chevrol-Benkeddache Y, Aubaniac JM: Modern unicompartmental knee arthroplasty with cement: A three to ten-year follow-up study. *J Bone Joint Surg Am* 2002;84: 2235-2239.
5. Keblish PA, Briard JL: Mobile-bearing unicompartmental knee arthroplasty: A 2-center study with an 11-year (mean) follow-up. *J Arthroplasty* 2004;19(suppl 2):87-94.
6. Naudie D, Guerin J, Parker DA, et al: Medial unicompartmental knee arthroplasty with the Miller-Galante prosthesis. *J Bone Joint Surg Am* 2004; 86:1931-1935.
7. Price AJ, Waite JC, Svard U: Long-term clinical results of the medial Oxford unicompartmental knee arthroplasty. *Clin Orthop Relat Res* 2005;435: 171-180.
8. Gesell MW, Tria AJ: MIS unicondylar knee arthroplasty: Surgical approach and early results. *Clin Orthop Relat Res* 2004;428:53-60.
9. Berger RA, Meneghini RM, Sheinkop MB, et al: The progression of patellofemoral arthrosis after medial unicompartmental replacement: Results at 11 to 15 years. *Clin Orthop Relat Res* 2004;428:92-99.
10. Hernigou P, Deschamps G: Posterior slope of the tibial implant and the outcome of unicompartmental knee arthroplasty. *J Bone Joint Surg Am* 2004;86:506-511.
11. Howe DJ, Taunton OD, Engh GA: Retained cement after unicondylar knee arthroplasty: A report of four cases. *J Bone Joint Surg Am* 2004;86: 2283-2286.
12. Swienckowski JJ, Pennington DW: Unicompartmental knee arthroplasty in patients sixty years of age or younger. *J Bone Joint Surg Am* 2004; 86(suppl 1 pt 2):131-142.
13. Squire MW, Callaghan JJ, Goetz DD, et al: Unicompartmental knee arthroplasty: A minimum fifteen year follow-up study. *Clin Orthop Relat Res* 1999;367:61-72.
14. Murray DW, Goodfellow JW, O'Connor JJ: The Oxford medial unicompartmental arthroplasty: A ten-year survival study. *J Bone Joint Surg Br* 1998;80:983-989.
15. Svard UCG, Price AJ: Oxford medial unicompartmental knee arthroplasty: A survival analysis of an independent series. *J Bone Joint Surg Br* 2001;83: 191-194.
16. Price AJ, Webb J, Topf H, et al: Rapid recovery after Oxford unicompartmental arthroplasty through a short incision. *J Arthroplasty* 2001;16:970-976.
17. Muller PE, Pellengahr C, Witt M, et al: Influence of minimally invasive surgery on implant positioning and the functional outcome for medial unicompartmental knee arthroplasty. *J Arthroplasty* 2004;19:296-301.
18. Pandit H, Jenkins C, Barker K, et al: The Oxford medial unicompartmental knee replacement using a minimally-invasive approach. *J Bone Joint Surg Br* 2006;88:54-60.
19. Robertsson O, Lidgren L: The short-term results of 3 common UKA implants during different periods in Sweden. *J Arthroplasty* 2008;23:801-807.

Video Reference

5.1: Della Valle CJ: Video. Medial unicompartmental knee arthroplasty utilizing an intramedullary guide, in Della Valle CJ, Stuchin SA, eds: *Surgical Techniques in Orthopaedics: Arthroplasty for Unicompartmental Arthritis*. DVD. Rosemont, IL, American Academy of Orthopaedic Surgeons, 2007.

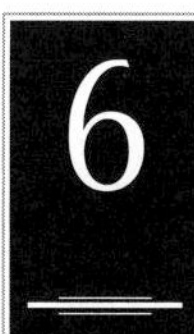

Mobile- Versus Fixed-Bearing Unicompartmental Knee Arthroplasty

Richard D. Scott, MD

Abstract

Unicompartmental knee arthroplasty using either a mobile- or fixed-bearing technique is an attractive alternative to osteotomy or total knee arthroplasty in selected patients with osteoarthritis. Both techniques appear to yield equivalent early results. Mobile-bearing articulations have the advantage of allowing a metal-backed component to be used with a composite thickness as thin as 6 mm. They also offer the potential for decreased long-term wear complications because of the high conformity of the articulation. The longevity of fixed-bearing components will likely be improved in the future with better prosthetic designs and improved polyethylene to minimize the incidence of late wear complications.

Instr Course Lect 2010;59:57-60.

In theory, unicompartmental knee arthroplasty (UKA) is an attractive alternative to osteotomy and total knee arthroplasty (TKA) in selected patients with osteoarthritis. The advantages of UKA over osteotomy include a higher initial success rate, fewer early complications, greater longevity, better cosmetic limb alignment, and easier conversion to TKA. Advantages of UKA over TKA include the preservation of both cruciate ligaments, which results in more normal knee kinematics and the potential for a higher level of performance. Bone stock is preserved in the opposite and patellofemoral compartments, allowing easier revision surgery in the future if necessary.

Despite these advantages, UKA has been a controversial procedure since its introduction in the early 1970s. Some initial reports regarding the use of UKA in the medial compartment were discouraging.[1,2] Other encouraging reports on the efficacy of UKA from the 1980s and 1990s established it as an acceptable arthroplasty procedure that is used to treat approximately 5% of patients with knee osteoarthritis in the United States.[3]

Evolution of UKA Designs

For the first decade after its introduction, revision rates after UKA remained competitive with those of TKA (approximately 1% per year). Follow-up of UKAs done in the 1970s, however, showed an increasing incidence of the need for revision in the second decade compared with reports documenting reoperation rates for TKA.[4] UKAs during this era usually failed because of wear, loosening, and degeneration of the opposite compartment. The metal-to-plastic articulation was often flat-on-flat; this highlighted the problem of edge loading as a cause of wear. Some wear problems also resulted from metal-backed components that had only 2 mm of polyethylene in the anterior and posterior areas of the articulation. Analysis of failed retrieved implants showed that the wear pattern of the polyethylene was anterior and peripheral.[5] It soon became apparent that the prosthetic unicompartmental wear pattern replicated the preoperative articulating pattern of the arthritic knee as described by White and associates.[6] All fixed-bearing UKA designs are subject to this wear pattern.

Dr. Scott or an immediate family member has received royalties from DePuy and serves as an unpaid consultant to DePuy.

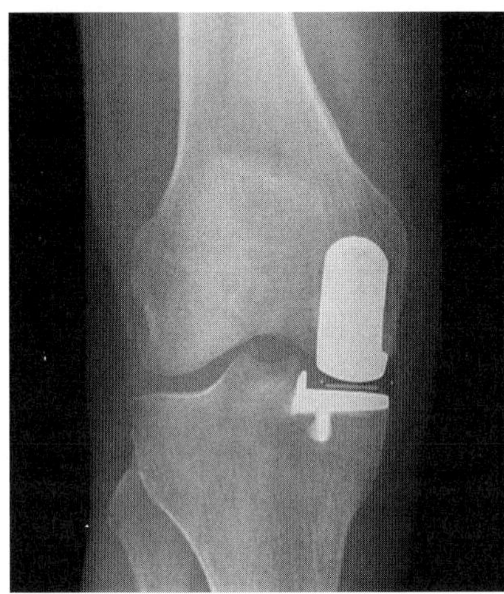

Figure 1 AP radiograph of a 6-mm composite mobile-bearing tibial component showing the conservation of tibial bone that is possible with a mobile-bearing UKA.

Attempts were made to correct the edge-loading problem and redirect the wear pattern by making the prosthetic articulation more conforming. These attempts to alter the wear pattern with a conforming fixed-bearing design created a kinematic conflict that led to an increased incidence of femoral and/or tibial component loosening caused by the increased force transmitted to the fixation interface. It became apparent that fixed-bearing UKA articulations must be nonconforming and remain round-on-relatively flat. A highly conforming articulation must be a mobile-bearing articulation to eliminate the adverse effects of constraint on the fixation interface.

Another advantage of a mobile-bearing articulation is the potential to provide a metal-backed component with a conservative composite thickness.[7-9] Fixed-bearing, metal-backed components are usually designed with a minimum of 6 mm of polyethylene. This design mandates a minimum composite thickness of 8 mm when added to a 2-mm thick metal backing; more often the metal backing is 3 mm, which increases the composite thickness to 9 mm. With the mobile-bearing knee, the Food and Drug Administration has approved a 3-mm polyethylene thickness because of improved wear characteristics and favorable long-term experience with this highly conforming articulation. The 3-mm metal backing allows a composite thickness as thin as 6 mm. One of the basic principles of UKA is the performance of an initial conservative tibial resection. This 6-mm composite allows this principle to be achieved (Figure 1). Until mobile-bearing knees were approved by the Food and Drug Administration, it was necessary to use an all-polyethylene tibial component to achieve a conservative tibial resection. Although an all-polyethylene tibial component is an acceptable alternative, especially in elderly patients, a metal-backed tibial component has potential advantages, such as modularity to facilitate the cementing process and allow an insert exchange to treat late wear. The metal backing may also distribute forces more uniformly than polyethylene and be preferable for use in younger, heavier, more active patients.

Surgical Technique

The basic UKA technique using the mobile-bearing Oxford Unicompartmental Knee System (Biomet Orthopedics, Warsaw, IN) consists of the following surgical principles: (1) The patient has a passively correctable varus knee deformity. (2) The initial bone is resected from the tibia. (3) A minimum 7-mm flexion gap is established. (4) The femur is sized. (5) The posterior condylar cutting jig is properly oriented and the posterior condyle resected. (6) An initial femoral reaming is performed using the "zero spigot." (7) The flexion gap space is confirmed and the differential between it and the extension gap is established. (8) The femur is reamed with the appropriate spigot that equalizes the gaps. (9) Trial components are inserted to confirm stability, orientation, and bearing thickness. (10) The components are implanted.

The author of this chapter has slightly modified some of these basic principles. There is some controversy as to whether the varus deformity must be passively correctable for the patient to be an appropriate candidate for unicompartmental replacement. In the author's experience, many varus knees can be passively corrected after the intraoperative removal of peripheral osteophytes from the femur and the tibia, allowing an intraoperative decision on whether the patient is an appropriate candidate for UKA. Controversy also exists regarding the size of the incision and the relative advantages of minimally invasive surgery. The key to a patient's rapid recovery is not the length of the incision but the ability to subluxate rather than evert the patella. Effective management of perioperative pain also is vital.

Preoperative planning is essential for UKA to fulfill the principle of achieving a conservative resection from the tibia (making any potential revision uncomplicated). A conservative resection line for a TKA that reflects the normal tibial resection appropriate for a bicompartmental knee replacement is drawn on the preoperative radiograph (Figure 2). The location where this line transects the periphery of the medial plateau is noted. This line represents a conservative initial resection so

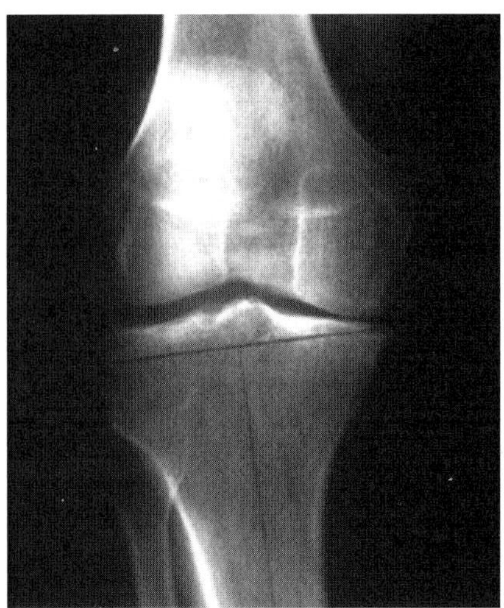

Figure 2 AP radiograph showing preoperative planning of a conservative tibial resection appropriate for bicompartmental arthroplasty.

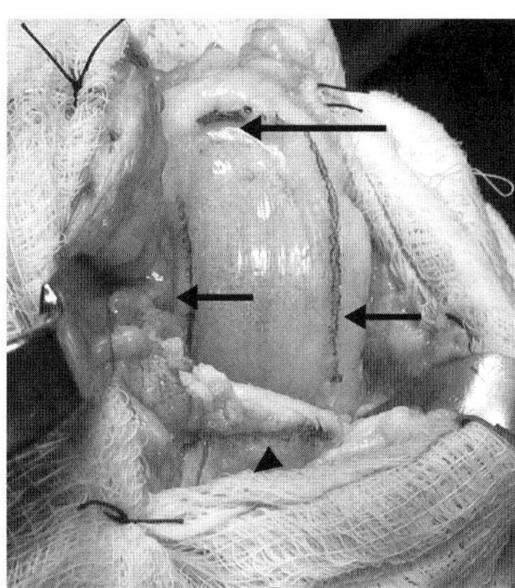

Figure 3 The anatomy of the medial compartment is defined showing the peripheral and intercondylar osteophytes (*short arrows*) and the tidemark (*long arrow*). A line is drawn on the tibia (*arrowhead*) indicating a conservative resection in proper alignment (perpendicular to the long axis of the tibia).

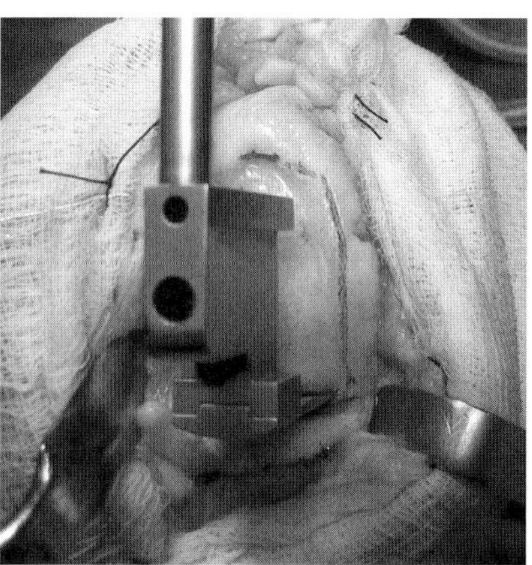

Figure 4 The top of the appropriately sized femoral jig usually rests 3 to 5 mm posterior to the tidemark.

that a standard tibial resection will be possible if conversion is needed.

Next, the anatomy of the femoral condyle is defined by removing intercondylar and peripheral osteophytes and defining the so-called tidemark (Figure 3). The tidemark is the junction between the eburnated bone on the distal condyle and the trochlear cartilage. This junction represents the point of full extension contact between the tibia and the femur. Removal of the intercondylar and peripheral osteophytes allows the true center of the femoral condyle to be defined. The removal of the intercondylar osteophytes creates a path for the tibial spine resection with a reciprocating saw. Removal of the peripheral osteophytes also allows passive correction of the deformity. A line is drawn on the anterior aspect of the tibia that defines the extent of tibial resection based on preoperative templating (Figure 3). The tibial resection is performed with the aid of a tibial alignment guide with the posterior slope between 3° and 7°, depending on the preoperative posterior slope. The resected tibial bone can be used as a template for sizing the tibial component. The tibial plateau should be capped as much as possible, but peripheral overhang of the metal should be avoided. It is sometimes necessary to move the tibial spine resection laterally to use the largest possible tibial component in the anteroposterior dimension and still avoid medial overhang. This is permissible if the anterior cruciate ligament is not compromised.

The flexion gap is then established. It should be a minimum of 7 mm as determined by the 7-mm spacer provided. If it is too tight, slightly more tibia can be resected; however, care must be taken not to overresect the tibia and compromise any future revision. As an alternative to more tibial resection, the author prefers to resect a small amount of posterior condylar cartilage to increase the flexion gap. This will move the femoral component the equivalent distance anteriorly. Moving the component anteriorly 1 or 2 mm does not compromise the kinematics of the articulation.

The femoral component can be sized with preoperative templating, but intraoperative sizing is simple and may be more accurate. In the appropriately sized component, the sizing guide (oriented in proper flexion) will rest approximately 3 to 5 mm posterior to the tidemark (Figure 4).

An intramedullary alignment guide is placed to establish the proper flexion/extension orientation as well as the varus/valgus angle of the femoral component. In the sagittal plane, the jig should be parallel to the top of the guide for proper flexion. In the varus/valgus coronal plane, the inner border of the jig should be parallel to the femoral alignment rod. Sometimes, it is preferable to err with a slight valgus orientation of the femoral component; varus placement should be avoided. A slightly valgus femoral component alignment decreases the chance of medial subluxation of the bearing.

The rotational alignment of the femoral jig can be established by

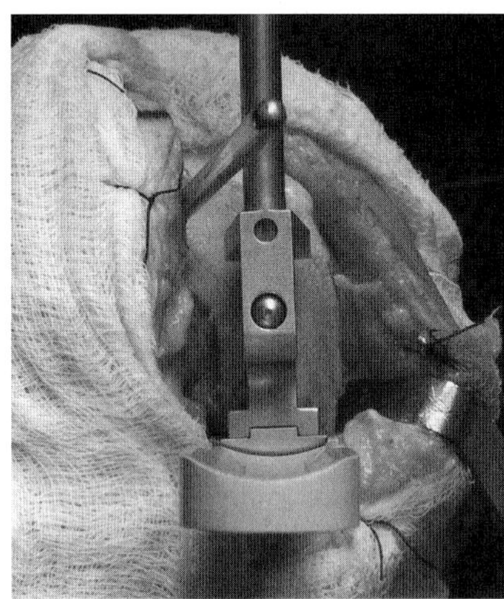

Figure 5 The larger lower hole of the femoral jig has been drilled in proper mediolateral, varus-valgus, and flexion-extension positioning, and the drill has been replaced with a 7-mm spigot. The jig can now be rotated internally or externally into proper congruency with the tibial trial spacer and secured by drilling the smaller upper hole.

placing a larger posterior drill hole centered over the center of the femoral condyle as established after removal of peripheral and intercondylar osteophytes. It is preferable to err toward slight lateral placement of this drill hole rather than medial placement to avoid peripheral tracking of the mobile bearing, which can cause soft-tissue impingement. Once this larger drill hole has been established in the proper orientation, a 7-mm spigot is used to replace the drill and stabilize the jig (W Fitz, MD, personal communication, Boston, MA, 2007). The jig can then be rotated internally or externally to establish the proper rotation of the femoral component (Figure 5). It is preferable to err with slight external rotation rather than internal rotation to maximize the stability of the bearing. Excessive internal rotation of the femoral component may also lead to overhanging of the mobile bearing from the periphery of the tibial tray causing painful soft-tissue impingement.

Comparative Clinical Experience

The author's most recently performed 101 UKAs with a minimum 2-year follow-up have been reviewed. Of these, 89 were medial and 12 were lateral arthroplasties. Of the 89 medial arthroplasties, 55 were mobile-bearing UKAs and 34 were fixed-bearing UKAs. Because the follow-up period ranged from a minimum of 2 years to a maximum of 3 years, long-term results cannot be assessed; however, it is possible to compare the two techniques for range of motion, patient satisfaction, and complications that occur during the first 2 years after surgery.

The range of motion using both techniques was equivalent. The average flexion of knees treated with mobile-bearing UKAs was 125° compared with 124° for the fixed-bearing UKAs. Patient satisfaction also was equivalent, with no patient dissatisfied with the procedure at a minimum 2-year follow-up.

Each technique resulted in one complication. In the mobile-bearing group there was one spontaneous hemarthrosis that occurred at 22 months, which was treated conservatively with no recurrence at 3 years postoperatively. In the fixed-bearing group, a painful osteophyte emanating from the medial aspect of the trochlea developed in one patient and resolved with arthroscopic débridement.

Summary

UKA, using either mobile- or fixed-bearing techniques, is an attractive alternative to osteotomy or TKA in selected osteoarthritic patients. Both techniques appear to yield equivalent early results. Mobile-bearing articulations have the advantage of allowing the use of a metal-backed component with a composite thickness as thin as 6 mm and offer the potential for decreased long-term wear complications. The longevity of fixed-bearing components will likely be improved in the future with better prosthetic designs and improved polyethylene to minimize the complications of long-term wear.

References

1. Insall J, Walker P: Unicondylar knee replacement. *Clin Orthop Relat Res* 1976;120:83-85.
2. Laskin RS: Unicompartmental tibiofemoral resurfacing arthroplasty. *J Bone Joint Surg Am* 1978;60:182-185.
3. Stern SH, Becker MW, Insall JN: Unicondylar knee arthroplasty: An evaluation of selection criteria. *Clin Orthop Relat Res* 1993;286:143-148.
4. Scott RD, Cobb AG, McQueary FG, Thornhill TS: Unicompartmental knee arthroplasty: Eight to twelve year follow-up evaluation with survivorship analysis. *Clin Orthop Relat Res* 1991;271:96-100.
5. McCallum JD, Scott RD: Duplication of medial erosion in unicompartmental knee arthroplasties. *J Bone Joint Surg Br* 1995;77:726-728.
6. White SH, Ludkowski PF, Goodfellow JW: Anteromedial osteoarthritis of the knee. *J Bone Joint Surg Br* 1991;73:582-586.
7. Bonutti PM, Dethmers DA: Contemporary unicompartmental knee arthroplasty: Fixed vs mobile bearing. *J Arthroplasty* 2008;23:24-27.
8. Murray DW: Mobile bearing unicompartmental knee replacement. *Orthopedics* 2007;30:768-769.
9. Price AJ, Dodd CA, Svard UG, Murray DW: Oxford medial unicompartmental knee arthroplasty in patients younger and older than 60 years of age. *J Bone Joint Surg Br* 2005;87:1488-1492.

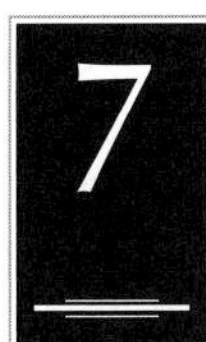

Bicompartmental Arthroplasty of the Knee

Alfred J. Tria Jr, MD

Abstract

Combined replacement of the patellofemoral and medial tibiofemoral joints has been performed in the past. The original approaches placed two separate implants during the same surgical procedure. Results were acceptable; however, with the increasing success of total knee arthroplasty, partial knee replacements lost favor. In the 1990s, a limited incision for unicondylar arthroplasty was introduced that encouraged interest in partial knee replacements. The newer implants combine the medial and patellofemoral articulations into a single femoral implant with a medial tibial tray and a polyethylene patella. The surgical technique and instruments are somewhat unique and training is helpful. Bicompartmental arthroplasty preserves all of the ligaments of the knee while replacing two compartments. The procedure is more complicated than unicompartmental knee arthroplasty, less invasive than total knee arthroplasty, and may have a place in replacement surgery.

Instr Course Lect 2010;59:61-73.

The McKeever and MacIntosh implants, which are no longer manufactured or sold, were designed in the 1950s and introduced the concept of partial knee arthroplasty.[1-4] Studies in the literature showed acceptable results at midterm follow-up for unicondylar knee arthroplasty (UKA) and patellofemoral arthroplasty (PFA) prostheses, which were developed in the late 1970s.[5-9] Some surgeons combined the UKA and PFA based on findings of the appropriate pathology at the time of the surgical procedure.[7] The early results were acceptable and provided the advantages of ligament preservation and improved proprioception. However, Argenson and associates[10] reported a 38% revision rate for the combined PFA and UKA procedures with a 5- to 23-year follow-up (mean, 12 years). They concluded that the high rate of revision was secondary to early experience with the surgical technique. No knee was revised for progression of disease in the remaining lateral compartment. Interest in the approach continued with the introduction of newer designs and instrumentation. As total knee arthroplasty (TKA) designs improved, there was declining interest in partial knee arthroplasty until Repicci introduced an approach that used a smaller incision for UKA.[11,12] Limited incisions for knee arthroplasty became more popular, and partial knee arthroplasty became more common.[13-15]

The bicompartmental replacements from the early 1970s had some recognized advantages over TKA, but the two separate implants required removal of a considerable amount of bone and the surgical procedure was complex. Rolston and associates[16] recognized these issues and developed a prosthesis that combined the two implant designs into a single unit called the Journey-Deuce Knee (Smith & Nephew, Memphis, TN). The new prosthesis required less bone removal and spared all of the ligaments of the knee. A custom device, the IDuo bicompartmental knee resurfacing device (ConforMIS, Burlington, MA), is similar to the Journey-Deuce Knee and is designed based on CT scans of the knee; it uses a resurfacing surgical technique with custom-designed cutting instruments.

The newer prosthetic designs and the surgical techniques combine technology from both UKA and

Dr. Tria or an immediate family member has received royalties from Zimmer and serves as a paid consultant to or is an employee of Smith & Nephew IMP.

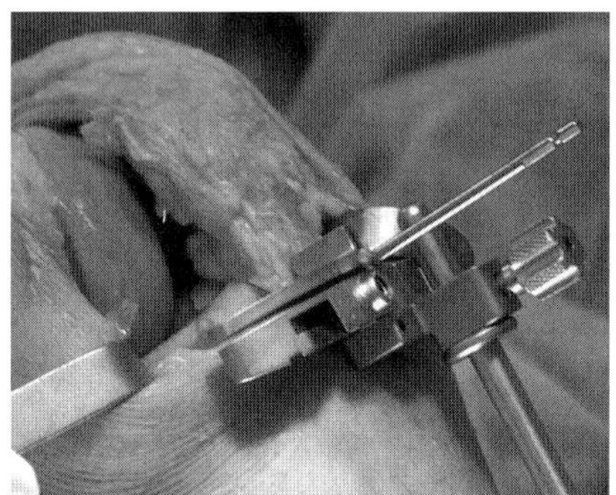

Figure 1 The extramedullary tibial guide references the medial tibial plateau surface.

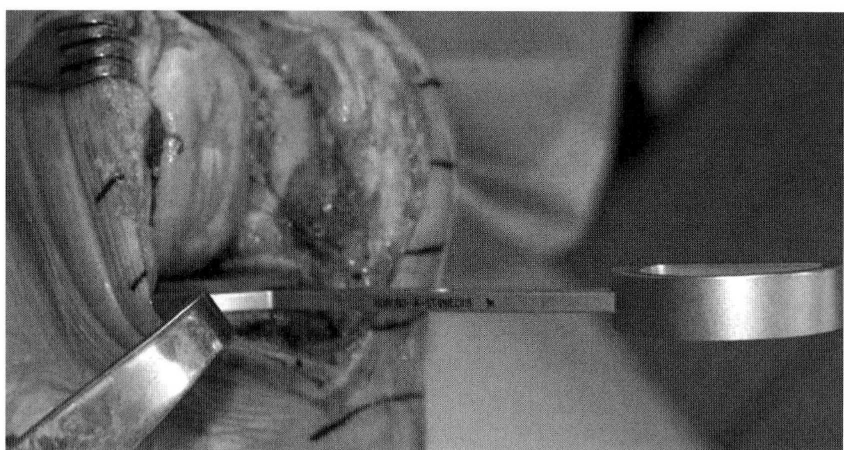

Figure 2 The spacer block is placed into the flexion gap and used as a reference for the extension gap.

TKA. It is hoped that the prosthetic modifications and instrument changes will improve the long-term results of bicompartmental arthroplasty and preserve its use in knee surgery.

Preoperative Evaluation

Patient selection is extremely important for bicompartmental knee arthroplasty. The patient history and physical examination and radiographic evaluation results should be considered. The patient should be able to describe the location of the pain in the knee and the duration with some clarity. If the entire knee is painful in a global fashion, bicompartmental replacement will not be successful despite the physical examination and radiographic findings.

The physical examination should correlate with the patient history. Most of the tenderness should be along the medial tibiofemoral joint line with extension to the medial patellofemoral articulation, but not to the lateral aspect of the knee. The clinical deformity should not exceed 10° of varus or flexion contracture. When the varus deformity corrects to neutral with valgus stress, the knee is more suited for the bicompartmental replacement procedure. A knee with a fixed deformity may require a slightly deeper tibial resection or even collateral ligament release; this will increase the difficulty of the operation. All ligaments should be clinically intact. Some degree of anterior laxity can be accepted, but grade IV laxity of any ligament is a contraindication. Inflammatory arthritis and knees with previous ligament reconstructions or osteotomies should be excluded.

It is preferable to obtain a full-length AP standing view of the entire limb before surgery; however, it is acceptable to use the standing radiograph of the knee, which should show an anatomic varus deformity that is less than 10° with minimal translocation of the tibia beneath the femur. Patellofemoral arthritic changes of any extent are acceptable. Lateral osteoarthritic changes are acceptable if they are mild. If there are changes in the lateral compartment, there should be no significant symptoms of pain or tenderness on physical examination.

Surgical Technique

Surgery is performed using a curvilinear medial incision with an associated similar medial arthrotomy. It is not necessary to limit the incision; however, a limited exposure is possible in most knees because it is only necessary to visualize the medial aspect of the knee.

The tibial plateau is treated first and an extramedullary guide is used to cut the surface 2 to 4 mm below the lowest point (Figure 1). The space is then evaluated using a spacer block with an 8-mm insert (Figure 2). The gap at 90° of flexion is compared with the gap in extension to plan the distal femoral resection. An intramedullary instrumentation system is used to make the femoral cuts. The anteroposterior axis is used for referencing proper external rotation. The first femoral guide sizes the femur from anterior to posterior and sets the anterior femoral resection depth and rotation (Figure 3). The distal femoral resection is performed by setting the depth on the medial side of the femur and referencing a point on the lateral side of the previously anterior cut surface where the edge of the prosthesis will meet the lateral aspect of the femoral cortex (Figure 4). The distal cut differs from the traditional TKA resection because the lateral femoral condyle surface is not removed. After the distal medial resection is completed, the space in full extension can be compared with the space in flexion and adjustments can be made before proceeding. If the flexion gap is too tight, it is easiest to increase the slope from anterior to posterior. If the extension gap is too tight, the distal femoral resection can be increased.

The finishing block for the femur is set on the cut surface and adjusted with reference to the medial femoral condyle and the lateral femoral cortex (Figure 5). The properly sized tibial tray is chosen with an attempt to cover the entire surface with cortical support but without any overhang in either the sagittal or coronal planes. The patellar surface is resected so that the final composite thickness of the implant and the remaining bone is 2 mm less than the original measurement. The resection can be completed either free hand with a power saw or with an instrument guide.

The trial components are inserted and the range of motion, tracking of the patella, tracking of the medial femoral condyle on the tibial polyethylene insert, and the laxity in full extension and 90° of flexion are evaluated (Figure 6). There should be 2 mm of laxity in full extension and at 90° of flexion. The components are then cemented. Surgical drains are inserted and the closure is performed in the standard fashion (Figure 7).

Video 7.1: Bicompartmental Replacement. Alfred J. Tria Jr, MD (28 min)

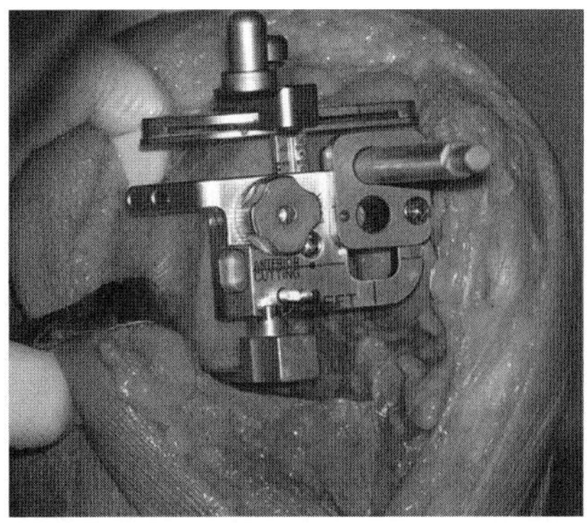

Figure 3 The first femoral guide references the posterior medial femoral condyle and sets the depth and rotation for the anterior cut.

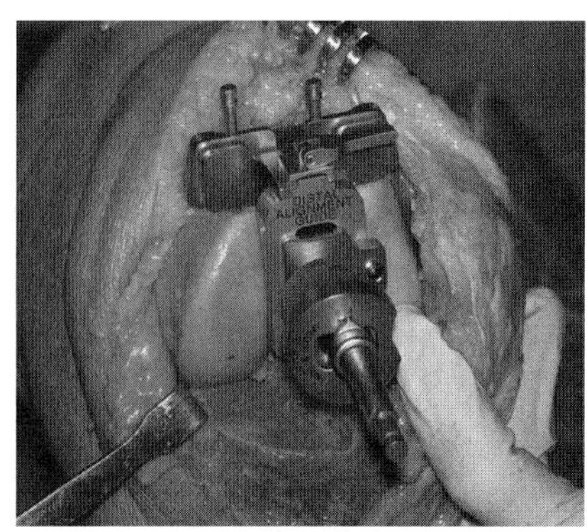

Figure 4 The distal femoral cut references the medial femoral condyle for the depth of resection and the lateral femoral cortex for proper angulation.

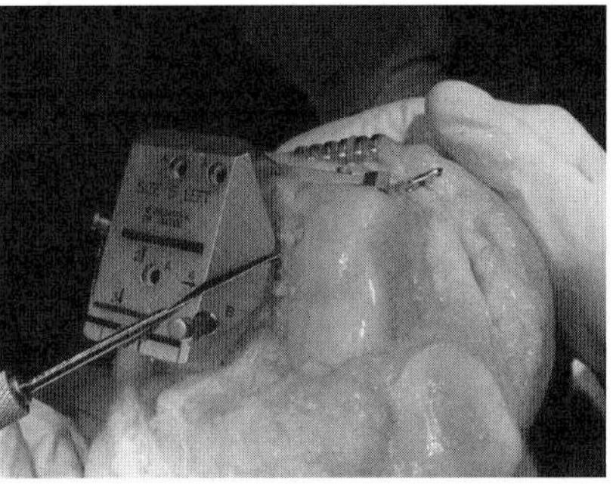

Figure 5 The femoral finishing block references the width of the medial femoral condyle and the lateral femoral cortex.

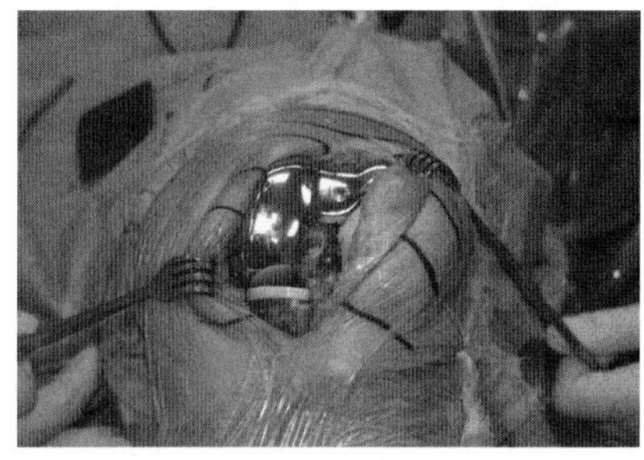

Figure 6 The trial components are set in place and the tracking, balance, and gap laxity are evaluated.

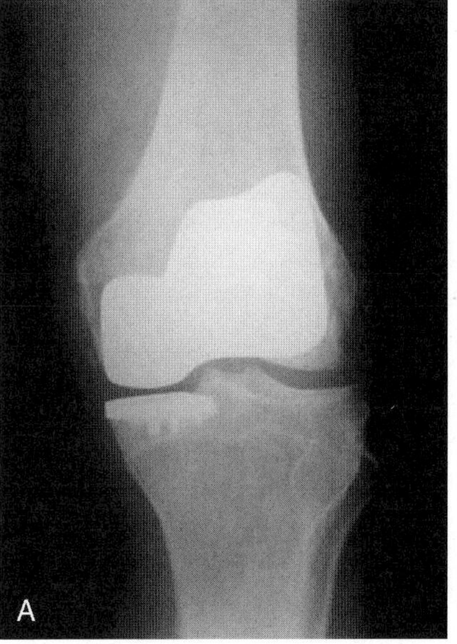

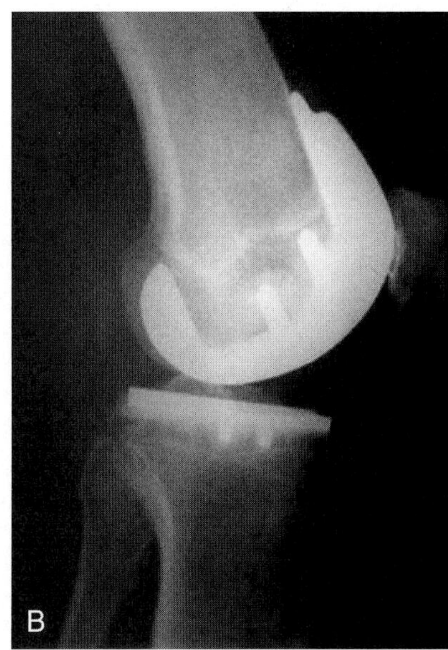

Figure 7 **A,** The AP radiograph of a left knee showing the Journey-Deuce knee implant in the proper position. **B,** Lateral radiograph of the left knee showing the correct implant sizing and slope for the tibial tray with the patella resurfaced.

Postoperative Management

Physical therapy and weight-bearing ambulation are started on the day of surgery. Prophylaxis with low-molecular-weight heparin is started 24 hours after surgery and is continued for 12 to 14 days. Most patients remain in the hospital for 1 or 2 days and continue outpatient physical therapy for approximately 6 weeks.

Outpatient follow-up visits are scheduled at 2 weeks after surgery, then at 6 weeks, 3 months, 6 months, and 1 year. Radiographs are taken at 2 weeks after surgery and then as necessary until 1 year after surgery when routine radiographs are repeated.

Results

The author of this chapter has performed 96 bicompartmental knee replacements with the Journey-Deuce Knee in the past 2 years. Although it is too early to make any definitive statements about the clinical results, some of the preliminary information is helpful. The mean age of the patients was 70 years (range, 49 to 89 years), the mean weight was 185 lb (range, 114 to 262 lb), and the mean body mass index was 30 (range, 20 to 42). The average surgical time (including surgery and anesthesia) was initially 114 minutes for the first 40 patients and decreased to 65 minutes with increasing experience. There have been no instances of pulmonary emboli, proximal thigh deep venous thromboses, myocardial infarctions, infections, mortalities, or revisions. A subluxating patella in deep flexion developed in one patient at 6 weeks after the surgery. The components were not malaligned or internally rotated and there was no disruption of the medial retinacular closure. The patient was returned to the operating room for a lateral release and had no further complications after more than 24 months of follow-up. All of the patients regained their preoperative range of motion by 2 months after surgery and no manipulations were performed. The Knee Society score improved from 49 to 84 and the function score improved from 57 to 81.

At this time, there are no reports of early results using the IDuo bicompartmental knee resurfacing device, but it is similar in design to the Journey-Deuce Knee prosthesis and should have similar short-term results.

Discussion

The indications for bicompartmental knee arthroplasty are evolving. Currently, there are two standards—one for younger patients and one for patients older than 75 years. Younger patients should have clear symptoms and physical examination findings that indicate involvement of the medial tibiofemoral and patellofemoral joints with no lateral tibiofemoral compartment involvement. Older patients can have some minimal involvement of the lateral tibiofemoral compartment.

It is important to determine if this type of an implant has a place in knee arthroplasty. The literature shows that bicompartmental replacement with separate implants can perform acceptably well in the first decade after surgery.[7,8] However, a recent report has shown a significant failure rate at longer term follow-up.[10] Most revisions were related to the tracking of the PFA and not to prosthetic loosening or arthritic progression. The authors concluded that the failures were related to the early surgical experience with a new technology and implied that the results might be improved with better instrumentation and more anatomic prosthetic designs. The single piece femoral component is an unusual design that requires unique instrumentation; however, it eliminates impingement and decreases the total amount of bone that is resected.

If the single piece femoral implant is considered a modified UKA, some authors would argue that the replacement of the patellofemoral joint is unnecessary because the reported incidence of patellofemoral complications is low.[6,15] If the implant is considered a less invasive modification of a TKA, it will be important to observe the progression of lateral joint arthritis after the surgery. The reported progression of arthritis in the lateral compartment of UKAs is low but may not be entirely comparable to this new implant design.[6,10] At the present time, the author of this chapter considers the single piece femoral implant more comparable to a UKA and uses those indications for the surgical procedure.

Summary

Bicompartmental knee arthroplasty using a combined single femoral component is a novel approach to treating medial knee arthritis. It is very early in the development and use of this type of prosthesis. Initial results are encouraging and should lead to component refinements and improved surgical techniques in the future. However, it is most likely that a combined single femoral component implant will be considered a modified UKA; therefore, it will have limited areas of application but excellent results when properly applied.

References

1. MacIntosh DL: Hemiarthroplasty of the knee using a space occupying prosthesis for painful varus and valgus deformities. *J Bone Joint Surg Am* 1958;40:1431.

2. MacIntosh DL: Arthroplasty of the knee in rheumatoid arthritis. *J Bone Joint Surg Br* 1966;48:179.
3. McKeever DC: Tibial plateau prosthesis. *Clin Orthop Relat Res* 1960;18: 86-95.
4. Emerson RH, Potter T: The use of the McKeever metallic hemiarthroplasty for unicompartmental arthritis. *J Bone Joint Surg Am* 1985;67:208-212.
5. Marmor L: Marmor modular knee in unicompartmental disease: Minimum four-year follow-up. *J Bone Joint Surg Am* 1979;61:347-353.
6. Goodfellow JW, Kershaw CJ, Benson MK, O'Connor JJ: The Oxford knee for unicompartmental osteoarthritis: The first 103 cases. *J Bone Joint Surg Br* 1988;70:692-701.
7. Cartier P, Sanouiller JL, Grelsamer R: Patellofemoral arthroplasty: 2-12 year follow-up study. *J Arthroplasty* 1990;5: 49-55.
8. Cartier P, Sanouiller JL, Khefacha A: Long-term results with the first patellofemoral prosthesis. *Clin Orthop Relat Res* 2005;436:47-54.
9. Argenson JN, Guillaume JM, Aubaniac JM: Is there a place for patellofemoral arthroplasty? *Clin Orthop Relat Res* 1995;321:162-167.
10. Parratte S, Pauly V, Aubaniac JM, Argenson JN: Survival of bicompartmental knee arthroplasty at 5 to 23 years [published online ahead of print August 8, 2009] *Clin Orthop Relat Res.* PMID: 19669384.
11. Repicci JA, Eberle RW: Minimally invasive surgical technique for unicondylar knee arthroplasty. *J South Orthop Assoc* 1999;8:20-22.
12. Romanowski MR, Repicci JA: Minimally invasive unicondylar arthroplasty: Eight year follow up. *J Knee Surg* 2002;15:17-22.
13. Chen AF, Alan RK, Redziniak DE, Tria AJ: Quadriceps sparing total knee arthroplasty: Initial experience with two to four year results. *J Bone Joint Surg Br* 2006;88:1448-1453.
14. Gesell MW, Tria AJ Jr: MIS unicondylar knee arthroplasty: Surgical approach and early results. *Clin Orthop Relat Res* 2004;428:53-60.
15. Price AJ, Webb J, Topf H, Dodd CAF, Goodfellow JW, Murray DW: Oxford Hip and Knee Group: Rapid recovery after Oxford unicompartmental arthroplasty through a short incision. *J Arthroplasty* 2001;16:970-976.
16. Rolston L, Bresch J, Engh G, et al: Bicompartmental knee arthroplasty: A bone sparing, ligament-sparing, and minimally invasive alternative for active patients. *Orthopedics* 2007;30(8 suppl):70-73.

Video Reference

7.1: Tria AJ Jr: Bicompartmental replacement, in Della Valle CJ, Stuchin SA, eds: *Surgical Techniques in Orthopaedics: Arthroplasty for Unicompartmental Arthritis.* DVD. Rosemont, IL, American Academy of Orthopaedic Surgeons, 2007.

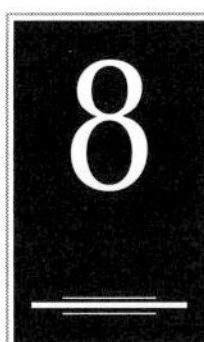

Patellofemoral Arthroplasty

Jess H. Lonner, MD

Abstract

Patellofemoral arthroplasty is an effective treatment for isolated arthritis of the anterior compartment of the knee. The best results are obtained when there is no patellar malalignment, the prosthesis is appropriately aligned, the soft tissues are balanced, and the implant has sound design features. The prevalence of patellofemoral dysfunction and failure caused by patellar maltracking and catching has been considerably reduced by the use of contemporary implant designs rather than earlier implant designs. Progressive tibiofemoral cartilage degeneration is the predominant failure mechanism; this factor underscores the importance of restricting the procedure to patients who do not have tibiofemoral chondromalacia or arthritis. Newer techniques that combine patellofemoral arthroplasty with autologous osteochondral transplantation or unicompartmental arthroplasty appear to be effective for patients with associated tibiofemoral chondromalacia.

Instr Course Lect 2010;59:67-84.

Isolated patellofemoral arthritis occurs in as many as 11% of men and 24% of women who are older than 55 years and have symptomatic osteoarthritis of the knee.[1] In most reports, approximately 75% of the patients receiving a patellofemoral arthroplasty are women.[2-15] This gender-related pattern undoubtedly is related to patellofemoral malalignment and dysplasia, which also are more common among women than men.

Patellofemoral arthroplasty increasingly is recognized as a legitimate, effective, and conservative alternative to total knee arthroplasty for a patient with isolated patellofemoral arthritis. In comparison with earlier implant designs, contemporary implants are geometrically better mated to the shape of the distal femora, leading to better patellar tracking, a lower incidence of patellofemoral complications, and improved outcomes.[9,12,16] The most common cause of failure is the eventual development of tibiofemoral arthritis. Careful patient selection is therefore important. A newer treatment strategy may be useful, such as combined patellofemoral arthroplasty and cartilage grafting or unicompartmental arthroplasty for treating associated tibiofemoral chondromalacia. A modular, bicompartmental arthroplasty system may be preferable to a monolithic system to allow the most accurate alignment and positioning of the trochlear and femoral components relative to the individual compartments they are resurfacing.

Indications and Contraindications

The success of patellofemoral arthroplasty partly depends on appropriate patient selection.[2,3,17] The procedure can be considered for patients with isolated patellofemoral osteoarthritis, posttraumatic arthritis, or advanced chondromalacia (Outerbridge grade IV) on either the trochlear or patellar surface or both. Although patellofemoral arthroplasty is effective in the presence of patellar or trochlear dysplasia,[8,13,17] onlay-style implant designs generally are preferable to others for the treatment of dysplasia.[9,11,12,16-18] Slight patellar tilt or subluxation, as observed on preoperative tangential radiographs or during surgery, usually can be effectively treated with a lateral retinacular release, medialization of the

Dr. Lonner or an immediate family member has received royalties from Zimmer; is a member of a speakers' bureau or has made paid presentations on behalf of Zimmer and MAKO Surgical; serves as a paid consultant to or is an employee of Zimmer and MAKO Surgical; serves as an unpaid consultant to Zimmer and MAKO Surgical; has received research or institutional support from Zimmer; and has received nonincome support (such as equipment or services), commercially derived honoraria, or other non–research-related funding (such as paid travel) from Wolters Kluwer Health–Lippincott Williams & Wilkins and Quadrant Health.

patellar component, and resection of the lateral patellar facet. The quadriceps (Q) angle is formed by the intersection of a line drawn from the center of the patella to the tibial tubercle and a line drawn from the center of the patella to the anterior superior iliac spine. A high Q angle (more than 20° in women and 15° in men) should be corrected before or during the patellofemoral arthroplasty to enhance patellar tracking. The patellofemoral prosthesis should not be expected to stabilize a highly malaligned patellofemoral articulation. The presence of a very high Q angle therefore is a relative contraindication to patellofemoral arthroplasty, unless a tibial tubercle anteromedialization is performed.

Patellofemoral arthroplasty also is contraindicated in patients who have considerable medial and lateral joint line pain. Any evidence of tibiofemoral arthritis, advanced chondromalacia, or chondrocalcinosis is a contraindication to isolated patellofemoral arthroplasty. Combining patellofemoral arthroplasty with chondral resurfacing for a focal defect of the weight-bearing condylar surfaces or with unicompartmental arthroplasty for more advanced tibiofemoral arthrosis is an emerging treatment strategy.[18,19] However, this treatment is not appropriate for patients with inflammatory arthritis. Severe coronal deformity may negatively affect patellar tracking and predispose the patient to developing tibiofemoral arthritis, unless it is corrected with a periarticular osteotomy. It is not known whether obesity or cruciate ligament insufficiency has a deleterious effect on the outcome of patellofemoral arthroplasty. There are no published data to determine whether younger and older patients have different results, provided that the articular cartilage is reasonably intact elsewhere in the joint.

Clinical Evaluation

History

Pain associated with patellofemoral arthritis is directly anterior, retropatellar, or immediately peripatellar, particularly during provocative activities that load the patellofemoral articulation (such as descending or ascending stairs, squatting, or kneeling). The pain is less severe during walking on level ground. The patient is more comfortable sitting with the knee straightened rather than flexed. Discomfort in the medial or lateral tibiofemoral compartment suggests a more diffuse pathology, which may not respond to treatment with isolated patellofemoral resurfacing. A history of recurrent atraumatic patellar dislocations raises the possibility that the patient has significant patellofemoral malalignment, which may need to be corrected before patellofemoral arthroplasty.[17]

Physical Examination

Patellar tracking and the Q angle are assessed first because these have an immediate impact on the decision to proceed with patellofemoral arthroplasty, as well as its ultimate outcome. Patellar tracking is observed with the patient seated on the edge of the examination table. The knee proceeds from 90° of flexion to extension with active quadriceps contraction. The presence of the J sign (visible lateral subluxation of the patella as the knee proceeds from flexion into the terminal 20° of extension) is characteristic of patellar malalignment or muscular imbalance. The Q angle is measured. Patellofemoral crepitus and pain with patellar inhibition testing or patellar compression are noted. Tenderness with palpation of the medial and lateral joint lines suggests more diffuse disease, which cannot be adequately treated with isolated patellofemoral arthroplasty. Investigation should exclude the possibility that the pain is emanating from another location, such as the quadriceps tendon, patellar ligament, pes anserinus bursa, lumbar spine, or hip. A planovalgus foot deformity can predispose the patient to patellar malalignment and maltracking, and the resulting patellofemoral pain may be improved by using a medial longitudinal arch support.[17]

Imaging Studies

All AP radiographs should be taken with the patient standing because radiographs taken with the patient supine can underestimate the extent of tibiofemoral arthritis (Figure 1). Mild squaring of the femoral condyles and small marginal osteophytes are acceptable radiographic findings provided that the patient has no medial or lateral joint pain with functional activities or on physical examination, and that chondral degeneration is minimal (as shown by arthroscopic views or during arthrotomy for patellofemoral arthroplasty). Posterior condylar wear, as seen on midflexion PA radiographs, is an indication for bicompartmental or total knee arthroplasty rather than isolated patellofemoral arthroplasty. Lateral radiographs are most useful in identifying patella alta or patella baja and, occasionally, patellofemoral osteophytes or joint space narrowing. Axial radiographs can reveal trochlear dysplasia, patellar tilt or subluxation, and the extent of patellofemoral arthritis. However, axial radiographs sometimes understate the severity of cartilage loss, particularly in a younger patient who may have relatively normal cartilage at the edges of the lesions.

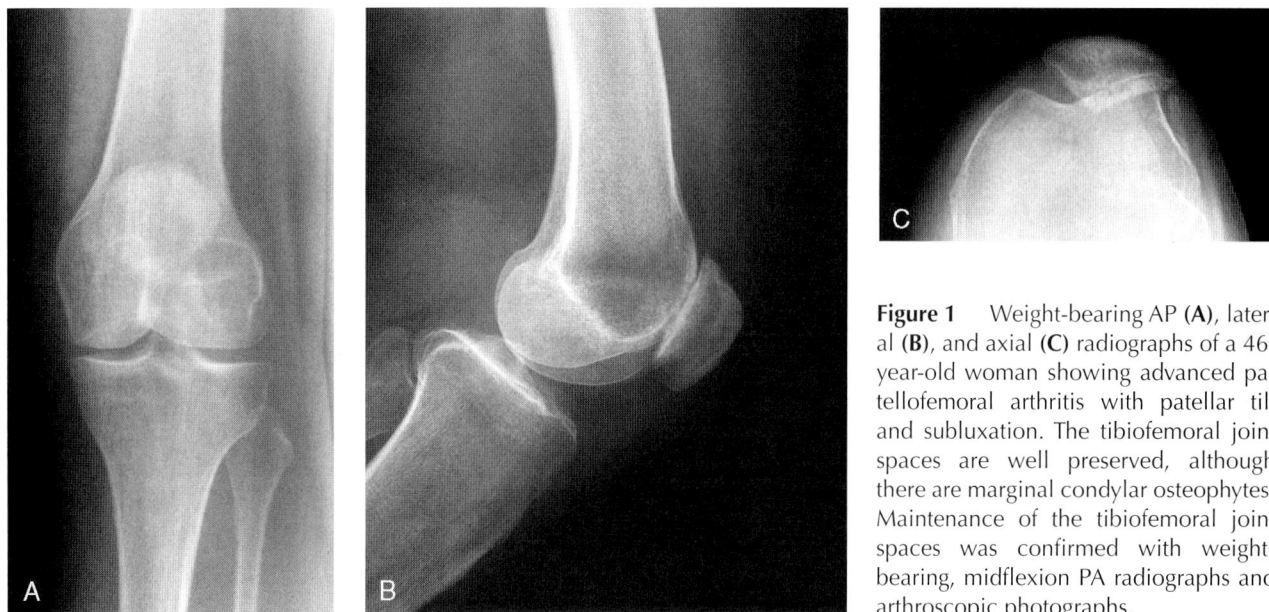

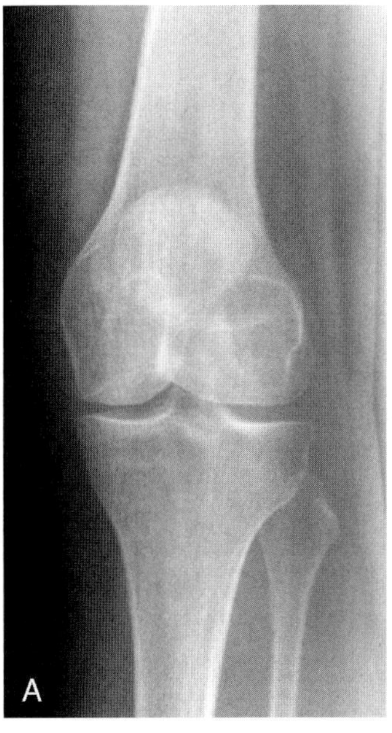

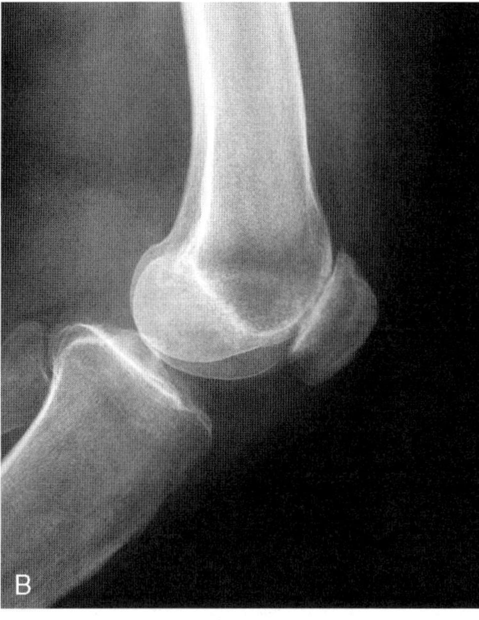

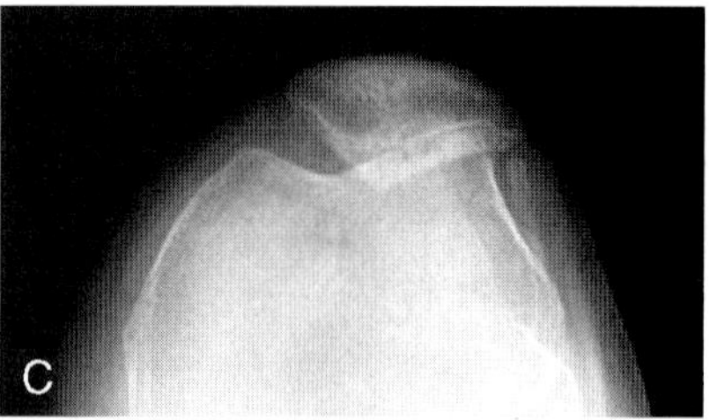

Figure 1 Weight-bearing AP **(A)**, lateral **(B)**, and axial **(C)** radiographs of a 46-year-old woman showing advanced patellofemoral arthritis with patellar tilt and subluxation. The tibiofemoral joint spaces are well preserved, although there are marginal condylar osteophytes. Maintenance of the tibiofemoral joint spaces was confirmed with weight-bearing, midflexion PA radiographs and arthroscopic photographs.

Axial CT scans have a role in assessing patellar tracking, but they are unnecessary for evaluating most patients with patellofemoral arthritis. Novel magnetic resonance techniques such as T1rho weighting or gadolinium enhancement may be useful for evaluating the quality of cartilage in the tibiofemoral compartments, despite an absence of findings on radiographs.[20] Arthroscopic views should be studied, if available.

Surgical Technique

The surgical approach should be utilitarian, so that it can be reused if later conversion to a total knee arthroplasty is necessary. Accidental incision into the normal articular cartilage, menisci, or intermeniscal ligament should be avoided during arthrotomy. The decision to proceed with patellofemoral arthroplasty is based on preoperative analysis and intraoperative inspection of the knee. The tibiofemoral compartments are evaluated for chondromalacia. It is then determined whether patellofemoral arthroplasty must be combined with biologic resurfacing of the femoral condyle[18,19] or with unicompartmental arthroplasty or if a total knee arthroplasty should be done instead of a patellofemoral arthroplasty.[17]

Specific surgical techniques vary slightly, depending on the use of an inlay or onlay implant design and the available instrumentation. The basic principles are consistent, however, regardless of the implant design. The patellar and trochlear components are appropriately aligned and positioned to optimize patellar tracking and enhance the likelihood that the patellofemoral arthroplasty will be successful.[17,18] Patellar tracking is optimized by rotational alignment of the trochlear component perpendicular to the AP axis of the distal femur (the Whiteside axis) or parallel to the epicondylar axis. The proximal edge of the trochlear implant should be flush with the anterior femoral cortex and not offset anteriorly; the intercondylar surfaces should be flush with or recessed 1 mm relative to the femoral condyles; and the medial and lateral edges should not extend past the femoral edges.[17,18] The patella is resurfaced using the same technique as for total knee arthroplasty, restoring the original patellar thickness and medializing the component. The exposed cut surface of the lateral patella that is not covered by the patellar prosthesis should be beveled or excised to avoid potentially painful articulation on the trochlear prosthesis or the lateral femoral condyle.[18]

Patellar tracking of the trial components is evaluated for tilt, subluxation, or catching. Tilt and mild subluxation usually can be remedied by a lateral retinacular release or recession of the retinaculum off the lateral edge of the patella. The position of the implant also should be scrutinized, and adjustments should be made if necessary. Uncorrected extensor mechanism malalignment (from a high Q angle) can compromise the tracking of the patellar component on the prosthetic trochlea. If the Q angle is higher than 20°

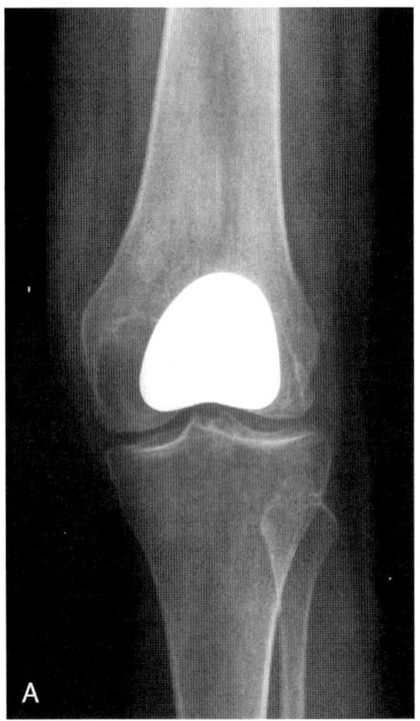

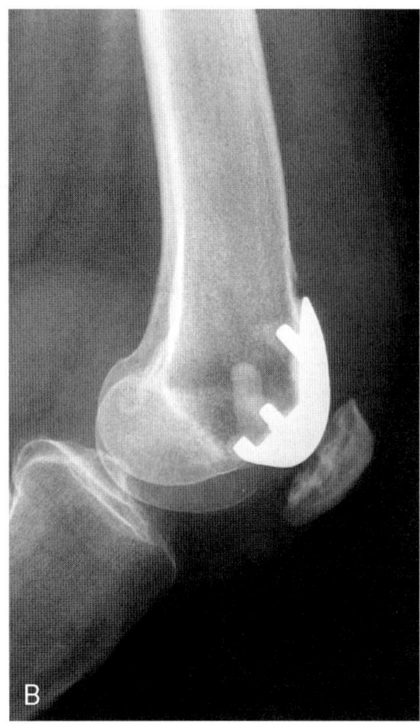

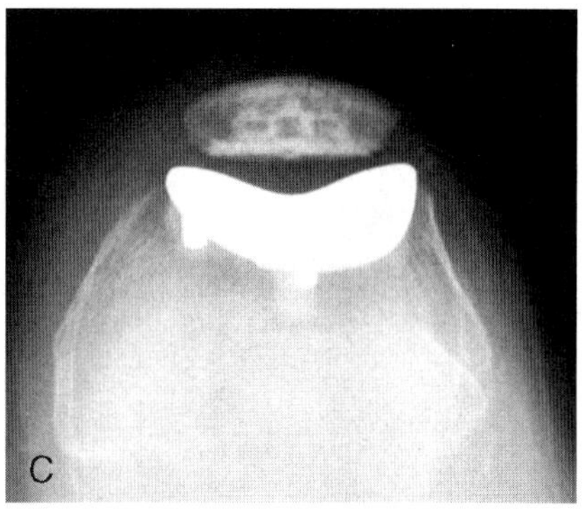

Figure 2 Postoperative AP (**A**), lateral (**B**), and axial (**C**) radiographs of the patient in Figure 1 after a successful cemented patellofemoral arthroplasty.

in a woman or 15° in a man, anteromedialization of the tibial tubercle should be done before or during the patellofemoral arthroplasty.[18]

Video 8.1: Patellofemoral Arthroplasty. Jess H. Lonner, MD (16 min)

Clinical Results

Most studies have reported that approximately 80% to 90% of patients have a good or excellent result at short-term or midterm follow-up. The clinical results of patellofemoral arthroplasty are affected by the trochlear component design features, as well as by patient selection and surgical technique.[2-4,9,13,16,17] Because of trochlear design improvements during the past 30 years, patient outcomes and patellofemoral performance have improved, and the need for secondary soft-tissue surgery to enhance patellar tracking after patellofemoral arthroplasty has decreased.[9,11,16] The radius of curvature, width, tracking angle, and extent of constraint of the trochlear component have been shown to affect patellar tracking and outcomes.[9,16] Contemporary designs have substantially reduced the incidence of patellofemoral complications (Figure 2). Tibiofemoral arthritis is now the most important source of failure of patellofemoral arthroplasties.

Blazina and associates[2] reported a satisfactory result in 81% of 57 knees less than 2 years after patellofemoral arthroplasty using a first-generation trochlear implant constrained with a sharp trochlear groove. Many of the patients required a subsequent procedure to realign the extensor mechanism or revise a malpositioned component. The investigators attributed the need for most of the secondary surgeries to technical errors; however, the trochlear constraint, an obtuse radius of curvature, and a narrow implant width certainly contributed to the failure rate.

Cartier and associates[4] reported good or excellent results after 61 of 72 first-generation patellofemoral arthroplasties (85%), at an average 4-year follow-up. Numerous concomitant surgical procedures were done to enhance patellar tracking, including soft-tissue realignment and tibial tubercle transfer. At a mean 10-year follow-up (range, 6 to 16 years), the investigators found that the results had deteriorated, primarily because of the development of tibiofemoral arthritis. The average patient age was 60 years at the time of the initial patellofemoral arthroplasty, so this finding is not surprising. At the most recent follow-up, 80% of the patients who had retained the patellofemoral prosthesis were pain free, and 20% had moderate or severe pain, primarily from tibiofemoral arthritis. Stair ambulation was considered normal in 91% of the patients. No patellar or trochlear loosening was identified. A peak in implant failures occurred 3 years after the initial surgery and was related to inappropriate patient selection and probably to patellar maltracking problems related to features of the implant design. A later peak in failures occurred during the 9th and 10th years after surgery, corresponding to the development of symptomatic tibiofemoral osteoarthritis. The implant survival rate after 11 years was 75%.[10] Kooijman and associates[14] reported an 86% long-term success rate after surgery using the same first-generation patellofemoral implant design, even though 18% of the patients required early secondary soft-tissue surgery and 16% required revision of the patellofemoral arthroplasty for catching, imbalance, or malposition.

A study of consecutive patellofemoral arthroplasties[9] in which 30 first-generation and 25 second-generation trochlear implants were used found that the results varied with the implant design. The incidence of patellofemoral dysfunction, subluxation, catching, and substantial pain was reduced from 17% when the first-generation design was used to less than 4% when the second-generation design was used. In another study,[21] the same first-generation patellofemoral implant was revised to a second-generation implant that had a more favorable topography for patellar tracking. The etiologies of failure of the primary procedure were component malposition, subluxation, polyethylene wear, and overstuffing. At a mean 5-year follow-up after revision, there was statistically significant improvement in knee scores and patellar tracking. Mild tibiofemoral arthritis (Ahlbach stage I) was predictive of a poorer clinical outcome. At the most recent follow-up, there was no evidence of wear, loosening, or subluxation. This study showed that, provided there is no tibiofemoral arthritis, significant improvement in patellar performance can be obtained by replacing a problematic trochlear implant with an implant having a more accommodating design.

Ackroyd and associates[11] reported on the results of 109 second-generation patellofemoral arthroplasties and found that patellar tracking was substantially better than when a first-generation implant was used. Patellar subluxation occurred after 3% of the arthroplasties, and residual anterior knee pain occurred after 4%. In 4%, revision to total knee arthroplasty was required, mostly because of tibiofemoral arthritis; none was necessitated by mechanical loosening or wear. Argenson and associates[8] reported the long-term results of 66 patellofemoral arthroplasties with a second-generation implant. The mean patient age at the time of the initial surgery was 57 years. At a mean 16-year follow-up, most patients had substantial and sustained pain relief. However, 39% of the patellofemoral arthroplasties had been revised to a total knee arthroplasty; the cause was tibiofemoral arthritis in 25% (at a mean 7.3 years after the patellofemoral arthroplasty) and aseptic loosening of the trochlear component in 14% (at a mean 4.5 years). Many of the replaced trochlear components were cementless. The best results occurred when the initial procedure was performed to treat posttraumatic patellofemoral arthritis or patellar subluxation-dysplasia; the least favorable results occurred in knees with primary degenerative arthritis. The most frequent cause of failure was the development of tibiofemoral arthritis. However, this finding is confounded by the fact that concomitant tibiofemoral osteotomies were performed for early arthritis in 14% of the initial patellofemoral arthroplasties. Among the patients who had a retained patellofemoral implant at most recent follow-up, there was a significant improvement in the Knee Society score. The authors promote patellofemoral arthroplasty as an intermediate procedure before total knee arthroplasty, in the absence of tibiofemoral arthritis or coronal plane malalignment.[8]

The development of tibiofemoral arthritis has been shown to be the most common failure mechanism after using either a contemporary implant design or an earlier design that avoids patellar instability. Tibiofemoral arthritis develops more commonly when the underlying diagnosis is primary osteoarthritis and less commonly when the diagnosis is patellofemoral dysplasia or posttraumatic arthritis.[8] If revision to total knee arthroplasty is necessary to treat progressive arthritis, the all-polyethylene patellar component typically can be retained if it is not worn or loose. Standard total knee components typically can be used without requiring stems, augments, or bone graft and without compromising the results.[22]

Summary

Patellofemoral arthroplasty is a treatment option for patellofemoral arthritis caused by primary osteoarthrosis, dysplasia, or trauma in patients who have normal or corrected patellofemoral alignment. Sparing of the tibiofemoral compartments, menisci, and cruciate ligaments preserves the normal kinematics better than total knee arthroplasty.

Some implant designs can lead to implant malpositioning, which also may contribute to failures from maltracking and mechanical catching of the patella. The use of newer implant designs has considerably reduced the incidence of patellofemoral complications. In addition, even a small loss of tibiofemoral cartilage can compromise the results. Progressive tibiofemoral arthritis probably is the primary failure mechanism when a newer implant is used.

Although only sparse long-term data are available, loosening of cemented trochlear and all-polyethylene patellar components appears to be uncommon. Further investigation is necessary to determine how these implants will perform into and beyond their second decade and whether younger patients can anticipate long-term success after patellofemoral arthroplasty when a newer implant design is used. For some patients who eventually develop tibiofemoral arthritis, patellofemoral arthroplasty is a bridging procedure, but it may be a permanent solution for other patients with isolated patellofemoral arthritis. Combining patellofemoral arthroplasty with autologous osteochondral grafting or unicompartmental arthroplasty is a reasonable alternative to total knee arthroplasty for the treatment of patellofemoral arthritis with associated medial or lateral compartment chondromalacia. Further study is necessary to determine the midterm and long-term success of these treatment methods.

References

1. McAlindon TE, Snow S, Cooper C, Dieppe PA: Radiographic patterns of osteoarthritis of the knee joint in the community: The importance of the patellofemoral joint. *Ann Rheum Dis* 1992;51:844-849.
2. Blazina ME, Fox JM, Del Pizzo W, Broukhim B, Ivey FM: Patellofemoral replacement. *Clin Orthop Relat Res* 1979;144:98-102.
3. Arciero RA, Toomey HE: Patellofemoral arthroplasty: A three- to nine-year follow-up study. *Clin Orthop Relat Res* 1988;236:60-71.
4. Cartier P, Sanouiller JL, Grelsamer R: Patellofemoral arthroplasty. *J Arthroplasty* 1990;5:49-55.
5. de Winter WE, Feith R, van Loon CJ: The Richards type II patellofemoral arthroplasty: 26 cases followed for 1-20 years. *Acta Orthop Scand* 2001;72: 487-490.
6. Tauro B, Ackroyd CE, Newman JH, Shah NA: The Lubinus patellofemoral arthroplasty: A five- to ten-year prospective study. *J Bone Joint Surg Br* 2001;83:696-701.
7. Krajca-Radcliffe JB, Coker TP: Patellofemoral arthroplasty: A 2- to 18-year follow up study. *Clin Orthop Relat Res* 1996;330:143-151.
8. Argenson JN, Flecher X, Parratte S, Aubaniac JM: Patellofemoral arthroplasty: An update. *Clin Orthop Relat Res* 2005;440:50-53.
9. Lonner JH: Patellofemoral arthroplasty: Pros, cons, and design considerations. *Clin Orthop Relat Res* 2004; 428:158-165.
10. Cartier P, Sanouiller JL, Khefacha A: Long-term results with the first patellofemoral prosthesis. *Clin Orthop Relat Res* 2005;436:47-54.
11. Ackroyd CE, Newman JH, Evans R, Eldridge JD, Joslin CC: The Avon patellofemoral arthroplasty: Five-year survivorship and functional results. *J Bone Joint Surg Br* 2007;89:310-315.
12. Sisto DJ, Sarin VK: Custom patellofemoral arthroplasty of the knee. *J Bone Joint Surg Am* 2006;88:1475-1480.
13. Argenson JN, Guillaume JM, Aubaniac JM: Is there a place for patellofemoral arthroplasty? *Clin Orthop Relat Res* 1995;321:162-167.
14. Kooijman HJ, Driessen AP, van Horn JR: Long-term results of patellofemoral arthroplasty: A report of 56 arthroplasties with 17 years of follow-up. *J Bone Joint Surg Br* 2003;85: 836-840.
15. Merchant AC: Early results with a total patellofemoral joint replacement arthroplasty prosthesis. *J Arthroplasty* 2004;19:829-836.
16. Lonner JH: Patellofemoral arthroplasty: The impact of design on outcomes. *Orthop Clin North Am* 2008;39: 347-354.
17. Lonner JH: Patellofemoral arthroplasty. *J Am Acad Orthop Surg* 2007;15: 495-506.
18. Lonner JH: Patellofemoral arthroplasty, in Lotke PA, Lonner JH, eds: *Master Techniques in Orthopaedic Surgery: Knee Arthroplasty*, ed 3. Philadelphia, PA, Wolters Kluwer Lippincott Williams and Wilkins, 2009, pp 343-360.
19. Lonner JH, Mehta S, Booth RE Jr: Ipsilateral patellofemoral arthroplasty and autogenous osteochondral femoral condylar transplantation. *J Arthroplasty* 2007;22:1130-1136.
20. Wheaton AJ, Casey FL, Gougoutas AJ, et al: Correlation of T1rho with fixed charge density in cartilage. *J Magn Reson Imaging* 2004;20: 519-525.
21. Hendrix MR, Ackroyd CE, Lonner JH: Revision patellofemoral arthroplasty: Three- to seven-year follow-up. *J Arthroplasty* 2008;23: 977-983.
22. Lonner JH, Jasko JG, Booth RE Jr: Revision of the failed patellofemoral arthroplasty to total knee arthroplasty. *J Bone Joint Surg Am* 2006;88: 2337-2342.

Video Reference

8.1: Lonner JH: Video. Patellofemoral arthroplasty, in Della Valle CJ, Stuchin SA, eds: *Surgical Techniques in Orthopaedics: Arthroplasty for Unicompartmental Arthritis*. DVD. Rosemont, IL, American Academy of Orthopaedic Surgeons, 2007.

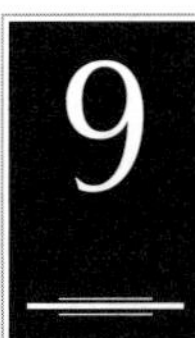

Scientific Evidence for Minimally Invasive Total Knee Arthroplasty

Michael A. Mont, MD
Michael G. Zywiel, MD
Mike S. McGrath, MD
Peter M. Bonutti, MD

Abstract

Total knee arthroplasty is often considered one of the most successful surgical operations, with implant survival rates as high as 95% reported over follow-up periods of 15 to 20 years. Despite these excellent reported results, some level of outcome dissatisfaction is reported in a considerable numbers of patients. Minimally invasive surgical techniques have been developed in an attempt to reduce or eliminate the surgical factors perceived to contribute to this dissatisfaction. An overview of minimally invasive total knee arthroplasty, with specific focus on level I (prospective, randomized) studies when available is presented along with an examination of how the published literature supports some of the more commonly stated benefits and drawbacks of minimally invasive techniques.

Minimally invasive total knee arthroplasty generally encompasses the following goals: reduced skin incision size, minimal or no incision of the extensor muscles and quadriceps tendon, minimal or no eversion of the patella, the use of downsized instrumentation, making bone cuts in situ, and minimal dislocation of the knee joint. Five principal surgical approaches have been developed that incorporate these aims, and, to date, four level I studies have been reported that compare the results of one or more of these techniques to traditional total knee arthroplasty. Three of these four studies showed no knee score differences at 3 months; one study showed higher scores at up to 9 months follow-up. In the opinion of the authors, these surgeons may have still been on their learning curve. Further studies that examine patients treated by surgeons who have mastered minimally invasive techniques may provide further insight into the true benefits and drawbacks of these techniques.

Instr Course Lect 2010;59:73-82.

Dr. Mont or an immediate family member has received royalties from Stryker; serves as a paid consultant to or is an employee of Stryker and Wright Medical Technology; and has received research or institutional support from Stryker Orthopaedics, Wright Medical Technology, Biomet, Brainlab, DePuy, Finsbury, Smith & Nephew, and Salient Surgical Technologies. Dr. Zywiel or an immediate family member has received research or institutional support from Stryker, Wright Medical Technology, Biomet, Brainlab, DePuy, Finsbury, Smith & Nephew, and Salient Surgical Technologies. Neither Dr. McGrath nor any immediate family member has received anything of value or owns stock in a commercial company or institution related directly or indirectly to the subject of this chapter. Dr. Bonutti or an immediate family member serves as a board member, owner, officer, or committee member of Joint Active Systems and Unity Ultrasonic Fixation; has received royalties from Styker, Arthrocare, and Biomet; is a member of a speakers' bureau or has made paid presentations on behalf of Stryker; and serves as a paid consultant to or is an employee of Stryker.

Total knee arthroplasty (TKA) is often considered one of the most successful orthopaedic surgical operations, with some authors reporting implant survivorship as high as 95% at follow-up times of 15 years.[1,2] Despite these excellent reported outcomes, a considerable number of patients have some level of dissatisfaction with pain, the duration of the rehabilitative period, and long-term functional limitations. Surgeon and patient assessment of the success of the procedure correlates poorly, with surgeon-centered objective assessment methods sometimes failing to recognize the factors that contribute to decreased patient satisfaction.[3]

Several authors have reported on factors that might contribute to the level of patient dissatisfaction. Mizner and associates[4] identified a profound loss of quadriceps muscle strength at 1 month after TKA when compared to preoperative functional level, and Silva and associates[5] reported that peak extension torque values remained up to 31% lower in patients more than 2 years after

TKA. Quadriceps muscle weakness substantially affects knee function during dependent movements such as walking or sitting to standing;[6] this may partly explain why Noble and associates[7] found that, at least 1 year after TKA, 52% of patients reported some degree of functional limitation compared with only 22% of matched control subjects with no previous knee disorders. Other factors included the duration of postoperative pain and the size of the skin incision.

To address patient dissatisfaction with TKA, several implant manufacturers and surgeons recently began developing implants, instruments, and surgical approaches (collectively known as minimally invasive surgery [MIS] techniques) that would reduce or eliminate surgical factors perceived to contribute to patient dissatisfaction. Some reports concerning the outcomes of these techniques suggest that their use is at least equivalent, if not favorable, when compared with traditional TKA techniques. Supporters of MIS have proposed benefits such as reduced postoperative pain, earlier return to function, and improved cosmetic appearance; however, some authors have reported an increased incidence of complications, including component malalignment or wound healing problems.

This chapter presents an overview of the field of minimally invasive total knee arthroplasty with specific focus on level I studies (prospective, randomized) when available. An examination of the published literature supports some of the more commonly stated benefits and drawbacks ascribed to these techniques, including the perception that strict exclusion criteria need to be applied; that they lead to a higher incidence of component malalignment; that MIS is more expensive than traditional arthroplasty; that patients experience lower postoperative pain and analgesia requirements; that MIS allows faster return to function and greater of range of motion (ROM); and that patients have higher rates of wound complications[8-27] (Table 1).

Techniques and Goals

Traditional TKA

Traditional TKA is typically performed through a medial parapatellar surgical approach. This approach provides excellent exposure of the knee joint, allowing direct visualization of the complete distal femur, proximal tibia, and patella. Ample room is provided for the relatively bulky alignment and cutting tools used in preparing the bone for implantation of the prosthesis components. Traditional TKA confers these benefits while allowing the surgeon to avoid any critical neurovascular structures. However, this approach involves a considerable incision of the quadriceps tendon, which may have long-term implications for muscle strength and knee function. Traditional TKA also involves lateral eversion of the patella, which has been reported to stretch the patellar tendon by as much as 16% and to have a significant correlation with longer time to straight leg raise and increased length of hospital stay after surgery.[28,29] More information on the medial parapatellar approach is available in chapter 10.

Minimally Invasive TKA

The definition of MIS TKA may differ between authors, but it usually involves a similar set of techniques for minimizing trauma to the joint and the surrounding soft tissue. These include a reduced size of the skin incision, minimal or no incision of the extensor muscles and quadriceps tendon, minimal or no eversion of the patella, the use of downsized instrumentation, making bone cuts in situ, and minimal dislocation of the knee joint. Different specific solutions have been developed for each of these aims and, over time, have developed into the five principal surgical approaches for MIS TKA: the mini medial parapatellar, quadriceps muscle-sparing, mini-midvastus, mini-subvastus, and direct lateral approaches. More information on these MIS approaches is available in chapter 10.

Study Results

Tremendous interest has developed in MIS TKA, with more than 200 peer-reviewed studies in the 5 years following the first report of this technique in 2003.[30] Although there is a large volume of data regarding short-term outcomes with MIS techniques, it is important to focus on studies that were performed with comparison groups and especially on those performed using a prospective design to better understand the scientific evidence that supports MIS. Reports have been published comparing MIS TKA to standard TKA using a medial parapatellar approach, including four prospective, randomized controlled, level I studies.[8-11]

Karachalios and associates[10] reported on 100 TKAs randomized to either a traditional parapatellar or mini-midvastus approach. The exact follow-up period is unknown because of inconsistencies in the reported data (reported as a mean of 23 months, with a range of 24 to 35 months) but is believed to encompass 2 to 3 years of follow-up. The authors reported significantly better Knee Society function scores in the MIS group at every interval as

Table 1
Comparative Studies of Minimally Invasive TKA

Authors	Year	Level of Evidence	Number of Knees and Approaches Used	Mean Length of Follow-up Period and Range (months)	Findings
Karachalios et al[10]	2008	Level I RCT	50 traditional versus 50 mini-midvastus	23 (24 to 35)*	Higher Knee Society and Oxford knee scores in MIS group up to 9-month follow-up; greater flexion in MIS group at early follow-up; no difference at final follow-up
Juosponis et al[9]	2008	Level I RCT	35 traditional versus 35 mini-midvastus	3	Higher Knee Society scores in MIS group at 6 weeks, no difference at 12 weeks; no difference in alignment
Kim et al[11]	2007	Level I RCT	120 traditional versus 120 quadriceps muscle-sparing in contralateral knee	14 (12 to 17)	Longer surgical time and higher rate of complications in quadriceps muscle-sparing group; no difference in Knee Society scores or ROM at 3 months or 1 year; no difference in alignment
Chin et al[8]	2007	Level I RCT	30 traditional versus 30 mini-midvastus versus 30 direct lateral	NR	Poorer femoral and tibial alignment in direct lateral group, no difference in alignment between mini-midvastus and traditional groups
Lin et al[24]	2008	Level I RCT	40 mini medial parapatellar versus 40 quadriceps muscle-sparing	2	No difference in muscle strength, postoperative pain, or functional outcomes; more varus alignment in quadriceps muscle-sparing group
Aglietti et al[25]	2006	Level I RCT	30 quadriceps muscle-sparing versus 30 mini-subvastus	3	Earlier straight leg raise in mini-subvastus group; no difference in pain, ROM, or alignment
Huang et al[22]	2007	Level II matched prospective comparative study	35 traditional versus 32 quadriceps muscle-sparing	24 (18 to 28)	Faster return to straight leg raise in quadriceps MIS group; greater knee flexion at 2 weeks; no difference in Knee Society scores at 6 weeks and 2 years; more poor alignment in MIS group
Tanvalee et al[26]	2007	Level II prospective comparative study	114 quadriceps muscle-sparing	24 (16 to 30)	Early ambulation significantly delayed with 3+ cm incision of quadriceps tendon compared with 0- to 2-cm incision
Kolisek et al[18]	2007	Level II non-blinded RCT	40 traditional versus 40 mini-midvastus	3	More delayed wound healing in MIS; no difference in blood loss, surgical time, Knee Society scores at 12 weeks; similar alignment
Boerger et al[17]	2005	Level II prospective comparative study	60 traditional versus 60 mini-subvastus	3	Earlier 90° flexion and straight leg raise in MIS; less pain on postoperative day 1 in MIS group; longer surgical time in MIS group with two intraoperative complications; good alignment except in one MIS treated tibia
Bonutti et al[13]	2004	Level II prospective comparative	216 mini-midvastus	24 minimum	97% good or excellent Knee Society scores at 2- to 4-year follow-up; six MUA, five reoperations
Bonutti et al[14]	In press	Level III retrospective comparative study	50 traditional versus 1,000 mini-midvastus	MIS Mean, NR (24 to 84), Traditional 36 (24 to 48)	6% complication rate first 200 knees, 1% in subsequent 800 knees; similar rate to comparison cohort of 50 traditional TKAs
Schroer et al[21]	2008	Level III retrospective and prospective comparative study	150 traditional versus 150 mini-subvastus	24	83% of patients in MIS group capable of straight leg raise on postoperative day 1; increased flexion in MIS group at up to 2-year follow-up; decreased need for skilled nursing or rehabilitation in MIS group; no difference in rate of complications

Table 1 (continued)
Comparative Studies of Minimally Invasive TKA

Authors	Year	Level of Evidence	Number of Knees and Approaches Used	Mean Length of Follow-up Period and Range (months)	Findings
McAllister and Stepanian[23]	2008	Level III retrospective comparative study	89 traditional versus 91 mini medial parapatellar	12	Higher flexion and extension in MIS group at 12 weeks; no difference at 52 weeks; fewer manipulations in MIS group; no differences in Knee Society scores or radiographic alignment at 1-year follow-up
Bonutti et al[35]	In press	Level III retrospective comparative study	25 traditional versus 25 mini-midvastus	Traditional (45 to 213), MIS (30 to 67)	Statistically improved quadriceps muscle strength in the MIS group at 3 months and 1 year postoperatively; better ROM in MIS group at 3 months and final follow-up: similar surgical time; similar postoperative radiographic alignment
Tashiro et al[20]	2007	Level III retrospective comparative study	25 traditional versus 24 mini medial parapatellar	16 (7 to 28)	Higher postoperative extensor torque in MIS group; lower pain and time to straight leg raise in MIS group; higher Knee Society scores at 3 weeks and 6 months in MIS group; no differences at 6 months; no differences in alignment or complication rate
King et al[16]	2007	Level III retrospective comparative study	50 traditional versus 100 quadriceps muscle-sparing	1.5	No difference in surgical time after first 25 MIS TKAs; shorter hospital stay, less need for inpatient rehabilitation, and less narcotic use at 2 and 6 weeks in MIS group; less need for ambulation assistance in MIS group
Kim et al[27]	2006	Level III retrospective comparative study	144 traditional versus 144 quadriceps muscle-sparing	22 (17 to 24)	No difference in Knee Society scores, complication rates, ROM, and alignment
Dalury and Dennis[15]	2005	Level III retrospective comparative study	30 traditional versus 30 mini medial parapatellar	3	Significantly shorter surgical time in MIS group; no difference in postoperative pain or ROM; four tibias in varus in MIS group versus none in traditional group
Tenholder et al[12]	2005	Level III retrospective cohort study	49 traditional versus 69 mini medial parapatellar	1.5	58% in mini medial parapatellar group did not require extending incision to traditional medial parapatellar incision; MIS group had smaller components and better postoperative flexion; no difference in complications or alignment problems
Laskin et al[19]	2004	Level III retrospective comparative study	26 traditional versus 32 mini-midvastus	3	Greater flexion in MIS group; greater Knee Society score improvements in MIS group at 6 weeks; lower pain medication in MIS group; no difference in alignment complications

*The exact follow-up period is unknown because of inconsistencies in the reported data.

MUA = manipulation under anesthesia, NR = not reported, RCT = randomized controlled trial, MIS = minimally invasive surgery, ROM = range of motion

well as at final follow-up (97 points for MIS versus 84 points for traditional TKA; $P = 0.01$). Knee Society total scores and Oxford knee scores were significantly better in the MIS group up to the 9-month follow-up (actual P values not reported; statistical significance set at $P < 0.05$) and were not significantly different at final follow-up. The mean postoperative flexion was significantly higher in the MIS group at up to 21-day follow-up (actual P value not reported) and remained 10.5° greater at final follow-up, although this difference was not significant ($P = 0.08$). Radiographic analysis at final follow-up showed six knees with malaligned tibial components (three with varus angle > 3° and three with anterior placement of components) in the MIS group, and nine knees with varus malalignment of the tibial component in the traditional approach group. No progressive lucencies were found in either group. There were four superficial wound healing complications in the MIS group and two in the traditional approach group. It is worth noting that a total of 34 MIS TKAs had been performed by the surgeons in Karachalios and associates'[10] department prior to the start of their study. Overall, this report presents evidence of earlier return of quadriceps muscle function and knee flexion in the MIS group, as well as the possibility of a long-lasting functional benefit with the MIS approach. No significant difference in the rate of complications between the two groups was found.

Chin and associates[8] randomized 90 knees treated with TKA to a traditional, mini-midvastus, or direct lateral approach and compared radiographic alignment between the approaches; clinical or functional outcomes were not reported. A significant difference was found in mean surgical time between the three approaches (92, 112, and 112 minutes for the traditional, mini-midvastus, and direct lateral approaches, respectively; $P < 0.001$), although it is not clear if the surgeons had any previous experience with minimally invasive approaches apart from practice in cadaver workshops. Standing radiographs taken at an unspecified follow-up time showed overall limb alignments within ±3° varus or valgus in 83% of the patients treated with the traditional approach, 83% of mini-midvastus patients, and 56% of direct lateral patients. The direct lateral approach had a significantly higher incidence ($P = 0.024$) of overall limb malalignment compared to both the traditional and mini-midvastus approaches, which had identical success rates. Overall, this report suggests that the mini-midvastus approach does not have a higher rate of malalignment than the traditional approach. Although the incidence of poor limb alignment was higher in the direct lateral group, this finding should be viewed with caution. The report suggested that the authors' experience with this approach was limited to 50 cadaver knees, raising the possibility that they were still within the learning curve for mastering the technique.

Kim and associates[11] performed bilateral TKAs on 120 patients, randomizing them to the quadriceps muscle-sparing approach in one knee and a traditional approach in the other. There were no significant differences ($P > 0.05$) in pain scores, Knee Society scores, ROM, or radiographic alignment between the two groups at any interval of follow-up or at a mean final follow-up of 1.8 years (range, 1.4 to 2 years). Surgical time was 6 minutes longer in the MIS group, which was significant ($P < 0.0001$) but not clinically relevant. It is worth noting that the operating surgeon had performed 25 TKAs with a quadriceps muscle-sparing approach prior to the start of this study, which may or may not be sufficient to achieve mastery of this technique.

Juosponis and associates[9] randomized 70 knees for treatment with TKAs through either a traditional or mini-midvastus approach. There was a significant difference between outcomes in the MIS and traditional groups in mean flexion (120° versus 110°, respectively; $P < 0.001$), the Knee Society mean objective score (85 points versus 65 points, respectively; $P < 0.001$), and Knee Society mean functional score (76 points versus 59 points, respectively; $P < 0.001$) at 6-week follow-up. Although all three of these measures remained better in the MIS group at 12-week follow-up, the differences were insignificant ($P = 0.075$ for ROM; $P = 0.055$ for the Knee Society objective score; $P = 0.77$ for the Knee Society functional score). No differences were found in component alignment, and no complications were reported in either group. The authors reported four lateralized patellae in the traditional approach group and none in the MIS group, although these were asymptomatic over the reported 12-week follow-up. The authors found a significantly longer mean surgical time in the MIS group (93 minutes versus 86 minutes, $P < 0.001$); however, they did not report their previous experience with the MIS technique used, making it impossible to speculate whether this difference could be related to relative inexperience with the surgical technique.

Overall, a review of the randomized controlled studies of MIS techniques for TKA demonstrates heterogeneity in the results. Function and ROM were either similar in both groups or better in the MIS group, whereas alignment was variable, depending on the study. Most importantly, the authors of three of these reports state that they had used MIS approaches for 25 to 50 knees prior to the commencement of the studies, whereas the fourth report does not mention the surgeons' experience; it is controversial whether this level of experience is sufficient to move beyond the learning curve.[14,16] Given that any new surgical technique is associated with a learning curve, studies that examine patients treated after surgeons have mastered the technique may provide further insight into the true benefits and drawbacks of MIS TKA.

Strict Exclusion Criteria

Some authors have suggested that the applicability of MIS TKA is limited by strict exclusion criteria, such as previous arthrotomy or knee infection, flexion contractures, obesity, considerable quadriceps muscle bulk, patella baja, or marked deformity of the knee, which need to be applied to ensure adequate exposure for component placement. Tenholder and associates[12] found that in 118 TKAs targeted for a mini medial parapatellar approach, intraoperative extension of the incision to a length of 14 cm or longer (the authors' maximum threshold to be considered a MIS approach) was necessary in 42% of patients. Shankar[31] reported that initially strict exclusion criteria, including previous open surgery, previous bone or soft-tissue trauma, previous infection of the knee, extreme obesity, osteoporosis, patella baja, reduced ROM, excessive deformity, and bone destruction after rheumatoid arthritis, limited the use of MIS quadriceps muscle-sparing approach to less than 20% of TKA patients. However, after using the technique for 1.5 years, the criteria could be sufficiently relaxed so that 70% of patients were being treated with a MIS approach. This is consistent with the evolutionary approach suggested by Bonutti and associates,[13] who recommend a gradual transition from a traditional to a minimally invasive incision, allowing a less abrupt progression through the learning curve. In a recent report of 1,000 consecutive knees, Bonutti and associates[14] reported that all TKA patients at their clinic are now treated using a minimally invasive approach, which is reflected in the mean body mass index of 31.2 kg/m^2 (range, 18 to 62 kg/m^2) of the reported cohort. The authors used a mini-midvastus approach for patients in their study, but the approach of the study's senior author (PMB) has since evolved to a modified mini-subvastus approach in which the distal 1 cm of the insertion of the vastus medialis obliquus muscle is peeled proximally together with the joint capsule.

Component Malalignment

Some authors have reported an increased incidence of component malalignment using MIS techniques when compared with a traditional approach, suggesting that minimal length incisions can increase the risk of such events for some surgeons.[15] However, most of these authors reported either their first experiences with the MIS technique or had only prior cadaver experience or minimal pilot-group experience. As with any new surgical procedure, the influence of a learning curve must be considered; however, the number of surgeries required to master MIS techniques is not completely clear. Based on surgical time alone, King and associates[16] suggested that the learning curve could be mastered after only 25 procedures. However, other authors reported a learning curve of up to 200 knees, based on a comparison of complication rates in 1,000 knees followed for a mean of 4 years (range, 2 to 7 years).[14] The actual learning curve will vary among surgeons and likely be reduced through awareness of and attention to avoiding the pitfalls and potential complications reported by the early adopter of MIS TKA. The authors believe that a gradual evolution from traditional techniques is crucial to minimizing complications through the learning curve and allows for successful adoption of minimally invasive techniques by both general orthopaedic surgeons and high-volume joint surgeons.

Cost Factors

MIS techniques require the use of downsized cutting blocks and alignment guides. As with traditional arthroplasty techniques, the instruments required for component implantation typically are provided without additional charge by the implant manufacturers, relieving the surgeon or hospital of the large, one-time cost of purchasing this equipment. Some surgeons may prefer to use retractors specifically designed to maximize visualization and reduce tissue trauma in MIS procedures; the purchase of these instruments represents a relatively minimal one-time investment. The largest potential recurring cost that could make MIS techniques more expensive is increased surgical time, which is associated with increased operating room and anesthesia costs, as well as the opportunity cost of being able to perform fewer surgeries during a given period of time. Although there have been some reports of higher surgical time with MIS techniques, other authors have reported no differences, or no differences after the early stages of the learning curve.[11,16-18] One author even reported a significantly shorter surgical time using MIS techniques (P = 0.003), although with a mean time difference of 3%, the practical implications of this difference are most likely minimal.[15] It is reasonable to expect that surgical times will be longer while surgeons are still relatively unfamiliar with a particular technique, so comparisons of surgical times between MIS and traditional techniques at similar experience levels are necessary for accurate assessment of this factor. A recent report compared the outcomes of MIS TKA using a mini-midvastus approach in 25 patients who had previously been treated with a TKA using a traditional approach in the contralateral knee performed by the same surgeon.[32] Although some of the MIS procedures were performed early in the surgeon's learning curve, many were done after gaining considerable experience with these techniques. The surgical time was found to be comparable, with a mean time from incision to wound closure of 63 minutes, (range, 45 to 120 minutes) in the minimally invasive group, and 64 minutes (range, 40 to 108 minutes) in the group treated with the traditional approach. Additional study results from experienced surgeons are needed to confirm this finding.

Pain Levels and Analgesia Requirements

One of the benefits promoted for MIS TKA is reduced postoperative pain and an associated decrease in postoperative analgesia requirements. Authors have reported lower pain levels in MIS knees in the immediate postoperative period; reports have been made of decreased analgesia requirements for up to 6 weeks after surgery.[16,17,19,20] The reason for decreased pain levels is not entirely clear, but may be related to decreased extensor mechanism trauma, reduced trauma to the posterior capsule because the knee is not dislocated during the procedure, or possibly the psychological expectation of decreased pain because of the smaller incision. Only one randomized controlled trial has reported on pain levels, finding no significant difference between approaches.[11] The earliest measurement of pain in this study was at 3-month follow-up, potentially missing a difference in pain level in the early postoperative period. Some authors have suggested additional benefits in terms of reduced pain with the direct lateral approach because of reduced incision stretching during knee motion in the immediate postoperative period and a less developed nerve plexus on the lateral aspect of the knee.[33,34] However, the authors of this chapter are not aware of any comparative reports that support or refute these suggestions.

Return to Function and Greater ROM

Several studies comparing outcomes between traditional TKA and minimally invasive techniques have examined postoperative ROM at serial follow-up periods. In a level I study, Kim and associates[11] reported no difference in ROM between traditional and quadriceps muscle-sparing approaches, although the earliest reported follow-up was 3 months postoperatively. In contrast, in level III studies, Schroer and associates[21] reported improved flexion in the MIS group at up to 2-year follow-up, and Bonutti and associates[35] reported significantly higher ROM at final follow-up in knees treated with MIS techniques (mean follow-up, 48 months; range, 30 to 47 months) compared with the contralateral knee treated using a traditional approach (mean follow-up, 115 months; range, 45 to 213 months). Several other authors have reported improved ROM with MIS TKA at early follow-up.[10,17,19,22,23] Although the duration of differences in postoperative ROM vary between reports, it appears that MIS techniques allow for greater ROM in the early follow-up period of up to 3 months, with some evidence suggesting that this difference persists for several years following the index arthroplasty.[10,17,19,22,23,35]

There are several reports of earlier return to function in knees treated with MIS techniques. Boerger and associates[17] and Tashiro and associates[20] both reported earlier achievement of straight leg raises in patients treated with MIS techniques. Seyler and associates[33] reported that 33 of 35 patients (94%) treated using a direct lateral approach achieved straight leg raises on postoperative day 1, whereas Schroer and associates[21] found the same achievement in 83% of patients treated with a mini-subvastus approach. Some authors have reported a decreased need for ambulation assistance and specialized rehabilitation in MIS patients, as well as a shorter time until discharge from hospital.[16,21] The authors of this chapter are not aware of any reports of poorer outcomes in MIS patients for these variables.

One concern in the rehabilitation of patients treated with TKA is ROM restoration. Patients are typically expected to regain most of their ROM within 6 weeks of surgery; failure to achieve at least 90° of flexion is a cause for concern and is typically an indication for manipulation under anesthesia in an attempt to increase ROM. Reports of the incidence of manipulation under anesthesia vary from approximately 2% to 20%, with several authors reporting rates of approximately 10%.[36-39] Although manipulation is usually successful in increasing knee ROM, these patients experience a delay in return to function, a return to the operating room, and must again undergo general anesthesia. Haas and associates[40] reported on manipulations under anesthesia in 8 of 391 TKAs (2%) performed with the mini-midvastus approach, and Bonutti and associates[14] reported 24 manipulations in 1,000 knees (2%). In a retrospective comparative study, McAllister and Stepanian[23] reported manipulation of 14% of knees treated with traditional techniques, compared with 2% of knees treated with a minimally invasive parapatellar approach ($P < 0.001$). These results suggest that MIS techniques may reduce the incidence of marked lasting postoperative reductions in ROM and the need for subsequent surgical procedures to improve function.

The reports to date suggest that MIS techniques result in better ROM in the early postoperative period, a quicker return to function, and decreased need for manipulation under anesthesia. Most studies do not show a significant clinical difference in Knee Society scores at final follow-up between MIS and traditional-approach TKAs.

Wound Complications

Some surgeons have expressed concern about the potential for wound edge necrosis and incision healing complications in patients treated with MIS techniques. In a comparison of 40 knees treated with a mini-midvastus approach and 40 knees treated with a traditional approach, Kolisek and associates[18] reported four superficial wound complications in the MIS group compared with one in the traditional group. Although not statistically significant, this difference raises the potential for healing complications in MIS patients because of prolonged, overzealous retraction in trying to maximize visualization through the shorter incision. The authors did not report on their experience level with the mini-midvastus approach, making it impossible to speculate on whether this finding was related to relative unfamiliarity with the reduced exposure of minimally invasive techniques. Experienced surgeons have discussed the importance of the creation of a mobile window and coordinated retraction techniques to optimize visualization without creating undue skin tension.[41,42] Specialized retractors designed for MIS surgery, which have an increased curvature to prevent the surgical assistant's hand from blocking the operative field, also can be used. In a recent report of 1,000 consecutive knees treated with minimally invasive techniques, Bonutti and associates[14] reported only two superficial wound complications, which resolved following local wound care. Although wound complications can occur with minimally invasive techniques, they may often result from improper retraction techniques rather than from an inherent feature of MIS approaches and can likely be avoided.

Summary

Current scientific evidence concerning MIS TKA suggests that in the hands of some surgeons these techniques may provide faster recovery and earlier return of function and ROM. Multiple studies also have reported less postoperative pain and decreased analgesia requirements, although this has not been confirmed by a randomized controlled trial. There have been some reports of an increased incidence of component malalignment and wound healing, but it is believed that these complications may be caused by surgeon inexperience with MIS techniques. There is no clear evidence of a difference in Knee Society scores at more than 2-year follow-up. Prospective randomized trials performed by surgeons experienced with MIS techniques are needed to definitively resolve concerns about the advantages and disadvantages of these approaches.

References

1. Ritter MA, Berend ME, Meding JB, Keatling EM, Faris PM, Crites BM: Long-term follow-up of anatomic graduated components posterior cruciate-retaining total knee replacement. *Clin Orthop Relat Res* 2001;388: 51-57.
2. Lachiewicz PF, Soileau ES: Fifteen-year survival and osteolysis associated with a modular posterior stabilized knee replacement: A concise follow-up of a previous report. *J Bone Joint Surg Am* 2009;91:1419-1423.
3. Bullens PH, van Loon CJ, de Waal Malefijt MC, Laan RF, Veth RP: Patient satisfaction after total knee arthroplasty: A comparison between subjective and objective outcome assessments. *J Arthroplasty* 2001;16: 740-747.
4. Mizner RL, Petterson SC, Stevens JE, Vandenborne K, Snyder-Mackler L: Early quadriceps strength loss after total knee arthroplasty: The contributions of muscle atrophy and failure of voluntary muscle activation. *J Bone Joint Surg Am* 2005;87:1047-1053.
5. Silva M, Shepherd EF, Jackson WO, Pratt JA, McClung CD, Schmalzried TP: Knee strength after total knee arthroplasty. *J Arthroplasty* 2003; 18:605-611.
6. Mizner RL, Snyder-Mackler L: Altered loading during walking and sit-to-stand is affected by quadriceps weakness after total knee arthroplasty. *J Orthop Res* 2005;23:1083-1090.
7. Noble PC, Gordon MJ, Weiss JM, Reddix RN, Conditt MA, Mathis KB: Does total knee replacement restore

normal knee function? *Clin Orthop Relat Res* 2005;431:157-165.

8. Chin PL, Foo LS, Yang KY, Yeo SJ, Lo NN: Randomized controlled trial comparing the radiologic outcomes of conventional and minimally invasive techniques for total knee arthroplasty. *J Arthroplasty* 2007;22:800-806.

9. Juosponis R, Tarasevicius S, Smailys A, Kalesinskas RJ: Functional and radiological outcome after total knee replacement performed with mini-midvastus or conventional arthrotomy: Controlled randomised trial. *Int Orthop*, in press.

10. Karachalios T, Giotikas D, Roidis N, Poultsides L, Bargiotas K, Malizos KN: Total knee replacement performed with either a mini-midvastus or a standard approach: A prospective randomised clinical and radiological trial. *J Bone Joint Surg Br* 2008;90: 584-591.

11. Kim YH, Kim JS, Kim DY: Clinical outcome and rate of complications after primary total knee replacement performed with quadriceps-sparing or standard arthrotomy. *J Bone Joint Surg Br* 2007;89:467-470.

12. Tenholder M, Clarke HD, Scuderi GR: Minimal-incision total knee arthroplasty: The early clinical experience. *Clin Orthop Relat Res* 2005;440: 67-76.

13. Bonutti PM, Mont MA, McMahon M, Ragland PS, Kester M: Minimally invasive total knee arthroplasty. *J Bone Joint Surg Am* 2004;86(suppl 2): 26-32.

14. Bonutti PM, Zywiel MG, Ulrich SD, McGrath MS, Mont MA. Minimally invasive total knee arthroplasty: Pitfalls and complications. *Am J Orthop*, in press.

15. Dalury DF, Dennis DA: Mini-incision total knee arthroplasty can increase risk of component malalignment. *Clin Orthop Relat Res* 2005;440: 77-81.

16. King J, Stamper DL, Schaad DC, Leopold SS: Minimally invasive total knee arthroplasty compared with traditional total knee arthroplasty: Assessment of the learning curve and the postoperative recuperative period. *J Bone Joint Surg Am* 2007;89:1497-1503.

17. Boerger TO, Aglietti P, Mondanelli N, Sensi L: Mini-subvastus versus medial parapatellar approach in total knee arthroplasty. *Clin Orthop Relat Res* 2005;440:82-87.

18. Kolisek FR, Bonutti PM, Hozack WJ, et al: Clinical experience using a minimally invasive surgical approach for total knee arthroplasty: Early results of a prospective randomized study compared to a standard approach. *J Arthroplasty* 2007;22:8-13.

19. Laskin RS, Beksac B, Phongjunakorn A, et al: Minimally invasive total knee replacement through a mini-midvastus incision: An outcome study. *Clin Orthop Relat Res* 2004;428: 74-81.

20. Tashiro Y, Miura H, Matsuda S, Okazaki K, Iwamoto Y: Minimally invasive versus standard approach in total knee arthroplasty. *Clin Orthop Relat Res* 2007;463:144-150.

21. Schroer WC, Diesfeld PJ, Reedy ME, LeMarr AR: Mini-subvastus approach for total knee arthroplasty. *J Arthroplasty* 2008;23:19-25.

22. Huang HT, Su JY, Chang JK, Chen CH, Wang GJ: The early clinical outcome of minimally invasive quadriceps-sparing total knee arthroplasty: Report of a 2-year follow-up. *J Arthroplasty* 2007;22:1007-1012.

23. McAllister CM, Stepanian JD: The impact of minimally invasive surgical techniques on early ROM after primary total knee arthroplasty. *J Arthroplasty* 2008;23:10-18.

24. Lin WP, Lin J, Horng LC, Chang SM, and Jiang CC: Quadriceps-sparing, minimal-incision total knee arthroplasty: A comparative study. *J Arthroplasty*. 2008. PMID: 18757172.

25. Aglietti P, Baldini A, Sensi L: Quadriceps-sparing versus mini-subvastus approach in total knee arthroplasty. *Clin Orthop Relat Res* 2006; 452:106-111.

26. Tanavalee A, Thiengwittayaporn S, Itiravivong P: Progressive quadriceps incision during minimally invasive surgery for total knee arthroplasty: The effect on early postoperative ambulation. *J Arthroplasty* 2007;22:1013-1018.

27. Kim YH, Sohn KS, Kim JS: Short-term results of primary total knee arthroplasties performed with a mini-incision or a standard incision. *J Arthroplasty* 2006;21:712-718.

28. Bonutti PM, Neal DJ, Kester MA: Minimal incision total knee arthroplasty using the suspended leg technique. *Orthopedics* 2003;26:899-903.

29. Walter F, Haynes MB, Markel DC: A randomized prospective study evaluating the effect of patellar eversion on the early functional outcomes in primary total knee arthroplasty. *J Arthroplasty* 2007;22:509-514.

30. Tria AJ Jr: Advancements in minimally invasive total knee arthroplasty. *Orthopedics* 2003;26(suppl 8):S859-S863.

31. Shankar NS: Minimally invasive technique in total knee arthroplasty: History, tips, tricks and pitfalls. *Injury* 2006:37(suppl 5):S25-S30.

32. Bonutti PM, Dethmers D, Ulrich SD, Seyler TM, Mont MA: Computer navigation-assisted minimally invasive TKA: Benefits and drawbacks. *Clin Orthop Relat Res* 2008; 466:2756-2762.

33. Seyler TM, Bonutti PM, Ulrich SD, Fatscher T, Marker DR, Mont MA: Minimally invasive lateral approach to total knee arthroplasty. *J Arthroplasty* 2007;22(7, suppl 3):21-26.

34. Bezwada HP, Mont MA, Bonutti PM, et al: Minimally invasive lateral approach to total knee arthroplasty, in Scuderi GR, Tria AJ Jr, Berger RA, eds: *MIS Techniques in Orthopedics*. New York, NY, Springer Science and Business Media, 2006, pp 339-348.

35. Bonutti PM, Seyler TM, Zywiel MG, et al: Minimally invasive total knee arthroplasty using the contralateral knee as a control group: A case-control study. *Int Orthop*, in press.

36. Fox JL, Poss R: The role of manipulation following total knee replacement. *J Bone Joint Surg Am* 1981;63: 357-362.

37. Keating EM, Ritter MA, Harty LD, et al: Manipulation after total knee arthroplasty. *J Bone Joint Surg Am* 2007; 89:282-286.

38. Esler CN, Lock K, Harper WM, Gregg PJ: Manipulation of total knee replacements: Is the flexion gained retained? *J Bone Joint Surg Br* 1999;81: 27-29.

39. Maloney WJ: The stiff total knee arthroplasty: Evaluation and management. *J Arthroplasty* 2002;17 (4, suppl 1):71-73.

40. Haas SB, Manitta MA, Burdick P: Minimally invasive total knee arthroplasty: The mini midvastus approach. *Clin Orthop Relat Res* 2006;452: 112-116.

41. Bonutti PM, Mont MA, Kester MA: Minimally invasive total knee arthroplasty: A 10-feature evolutionary approach. *Orthop Clin North Am* 2004; 35:217-226.

42. Tria AJ Jr, Coon TM: Minimal incision total knee arthroplasty: Early experience. *Clin Orthop Relat Res* 2003; 416:185-190.

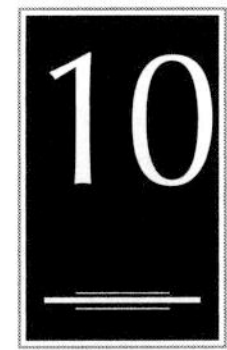

Surgical Techniques for Minimally Invasive Exposures for Total Knee Arthroplasty

Peter M. Bonutti, MD
Michael G. Zywiel, MD
Mike S. McGrath, MD
Michael A. Mont, MD

Abstract

The anterior medial parapatellar approach has long been the standard approach for total knee arthroplasty. Although this approach uses a simple, reproducible technique, some patients have reported lasting functional limitations after the surgery. Recently, marked interest has arisen in developing minimally invasive surgical approaches, implants, and instruments with the aim of improving patient outcomes. Five principal surgical approaches—the mini medial parapatellar, the quadriceps muscle-sparing, the mini-midvastus, the mini-subvastus, and the direct lateral—are most commonly used with minimally invasive techniques. Understanding the benefits and drawbacks of each approach as well as the reported results will aid orthopaedic surgeons in selecting the best treatment option for their patients.

Instr Course Lect 2010;59:83-91.

The anterior medial parapatellar approach, first described in 1945 by Abbott and Carpenter,[1] has long been the standard approach used for total knee arthroplasty (TKA). This approach is simple and reproducible and allows excellent exposure of the knee joint, which provides obvious benefits in terms of visualizing the surgical field and allowing unencumbered use of the large and bulky cutting jigs traditionally required for TKA procedures. The long incision used with this approach contributed to the surgeons' ability to properly align and fix the implants while maintaining a safe distance from any critical neurovascular structures. Although surgeons were satisfied with this technique, some studies that measured subjective outcomes suggested that patients were less pleased with the results.[2] Although the impact of the cosmetic appearance of the incision on patient satisfaction is equivocal, there have been reports of both short-term and lasting deficits in quadriceps function resulting from soft-tissue trauma related to the extensive exposure of the standard parapatellar approach.[3,4] A recent report also has implicated patellar eversion as a cause of poorer outcomes in TKA.[5] Minimally invasive surgery (MIS) was developed to limit soft-tissue trauma and the potential associated functional deficits.

Although MIS techniques are relatively new, with the first report published in 2003, there are now close to 300 reports in the literature. With various groups developing different strategies for MIS TKA, five

Dr. Bonutti or an immediate family member serves as a board member, owner, officer, or committee member of Joint Active Systems and Unity Ultrasonic Fixation; has received royalties from Styker, Arthrocare, and Biomet; is a member of a speakers' bureau or has made paid presentations on behalf of Stryker; and serves as a paid consultant to or is an employee of Stryker. Dr. Zywiel or an immediate family member has received research or institutional support from Stryker, Wright Medical Technology, Biomet, Brainlab, DePuy, Finsbury, Smith & Nephew, and Salient Surgical Technologies. Neither Dr. McGrath nor any immediate family member has received anything of value or owns stock in a commercial company or institution related directly or indirectly to the subject of this chapter. Dr. Mont or an immediate family member has received royalties from Stryker; serves as a paid consultant to or is an employee of Stryker and Wright Medical Technology; and has received research or institutional support from Stryker Orthopaedics, Wright Medical Technology, Biomet, Brainlab, DePuy, Finsbury, Smith & Nephew, and Salient Surgical Technologies.

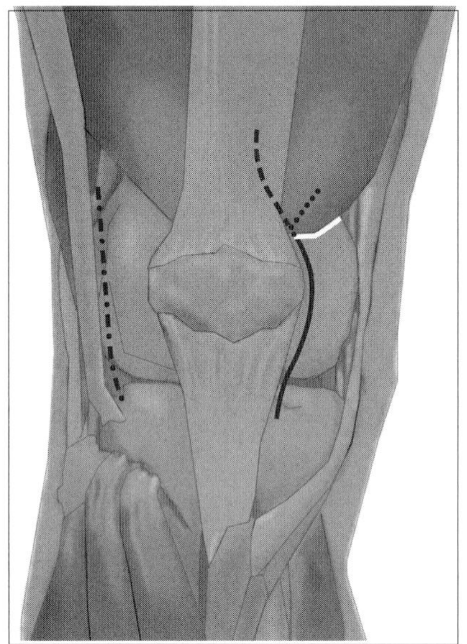

Figure 1 Illustration of the five different arthrotomy incisions used with the five principal surgical approaches for MIS TKA. Direct lateral = dotted-dashed line; mini medial parapatellar = black line + dashed line; mini-midvastus = black line + dotted line; mini-subvastus = black line + white line, quadriceps-sparing = black line.

surgical approaches—the mini medial parapatellar, the quadriceps-sparing, the mini-midvastus, the mini-subvastus, and the direct lateral—have emerged as the most commonly used techniques (Figure 1). This chapter will review these five approaches in detail, along with their reported benefits, drawbacks, and outcome results.

Mini Medial Parapatellar Approach

The mini medial parapatellar approach is similar to the standard medial parapatellar approach but with a reduced skin and arthrotomy incision length. As the surgeon gains experience with the standard TKA technique, the incision length can be gradually reduced, providing a smooth transition to the minimally invasive version of this approach.

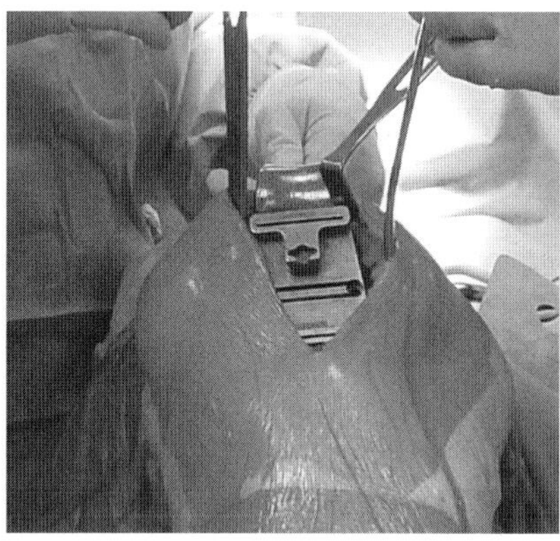

Figure 2 Specialized MIS instruments, such as this downsized femoral cutting block, are needed to fit through the reduced exposure window.

Technique

With the patient supine on the operating room table and the leg in full extension, a 10- to 14-cm incision is made in the typical location from the level of the superior pole of the patella to the tibial tubercle. A generous subcutaneous dissection should be performed to create a mobile window. By synchronizing retraction to ensure that tension is placed on only one side of the incision at a given time, greater visualization can be achieved than by retracting in all directions at once. After releasing the fascia, a minimal incision is made in the quadriceps tendon to allow lateral displacement of the patella without eversion. Typically, a 2- to 4-cm incision in the tendon, followed by lateral retraction and flexion of the knee, should suffice to subluxate the patella. If the patellar tendon is under excessive tension or at risk of rupture, the incision can be extended proximally until sufficient exposure is gained.

Bone cuts can now be made in the order that the surgeon prefers, although it has been suggested that starting with a tibial resection provides laxity that greatly facilitates subsequent placement of the femoral cutting guides.[6] Placement of the tibial cutting guide can be aided by hyperflexion and external rotation of the joint, causing the tibial plateau to protrude proud of the incision. As with the standard technique, retractors should be strategically placed to protect the collateral ligaments, patellar tendon, and skin edges from oscillating saw damage. Coordinated medial retraction can be used during resection of the corresponding tibial plateau, with the mobile window then moved laterally when cutting the remaining tibial bone. Regardless of the exact order of resection, downsized cutting blocks are needed to fit through the reduced size of the exposure window (Figure 2). The knee is kept in flexion, and with the assistance of tibial distraction, the femoral guide can be placed and bone cuts can be made. With both tibial and femoral cuts complete, there is significant laxity in the knee, and the patella can now be briefly everted with the leg in extension, allowing preparation of the articular surface while placing minimal stress on the extensor mechanism. After component trialing and bone preparation, the prosthesis is fixed in the typical manner. Just as with the bony resections, it is recommended that the tibia be addressed first. Soft-tissue balancing is performed according to the same principles as used in standard techniques. Once the components are well fixed and the knee has been adequately balanced, the soft tissues can be closed.

Benefits, Drawbacks, and Results

The benefits of the medial parapatellar approach include (1) a surgical approach that is fundamentally similar to the standard parapatellar approach, enabling a smooth transition to minimally invasive techniques; and (2) no critical neurovascular structures in proximity to the surgical field. However, the principal drawback is that surgeons and assistants may try to achieve a similar level of exposure as with standard techniques and may be overly enthusiastic with their retraction. In addition to potentially causing skin tearing or bruising as a result of excessive soft-tissue tension, there is the possibility for compromise or even avulsion of the patellar tendon. This can be avoided by extending the skin and/or tendon incisions if the exposure is deemed insufficient.

In a recent comparison of 89 TKAs performed with traditional techniques and 91 TKAs performed with a mini medial parapatellar approach, McAllister and Stepanian[7] reported significantly better flexion and extension at 12 weeks in the MIS group ($P < 0.0001$) and a significantly decreased need for manipulation over a 1-year follow-up period ($P < 0.001$). However, the authors reported no significant difference in range of motion, functional outcome, or complication rates at 1 year follow-up in these two groups. Tenholder and associates[8] reported on 118 consecutive primary TKAs treated with a mini parapatellar approach, with the intraoperative incision extended as necessary to facilitate exposure. The authors reported that the mini incision provided sufficient exposure to complete the procedure in 58% of patients and judged it to be particularly suitable in thin women with a low body mass index and a narrow femur. Other authors have reported encouraging results with this technique.[9-11]

Quadriceps Muscle-Sparing Approach

The quadriceps muscle-sparing approach is a modification of the technique first reported by Repicci and Eberle[12] for unicondylar knee arthroplasty. Several surgeons began using the approach for MIS TKA earlier this decade,[13-15] with the first results with minimum 2-year follow-up reported in 2006 by Chen and associates.[16]

Technique

With the knee in flexion, the quadriceps muscle-sparing approach is started with a curved skin incision medial to the patella, extending from the level of the superior pole to approximately 2 cm below the tibial joint line. The capsule is incised following a similar path, from the insertion of the vastus medialis muscle to below the tibial joint line. The vastus medialis tendon is preserved if possible, but because of anatomic variations in the insertion point on the patella, it may be necessary to extend the arthrotomy proximally to gain sufficient exposure. The knee is then placed in extension, the patellar fat pad is removed, and the articular surface of the patella is removed with a saw to gain additional exposure. After subluxating the patella laterally, the knee is returned to the flexed position, and the distal femoral cuts are made with the assistance of downsized instrumentation. Attention is then directed to the tibia. Because this surgical approach typically limits intraoperative flexion to less than 90°, it is not possible to force the tibia out of the incision through hyperflexion and external rotation at the knee. With exposure of the tibia limited, it is generally recommended that the medial tibial cut be made first, and the medial bone removed, before resecting the lateral plateau. This staged approach improves visualization of the lateral compartment and should reduce the chance for unintended soft-tissue trauma during the lateral cut. Next, the femoral cuts are completed, followed by preparation of the patella, component trialing, balancing the knee, fixation of the prosthetic components, and tissue closure.

Benefits, Drawbacks, and Results

The primary benefit of the quadriceps muscle-sparing approach is that when properly performed, the extensor mechanism should be wholly spared from trauma, possibly improving postoperative quadriceps muscle strength and speeding the recovery process.[13] However, anatomic variation of the insertion of the tendon on the patella has been noted, and a sizable proportion of the population may have a low insertion point extending as far distally as the inferior pole of the patella.[17] In a study of MRI scans and cadaver specimens of the vastus medialis tendon, Holt and associates[18] reported insertion in the distal 40% of the patella in 25% of patients. In these patients, it is typically necessary to violate the tendon insertion during the arthrotomy to gain sufficient exposure; therefore, the approach is not truly a quadriceps muscle-sparing approach. Although Tanavalee and associates[19] reported that patients with vastus medialis tendon incisions 2 cm in length or shorter have significantly improved early ambulation compared with those with 3-cm incisions, it is not clear to what extent the tendon can be incised before the benefits of this surgical approach are markedly attenuated.

Lin and associates[10] recently compared 80 patients treated with TKAs

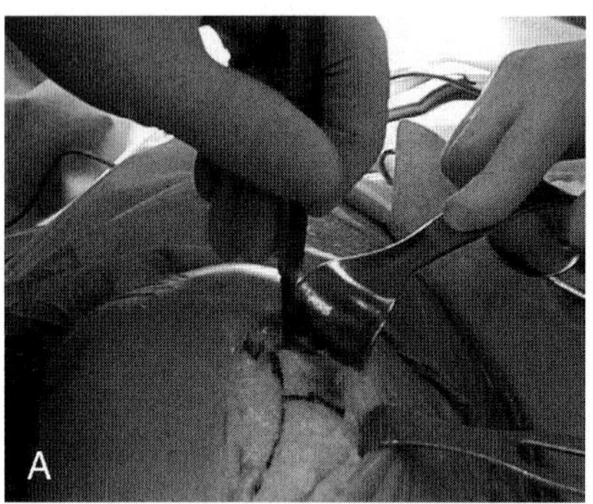

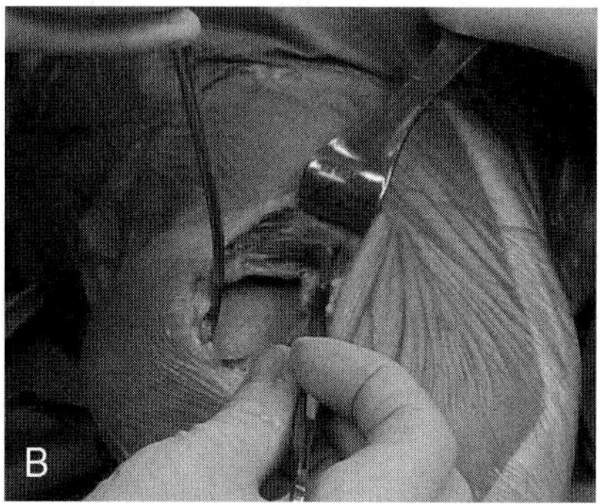

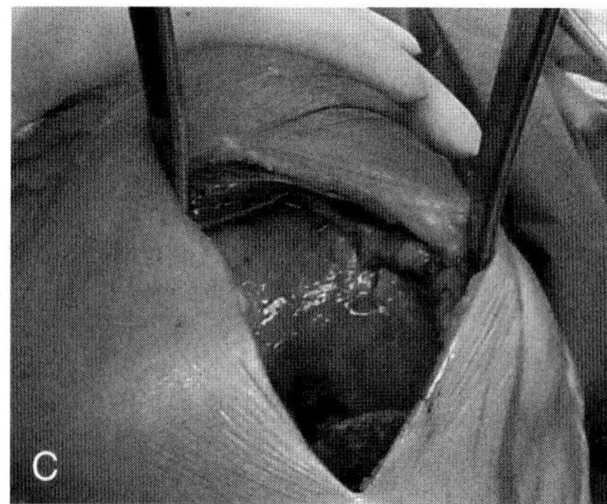

Figure 3 Intraoperative photographs of the mini-midvastus approach. **A,** The vastus medialis obliquus muscle is incised proximally along the length of the muscle fibers. **B,** The arthrotomy is then extended distally medial to the patella. **C,** The intra-articular cavity is exposed.

who were randomized to either the quadriceps muscle-sparing approach or the mini medial parapatellar approach. The authors found the hip-knee-ankle axis to be more varus in patients treated with the quadriceps muscle-sparing approach but found no significant short-term difference in pain level or functional outcome. Aglietti and associates[20] compared two groups of 30 patients treated with either a quadriceps muscle-sparing or mini-subvastus approach. Straight leg raising was achieved at mean of one half day earlier in the mini-subvastus group, but there was no significant difference in postoperative pain or maximum flexion between the two groups at 1 week, 1 month, or 3 months postoperatively. Other studies of this technique have reported excellent results.[13,21-23]

Mini-Midvastus Approach

The mini-midvastus approach combines the familiarity of the medial parapatellar approach to the knee with a markedly reduced incision length. The vastus medialis obliquus muscle is split along the length of the muscle fibers to enhance exposure of the knee joint while minimizing trauma to the extensor mechanism.

Technique

The patient is positioned and draped in a standard manner. With the knee in flexion, an incision is made medial to the patella starting at the superior pole and extending just proximal to the tibial tubercle. This incision can be extended later if necessary, although using the mobile window techniques described previously should limit this need. The arthrotomy is performed along the same incision, with the addition of a 2-cm cut of the vastus medialis obliquus muscle extending proximally in line with the muscle fibers from the level of the superior pole of the patella (Figure 3). If at any point during the procedure the exposure is judged to be insufficient, the incision of the vastus medialis can be extended.

The patella is then retracted with the knee in extension. An inferior capsular release is performed with excision of the fat pad, followed by a superior capsular release. This should provide sufficient laxity to subluxate the patella laterally, exposing the joint space. After performing the necessary tibial releases and returning the knee to flexion, the tibial cut can be made in situ using an extramedullary referencing system. Attention is then turned to the femur. The rotational plane of the femoral bone cuts is carefully established using appropriate MIS instrumentation, which initially can be more challenging compared with a standard approach because of the reduced capacity for direct visualization. After making the anterior cut, intramedullary referencing is used for the distal cut, and the remaining cuts are made using a downsized block. If the patella is being resurfaced, the cuts and holes can be made in extension without the need for eversion.

A thorough assessment of bone cuts, osteophytes, loose fragments, and excess soft tissue should be made through both direct visualization and manual palpation of all compartments and gutters. The leg can be distracted in full extension to allow a more thorough examination. Next, component trialing and ligament balancing is performed in the typical fashion. Cementing of the final components can sometimes be challenging because of the reduced exposure, and care should be taken to use proper cementing techniques, with flexion, extension, and retraction as necessary to ensure proper component positioning and impaction. Great care should be taken to remove excess cement, with frequent manual palpation in the lateral compartments because of the reduced visualization. Closure proceeds in the typical manner, with a single stitch in the vastus medialis obliquus muscle split.

Video 10.1: Minimally Invasive Total Knee Arthroplasty: The Mini-Midvastus Approach. Peter M. Bonutti, MD; Michael A. Mont, MD; Thorsten M. Seyler, MD; Johannes F. Plate, BS (11 min)

Benefits, Drawbacks, and Results

The principal advantages of the mini-midvastus approach include reduced postoperative pain and extensor mechanism trauma resulting from a muscle incision that is kept parallel to the muscle fibers and offers the flexibility to extend the incision and provide the generous exposure that may be necessary in more obese or muscular patients, or those with deformities about the knee. Cooper and associates[24] studied the midvastus approach in cadavers, finding that a mean vastus medialis obliquus muscle split of 8.8 cm could be performed before approaching the popliteal vessels. Disadvantages of this technique include the potential for skin or quadriceps trauma secondary to excessive retraction; the possibility of retained fragments, cement, or soft-tissue impingement in the lateral compartment if adequate manual palpation is not performed; and the possibility of damage to the lateral femoral condyle by the tibial component resulting from difficult keel implantation.

Karachalios and associates[25] recently reported a prospective, randomized comparison of the mini-midvastus versus standard parapatellar approach for TKA. The authors found a significantly better functional outcome in the mini-midvastus group ($P = 0.05$) up to 9 months postoperatively, as measured by the Knee Society and Oxford knee scores. Bonutti and associates[26] reported on a series of 1,000 consecutive TKAs performed using the mini-midvastus approach. Although the authors suggested the learning curve may be up to 200 surgeries, the overall revision rate was 2%, dropping to 1% when the first 200 knees are excluded, over a follow-up range of 2 to 7 years. More information on these studies is available in chapter 9. Other authors reported that this approach is associated with rapid functional recovery and substantial gains in range of motion.[27,28] These results suggest that when proper techniques are used, the mini-midvastus approach can provide excellent results in TKA. Additional reports have been made of results that are consistent with these conclusions.[29-31]

Mini-Subvastus Approach

The mini-subvastus approach to the knee was originally described by Hoffman and associates[32] as an alternative, quadriceps muscle-sparing approach for standard TKA. Because of difficulties with everting the patella using this approach, adoption for standard techniques was limited; however, it has proven useful for MIS TKA, where patellar eversion is typically avoided.

Technique

The patient is positioned and draped in a standard manner. A skin incision is made slightly medial to the midline, from the superior pole of the patella to the top of the tibial tubercle. Dissecting down to the fascia, the inferior border of the vastus medialis muscle is identified approximately 5 cm medial to the patella (Figure 4), and a stab incision is made in the fascia. Using a combination of blunt dissection and electrocautery, the vastus medialis muscle is separated from the medial retinaculum, taking care to preserve a cuff of fascia on the muscle for later repair, and leaving the tendinous insertion onto the patella intact. An arthrotomy is then performed on the underlying capsule, starting along the inferior border of the vastus medialis muscle and continuing inferiorly along the medial aspect of the patella and patellar tendon to the proximal tibia. A retractor is placed into the lateral gutter, and with levering against the insertion of the vastus medialis muscle, the extensor mechanism and patella is subluxated laterally. The knee is then flexed, with soft-tissue releases performed as necessary, leaving the patella resting in the lateral gutter and exposing the articular surfaces of the femur and tibia. Beginning with resection of the fat pad, the remainder of the arthroplasty is performed similarly to the methods described for the

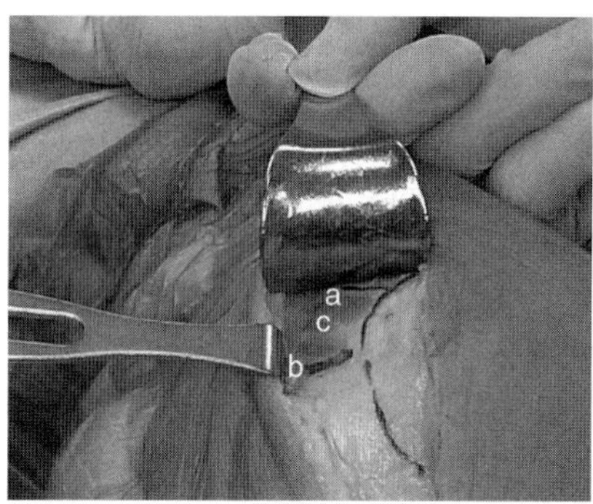

Figure 4 Photograph showing the different arthrotomy incisions used for the mini-midvastus (a) and subvastus (b) approaches. The vastus medialis obliquus muscle (c) can be seen through the overlying fascia.

mini medial parapatellar approach. After final fixation of the components, it is important to deflate the tourniquet to ensure excellent hemostasis. The vastus medialis muscle contains small vessels that are susceptible to rupture after more vigorous mobilization of the muscle, which can lead to the development of a subvastus hematoma if bleeding vessels are not cauterized before closure.

Video 10.2: Minimally Invasive Total Knee Arthroplasty: The Mini-Subvastus Approach. Peter M. Bonutti, MD; Michael A. Mont, MD; Thorsten M. Seyler, MD; Johannes F. Plate, BS (21 min)

Benefits, Drawbacks, and Results

The advantages of the mini-subvastus approach are that it is a potentially muscle-sparing approach, with no incision in the extensor mechanism. Additionally, it may confer some theoretic benefit by preserving blood supply to the patella by leaving the medial retinaculum and retinacular artery intact.[33] Disadvantages of this approach include marked stretching forces on the vastus medialis muscle, which put it at risk for hematoma formation. Additionally, visualization of the anterior femur is limited with this approach because it remains partially covered by the extensor mechanism even with maximal retraction of the patella. This can make it more challenging to accurately align the cutting guide, especially for surgeons less experienced with the technique. Another concern is the proximity of the saphenous nerve and branch of the femoral artery to the inferior margin of the vastus medialis muscle, raising the potential for injury to these structures during the approach.[34]

Schroer and associates[35] compared 150 patients treated with a mini-subvastus approach and 150 patients treated with a standard parapatellar incision. The authors found that the MIS group could perform a straight leg raise significantly earlier and had a shorter hospital stay than the group treated with the standard approach. The MIS group also had significantly higher mean flexion than the traditional group throughout the first 2 years of follow-up. No significant increase in complication rates was found with the MIS group, although another study reported an increased incidence of patella clunk syndrome in patients treated with the MIS approach.[36] This finding was ascribed to increased postoperative knee flexion rather than the surgical approach itself and was found to decrease in association with a posterior stabilized prosthesis. Boerger and associates[37] reported on 120 knees randomized to either a mini-subvastus or standard parapatellar approach. They found that the MIS group had better pain scores on postoperative day 1, faster time to 90° flexion, and slightly better flexion in the first 90 postoperative days. However, the authors reported a higher complication rate in the MIS group and only short-term benefits with the MIS approach. Other studies have consistently reported improved early extensor muscle function in patients treated with the mini-subvastus approach.[20,38]

Direct Lateral Approach

The direct lateral approach is a new technique that brings the benefits of MIS to TKA. It is unique compared to the other common MIS techniques because it avoids any disruption of the anterior aspect of the knee (including the skin, anterior capsule, and the extensor mechanism) by approaching the knee through the lateral skin and the iliotibial band.

Technique

The patient is placed supine on the operating table. A rest can be placed against the lateral thigh to assist in opening the medial compartment during the procedure. With the knee in extension, an incision is made on the lateral aspect of the knee from the lateral femoral epicondyle to just distal to the Gerdy tubercle, exposing the iliotibial band. The distal femur and proximal tibia are then exposed, followed by resection of the fat pad and anterior horn of the lateral meniscus. With the assistance of medial retraction of the patellar tendon, any additional soft-tissue releases can be performed to visualize the medial meniscus and resect the anterior horn. With the assistance of selective retraction, the suprapatellar pouch is exposed, and soft tissues are dissected to expose the anterior aspect of the femur. At this point, the patella should be sufficiently mobile to allow medial subluxation.

Specialized side-cutting blocks are used, starting with resection of the distal femur, followed by the tibial cut (Figure 5). The knee should have sufficient laxity to make the tibial and femoral holes, as well as the patellar cuts and holes, without the need to evert the patella. Component trialing and soft-tissue balancing then can be performed, followed by component fixation and final evaluation of the knee kinematics.

Benefits, Drawbacks, and Results

The principal advantage of the lateral approach to the knee is the com-

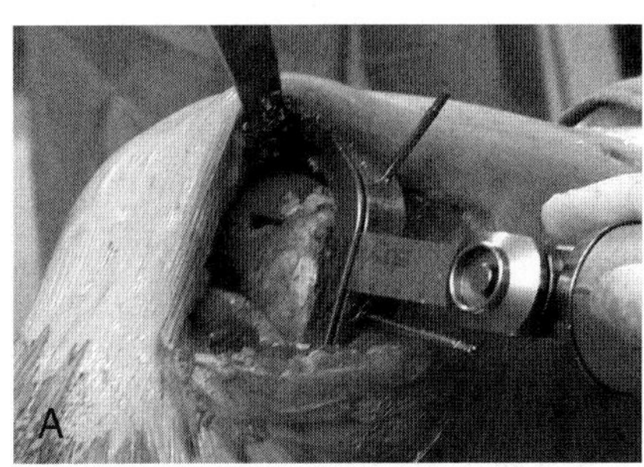

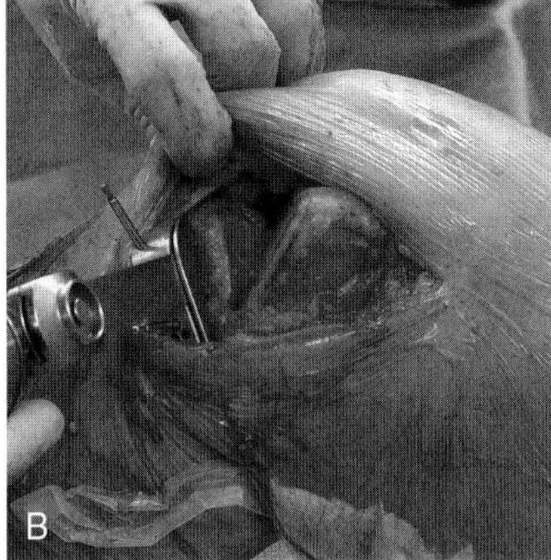

Figure 5 Intraoperative photographs of the side-cutting blocks used in the direct lateral approach, starting with resection of the distal femur **(A)** followed by the tibial plateau **(B)**.

plete avoidance of any muscle splitting, with all incisions made clear of the extensor mechanism. Combined with the reduced tension on the healing incision as a result of it being displaced away from the extensor aspect of the knee, this can result in a rapid return of knee motion and function. Seyler and associates[39] reported that 33 of 35 patients (94%) treated with TKA using the lateral approach were able to perform an independent straight leg raise on postoperative day 1, and all 35 patients were able to do so by postoperative day 3. An additional benefit of this approach is that the knee is not dislocated, which reduces soft-tissue trauma.

At a mean follow-up of 3.8 years, the cohort reported by Seyler and associates[39] had mean Knee Society functional scores of 92 points (range, 72 to 98 points) and a mean range of motion of 120° (range, 95° to 125°). However, three knees had an anatomic valgus alignment of greater than 7° at final follow-up, making them susceptible to early failure, and one knee required revision for aseptic loosening of the tibial component. The authors postulated that this failure rate reflects the early learning curve for this approach. Chin and associates[40] compared outcomes of 90 TKAs randomized to either the standard, the mini-midvastus, or the direct lateral approach. These authors reported significantly poorer femoral implant placement ($P = 0.028$) and overall limb alignment ($P = 0.024$) in the direct lateral group compared with the groups treated with the other two approaches. The authors of this chapter are not aware of any other current reports on the direct lateral technique.

Summary

Although MIS techniques have only recently begun to be used in TKA, their use has resulted in tremendous interest. Five distinct surgical approaches have evolved for this procedure, each with unique benefits and drawbacks. Although reports have been made of clinical and functional results for each of these approaches, they are all limited by relatively short follow-up periods. (Please see chapter 9 for a table presenting the findings of comparative studies of MIS TKAs.) As greater numbers of patients are treated using MIS techniques and longer-term follow-up data becomes available, the advantages and disadvantages of these approaches will be better understood.

Acknowledgment

The authors would like to thank Joe Michalski for his assistance with the preparation of the artwork for this manuscript.

References

1. Abbott LC, Carpenter WF: Surgical approaches to the knee joint. *J Bone Joint Surg Am* 1945;27:277-310.
2. Bullens PH, van Loon CJ, de Waal Malefijt MC, Laan RF, Veth RP: Patient satisfaction after total knee arthroplasty: A comparison between subjective and objective outcome assessments. *J Arthroplasty* 2001;16:740-747.
3. Mizner RL, Petterson SC, Stevens JE, Vandenborne K, Snyder-Mackler L: Early quadriceps strength loss after total knee arthroplasty: The contributions of muscle atrophy and failure of voluntary muscle activation. *J Bone Joint Surg Am* 2005;87:1047-1053.
4. Silva M, Shepherd EF, Jackson WO, Pratt JA, McClung CD, Schmalzried TP: Knee strength after total knee arthroplasty. *J Arthroplasty* 2003;18:605-611.
5. Walter F, Haynes MB, Markel DC: A randomized prospective study evaluating the effect of patellar eversion on the early functional outcomes in primary total knee arthroplasty. *J Arthroplasty* 2007;22:509-514.
6. Scuderi GR: Total knee arthroplasty with a limited medial parapatellar arthrotomy, in Scuderi GR, Tria AJ Jr, Berger RA, eds: *MIS Techniques in Orthopedics*. New York, NY, Springer Science and Business Media, 2006, pp 303-314.
7. McAllister CM, Stepanian JD: The impact of minimally invasive surgical techniques on early range of motion after primary total knee arthroplasty. *J Arthroplasty* 2008;23:10-18.
8. Tenholder M, Clarke HD, Scuderi GR: Minimal-incision total knee arthroplasty: The early clinical experience. *Clin Orthop Relat Res* 2005;440:67-76.

9. Tashiro Y, Miura H, Matsuda S, Okazaki K, Iwamoto Y: Minimally invasive versus standard approach in total knee arthroplasty. *Clin Orthop Relat Res* 2007;463:144-150.

10. Lin WP, Lin J, Horng LC, Chang SM, Jiang CC: Quadriceps-sparing, minimal-incision total knee arthroplasty: A comparative study. *J Arthroplasty* 2009;24:1024-1032.

11. Dalury DF, Dennis DA: Mini-incision total knee arthroplasty can increase risk of component malalignment. *Clin Orthop Relat Res* 2005;440: 77-81.

12. Repicci JA, Eberle RW: Minimally invasive surgical technique for unicondylar knee arthroplasty. *J South Orthop Assoc* 1999;8:20-27.

13. Huang HT, Su JY, Chang JK, Chen CH, Wang GJ: The early clinical outcome of minimally invasive quadriceps-sparing total knee arthroplasty: Report of a 2-year follow-up. *J Arthroplasty* 2007;22:1007-1012.

14. Tria AJ Jr: Minimally invasive total knee arthroplasty using the quadriceps-sparing approach, in Scuderi GR, Tria AJ Jr, Berger RA, eds: *MIS Techniques in Orthopedics*. New York, NY, Springer Science and Business Media, 2006, pp 349-364.

15. Kim YH, Sohn KS, Kim JS: Short-term results of primary total knee arthroplasties performed with a mini-incision or a standard incision. *J Arthroplasty* 2006;21:712-718.

16. Chen AF, Alan RK, Redziniak DE, Tria AJ Jr: Quadriceps sparing total knee replacement: The initial experience with results at two to four years. *J Bone Joint Surg Br* 2006;88:1448-1453.

17. Roberts VI, Mereddy PK, Donnachie NJ, Hakkalamani S: Anatomical variations in vastus medialis obliquus and its implications in minimally-invasive total knee replacement: An MRI study. *J Bone Joint Surg Br* 2007; 89:1462-1465.

18. Holt G, Nunn T, Allen RA, Forrester AW, Gregori A: Variation of the vastus medialis obliquus insertion and its relevance to minimally invasive total knee arthroplasty. *J Arthroplasty* 2008;23:600-604.

19. Tanavalee A, Thiengwittayaporn S, Itiravivong P: Progressive quadriceps incision during minimally invasive surgery for total knee arthroplasty: The effect on early postoperative ambulation. *J Arthroplasty* 2007;7:1013-1018.

20. Aglietti P, Baldini A, Sensi L: Quadriceps-sparing versus mini-subvastus approach in total knee arthroplasty. *Clin Orthop Relat Res* 2006; 452:106-111.

21. Kim YH, Kim JS, Kim DY: Clinical outcome and rate of complications after primary total knee replacement performed with quadriceps-sparing or standard arthrotomy. *J Bone Joint Surg Br* 2007;89:467-470.

22. Yu JK, Yu CL, Ao YF, et al: Comparative study on early period of recovery between minimally invasive surgery total knee arthroplasty and minimally invasive surgery-quadriceps sparing total knee arthroplasty in Chinese patients. *Chin Med J (Engl)* 2008;121: 1353-1357.

23. King J, Stamper DL, Schaad DC, Leopold SS: Minimally invasive total knee arthroplasty compared with traditional total knee arthroplasty: Assessment of the learning curve and the postoperative recuperative period. *J Bone Joint Surg Am* 2007;89:1497-1503.

24. Cooper RE Jr, Trinidad G, Buck WR: Midvastus approach in total knee arthroplasty: A description and a cadaveric study determining the distance of the popliteal artery from the patellar margin of the incision. *J Arthroplasty* 1999;14:505-508.

25. Karachalios T, Giotikas D, Roidis N, Poultsides L, Bargiotas K, Malizos KN: Total knee replacement performed with either a mini-midvastus or a standard approach: A prospective randomised clinical and radiological trial. *J Bone Joint Surg Br* 2008;90: 584-591.

26. Bonutti PM, Zywiel MG, Ulrich SD, McGrath MS, Mont MA: Minimally invasive total knee arthroplasty: Pitfalls and complications. *Amer J Orthop,* in press.

27. Haas SB, Manitta MA, Burdick P: Minimally invasive total knee arthroplasty: The mini midvastus approach. *Clin Orthop Relat Res* 2006;452: 112-116.

28. Laskin RS, Beksac B, Phongjunakorn A, et al: Minimally invasive total knee replacement through a mini-midvastus incision: An outcome study. *Clin Orthop Relat Res* 2004; 428: 74-81.

29. Kolisek FR, Bonutti PM, Hozack WJ, et al: Clinical experience using a minimally invasive surgical approach for total knee arthroplasty: Early results of a prospective randomized study compared to a standard approach. *J Arthroplasty* 2007;22:8-13.

30. Juosponis R, Tarasevicius S, Smailys A, Kalesinskas RJ: Functional and radiological outcome after total knee replacement performed with mini-midvastus or conventional arthrotomy: Controlled randomised trial. *Int Orthop* 2009;33:1233-1237.

31. Bonutti PM, Mont MA, McMahon M, Ragland PS, Kester M: Minimally invasive total knee arthroplasty. *J Bone Joint Surg Am* 2004;86:26-32.

32. Hofmann AA, Plaster RL, Murdock LE: Subvastus (Southern) approach for primary total knee arthroplasty. *Clin Orthop Relat Res* 1991;269: 70-77.

33. Kayler DE, Lyttle D: Surgical interruption of patellar blood supply by total knee arthroplasty. *Clin Orthop Relat Res* 1988;229:221-227.

34. Scheibel MT, Schmidt W, Thomas M, von Salis-Soglio G: A detailed anatomical description of the subvastus region and its clinical relevance for the subvastus approach in total knee arthroplasty. *Surg Radiol Anat* 2002;24:6-12.

35. Schroer WC, Diesfeld PJ, Reedy ME, LeMarr AR: Mini-subvastus approach for total knee arthroplasty. *J Arthroplasty* 2008;23:19-25.

36. Schroer WC, Diesfeld PJ, Reedy ME, Lemarr A: Association of increased knee flexion and patella clunk syndrome after mini-subvastus total knee arthroplasty. *J Arthroplasty* 2009;24: 281-287.

37. Boerger TO, Aglietti P, Mondanelli N, Sensi L: Mini-subvastus versus medial parapatellar approach in total knee arthroplasty. *Clin Orthop Relat Res* 2005;440:82-87.

38. Pagnano MW, Meneghini RM: Minimally invasive total knee arthroplasty with an optimized subvastus approach. *J Arthroplasty* 2006;21:22-26.

39. Seyler TM, Bonutti PM, Ulrich SD, Fatscher T, Marker DR, Mont MA: Minimally invasive lateral approach to total knee arthroplasty. *J Arthroplasty* 2007;22:21-26.

40. Chin PL, Foo LS, Yang KY, Yeo SJ, Lo NN: Randomized controlled trial comparing the radiologic outcomes of conventional and minimally invasive techniques for total knee arthroplasty. *J Arthroplasty* 2007;22:800-806.

Video References

10.1: Bonutti PM, Mont MA, Seyler TM, Plate JF: Video. *Minimally Invasive Total Knee Arthroplasty: The Mini-Midvastus Approach.* Effingham, IL, 2008.

10.2: Bonutti PM, Mont MA, Seyler TM, Plate JF: Video. *Minimally Invasive Total Knee Arthroplasty: The Mini-Subvastus Approach.* Effingham, IL, 2008.

Avoiding Pitfalls in Minimally Invasive Total Knee Arthroplasty

Alfred J. Tria Jr, MD

Abstract

Minimally invasive total knee arthroplasty started in the early 1990s with the introduction of unicondylar knee arthroplasty using a limited surgical incision. The techniques were initially received with remarkable enthusiasm; however, enthusiasm waned when results were compromised by the limited visibility of the approaches. Minimally invasive total knee arthroplasty can produce better early results than the traditional approach and can increase the final range of motion of the knee. The techniques are somewhat demanding, and the results can be improved with more careful patient selection, a thorough review of the preoperative radiographs, appropriate choice of the prosthesis, strict attention to the surgical technique, and an aggressive postoperative rehabilitation program.

Instr Course Lect 2010;59:93-97.

Minimally invasive total knee arthroplasty (TKA) dates back to the early 1990s when unicondylar knee arthroplasty was first performed using a limited incision.[1,2] This was followed by approaches to TKA that decreased the length of the skin incision and the incision into the extensor mechanism.[2-8] The initial enthusiasm for the procedures was tempered when it became evident that the operations were not simple procedures and required more surgical time and more extensive surgical skills.[9-12] Some authors also reported that changes in the protocols for the perioperative management of the patient led to benefits that were unrelated to the modifications in surgical technique.[13,14]

Avoiding complications with minimally invasive TKA involve careful attention to patient selection, radiographic evaluation, the selection of the prosthetic device, the surgical technique, and the rehabilitation program. A problem in any of these five areas can compromise surgical results. It is possible to achieve excellent results with the newer, limited surgical approaches, but patients must be carefully selected, and the surgery must be performed in a meticulous manner.

Dr. Tria or an immediate family member has received royalties from Zimmer and serves as a paid consultant to or is an employee of Smith & Nephew IMP.

Five Factors That Influence Outcomes

Patient Selection

The patient should be well motivated and understand the chosen procedure. Most surgeons have an associated protocol for the procedure; the patient should understand the goals. These protocols are used for all patients undergoing TKA and are not unique to minimally invasive TKA surgery. The surgeon should explain the chosen surgical technique and the possibilities that it will be modified or abandoned depending on the progress of the procedure in the operating room. The goal is a successful, well-aligned implant that will have long-term survival.

On physical examination, the patient should weigh less than 225 lb and should have a range of motion of at least 105° with no more than 10° of varus, 15° of valgus, or 10° of knee flexion contracture. Passively correctable deformity is ideal.[7] The weight limitation is somewhat arbitrary. Simple weight and body mass index have not proved entirely helpful in determining appropriate candidates for the minimally invasive approach; the overall appearance of the lower limb is the most

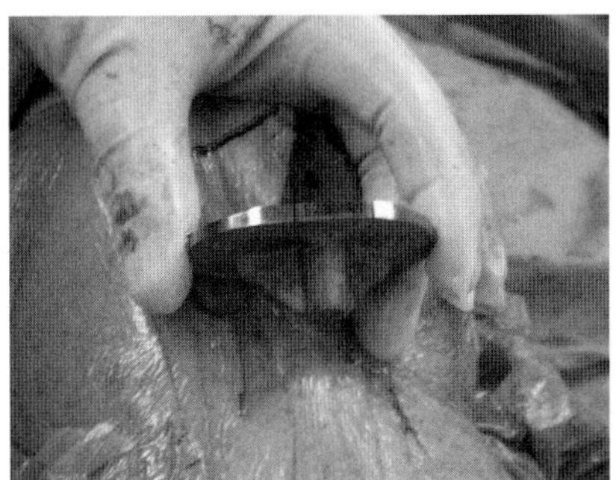

Figure 1 A tibial component designed with an abbreviated intramedullary stem for ease of insertion with a limited surgical approach.

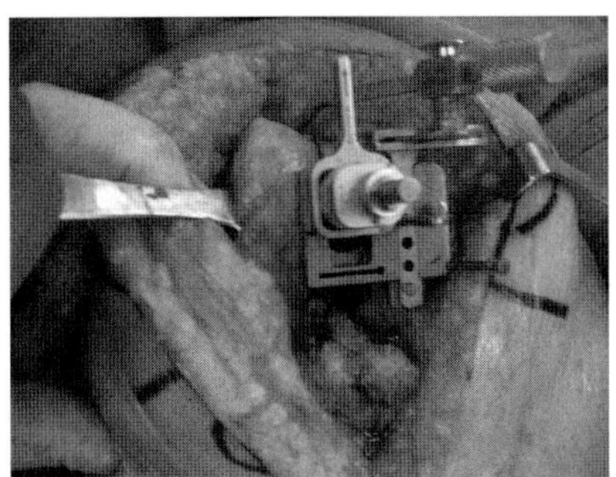

Figure 3 A standard intramedullary femoral cutting guide that has been cut down on one side; the anterior cortical probe is also abbreviated.

important finding. The author of this chapter has used a clinical ratio of the length of the thigh (measured from the anterior superior iliac spine of the pelvis to the middle of the patella with the patient supine) divided by the circumference of the knee at the level of the midpatella. If this ratio is greater than 2.5, it will be easier to treat the knee with minimally invasive TKA.

Previous arthrotomy incisions, osteotomies, and inflammatory arthritis are relative contraindications. A medial or lateral thrust of the femur on the tibia through the stance phase of gait correlates with laxity of the ligaments and helps to improve visualization because the exposure is easier with ligamentous laxity.

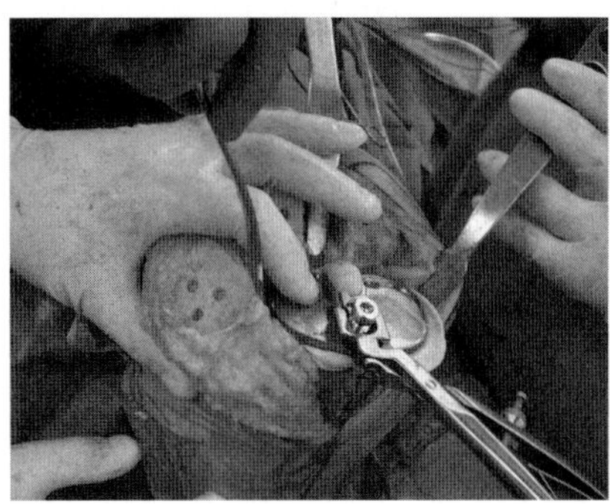

Figure 2 A tibial component with a stem that is screwed through the base plate for use with a limited incision. The extended exposure with patella eversion shown here was used in the early development of the prosthesis.

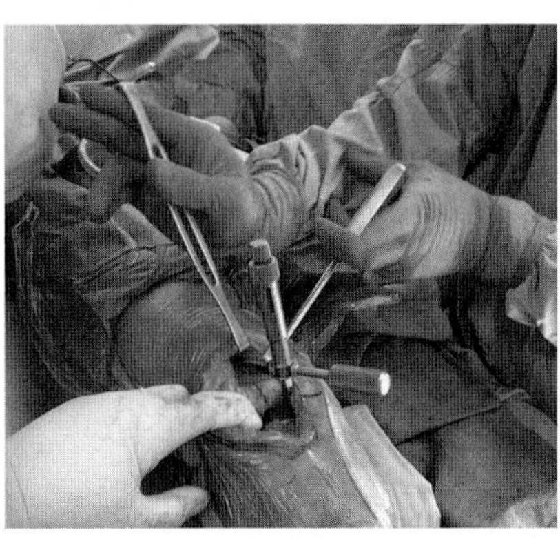

Figure 4 A femoral guide that is designed specifically for minimally invasive knee surgery and references the anterior cortex in 30° of knee flexion.

Radiographic Evaluation

The radiographic evaluation should include a standard weight-bearing AP view, ideally full length, to identify the mechanical axis of the limb. A lateral radiograph will identify the preexisting tibial slope, and a skyline radiograph will indicate any patellofemoral malalignment. The radiographic deformities should correlate with the physical examination and should not exceed the previously outlined limits. Patella baja is a relative contraindication because exposing the lateral aspect of the knee is more difficult.

Choice of Prosthesis

The surgeon should choose a familiar prosthesis so that the surgery is as simple as possible. There are minimally invasive tibial components that can facilitate the surgery (Figure 1). Some tibiae have shortened intramedullary stems that help to decrease the overall component size without compromising biomechanical stability. Other tibiae are modular with a limited tray and an attachable intramedullary stem (Figure 2). The latter design adds extra interfaces but thus far has not led to increased debris in the knee.[9] Ideally, the surgeon should implant a standard TKA design and manipulate the soft tissues to accept it.

Surgery

The pitfalls in the surgical procedure can be analyzed with respect to the exposure, the instruments, the prosthetic insertion, and the closure.

The surgical approach leads to the greatest number of complications—the surgeon's experience and the ability to visualize the entire joint are the limiting factors. As the surgical exposure is decreased, it is often helpful to use modified instruments that are designed for smaller incisions. If used, the surgeon should be familiar with the modified instruments before proceeding. Some instruments are standard designs that have merely been abbreviated (Figure 3); other instruments are completely new and require a change in the actual surgical technique (Figure 4).

There are four major surgical techniques: the limited medial parapatellar, the mini-midvastus, the subvastus, and the quadriceps muscle-sparing approaches.[3,4,6,9] The limited medial parapatellar arthrotomy is the most familiar and easiest technique. Some authors have reported that limiting the quadriceps incision to 4 cm above the patella enables the use of a smaller skin incision and achieves results that rival those of other approaches. Scuderi and associates[4] reported a decrease in blood loss and no decrease in accuracy compared with TKA using a longer standard approach. Tanavalee and associates[15] found that a 2-cm incision into the quadriceps tendon produced results that were equal to other limited approaches; however, further extension of the incision achieved results more like those of the standard approach. The medial incision can be completed without everting the patella and limits injury to the extensor mechanism. Floren and associates[16] reported that patellar eversion leads to patella baja and a less desirable result. All of the limited approaches emphasize the treatment of the extension mechanism while avoiding patellar eversion. The medial approach is a good introduction to limited incision TKA and can be performed with a skin incision of approximately 12 cm in length. The increased amount of soft tissue about the knee makes patellar subluxation difficult, and it is difficult to see the lateral side of the knee, especially the posterolateral aspect of the tibia. This limitation can lead to inadequate cementing and subsequent loosening of the tibial implant.

The mini-midvastus, the most popular approach, has an extensive history in the literature. An early description of the approach by Engh and associates[17] reviewed the possibility of denervation of the distal portion of the vastus medialis and suggested that the incision be limited to the lower one third of the muscle, which would preserve the innervation posteriorly. The revised approach of Laskin and associates[8] limited the length of the incision into the muscle and is called the mini-midvastus approach. The two major complications of this approach are denervation and hematoma. A denervated muscle can lead to medial quadriceps weakness and lateral patellar subluxation because of muscle imbalance. The hematoma can be the result of an extended incision into the muscle that violates the penetrating vessels posteriorly. The resultant swelling cannot be surgically evacuated because it spreads within the medial muscle fibers, which can result in increased pain and subsequent loss of range of motion after the TKA. If the swelling occurs in the first few days after surgery, the knee should be iced, and aggressive physical therapy should be started to maintain motion.

The limited subvastus approach is the only approach that truly avoids invasion of the quadriceps muscle and can be called a quadriceps muscle-sparing approach. The original description by Hofmann and associates[18] in the early 1990s used a standard skin incision. Other authors have evaluated the limited subvastus approach in association with a limited skin incision and a limited incision beneath the muscle. Aglietti and associates[12] recognized the benefits of the approach but believed that it was too difficult and time consuming in the operating room. Pagnano and Meneghini[6] were more supportive of the approach and believed that it could be applied to nearly all patients. Lifting the quadriceps muscle over the anterior aspect of the femur is difficult in an obese patient, and a hematoma can occur if the subvastus incision is extended proximately to facilitate the exposure. If there is a preexisting patella baja, this approach is difficult and the exposure of the posterolateral aspect of the knee can be compromised.

The quadriceps muscle-sparing approach is the most limited and difficult of the approaches because of its steep learning curve for surgeons using the procedure; however, documented evidence shows improvement in early results and long-term range of motion.[9,19,20] The approach extends from the superior pole of the patella to 2 cm beneath the level of the joint line. The name "quadriceps muscle-sparing" is not anatomically correct because the arthrotomy incision does separate the insertion of the vastus medialis from the medial aspect of the patella. The approach limits visualization of the joint and makes prosthetic insertion difficult. The minimally invasive tibial components with abbreviated stems can facilitate prosthetic insertion but are not typically necessary if the correct patient is chosen for the procedure. The main complication of the surgery is component malalignment with subsequent prosthetic loosening, which is most common on the tibial side. On occasion, the components may be well aligned, but loosening can occur because of difficulty in cementing the tibial tray with poor mantle coverage at the posterolateral tibial surface (Figure 5). This approach should be used with careful evaluation of the knee. It is best suited for patients with a lower than average body mass index, with range of motion greater than 110°, with deformity less than 10° in all planes, and with a mobile extensor mechanism. The surgeon should have some experience with the approach and facility with the surgical instruments.

All of the limited approaches are facilitated with smaller instruments.[21] The best instruments are

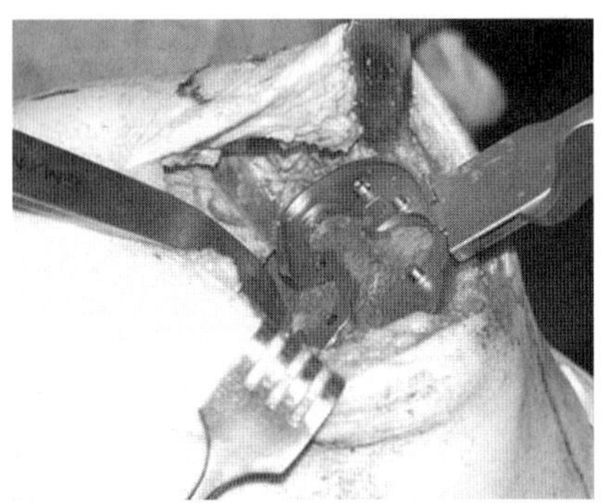

Figure 5 A quadriceps muscle-sparing exposure can be used to visualize the posterolateral side of the tibia for proper positioning and cementing.

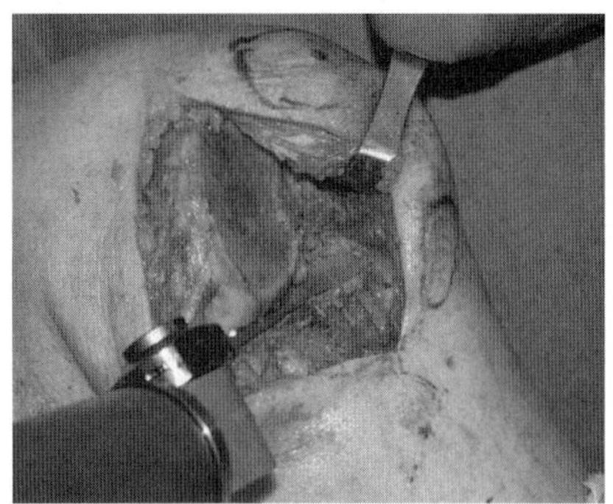

Figure 6 The quadriceps muscle-sparing incision is moved medially as a mobile window for exposing the tibial plateau resection.

those that are modified from traditional instruments as opposed to completely new designs that may introduce another element to the learning curve. The margins of the skin should be protected at all times, and the incision should be moved as a mobile window to visualize each area of the knee as it becomes necessary (Figure 6). The retractors should be modified so that the overall size is reduced for easy insertion into the wound.

The implants should be inserted with proper retraction so that alignment can be confirmed. If there is any compromise in the exposure, the arthrotomy should be extended as necessary. The components can be cementless or cemented designs. The cement is easier to work with if it has a short liquid phase and a longer doughy phase, such as Palacos bone cement (Zimmer, Warsaw, IN). These properties allow more time for insertion and positioning of the implant. The cement should be placed on the cut tibial surface, not on the implant surface, because this assures a more uniform mantle. When the implant is fully seated, it is critical to confirm that the cement extravasates outward from beneath all margins. This extravasation assures that the cement mantle is uniform.

The femoral component is easier to insert than the tibial component with either a cementless or cemented design. The cement can be used on either the bone surface or the implant with little difference in the surgical result.

The closure of the arthrotomy and the skin incision should proceed in a normal fashion if the soft tissues have been respected throughout the surgical procedure. This can be completed either in full extension or flexion depending on the surgeon's preference. The position of the closure does not appear to affect the clinical result.

Rehabilitation

Many surgeons believe that the accelerated recovery and benefits of minimally invasive procedures are associated with changes in the rehabilitation protocol and modifications in pain management rather than with the surgical approach itself. Ranawat and Ranawat[13] reported accelerated recovery and decreased pain with a combination of regional anesthesia, preemptive analgesia, nerve blocks, and local periarticular injections. Dorr and associates[14] reported improved results with a multimodal analgesic protocol and avoided parenteral narcotics. These regimens are helpful but also have associated complications, including hypotension, pruritus, quadriceps muscle weakness, and emesis. Each protocol should be designed for the particular patient, hospital setting, and surgical approach.

Conclusions

All minimally invasive TKA approaches have reported benefits to the patient in the early postoperative period; however, complications and shortcomings can compromise the results. Kolisek and associates[22] reported on 80 knees treated with TKA and found delayed wound healing in 4 knees treated with a minimally invasive approach and 1 knee treated with a standard approach. Outcomes were otherwise the same, leading the authors to conclude that the minimally invasive approach did not have a significant benefit. Laskin and associates[8] did not report significant complications with the mini-midvastus approach but reported that patients were individually selected for the minimally invasive procedure. Bonutti and associates[23] reported that in 17 revision TKAs treated with a minimally invasive approach, there was only 1 complication involving retained cement. Chen and associates[9] reported on the quadriceps muscle-sparing approach and described an increase in outliers in patients treated with the minimally invasive approach (13 versus 5 for the standard TKA). Haas and associates[24] reported on 391 knees treated with the mini-midvastus approach and found no increase in the complication rate.

Most of the reports on minimally invasive techniques are from surgeons who designed the approaches and have extensive surgical experience. Their complication rates are not significantly higher than those of surgeons using traditional TKA; however, it may not be appropriate for all surgeons to adopt these techniques and expect similar results.

Summary

Minimally invasive TKA is a surgical technique that can improve the clinical result of standard knee replacement surgery. There are four different approaches, each with its own benefits and disadvantages. It is important to maximize the opportunity for a successful outcome with appropriate patient selection, a thorough review of radiographic studies, the selection of an appropriate prosthetic design, strict attention to surgical technique, and an aggressive rehabilitation program.

References

1. Repicci JA, Eberle RW: Minimally invasive surgical technique for unicondylar knee arthroplasty. *J South Orthop Assoc* 1999;8:20-27.
2. Romanowski MR, Repicci JA: Minimally invasive unicondylar arthroplasty: Eight-year follow-up. *J Knee Surg* 2002;15:17-22.
3. Haas SB, Cook S, Beksac B: Minimally invasive total knee replacement through a mini midvastus approach. *Clin Orthop Relat Res* 2004;428:68-73.
4. Scuderi GR, Tenholder M, Capeci C: Surgical approaches in mini-incision total knee arthroplasty. *Clin Orthop Relat Res* 2004;428:61-67.
5. Scuderi GR, Tria AJ Jr: Minimal incision total knee arthroplasty. *Tech Knee Surg* 2004;3:97-104.
6. Pagnano MW, Meneghini RM: Minimally invasive total knee arthroplasty with an optimized subvastus approach. *J Arthroplasty* 2006;21 (suppl 4):22-26.
7. Tria AJ Jr, Coon TM: Minimal incision TKA: Early experience. *Clin Orthop Relat Res* 2003;416:185-190.
8. Laskin RS, Beksac B, Phongjunakorn A, et al: Minimally invasive total knee replacement through a mini-midvastus incision: An outcome study. *Clin Orthop Relat Res* 2004;428: 74-81.
9. Chen AF, Alan RK, Redziniak DE, Tria AJ Jr: Quadriceps sparing total knee replacement. *J Bone Joint Surg Br* 2006;88:1448-1453.
10. Dalury DF, Dennis DA: Mini-incision total knee arthroplasty can increase risk of component malalignment. *Clin Orthop Relat Res* 2005;440: 77-81.
11. Aglietti P, Baldini A, Giron F, Sensi L: Minimally invasive total knee arthroplasty: Is it for everybody? *HSS J* 2006;2:22-26.
12. Aglietti P, Baldini A, Sensi L: Quadriceps-sparing versus mini-subvastus approach in total knee arthroplasty. *Clin Orthop Relat Res* 2006; 452:106-111.
13. Ranawat AS, Ranawat CS: Pain management and accelerated rehabilitation for total hip and total knee arthroplasty. *J Arthroplasty* 2007;22 (7, suppl 3):12-15.
14. Dorr LD, Raya J, Long WT, Boutary M, Sirianni LE: Multimodal analgesia without parenteral narcotics for total knee arthroplasty. *J Arthroplasty* 2008;23:502-508.
15. Tanavalee A, Thiengwittayaporn S, Itiravivong P: Progressive quadriceps incision during minimally invasive surgery for total knee arthroplasty: The effect on early postoperative ambulation. *J Arthroplasty* 2007;22:1013-1018.
16. Floren M, Davis J, Peterson MG, Laskin RS: A mini-midvastus capsular approach with patellar displacement decreases the prevalence of patella baja. *J Arthroplasty* 2007;22 (6 suppl 2):51-57.
17. Engh GA, Holt BT, Parks NL: A midvastus muscle-splitting approach for total knee arthroplasty. *J Arthroplasty* 1997;12:322-331.
18. Hofmann AA, Plaster RL, Murdock LE: Subvastus (southern) approach for primary total knee arthroplasty. *Clin Orthop Relat Res* 1991;269: 70-77.
19. King J, Stamper DL, Schaad DC, Leopold SS: Minimally invasive total knee arthroplasty compared with traditional total knee arthroplasty: Assessment of the learning curve and the postoperative recuperative period. *J Bone Joint Surg Am* 2007;89:1497-1503.
20. Huang HT, Su JY, Chang JK, Chen CH, Wang GJ: The early clinical outcome of minimally invasive quadriceps-sparing total knee arthroplasty: Report of a 2-year follow-up. *J Arthroplasty* 2007;22:1007-1012.
21. Tria AJ Jr: The importance of instrumentation. *Orthop Clin North Am* 2004;35:227-234.
22. Kolisek FR, Bonutti PM, Hozack WJ, et al: Clinical experience using a minimally invasive surgical approach for total knee arthroplasty: Early results of a prospective randomized study compared to a standard approach. *J Arthroplasty* 2007;22:8-13.
23. Bonutti PM, Seyler TM, Kester M, McMahon M, Mont MA: Minimally invasive revision total knee arthroplasty. *Clin Orthop Relat Res* 2006;446: 69-75.
24. Haas SB, Manitta MA, Burdick P: Minimally invasive total knee arthroplasty: The mini midvastus approach. *Clin Orthop Relat Res* 2006;452: 112-116.

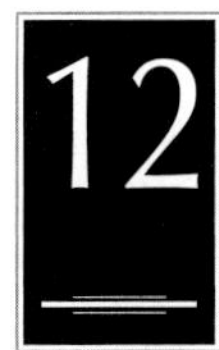

Contemporary Pain Management Strategies for Minimally Invasive Total Knee Arthroplasty

Aaron J. Krych, MD
Terese T. Horlocker, MD
James R. Hebl, MD
Mark W. Pagnano, MD

Abstract

The introduction of minimally invasive total knee arthroplasty has been accompanied by substantial changes in anesthesia and analgesia techniques. It is well recognized that the goals of minimally invasive surgery, which include rapid rehabilitation and improved patient function, cannot be achieved without excellent postoperative analgesia. Traditional postoperative pain management has been associated with high rates of suboptimal pain control, however. The conventional options for early postsurgical pain management include indwelling epidural catheters, which require changes in postoperative prophylaxis for thromboembolism, and patient-controlled analgesia pumps, which are associated with fluctuating pain levels and inconsistent pain relief. Numerous adverse effects are associated with traditional opioid medications, including respiratory depression, urinary retention, nausea, sedation, constipation, and pruritus. Safe, effective, and well-tolerated early pain relief after a minimally invasive knee replacement can be accomplished using a multimodal oral pain regimen, peripheral nerve blocks, and local injections.

Instr Course Lect 2010;59:99-109.

The long-term beneficial effects of total knee arthroplasty (TKA) are restoration of mobility and function, relief of disabling joint pain, and improved quality of life.[1] The goal is to allow patients the most rapid and effective rehabilitation and recovery possible, but achieving this goal has been difficult with traditional surgical techniques. TKA generates intense early postoperative pain, and effective analgesia is vital. Some researchers report less postoperative pain with the more recent minimally invasive techniques, including the subvastus approach, than with the traditional medial parapatellar approach.[2] Optimal analgesia remains a key to controlling a patient's pain.

The introduction of minimally invasive knee techniques has been accompanied by substantial improvements in anesthesia and analgesia techniques, rapid rehabilitation protocols, and changes in patient education and expectations. The optimal method for analgesia following a minimally invasive TKA maximizes pain control while minimizing narcotic adverse effects. One such method is a multimodal pathway that centers on nerve blocks and is augmented by oral analgesics and local periarticular injections placed at the time of surgery. The concept of multimodal analgesia is receiving increasing attention.[3-5] In one study, the incidence of arthrofibrosis re-

Neither Dr. Krych nor an immediate family member has received anything of value from or own stock in a commercial company or institution related directly or indirectly to the subject of this chapter. Dr. Horlocker or an immediate family member has received nonincome support (such as equipment or services), commercially derived honoraria, or other non–research-related funding (such as paid travel) from Anesthesia and Analgesia. Dr. Hebl or an immediate family member serves as a board member, owner, officer, or committee member of the Minnesota Society of Anesthesiologists. Dr. Pagnano or an immediate family member has received royalties from DePuy and Zimmer and has received research or institutional support from DePuy, the Musculoskeletal Transplant Foundation, the National Institutes of Health (National Institute of Arthritis, Musculoskeletal and Skin Diseases; National Institute of Child Health and Human Development), Stryker, and Zimmer.

Table 1
Intravenous Opioids for PCA

Agent (Standard Concentration)*	Bolus Dosage	Lockout Interval	4-Hour Maximum Dosage	Infusion Rate (per Hour)†
Fentanyl (10 μg/mL)	10-20 μg	5-10 min	300 μg	20-100 μg
Hydromorphone (0.2 mg/mL)	0.1-0.2 mg	5-10 min	3 mg	0.1-0.2 mg
Morphine sulfate (1 mg/mL)	0.5-2.5 mg	5-10 min	30 mg	1-20 mg

*Meperidine is no longer considered an appropriate opioid for perioperative analgesia because of inconsistent analgesic effect and high toxicity.
†A background infusion rate is not recommended for opioid-naïve patients.
(Adapted with permission from the Mayo Foundation for Medical Education and Research, Rochester, MN.)

quiring manipulation decreased from 4.75% with the traditional pain control approach to 2.24% with multimodal pain management.[6]

Traditional Analgesic Methods

Traditional postoperative pain management includes neuraxial analgesia with indwelling epidural catheters and parenteral opioid analgesia with patient-controlled analgesia (PCA) pumps. The primary advantage of both methods is their simplicity and ease of implementation. However, these conventional methods can have adverse effects, and studies have found that most patients receive suboptimal pain control.[7]

Neuraxial Analgesia

Neuraxial analgesia is provided using a spinal or epidural technique and a single-dose or continuous infusion. Adverse effects may be more common and more prolonged with neuraxial analgesia than with systemic opioids.[8] In a study of almost 6,000 patients who had neuraxial analgesia, the frequency of pruritus was 37%; nausea and vomiting, 25%; and respiratory depression, 3%.[9] A systematic Cochrane review of 14 studies with almost 600 patients found no difference between epidural and systemic analgesia in the frequency of nausea and vomiting or respiratory depression.[10] Urinary retention, pruritus, and hypotension were more frequent with epidural analgesia, but sedation was less frequent. Compared with systemic analgesia, epidural analgesia was associated with lower at-rest pain scores 4 to 6 hours after surgery and lower scores with ambulation or leg movement 18 to 24 hours after surgery.

The most important limitation of an indwelling epidural catheter for postoperative analgesia is that it cannot be used when the patient is receiving low-molecular-weight heparin, warfarin, or fondaparinux for the prevention of deep venous thrombosis. The use of an epidural catheter with low-molecular-weight heparin for thromboprophylaxis was found to increase by as much as 50 times the risk of epidural hematoma and irreversible nerve damage.[11-13] Current anesthesia management guidelines recommend removal of an epidural catheter before initiation of thromboprophylaxis with low-molecular-weight heparin or fondaparinux.[14]

Parenteral Opioids

Systemic opioids can be delivered intravenously, intramuscularly, or orally. The most common regimen is to use intravenous PCA with a later transition to oral opioids. The PCA pump can be programmed for a bolus dose, a lockout interval, a maximal dosage, and an infusion rate (Table 1).

Achieving adequate pain control with parenteral opioids alone often requires a dosage large enough to cause substantial adverse effects, including sedation, nausea, and pruritus, all of which undermine the patient's recovery from surgery. The level of pain control varies, even with customized settings; some patients are undermedicated, some are overmedicated, and the level of pain control fluctuates in others. The result is a moderate or severe pain score with ambulation during the first 2 days after surgery.[10,15] In a systematic review, gastrointestinal adverse effects including nausea, ileus, and vomiting were found to be present in 37% of patients; cognitive adverse effects such as disorientation and somnolence, in 34%; urinary retention, in 16%; pruritus, in 15%; and respiratory depression, in 2%.[16]

The Multimodal Analgesic Regimen

Peripheral Nerve Block

Peripheral nerve blocks often are underused, but they can be considered the hallmark of the comprehensive anesthesia protocol.[3] Lower extremity blocks are technically difficult because the nerves supplying the lower extremity are not clustered as they are in the brachial plexus. These blocks traditionally have been done using loss of resistance, paresthesias, or field block techniques, with variable success. However, advances in nerve-stimulating needles and ultrasonography have made the localization of neural structures more reliable and nerve block techniques more reproducible.[17] The unilateral nature of peripheral nerve blocks makes them ideal for use after minimally invasive TKA because patients can use the contralateral limb for ambulation during the early postoperative period.

The recent application of peripheral nerve block techniques in conjunction with an indwelling peripheral catheter has allowed prolonged and effective postoperative analgesia.[3,4,15] Two studies suggested that patients who receive a continuous femoral nerve block or epidural anesthesia have lower pain scores, earlier ambulation, better knee flexion, and shorter hospital stays than patients who receive PCA with intravenous morphine.[15,18] In both studies the preferred analgesic method was the continuous femoral nerve block because it is simple to use and has fewer adverse effects than the epidural nerve block. In two other studies, the continuous-infusion femoral nerve block also was associated with significant improvement in knee flexion and earlier ambulation when compared with a placebo or no treatment.[19,20] The primary risks associated with peripheral nerve blocks are neurologic dysfunction and inadvertent intravascular injection. In a study of more than 50,000 peripheral blocks, only 12 nerve injures were reported (0.02%), and most of the complications were transient.[21]

The lumbar plexus can be blocked for minimally invasive TKA through a psoas, femoral, or fascia iliaca approach. The psoas blockade anesthetizes the entire lumbar plexus (the femoral, obturator, and lateral femoral cutaneous nerves).[22] The femoral and fascia iliaca blockades reliably anesthetize the femoral nerve but not the obturator or lateral femoral cutaneous nerves.[22] Both femoral and obturator peripheral nerve blocks may be helpful in providing pain relief following TKA. Kardash and associates[23] found that a single-injection femoral block improved analgesia after spinal anesthesia, but an obturator nerve block alone was of no benefit to patients. A complete unilateral lower extremity block can be obtained by combining a lumbar plexus technique with a sciatic nerve block.

Regional anesthesia is preferred for minimally invasive TKA, using the distal femoral (Figure 1) or fascia iliaca (Figure 2) approach. A sciatic block is a useful supplement because it blocks sensation to the posterior thigh and leg, except for the saphenous nerve distribution (Figure 3), and it ensures blocking of the posterior femoral cutaneous nerve, which is beneficial immediately after TKA, when posterior knee pain is common. If a supplemental sciatic block cannot be done, an additional local periarticular injection is recommended for blocking the posterior structures.

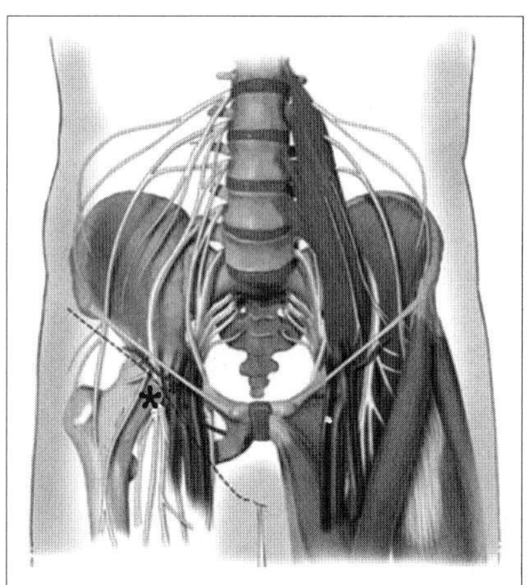

Figure 1 The femoral nerve block. The needle is inserted 1 to 2 cm lateral to the femoral arterial pulsation at the level of the inguinal crease. A 5-cm needle is advanced until a quadriceps response is noted, and 25 mL of local anesthetic is incrementally injected. Asterisk = the femoral nerve, dashed line = the inguinal crease. (Adapted with permission from the Mayo Foundation for Medical Education and Research, Rochester, MN.)

Local Periarticular Injection

The local delivery of analgesia directly to the surgical area is an appealing method of controlling postoperative pain with minimal systemic adverse effects. However, the true efficacy of locally injected analgesics after knee surgery remains controversial. Continuous infusion of bupivacaine and opioids was shown to provide effective pain control but caused prolonged knee drainage in a significant number of patients.[24] Two retrospective studies found that intra-articular injections were of equivocal benefit.[25,26] Other studies found that a periarticular injection of local analgesics following knee surgery not only reduced postoperative analgesia requirements but also led to earlier hospital discharge.[27-29] Two prospective, randomized studies supported these findings.[30,31] Of 64 patients who underwent TKA with a standard medial parapatellar approach, those who received injected epinephrine, epimorphine (an opioid), ketorolac (a nonsteroidal anti-inflammatory drug [NSAID]), and ropivacaine (a long-acting local anesthetic) were found to use significantly less PCA at 6, 12, and 24 hours after surgery than patients in the control group. In addition, the patients who re-

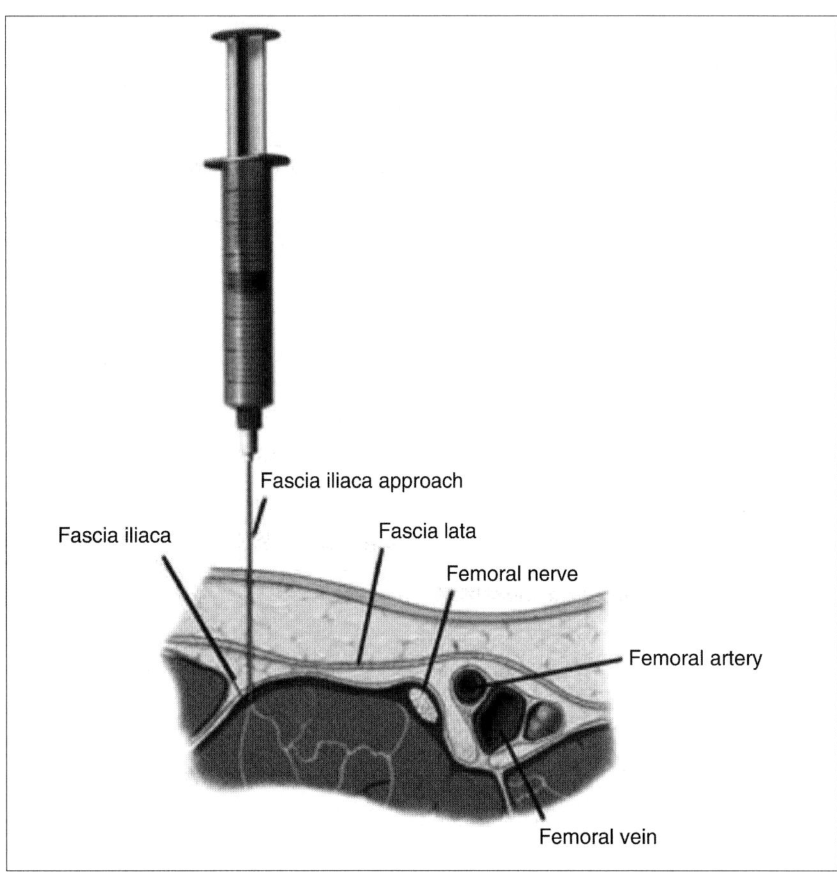

Figure 2 The fascia iliaca approach to femoral nerve block. The inguinal ligament is identified, the junction of its lateral one third with its medial two thirds is determined, and a 17-gauge Tuohy needle is inserted 1 cm below this point. An initial loss of resistance is noted as the needle penetrates the fascia lata, and a second loss of resistance is felt as the needle penetrates the fascia iliaca; 30 mL of local anesthetic is incrementally injected. (Adapted with permission from the Mayo Foundation for Medical Education and Research, Rochester, MN.)

ceived the injections had significantly lower pain scores and higher satisfaction scores. No toxicity or adverse effects were observed. The injections were into the posterior capsule and collateral ligaments just before implantation of the component, into the retinacular tissues and quadriceps mechanism during cement curing, and finally into the fat and subcutaneous tissues.[30] A similar injection protocol can be used for minimally invasive TKA with a subvastus approach.

Similar findings were reported in a prospective study of 60 patients who underwent TKA and were randomly assigned to receive a periarticular injection of bupivacaine, morphine sulfate, epinephrine, methylprednisolone acetate, cefuroxime, and normal saline; or PCA with a femoral block.[31] The group receiving the intraoperative injection had less narcotic usage, fewer adverse effects, and better early functional recovery. The researchers concluded that the use of a combination of pharmacologic agents with different mechanisms of action results in superior pain control with fewer adverse effects. They also suggested that administering the injection before the height of the physiologic pain response is important for preemptive analgesia.

Other studies support the synergistic effect of a pharmacologic cocktail. Morphine has analgesic properties through its effect on opioid receptors. Opioid receptors are present in inflamed peripheral tissues[32] and are expressed hours after surgical trauma through afferent sensory input to the central nervous system.[33] Locally administered morphine has been shown to reduce pain after TKA.[34] NSAIDs such as ketorolac inhibit the eicosanoid pathway that produces the inflammatory mediators causing peripheral sensitization and activation of nociceptors.[35] The use of long-acting local anesthetics such as ropivacaine allows the administration of larger doses with less cardiac and central nervous system toxicity because of more favorable pharmacodynamic enantioselectivity than with short-acting local anesthetics.[36] By decreasing systemic absorption, epinephrine, with its α-adrenergic–mediated vasoconstriction, reduces the toxicity of the local anesthetic and prolongs the action of the local agents;[37] in addition, it may decrease postoperative bleeding and hematoma.[31] Corticosteroids are well known for their local anti-inflammatory effects and are often used in intra-articular injections. A negative effect on wound healing has not been reported, although it is a theoretic concern.[38] If local periarticular injections are used in combination with peripheral nerve blocks and spinal anesthesia, it is important to avoid exceeding the recommended total dosage. However, there is some controversy about these dosages.[39]

The Multimodal Oral Pain Regimen

The use of both nonopioid and opioid medications has been affected by advances in the multimodal oral analgesic regimen for minimally invasive TKA. Many adverse effects of analgesics are related to the systemic administration of opioids and specifically to the dosage. These adverse effects are among the most important factors in patient satisfaction during the postoperative hospital stay.[40] Therefore, a guiding principle of the multimodal approach is to limit the use of all opioids (and of parenteral opioids in particular). The use of nonopioid analgesics decreases the likelihood of adverse effects, especially nausea and vomiting. The multimodal effect is maximized by selecting analgesics that have complementary mechanisms of action, and a multimodal regimen has been shown to improve the overall level of analgesia.

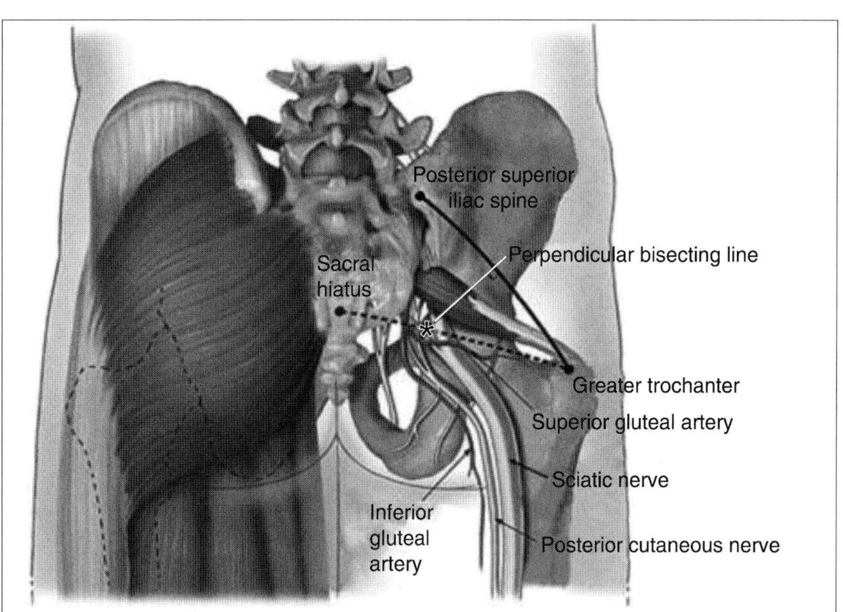

Figure 3 The classic posterior approach to sciatic nerve block. The needle insertion (asterisk) is 5 cm along the perpendicular line (white line) that bisects a line connecting the greater trochanter and posterosuperior iliac spine (black line). The needle insertion is confirmed by the intersection of the perpendicular bisecting line and a second line connecting the greater trochanter and sacral hiatus (black dashed line). A 10-cm stimulating needle is advanced until a tibial or peroneal motor response is elicited, then 20 to 30 mL of local anesthetic is incrementally injected. Light dashed lines = underlying osseous anatomy, light solid lines = gluteal fold. (Adapted with permission from the Mayo Foundation for Medical Education and Research, Rochester, MN.)

The nonopioid analgesics are acetaminophen, the NSAIDs, and tramadol (Table 2). Acetaminophen is believed to act primarily by inhibiting prostaglandin synthesis in the central nervous system, although the exact mechanism has never been fully elucidated. Acetaminophen has very few adverse affects if the daily dosage is limited to 4,000 mg. To maximize the analgesic effect, acetaminophen should be given on a scheduled, rather than an as-needed, basis. Many opioid preparations include acetaminophen. However, the opioid dose that can be administered through such a preparation is limited by the allowable acetaminophen dose. To maintain the greatest flexibility in the dosing schedule, it is best to avoid these preparations.

NSAIDs block prostaglandin synthesis through the cyclooxygenase (COX) enzymatic pathways. Both the COX-1 and COX-2 pathways generally are inhibited with NSAID use. The COX-1 pathway is involved in gastric mucosal protection mediated by prostaglandin E_2 and in thromboxane effects on coagulation. Medications that are selective for COX-2 block only the prostaglandins involved in pain and fever; they do not affect platelet function or coagulation and do not cause adverse gastrointestinal and hematologic effects. Perioperative use of a COX-2 inhibitor was shown to reduce opioid consumption, pain, vomiting, and sleep disturbance following TKA,[41] and a significant increase in perioperative bleeding after TKA was not found.[42] COX-2 inhibitors were associated with lower pain scores than a matching placebo as late as 3 days after surgery, and a reliable reduction in supplemental analgesic use was found.[41,43,44] Celecoxib (Celebrex; Pfizer, New York, NY) currently is the only COX-2 inhibitor available in the United States. Other COX-2 medications were withdrawn because of adverse cardiac events after prolonged use. There is no evidence that COX-2 inhibitors have a clinically important effect on bone ingrowth to cementless knee implants after TKA.

Ketorolac is the only NSAID that can be delivered parenterally as well as orally. A 10- to 30-mg parenteral dose was found to have an efficacy similar to that of 10 to 12 mg of intravenous morphine and to be effective in reducing postoperative opi-

Table 2
Oral Nonopioid Analgesics

Analgesic	Oral Dose (mg)	Dosing Interval (Hours)	Maximum Daily Dosage (mg)	Comments
Acetaminophen	500-1,000	4-6	4,000	As effective as aspirin. 1,000 mg may be more effective than 650 mg.
NSAID				
Celecoxib	400 initially, then 200	12	800	The only COX-2 inhibitor available in North America.
Aspirin	325-1,000	4-6	4,000	Has the most potent antiplatelet effect.
Ibuprofen	200-400	4-6	3,200	200 mg are equivalent to 650 mg of aspirin or acetaminophen.
Naproxen	500	12	1,000	250 mg are equivalent to 650 mg of aspirin, with longer duration.
Ketorolac	15-30	4-6	60	15-30 mg are comparable to 10 mg morphine. Lower dosage for patient who weighs less than 50 kg or has renal impairment. Total duration of administration is 5 days. Also can be administered intramuscularly or intravenously.
Tramadol	50-100	6	400*	Tramadol-acetaminophen combination product is available.

*Lower dosage for patient with renal or hepatic disease.
(Adapted with permission from the Mayo Foundation for Medical Education and Research, Rochester, MN.)

oid consumption by 36%.[45] Ketorolac and all other NSAIDs can cause severe renal impairment. Although inhibition of the COX enzyme may have only a minor effect in patients with healthy kidneys, the effect can be serious in patients with low creatinine clearance or volume depletion secondary to blood loss.[42]

Tramadol is a centrally acting analgesic that is structurally related to morphine and codeine. It acts by binding opioid receptors and blocking the reuptake of norepinephrine and serotonin. Adverse effects such as respiratory depression and constipation, as well as the potential for abuse of the drug, are uncommon with tramadol. Nausea is less common than with equivalent opioid medications. However, when tramadol is combined with selective serotonin reuptake inhibitors or tricyclic antidepressants, the seizure threshold is decreased. Therefore, tramadol should be avoided in patients taking a selective serotonin reuptake inhibitor or a tricyclic antidepressant.

The oral opioid analgesics include extended-release oxycodone, extended-release morphine, oxycodone, hydromorphone, hydrocodone, and codeine (Table 3). The adverse effects of oral opioids are substantially less than those of intravenous opioids; nausea or vomiting and constipation are the most common. Controlled-release oxycodone may be useful for opioid-tolerant patients who have substantial postoperative pain. When administered postoperatively, controlled-release oxycodone improves analgesia and is associated with less opioid-associated bowel dysfunction than oxycodone administered on an as-needed basis.[46]

A multimodal regimen designed to maximize analgesia and decrease adverse effects could include scheduled administration of controlled-release oxycodone combined with as-needed administration of oxycodone for breakthrough pain. When a combination of a continuous peripheral nerve block and a multimodal oral regimen was used, with no intravenous opioids, 90% of patients were ready for hospital discharge 48 hours after minimally invasive TKA.[3]

Preemptive Analgesia

Preemptive analgesia is administered before noxious stimuli begin, and it is important to overall pain control during TKA. Surgical trauma changes the responsiveness of the central nervous system by increasing the excitability of spinal neurons and reducing the threshold for afferent nociceptive neurons. These modifications together contribute to postoperative pain hypersensitivity by decreasing the pain threshold at both the injured and surrounding uninjured tissue and by increasing the response to unpleasant stimuli. Preemptive analgesia prevents sensitization of the central nervous system and thereby improves postoperative pain control.[47,48]

Animal studies suggest that preemptive analgesia is a powerful adjunct to pain control regimens. However, it is unclear whether preemptive analgesic regimens are more effective than traditional

Table 3
Oral Opioid Analgesics

Analgesic	Oral Dose (mg)	Dosing Interval (Hours)	Comments
Extended-release oxycodone	10-20	12	Should be limited to a total of four doses to avoid accumulation and opioid-related adverse effects.
Extended-release morphine	15-30	8-12	Should be limited to a total of four doses to avoid accumulation and opioid-related adverse effects.
Oxycodone	5-10	4-6	Oxycodone-acetaminophen and oycodone-aspirin combination products are available.
Hydromorphone	2-4	4-6	Also available as a suppository (3 mg) with a 6- to 8-hour effect.
Hydrocodone	5-10	4-6	All preparations contain acetaminophen.
Codeine	30-60	4	Codeine-acetaminophen and codeine-aspirin combination products are available.

(Adapted with permission from the Mayo Foundation for Medical Education and Research, Rochester, MN.)

methods for reducing patients' postoperative pain. A meta-analysis of 66 studies with 3,261 patients found that patients who received preemptive epidural analgesia had decreased total analgesic consumption, more time before the first rescue dose of opioids was administered, and lower postoperative pain scores.[49] The time before the first rescue dose of opioids also was increased when the preemptive analgesic was administered with the local anesthesia and before the skin incision and NSAID administration. Although opioids have less preemptive efficacy than local anesthesia before skin incision and NSAID administration, a study of patients undergoing TKA found that the preemptive use of sustained-release oxycodone led to better pain control than as-needed oxycodone used alone.[50]

Nonpharmacologic Modalities

Some nonpharmacologic measures can be effective in reducing postoperative pain levels when used in addition to a multimodal oral pain regimen, peripheral nerve block, or local injections. A recent prospective, randomized, blinded, placebo-controlled clinical study found that the use of intraoperative music significantly reduced postoperative pain.[51] Two studies found that the use of narcotics decreased when postoperative compression and cooling techniques were used.[52,53] Greater pain relief during the early postoperative period also may be achieved by teaching the patient pain communication skills and providing pain management information before surgery.[54] A prospective, randomized, double-blind study found an association among tourniquet release before suturing, improved postoperative pain control, and earlier quadriceps function.[55]

In contrast, transcutaneous electrical nerve stimulation has not been shown to have a significant effect on postoperative pain control,[56] and multiple studies found that continuous passive motion had no significantly beneficial effect on patients' pain scores after TKA.[57-59]

The Preferred Pain Management Algorithm

The multimodal pain regimen preferred by the senior author (MWP) for minimally invasive TKA is outlined in Table 4. A preoperative discussion is essential for informing the patient of the pain control regimen and the perioperative rehabilitation protocol. Preemptive analgesia, which is administered in the surgical preparation room, includes 10 to 20 mg of oxycodone (OxyContin; Purdue Pharma, Stamford, CT), which often is withheld for patients older than 75 to 80 years; 600 mg of gabapentin; and 400 mg of celecoxib. Nerve blocks also are placed at this time; an indwelling femoral catheter with an additional single-injection sciatic block is most routinely used. For intraoperative anesthesia, a short-acting spinal anesthetic is preferred to a general anesthetic.

If no sciatic block was done, a local periarticular injection with 0.25% bupivacaine is administered just before cementing, preferentially into the posterior structures. Avoiding hematoma formation is critical to postoperative pain control and early rehabilitation. Therefore, the tourniquet is routinely released after cementing, and tranexamic acid is used before the incision and after the tourniquet release to control bleeding; drains are placed, and a compressive dressing and ice are used postoperatively.

Immediately after the patient's arrival in the postanesthesia care unit, a

Table 4
The Preferred Multimodal Regimen for Pain Management in Minimally Invasive TKA

Preemptive analgesia (surgical preparation room)
- Oxycodone (10 to 20 mg by mouth; often withheld for patients older than 75 to 80 years)
- Gabapentin (600 mg by mouth)
- Celecoxib (400 mg by mouth)
- Nerve blocks
  - Femoral catheter
  - Sciatic block

Intraoperative anesthesia
- Spinal anesthesia is preferred to general anesthesia.

Minimally invasive surgical technique
- Local periarticular injection with 0.25% bupivacaine (if no sciatic block was done)
- Tourniquet release after cementing
- Hematoma risk minimized with tranexamic acid, drains, compressive dressing, and postoperative ice

Postoperative analgesia (postanesthesia care unit)
- Peripheral nerve catheter
- Bolus (10 mL) of 0.2% bupivacaine upon arrival in unit
- Continuous infusion of 0.2% bupivacaine (10 mL/h)
- Postoperative day 1: continuous infusion of 0.1% bupivacaine (12 mL/h)

Postoperative analgesia (patient care unit)
- Femoral catheter removed (after a total of 36 to 48 hours)
- Multimodal nonopioid oral regimen
  - Celecoxib (200 mg twice daily)
  - Acetaminophen (1,000 mg every 6 hours [8 am, 2 pm, 8 pm])
  - Tramadol (50-100 mg every 6 hours; tramadol or acetaminophen is administered every 3 hours), as needed for pain
- Oxycodone (5-10 mg by mouth every 4 hours) as needed for breakthrough pain

Patient mobilization as related to pain management
- Sit in chair the evening of surgery.
- Ambulate with toe-touch weight bearing on postoperative day 1.
- Ambulate and climb stairs on postoperative day 2, with weight bearing as tolerated immediately after block is resolved.
- Transfer in and out of bed with minimal help, climb several stairs using walker or crutches, control pain with oral medications; discharge from hospital.

10-mL bolus of 0.2% bupivacaine is administered through the indwelling femoral nerve catheter, and a continuous infusion of 0.2% bupivacaine at 10 mL per hour is initiated. At 6 am the following day (postoperative day 1), 0.1% bupivacaine at 12 mL per hour is substituted in the continuous infusion. The continuous infusion is used for a total of 36 to 48 hours, with the catheter removed on the patient care unit at 6 am of postoperative day 2. The infusion dosage can be gradually decreased over the 36- to 48-hour period to ensure complete resolution of the block before hospital discharge.

With the indwelling femoral nerve catheter, a multimodal oral pain regimen that maximizes nonopioid medications is used. The patient receives 200 mg of celecoxib twice daily by mouth while in the hospital and ideally continuing for a 2-week course. Acetaminophen (1,000 mg) and tramadol (50 to 100 mg) are given alternately every 3 hours by mouth while the patient is awake. Oxycodone (5 to 10 mg) is given every 4 hours by mouth, as needed to control breakthrough pain. With this regimen, most patients have good pain control, and limiting the use of opioids minimizes the risk of adverse effects.

Patients can begin postoperative mobilization by sitting in a chair the evening of the surgery. This practice is believed to preclude the possibility that the physical therapy session scheduled for the next morning will be delayed because of lightheadedness or dizziness. The patient ambulates with toe-touch weight bearing on postoperative day 1, using a walker or crutches to protect against a fall caused by quadriceps weakness from the indwelling femoral nerve catheter. After the block wears off on postoperative day 2, the patient is allowed to ambulate with weight bearing as tolerated and climb stairs. The criteria for discharge are the ability to transfer into and out of bed with minimal help, climb several stairs using a walker or crutches, and to control pain with oral medications. Most patients meet these criteria 48 hours after surgery.

Summary

The introduction of techniques for minimally invasive TKA has been accompanied by substantial changes in techniques for perioperative anesthesia and analgesia. The goal of minimally invasive TKA is rapid rehabilitation, which cannot be achieved without effective postoperative analgesia. The combination of unilateral nerve blocks, local periarticular injections, and a multimodal oral regimen that limits the adverse effects of opioids and provides excellent analgesia is safe for patients and allows them to achieve a rapid rehabilitation.

References

1. Räsänen P, Paavolainen P, Sintonen H, et al: Effectiveness of hip or knee replacement surgery in terms of quality-adjusted life years and costs. *Acta Orthop* 2007;78:108-115.
2. Roysam GS, Oakley MJ: Subvastus approach for total knee arthroplasty: A prospective, randomized, and observer-blinded trial. *J Arthroplasty* 2001;16:454-457.

3. Hebl JR, Kopp SL, Ali MH, et al: A comprehensive anesthesia protocol that emphasizes peripheral nerve blockade for total knee and total hip arthroplasty. *J Bone Joint Surg Am* 2005;87:63-70.

4. Horlocker TT, Kopp SL, Pagnano MW, Hebl JR: Analgesia for total hip and knee arthroplasty: A multimodal pathway featuring peripheral nerve block. *J Am Acad Orthop Surg* 2006;14:126-135.

5. Vendittoli PA, Makinen P, Drolet P, et al: A multimodal analgesia protocol for total knee arthroplasty: A randomized, controlled study. *J Bone Joint Surg Am* 2006;88:282-289.

6. Lavernia C, Cardona D, Rossi MD, Lee D: Multimodal pain management and arthrofibrosis. *J Arthroplasty* 2008; 23:74-79.

7. Filos K, Lehmann K: Current concepts and practice in postoperative pain management: Need for a change? *Eur Surg Res* 1999;31:97-107.

8. Chaney MA: Side effects of intrathecal and epidural opioids. *Can J Anaesth* 1995;42:891-903.

9. Gwirtz KH, Young JV, Byers RS, et al: The safety and efficacy of intrathecal opioid analgesia for acute postoperative pain: Seven years' experience with 5969 surgical patients at Indiana University Hospital. *Anesth Analg* 1999;88:599-604.

10. Choi PT, Bhandari M, Scott J, Douketis JD: Epidural analgesia for pain relief following hip or knee replacement. *Cochrane Database Syst Rev* 2003;3:CD003071.

11. Heit J: Low-molecular-weight heparin: Biochemistry, pharmacology, and concurrent drug precautions. *Reg Anesth Pain Med* 1998;23:135-139.

12. Leclerc JR, Geerts WH, Desjardins L, et al: Prevention of venous thromboembolism after knee arthroplasty: A randomized, double-blind trial comparing enoxaparin with warfarin. *Ann Intern Med* 1996;124: 619-626.

13. Schroeder DR: Statistics: Detecting a rare adverse drug reaction using spontaneous reports. *Reg Anesth Pain Med* 1998;23:183-189.

14. Horlocker TT, Wedel DJ, Benzon H, et al: Regional anesthesia in the anticoagulated patient: Defining the risks (the second ASRA Consensus Conference on Neuraxial Anesthesia and Anticoagulation). *Reg Anesth Pain Med* 2003;28:172-197.

15. Capdevila X, Barthelet Y, Biboulet P, Ryckwaert Y, Rubenovitch J, d'Athis F: Effects of perioperative analgesic technique on the surgical outcome and duration of rehabilitation after major knee surgery. *Anesthesiology* 1999;91:8-15.

16. Wheeler M, Oderda GM, Ashburn MA, Lipman AG: Adverse events associated with postoperative opioid analgesia: A systematic review. *J Pain* 2002;3:159-180.

17. Birnbaum J, Kip M, Spies CD, et al: The effect of stimulating versus nonstimulating catheters for continuous interscalene plexus blocks in short-term pain management. *J Clin Anesth* 2007;19:434-439.

18. Chelly JE, Greger J, Gebhard R, et al: Continuous femoral blocks improve recovery and outcome of patients undergoing total knee arthroplasty. *J Arthroplasty* 2001;16:436-445.

19. Singelyn FJ, Deyaert M, Joris D, Pendeville E, Gouverneur JM: Effects of intravenous patient-controlled analgesia with morphine, continuous epidural analgesia, and continuous three-in-one block on postoperative pain and knee rehabilitation after unilateral total knee arthroplasty. *Anesth Analg* 1998;87:88-92.

20. Ganapathy S, Wasserman RA, Watson JT, et al: Modified continuous femoral three-in-one block for postoperative pain after total knee arthroplasty. *Anesth Analg* 1999;89:1197-1202.

21. Auroy Y, Benhamou D, Bargues L, et al: Major complications of regional anesthesia in France: The SOS Regional Anesthesia Hotline Service. *Anesthesiology* 2002;97:1274-1280.

22. Awad IT, Duggan EM: Posterior lumbar plexus block: Anatomy, approaches, and techniques. *Reg Anesth Pain Med* 2005;30:143-149.

23. Kardash K, Hickey D, Tessler MJ, Payne S, Zukor D, Velly AM: Obturator versus femoral nerve block for analgesia after total knee arthroplasty. *Anesth Analg* 2007;105:853-858.

24. DeWeese FT, Akbari Z, Carline E: Pain control after knee arthroplasty: Intraarticular versus epidural anesthesia. *Clin Orthop Relat Res* 2001;392: 226-231.

25. Mauerhan DR, Campbell M, Miller JS, Mokris JH, Gregory A, Kiebzak GM: Intra-articular morphine and/or bupivacaine in the management of pain after total knee arthroplasty. *J Arthroplasty* 1997;12:546-552.

26. Klasen JA, Opitz SA, Melzer C, Thiel A, Hempelmann G: Intraarticular, epidural, and intravenous analgesia after total knee arthroplasty. *Acta Anaesthesiol Scand* 1999;43:1021-1026.

27. Allen GC, St Amand MA, Lui AC, Johnson DH, Lindsay MP: Postarthroscopy analgesia with intraarticular bupivacaine/morphine: A randomized clinical trial. *Anesthesiology* 1993; 79:475-480.

28. Osborne D, Keene G: Pain relief after arthroscopic surgery of the knee: A prospective, randomized, and blinded assessment of bupivacaine and bupivacaine with adrenaline. *Arthroscopy* 1993;9:177-180.

29. Smith I, Van Hemelrijck J, White PF, Shively R: Effects of local anesthesia on recovery after outpatient arthroscopy. *Anesth Analg* 1991;73:536-539.

30. Busch CA, Shore BJ, Bhandari R, et al: Efficacy of periarticular multimodal drug injection in total knee arthroplasty: A randomized trial. *J Bone Joint Surg Am* 2006;88:959-963.

31. Parvataneni HK, Shah VP, Howard H, Cole N, Ranawat AS, Ranawat CS: Controlling pain after total hip and knee arthroplasty using a multimodal protocol with local periarticular injec-

tions: A prospective randomized study. *J Arthroplasty* 2007;22:33-38.

32. Stein C: The control of pain in peripheral tissue by opioids. *N Engl J Med* 1995;332:1685-1690.

33. Stein C: Peripheral mechanisms of opioid analgesia. *Anesth Analg* 1993; 76:182-191.

34. Tanaka N, Sakahashi H, Sato E, Hirose K, Ishii S: The efficacy of intra-articular analgesia after total knee arthroplasty in patients with rheumatoid arthritis and in patients with osteoarthritis. *J Arthroplasty* 2001;16: 306-311.

35. McCormack K, Brune K: Dissociation between the antinociceptive and anti-inflammatory effects of the nonsteroidal anti-inflammatory drugs: A survey of their analgesic efficacy. *Drugs* 1991;41:533-547.

36. Denson D, Myers J, Hartrick C, Pither C, Coyle D, Raj P: The relationship between free bupivacaine concentration and central nervous system toxicity. *Anesthesiology* 1984;61: 211.

37. Solanki DR, Enneking FK, Ivey FM, Scarborough M, Johnston RV: Serum bupivacaine concentrations after intraarticular injection for pain relief after knee arthroscopy. *Arthroscopy* 1992; 8:44-47.

38. Salerno A, Hermann R: Efficacy and safety of steroid use for postoperative pain relief: Update and review of the medical literature. *J Bone Joint Surg Am* 2006;88:1361-1372.

39. Rosenberg PH, Veering BT, Urmey WF: Maximum recommended doses of local anesthetics: A multifactorial concept. *Reg Anesth Pain Med* 2004;29:564-575.

40. Dorr LD, Chao L: The emotional state of the patient after total hip and knee arthroplasty. *Clin Orthop Relat Res* 2007;463:7-12.

41. Buvanendran A, Kroin JS, Tuman KJ, et al: Effects of perioperative administration of a selective cyclooxygenase 2 inhibitor on pain management and recovery of function after knee replacement: A randomized controlled trial. *JAMA* 2003;290: 2411-2418.

42. Stephens JM, Pashos CL, Haider S, Wong JM: Making progress in the management of postoperative pain: A review of the cyclooxygenase 2-specific inhibitors. *Pharmacotherapy* 2004;24:1714-1731.

43. Hubbard RC, Naumann TM, Traylor L, Dhadda S: Parecoxib sodium has opioid-sparing effects in patients undergoing total knee arthroplasty under spinal anaesthesia. *Br J Anaesth* 2003;90:166-172.

44. Reynolds LW, Hoo RK, Brill RJ, North J, Recker DP, Verburg KM: The COX-2 specific inhibitor, valdecoxib, is an effective, opioid-sparing analgesic in patients undergoing total knee arthroplasty. *J Pain Symptom Manage* 2003;25:133-141.

45. Macario A, Lipman AG: Ketorolac in the era of cyclo-oxygenase-2 selective nonsteroidal anti-inflammatory drugs: A systematic review of efficacy, side effects, and regulatory issues. *Pain Med* 2001;2:336-351.

46. Vondrackova D, Leyendecker P, Meissner W, et al: Analgesic efficacy and safety of oxycodone in combination with naloxone as prolonged release tablets in patients with moderate to severe chronic pain. *J Pain* 2008;9: 1144-1154.

47. Ringrose NH, Cross MJ: Femoral nerve block in knee joint surgery. *Am J Sports Med* 1984;12:398-402.

48. Woolf CJ, Chong MS: Preemptive analgesia: Treating postoperative pain by preventing the establishment of central sensitization. *Anesth Analg* 1993;77:362-379.

49. Ong CK, Lirk P, Seymour RA, Jenkins BJ: The efficacy of preemptive analgesia for acute postoperative pain management: A meta-analysis. *Anesth Analg* 2005;100:757-773.

50. Cheville A, Chen A, Oster G, McGarry L, Narcessian E: A randomized trial of controlled-release oxycodone during inpatient rehabilitation following unilateral total knee arthroplasty. *J Bone Joint Surg Am* 2001;83: 572-576.

51. Simcock XC, Yoon RS, Chalmers P, Geller JA, Kiernan HA, Macaulay W: Intraoperative music reduces perceived pain after total knee arthroplasty: A blinded, prospective, randomized, placebo-controlled clinical trial. *J Knee Surg* 2008;21:275-278.

52. Holmström A, Härdin BC: Cryo/cuff compared to epidural anesthesia after knee unicompartmental arthroplasty: A prospective, randomized, and controlled study of 60 patients with a 6-week follow-up. *J Arthroplasty* 2005;20:316-321.

53. Webb JM, Williams D, Ivory JP, Day S, Williamson DM: The use of cold compression dressings after total knee replacement: A randomized controlled trial. *Orthopedics* 1998;21:59-61.

54. McDonald DD, Molony SL: Postoperative pain communication skills for older adults. *West J Nurs Res* 2004;26: 836-859.

55. Barwell J, Anderson G, Hassan A, Rawlings I: The effects of early tourniquet release during total knee arthroplasty: A prospective randomized double-blind study. *J Bone Joint Surg Br* 1997;79:265-268.

56. Angulo DL, Colwell CW: Use of postoperative TENS and continuous passive motion following total knee replacement. *J Orthop Sports Phys Ther* 1990;11:599-604.

57. Can F, Alpaslan M: Continuous passive motion on pain management in patients with total knee arthroplasty. *Pain Clin* 2003;15:479-485.

58. Harms M, Engstrom B: Continuous passive motion as an adjunct to treatment in the physiotherapy management of the total knee arthroplasty patient. *Physiotherapy* 1991;77: 301-307.

59. Montgomery F, Eliasson M: Continuous passive motion compared to active physical therapy after knee arthroplasty: Similar hospitalization times in a randomized study of 68 patients. *Acta Orthop Scand* 1996;67:7-9.

Primary Total Knee Arthroplasty: A Comparison of Computer-Assisted and Manual Techniques

Wendy M. Novicoff, PhD
Khaled J. Saleh, MD, MSc, FRCSC
William M. Mihalko, MD, PhD
Xin-Qun Wang, MS
Hanns-Peter Knaebel, MD, MBA

Abstract

Total knee arthroplasty has proven to be successful in improving a patient's quality of life. Traditional total knee instrumentation aligns 80% of knees within 3° of neutral alignment, leaving 20% with outliers with more than 3° of deformity. Computer-assisted surgery in total knee arthroplasty is a relatively new technique for decreasing these alignment outliers.

Database searches from January 1990 through April 2008 were used to review studies comparing manual and computer-assisted techniques in total knee arthroplasty. A multistage assessment was used to ensure the broadest coverage. Potential articles were identified and further examined. Full data extraction was performed on 52 articles using a standardized data collection tool. Analysis of 22 randomized controlled studies showed a clear advantage in terms of alignment for computer-assisted surgery versus manual surgery; however, no studies evaluated the associations between patient characteristics and outcomes or measured functional outcome beyond the degree of malalignment within a short period after the surgery. There is a need for studies that examine functional outcomes more than 1 year postoperatively using standardized assessment tools, especially because malalignment is an intermediate outcome measure that cannot be linked causally in all cases of eventual implant failure.

Instr Course Lect 2010;59:109-117.

Dr. Novicoff or an immediate family member has received research or institutional support from Aesculap/B. Braun, DePuy, Smith & Nephew, Stryker, and Zimmer. Dr. Saleh or an immediate family member has received royalties from Smith & Nephew; is a member of a speakers' bureau or has made paid presentations on behalf of Aesculap/B. Braun, Stryker, OMNI, and Kimberly Clark; serves as a paid consultant to or is an employee of Aesculap/B. Braun, Stryker, and OMNI; has received research or institutional support from the Journal of Bone and Joint Surgery–American*, Stryker, EKR Therapeutics, and Aesculap; and has received nonincome support (such as equipment or services), commercially derived honoraria, or other non–research-related funding (such as paid travel) from Blue Cross Blue Shield and Kimberly Clark. Dr. Mihalko or an immediate family member has received royalties from Elsevier; is a member of a speakers' bureau or has made paid presentations on behalf of Ethicon and Aesculap/B. Braun; serves as a paid consultant to or is an employee of Aesculap/B. Braun, Ethicon, Johnson & Johnson, and Stryker; and has received research or institutional support from the* Journal of Bone and Joint Surgery–American*, Smith & Nephew, and Aesculap/B. Braun. Dr. Knaebel or an immediate family member serves as a paid consultant to or is an employee of Aesculap/B. Braun. Neither Xin Wang nor an immediate family member has received anything of value from or owns stock in a commercial company or institution related directly or indirectly to the subject of this chapter.*

Each year, knee pain from multiple causes decreases the quality of life for millions of patients.[1,2] In 2002, the American Academy of Orthopaedic Surgeons predicted that the number of total knee arthroplasties (TKAs) performed in the United States would reach nearly 500,000 per year by 2030. It is clear that these estimates were too low because more than 533,000 procedures were performed in 2005. Newer studies have shown that the demand will be approximately 3 million procedures per year by 2030.[3,4] The rapid increase in the number of TKAs performed each year can be attributed to the increasing average age of the US population and the increasing prevalence of arthritis and other factors that lead to the need for these procedures.[5,6] The perceived success of TKA—improved functional status, pain relief, low perioperative morbidity and mortality, and good implant survivorship—has expanded demand among all population segments.[7-16]

There are many different surgical approaches and options available in TKA. The emergence of new technology over the previous 20 years has led to new surgical advances in the field, which now includes minimally invasive surgery and computer-assisted surgery (CAS). Minimally invasive surgery encompasses several techniques designed to decrease postoperative morbidity through the use of smaller incisions, smaller instruments, less strain on the quadriceps mechanism, and less patellar eversion. CAS was first introduced in the late 1990s as an alternative surgical method designed to improve alignment of knee replacements and lead to potentially better outcomes for patients. In CAS, various guides are used to monitor where and how cuts are made during surgery with the ultimate goal of improving longevity of the prosthesis for the individual patient. There is no consensus among surgeons as to which surgical technique (CAS, conventional, or minimally invasive) is best.[17]

Because of the increasing use of CAS since its introduction, it is important to compare and contrast its risks and benefits with those of manual techniques. Two recent meta-analyses have been published on this topic.[18,19] Bauwens and associates[18] reported that CAS provided few advantages compared with conventional surgery. They found that CAS increased the length of surgery by 23% and did not significantly increase mean mechanical axes alignment; however, CAS did decrease the risk of a malalignment that was more than 2° or 3° from normal. In contrast, Mason and associates[19] focused on the benefits of CAS for decreasing malalignment and concluded that CAS showed a sufficient advantage over manual techniques to recommend its regular use. Both studies mentioned the limitations in the available literature on the subject—small sample sizes, short follow-up periods, no measurement of functional outcomes, and the use of malalignment as the primary outcome of interest. Although decreasing the degree of malalignment should lead to better outcomes for patients, the actual relationship between the degree of malalignment and overall patient outcome is still debated. Some studies have shown better implant survival rates and functional outcomes resulting from better alignment,[20,21] whereas other studies have shown that malalignment may be just one of many factors that can influence implant survival rates.[22,23]

Because of the differing conclusions of these two prior meta-analyses, and because there were significant methodological differences in how studies were chosen for inclusion in the two articles (including the use of studies with lower levels of evidence), the authors decided to undertake a more recent systematic review and meta-analysis that could combine the results of the two prior meta-analyses with the results of more recently published studies. It was hypothesized that using computer navigation in TKA would significantly improve postoperative alignment, particularly in reducing the risk of malalignment of the mechanical axis more than 3° away from normal. Current studies also were examined to determine if other conclusions could be made concerning the risks and benefits of CAS.

Materials and Methods

Systematic Review

Procedures for this review followed established methods for systematic review research.[24] A written protocol and standardized data collection tool were used. A search strategy was used that encompassed Medline, PubMed, and Cochrane databases, with no restriction on language. All studies reporting clinical trials comparing CAS in TKA with manual techniques published between January 1986 and April 2008 were eligible for inclusion. All studies cited in the two prior meta-analyses were included, and other sources of information were searched (including the Internet) for additional reports or studies that could potentially provide information on this subject. In addition, manual reference checks of all articles were performed to supplement electronic searches with any additional relevant studies.

Inclusion Criteria

In the first article review, all study inclusion criteria used by Mason and associates[19] were applied. The study had to report on primary TKA using CAS, had to report postoperative implant and limb alignment outcomes, and had at least 10 patients in the treatment group. After the initial review, a second-level review was done to ensure inclusion of and focus on randomized controlled clinical trials (RCTs) that were part of the previous meta-analyses or had been published from January 31, 2007 (the cut off for the most recent prior meta-analysis) through April 30, 2008. All eligible studies were rated for level of evidence using the Center for Evidence-Based Medicine rating scale.[25] Studies reserved for further analysis either had to be included in the prior meta-analyses or be classified as RCTs not previously included and had to report on postoperative alignment. All data elements were abstracted by two researchers and confirmed by a third party in terms of agreement with each other and with the original publication. Any discrepancies were resolved before data analysis. In keeping with the methods of the previous meta-analyses, all available data were extracted, including demographics, baseline comorbidities, and surgical and functional outcomes.

Statistical Analysis

Data elements were entered into a relational database and analyzed using SAS version 9.1 (SAS Institute, Cary, NC). The primary outcome of interest was postoperative implant and limb alignment, but data were also examined for other potential outcomes of interest. In an attempt to increase the number of well-controlled studies in the analysis, a comparison was made among the postoperative degree of alignment of the mechanical axis reported in the study by Mason and associates[19] (pooled results), individual results from the RCTs referenced in Bauwens and associates[18] and Mason and associates,[19] and the results from the more recent RCTs. Odds ratios were calculated using Fisher's Exact Test and were plotted for all studies with the exception of the pooled results from Bauwens and associates.[18] This meta-analysis presented risk ratios, which could not be directly compared.

As was done by Bauwens and associates,[18] an attempt was made to define statistical models using multiple logistic regression techniques to identify which patient characteristics or other variables might predict which patients would have better outcomes based on the type of surgery. However, as was concluded in the prior analyses,[18,19] the current available studies do not provide sufficient data on functional outcomes (few reported any outcomes other than degree of malalignment) or sufficient follow-up periods to provide the power needed to detect differences.

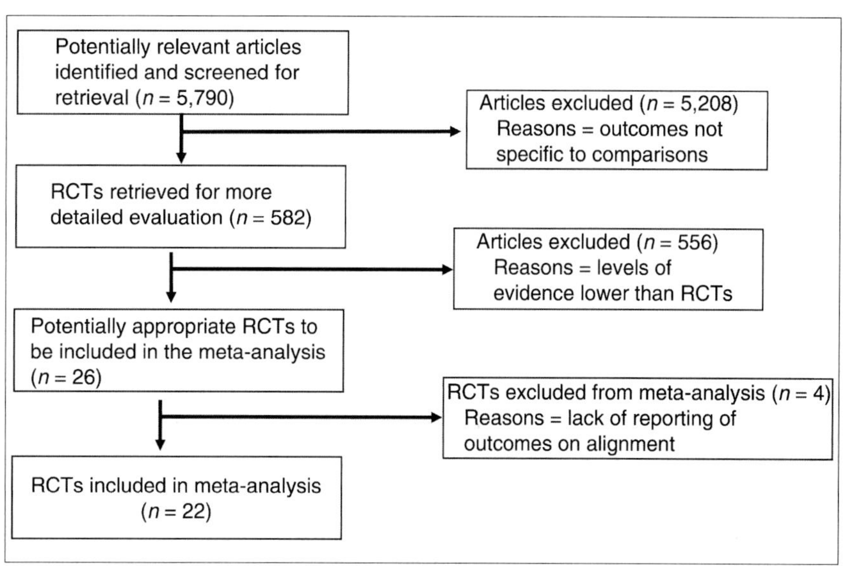

Figure 1 Quorum diagram for systematic review for comparing CAS to conventional surgery for TKA.

Results

A total of 5,790 studies met initial inclusion criteria; 582 were selected for further analysis. There were 127 studies representing all levels of evidence on the use of computer navigation in TKA that had been published from January 31, 2007 through April 30, 2008. A total of 52 studies met all criteria and were fully analyzed. Forty-one of these studies had been included in the prior meta-analyses, and 11 were RCTs that were published recently or had not been included in the prior analyses.[26-36] This process resulted in an additional 11 studies being added to the original analysis[37-47] for a total of 22 RCTs in the final analysis (Figure 1, Table 1). Four other RCTs were identified that could not be included because of a lack of specific reporting of malalignment outcomes that could be matched to other studies or because the focus of the studies was on another comparison aspect of the two techniques, such as blood loss or development of emboli.[48-51] In their outcome of interest, each of the four studies that could not be included showed the superior performance of CAS compared with manual techniques.

All plotted studies, including the result of the meta-analysis by Mason and associates,[19] produced odds ratios that showed a decreased risk of having a mechanical axis alignment more than 3° away from normal with the use of CAS compared with conventional surgery (Figure 2). Thirteen RCTs produced odds ratios that significantly favored CAS over conventional surgery.[26-28,30-33,37,38,43,45-47] Table 1 shows specific information for each of the RCTs included in the analysis, and Table 2 shows the odds ratios and 95% confidence interval (CI).

Most of the studies were from European or Asian centers, primarily single-site studies, and had relatively low sample sizes.[18,19] These

Table 1
Numbers of Patients in Each Treatment Group and Number of TKAs Malaligned More Than 3° Postoperatively

Study Authors	Publication Year	Conventional Surgery (*n*)	Conventional Surgery: Malalignment (*n*)	CAS (*n*)	CAS: Malalignment (*n*)
Meta-analysis:					
Mason et al[19]	2007	1,376	438	1,418	127
Most recent studies:					
Macule-Beneyto et al[30]	2006	84	59	102	53
Cobb et al[26]	2006	14	6	13	0
Ensini et al[28]	2006	60	12	60	1
Seon et al[36]	2007	42	8	42	2
Park and Lee[34]	2007	30	9	32	3
Mullaji et al[33]	2007	185	40	282	26
Martin et al[31]	2007	100	24	100	8
Kim et al[29]	2007	100	35	100	28
Matziolis et al[32]	2007	28	7	32	1
Seon and Song[35]	2006	53	6	49	3
Dutton et al[27]	2008	56	18	52	4
RCTs from Bauwens et al:[18]					
Chauhan et al[39]	2004	30	10	34	5
Chin et al[40]	2005	60	22	30	6
Decking et al[41]	2005	25	16	27	13
Keene et al[42]	2006	20	8	20	3
Saragaglia et al[44]	2001	25	6	25	4
Victor and Hoste[47]	2004	49	13	48	0
Additional RCTs from Mason et al:[19]					
Bäthis et al[37]	2004	80	18	80	3
Böhling et al[38]	2005	50	27	50	3
Oberst et al[43]	2003	13	5	12	0
Sparmann et al[45]	2003	120	16	120	0
Stulberg et al[46]	2000	15	5	15	0

shortcomings also were prevalent in the newer RCTs; however, sample sizes and follow-up times were somewhat increased, with three recent RCTs each reporting results from more than 200 patients.[29,31,33] Patient characteristics were usually not well described, and the choice of implants and cementing techniques was not uniform.

Discussion

The chapter authors' study showed that using CAS in TKA improves postoperative alignment, particularly in reducing the risk of malalignment of the mechanical axis by more than 3°. Although prior studies have reported this result, combining all results from RCTs included in the prior meta-analyses and newer RCTs provides an even greater confidence in this conclusion.[52,53]

The role of knee alignment and its effect on both short- and long-term outcomes has been well explored. The degree of coronal alignment has been shown to be an important factor in preventing implant loosening.[54-56] Malalignment in the axial rotation has been shown to be detrimental, whereas well-aligned knees increase articular conformity and reduce polyethylene contact stresses, leading to better implant survivorship.[57] Patients with good femoral and tibial alignment report better functional outcomes, with quicker rehabilitation, shorter hospital stays, and better Knee Society scores at 1 year.[58] Similar results have been reported in patients undergoing unicompartmental knee arthroplasty, in which

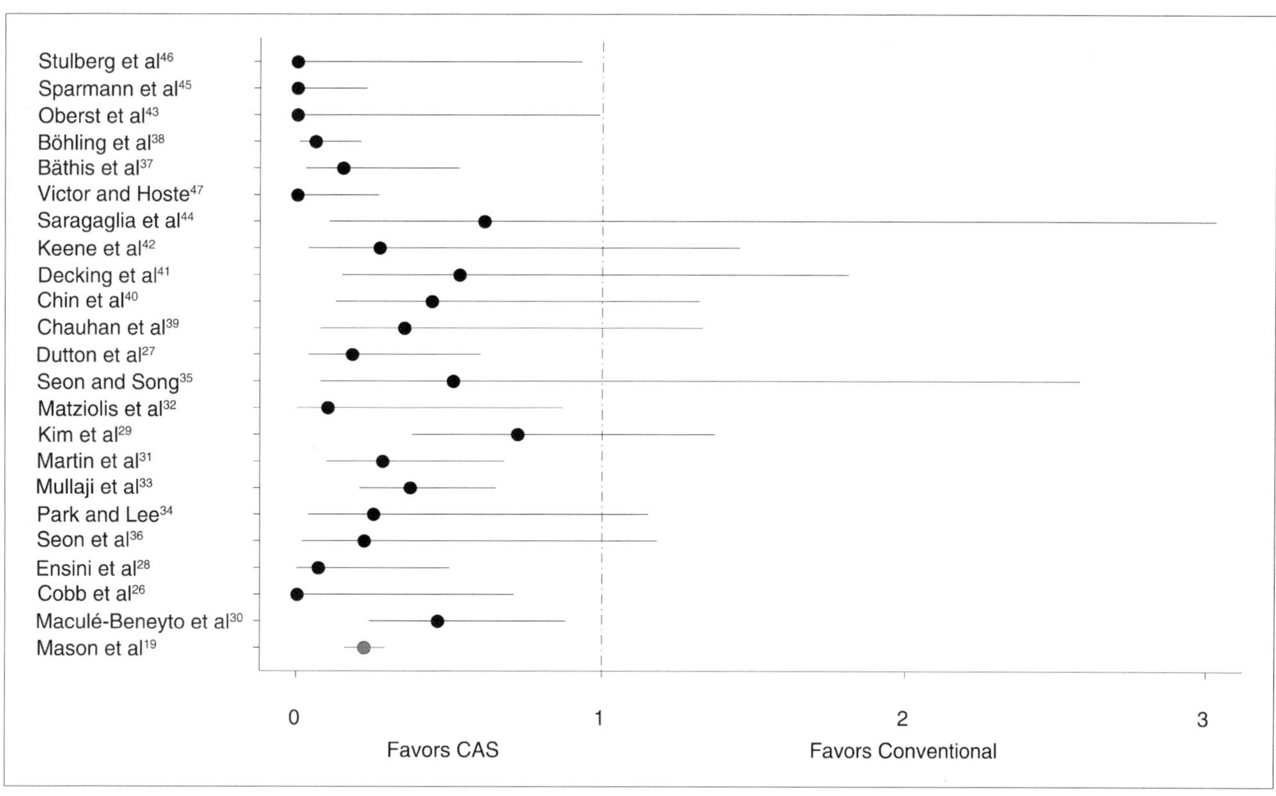

Figure 2 Comparison of computer-assisted and conventional knee arthroplasty with respect to odds ratio of greater than 3° of malalignment, with a 95% CI. The vertical dashed line is a reference line of no effect. All results except those of Mason et al were estimated using the Fisher exact test. The result for the meta-analysis by Mason and associates was estimated using a random effect model.

proper alignment of the implant led to improved surgical outcomes.[59] There also are multiple biomechanical studies that show the increase in loads to the tibial baseplate with increasing malalignment of more than 3°.[60] Other studies associate immediate postoperative malalignment with other important factors, such as soft-tissue balancing and alignment deterioration after surgery.[23,55,61] Alignment is not the only factor that can impact implant longevity and wear.[62] Soft-tissue balances and muscle forces also play a role in how forces are distributed across the knee joint.

It remains to be determined if better alignment reported in the current literature will translate into better long-term outcomes and implant survival rates. Although two recent case-controlled studies with longer follow-up periods (5 years and 2 years) concluded that there were no significant differences in functional outcomes despite better alignment in the CAS group, this does not discount the possibility that CAS could be a cost-effective alternative to conventional techniques over a longer period of time.[63,64] Two studies on the cost-effectiveness of CAS concluded that CAS is cost-effective in terms of additional quality adjusted life years gained.[65,66] In one of the studies, the probability of revision knee surgery was calculated with neutral alignment (4.7%) versus malalignment (54%).[66] This finding gives more credence to the belief that because CAS provides superior postoperative alignment, the rate of revision surgeries may decrease as the rate of CAS increases.

As with any study, the chapter authors' study had important limitations. Not all studies published since January 31, 2007 were included because it was believed that one of the shortcomings of the prior analyses was the inclusion of studies with lower levels of evidence. Because the RCT is considered the gold standard for determining the efficacy of a treatment, pooling the results from the RCTs was considered a reasonable method for making stronger conclusions about the advantages of CAS.

The chapter authors' study was not able to produce predictive

Table 2
Odds Ratios, 95% CIs, and *P* Values for Each Study

Study Authors	Odds Ratio	Lower 95% CI	Upper 95% CI	*P* value
Meta-analysis:				
Mason et al[19]	0.22	0.16	0.29	0.0001
Most recent studies:				
Maculé-Beneyto et al[30]	0.46	0.24	0.88	0.0158
Cobb et al[26]	0.00	0.00	0.71	0.0159
Ensini et al[28]	0.07	0.002	0.50	0.0020
Seon et al[36]	0.22	0.02	1.18	0.0882
Park and Lee[34]	0.25	0.04	1.15	0.0555
Mullaji et al[33]	0.37	0.21	0.65	0.0002
Martin et al[31]	0.28	0.10	0.68	0.0033
Kim et al[29]	0.72	0.38	1.37	0.3611
Matziolis et al[32]	0.10	0.002	0.87	0.0201
Seon and Song[35]	0.51	0.08	2.58	0.4907
Dutton et al[27]	0.18	0.04	0.60	0.0018
RCTs from Bauwens et al:[18]				
Chauhan et al[39]	0.35	0.08	1.33	0.1379
Chin et al[40]	0.44	0.13	1.32	0.1480
Decking et al[41]	0.53	0.15	1.81	0.2781
Keene et al[42]	0.27	0.04	1.45	0.1552
Saragaglia et al[44]	0.61	0.11	3.03	0.7252
Victor and Hoste[47]	0.00	0.00	0.27	< 0.0001
Additional RCTs from Mason et al:[19]				
Bäthis et al[37]	0.15	0.03	0.53	0.0008
Böhling et al[38]	0.06	0.01	0.21	< 0.0001
Oberst et al[43]	0.00	0.00	0.99	0.0391
Sparmann et al[45]	0.00	0.00	0.23	< 0.0001
Stulberg et al[46]	0.00	0.00	0.93	0.0422

models based on the evidence presented in the current literature, so definitive conclusions could not be made about the risks and benefits of CAS beyond superior alignment. This lack of evidence is a significant shortcoming for the acceptance of CAS by surgeons. A recent survey showed that only 33.1% of physicians use computer navigation for at least 50% of their TKAs, and only 25% report using it in 75% or more of their TKAs.[67] The most common reason cited for using CAS was improvement in the alignment of the prosthesis, whereas the most common reasons for not using the a navigation system were increased surgical time and risk of infection.

Other interested parties, including payers, are demanding more evidence that proves CAS will produce better patient outcomes than conventional surgery, especially because studies have shown that CAS adds several minutes to surgical time and requires specialized equipment.[18,19] Other studies have reported that, despite longer surgical times, blood loss and the development of systemic emboli are reduced with CAS compared with conventional techniques.[49,50] Surgeons also must decide whether to use technology that has not been definitively proven to be effective. Medical liability cases have been pursued previously in orthopaedic surgery because no set standard exists for the use of new technology, implants, and surgical approaches.[68-70]

Summary

Because the risk of revision surgery and early TKA failure is a multifactorial equation, further study is needed. To produce sound evidence about the advantages and disadvantages of CAS, it is necessary to ascertain the kinematic patterns and soft-tissue gap kinematics of patients before and after surgery, patient comorbidities, and surgical and implant variables. Future trials should have high methodological standards (including randomization); have longer and more standard follow-up periods; have better control of preoperative, intraoperative, and postoperative care and focus on outcomes that are meaningful to assess functional recovery and quality of life. Studies also should include financial end points, such as length of hospital stay and risk for readmission, both of which are increasingly important aspects of patient management for the orthopaedic surgeon but have not been definitively explored in relationship to CAS. Without such studies, there will be no method to fully assess the benefits (and associated risks) of using CAS as the predominant surgical approach for primary TKA.

Acknowledgments

The authors would like to thank Harris Slone, MD; Timothy Craft, MD; and Vincent Gomez, BS for their assistance in preparing this manuscript.

References

1. American Academy of Orthopaedic Surgeons Website. Data analyzed from National Hospital Discharge Survey, 1991–2004. http://www.aaos.org/Research/stats/Total%20Knee%20Replacement%20Chart.pdf. Accessed May 26, 2008.
2. Elders M: The increasing impact of arthritis on public health. *J Rheumatol Suppl* 2000;60:6-8.
3. Kurtz S, Ong K, Lau E, Mowat F, Halpern M: Projections of primary and revision hip and knee arthroplasty in the United States from 2005 to 2030. *J Bone Joint Surg Am* 2007;89:780-785.
4. Mahomed NN, Barrett J, Katz JN, Baron JA, Wright J, Losina E: Epidemiology of total knee replacement in the United States Medicare population. *J Bone Joint Surg Am* 2005;87:1222-1228.
5. Acheson RM, Collart AB: New Haven survey of joint diseases: XVII. Relationship between some systemic characteristics and osteoarthrosis in a general population. *Ann Rheum Dis* 1975;34:379-387.
6. Peyron JG: Osteoarthritis: The epidemiologic viewpoint. *Clin Orthop Relat Res* 1986;213:13-19.
7. Callahan CM, Drake BG, Heck DA, Dittus RS: Patient outcomes following tricompartmental total knee replacement: A meta-analysis. *JAMA* 1994;271:1349-1357.
8. Crowninshield RD, Rosenberg AG, Sporer SM: Changing demographics of patients with total joint replacement. *Clin Orthop Relat Res* 2006;443:266-272.
9. Deshmukh RV, Scott RD: Unicompartmental knee arthroplasty: Long-term results. *Clin Orthop Relat Res* 2001;392:272-278.
10. Ethgen O, Bruyère O, Richy F, Dardennes C, Reginster JY: Health-related quality of life in total hip and total knee arthroplasty: A qualitative and systematic review of the literature. *J Bone Joint Surg Am* 2004;86:963-974.
11. Hawker G, Wright J, Coyte P, et al: Health-related quality of life after knee replacement. *J Bone Joint Surg Am* 1998;80:163-173.
12. Heck DA, Robinson RL, Partridge CM, Lubitz RM, Freund DA: Patient outcomes after knee replacement. *Clin Orthop Relat Res* 1998;356:93-110.
13. Kane RL, Saleh KJ, Wilt TJ, Bershadsky B: The functional outcomes of total knee arthroplasty. *J Bone Joint Surg Am* 2005;87:1719-1724.
14. Rand JA, Ilstrup DM: Survivorship analysis of total knee arthroplasty: Cumulative rates of survival of 9200 total knee arthroplasties. *J Bone Joint Surg Am* 1991;73:397-409.
15. Räsänen P, Paavolainen P, Sintonen H, et al: Effectiveness of hip or knee replacement surgery in terms of quality-adjusted life years and costs. *Acta Orthop* 2007;78:108-115.
16. Shields RK, Enloe LJ, Leo KC: Health related quality of life in patients with total hip or knee replacement. *Arch Phys Med Rehabil* 1999;80:572-579.
17. Ulrich SD, Bonutti PM, Seyler TM, Marker DR, Jones LC, Mont MA: Scientific evidence supporting computer-assisted surgery and minimally invasive surgery for total knee arthroplasty. *Expert Rev Med Devices* 2007;4:873-883.
18. Bauwens K, Matthes G, Wich M, et al: Navigated total knee replacement: A meta-analysis. *J Bone Joint Surg Am* 2007;89:261-269.
19. Mason JB, Fehring TK, Estok R, Banal D, Fahrbach K: Meta-analysis of alignment outcomes in computer-assisted total knee arthroplasty surgery. *J Arthroplasty* 2007;22:1097-1106.
20. Ritter MA, Faris PM, Keating EM, Meding JB: Postoperative alignment of total knee replacement: Its effect on survival. *Clin Orthop Relat Res* 1994;299:153-156.
21. Wasielewski RC, Galante JO, Leighty RM, Natarajan RN, Rosenberg AG: Wear patterns on retrieved polyethylene inserts and their relationship to technical considerations during total knee arthroplasty. *Clin Orthop Relat Res* 1994;299:31-43.
22. Mulhall KJ, Ghomrawi HM, Scully S, Callaghan JJ, Saleh KJ: Current etiologies and modes of failure in total knee arthroplasty revision. *Clin Orthop Relat Res* 2006;446:45-50.
23. Sharkey PF, Hozack WJ, Rothman RH, Shastri S, Jacoby SM: Why are total knee arthroplasties failing today? *Clin Orthop Relat Res* 2002;404:7-13.
24. Cook DJ, Mulrow CD, Haynes RB: Systematic reviews: Synthesis of best evidence for clinical decisions. *Ann Intern Med* 1997;126:376-380.
25. Oxford Center for Evidence-Based Medicine Website. http://www.cebm.net. Accessed March 24, 2009.
26. Cobb J, Henckel J, Gomes P, et al: Hands-on robotic unicompartmental knee replacement: A prospective, randomized controlled study of the acrobat system. *J Bone Joint Surg Br* 2006;88:188-197.
27. Dutton AQ, Yeo SJ, Yang KY, Lo NN, Chia KU, Chong HC: Computer-assisted minimally invasive total knee arthroplasty compared with standard total knee arthroplasty: A prospective, randomized study. *J Bone Joint Surg Am* 2008;90:2-9.
28. Ensini A, Catani F, Leardini A, Romagnoli M, Giannini S: Alignments and clinical results in conventional and navigated total knee arthroplasty. *Clin Orthop Relat Res* 2006;457:156-162.
29. Kim YH, Kim JS, Yoon SH: Alignment and orientation of the components in total knee replacement with and without navigation support: A

prospective, randomized study. *J Bone Joint Surg Br* 2007;89:471-476.

30. Maculé-Beneyto F, Hernández-Vaquero D, Segur-Vilalta JM, et al: Navigation in total knee arthroplasty: A multicenter study. *Int Orthop* 2006; 30:536-540.
31. Martin A, Wohlgennannt O, Prenn M, Oelsch C, von Strempel A: Imageless navigation for TKA increases implantation accuracy. *Clin Orthop Relat Res* 2007;460:178-184.
32. Matziolis G, Krocker D, Weiss U, Tohtz S, Perka C: A prospective, randomized study of computer-assisted and conventional total knee arthroplasty: Three-dimensional evaluation of implant alignment and rotation. *J Bone Joint Surg Am* 2007;89:236-243.
33. Mullaji A, Kanna R, Marawar S, Kohli A, Sharma A: Comparison of limb and component alignment using computer-assisted navigation versus image intensifier-guided conventional total knee arthroplasty: A prospective, randomized, single-surgeon study of 467 knees. *J Arthroplasty* 2007; 22:953-959.
34. Park SE, Lee CT: Comparison of robotic-assisted and conventional manual implantation of a primary total knee arthroplasty. *J Arthroplasty* 2007;22:1054-1059.
35. Seon JK, Song EK: Navigation-assisted less invasive total knee arthroplasty compared with conventional total knee arthroplasty: A randomized prospective trial. *J Arthroplasty* 2006;21:777-782.
36. Seon JK, Song EK, Yoon TR, Park SJ, Bae BH, Cho SG: Comparison of functional results with navigation-assisted minimally invasive and conventional techniques in bilateral total knee arthroplasty. *Comput Aided Surg* 2007;12:189-193.
37. Bäthis H, Perlick L, Tingart M, Lüring C, Zurakowski D, Grifka J: Alignment in total knee arthroplasty: A comparison of computer-assisted surgery with the conventional technique. *J Bone Joint Surg Br* 2004;86: 682-687.
38. Böhling U, Schamberger H, Grittner U, Scholz J: Computerized and technical navigation in total knee-arthroplasty. *J Orthopaed Traumatol* 2005;6:69-75.
39. Chauhan SK, Scott RG, Breidahl W, Beaver RJ: Computer-assisted knee arthroplasty versus a conventional jig-based technique: A randomized, prospective trial. *J Bone Joint Surg Br* 2004;86:372-377.
40. Chin PL, Yang KY, Yeo SJ, Lo NN: Randomized control trial comparing radiographic total knee arthroplasty implant placement using computer navigation versus conventional technique. *J Arthroplasty* 2005;20:618-626.
41. Decking R, Markmann Y, Fuchs J, Puhl W, Scharf HP: Leg axis after computer-navigated total knee arthroplasty: A prospective randomized trial comparing computer-navigated and manual implantation. *J Arthroplasty* 2005;20:282-288.
42. Keene G, Simpson D, Kalairajah Y: Limb alignment in computer-assisted minimally-invasive unicompartmental knee replacement. *J Bone Joint Surg Br* 2006;88:44-48.
43. Oberst M, Bertsch C, Würstlin S, Holz U: CT analysis of leg alignment after conventional vs. navigated knee prosthesis implantation: Initial results of a controlled, prospective and randomized study. *Unfallchirurg* 2003; 106:941-948.
44. Saragaglia D, Picard F, Chaussard C, Montbarbon E, Leitner F, Cinquin P: Computer-assisted knee arthroplasty: Comparison with a conventional procedure. Results of 50 cases in a prospective randomized study. *Rev Chir Orthop Reparatrice Appar Mot* 2001;87: 18-28.
45. Sparmann M, Wolke B, Czupalla H, Banzer D, Zink A: Positioning of total knee arthroplasty with and without navigation support: A prospective, randomized study. *J Bone Joint Surg Br* 2003;85:830-835.
46. Stulberg DS, Picard F, Saragaglia D: Computer-assisted total knee replacement arthroplasty. *Oper Tech Ortho* 2000;10:25.
47. Victor J, Hoste D: Image-based computer-assisted total knee arthroplasty leads to lower variability in coronal alignment. *Clin Orthop Relat Res* 2004;428:131-139.
48. Hernandez-Vaquero D, Suarez-Vazquez A, Garcia-Sandoval MA, Fernandez-Carreira JM, Perez-Hernandez D: Computer-assisted implant in knee endoprosthesis with a wireless system. *J Bone Joint Surg Br* 2004;86:227.
49. Kalairajah Y, Simpson D, Cossey AJ, Verrall GM, Spriggins AJ: Blood loss after total knee replacement: Effects of computer-assisted surgery. *J Bone Joint Surg Br* 2005;87:1480-1482.
50. Kalairajah Y, Cossey AJ, Verrall GM, Ludbrook G, Spriggins AJ: Are systemic emboli reduced in computer-assisted knee surgery? A prospective, randomized, clinical trial. *J Bone Joint Surg Br* 2006;88:197-202.
51. Stöckl B, Nogler M, Rosiek R, Fischer M, Krismer M, Kessler O: Navigation improves accuracy of rotational alignment in total knee arthroplasty. *Clin Orthop Relat Res* 2004; 426:180-186.
52. Mason JB, Fehring R, Fahrback K: Navigated total knee replacement. *J Bone Joint Surg Am* 2007;89:2547-2548.
53. Katz JN, Losina E: Navigated total knee replacement. *J Bone Joint Surg Am* 2007;89:2548-2550.
54. Jeffery RS, Morris RW, Denham RA: Coronal alignment after total knee replacement. *J Bone Joint Surg Br* 1991; 73:709-714.
55. Berend ME, Ritter MA, Meding JB, et al: Tibial component failure mechanisms in total knee arthroplasty. *Clin Orthop Relat Res* 2004; 428 :26-34.
56. Collier MB, Engh CA Jr, McAuley JP, Engh GA: Factors associated with the loss of thickness of polyethylene tibial bearings after knee arthroplasty. *J Bone Joint Surg Am* 2007;89: 1306-1314.

57. D'Lima DD, Chen PC, Colwell CW Jr: Polyethylene contact stresses, articular congruity, and knee alignment. *Clin Orthop Relat Res* 2001;392: 232-238.

58. Longstaff LM, Sloan K, Stamp N, Scaddan M, Beaver R: Good alignment after total knee arthroplasty leads to faster rehabilitation and better function. *J Arthroplasty* 2009;24: 570-578.

59. Kasodekar VB, Yeo SJ, Othman S: Clinical outcome of unicompartmental knee arthroplasty and influence of alignment on prosthesis survival rate. *Singapore Med J* 2006;47:796-802.

60. Werner FW, Ayers DC, Maletsky LP, Rullkoetter PJ: The effect of valgus/varus malalignment on load distribution in total knee replacements. *J Biomech* 2005;38:349-355.

61. Tew M, Waugh W: Tibiofemoral alignment and the results of knee replacement. *J Bone Joint Surg Br* 1985; 67:551-556.

62. Callaghan JJ, Liu SS, Warth LC: Computer-assisted surgery: A wine before its time. In the affirmative. *J Arthroplasty* 2006;21(4, suppl 1): 27-28.

63. Molfetta L, Caldo D: Computer navigation versus conventional implantation for varus knee total arthroplasty: A case-control study at 5 years follow-up. *Knee* 2008;15:75-79.

64. Spencer JM, Chauhan SK, Sloan K, Taylor A, Beaver RJ: Computer navigation versus conventional total knee replacement: No difference in functional results at two years. *J Bone Joint Surg Br* 2007;89:477-480.

65. Dong H, Buxton M: Early assessment of the likely cost-effectiveness of a new technology: A Markov model with probabilistic sensitivity analysis of computer-assisted total knee replacement. *Int J Technol Assess Health Care* 2006;22:191-202.

66. Novak EJ, Silverstein MD, Bozic KJ: The cost-effectiveness of computer-assisted navigation in total knee arthroplasty. *J Bone Joint Surg Am* 2007; 89:2389-2397.

67. Friederich N, Verdonk R: The use of computer-assisted orthopedic surgery for total knee replacement in daily practice: A survey among ESSKA/SGO-SSO members. *Knee Surg Sports Traumatol Arthrosc* 2008;16:536-543.

68. Dorr LD, Sirianni L: The risk of product liability: Orthopaedic surgeons can be trapped. *Clin Orthop Relat Res* 2003;407:50-53.

69. Goldstein WM, Gordon A, Branson JJ: Leg length inequality in total hip arthroplasty. *Orthopedics* 2005;28: S1037-S1040.

70. Attarian DE, Vail TP: Medicolegal aspects of hip and knee arthroplasty. *Clin Orthop Relat Res* 2005;433:72-76.

Quadriceps Strength in Relation to Total Knee Arthroplasty Outcomes

Khaled J. Saleh, MD, MSc, FRCSC
Laura W. Lee, MD, MBA
Rajiv Gandhi, MD, FRCSC
Christopher D. Ingersoll, PhD, ATC, FACSM
Nizar N. Mahomed, MD, ScD, FRCSC
Shahin Sheibani-Rad, MD
Wendy M. Novicoff, PhD
William M. Mihalko, MD, PhD

Abstract

After total knee arthroplasty, quadriceps femoris muscle strength is an important determinant of physical function. Quadriceps weakness is often present in the osteoarthritic limb and worsens after total knee arthroplasty. Although some quadriceps strength is regained, it may take more than 2 years to achieve preoperative levels, and it is unclear if quadriceps strength in the operated limb ever reaches that of the nondiseased contralateral limb or the quadriceps strength of healthy controls. Studies point to volitional muscle activation rather than muscle atrophy or joint pain as the cause of the weakness. The unresolved challenge lies in clarifying the optimal surgical and rehabilitation course that will reverse the weakness early or prevent its occurrence. Studies suggest that progressive resistive strengthening exercises and neuromuscular electrical stimulation, possibly along with "prehabilitation," improve quadriceps volitional force output. Well-designed, controlled studies are necessary to determine efficacy. Because knee osteoarthritis and total knee arthroplasty are highly prevalent, improving quadriceps weakness is an important goal for orthopaedic surgeons and rehabilitation specialists.

Instr Course Lect 2010;59:119-130.

Total knee arthroplasty (TKA) remains one of the most commonly performed and universally successful surgical procedures for patients with osteoarthritis (OA) and other knee disorders, with more than 600,000 procedures performed in 2007.[1] However, it remains to be determined if all aspects of gait and functional recovery normalize over time when compared with healthy cohorts.[2] Studies have shown that clinical measures of knee function, lower limb kinematics, and joint moments improve following TKA, but a lack of quadriceps strength may lead to long-lasting deficits in

Dr. Saleh or an immediate family member has received royalties from Smith & Nephew; is a member of a speakers' bureau or has made paid presentations on behalf of Aesculap/B. Braun, Stryker, OMNI, and Kimberly Clark; serves as a paid consultant to or is an employee of Aesculap/B. Braun, Stryker, and OMNI; has received research or institutional support from Stryker, EKR Therapeutics, and Aesculap/B. Braun; and has received nonincome support (such as equipment or services), commercially derived honoraria, or other non–research-related funding (such as paid travel) from Blue Cross Blue Shield and Kimberly Clark. Dr. Lee or an immediate family member has stock or stock options held in retirement stock accounts, companies undisclosed. Neither Dr. Gandhi, Dr. Ingersoll, Dr. Sheibani-Rad nor any immediate family members have received anything of value from or own stock in a commercial company or institution related directly or indirectly to the subject of this chapter. Dr. Mahomed or an immediate family member is a member of a speakers' bureau or has made paid presentations on behalf of Smith & Nephew; serves as a paid consultant to or is an employee of Smith & Nephew; and has received research or institutional support from Smith & Nephew. Dr. Novicoff or an immediate family member has received research or institutional support from Aesculap/B. Braun, DePuy, Smith & Nephew, Stryker, and Zimmer. Dr. Mihalko or an immediate family member has received royalties from Elsevier; is a member of a speakers' bureau or has made paid presentations on behalf of Ethicon and Aesculap/B. Braun; serves as a paid consultant to or is an employee of Aesculap/B. Braun, Ethicon, Johnson & Johnson, and Stryker; and has received research or institutional support from Smith & Nephew and Aesculap/B. Braun.

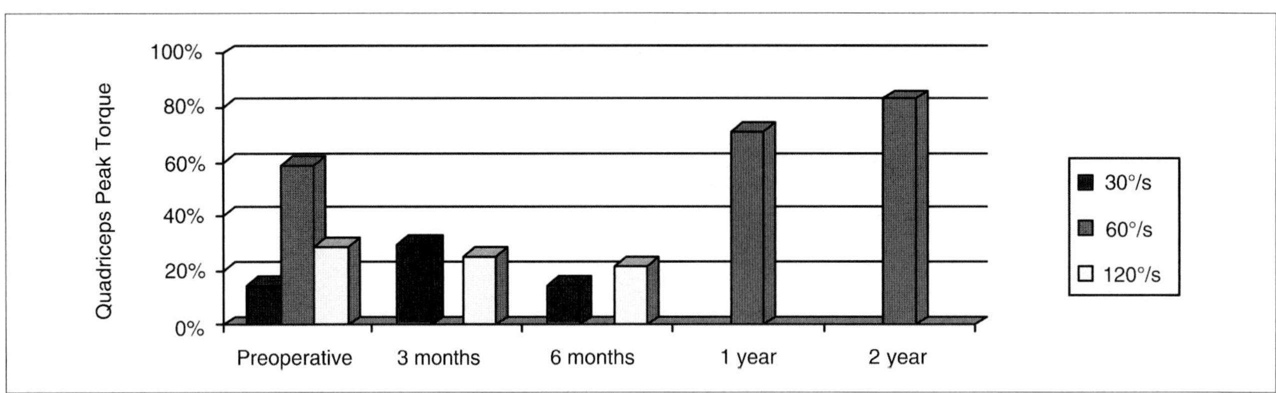

Figure 1 Graph showing the percentage of quadriceps peak torque values during isokinetic testing in patients treated with TKA compared with control subjects.

the gait pattern.[3-6] This chapter provides an overview of the surgical options and implant designs available for decreasing the impact of reduced quadriceps strength after TKA and discusses the potential for rehabilitation regimens to maximize improvement of quadriceps strength.

Epidemiology of Quadriceps Weakness after TKA

Quadriceps femoris muscle strength after TKA is an important determinant of physical function and gait. Quadriceps weakness, a common complication after TKA, can persist for long periods after surgery and postoperative rehabilitation.[3,4,7-11] One study reported that 31% of complications after TKA in patients with difficult courses of rehabilitation were related to quadriceps weakness, which occurred second in frequency only to knee flexion contractures.[12] Several studies have shown that quadriceps strength is reduced in the problematic knee of patients needing TKA (both before and for the 2-year period after surgery) compared with knee strength in healthy control subjects.[6,8,10,13-15] These studies reported significantly lower knee extension torques on isometric and isokinetic dynamometer testing for the operated knee compared with the nonoperated/uninvolved side. The ratio of knee flexion-to-extension peak torque values remained abnormal as flexion peak torque values approached control levels within 1 year of TKA.[8] The extension torque values remained abnormal for 2 years, even as pain resolved (compared with healthy control subjects, the average isometric extension peak torque values in patients 2 years after TKA were reduced by up to 30.7%).[8] Studies differ on when knee extension torque values start improving after initially worsening after surgery, with improvements beginning from 1 to 3 months postoperatively (Figure 1).

Women, those with rheumatoid arthritis, obese people, and possibly older adults with weaker than normal quadriceps strength and force are more vulnerable to quadriceps weakness after TKA.[8,13-16] A study by de Amorim Aguino and associates[17] reported that female patients who were tested for quadriceps muscle strength 1 to 3 years after TKA had significantly reduced maximum extensor and flexor torques compared with age-matched control subjects. Another study of women found that muscle strength was reduced approximately 20% in the arthritic limb compared with the contralateral nonarthritic limb, although lean muscle mass was only 3% less in the arthritic limb.[18] Gapeyeva and associates[19] reported that women had a maximal voluntary isometric contraction force of the quadriceps that was 48% lower before their TKA and 44% lower 6 months after the TKA (with reduced voluntary activation and delayed half-time relaxation after surgery) compared with age- and gender-matched controls.

It has long been believed that quadriceps weakness results from disuse atrophy secondary to pain and swelling in the involved joint both before and after TKA, given that OA changes muscle fiber composition.[20] However, findings suggest that pain and atrophy alone cannot account for the quadriceps weakness in patients treated with TKA because the weakness persists after the pain and swelling subside.[13,21,22] Studies have indicated that patients with knee arthroplasty demonstrate an impaired ability to fully activate (for example, a reduced voluntary contraction force) their quadriceps musculature, a phenomenon referred to as arthrogenic muscle inhibition (AMI).[21,22] Quadriceps inhibition is typically estimated using interpolated twitch and burst superimposition protocols in which an electrical stimulus or stimuli are superimposed on a voluntary quadriceps contraction.[23,24] The premise behind these measurement techniques is that if the muscle is not inhibited, the electrical stimulation will not generate any additional force above that recorded during the voluntary contraction. However, if muscle inhibition is present, then the electrical stimulation will produce additional force beyond that of the voluntarily generated force. The generation of maximum force during muscle contraction requires complete motor unit activation and optimal motor unit firing patterns. Increased recruitment during volitional activity leaves fewer motor units available to be activated by the electrical stimulus, thus reducing the force generated during electrical stimulation.

The interpolated twitch and burst superimposition techniques differ in the type of stimuli delivered to the voluntary force and how the measurements are normalized. The interpolated twitch technique typically involves applying a single or double pulse on varying levels of maximal voluntary effort, as well as to the resting muscle.[25] The force generated by the stimulus applied to the resting muscle, referred to as the resting twitch, is used to normalize the peak force generated by the twitch applied on top of the contraction. In contrast, the burst superimposition technique superimposes a train of pulses on a maximal isometric voluntary contraction.[26] The maximum voluntary contraction produced without the added stimulus is compared with the peak force generated by imposing the stimulus on the maximum voluntary contraction.

AMI has been reported in patients with knee OA before TKA and at an increased level of severity after the procedure. In a study of 123 patients who were candidates for TKA with unilateral Kellgren-Lawrence grade IV knee OA, quadriceps strength in both limbs was assessed with volitional muscle activation using a burst superimposition test; the lean muscle cross-sectional area was assessed with MRI. Regression analysis showed that in the limb with OA, volitional muscle activation was the primary determinant (40% of variance versus 27% for the lean muscle cross-sectional area) of quadriceps strength, whereas in the nondiseased limb, lean muscle cross-sectional area was the primary determinant (41% of variance versus 17% for volitional muscle activation).[27] Hurley and Newham[28] examined 10 patients with unilateral joint degeneration who had no reported pain or signs of joint effusion. Patients were referred to outpatient physical therapy clinics to increase quadriceps strength and improve function. Using the interpolated twitch technique to quantify quadriceps activation, they found that, on average, patients were unable to activate 19% of their quadriceps muscle in the affected limb and 6% in their unaffected limb. In a subsequent investigation using similar procedures to quantify muscle inhibition, Hurley and associates[29] found that 103 patients diagnosed with knee OA were unable to completely activate their quadriceps; they also reported that quadriceps activation was less in the affected limb in patients with knee OA compared to the limbs of healthy control subjects. Similar results were found in a study of 97 patients with knee OA who were evaluated with the interpolated twitch test to assess the presence of AMI. Results showed quadriceps inhibition (AMI = 27.25%) in all patients at the time of testing, with no reported gender differences.[30]

Machner and associates[31] studied patients before and at 18 months following unicompartmental knee arthroplasty. They found that quadriceps inhibition was reduced in the operated limb following surgery and postoperative rehabilitation (preoperative AMI = 33.6%; postoperative AMI = 23.1%) and also in the nonoperated limb (preoperative AMI = 33.4%; postoperative AMI = 21.5%). Quadriceps strength improved postoperatively in the operated limb (preoperative strength = 50.3 Nm; postoperative strength = 70.4 Nm) and in the nonoperated limb (preoperative strength = 66.91 Nm; postoperative strength = 77.2 Nm). Mizner and associates[22] evaluated 20 patients treated with tricompartmental cemented TKA at an average of 10 days before TKA and approximately 1 month after TKA. Using a burst-superimposition testing technique, they found that the involved limb had a postoperative 62% decrease in quadriceps strength and impaired volitional activation (AMI = 17%). Although the maximal cross-sectional area showed a 10% loss compared with preoperative values, regression analysis showed that the failure of voluntary activation contributed nearly twice as much to the loss of quadriceps strength as did muscle atrophy.

Stevens and associates[32] examined 28 patients approximately 10 days before and approximately 26 days after TKA. Following surgery, quadriceps volitional activation decreased in the involved limb (preoperative AMI = 15%; postoperative AMI = 31%) but remained unchanged postoperatively in the uninvolved limb (preoperative AMI = 9%; postoperative AMI = 9%).

Implant Design and Quadriceps Weakness

Implant design plays an important role in functional outcome after TKA and in the resulting quadriceps weakness. The kinematics theory of knee function has shown that flexion and extension occur around a changing instant center of rotation.[33] This theory is the basis for multiradius femoral components. Previous data have shown that TKA using a multiradius femoral component does not restore extensor mechanism moment arms to normal values.[34,35] The greatest reduction in quadriceps force occurs in 30° of extension. Shorter extensor mechanism moment arms after TKA are caused by the anterior axis of rotation.

The moment arm of the extensor mechanism is a determinant of the required force for knee extension.[36] The moment arm is the perpendicular distance from the center of flexion to the line of application of force at the patella. It is also the result of the transfer of force from the quadriceps tendon articulating with the trochlear groove. The single radius design axis is more posterior than the axis of a multiradius implant. In cadaver studies, the single radius design axis has been shown to increase the quadriceps moment arm.[37] In a study of quadriceps moment arm and forces, D'Lima and associates[37] showed that the greater quadriceps moment arm length in the single radius design resulted in a reduced amount of quadriceps muscle force needed to generate 40 Nm compared with a multiradius prosthesis. The single radius design also allows for femoral rollback, reduced patellofemoral joint forces, and improved quadriceps muscle efficiency. In the single radius design, because the knee flexion-knee extension axis is fixed to the femur, it simultaneously rotates with the femur during internal and external rotation. The knee flexion-extension axis of single radius implants is located more posteriorly by 2.5 to 3.5 mm.[38] Single radius implants also demonstrated increased mediolateral stability during flexion compared with multiradius implants, exhibiting less abduction angular displacement and an earlier abduction peak.

Normally, quadriceps muscle force is greatest in full extension. Extensor mechanism function is a major factor in the patient's ability to perform daily activities after TKA. One of the most common reasons for TKA revision is the inability to rise from a chair, climb stairs, or walk because of weak knee extension.[39] Better quadriceps function, which is dependent on extensor mechanism function, is associated with better functional outcome after TKA.[8] Fuchs and associates[40] showed that patients treated with TKA were able to improve their preoperative extension torque up to 50% but were not able to reach the same functional level as healthy subjects. The results indicate that higher quadriceps forces are needed after TKA to extend the knee at the same extension moment. A study by Mahoney and associates[41] reported that more patients with single radius implants can rise from a sitting position at 6 weeks postoperatively than can patients with multiradius implants. This finding was confirmed in a study by Wang and associates[42] in which patients with a single radius implant took significantly less time to rise from a sitting to a standing position (sit-to-stand movement) compared with those with a multiradius implant. This benefit of single radius implants results from the longer quadriceps moment arm in the single radius design compared with the multiradius design. Greater muscle force is required for rising from a chair in those with multiradius implants. It was hypothesized that the faster sit-to-stand time for patients with single radius implants was secondary to the ability of the implant to generate greater torque and greater knee flexion deceleration.[38] During sit-to-stand movements, those with single radius implants completed flexion movements more quickly than those with multiradius implants.

Kinematics analysis has shown that during knee flexion, there is a progressive posterior translation of the femorotibial contact area (posterior femoral rollback) as well as internal tibial rotation.[43] Femoral rollback maintains the anterior displacement of the quadriceps from the center of rotation of the knee. This creates a longer moment arm and a more efficient quadriceps function. An absent or malfunctioning posterior cruciate ligament (PCL) will diminish femoral rollback. In a study by Dennis and associates,[44] it was observed that PCL-substituting implants had a 6-mm rollback, whereas PCL-retaining implants had an erratic pattern of rollback. Normal knees have a 14-mm rollback. In the last decade, there has been a shift toward using PCL-substituting implants. In the 1990s, PCL-substituting implants accounted for less 20% of all TKAs, but by 2001 they were used in nearly 50% of TKAs.[45]

Early PCL-retaining implants with porous-coated anatomic prostheses showed a high rate of polyethylene wear and a high failure rate at 5- to 10-year follow-up.[46-48] Current studies show that newer implant designs have an approximate 99% success rate at 10-year follow-up.[49,50] Most clinical studies have shown no difference in short-term clinical outcomes between PCL-substituting and PCL-retaining implants. Hirsch and associates[51] and Lombardi and associates[52] showed no difference in revision rates between PCL-substituting and PCL-retaining implants. Victor and associates[53] showed that although the clinical outcomes of PCL-retaining and PCL-substituting implants are similar, their kinematics were significantly different. Kinematics studies have shown that PCL-substituting implants provide a more reliable rollback than PCL-retaining implants.[54] Weight-bearing kinematics proved that posterior femoral translation during flexion occurs more reliably with PCL-substituting implants, leading to an increase in maximal knee flexion under weight-bearing conditions.[55,56] A study by Dennis and associates[57] showed that, under weight-bearing conditions, patients implanted with a PCL-substituting TKA had a greater mean range of motion (ROM) than those with PCL-retaining implants. This finding was believed to result from the anterior translation of the femorotibial contact position with progressive knee flexion. A 2008 study by Hall and associates[58] reported no difference in the ability of patients with PCL-retaining designs to rise from a chair in those with single radius and multiradius implants. This is believed to result from the fact that the lowest point on the articular surface is located posterior to the center of the tray inducing femoral rollback, which is provided by PCL-substituting implants.[59] This rollback may cause a longer extensor mechanism moment arm, resulting in equal performance in chair rising ability. A randomized clinical trial by Harato and associates[60] reported no significant differences in groups treated with PCL-retaining or PCL-substituting implants at 5-year follow-up based on the total Knee Society score, the Western Ontario and McMaster Universities Osteoarthritis index, the Medical Outcomes Study 12-Item Short Form score, or radiologic outcomes. The PCL-substituting group had a significant improvement in flexion and ROM compared with the PCL-retaining group at 5-year follow-up.

Rotating-platform implants were created to maximize the contact area throughout ROM. When compared with fixed-bearing implants, rotating-platform designs have higher contact areas, which produce a significant reduction in contact stresses.[61] Polyethylene contact stress is inversely proportional to the contact area for a given load.[62] The increased conformity of the implant is believed to increase contact surface area and reduce contact stresses, thus reducing the rate of polyethylene wear. Rotating-platform implants have been reported to have a 99% survival rate at 9- to 12-year follow-up.[63] Callaghan[64] showed that mobile-bearing TKAs achieve a comparable clinical result to those of fixed-bearing TKAs. In a comparison of rotating-platform implants and fixed-bearing implants, the mean range of postoperative flexion in the rotating-platform group was 116° compared with 113° in the fixed-bearing TKA group; full extension was achieved in both groups.[65] In a recent study by Bhan and associates,[66] the mean postoperative flexion was 107° in the rotating-platform group compared with 105° in the fixed-bearing group. Ranawat and associates[67] found no significant difference in terms of ROM, overall satisfaction, or Knee Society scores between the patients treated with rotating-platform or fixed-bearing implant designs. Clinically, both implant designs produce similar results.

Surgical Factors and Quadriceps Weakness

Surgical factors in TKA that affect quadriceps muscle strength include the surgical approach, restoration of a normal patellofemoral articulation, and tibial slope. Improved quadriceps strength after TKA may translate into improved short-term and long-term outcomes and a shorter length of stay in the hospital.[3,8,68] Most studies on this topic use the straight-leg raise (SLR) test or electromyographic testing to evaluate quadriceps strength after knee replacement surgery.

Minimally invasive surgery using the mini-subvastus and mini-midvastus approaches spare the quadriceps tendon compared with the traditional quadriceps-splitting medial parapatellar approach.[5,6,22] The mini-subvastus approach uses an anterior incision through the medial intermuscular septum, leaving the innervation of the vastus medialis intact in contrast to the midvastus approach.[69] The medial parapatellar approach may increase postoperative pain, require a longer rehabilitation period, and cause quadriceps lag when compared with minimally invasive approaches.[69-71]

In a randomized study by Bäthis and associates,[71] patients treated with a midvastus approach showed significantly improved quadriceps strength (as measured by a dynamometer) at 3 and 6 weeks postoperatively when compared with patients treated with a traditional medial parapatellar approach. Similarly, a study by Schroer and associates[72] reported that on the first postoperative day, 83% of patients in the mini-subvastus group could perform a SLR compared with no patients in the group treated with a traditional approach. In another randomized study, the mini-subvastus group achieved an earlier ability to perform SLRs (1.4 ± 1.3 days) when compared with the group treated with the medial parapatellar approach (1.9 ± 1.5 days); however, the authors did not consider this difference clinically significant.[73] In comparing the midvastus and subvastus approaches, Berth and associates[74] used the twitch-interpolation technique for measuring quadriceps strength and found no differences in maximum voluntary contraction between the two cohorts at 3 and 6 months postoperatively.

The limitation of minimally invasive approaches is the increased level of surgical complexity caused by the smaller operating window, particularly in obese or highly muscular patients.[73,74] Despite the earlier return of quadriceps function with minimally invasive surgery, final quadriceps strength and functional outcome scores measured at 3 months and 1 year after surgery are equivalent to those of patients treated with a traditional approach.[15,69,73,75] It is yet unknown if mini-incision techniques result in a higher complication rate than traditional approaches.

Patellofemoral Articulation

Restoration of a normal patellofemoral joint, including patellar height, thickness, and alignment, will result in a greater mechanical advantage for the quadriceps tendon through a properly tensioned moment arm. Patellar resurfacing versus patelloplasty was not shown to be a significant predictor of improved extensor mechanism strength in a 2-year follow-up study.[76] However, a randomized controlled trial by Walter and associates[68] showed that avoidance of patellar eversion during surgery may lead to improved quadriceps strength after surgery. Patellectomies have been clearly linked to quadriceps lag following surgery.[77]

Femoral Rollback and Tibial Slope

Femoral rollback on the tibia is an important component in optimizing extensor mechanism efficiency after surgery. To achieve flexion greater than 105°, posterior displacement of the femur allows for clearance of the posterior margin of the tibia and also lengthens the level arm of the quadriceps.[78] In fluoroscopic studies by Yoshiya and associates[79] and Barnes and Sledge,[80] cruciate-retaining femoral designs showed a paradoxical roll forward of the femur on the tibia, with flexion compared with more physiologic movements with cruciate-substituting implants. Loss of this rollback results in the need for increased quadriceps force to accomplish daily activities and the potential for increased anterior knee pain. Accurate flexion and extension gap balancing also help to ensure proper knee mechanics.[79] Ostermeier and associates[81] showed that posterior tibial slope can result in improved quadriceps force when compared with a neutral slope. However, this study evaluated only seven patients and did not provide details on the normal tibial slopes of the patients before surgery.

Outcome Measurements

A critical evaluation of the existing literature on quadriceps strength following TKA shows that the SLR test is the most often cited outcome measure; however, this measure is likely confounded by the patient's level of pain. The SLR test evaluated as a binary outcome fails to distinguish the height that the leg is raised and the ability of the patient to hold up the leg with a constant contraction. Using electromyographic study results as the outcome measure with a clinically relevant defined threshold may be of greater value. In addition, many studies do not include preoperative measures of quadriceps strength, which should be used as a baseline reference for each patient. Tibial slope, femoral component rotation, and alignment are all factors believed to affect quadriceps strength after TKA; however, there are few data on these variables.[81-83]

Rehabilitation of Quadriceps Weakness

Quadriceps inhibition is reduced during postoperative rehabilitation; although improvements occur with time, quadriceps weakness can persist for years after surgery. Currently, rehabilitation regimens following TKA are designed to help patients resume the activities of daily living and return to functional activity (Figure 2). The rehabilitation exercises are usually started immediately following TKA, with the goals of controlling pain, improving ambulation and muscle strength, and maximizing ROM.[84] Few data are available comparing the effectiveness of specific rehabilitation protocols on quadriceps weakness in patients following TKA. Kramer and associates[85] compared a clinic- and home-based rehabilitation protocol designed to improve ROM and strength after TKA and found no difference in scores on the Knee Society scale and Western Ontario and

McMaster Universities Osteoarthritis index or any differences in ROM, distance walked, and time to ascend/descend stairs. Frost and associates[86] performed a randomized controlled study to evaluate 47 patients treated with TKA (except for 1 patient treated with a unicompartmental knee arthroplasty) and an inpatient rehabilitation program, followed by either a home-based traditional strengthening program or a functional strengthening exercise program. Leg extension power (force × velocity of contraction) did not significantly increase in the functional exercise group; however, interpretation of the study data were hampered by a high dropout rate, especially in patients with low motivation. Some evidence is available suggesting that rehabilitation protocols containing aerobic, resistance, and proprioceptive exercises have beneficial effects (increased ROM, improved sensorimotor function, decreased quadriceps inhibition, improved functional status) in patients with osteoarthritis, including older adults.[29,30,87,88]

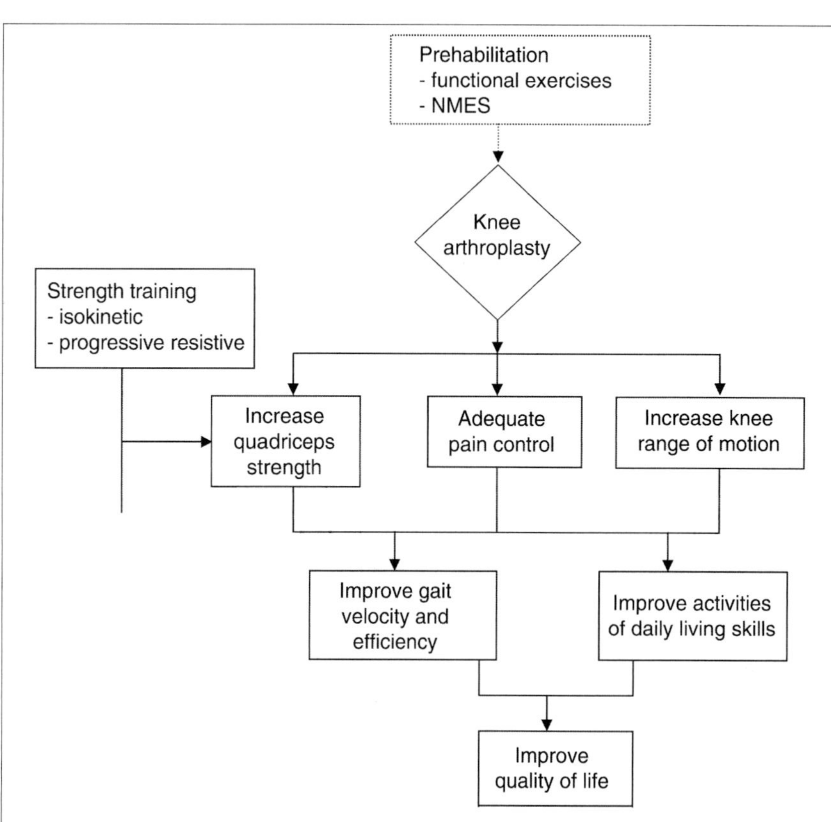

Figure 2 The rehabilitation pathway after TKA. NMES = neuromuscular electrical stimulation.

Because of the association of quadriceps weakness with functional and gait abnormalities, such as a larger hip extension and anterior trunk lean during stance as compensating mechanisms, developing effective strategies to improve strength is paramount.[6,12] A study by Mizner and associates[21] found that 3 to 4 weeks after TKA, one group of older adults had a 64% lower average normalized knee extension force than control subjects, and the average volitional activation deficit was four times greater (26% versus 6%) than that of the control subjects who were slightly older (64.9 ± −7.7 versus 72.2 ± −5.3 years, respectively). The authors surmised that volitional activation was highly correlated with knee extension force production, and rehabilitation programs that focused on volitional exercise alone after TKA without attempting to correct the early quadriceps muscle inhibition would be unlikely to overcome the lack of activation. Highly intense strengthening exercise protocols have been mentioned in the literature as an effective method for increasing quadriceps strength and volitional activation. Tal-Akabi and associates[89] reported on a randomized controlled study of 62 elderly patients treated with a lower extremity orthopaedic procedure (of these procedures, 23 were TKAs) approximately 12 days previously. For 3 weeks, the patients participated in a high- or regular-intensity strengthening program for the non-operated limb. The high-intensity program consisted of progressively resistive closed-chain exercises, whereas the regular-intensity program involved exercise with low weight resistance. Both groups exercised five times per week. Although results showed an increase in quadriceps concentric torque and isometric force, the applicability of these results to patients after TKA is unclear. Rossi and associates[90] evaluated 38 elderly patients treated with a unilateral tricompartmental knee arthroplasty by the same surgeon. All patients had an identical rehabilitation course with transfer to acute rehabilitation on postoperative day 3 and transition to outpatient rehabilitation on postoperative day 10. During the next 8 weeks, the patients participated in physical therapy three times per week, including an isokinetic resistive strengthening program 2 weeks after surgery, ROM exercises, and transfer and stair training. The results showed statistically significant improvement, with the knee extensors of the operated limb producing 65% and 74% (at 60°/s and 180°/s, respectively) of uninvolved limb isokinetic force preoperatively ($P = 0.001$) and 67% and 78% at postoperative day 30 compared with preoperative results ($P = 0.001$), and 91% and 99% at postoperative day 60 compared with preoperative force testing results. Nonetheless, even at postoperative day 60, the extensor force values were not closely comparable to the nondiseased side. Although there was no control group in this study, the trajectory of improvement appears better than that reported in the previously mentioned observational studies in which the rehabilitation phase was not identical among patients.

Application of neuromuscular electrical stimulation (NMES) over the quadriceps has been advocated in conjunction with strengthening exercises and in some instances with biofeedback.[12,91] NMES following TKA has been shown to improve knee extensor lag and decrease the length of the hospital stay.[92] Even for patients with residual quadriceps weakness at least 2.5 months after TKA, NMES has demonstrated efficacy in isokinetic strength testing.[91] NMES may improve muscle activation and AMI in addition in improving overall strength. Case studies have shown that when NMES is added to an active rehabilitation program, deficits in quadriceps muscle strength and activation resolve more quickly after TKA when compared with rehabilitation exercise alone.[93,94] A 25% improvement in quadriceps volitional force output was reported following 16 NMES treatments and volitional strength training over a 6-week period, with a central activation ratio improvement from 0.83 to 0.97.[94] NMES has produced improvements in quadriceps strength in elderly patients, and the treatment is well tolerated.[89,95] The use of NMES in female patients improves quadriceps activation and performance on functional tests.[96] Avramidis and associates[97] randomly assigned 30 patients for therapy with NMES of the vastus medialis plus standard physical therapy for 4 hours per day for 6 weeks postoperatively or to a control group who had physical therapy alone. The NMES group had a statistically significant increase in walking speed, although there was no statistically significant improvement in the Hospital for Special Surgery knee score. The improvement in walking speed compared with the control group was still evident at 12 weeks after surgery. In another study, 50 female patients with OA who had not yet been treated with TKA participated in either a NMES program or a biofeedback-assisted isometric exercise program for 5 days a week for 4 weeks.[98] Both groups had statistically significant improvements in pain, physical function, walking and stair climbing time, and quadriceps strength, showing that NMES is just as effective as regular exercise in improving patient outcomes.

The question arises that if postoperative exercise training improves quadriceps strength, will exercise training or NMES treatment before TKA benefit patients who can tolerate the pain? Quadriceps force torque seems to be improved by general functional exercises, although there is no significant improvement from focused isokinetic or aquatic exercises in people with OA.[99] However, there is conflicting evidence on whether prehabilitation leads to long-term benefits after TKA.[100,101]

Summary

Quadriceps weakness is often present in the osteoarthritic limb and worsens after TKA. Although quadriceps strength is regained, it may take more than 2 years to achieve preoperative levels. It is unclear if quadriceps strength in the operated limb ever reaches that of the nondiseased side or the level of strength in healthy control subjects. In examining quadriceps weakness, studies point to volitional muscle activation rather than muscle atrophy or joint pain as the cause of the weakness. The unresolved challenge lies in clarifying the optimal surgical and rehabilitation course that will result in an early reversal of quadriceps weakness or prevent its occurrence. Studies suggest that progressive resistive strengthening exercises and NMES, possibly along with prehabilitation, improve quadriceps volitional force output; however, well-designed, controlled studies are necessary to determine efficacy. Given that knee OA and TKA are highly prevalent in the healthcare system, improving quadriceps strength is an important goal for orthopaedic rehabilitation specialists.

References

1. 2008 Hip and Knee Implant Review. *Orthopedic Network News* 2008;19:1-20.
2. Finch E, Walsh M, Thomas SG, Woodhouse LJ: Functional ability perceived by individuals following total knee arthroplasty compared to age-matched individuals without knee disability. *J Orthop Sports Phys Ther* 1998;27:255-263.

3. Mizner RL, Petterson SC, Snyder-Mackler L: Quadriceps strength and the time course of functional recovery after total knee arthroplasty. *J Orthop Sports Phys Ther* 2005;35:424-436.

4. Mizner RL, Petterson SC, Stevens JE, Axs MJ, Snyder-Mackler L: Preoperative quadriceps strength predicts functional ability one year after total knee arthroplasty. *J Rheumatol* 2005; 32:1533-1539.

5. Mizner RL, Snyder-Mackler L: Altered loading during walking and sit-to-stand is affected by quadriceps weakness after total knee arthroplasty. *J Orthop Res* 2005;23:1083-1090.

6. Yoshida Y, Mizner RL, Ramsey DK, Snyder-Mackler L: Examining outcomes from total knee arthroplasty and the relationship between quadriceps strength and knee function over time. *Clin Biomech (Bristol, Avon)* 2008;23:320-328.

7. Lamb SE, Frost H: Recovery of mobility after knee arthroplasty: Expected rates and influencing factors. *J Arthroplasty* 2003;18:575-582.

8. Silva M, Shepherd EF, Jackson WO, Pratt JA, McClung CD, Schmalzried TP: Knee strength after total knee arthroplasty. *J Arthroplasty* 2003; 18:605-611.

9. Walsh M, Woodhouse LJ, Thomas SG, Finch F: Physical impairments and functional limitations: A comparison of individuals 1 year after total knee arthroplasty with control subjects. *Phys Ther* 1998;78:248-258.

10. Berman AT, Bosacco SJ, Israelite C: Evaluation of total knee arthroplasty using isokinetic testing. *Clin Orthop Relat Res* 1991;271:106-113.

11. Ouellet D, Moffet H: Locomotor deficits before and two months after knee arthroplasty. *Arthritis Rheum* 2002;47:484-493.

12. Bhave A, Mont M, Tennis S, Nickey M, Starr R, Etienne G: Functional problems and treatment solutions after total hip and knee joint arthroplasty. *J Bone Joint Surg Am* 2005;87(suppl):9-21.

13. Lorentzen JS, Petersen MM, Brot C, Madsen OR: Early changes in muscle strength after total knee arthroplasty: A 6-month follow-up of 30 knees. *Acta Orthop Scand* 1999;70:176-179.

14. Rossi MD, Brown LE, Whitehurst M: Knee extensor and flexor torque characteristics before and after unilateral total knee arthroplasty. *Am J Phys Med Rehabil* 2006;85:737-746.

15. Fauré BT, Benjamin JB, Lindsey B, Volz RG, Schutte D: Comparison of the subvastus and paramedian surgical approaches in bilateral knee arthroplasty. *J Arthroplasty* 1993;8:511-516.

16. Hernàndez-Vaquero D, Fernández-Carreira JM, Perez-Hernàndez D, Fernández-Lombardía J, García-Sandoval MA: Total knee arthroplasty in the elderly: Is there an age limit? *J Arthroplasty* 2006;21:358-361.

17. de Amorim Aquino M, Leme LE: Isokinetic dynamometry in elderly women undergoing total knee arthroplasty: A comparative study. *Clinics (Sao Paulo)* 2006;61:215-222.

18. Madsen OR, Brot C, Petersen MM, Sørensen OH: Body composition and muscle strength in women scheduled for a knee or hip replacement: A comparative study of two groups of osteoarthritic women. *Clin Rheumatol* 1997;16:39-44.

19. Gapeyeva H, Buht N, Peterson K, Ereline J, Haviko T, Pääsuke M: Quadriceps femoris muscle voluntary isometric force production and relaxation characteristics before and 6 months after unilateral total knee arthroplasty in women. *Knee Surg Sports Traumatol Arthrosc* 2007;15: 202-211.

20. Fink B, Egl M, Singer J, Fuerst M, Bubenheim M, Neuen-Jacob E: Morphologic changes in the vastus medialis muscle in patients with osteoarthritis of the knee. *Arthritis Rheum* 2007;56:3626-3633.

21. Mizner RL, Stevens JE, Snyder-Mackler L: Voluntary activation and decreased force production of the quadriceps femoris muscle after total knee arthroplasty. *Phys Ther* 2003;83: 359-365.

22. Mizner RL, Petterson SC, Stevens JE, Vandenborne K, Synder-Mackler L: Early quadriceps strength loss after total knee arthroplasty: The contributions of muscle atrophy and failure of voluntary muscle activation. *J Bone Joint Surg Am* 2005;87:1047-1053.

23. Behm DG, St-Pierre DM, Perez D: Muscle inactivation: Assessment of interpolated twitch technique. *J Appl Physiol* 1996;81:2267-2273.

24. Stackhouse SK, Dean JC, Lee SC, Binder-MacLeod SA: Measurement of central activation failure of the quadriceps femoris in healthy adults. *Muscle Nerve* 2000;23:1706-1712.

25. Oskouei MA, Van Mazijk BC, Schuiling MH, Herzog W: Variability in the interpolated twitch torque for maximal and submaximal voluntary contractions. *J Appl Physiol* 2003;95: 1648-1655.

26. Lewek MD, Rudolph KS, Snyder-Mackler L: Quadriceps femoris muscle weakness and activation failure in patients with symptomatic knee osteoarthritis. *J Orthop Res* 2004; 22:110-115.

27. Petterson SC, Barrance P, Buchanan T, Binder-Macleod S, Snyder-Mackler L: Mechanisms underlying quadriceps weakness in knee osteoarthritis. *Med Sci Sports Exerc* 2008;40: 422-427.

28. Hurley MV, Newham DJ: The influence of arthrogenous muscle inhibition on quadriceps rehabilitation of patients with early, unilateral osteoarthritic knees. *Br J Rheumatol* 1993;32: 127-131.

29. Hurley MV, Scott DL, Rees J, Newham DJ: Sensorimotor changes and functional performance in patients with knee osteoarthritis. *Ann Rheum Dis* 1997;56:641-648.

30. Hurley MV, Scott DL: Improvements in quadriceps sensorimotor function and disability of patients with knee osteoarthritis following a clinically practicable exercise regime. *Br J Rheumatol* 1998;37:1181-1187.

31. Machner A, Pap G, Awiszus F: Evaluation of quadriceps strength and voluntary activation after unicompartmental arthroplasty for medial osteoarthritis of the knee. *J Orthop Res* 2002;20:108-111.

32. Stevens JE, Mizner RL, Snyder-Mackler L: Quadriceps strength and volitional activation before and after total knee arthroplasty for osteoarthritis. *J Orthop Res* 2003;21:775-779.

33. Reauleaux F: *The Kinematics Machinery: Outline of a Theory of Machines.* London, United Kingdom, Macmillan, 1960.

34. Huang CH, Cheng CK, Lee YT, Lee KS: Muscle strength after successful total knee replacement: A 6- to 13-year followup. *Clin Orthop Relat Res* 1996;328:147-154.

35. Lewandowski PJ, Askew MJ, Lin DF, Hurst FW, Melby A: Kinematics of posterior cruciate ligament-retaining and -sacrificing mobile bearing total knee arthroplasties: An in vitro comparison of the New Jersey LCS meniscal bearing and rotating platform prostheses. *J Arthroplasty* 1997;12: 777-784.

36. Insall JN, Lachiewicz PF, Burstein AH: The posterior stabilized condylar prosthesis: A modification of the total condylar design. Two to four-year clinical experience. *J Bone Joint Surg Am* 1982;64:1317-1323.

37. D'Lima DD, Poole C, Chadha H, Hermida JC, Mahar A, Coldwell CW Jr: Quadriceps moment arm and quadriceps forces after total knee arthroplasty. *Clin Orthop Relat Res* 2001; 392:213-220.

38. Wang H, Simpson KJ, Chamnogkich S, Kinsey T, Mahoney OM: A biomechanical comparison between the single-axis and multi-axis total knee arthroplasty systems for the stand-to-sit movement. *Clin Biomech (Bristol, Avon)* 2005;20:428-433.

39. Rand JA: The patellofemoral joint in total knee arthroplasty. *J Bone Joint Surg Am* 1994;76:612-620.

40. Fuchs S, Tibesku CO, Jerosch J: Isokinetic measurements in total knee arthroplasty patients compared to healthy volunteers, in *Proceedings of the 8th Congress of the European Society of Sports Traumatology, Knee Surgery, and Arthroscopy.* Luxenbourg, ESSKA, 1998.

41. Mahoney OM, Kinesey TL, Casto SR, et al: Laboratory demonstration of mechanical and functional advantages of a single-radius TKA design. *69th Annual Meeting Proceedings.* Rosemont, IL, American Academy of Orthopaedic Surgeons, 2002, p 442.

42. Wang H, Simpson KJ, Ferrara MS, Chamnongkich S, Kinsey T, Mahoney OM: Biomechanical differences exhibited during sit-to-stand between total knee arthroplasty designs of varying radii. *J Arthroplasty* 2006;21:1193-1199.

43. Pinskerova V, Johal P, Nakagawa S, et al: Does the femur roll-back with flexion? *J Bone Joint Surg Br* 2004;86: 925-931.

44. Dennis DA, Komistek RD, Hoff WA, Gabriel SM: In vivo knee kinematics derived using an inverse perspective technique. *Clin Orthop Relat Res* 1996; 331:107-117.

45. Hip and Knee Replacement Market Report: Report DMHC2264. Datamonitor Website. http://www.datamonitor.com/store/browse/?ntt=dmhc2264. Accessed October 2009.

46. Tsao A, Mintz L, McRae CR, Stulberg SD, Wright T: Failure of the porous-coated anatomic prosthesis in total knee arthroplasty due to severe polyethylene wear. *J Bone Joint Surg Am* 1993;75:19-26.

47. Wright TM, Rimnac CM, Faris PM, Bansal M: Analysis of surface damage in retrieved carbon fiber-reinforced and plain polyethylene tibial components from posterior stabilized total knee replacements. *J Bone Joint Surg Am* 1988;70:1312-1319.

48. Knight JL, Gorai PA, Atwater RD, Grothaus L: Tibial polyethylene failure after primary porous-coated anatomic total knee arthroplasty: Aids to diagnosis and revision. *J Arthroplasty* 1995;10:748-757.

49. Ritter MA, Berend ME, Medling JB, Keating EM, Faris PM, Crites BM: Long-term followup of anatomic graduated components posterior cruciate-retaining total knee replacement. *Clin Orthop Relat Res* 2001; 388:51-57.

50. Gill GS, Joshi AB: Long-term results of cemented, posterior cruciate ligament-retaining total knee arthroplasty in osteoarthritis. *Am J Knee Surg* 2001;14:209-214.

51. Hirsch HS, Lotke PA, Morrison LD: The posterior cruciate ligament in total knee surgery: Save, sacrifice, or substitute? *Clin Orthop Relat Res* 1994; 309:64-68.

52. Lombardi AV Jr, Mallory TH, Fada RA, et al: An algorithm for the posterior cruciate ligament in total knee arthroplasty. *Clin Orthop Relat Res* 2001;392:75-87.

53. Victor J, Banks S, Bellemans J: Kinematics of posterior cruciate ligament-retaining and -substituting total knee arthroplasty: A prospective randomised outcome study. *J Bone Joint Surg Br* 2005;87:646-655.

54. Banks S, Bellemans J, Nozaki H, Whiteside LA, Harman M, Hodge WA: Knee motions during maximum flexion in fixed and mobile-bearing arthroplasties. *Clin Orthop Relat Res* 2003;410:131-138.

55. Dennis DA, Komistek RD, Colwell CE Jr, et al: In vivo anteroposterior femorotibial translation of total knee arthroplasty: A multicenter analysis. *Clin Orthop Relat Res* 1998; 356:47-57.

56. Dennis DA, Komistek RD, Mahfouz MR, Haas BD, Stiehl JB: Multicenter determination of in vivo kinematics after total knee arthroplasty. *Clin Orthop Relat Res* 2003;416:37-57.

57. Dennis DA, Komistek RD, Scuderi GR, Zingde S: Factors affecting flexion after total knee arthroplasty. *Clin Orthop Relat Res* 2007;464:53-60.

58. Hall J, Copp SN, Adelson WS, D'Lima DD, Colwell CW Jr: Extensor mechanism function in single-radius vs multiradius femoral compo-

nents for total knee arthroplasty. *J Arthroplasty* 2008;23:216-219.

59. Dennis DA, Mahfouz MR, Komistek RD, Hoff W: In vivo determination of normal and anterior cruciate ligament-deficient knee kinematics. *J Biomech* 2005;38:241-253.

60. Harato K, Bourne RB, Victor J, Snyder M, Hart J, Ries MD: Midterm comparison of posterior cruciate-retaining versus -substituting total knee arthroplasty using the Genesis II prosthesis: A multicenter prospective randomized clinical trial. *Knee* 2008; 15:217-221.

61. Buechel FF, Pappas MJ: The New Jersey Low-Contact-Stress Knee Replacement System: Biomechanical rationale and review of the first 123 cemented cases. *Arch Orthop Trauma Surg* 1986;105:197-204.

62. Bartel DL, Bicknell VL, Wright TM: The effect of conformity, thickness, and material on stresses in ultra-high molecular weight components for total joint replacement. *J Bone Joint Surg Am* 1986;68:1041-1051.

63. Callaghan JJ, Squire MW, Goetz DD, Sullivan PM, Johnston RC: Cemented rotating-platform total knee replacement: A nine to twelve-year follow-up study. *J Bone Joint Surg Am* 2000;82:705-711.

64. Callaghan JJ: Mobile-bearing knee replacement: Clinical results. A review of the literature. *Clin Orthop Relat Res* 2001;392:221-225.

65. Evans MC, Parsons EM, Scott RD, Thornhill TS, Zurakowski D: Comparative flexion after rotating-platform vs fixed-bearing total knee arthroplasty. *J Arthroplasty* 2006;21: 985-991.

66. Bhan S, Malhotra R, Kiran EK, Shukla S, Bijjawara M: A comparison of fixed-bearing and mobile-bearing total knee arthroplasty at a minimum follow-up of 4.5 years. *J Bone Joint Surg Am* 2005;87:2290-2296.

67. Ranawat AS, Rossi R, Loreti I, Rasquinha VJ, Rodriguez JA, Ranawat CS: Comparison of the PFC Sigma fixed-bearing and rotating-platform total knee arthroplasty in the same patient: Short-term results. *J Arthroplasty* 2004;19:35-39.

68. Walter F, Haynes MB, Markel DC: A randomized prospective study evaluating the effect of patellar eversion on the early functional outcomes in primary total knee arthroplasty. *J Arthroplasty* 2007;22:509-514.

69. Chang CH, Chen KH, Yang RS, Liu TK: Muscle torques in total knee arthroplasty with subvastus and parapatellar approaches. *Clin Orthop Relat Res* 2002;398:189-195.

70. Huang HT, Su JY, Chang JK, Chen CH, Wang GJ: The early clinical outcome of minimally invasive quadriceps-sparing total knee arthroplasty: Report of a 2-year follow-up. *J Arthroplasty* 2007;22:1007-1012.

71. Bäthis H, Perlick L, Blum C, Lüring C, Perlick C, Girfka J: Midvastus approach in total knee arthroplasty: A randomized, double-blinded study on early rehabilitation. *Knee Surg Sports Traumatol Arthrosc* 2005;13: 545-550.

72. Schroer WC, Diesfeld PJ, Reedy ME, LeMarr AR: Mini-subvastus approach for total knee arthroplasty. *J Arthroplasty* 2008;23:19-25.

73. Aglietti P, Baldini A, Sensi L: Quadriceps-sparing versus mini-subvastus approach in total knee arthroplasty. *Clin Orthop Relat Res* 2006; 452:106-111.

74. Berth A, Urbach D, Neumann W, Awiszus F: Strength and voluntary activation of quadriceps femoris muscle in total knee arthroplasty with midvastus and subvastus approaches. *J Arthroplasty* 2007;22:83-88.

75. Kelly MJ, Rumi MN, Kothari M, et al: Comparison of the vastus-splitting and median parapatellar approaches for primary total knee arthroplasty: A prospective, randomized study. *J Bone Joint Surg Am* 2006; 88:715-720.

76. Bourne RB, Rorabeck CH, Vaz M, Kramer J, Hardie R, Robertson D: Resurfacing versus not resurfacing the patella during total knee replacement. *Clin Orthop Relat Res* 1995; 321:156-161.

77. Chang MA, Rand JA, Trousdale RT: Patellectomy after total knee arthroplasty. *Clin Orthop Relat Res* 2005;440: 175-177.

78. Mahoney OM, Noble PC, Rhoads DD, Alexander JW, Tullos HS: Posterior cruciate function following total knee arthroplasty: A biomechanical study. *J Arthroplasty* 1994; 9:569-578.

79. Yoshiya S, Matsui N, Komistek RD, Dennis DA, Mahfouz M, Kurosaka M: In vivo kinematic comparison of posterior cruciate-retaining and posterior stabilized total knee arthroplasties under passive and weight-bearing conditions. *J Arthroplasty* 2005;20:777-783.

80. Barnes CL, Sledge CB: Total knee arthroplasty with posterior cruciate ligament retention designs, in Insall JN, Windsor RE, Scott WN, et al, eds: *Surgery of the Knee*, ed 2. New York, NY, Churchill Livingstone, 1993, vol 2, pp 815-827.

81. Ostermeier S, Huschler C, Windhagen H, Stukenborg-Colsman C: In vitro investigation of the influence of tibial slope on quadriceps extension force after total knee arthroplasty. *Knee Surg Sports Traumatol Arthrosc* 2006;14:934-939.

82. He Y, Wang C: The influence of changes in patellar and femoral prosthesis on knee extensor mechanism after TKA. *Conf Proc IEEE Eng Med Biol Soc* 2005;6:6180-6183.

83. Miller MC, Berger RA, Petrella AJ, Karmas A, Rubash HE: Optimizing femoral component rotation in total knee arthroplasty. *Clin Orthop Relat Res* 2001;392:38-45.

84. Ranawat CS, Ranawat AS, Mehta A: Total knee arthroplasty rehabilitation protocol: What makes the difference? *J Arthroplasty* 2003;18:27-30.

85. Kramer JF, Speechley M, Bourne R, Rorabeck C, Vaz M: Comparison of clinic- and home-based rehabilitation programs after total knee arthroplasty.

Clin Orthop Relat Res 2003;410: 225-234.

86. Frost H, Lamb SE, Robertson S: A randomized controlled trial of exercise to improve mobility and function after elective knee arthroplasty: Feasibility, results and methodological difficulties. *Clin Rehabil* 2002;16: 200-209.

87. van Baar ME, Dekker J, Oostendorp RA, et al: The effectiveness of exercise therapy in patients with osteoarthritis of the hip or knee: A randomized clinical trial. *J Rheumatol* 1998;25:2432-2439.

88. Ettinger WH Jr, Burns R, Messier SP, et al: A randomized trial comparing aerobic exercise and resistance exercise with a health education program in older adults with knee osteoarthritis: The Fitness Arthritis and Seniors Trial (FAST). *JAMA* 1997;277:25-31.

89. Tal-Akabi A, Steiger U, Villiger PM: Neuromuscular adaptation to early post-operative, high-intensity, short resistance training of non-operated lower extremity in elderly patients: A randomized controlled trial. *J Rehabil Med* 2007;39:724-729.

90. Rossi MD, Brown LE, Whitehurst M: Early strength response of the knee extensors during eight weeks of resistive training after unilateral total knee arthroplasty. *J Strength Cond Res* 2005; 19:944-949.

91. Ulrich SD, Bhave A, Marker DR, Seyler TM, Mont MA: Focused rehabilitation treatment of poorly functioning total knee arthroplasties. *Clin Orthop Relat Res* 2007;464:138-145.

92. Gotlin RS, Hershkowitz S, Juris PM, Gonzalez EG, Scott WN, Insall JN: Electrical stimulation effect on extensor lag and length of hospital stay after total knee arthroplasty. *Arch Phys Med Rehabil* 1994;75:957-959.

93. Stevens JE, Mizner RL, Snyder-Mackler L: Neuromuscular electrical stimulation for quadriceps muscle strengthening after bilateral total knee arthroplasty: A case series. *J Orthop Sports Phys Ther* 2004;34:21-29.

94. Petterson S, Snyder-Mackler L: The use of neuromuscular electrical stimulation to improve activation deficits in a patient with chronic quadriceps strength impairments following total knee arthroplasty. *J Orthop Sports Phys Ther* 2006;36:678-685.

95. Lewek M, Stevens J, Snyder-Mackler L: The use of electrical stimulation to increase quadriceps femoris muscle force in an elderly patient following a total knee arthroplasty. *Phys Ther* 2001;81:1565-1571.

96. Mintken PE, Carpenter KJ, Eckhoff D, Kohrt WM, Stevens JE: Early neuromuscular electrical stimulation to optimize quadriceps muscle function following total knee arthroplasty: A case report. *J Orthop Sports Phys Ther* 2007;37:364-371.

97. Avramidis K, Strike PW, Taylor PN, Swain ID: Effectiveness of electric stimulation of the vastus medialis muscle in the rehabilitation of patients after total knee arthroplasty. *Arch Phys Med Rehabil* 2003;84:1850-1853.

98. Durmuş D, Alayli G, Cantürk F: Effects of quadriceps electrical stimulation program on clinical parameters in the patients with knee osteoarthritis. *Clin Rheumatol* 2007;26:674-678.

99. Ottawa panel evidence-based clinical practice guidelines for therapeutic exercises and manual therapy in the management of osteoarthritis. *Phys Ther* 2005;85:907-971.

100. Rooks DS, Huang J, Bierbaum BE, et al: Effect of preoperative exercise on measures of functional status in men and women undergoing total hip and knee arthroplasty. *Arthritis Rheum* 2006;55:700-708.

101. Jaggers JR, Simpson CD, Frost KL, et al: Prehabilitation before knee arthroplasty increases postsurgical function: A case study. *J Strength Cond Res* 2007;21:632-634.

Decolonization of Drug-Resistant Organisms Before Total Joint Arthroplasty

Javad Parvizi, MD, FRCS
Wadih Y. Matar, MD, MSc, FRCSC
Khaled J. Saleh, MD, MSc, FRCSC
Thomas P. Schmalzried, MD
William M. Mihalko, MD, PhD

Abstract

Periprosthetic joint infection is now the leading cause of failure after a total knee arthroplasty, and Staphylococcus aureus, *most commonly from the patient's own flora, typically is the infective agent. Several preoperative screening tests have been developed to identify patients who are carrying methicillin-resistant* S aureus. *Testing and decolonization programs have generally been effective in decreasing the incidence of surgical site infections, but the role of such programs in total joint arthroplasty has not been thoroughly investigated. Although recent studies found a tendency toward fewer methicillin-resistant* S aureus *infections after total joint arthroplasty when a testing and decolonization program was used, most of these studies were underpowered. Larger, randomized, controlled studies are needed.*

Instr Course Lect 2010;59:131-137.

The incidence of periprosthetic joint infection has been slowly increasing, and it now is the most common reason for revision surgery after total knee arthroplasty in the United States.[1-3] Bozic and associates[1] studied data from the Nationwide Inpatient Sample on 60,355 revision total knee arthroscopies done during 2005 and 2006, finding that a revision procedure was most commonly required because of infection (25.2%) or mechanical loosening (16.1%). The demand for primary total knee arthroplasty is projected to grow 673% (to 3.48 million) from 2005 to 2030, and the demand for revision surgery is projected to grow 601% (to 1.3 million procedures).[2]

Both patient- and pathogen-specific factors are implicated in the increased incidence of infection. In general, patients are living longer, are more likely to be immunocompromised, and are more likely to receive care that violates the natural

Dr. Parvizi or an immediate family member serves as a board member, owner, officer, or committee member of the American Association of Hip and Knee Surgeons, the American Board of Orthopaedic Surgery, the British Orthopaedic Association, the Orthopaedic Research and Education Foundation, and SmartTech; serves as a paid consultant to or is an employee of Stryker; and has received research or institutional support from KCI, the Musculoskeletal Transplant Foundation, Smith & Nephew, and Stryker. Neither Dr. Matar nor any immediate family members have received anything of value from or own stock in a commercial company or institution related directly or indirectly to the subject of this chapter. Dr. Saleh or an immediate family member has received royalties from Smith & Nephew; is a member of a speakers' bureau or has made paid presentations on behalf of Aesculap/B. Braun, Stryker, OMNI, and Kimberly Clark; serves as a paid consultant to or is an employee of Aesculap/B. Braun, Stryker, and OMNI; has received research or institutional support from the Journal of Bone and Joint Surgery–American, *Stryker, EKR Therapeutics, and Aesculap/B. Braun; and has received nonincome support (such as equipment or services), commercially derived honoraria, or other non–research-related funding (such as paid travel) from Blue Cross Blue Shield and Kimberly Clark. Dr. Schmalzried or an immediate family member serves as a board member, owner, officer, or committee member of the Orthopaedic Research and Education Foundation; has received royalties from DePuy and Stryker; serves as a paid consultant to or is an employee of Stryker; has received research or institutional support from DePuy and Stryker; and has stock or stock options held in Johnson & Johnson, Smith & Nephew, Stryker, and Zimmer. Dr. Mihalko or an immediate family member has received royalties from Elsevier; is a member of a speakers' bureau or has made paid presentations on behalf of Ethicon and Aesculap/B.Braun; serves as a paid consultant to or is an employee of Aesculap/B.Braun, Ethicon, Johnson & Johnson, and Stryker; and has received research or institutional support from the* Journal of Bone and Joint Surgery–American, *Smith & Nephew, and Aesculap/B. Braun.*

barrier of the skin and allows bacterial invasion.[4,5] The liberal use of wide-spectrum antibiotics is directly associated with the emergence of antibiotic-resistant strains of bacteria.[6,7]

Drug-Resistant Organisms

Staphylococcus aureus is the cause of approximately 60% of all prosthetic joint infections, and *Staphylococcus epidermidis* is responsible for 20% to 25%; both are gram-positive organisms.[5] In 1947, 4 years after penicillin became commercially available, *S aureus* became the first bacteria to develop resistance to it. In 1961, 2 years after the introduction of methicillin to treat infections caused by penicillin-resistant *S aureus*, *S aureus* methicillin resistance was first reported.[8] Methicillin-resistant *S aureus* (MRSA) was first reported in England, but it soon appeared in other European countries, Japan, Australia, and the United States.[9,10] In 1975, health care–associated MRSA (HA-MRSA) accounted for 2.4% of all infections in US hospitals, and the incidence rose to 29% by 1991.[11] *S aureus* resistance to β-lactam compounds was found in more than 50% of isolates from US hospitals in 2003, and it now is also commonly found in community associated MSRA (CA-MRSA) infections.[6,12] Outbreaks of CA-MRSA most frequently involve members of sports teams, people who use locker rooms, children who attend day care centers, and prison inmates. The incidence of HA-MRSA has increased in many European countries during the past two decades. *S aureus* resistance has become a global challenge.[13]

The US Centers for Disease Control and Prevention investigated 8,987 reports of MRSA infection from nine US communities during 2005.[14] The incidence was determined to be 31.8 MRSA infections per 100,000 population. HA-MRSA accounted for 85.0% of the infections, CA-MRSA accounted for 13.7%, and 1.3% was unclassifiable. Those at highest risk for HA-MRSA were patients who had a culture obtained more than 48 hours after admission to a nursing home, were receiving dialysis, had a history of MRSA infection or colonization, had an invasive device such as a gastric feeding tube, or had an earlier surgical procedure or hospitalization. Two thirds of the instances of HA-MRSA were classified as community onset (in which the patient had a health care risk factor and a culture was obtained more than 48 hours after admission), and one third of the instances were classified as hospital onset (in which a culture was obtained more than 48 hours after admission). The MRSA strains usually associated with CA-MRSA were isolated from patients with both community-onset and hospital-onset HA-MRSA.

S aureus is continuing to evolve. Strains of MRSA have been isolated with an intermediate or high level of resistance to vancomycin; these strains are called vancomycin intermediate-sensitive *S aureus* and vancomycin-resistant *S aureus.* Fortunately, these isolates have a low level of dissemination and are infrequently found. *S epidermidis* also has developed resistance to methicillin; from 1980 to 1989, the incidence of methicillin-resistant *S epidermidis* increased from 20% to 60% of nosocomial infections in which *S epidermidis* was isolated.[15] Antibiotic resistance has been reported among bacteria other than staphylococci; vancomycin-resistant *Enterococcus* is an example.[16]

Drug-Resistant Organisms in Prosthetic Joint Infections

The percentage of prosthetic joint infections caused by a drug-resistant organism is increasing.[17,18] Parvizi and associates[5] recently reported that the incidence of MRSA and methicillin-resistant *S epidermidis* isolated from prosthetic joint infections increased from 27% in 1999 to 55% in 2005 and 62% in 2006; therefore, most prosthetic joint infections in the more recent years of the study were caused by drug-resistant staphylococci. The incidence of vancomycin-resistant *Enterococcus* remained low, at 1.3%.

The increase in the rate of infections caused by drug-resistant organisms has worrisome clinical and economic implications. Several studies reported lower success rates after treatment for prosthetic joint infection caused by a resistant organism.[19-25] Success rates of 11% to 29% were reported after irrigation and débridement with implant retention.[19-21] Success rates of 12% to 76% were reported after two-stage exchange arthroplasty to treat infection caused by a resistant organism; similar procedures to treat infection caused by a nonresistant organism were considerably more successful.[21-23] Higher rates of un successful treatment are accompanied by higher rates of reoperation and longer hospitalizations.[19] In a recent report by Walls and associates,[26] 12 of 16 MRSA surgical site infections (75%) in 15 patients after primary total hip arthroplasty were early infections. The cumulative hospital stay of the patients in the study was 11 times higher than that of a comparable group of patients without MRSA surgical site infection. The economic impact of surgical site infections, including those caused by MRSA, has been well documented.[27-29] Under US federal regulations, the cost of treating some nosocomial infections is not separately reimbursable, and the list of nonreimbursable nosocomial infections is expanded every year. However, the treatment is reimbursable if the patient can be shown to have the infectious agent before hospital admission. Therefore, for purposes of reimbursement, it may become important to identify carriers of MRSA.

Because of the poor success rates of treatment for prosthetic joint infections caused by a drug-resistant organism and the higher cost of treating these infections, some surgeons prefer to use vancomycin as prophylaxis during total joint arthroplasty, if the patient is at high risk. Other surgeons prefer to reserve vancomycin prophylaxis for patients who are known to be colonized by MRSA or another resistant organism.[30-32]

Preoperative Screening

The rationale for preoperative screening is the belief that the most common source of infection is the patient's own flora. Identifying resistant flora and implementing appropriate strategies are likely to reduce the patient's risk of infection.[33,34] Perl and Golub[31] found that in 30% of patients with MRSA infection, the infective strain originated in the patient's own flora.

Several commercial tests are available to screen for MRSA using a conventional culture (with or without enrichment) or a molecular method. Traditionally, MRSA is cultured from a swab gently manipulated deep within the patient's nares for several seconds or from swabs used at several superficial sites, such as the nose, throat, or perineum.[35] The reported sensitivity of nasal swabbing is 80%, and it can be increased to 95% with the addition of swabbing from other superficial sites.[36] The swab is selectively cultured on a liquid or solid agar medium, or both. The culture medium usually contains a MRSA indicator such as mannitol, as well as phenol red (a pH indicator). A chromographic indicator identifies possible MRSA colonies. The culture medium also contains an inhibitory substance to help in distinguishing *S aureus* from other bacteria. Methicillin, oxacillin, or cefoxitin is added to determine the specific MRSA strain. This conventional approach can be labor intensive, and it usually requires more time than a readily available molecular test. As long as 48 hours may be needed for confirmation of a positive result, although culturing with a readily available chromogenic medium requires considerably less time.[37] The sensitivity and specificity indicated by conventional culturing must be interpreted cautiously because they are greatly affected by the gold standard to which the test is compared, as well as the local behavior of each MRSA strain.[35] The sensitivity of the test can be increased 15% to 30% by enriching the bacteria, either with overnight incubation to allow small numbers of MRSA to grow before subculturing or with the use of a multibroth, in which several swabs from the same patient are placed together into one enrichment broth before being placed in the culture medium.[35,36,38,39] However, enrichment increases the cost of culturing and can delay obtaining the results by as long as 18 to 24 hours.

Molecular DNA-based tests, including commercial and in-house nucleic acid amplification assays, have recently come into use for detecting MRSA within 24 hours.[35,40-42] Most of these tests use polymerase chain reaction (PCR) to detect a specific sequence of *S aureus* and the *mecA* gene responsible for encoding methicillin resistance. Although these newer tests are considerably more rapid than conventional methods, their cost is much greater. Few studies have compared the effectiveness of conventional and molecular tests.[36] Two recent European studies did not find that the universal use of PCR for rapid detection of MRSA was beneficial in reducing the incidence of nosocomial or surgical site MRSA infection.[43,44] Additional cost-effectiveness studies are needed, however. A US study using a budget impact model found a 64.5% probability of cost savings when patients undergoing elective surgery received rapid PCR testing for MRSA colonization, with subsequent decolonization therapy.[45]

Decolonization Protocols

People who carry MRSA are 10 times more likely to become infected with the colonizing strain than people who carry methicillin-susceptible *S aureus* (MSSA).[46] Investigations of the efficacy of preventing the person-to-person spread of MRSA and using decolonization protocols have had differing results.[46-49] Protocols to prevent the spread of MRSA focus on hand washing and environmental hygiene, patient isolation, and carrier decolonization.[47] MRSA is spread from patient to patient primarily via the hands of health care workers, and good hand hygiene therefore is of prime importance in preventing MRSA spread. The ability of MRSA to survive for months in a dry environment, as is found on a door handle or bed,[47] provides further justification for isolation and environmental hygiene protocols aimed at decreasing MRSA transmission. The use of isolation rooms can hinder the spread of MRSA by physically separating a patient who is a MRSA carrier from other patients and serving as a continual reminder to health care workers of the importance of hand hygiene.

Attempts to decolonize MRSA using chemotherapeutic agents have had conflicting results, and many authors have pointed out the lack of high-quality studies.[48,49] Topical agents including mupirocin, bacitracin, neomycin, povidone-iodine, and retapamulin have been used.[47-49] Mupirocin, the most widely studied agent, is applied topically to the anterior nares two or three times a day for 5 days. A randomized, controlled study of two groups of patients living in a long-term facility found a 93% rate of decolonization 6 months after mupirocin was used.[50] A meta-analysis of 2,445 patients found that nosocomial infection rates decreased when mupirocin was used.[51] However, preventing the emergence of mupirocin-resistant organisms is a concern. It is recommended that mupirocin be used only in patients who are receiving an implanted device or an organ or stem cell transplant, as well as other patients who are immunocompromised.[52-54]

Multisite colonization is common. To increase the success of the eradication strategy, whole-body antiseptic soap or skin cleanser is used to supplement the topical agents.[49,51] Most commonly, the patient receives a daily chlorhexidine bath or shower in conjunction with mupirocin. If topical agents fail to decolonize the organism, oral antibiotics can be added to the regimen. Vancomycin, rifampin, trimethoprim-sulfamethoxazole, doxycycline, and minocycline have been used, but no agent has been established as superior to the others.[49] Oral antibiotics should not be used alone, as they may not become sufficiently concentrated in nasal secretions to eradicate MRSA from the nares.[49] Additional randomized, controlled studies are needed to establish the optimal decolonization regimen and determine whether its use reduces the rate of infection.

Results in Total Joint Arthroplasty

Several reports have documented the efficacy of MRSA decolonization in patients undergoing surgery.[34,55] In a randomized, double-blind, placebo-controlled study of 614 patients undergoing an orthopaedic procedure, Kalmeijer and associates[31] found that *S aureus* was eradicated in 83.5% of patients who received mupirocin nasal ointment, compared with 27.8% of patients who received a placebo, and that the rate of infections caused by endogenous *S aureus* was five times lower among patients in the treatment group than among patients in the placebo group. Possibly because of the small sample size, these results were not correlated with reductions in the rate of surgical site infection or the average length of hospital stay.

Two studies investigated the efficacy and cost-effectiveness of mupirocin used for *S aureus* decolonization in patients undergoing total joint arthroplasty. In a prospective observational study, Rao and associates[56] screened 636 patients 2 to 4 weeks before elective total joint arthroplasty. Nasal carriage of *S aureus* was found in 164 (26%), of whom 147 (23% of all patients) had MSSA and 17 (3%) had MRSA. The patients identified as MSSA or MRSA carriers received a decolonization treatment consisting of topical mupirocin and a chlorhexidine body wash 1 week before surgery, as well as perioperative antibiotic prophylaxis. Cefazolin was administered to the patients who were carriers of MSSA, except for patients with a type I allergy to penicillin or a history of MRSA. These patients and those identified as carriers of MRSA received vancomycin. No *S aureus* infections were reported among the patients in the intervention group. In contrast, there were 12 infections among the 1,330 patients in the control group; by assuming that all *S aureus* infections in the control group occurred in patients who were nasal carriers, the authors calculated an infection rate of 3.5% in the control group, compared with 0% in the intervention group. More importantly, the infection rate among all patients of surgeons who had some patients enrolled in the study decreased from 2.6% during the preintervention period to 1.5% during the intervention period. The authors found that lowering the infection rate led to an overall reduction in hospital costs. The study was limited by a lack of randomization and the use of historical patient data to assemble a control group. The refusal of some patients to participate in the study added a possible selection bias.

Hacek and associates[57] also investigated the role of mupirocin in lowering the rate of surgical site infection among patients undergoing total joint arthroplasty. A molecular test to detect *S aureus* was used 2 to 4 weeks before surgery, and patients with a positive nasal screening were treated with mupirocin for 5 days. Patients undergoing total hip arthroplasty received cefazolin as well as a chlorhexidine bath the day of surgery; those undergoing total knee arthroplasty received vancomycin. This screening and decolonization protocol was successful in reducing the rate of surgical site infection among patients identified as carriers of *S aureus*; the rate among surgical patients was four times higher. However, the overall reduction in the rate of surgical site infection was not statistically significant. This study of 1,495 patients was underpowered; the authors calculated that a total of 7,000 patients would constitute an adequate sample size.

Table 1
Recommended Screening and Decolonization Treatment for Drug-Resistant Organisms

Elective Total Joint Arthroplasty
All patients
The patient receives a chlorhexidine shower 24 hours before surgery.
Additional chlorhexidine scrubbing is done early on the day of surgery and during preoperative preparation.
Patients at high risk
The patient is screened at least 2 weeks before the scheduled surgery, using a nasal culture or molecular (PCR) method.
If MRSA is identified, the patient receives nasal mupirocin for 1 week.
A second screening is done at the conclusion of the mupirocin regimen, using a nasal culture or molecular (PCR) method.
If MRSA is identified, the patient is cared for before and after surgery in an isolation unit.
Emergency Surgery
Patients with a positive MRSA culture
Patients at high risk who cannot be quickly screened
The patient receives 1 g of vancomycin before surgery and for a period of 24 hours after surgery.
If MRSA is identified, the patient is cared for before and after surgery in an isolation unit.

Recommendations

Screening of patients at high risk for developing a surgical site infection is advisable before elective total joint arthroplasty, as outlined in Table 1. Patients at high risk include those who live in an institution (particularly a nursing home), frequently receive an outpatient treatment such as dialysis, work in a hospital, or have a history of MRSA.

Summary

Resistant organisms such as MRSA continue to be a leading cause of infection after total joint arthroplasty. Advances have been made during the past decade in identifying potential carriers through preoperative screening. Although several decolonization protocols have been established, none has been established as superior. Strong recent evidence suggests that decolonization treatment for patients identified as *S aureus* nasal carriers leads to lower rates of infection after total joint arthroplasty. However, the studies were underpowered, given the low rates of infection after total joint arthroplasty, and larger randomized controlled studies are needed. Screening and decolonization programs can be quite costly, but strong evidence suggests that they result in an overall lowering of cost to the health care system.

References

1. Bozic K, Kurtz S, Lau E, et al: The epidemiology of revision total knee arthroplasty in the United States. [published online ahead of print June 25, 2009]. *Clin Orthop Relat Res.* PMID: 19554385 .
2. Kurtz S, Ong K, Lau E, Mowat F, Halpern M: Projections of primary and revision hip and knee arthroplasty in the United States from 2005 to 2030. *J Bone Joint Surg Am* 2007;89: 780-785.
3. Kurtz SM, Lau E, Schmier J, Ong KL, Zhao K, Parvizi J: Infection burden for hip and knee arthroplasty in the United States. *J Arthroplasty* 2008;23: 984-991.
4. Mihalko WM, Manaswi A, Brown TE, Parvizi J, Schmalzried TP, Saleh KJ: Infection in primary total knee arthroplasty: Contributing factors. *Instr Course Lect* 2008;57:317-325.
5. Parvizi J, Bender B, Saleh KJ, Brown TE, Schmalzried TP, Mihalko WM: Resistant organisms in infected total knee arthroplasty: Occurrence, prevention, and treatment regimens. *Instr Course Lect* 2009;58: 271-278.
6. Arias CA, Murray BE: Antibiotic-resistant bugs in the 21st century: A clinical super-challenge. *N Engl J Med* 2009;360:439-443.
7. Soulsby EJ: Resistance to antimicrobials in humans and animals. *BMJ* 2005;331:1219-1220.
8. Jevons MP, Coe AW, Parker MT: Methicillin resistance in staphylococci. *Lancet* 1963;1:904-907.
9. Ayliffe GA: The progressive intercontinental spread of methicillin-resistant Staphylococcus aureus. *Clin Infect Dis* 1997;24:S74-S79.
10. Enright MC, Robinson DA, Randle G, Feil EJ, Grundmann H, Spratt BG: The evolutionary history of methicillin-resistant Staphylococcus aureus (MRSA). *Proc Natl Acad Sci USA* 2002;99:7687-7692.
11. Panlilio AL, Culver DH, Gaynes RP, et al: Methicillin-resistant Staphylococcus aureus in U.S. hospitals: 1975-1991. *Infect Control Hosp Epidemiol* 1992;13:582-586.

12. Maree CL, Daum RS, Boyle-Vavra S, Matayoshi K, Miller LG: Community-associated methicillin-resistant Staphylococcus aureus isolates causing healthcare-associated infections. *Emerg Infect Dis* 2007;13: 236-242.

13. Struelens MJ: The epidemiology of antimicrobial resistance in hospital acquired infections: Problems and possible solutions. *BMJ* 1998;317: 652-654.

14. Klevens RM, Morrison MA, Nadle J, et al: Invasive methicillin-resistant Staphylococcus aureus infections in the United States. *JAMA* 2007;298: 1763-1771.

15. Schaberg DR, Culver DH, Gaynes RP: Major trends in the microbial etiology of nosocomial infection. *Am J Med* 1991;91:72S-75S.

16. Ries MD: Vancomycin-resistant Enterococcus infected total knee arthroplasty. *J Arthroplasty* 2001;16:802-805.

17. Fulkerson E, Valle CJ, Wise B, Walsh M, Preston C, DiCesare PE: Antibiotic susceptibility of bacteria infecting total joint arthroplasty sites. *J Bone Joint Surg Am* 2006;88:1231-1237.

18. Ip D, Yam SK, Chen CK: Implications of the changing pattern of bacterial infections following total joint replacements. *J Orthop Surg (Hong Kong)* 2005;13:125-130.

19. Salgado CD, Dash S, Cantey JR, Marculescu CE: Higher risk of failure of methicillin-resistant Staphylococcus aureus prosthetic joint infections. *Clin Orthop Relat Res* 2007;461:48-53.

20. Barberán J, Aguilar L, Carroquino G, et al: Conservative treatment of staphylococcal prosthetic joint infections in elderly patients. *Am J Med* 2006;119:993.

21. Kilgus DJ, Howe DJ, Strang A: Results of periprosthetic hip and knee infections caused by resistant bacteria. *Clin Orthop Relat Res* 2002;404: 116-124.

22. Hirakawa K, Stulberg BN, Wilde AH, Bauer TW, Secic M: Results of 2-stage reimplantation for infected total knee arthroplasty. *J Arthroplasty* 1998;13:22-28.

23. Mittal Y, Fehring TK, Hanssen A, Marculescu C, Odum SM, Osmon D: Two-stage reimplantation for periprosthetic knee infection involving resistant organisms. *J Bone Joint Surg Am* 2007;89:1227-1231.

24. Hart WJ, Jones RS: Two-stage revision of infected total knee replacements using articulating cement spacers and short-term antibiotic therapy. *J Bone Joint Surg Br* 2006;88:1011-1015.

25. Volin SJ, Hinrichs SH, Garvin KL: Two-stage reimplantation of total joint infections: A comparison of resistant and non-resistant organisms. *Clin Orthop Relat Res* 2004;427:94-100.

26. Walls RJ, Roche SJ, O'Rourke A, McCabe JP: Surgical site infection with methicillin-resistant Staphylococcus aureus after primary total hip replacement. *J Bone Joint Surg Br* 2008;90: 292-298.

27. Cosgrove SE, Carmeli Y: The impact of antimicrobial resistance on health and economic outcomes. *Clin Infect Dis* 2003;36:1433-1437.

28. Engemann JJ, Carmeli Y, Cosgrove SE, et al: Adverse clinical and economic outcomes attributable to methicillin resistance among patients with Staphylococcus aureus surgical site infection. *Clin Infect Dis* 2003;36: 592-598.

29. Whitehouse JD, Friedman ND, Kirkland KB, Richardson WJ, Sexton DJ: The impact of surgical-site infections following orthopedic surgery at a community hospital and a university hospital: Adverse quality of life, excess length of stay, and extra cost. *Infect Control Hosp Epidemiol* 2002;23: 183-189.

30. Kluytmans J, van Belkum A, Verbrugh H: Nasal carriage of Staphylococcus aureus: Epidemiology, underlying mechanisms, and associated risks. *Clin Microbiol Rev* 1997;10: 505-520.

31. Perl TM, Golub JE: New approaches to reduce Staphylococcus aureus nosocomial infection rates: Treating S. aureus nasal carriage. *Ann Pharmacother* 1998;32:S7-S16.

32. Kalmeijer MD, Coertjens H, van Nieuwland-Bollen E, et al: Surgical site infections in orthopaedic surgery: The effect of mupirocin nasal ointment in a double-blind, randomized, placebo controlled study. *Clin Infect Dis* 2002;35:353-358.

33. Nixon M, Jackson B, Varghese P, Jenkins D, Taylor G: Methicillin-resistant Staphylococcus aureus on orthopaedic wards: Incidence, spread, mortality, cost and control. *J Bone Joint Surg Br* 2006;88:812-817.

34. Hassan K, Koh C, Karunaratne D, Hughes C, Giles SN: Financial implications of plans to combat methicillin-resistant Staphylococcus aureus (MRSA) in an orthopaedic department. *Ann R Coll Surg Engl* 2007; 89:668-671.

35. Brown DF, Edwards DI, Hawkey PM, et al: Guidelines for the laboratory diagnosis and susceptibility testing of methicillin-resistant Staphylococcus aureus (MRSA). *J Antimicrob Chemother* 2005;56:1000-1018.

36. Struelens MJ, Hawkey PM, French GL, Witte W, Tacconelli E: Laboratory tools and strategies for methicillin-resistant Staphylococcus aureus screening, surveillance and typing: State of the art and unmet needs. *Clin Microbiol Infect* 2009;15: 112-119.

37. Malhotra-Kumar S, Haccuria K, Michiels M, et al: Current trends in rapid diagnostics for methicillin-resistant Staphylococcus aureus and glycopeptide-resistant enterococcus species. *J Clin Microbiol* 2008;46:1577-1587.

38. Nonhoff C, Denis O, Brenner A, et al: Comparison of three chromogenic media and enrichment broth media for the detection of methicillin-resistant Staphylococcus aureus from mucocutaneous screening specimens: Comparison of MRSA chromogenic media. *Eur J Clin Microbiol Infect Dis* 2009;28:363-369.

39. Böcher S, Smyth R, Kahlmeter G, Kerremans J, Vos MC, Skov R: Evaluation of four selective agars and two enrichment broths in screening for methicillin-resistant Staphylococcus aureus. *J Clin Microbiol* 2008;46:3136-3138.

40. Huletsky A, Giroux R, Rossbach V, et al: New real-time PCR assay for rapid detection of methicillin-resistant Staphylococcus aureus directly from specimens containing a mixture of staphylococci. *J Clin Microbiol* 2004;42:1875-1884.

41. Francois P, Pittet D, Bento M, et al: Rapid detection of methicillin-resistant Staphylococcus aureus directly from sterile or nonsterile clinical samples by a new molecular assay. *J Clin Microbiol* 2003;41:254-260.

42. Struelens MJ, Denis O: Rapid molecular detection of methicillin-resistant Staphylococcus aureus: A cost-effective tool for infection control in critical care? *Crit Care* 2006; 10:128.

43. Harbarth S, Fankhauser C, Schrenzel J, et al: Universal screening for methicillin-resistant Staphylococcus aureus at hospital admission and nosocomial infection in surgical patients. *JAMA* 2008;299:1149-1157.

44. Jeyaratnam D, Whitty CJ, Phillips K, et al: Impact of rapid screening tests on acquisition of methicillin resistant Staphylococcus aureus: Cluster randomised crossover trial. *BMJ* 2008; 336:927-369.

45. Noskin GA, Rubin RJ, Schentag JJ, et al: Budget impact analysis of rapid screening for Staphylococcus aureus colonization among patients undergoing elective surgery in US hospitals. *Infect Control Hosp Epidemiol* 2008; 29:16-24.

46. Davis KA, Stewart JJ, Crouch HK, Florez CE, Hospenthal DR: Methicillin-resistant Staphylococcus aureus (MRSA) nares colonization at hospital admission and its effect on subsequent MRSA infection. *Clin Infect Dis* 2004;39:776-782.

47. Humphreys H, Grundmann H, Skov R, Lucet JC, Cauda R: Prevention and control of methicillin-resistant Staphylococcus aureus. *Clin Microbiol Infect* 2009;15:120-124.

48. Loveday HP, Pellowe CM, Jones SR, Pratt RJ: A systematic review of the evidence for interventions for the prevention and control of methicillin-resistant Staphylococcus aureus (1996-2004): Report to the Joint MRSA Working Party (Subgroup A). *J Hosp Infect* 2006;63: S45-S70.

49. McConeghy KW, Mikolich DJ, LaPlante KL: Agents for the decolonization of methicillin-resistant Staphylococcus aureus. *Pharmacotherapy* 2009;29:263-280.

50. Mody L, Kauffman CA, McNeil SA, Galecki AT, Bradley SF: Mupirocin-based decolonization of Staphylococcus aureus carriers in residents of 2 long-term care facilities: A randomized, double-blind, placebo-controlled trial. *Clin Infect Dis* 2003; 37:1467-1474.

51. Tacconelli E, Carmeli Y, Aizer A, Ferreira G, Foreman MG, D'Agata EM: Mupirocin prophylaxis to prevent Staphylococcus aureus infection in patients undergoing dialysis: A meta-analysis. *Clin Infect Dis* 2003;37:1629-1638.

52. Walker ES, Levy F, Shorman M, David G, Abdalla J, Sarubbi FA: A decline in mupirocin resistance in methicillin-resistant Staphylococcus aureus accompanied administrative control of prescriptions. *J Clin Microbiol* 2004;42:2792-2795.

53. Fawley WN, Parnell P, Hall J, Wilcox MH: Surveillance for mupirocin resistance following introduction of routine peri-operative prophylaxis with nasal mupirocin. *J Hosp Infect* 2006;62:327-332.

54. Cookson BD: The emergence of mupirocin resistance: A challenge to infection control and antibiotic prescribing practice. *J Antimicrob Chemother* 1998;41:11-18.

55. Kallen AJ, Wilson CT, Larson RJ: Perioperative intranasal mupirocin for the prevention of surgical-site infections: Systematic review of the literature and meta-analysis. *Infect Control Hosp Epidemiol* 2005;26:916-922.

56. Rao N, Cannella B, Crossett LS, Yates AJ Jr, McGough R III: A preoperative decolonization protocol for staphylococcus aureus prevents orthopaedic infections. *Clin Orthop Relat Res* 2008;466:1343-1348.

57. Hacek DM, Robb WJ, Paule SM, Kudrna JC, Stamos VP, Peterson LR: Staphylococcus aureus nasal decolonization in joint replacement surgery reduces infection. *Clin Orthop Relat Res* 2008;466:1349-1355.

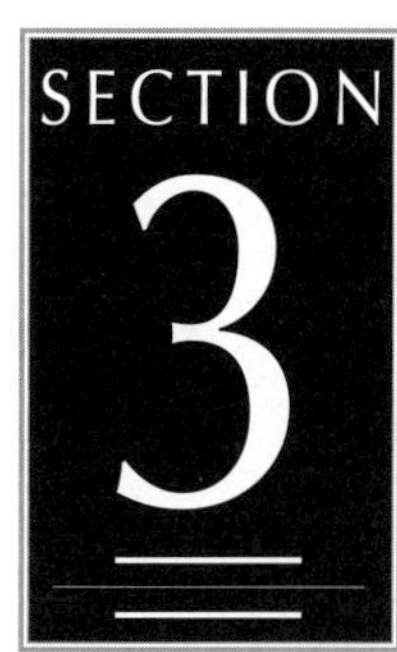

Sports Medicine

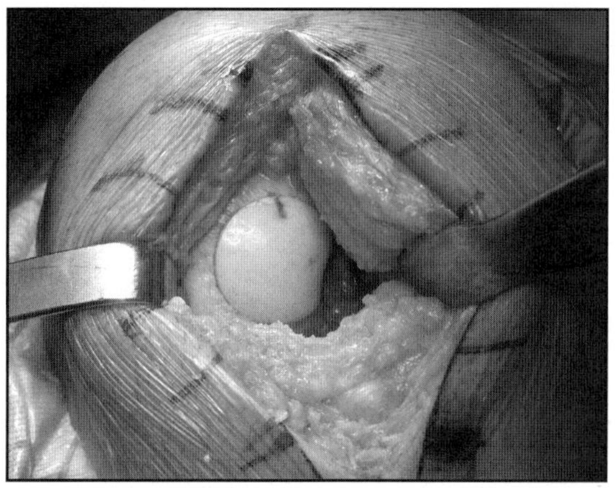

Arthroscopic Management of Shoulder Instabilities: Anterior, Posterior, and Multidirectional

Jeffrey S. Abrams, MD
James P. Bradley, MD
Richard L. Angelo, MD
Robert Burks, MD

Abstract

Arthroscopy is considered a relatively new technique for the surgical repair of an unstable shoulder. Shoulder arthroscopy has grown in popularity and is considered the gold standard for treating carefully selected patients. Despite its increasing popularity, the procedure has a significant learning curve and has resulted in early higher recurrence rates when compared with patients treated with open techniques. With the addition of newer instrumentation, the refinement of techniques, and additional capsular plication and tensioning, outcomes for patients treated with shoulder arthroscopy should continue to improve.

A major distinguishing feature in selecting appropriate candidates for shoulder arthroscopy is whether there have been significant bone changes resulting from dislocation recurrence. Recurrent anterior dislocation may create an anterior glenoid rim fracture, erosion loss from multiple recurrences, and an impression defect on the posterior aspect of the humeral head. The loss of contact area between the "ball and cup" may compromise the results of techniques that restore the anatomic restraints of soft tissues. Early intervention is becoming recognized as an important factor in patient selection for arthroscopic treatment. Imaging studies after traumatic injuries include radiographs, CT scans, possible articular contrast studies, and MRIs. These studies can identify and quantify rim fractures and the remaining articular contact in patients with recurrent subluxations, allowing for earlier appropriate intervention.

Patients with significant bone loss may be best treated with an open procedure that allows grafting of the deficiency. Arthroscopic techniques to repair fractures or graft deficiencies continue to evolve. Rim fractures can be anatomically repaired with a suture anchor technique when recognized early. Rim erosion from chronic recurrent dislocations may require a combination of soft-tissue reattachment and coracoid grafting. Humeral head defects may require either soft-tissue or bone grafting to avoid engagement with the anterior edge of the glenoid. These techniques require arthroscopic skill and experience and are currently being performed as open procedures. In the future, it is likely that arthroscopy will be involved in the entire spectrum of treatment for shoulder instability.

Instr Course Lect 2010;59:141-155.

Dr. Abrams or an immediate family member serves as a board member, owner, officer, or committee member of the Orthopaedic Learning Center, the American Shoulder and Elbow Surgeons, and the Arthroscopy Association of North America; has received royalties from CONMED Linvatec; is a member of a speakers' bureau or has made paid presentations on behalf of the Orthopaedic Scientific Research Foundation; serves as a paid consultant to or is an employee of Arthrocare, CONMED Linvatec, and Wright Medical Technology; serves as an unpaid consultant to KFx Medical; has stock or stock options held in Arthrocare, KFx Medical, Cayenne Medical, and Ingen Medical; and has received nonincome support (such as equipment or services), commercially derived honoraria, or other non–research-related funding (such as paid travel) from Springer. Dr. Angelo or an immediate family member serves as a board member, owner, officer, or committee member of the Arthroscopy Association of North America; is a member of a speakers' bureau or has made paid presentations on behalf of Mitek; and serves as a paid consultant to or is an employee of Mitek. Dr. Burks or an immediate family member has received royalties from Arthrex and has received research or institutional support from AO, Arthrex, Biomet, DePuy, Stryker, and Synthes. Dr. Bradley or an immediate family member has received royalties from Arthrex; has received research or institutional support from Arthrex; and has stock or stock options held in Arthrex.

Arthroscopy is considered a relatively new technique to surgically repair an unstable shoulder. When selecting a patient for shoulder arthroscopy, it is important to determine if there have been significant bone changes resulting from recurrent dislocations. Recurrent anterior dislocation may create an anterior glenoid rim fracture, erosion loss in instances of multiple recurrences, and an impression defect on the posterior aspect of the humeral head. The loss of contact area between the "ball and cup" may compromise the results of techniques that restore soft-tissue anatomic restraints. Early intervention is recognized as an important factor in arthroscopic treatment. Following traumatic injuries, the results of imaging studies such as radiographs, CT scans, and possible articular contrast studies, along with a patient's profile, may suggest the need for early arthroscopic repair.

Shoulder arthroscopy has advantages in managing disorders of the overhead athlete. Stiffness has been reported to be less frequent in arthroscopically treated patients, possibly because of an intact rotator cuff insertion and the use of an anatomic approach to the avulsed capsule and labrum.[1,2] Complications involving the subscapularis that are associated with an open approach are avoided using the arthroscopic articular approach.

This chapter will describe the current state of the art of arthroscopic stabilization, including treatment of anterior instability in high-risk athletes, posterior instability caused by recurrent subluxation, repairing shoulders with multidirectional instability (MDI), and evaluating and treating patients in whom prior shoulder stabilization procedures have failed.

Anterior Shoulder Instability in Contact and Collision Athletes

Anterior shoulder instability is a common condition in athletic participants, with collision and contact athletes having a higher risk of recurrence. Collision sports are defined as those in which athletes purposely hit or collide with each other or inanimate objects (including the ground). Contact sports are defined as those in which athletes routinely make contact with each other. Taylor and Arciero[3] evaluated 63 patients between the ages of 17 and 24 years after acute shoulder dislocations and found 97% had Bankart lesions with no gross capsular injury. McMahon and associates[4] reported only 0.8 mm of irrecoverable deformation at the glenoid insertion site of the anterior band of the inferior glenohumeral ligament in the setting of a Bankart lesion.

Collision and contact athletes as well as patients younger than age 20 years experience additional physical demands that put them at increased risk for instability. Sachs and associates[5] reported on a study of 131 patients (ages 12 to 82 years) with anterior shoulder instability who were followed for a mean of 4 years. The authors reported that approximately 25% of the patients selected surgical repair following the dislocation, whereas the others choose to continue their activity without surgery or made lifestyle adjustments to reduce the risk of subluxations. Bottoni and associates[6] reported the development of recurrent instability in 75% of cadets with anterior instability who were treated nonsurgically. Subsequent instability develops in 90% to 95% of collision athletes and patients younger than 20 years after a shoulder dislocation.[7,8] These findings emphasize the need to evaluate each patient individually regarding age, type of sport and position played, and timing of the injury with respect to the athletic season.

Clinical Evaluation

The evaluation of an athlete with suspected anterior shoulder instability begins with a thorough history and physical examination. Inquiries should be made concerning prior dislocations, the specific mechanism of injury (including the position of the arm at the time of injury), whether the injury involved a true dislocation or a subluxation, the treatment provided (including reduction maneuvers), the extent of associated injuries, current reports of subjective instability, the types of activities that reproduce pain, the sports the athlete is interested in playing, and the timing of the injury with respect to the athletic season. The physical examination of the shoulder should evaluate anterior and posterior shoulder translation with load-and-shift testing, evidence of inferior shoulder instability, rotator cuff strength, associated biceps tendon pathology, and neurovascular status (Figure 1).

Musculoskeletal imaging is important in determining the most appropriate treatment option. All patients should have at least three orthogonal radiographs of the shoulder, including AP, lateral in the scapular plane, and axillary views. These images are critical to ensure appropriate glenohumeral joint reduction and to rule out proximal humerus or scapula fractures. Other views, such as a West Point view, may assist in evaluating for bony Bankart lesions of the glenoid (Figure 2). If a significant bony defect is suspected on either the glenoid or

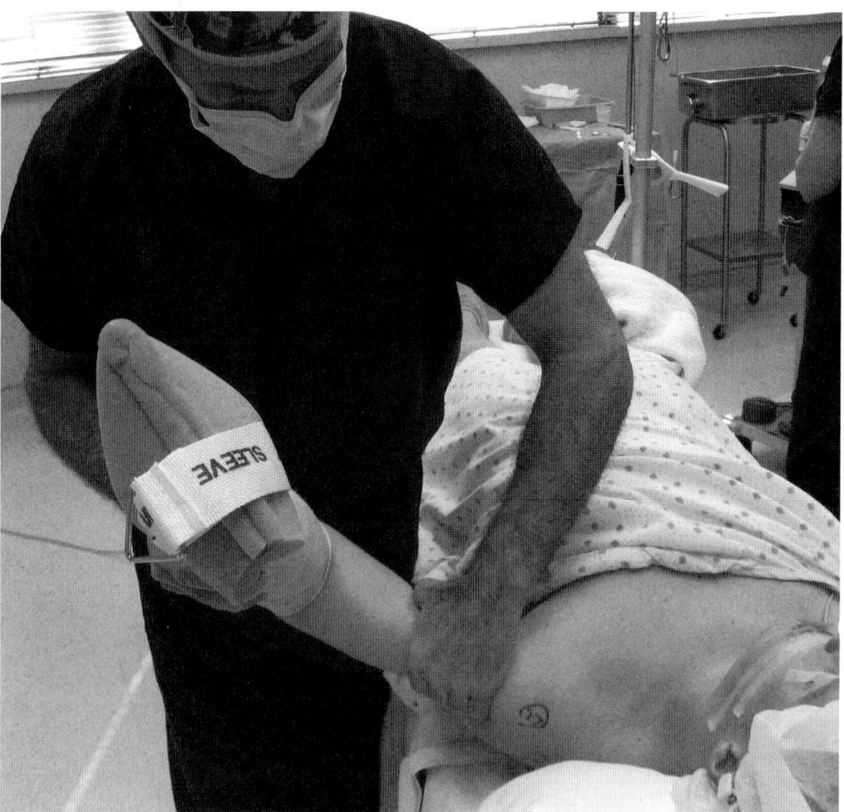

Figure 1 Load-and-shift translation testing of the anterior restraints in a provocative position.

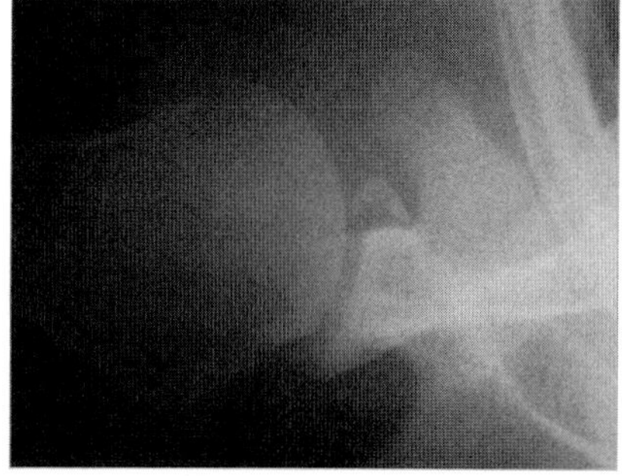

Figure 2 A West Point radiographic view can show anterior glenoid rim injury.

the proximal humerus, CT may help delineate the extent of the injury. Bony Bankart lesions that involve greater than 25% of the glenoid, an inverted pear-shaped glenoid, and Hill-Sachs lesions that engage with the glenoid in the functional range of motion are all structural changes that influence treatment options. MRI is helpful in determining soft-tissue injury to the labrum, capsule, and glenohumeral ligaments, as well as biceps, chondral, or rotator cuff pathology. Identifying associated pathology may help determine the best course of treatment.

Treatment Options

Nonsurgical management involves a period of immobilization followed by a structured rehabilitation program. The goals are to regain range of motion and strengthen the dynamic stabilizers (the rotator cuff and periscapular muscles) of the glenohumeral joint. Historically, patients have been immobilized in a sling that keeps the affected arm in internal rotation. Itoi and associates[9] challenged this approach with an MRI study that found significantly less separation and displacement of a Bankart lesion from the glenoid neck when the arm was held in external rotation. A clinical study evaluating patients treated nonsurgically with a minimum 2-year follow-up reported that patients immobilized with a sling in full internal rotation had a recurrence rate of 42%, whereas a second group immobilized with a sling in 10° of external rotation had a recurrence rate of 26%.[10]

Nonsurgical treatment using a harness can be successful in managing athletes during their playing season. Buss and associates[11] evaluated the results of nonsurgically treating 30 in-season athletes with anterior instability. They found that athletes missed an average of 10.2 days of play (range, 0 to 30 days); 26 of 30 athletes (87%) were able to complete the season, 10 of 27 (37%) had at least one episode of instability in-season, and 16 of 30 (53%) had surgery after the season. No short-term injuries related to shoulder instability occurred during play that affected the surgical options available at the end of the season.

Arthroscopic shoulder procedures have advantages compared with similar open procedures. Specifically, arthroscopy allows accurate identification and treatment of associated intra-articular pathology (rotator interval lesions, superior labrum anterior and posterior tears, capsular rents), causes less iatrogenic damage to normal tissues (subscapularis insertion), and patients have fewer motion limitations and less postoperative pain. Recent improvements in arthroscopy have led some authors to believe that arthroscopic techniques are now comparable to open techniques in patients at high risk for treatment failure.[12-14]

Arthroscopic anterior shoulder stabilization may involve Bankart repair, capsular shift, capsulolabral repair, and rotator interval closure. A Cochran review of four randomized controlled trials reported that highly active young adult men are less likely to have subsequent instability when treated surgically after an acute anterior shoulder dislocation.[15]

As arthroscopic techniques have evolved, the recurrence rate following arthroscopic stabilization has improved.[16] Using modern suture anchors, the rates of recurrent instability in athletes of all types of sports have been reported between 0% and 10%.[17-19] Studies comparing failure rates of arthroscopic and open techniques have shown comparable rates. In a prospective randomized controlled study by Bottoni and associates,[12] 29 patients treated with open stabilization were compared with 32 patients treated with arthroscopic techniques. After a mean follow-up of 32 months, there were no differences in the rate of recurrent dislocations, but there was a greater mean loss of motion in the group treated with open stabilization.

The improved results achieved with arthroscopic stabilization in the general athletic population have encouraged some authors to use these techniques in collision and contact athletes.[20] Ide and associates[1] found the recurrence rate in contact athletes was 9.5%, which was not significantly different than the 6% rate found in noncontact athletes. Mazzocca and associates[14] studied 13 collision and 5 contact athletes younger than 20 years with anterior shoulder instability who were treated arthroscopically. After an average follow-up of 37 months, the authors reported an overall recurrence rate of 11%; all recurrences occurred in collision athletes. The authors concluded that arthroscopic stabilization is a viable treatment option in contact and collision athletes. Larrain and associates[13] evaluated 204 rugby players treated with arthroscopic stabilization and reported a recurrent dislocation rate of 5%, which was comparable to previously published results for open techniques.

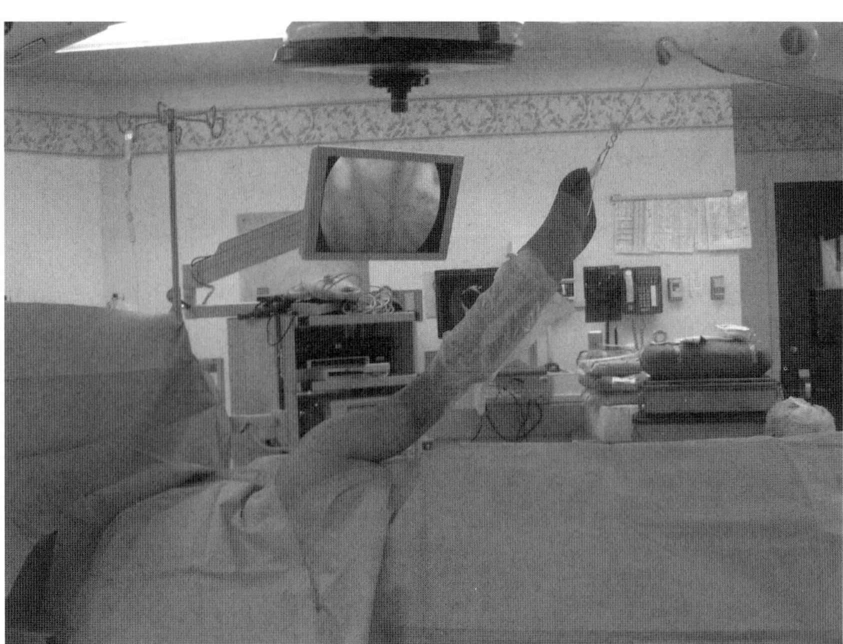

Figure 3 The lateral decubitus position with the arm suspended with gentle traction.

Some authors believe that arthroscopic surgery is contraindicated when certain associated pathology is present. Bony injury to the glenohumeral joint (including an inverted pear-shaped glenoid), a significant bony Bankart lesion (> 25%), or an engaging Hill-Sachs lesion in the functional position of abduction and external rotation have been shown to increase the risk of recurrent instability.[21,22] Burkhart and De Beer[21] evaluated 194 consecutive arthroscopic Bankart repairs, 101 of which occurred in contact athletes. In the contact athletes, there was a 6.5% recurrence rate in patients without significant bony defects and an 89% recurrence rate in patients with a significant bony defect. In a biomechanical study, Itoi and associates[22] found that an osseous defect of at least 21% of the glenoid length is needed to cause instability. Other factors that may support an open surgical approach include patients with multiple recurrences, abnormal laxity patterns, a large humeral capsular avulsion adjacent to an area where iatrogenic neurologic injury could result from arthroscopic repair, and failed prior arthroscopic Bankart surgery.[23]

Arthroscopic Anterior Stabilization

The patient is positioned supine on the operating table and administered general anesthesia and preoperative antibiotics. An evaluation of the shoulder is performed under anesthesia to confirm the findings of isolated anterior instability. The patient is then placed in the lateral decubitus position with the operative extremity placed in 10 lb of traction (Figure 3). The joint is insufflated with 50 mL of 8.25% bupivacaine and 1:200,000 epinephrine, and a standard posterior portal is established. Dual anterior portals are established, and diagnostic arthroscopy is then performed to evaluate the intra-articular pathology.

Anterior stabilization is performed by mobilizing the labrum with an elevator (Figure 4). The bony bed of the glenoid is prepared with a rasp and burr. The patulous capsule directly anterior to the labrum is roughened with a rasp. The drill guide is then inserted through the anteroinferior portal, and the anchors are positioned at a 45° angle to the face of the glenoid. A curved 45° right or left suture hook is inserted in the anteroinferior portal and used to pass a monofilament suture through a portion of capsule anterior to the labrum, under the labrum, and into the glenohumeral joint at or inferior to the level of the previously placed anchor. Using a suture grasper, the anchor stitch closest to the labrum is retrieved along with the monofilament suture and pulled together through the anterosuperior or posterior portals. This move will untangle the sutures in the cannula and prevent "suture spaghetti." The sutures are tied together and pulled under the labrum and back out of the cannula. Both ends of the suture are then secured with a sliding locking knot. This sequence is repeated as necessary to repair the labrum; typically it requires three to four suture anchors to achieve an acceptable construct (Figure 5). If additional laxity is present after capsulolabral reconstruction, rotator interval pathology and additional capsular patholaxity are treated with imbrication sutures passed in between the suture anchors.

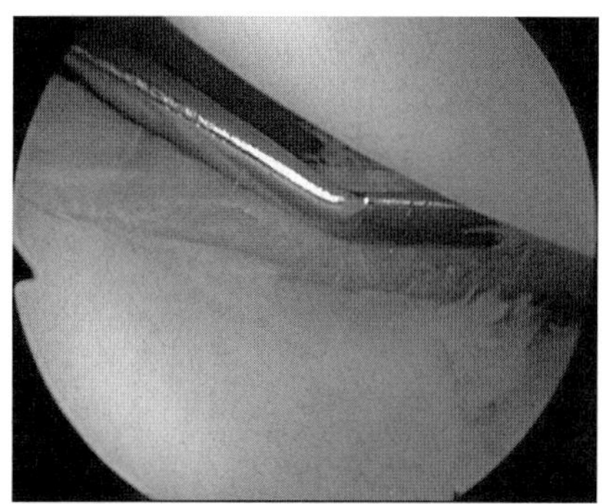

Figure 4 An elevator is introduced in the anterior portal to mobilize the labrum and the capsule.

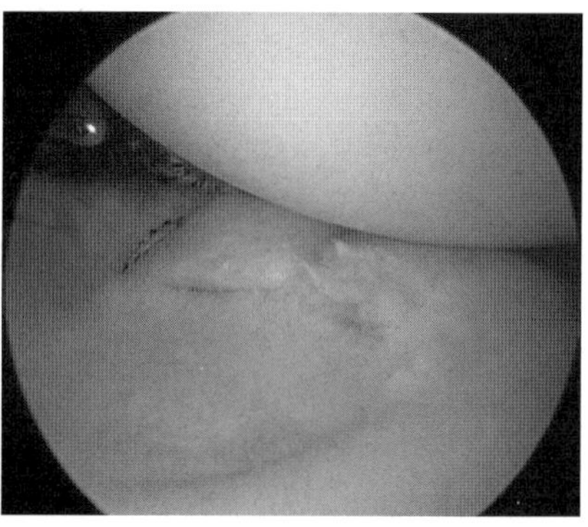

Figure 5 The suture anchor repair replaces the labrum on top of the glenoid and tensions the inferior capsular structures.

The postoperative rehabilitation program includes 6 weeks of immobilization in a sling with early controlled range-of-motion activities. Once use of the sling is discontinued, a progressive, structured rehabilitation program that includes range-of-motion and strengthening exercises is encouraged. A return to full activity is anticipated approximately 6 months after surgery.

Posterior Shoulder Instability

Posterior shoulder instability is a challenging pathologic entity to successfully manage. Recent advances in the understanding of the pathophysiology of posterior instability have led to substantial improvements in patient outcomes. Arthroscopic suture anchor repair for posterior Bankart lesions has achieved success rates in patients (including contact athletes) from 89% to 92%.[24-26]

Indications for surgery include disabling or recurrent posterior subluxation that is unresponsive to comprehensive conservative treatment, traumatic reverse Bankart lesions, or posterior humeral avulsion of the glenohumeral ligaments. A distinct history of trauma is present in approximately 50% of patients. The consistent shoulder position of jeopardy includes flexion, adduction, and internal rotation. Posterior shoulder pain is typical, although apprehension is not. Important examination findings include the magnitude of translational laxity determined on the load-and-shift test. Patients are often misclassified as having MDI when they have symptomatic posterior instability with asymptomatic multidirectional laxity, which may include a positive sulcus sign. A positive jerk test for posterior subluxation and reduction is usually painful.

An arthroscopic repair is contraindicated in patients with truly pathologic collagen tissue exemplified by very elastic skin, hypermobile joints (thumbs, elbows, patellas), and significant bone loss or excessive retroversion.

Diagnostic Arthroscopy and Pathologic Findings

An examination under anesthesia should be performed to assess range of motion and translational laxity. Patient positioning is determined by the surgeon's preference; however, the lateral decubitus orientation often provides easier access to the posterior aspect of the joint. A 10-lb weight is affixed to the arm sleeve and provides "suspension" rather than traction to the distal arm. An arm position of 45° abduction and 20° flexion will offer adequate access to all regions of the glenohumeral joint.

The narrowness of the posterior glenoid rim and the normal glenoid version make it difficult to place suture anchors through the posterior portal without skiving along the articular cartilage. The entry site for the posterior portal must be adjusted 1 cm lateral to the standard placement (directly in line with the posterolateral corner of the acromion). The entry for a midanterior portal begins 1.5 cm lateral and 1.5 cm inferior to the coracoid tip. A spinal needle identifies the appropriate course and an obturated cannula is inserted. The anterosuperior portal is created 1 cm lateral to the anterolateral corner of the acromion and provides an optimal view of the posterior glenoid. If access to the axillary capsule is needed, a posteroinferior portal is created 2 cm inferior and 1 cm lateral to the initial posterior portal. Additional suture anchor portals can be placed percutaneously from a more lateral entry point to gain a favorable angle of entry.

A thorough diagnostic survey is then completed to determine which pathologic components must be corrected. Evaluation begins with the posterior labrum, which may be cracked, fissured, or flattened as a result of recurrent humeral head subluxation. A Kim lesion, a hidden posterior Bankart lesion beneath a split but substantially intact labrum, may be identified on a preoperative MRI. A posterior Bankart lesion with capsulolabral separation from the glenoid is palpated. A patulous or redundant posterior capsule and associated incompetent posterior band of the glenohumeral ligament may be the primary pathology responsible for posterior shoulder instability. Avulsion of the glenohumeral ligaments from the humeral neck can result from posterior instability. A reverse Hill-Sachs lesion is sometimes present and may impact treatment decisions if excessive bone loss is discovered.

Posterior Bankart Repair

If a frank capsulolabral detachment is evident, a suture anchor repair is performed.[24,26-28] While viewing from the anterosuperior portal, a full-radius synovial resector is introduced through the posterior portal to débride the ragged, unstable margins of labrum and articular cartilage. Using a liberator elevator, the scar tissue tethering the capsulolabral tissue to the glenoid neck is released inferiorly at least to the 6 o'clock position. Adequate release is confirmed by free mobility of the capsular tissue and visibility of the infraspinatus muscle. A drill guide is then securely seated 2 to 3 mm onto the rim of the glenoid at the 7 o'clock position. The drill should approach the glenoid approximately at a 45° angle. The anchor is inserted and tested for security, and the sutures are retrieved posteriorly. A cannulated suture hook is introduced through the posterior portal and enters the capsulolabral tissue 1 cm inferior and 1 cm lateral to the anchor site to superiorly advance and medially plicate the posterior capsule. With the hook embedded in the capsule, firm superior tension is applied and brought superior to the anchor site to retension the tissue. A separate monofilament traction suture can be used if it is necessary to reduce the capsule prior to introducing the suture-passing device. A monofilament (nylon) suture is delivered through the suture hook and retrieved out of the midanterior cannula. An effective shuttle is created by tying a simple overhand knot in the anterior limb of monofilament suture around the inferior limb of anchor suture that exits the midanterior portal. Traction is applied to the posterior limb of the nylon suture to deliver the anchor suture from anterior to posterior through the capsulolabral tissue and out of the posterior cannula. This capsular limb becomes the post for a sliding knot, which is secured by adding three or four half-hitches. As the knot is tightened, it will advance the tissue superiorly as well as up onto the glenoid rim. A pseudolabrum is created and deepens the glenoid concavity. Additional anchors are placed at the 8:30 o'clock and 10 o'clock positions along the posterior glenoid, and the repair is completed. Occasionally, four anchors are required to create secure fixation of the capsule to the posterior glenoid (Figure 6).

Posterior Capsular Plication

When posterior capsular laxity is present along with a substantially intact labrum, a posterior capsular plication is performed.[29-31] While viewing from the anterosuperior portal, a rasp or full-radius shaver with the suction turned off is introduced through one of the posterior portals to excoriate the posterior and inferior capsule and adjacent labrum to stimulate a healing response. If the inflow of irrigant is shut off following the capsular abrasion, punctate bleeding can often be observed. A 45° cannulated suture hook is introduced through a posterior portal to create a "pinch-tuck" plication of the capsule. Beginning at the 6 o'clock position, the hook tip is in-

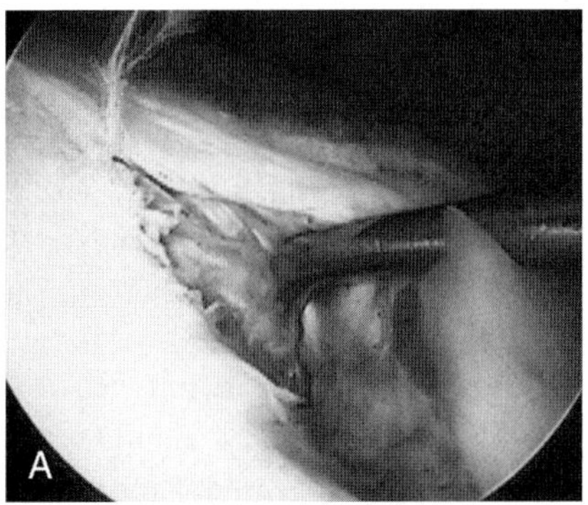

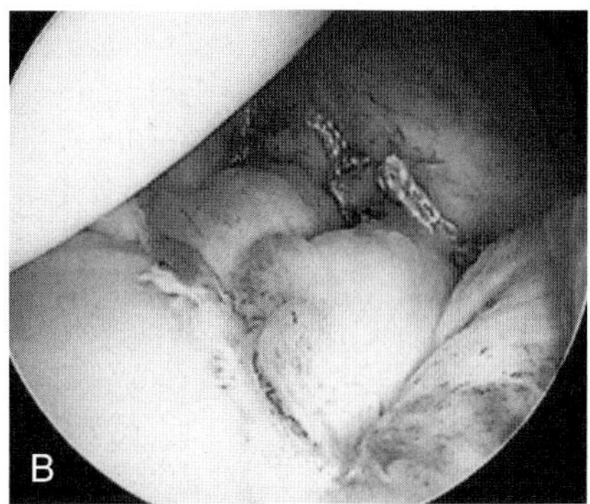

Figure 6 **A,** A posterior Bankart labral detachment. **B,** A repaired labrum with suture anchors.

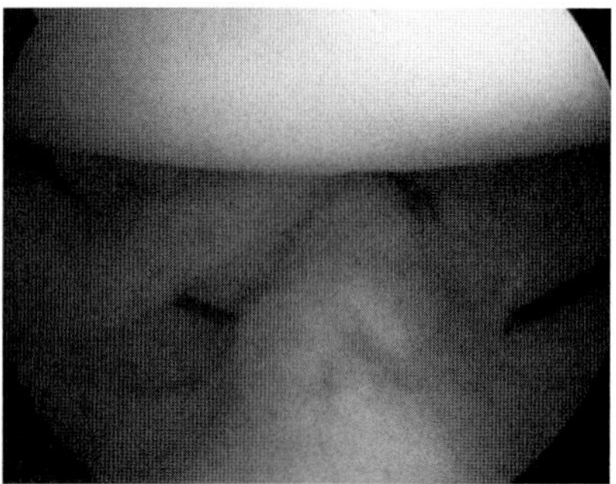

Figure 7 Posterior capsular plication is used to repair an insufficient capsular restraint.

troduced perpendicular to the capsule approximately 12 mm lateral to the labral rim. After penetrating the capsule, it is then passed beneath and parallel to the capsule to avoid encircling subjacent tissue, particularly the axillary nerve. The tip exits the capsule 7 mm from the glenoid rim. The hook tip is then brought toward the glenoid and passed beneath the annular fibers of the entire labrum to exit on the articular surface. In doing so, a pleat or dart of capsule is created (Figure 7). A polydioxanone suture is delivered and retrieved out the midanterior cannula. The polydioxanone suture can be used as the definitive repair suture or, alternatively, used to shuttle a No. 2 permanent braided suture back through the capsule and out of the posterior cannula. The posterior limb, which exits the capsule laterally, is identified as the post, and a sliding knot is delivered and backed up with three half-hitches. A total of three to five sutures are placed in a similar manner. Care must be taken to avoid creating a progressively larger pleat as the repair progresses superiorly. A hook probe is then used to verify the security of the suture loops and assess capsular tension. When the posterior labrum has insufficient integrity, suture anchors are used to improve the fixation of the capsulolabral tissue to the glenoid rim.

Traditionally, a rotator interval closure in some fashion has been added in an effort to enhance posteroinferior stability.[32,33] Recent studies indicate that interval closures in this manner may do little to change the dimensions of the rotator interval or improve posterior stability.[34-36] If the residual anterior laxity is deemed excessive on load-and-shift testing, anterior plication sutures can be placed in an attempt to balance the capsule.

Repair of a Posterior Humeral Avulsion of the Glenohumeral Ligament

Arthroscopic reattachment of the glenohumeral ligaments to the posterior neck of the humerus offers a secure repair without the morbidity of an open approach.[37] The arthroscope is placed in the anterosuperior portal. The posterior cannula is effectively extra-articular because it does not penetrate the posterior veil of capsule that has fallen medially. Through the posterior portal, a burr is introduced to excoriate the humeral neck. Typically, two double-loaded suture anchors are sufficient. After appropriate bone preparation, the posteroinferior anchor is inserted into the humeral neck through a 5-mm stab incision just lateral to the posterior cannula. A loop grasper is used to retrieve one limb of suture out of the posterior cannula. The suture is then loaded into an antegrade suture passer, which is introduced through the posterior cannula and used to grasp and reduce the capsule. The initial suture is placed 2 to 3 mm medial to the torn capsular margin at the inferior extent of the tear. Once delivered, the loop of suture is grasped with the passing device and delivered through the posterior cannula. In a similar manner, each of the additional three limbs of the two folded sutures is passed in a horizontal mattress fashion. The cannula is withdrawn and reinserted, placing the sutures outside the cannula. The most inferior mattress pair is retrieved through the posterior cannula and securely tied with an arthroscopic knot with appropriate half-hitch backups. The second mattress suture is tied to complete the repair.

Rehabilitation

The shoulder is immobilized in a sling and swath for 4 weeks, and rotator cuff and periscapular isomet-

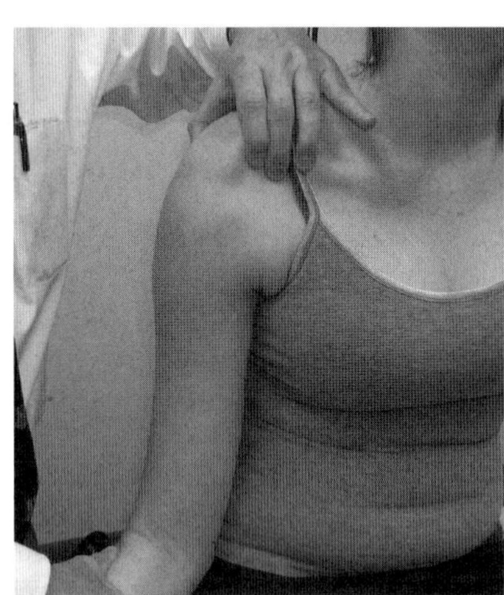

Figure 8 A sulcus test shows excessive inferior translation of the humerus.

rics are performed. Patients are permitted light activities with the affected extremity in front of the body from the waist to the face. At 4 to 6 weeks, gentle passive range-of-motion exercises are initiated, avoiding internal rotation. Full motion is expected at 12 weeks with the exception of internal rotation. Postoperatively, active and passive internal rotation are avoided and allowed to gradually return. If significant restrictions are present at 10 weeks, gentle passive motion is initiated. At 10 to 12 weeks, light progressive resistive cuff, periscapular, and deltoid strengthening are begun. Return-to-sports activities are permitted at 6 months if shoulder strength is sufficient.

Multidirectional Instability

Diagnosis

In treating MDI of the shoulder, one of the most significant challenges is achieving an accurate diagnosis. Neer and Foster[38] described MDI as uncontrollable and involuntary inferior subluxation or dislocation associated with both anterior and posterior dislocation or subluxation. Cooper and Brems[39] reported that more than 50% of their patients with MDI also had signs of ligamentous laxity, and 70% of their patients had bilateral shoulder laxity, even if only one shoulder was symptomatic. Misamore and associates[40] described MDI as a grade 2 translation with reproduction of symptoms in at least two directions. This description is fairly consistent with recent descriptions of MDI and for practical purposes is probably used by many surgeons.

Other difficulties in diagnosing MDI are the variability of findings on physical examinations and differentiating laxity and instability. Lintner and associates[41] evaluated 76 asymptomatic athletes and reported that many had significant translation of the shoulder. McFarland and associates[42] evaluated asymptomatic athletes and reported that 9% of females with a grade III sulcus had significant posterior translation. The physician must be sure that a particular laxity truly causes symptoms to make an MDI diagnosis. Therefore, a patient with MDI would have symptomatic instability in at least two directions; laxity in all three directions with a sulcus of at least grade II and the ability to translate the humeral head at least onto the rim anteriorly and posteriorly; a contralateral shoulder that likely has increased translation with a positive sulcus examination, although that shoulder may be asymptomatic; and associated signs of ligamentous laxity.

Patients with MDI may report that the instability can be voluntary, which does not necessarily imply a psychiatric issue. There are also a significant number of patients who can demonstrate instability; these are often situations in which the shoulder is felt to be subluxated but then self-reduces. Patients also can have significant pain or neurologic symptoms, which can be magnified when carrying objects.

Physical Examination

The physical examination of a patient with suspected MDI includes a seated or supine load-and-shift test to palpate anterior and posterior translation of the glenohumeral joint and reproduce symptoms. Apprehension testing done for common anterior instability also is performed; a relocation test can be added to improve the sensitivity of the examination. The Gagey hyperabduction test has been proposed as a test for inferior glenohumeral laxity of the shoulder and is believed to be positive if there is more than 105° of abduction between the humerus and scapula. The hallmark of testing for MDI is the sulcus test (Figure 8). This test is typically performed with the patient's arm at his or her side. A grade 1 translation is up to 1 cm, a grade 2 is 1 to 2 cm, and a grade 3 translation is more than 2 cm. The examination is repeated with the arm in external rotation because classic MDI sulcus signs remain unchanged with the arm in external rotation. The inferior capsule also can be tested in an abducted position with the arm held at approximately 90° of abduction; the proximal humerus is levered inferiorly to detect the inferior translation in an abducted position. It is important to question the patient to ascertain which direction(s) best reproduce symptoms. For example, the shoulder may have a significantly increased anterior translation, but it is the posterior and inferior translation that actually reproduces the patient's symptoms. Winging issues or substantial scapular dysfunction can aggravate shoulder stability, and it is important to determine if this is a compensatory issue or may contribute to the unstable glenohumeral joint.

Imaging

Standard radiographs consisting of a true AP view of the glenohumeral joint, and outlet, axillary, and acromioclavicular joint views are obtained. Occasionally abnormalities are noted, but radiographs usually appear normal. It is believed that MRI with intra-articular contrast to enhance the sensitivity of the imaging will show an increased capsular volume along with a significant axillary recess.

Treatment Options

At 2-year follow-up, Burkhead and Rockwood[43] reported 88% good to excellent results in patients after participation in an MDI exercise program. Rook and associates[44] reported satisfactory results in 90% of patients treated with 6 months of rehabilitation for MDI. In contrast to these promising results, Misamore and associates[40] reported that 40 of 57 patients (70%) with MDI in their study who were available for final follow-up either had required surgical treatment or had fair or poor ratings on the Rowe grading scale with nonsurgical treatment. The authors believed that most of the patients treated with physical therapy showed improvement within 3 months; therefore, prolonged nonsurgical treatment was not beneficial.

Until recently, the open capsular shift procedure as described by Neer and Foster[38] was considered the gold standard for treating MDI of the shoulder. The shift was placed on the side of the shoulder with the primary symptomatic direction of instability. Neer and Foster[38] reported on 1 failure in 40 shoulders treated with the procedure. Cooper and Brems[39] reported on 39 shoulders with 4 failures, and Pollock and associates[45] reported on 52 shoulders with 3 failures. Although the results of these open repairs appear good, arthroscopy has become more prominent in the treatment of MDI of the shoulder. It should be noted in the original Neer and Foster[38] study, 7 of 40 shoulders were treated with both anterior and posterior approaches, which would result in significant morbidity for the patient. Both sides of the shoulder could be treated in a much less invasive manner using arthroscopy. In reviewing the results of MDI treated arthroscopically, Treacy and associates[46] reported 88% satisfactory outcomes at 5 years, and Gartsman and associates[47] reported 44 of 47 good to excellent results (94%) at 3-year follow-up.

At the time of surgery, an examination is performed with the patient under anesthesia to confirm the levels and directions of translation. The patient is positioned in a lateral decubitus position with the arm in balanced suspension in approximately 20° to 30° of abduction and lateral suspension on the proximal humerus. A standard posterior portal is made and the shoulder is evaluated with the standard diagnostic approach. If it is necessary to place suture anchors and capsular plication sutures, auxiliary anterior or posterior portals may be added to the procedure. The synovium is rasped in the areas where plication will be placed, and areas are débrided where the labrum needs to be advanced to a fresh bony bed. In general, the area of primary instability or the side that will require labral repair along with capsular plication is treated first. Capsular plication sutures are usually placed with a curved suture hook that passes a monofilament suture through the capsule approximately 1 cm from the labrum or anchor. The hook is then advanced anterosuperiorly or posterosuperiorly depending on which side of the shoulder requires superior advancement of the capsule to either the labrum or an anchor when the labrum appears insufficient. The monofilament suture is passed through and shuttled to a permanent suture for tying, although no suture type has been shown to produce superior results. Typically, the sutures are started near the 6 o'clock position and worked progressively superior on the anterior or posterior aspect of the shoulder (Figure 9). It is not necessary to tie all of these sutures as they are placed. Once the inferior capsule has been advanced and the anterior or posterior side has been treated, the contralateral side then can be plicated depending on the perceived level of laxity determined by the patient's physical examination and arthroscopic evaluation.

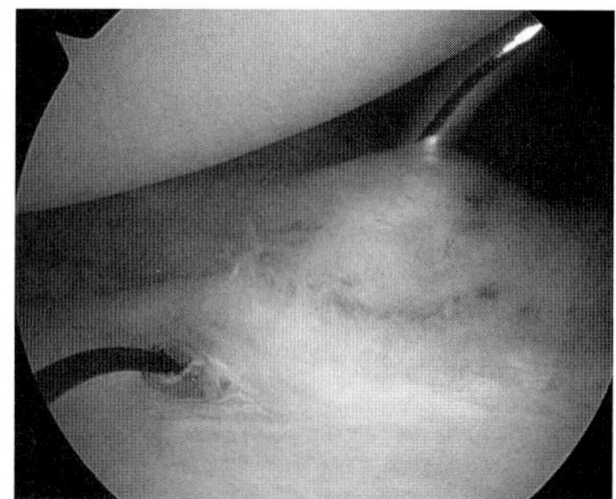

Figure 9 Inferior capsular plication can reduce the size and volume of the pouch.

Historically, either laser or thermal probes for capsular shrinkage were part of the treatment.[48-50] The preponderance of evidence suggests that thermal treatment of the capsule as an isolated procedure is not the treatment of choice for MDI of the shoulder, and suture capsulorrhaphy is the preferred approach.[51]

Treatment of the rotator interval must also be considered. Harryman and associates[32] popularized the notion that rotator interval closure will check inferior translation in adduction and provide additional posterior stability. This clearly would be of benefit in most MDI surgeries. Harryman and associates[32] described a mediolateral directed closure that included the coracohumeral ligament and clearly had the potential to significantly affect motion and translation. Basic science studies indicate that arthroscopically performed rotator interval closure does not have as great an effect on inferior translation and posterior translation.[34,36] Most authors have found some decrease in anterior translation at various arm angles along with a significant loss of external rotation.[52,53] However, patients with MDI who typically have substantial preoperative external rotation as a normal finding have significantly increased capsular volume; therefore, it would be reasonable to close the rotator interval in these patients.[33,35]

Rehabilitation

Patients usually wear a sling for 4 to 6 weeks after surgery. The sling is removed daily when the patient performs simple Codman-type exercises to increase elbow, hand, and wrist motion. In patients with primary posterior instability, an external rotation brace may be a considered to keep the arm in a more neutral position. After surgery, it is believed to be important to perform serial checks for potential shoulder stiffness rather than waiting a significant period of time and potentially recognizing this complication after a delay. Early implementation of scapular stabilizing exercises is important in the rehabilitation program; after 6 to 8 weeks a standard rotator cuff rehabilitation program can be started. Because regaining absolute symmetric range of motion is not usually the necessary endpoint, pushing the extremes of abduction and external rotation, cross arm adduction, or internal rotation behind the back need not be done for at least 3 months to allow as much healing of the capsule as possible.

Complications and Revision Surgery

One of the goals of a sports medicine physician is returning athletes to sports participation at a level comparable to their preinjury state. There is always the risk of recurrence of shoulder instability. Because shoulder injuries can occur throughout an athlete's career, the treating physician should be familiar with managing symptomatic shoulders that develop after surgical repair.

Instability Recurrence

The potential for a shoulder to subluxate after surgery has been well documented.[54,55] The initial reports on surgical treatments used the absence of dislocation as a benchmark for successful stabilization. Subluxation with spontaneous reduction, continued apprehension, and the inability or choice to avoid athletic participation was not included in the parameters that defined the success and failure of open treatment. Arthroscopic treatment to achieve anterior stabilization uses a similar but not identical technique as open surgical repair. Several differences in open treatment include the subscapularis detachment or split, the lateral capsular detachment allowing for a second location for retensioning, overlapping capsular flaps creating a thickened capsule along the anterior band of the inferior glenohumeral ligament, and tying the labral repair knots on the exterior of the capsule.[56-58] Considering the differences in managing the subscapularis and potential stiffness, the arthroscopic approach is preferable for an overhead athlete, and an open or arthroscopic approach would be suitable for a contact athlete depending on the goals of the athlete.[2,59-61]

Patient selection for arthroscopic revision surgery is equally as important as patient selection for the initial procedure.[62-65] The treating physician should determine the reason for the recurrence and whether a better approach can be applied to the revision surgery. Results of revision surgery for shoulder instability have not been as successful, possibly because of bone changes, soft-tissue deterioration, hardware complications, and joint degenerative changes.[23,66]

The ideal candidate for arthroscopic revision surgery following recurrence of shoulder instability will have a normal articular surface with minimal bone loss from the glenoid or humeral head, acute rim fractures that are reparable, robust labral and capsular tissue that can be mobilized and repaired, and the willingness to comply with a reasonable schedule for proper rehabilitation and recovery. Patients initially may have been treated with open surgery or an arthroscopic procedure. Some open surgeries may not have treated the glenoid soft-tissue avulsion and can be arthroscopically revised without removal of the bone block. If a surgeon chooses revision surgery for a patient treated with an arthroscopic Bankart repair, the original procedure should be evaluated to determine what changes are needed to avoid the risk of recurrence. In the authors' experience, a greater degree of tissue mobilization, increased tensioning, and additional surgical fixation has produced short-term and midterm successful outcomes.

Recurrence of instability resulting from trauma often re-creates a labral avulsion and possibly a rim fracture that is favorable to arthroscopic repair. Multiple recurrences with glenoid rim erosion may have a poorer prognosis with arthroscopic revision. Researchers do not agree on the amount of glenoid deficiency that causes a significant risk of failure, with estimates ranging from 20% to 30% of the width of the glenoid.[21,22,67] The presence of a Hill-Sachs lesion must be considered when calculating bone loss. Treatment options in patients with excessive bone loss include open capsular labral repair and bone grafting to the anterior glenoid rim.[68]

Technical Pearls

Arthroscopic anterior stabilization was previously discussed; however, several steps may deserve additional emphasis when considering revision surgery. Patient selection is considered based on a review of the history prior to and including the initial surgery, a description of the new traumatic event, the physical examination, and imaging studies. Important factors include the age of the athlete, type of sport played, desired activities for future participation, and evaluation of translation using a load-and-shift examination. Shoulders with grade 3 translation and those that remain dislocated after translation forces are relaxed suggest excessive bone loss of the glenoid and humeral articular surface. The choice for arthroscopic versus open revision most often is determined preoperatively, but occasionally is altered during the arthroscopic examination.[2] If a compromised glenoid width is identified or there is a significant capsular tear adjacent to the axillary nerve, it may be preferable to convert to open surgery.

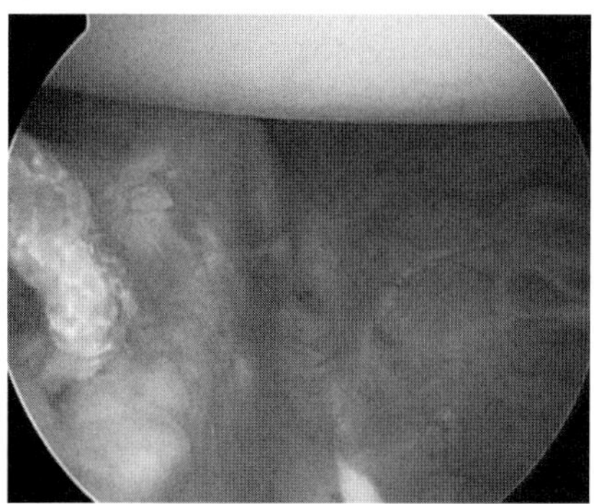

Figure 10 An anterior capsule and labrum detached from the glenoid edge and healed to the subscapularis tendon.

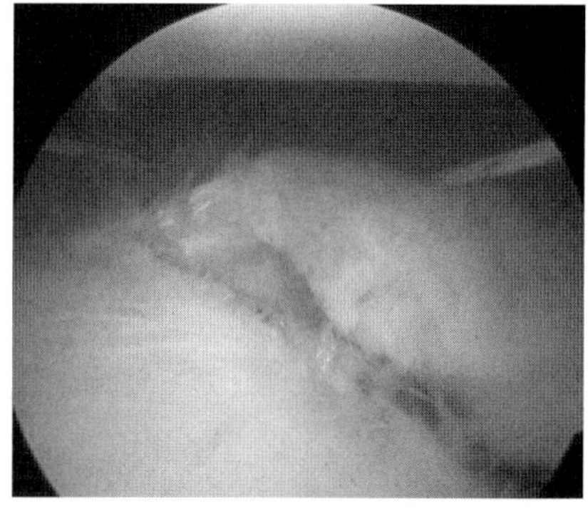

Figure 11 A mattress suture through a posterior portal may improve inferior capsular fixation.

Tissue mobilization is important for creating a sturdy repair. The capsule and labrum is not only elevated from the glenoid but also separated from the subscapularis. This may be challenging, especially in patients with an anterior periosteal sleeve avulsion lesion in which the capsule has reattached medially along the glenoid neck (Figure 10). The separation of the anteroinferior capsule permits improved repositioning along the glenoid rim. Because the axillary nerve rests along the inferior border of the subscapularis, special care during dissection should be taken to avoid inadvertent nerve injury.

Anchor placement should be dictated by the extent of labral detachment. Recurrence may extend the injury more posteriorly. With the arthroscope in the anterosuperior portal and looking posteriorly, an anchor can be placed through a posterolateral puncture into the inferior glenoid. If the labrum is intact, plication sutures incorporating the capsule and labrum can be placed and tied.

Use of the posterior portal may include introduction of curved suture hooks that provide a better angle for reducing the pouch and shifting tissues.[2] The important anteroinferior anchor is responsible for pouch reduction and re-creation of a labral buttress. The posterior cannula can deliver the curved hook to ensure that the tissue bite is inferior and posterior to the lesion. Using a second hook anteriorly creates a mattress suture, allowing improved tissue transfer and security against the abraded glenoid neck. It is common to use three or four anchors in arthroscopic revision surgery (Figure 11).

The capsular pouch is reduced with either suture anchor stitches or independent sutures placed within the capsule. Tissue transfers from inferior to superior will limit the amount of rotation lost in the overhead athlete. The capsule can be thickened with plication sutures placed in the midcapsular regions, and absorbable and braided sutures can be used.

In most revision surgeries, the rotator capsular interval is closed to further reinforce the anterior buttress.[35] A balanced repair with sutures on both sides minimizes the risk of creating symptoms in the opposite direction, particularly with patients with multidirectional laxity.

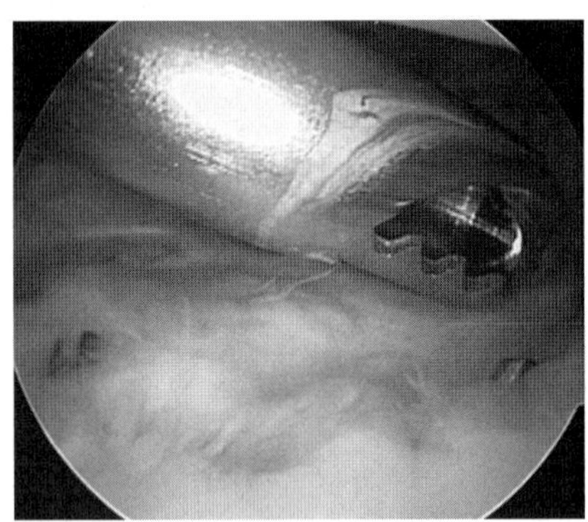

Figure 12 Prominent hardware can cause significant pain and alter adjacent cartilage.

A balanced repair centers the humeral head, retensions the capsule, and reduces the inferior sulcus.

Postoperative treatment and healing of the repaired capsule and labrum are critical to the surgical outcome. Immobilization in a pillow in neutral rotation or slight internal rotation is helpful. Gentle shoulder shrugs, elbow flexion and extension, and early grip strength may limit tissue changes about the shoulder. Flexibility stretching can begin at 3 weeks but should progress slowly over 3 to 4 months. Scapular muscle retraining is often emphasized at 8 weeks, and positions that are provocative to shoulder instability are delayed until 4 months. Sports-specific training can begin at 3 months and is often continued for approximately 1 year, even if the athlete returns to competition.

Video 16.1: Arthroscopic Management of Shoulder Instabilities: Technical Pearls. Jeffrey S. Abrams, MD (6 min)

The Painful Stable Shoulder

Certain shoulders can become painful after surgery even in the absence of instability recurrence. Hawkins and Angelo[69] reported on degenerative changes that developed in patients from overtensioning of the glenohumeral articulation. Another possible cause of pain is hardware placed along the glenoid rim. Prominent anchors may not be detectable on radiographs and other imaging studies. If hardware placement is suspected as the cause of the pain, an arthroscopic evaluation should be performed to determine if possible anchor removal or exchange is needed (Figure 12).

Suture knots also can create a foreign body response. Sliding knots placed along the nonpost arm of the suture often migrate toward the anchor eyelet. Here the knots abrade along the glenoid articular cartilage and possibly the humeral head. The "squeaky" shoulder is a concern. Previously placed softer and weaker sutures may correct this situation with time. Reinforced sutures are not as likely to resolve and may require arthroscopic evaluation and removal.

Articular cartilage complications may be painful. Labral transfers over full-thickness glenoid defects may be helpful in alleviating shearing forces and contact pressure, which anecdotally have been shown to be more effective in anterior instability than in posterior instability. Labral transfer is performed by placing an anchor on the abraded lesion and creating a mattress suture deep to the labrum. As the knot is tied, the tissue shifts over the lesion. Biologic resurfacing has been performed but has shown greater success when combined with arthroscopic stabilization.

The most significant cartilage complication is chondrolysis, which can occur after arthroscopic stabilization procedures and produces a global loss of cartilage during the early postoperative period. Although multiple factors probably contribute to chondrolysis, thermal treatment, pain pumps with bupivacaine, and certain suture materials have been hypothesized as the cause. Arthroscopic revision or release may be attempted, but most patients require more significant open procedures.

Summary

Athletes often want to return to the activities that produce an unstable shoulder. Certain genetic traits such as laxity, combined with a young age and demanding sport, continue to place the shoulder at risk for recurrent instability. Arthroscopy can be used to assess the trauma and perform revision surgery in selected patients. Critical issues include the quality of the soft tissues, the location of the tear, the amount of articular surface involved, the presence of acute rim fractures, and a well-planned postoperative rehabilitation plan. In patients with appropriate characteristics and pathology, arthroscopy can be successful in the treatment of anterior, posterior, multidirectional, and recurrent instability.

References

1. Ide J, Maeda S, Takagi K: Arthroscopic Bankart repair using suture anchors in athletes: Patient selection and postoperative sports activity. *Am J Sports Med* 2004;32:1899-1905.
2. Abrams JS: Role of arthroscopy in treating anterior instability of the athlete's shoulder. *Sports Med Arthrosc* 2007;15:230-238.
3. Taylor DC, Arciero RA: Pathologic changes associated with shoulder dislocations: Arthroscopic and physical examination findings in first-time, traumatic anterior dislocations. *Am J Sports Med* 1997;25:306-311.
4. McMahon PJ, Tibone JE, Cawley PW, et al: The anterior band of the

inferior glenohumeral ligament: Biomechanical properties from tensile testing in the position of apprehension. *J Shoulder Elbow Surg* 1998;7: 467-471.

5. Sachs RA, Lin D, Stone ML, Paxton E, Kuney M: Can the need for future surgery for acute traumatic anterior shoulder dislocation be predicted? *J Bone Joint Surg Am* 2007; 89:1665-1674.
6. Bottoni CR, Wilckens JH, DeBerardino TM, et al: A prospective, randomized evaluation of arthroscopic stabilization versus nonoperative treatment in patients with acute, traumatic, first-time shoulder dislocations. *Am J Sports Med* 2002;30: 576-580.
7. Postacchini F, Gumina S, Cinotti G: Anterior shoulder dislocation in adolescents. *J Shoulder Elbow Surg* 2000;9: 470-474.
8. Larrain MV, Botto GJ, Montenegro HJ, Mauas DM: Arthroscopic repair of acute traumatic anterior shoulder dislocation in young athletes. *Arthroscopy* 2001;17:373-377.
9. Itoi E, Sashi R, Minagawa H, Shimizu T, Wakabayashi I, Sato K: Position of immobilization after dislocation of the glenohumeral joint: A study with use of magnetic resonance imaging. *J Bone Joint Surg Am* 2001;83:661-667.
10. Itoi E, Hatakeyama Y, Sato T, et al: Immobilization in external rotation after shoulder dislocation reduces the risk of recurrence: A randomized controlled trial. *J Bone Joint Surg Am* 2007;89:2124-2131.
11. Buss DD, Lynch GP, Meyer CP, Huber SM, Freehill MQ: Nonoperative management for in-season athletes with anterior shoulder instability. *Am J Sports Med* 2004;32:1430-1433.
12. Bottoni CR, Smith EL, Berkowitz MJ, Towle RB, Moore JH: Arthroscopic versus open shoulder stabilization for recurrent anterior instability: A prospective randomized clinical trail. *Am J Sports Med* 2006;34: 1730-1737.
13. Larrain MV, Montenegro HJ, Mauas DM, Collazo CC, Pavon F: Arthroscopic management of traumatic anterior shoulder instability in collision athletes: Analysis of 204 cases with a 4- to 9-year follow-up and results with the suture anchor technique. *Arthroscopy* 2006;22:1283-1289.
14. Mazzocca AD, Brown FM Jr, Carreira DS, Hayden J, Romeo AA: Arthroscopic anterior shoulder stabilization of collision and contact athletes. *Am J Sports Med* 2005;33:52-60.
15. Handoll HH, Almaiyah MA, Rangan A: Surgical versus non-surgical treatment for acute anterior shoulder dislocation. *Cochrane Database Syst Rev* 2004;1:CD004325.
16. Kim SH, Ha KI, Cho YB, Ryu BD, Oh I: Arthroscopic anterior stabilization of the shoulder: Two to six-year follow-up. *J Bone Joint Surg Am* 2003; 85-A:1511-1518.
17. Fabbriciani C, Milano G, Demontis A, Fadda S, Ziranu F, Mulas PD: Arthroscopic versus open treatment of Bankart lesion of the shoulder: A prospective randomized study. *Arthroscopy* 2004;20:456-462.
18. Carreira DS, Mazzocca AD, Oryhon J, Brown FM, Hayden JK, Romeo AA: A prospective outcome evaluation of arthroscopic Bankart repairs: Minimum 2-year follow-up. *Am J Sports Med* 2006;34:771-777.
19. Marquardt B, Witt KA, Liem D, Steinbeck J, Potzl W: Arthroscopic Bankart repair in traumatic anterior shoulder instability using a suture anchor technique. *Arthroscopy* 2006;22: 931-936.
20. Rhee YG, Ha JH, Cho NS: Anterior shoulder stabilization in collision athletes: Arthroscopic versus open Bankart repair. *Am J Sports Med* 2006;34: 979-985.
21. Burkhart SS, De Beer JF: Traumatic glenohumeral bone defects and their relationship to failure of arthroscopic Bankart repairs: Significance of the inverted-pear glenoid and the humeral engaging Hill-Sachs lesion. *Arthroscopy* 2000;16:677-694.
22. Itoi E, Lee SB, Berglund LJ, Berge LL, An KN: The effect of a glenoid defect on anteroinferior stability of the shoulder after Bankart repair: A cadaveric study. *J Bone Joint Surg Am* 2000;82:35-46.
23. Marquardt B, Garmann S, Schulte T, Witt KA, Steinbeck J, Potzl W: Outcome after failed traumatic anterior shoulder instability repair with and without surgical revision. *J Shoulder Elbow Surg* 2007;16:742-747.
24. Savoie FH III, Holt MS, Field LD, Ramsey JR: Arthroscopic management of posterior instability: Evolution of technique and results. *Arthroscopy* 2008;24:389-396.
25. Radkowski CA, Chhabra A, Baker CL III, et al: Arthroscopic capsulolabral repair for posterior shoulder instability in throwing athletes compared with nonthrowing athletes. *Am J Sports Med* 2008;36:693-699.
26. Bradley JP, Baker C III, Kline A, et al: Arthroscopic capsulolabral reconstruction for posterior instability of the shoulder: A prospective study of 100 shoulders. *Am J Sports Med* 2006; 34:1061-1071.
27. Williams RJ III, Strickland S, Cohen M, et al: Arthroscopic repair for traumatic posterior shoulder instability. *Am J Sports Med* 2003;31:203-209.
28. Bottoni CR, Franks BR, Moore J, DeBerardino TM, Taylor DC, Arciero RA: Operative stabilization of posterior shoulder Instability. *Am J Sports Med* 2005;33:996-1002.
29. Antoniou J, Duckworth DT, Harryman DT II: Capsulolabral augmentation for the management of posteroinferior instability of the shoulder. *J Bone Joint Surg* 2000;82:1220-1230.
30. Kim SH, Ha KI, Park JH, et al: Arthroscopic posterior labral repair and capsular shift for traumatic unidirectional posterior subluxation of the shoulder. *J Bone Joint Surg* 2003;85: 1479-1487.
31. Metcalf MH, Pond JD, Harryman DT II , Loutzenheiser T, Sidles JA: Capsulolabral augmentation in-

creases glenohumeral stability in the cadaver shoulder. *J Shoulder Elbow Surg* 2001;10:532-538.

32. Harryman DT III, Sidles JA, Harris SL, et al: The role of the rotator interval capsule in passive motion and stability of the shoulder. *J Bone Joint Surg Am* 1992;74:53-66.

33. Dewing CB, McCormick F, Bell SJ, et al: An analysis of capsular area in patients with anterior, posterior, and multidirectional shoulder instability. *Am J Sports Med* 2008;36:515-522.

34. Provencher MT, Mologne TS, Hongo M, Zhao K, Tasto JP, An KN: Arthroscopic versus open rotator interval closure: Biomechanical evaluation of stability and motion. *Arthroscopy* 2007;23:583-592.

35. Mologne TS, Zhao K, Hongo M, et al: The addition of rotator interval closure after arthroscopic repair of either anterior or posterior shoulder instability: Effect on glenohumeral translation and range of motion. *Am J Sports Med* 2008;36:1123-1131.

36. Plausinis D, Bravman JT, Heywood CH, et al: Arthroscopic rotator interval closure: Effect of sutures on glenohumeral motion and anterior-posterior translation. *Am J Sports Med* 2006;34:1656-1661.

37. Castagna A, Snyder S, Conti M, et al: Posterior humeral avulsion of the glenohumeral ligaments: A clinical review of 9 cases. *Arthroscopy* 2007;23:809-815.

38. Neer CS, Foster CR: Inferior capsular shift for involuntary inferior and multidirectional instability of the shoulder: A preliminary report. *J Bone Joint Surg Am* 1980;62:897-908.

39. Cooper RA, Brems JJ: The inferior capsular-shift procedure for multidirectional instability of the shoulder. *J Bone Joint Surg Am* 1992;74:1516-1521.

40. Misamore GW, Sallay PI, Didelot W: A longitudinal study of patients with multidirectional instability of the shoulder with seven to ten-year follow-up. *J Shoulder Elbow Surg* 2005;14:466-470.

41. Lintner SA, Levy AS, Kenter K, Speer KP: Glenohumeral translation in the asymptomatic athlete's shoulder and its relationship to other clinically measurable anthropometric variables. *Am J Sports Med* 1996;24:716-720.

42. McFarland EG, Campbell G, McDowell J: Posterior shoulder laxity in asymptomatic athletes. *Am J Sports Med* 1996;24:468-471.

43. Burkhead WZ, Rockwood CA: Treatment of instability of the shoulder with an exercise program. *J Bone Joint Surg Am* 1992;74:890-896.

44. Rook RT, Savoie FH III, Field LD: Arthroscopic treatment of instability attributable to capsular injury or laxity. *Clin Orthop Relat Res* 2001;390:52-58.

45. Pollock RG, Owens JM, Flatow EL, Bigliani LU: Operative results of the inferior capsular shift procedure for multidirectional instability of the shoulder. *J Bone Joint Surg Am* 2000;82:919-928.

46. Treacy SH, Savoie FH III, Field LD: Arthroscopic treatment of multidirectional instability. *J Shoulder Elbow Surg* 1999;8:345-350.

47. Gartsman GM, Roddey TS, Hammerman SM: Arthroscopic treatment of multidirectional glenohumeral instability: 2- to 5-year follow-up. *Arthroscopy* 2001;17:236-243.

48. Lyons TR, Griffith PL, Savoie FH III, Field LD: Laser-assisted capsulorrhaphy for multidirectional instability of the shoulder. *Arthroscopy* 2001;17:25-30.

49. Miniaci A, McBirnie J: Thermal capsular shrinkage for treatment of multidirectional instability of the shoulder. *J Bone Joint Surg Am* 2003;85:2283-2287.

50. D'Alessandro DF, Bradley JP, Fleischli JE, Connor PM: Prospective evaluation of thermal capsulorrhaphy for shoulder instability. *Am J Sports Med* 2004;32:21-33.

51. Abrams JS: Thermal capsulorrhaphy for instability of the shoulder: Concerns and applications of the heat probe. *Instr Course Lect* 2001;50:29-36.

52. Yamamoto N, Itoi E, Tuoheti Y, et al: Effect of rotator interval closure onglenohumeral stability and motion: A cadaveric study. *J Shoulder Elbow Surg* 2006;15:750-758.

53. Shafer BL, Mihata T, McGarry MH, et al: Effects of capsular plication and rotator interval closure in simulated multidirectional shoulder instability. *J Bone Joint Surg Am* 2008;90:136-144.

54. Rowe CR, Zarins B, Ciullo JV: Recurrent anterior dislocation of the shoulder after surgical repair. *J Bone Joint Surg Am* 1954;66:159-168.

55. Hawkins RH, Hawkins RJ: Failed anterior reconstruction for shoulder instability. *J Bone Joint Surg Br* 1985;67:709-714.

56. Burkhead WZ, Richie MF: Revision of failed shoulder reconstruction. *Contemp Orthop* 1992;24:126-133.

57. Zabinski SJ, Callaway GH, Cohen S, Warren RF: Revision shoulder stabilization: 2- to 10-year results. *J Shoulder Elbow Surg* 1999;8:58-65.

58. Levine WN, Arroyo JS, Pilock RG, Flatow EL, Bigliani LU: Open revision stabilization surgery for recurrent anterior glenohumeral instability. *Am J Sports Med* 2000;28:156-160.

59. Kim SH, Ha KI, Kim SH: Bankart repair in traumatic anterior shoulder instability: Open versus arthroscopic technique. *Arthroscopy* 2002;18:755-763.

60. Abrams JS: Innovations in arthroscopic surgery of the shoulder: Advances in arthroscopic shoulder stabilization. *Arthroscopy* 2003;19 (10 supp 1):106-108.

61. Sekiya JK, Willobee JA, Miller MD: Arthroscopic multi-pleated capsular plication compared with open inferior capsular shift for reduction of shoulder volume in a cadaveric mode. *Arthroscopy* 2007;23:1145-1151.

62. Creighton RA, Romeo AA, Brown FM, Hayden JK, Verma NN: Revision arthroscopic shoulder instability repair. *Arthroscopy* 2007;23:703-709.

63. Kim SH, Swon-Ick H, Kim YM: Arthroscopic revision Bankart repair: A prospective outcome study. *Arthroscopy* 2002;18:469-482.

64. Neri BR, Tuckman DV, Bravman JT, Yim D, Sahajpal DT, Rokito AS: Arthroscopic revision of Bankart repair. *J Shoulder Elbow Surg* 2007;16: 419-424.

65. Boileau P, Richou J, Lisai A, Balestro JC, Bicknell R, Jacquot N: Arthroscopic revision of failed open anterior stabilization of the shoulder, in Boileau P, ed: *Shoulder Arthroscopy & Arthroplasty, Current Concepts 2006.* Montpellier, France, Sauramps Medical, 2006, pp 117-130.

66. Meehan RS, Petersen SA: Results and factors affecting outcome of revision surgery for shoulder instability. *J Shoulder Elbow Surg* 2005;14:31-37.

67. Montgomery WH Jr, Wahl M, Hettrich C, Itoi E, Lippitt SB, Matsen FA III: Anteroinferior bone-grafting can restore stability in osseous glenoid defects. *J Bone Joint Surg Am* 2005;87:1972-1977.

68. Burkhart SS, De Beer JF, Barth JR, Cresswell T, Roberts C, Richards DP: Results of modified Latarjet reconstruction in patients with anteroinferior instability and significant bone loss. *Arthroscopy* 2007;23: 1033-1041.

69. Hawkins RJ, Angelo RL: Glenohumeral osteoarthritis: A late complication of the Putti-Platt repair. *J Bone Joint Surg Am* 1990;72:1193-1196.

Video Reference

16.1: Abrams JS: Video. *Arthroscopic Management of Shoulder Instabilities: Technical Pearls.* Princeton, NJ, 2009.

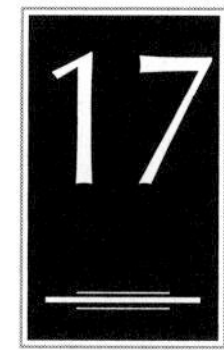

Current Strategies for Nonsurgical, Arthroscopic, and Minimally Invasive Surgical Treatment of Knee Cartilage Pathology

Nicholas A. Sgaglione, MD
Eli Chen, MD, PhD
Jack M. Bert, MD
Annunziato Amendola, MD
William D. Bugbee, MD

Abstract

The current approaches to treating articular cartilage defects in the knee comprise a spectrum from pharmacologic therapies to total knee arthroplasty. Nonsurgical treatment can include anti-inflammatory medications, bracing, and physical therapy. Surgical treatments include reconstructive repair of a small or large defect using microfracture, osteochondral autograft transplantation, autologous chrondrocyte transplantation, or osteochondral allograft transplantation; realignment procedures including osteotomies; and unicompartmental arthroplasty. A comprehensive algorithm can be used to determine the appropriate treatment for knee defects.

Instr Course Lect 2010;59:157-180.

Osteoarthritis (OA), the most common type of arthritis, affects approximately 27 million people in the United States.[1] Arthritis and related conditions cost the US economy approximately $86 billion per year in medical care and lost wages and production.[2] The lifetime risk of symptomatic knee OA approaches 45%, with higher levels for people who have had a knee injury or are obese.[3] Articular cartilage damage is ob-

Dr. Sgaglione or an immediate family member serves as a board member, owner, officer, or committee member of the Arthroscopy Association of North America and serves as a paid consultant to or is an employee of Smith & Nephew, Arthrocare, Conmed Linvatec, and Biomet Sports Medicine. Dr. Bert or an immediate family member serves as a board member, owner, officer, or committee member of the Arthroscopy Association of North America and serves as a paid consultant to or is an employee of Exactech, Genzyme, Regen Biologics, and Wright Medical Technology. Dr. Amendola or an immediate family member serves as a board member, owner, officer, or committee member of the International Society of Arthroscopy, Knee Surgery, and Orthopaedic Sports Medicine, the American Board of Orthopaedic Surgery, and the Iowa Donor Network; has received royalties from Arthrex; serves as a paid consultant to or is an employee of Arthrex and Arthrosurface; and owns stock or stock options in Arthrosurface. Dr. Bugbee or an immediate family member serves as a board member, owner, officer, or committee member of the AAOS Biologic Implants Committee Advanced Biohealing; has received royalties from Smith & Nephew and Zimmer; serves as a paid consultant to or is an employee of Arthrex, DePuy, Smith & Nephew, Zimmer, and the Joint Restoration Foundation; and has recieved research or institutional support from OREF. Neither Dr. Chen nor any immediate family member has received anything of value or owns stock in a commercial company or institution related directly or indirectly to the subject of this chapter.

Portions of this chapter adapted with permission from Bert JM: Unicompartmental arthroplasty for unicompartmental knee arthritis. Techniques in Knee Surgery *2008; 7:51-60.*

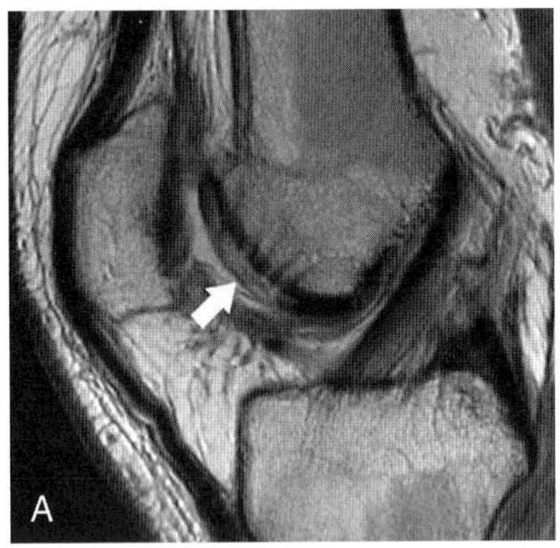

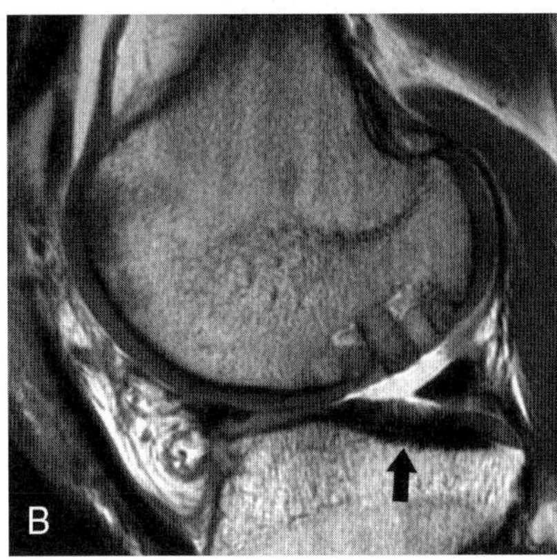

Figure 1 Cartilage-sensitive FSE MRIs of the knee. **A,** Sagittal image showing hyperintense repair cartilage (*arrow*) 5 months after microfracture in a 30-year-old woman. Reparative fibrocartilage is hyperintense owing to a less organized matrix and increased mobility of water. **B,** Sagittal image showing restoration of the condylar radius of curvature after osteochondral autograft transplantation (OAT) in a 21-year-old man with a large osteochondral defect of the lateral femoral condyle. Mild thinning of cartilage over the more posterior plugs as well as fibrillation of cartilage over the corresponding tibial plateau (*arrow*) is shown. (Reproduced with permission from Potter HG, Foo LF: Magnetic resonance imaging of articular cartilage: Trauma, degeneration, and repair. *Am J Sports Med* 2006;34:661-677.)

served during at least 60% of arthroscopic knee procedures,[4,5] appearing as a focal traumatic osteochondral defect, an osteochondritis dissecans (OCD) lesion, an early isolated degenerative lesion, or diffuse degenerative disease.

Multiple clinical and patient-specific factors must be considered in the evaluation and treatment of a patient with articular cartilage pathology. The timing and mechanism of an injury can be used in predicting the extent of cartilage damage. Any earlier surgical intervention must be documented. The size, depth, age, and location of cartilage defects and the extent of the underlying degenerative joint disease can shape the treatment approach. The patient's age, level of function, body mass index, and goals can be used to select articular cartilage treatments.

The development of higher resolution MRI and new, cartilage-specific protocols allow the detection of subclinical traumatic lesions and more accurate evaluation of cartilage morphology and the efficacy of cartilage repairs. Potter and Foo[6] reviewed several studies comparing diagnostic MRI to arthroscopic visualization of articular surfaces; they concluded that fat-suppressed, fast spin-echo (FSE) MRI had the least interobserver variability and the greatest sensitivity and specificity. FSE MRI provides a differential contrast of fluid, subchondral bone, and meniscus; in addition, based on different levels of water sequestration, it allows articular cartilage, fibrocartilage, and synovial fluid to be identified. FSE MRI yields valuable information about structural defects and their repair, including the viability of the repair site, the tissue fill volume, the surface congruence, the status of underlying subchondral bone, and the perimeter integration (Figure 1). Other cartilage-specific sequences are available, including T1-weighted FSE; T1 three-dimensional, gadolinium-enhanced MRI of cartilage (known as dGEMRIC); gradient-refocused acquisition in the steady state and iterative decomposition of water and fat with echo asymmetry and least-squares estimation (GRASS-IDEAL); isotropic, three-dimensional, steady-state free procession (SSFP); and driven equilibrium Fourier transform (DEFT).

The treatment options for symptomatic articular cartilage defects in the knee include nonsurgical management, reconstruction or repair, realignment, and arthroplasty.

Nonsurgical Management

Cartilage with OA exhibits characteristic changes, including lower concentrations and molecular weights of hyaluronic acid and loss of glycosaminoglycans. The result is decreased resiliency and increased brittleness.[7] A patient with an articular cartilage defect is treated to relieve the symptoms and limit the progression of the pathology. The nonsurgical treatment possibilities include the use of nonsteroidal anti-inflammatory drugs (NSAIDs), cyclooxygenase-2 (COX-2) inhibitors, corticosteroid injections, viscosupplementation injections, nutritional supplements, bracing, muscle strengthening, topical medications, acupuncture, and pulsed electrical stimulation.

Acetaminophen and NSAIDs

Acetaminophen is the most commonly prescribed first-line analgesic for the treatment of arthritis symptoms. It is safer to use than NSAIDs and has similar efficacy. The dosage can be as high as 4,000 mg per day. Hepatic dysfunction and renal toxicity secondary to acetaminophen overdosage have been reported but are uncommon.

NSAIDs are the most widely prescribed drugs for the treatment of degenerative joint disease, although adverse effects lead to the hospitalization of more than 100,000 patients annually. The adverse effects of NSAIDs, including gastrointestinal bleeding and toxicity, account for as much as 33% of the overall expense of treating OA in the United States.[8] NSAIDs work by inhibiting the enzyme cyclooxygenase, resulting in a decrease in prostaglandin synthesis. Prostaglandins mediate the inflammatory response and also protect the gastric mucosa. NSAIDs appear to stimulate collagen synthesis, which may have a beneficial effect on soft-tissue healing,[9] but NSAIDs also were found to delay fracture healing and bone ingrowth.[10] A meta-analysis comparing the effectiveness of topical and oral NSAIDs to a placebo found that topical NSAIDs were effective only for approximately 2 weeks and caused a rash, itching, and burning.[11]

Cyclooxygenase is present as two isoforms that catalyze the same reaction but differ in expression and regulatory patterns. Cyclooxygenase-1 is constitutively expressed in most tissues, including gastric mucosa and platelets. COX-2 is constitutively expressed in the brain and kidney, and it is inducible elsewhere, including areas of inflammation. Selective COX-2 inhibitors have been promoted for their ability to avoid the gastrointestinal adverse effects of other NSAIDs, including toxicity and bleeding, while maintaining therapeutic efficacy for OA.[12] A large randomized controlled study found lower rates of upper gastrointestinal ulcer complications with a selective COX-2 inhibitor (celecoxib) than with conventional NSAIDs.[13] A more recent Cochrane review compared data from all studies published through 2006 on the gastrointestinal effects of conventional NSAIDs and COX-2 inhibitors. COX-2 inhibitors were found to produce significantly fewer gastroduodenal ulcers (relative risk, 0.26) and other clinically important ulcers (relative risk, 0.39).[14] Because COX-2 inhibitors do not act on platelets, the risk of bleeding is lower than with other NSAIDs.[15] However, COX-2 is induced in the setting of inflammation, and COX-2 inhibitors therefore have a more deleterious effect on bone healing than other NSAIDs.[16]

Corticosteroid Injections

Intra-articular injections of corticosteroids can provide transient relief of inflammation in patients with OA. The most commonly used agents are methylprednisolone and triamcinolone, which are depot formulations with low solubility and a relatively long duration of activity.[17] The adverse effects of corticosteroid injections include a postinjection flare characterized by facial flushing and skin or fat atrophy. Animal studies suggesting that corticosteroid injections are toxic to articular cartilage have not been corroborated in humans.[18-20] In a randomized controlled double-blind study comparing triamcinolone and saline injections into the knee every 3 months for as long as 2 years, the patients treated with triamcinolone had improved range of motion and no progression of joint space narrowing compared with the patients who received a placebo.[21] The systemic effects of injected corticosteroids generally are mild and transient; they include effects on bone formation, serum cortisol levels, and glucose metabolism.

Viscosupplementation

Viscosupplementation is the injection of exogenous hyaluronan into a joint for the purpose of restoring the mechanical and physiochemical functions of synovial fluid and thus decreasing the symptoms of OA. Endogenous hyaluronan, the major hydrodynamic component of joint synovial fluid, is produced by type B synoviocytes and fibroblasts of the synovial membrane; its molecular weight is 5 to 7 $\times$ 10^6 daltons. Subsequent to the series of injections, viscosupplementation enhances chondrocyte metabolism, increases endogenous hyaluronan levels, and improves the viscous and elastic moduli of the synovial fluid.[22] A review of 20 randomized controlled studies comparing hyaluronan injections to a placebo found significant improvement in pain and functional outcome in the patients who received hyaluronan.[23] Patients older than 65 years and patients with radiographically identified advanced degenerative joint disease benefited the least. All of the hyaluronan preparations used in the study were derived from avian-derived fractionated hyaluronans.

Most proprietary hyaluronan products are extracted from avian combs, with the exception of Euflexxa (Ferring Pharmaceuticals, Parsippany, NJ), which is produced using a bacterial fermentation process. Hylan G-F 20 (Synvisc; Genzyme, Cambridge, MA) is the only form of injectable hyaluronan available in the United States that has cross-linked hyaluronan, which increases the average molecular weight but can cause hypersensitivity.[24]

Recent prospective randomized studies have shown statistically improved outcomes when hyaluronan was added to a postarthroscopy treatment regimen.[25] Hyaluronan also was used after anterior cruciate ligament (ACL) reconstruction and mosaicplasty.[26,27] There is some evidence that hylan G-F 20 can delay the need for total knee arthroplasty (TKA) by 2 to 7 years.[28] The adverse effects of hyaluronan include erythema and irritation, which were reported in as many as 8.5% of patients after a second hylan G-F 20 injection.[29]

Nutritional Supplements

Glucosamine and chondroitin sulfate are among the most extensively studied nutritional supplements. Glucosamine, a constituent of glycosaminoglycan, has been shown to stimulate the synthesis of proteoglycans.[30] Chondroitin sulfate is a glycosaminoglycan that contains a significant amount of aggrecan, the major structural component of cartilage. Both glucosamine and chondroitin sulfate have been implicated in the inhibition of inflammatory mediators and attenuation of matrix metalloproteinases and the other proteolytic enzymes.[31] Several clinical studies have examined the effects of glucosamine and chondroitin sulfate alone or in combination. A meta-analysis of glucosamine and chondroitin sulfate supplementation found some benefit to their use, although there were concerns with the study design.[32] The most recent Cochrane review of glucosamine supplementation found no overall improvement in pain or function after 2 to 3 months of use, although there is some variation between preparations, and preparation potency and variability differences have been cited.[33] A multicenter double-blind study compared glucosamine and chondroitin sulfate, used alone or together, with celecoxib and a placebo. After 24 weeks, combined glucosamine and chondroitin sulfate supplementation was found to provide symptomatic relief similar to that provided by the placebo and less than that of celecoxib.[34]

Other nutritional supplements being studied include *S*-adenosylmethionine, which enhances the synthesis of proteoglycan; collagen hydrolysate, which synthesizes collagen; diacerein, which decreases interleukin; oxaceprol, which decreases leukocyte adhesion; and avocado-soybean unsaponifiables, which decrease the inflammatory mediators of articular cartilage. Green tea polyphenols reduce the expression of inflammatory mediators. Catechin, an active component of green tea, inhibits the induction of nitric oxide synthase by interleukin-1β, ultimately reducing the production of nitric oxide, which is a free radical implicated in the pathophysiology of articular cartilage breakdown.[35]

Bracing

Early degenerative changes most commonly occur in the medial compartment of the knee. Medial unloader braces correct the varus alignment by shifting part of the weight-bearing surface to the unaffected lateral compartment. Studies found that pain improved in more than 75% of patients with bracing.[36,37] An 11% reduction in the load of the medial compartment was found to occur, as well as a 13% reduction of the varus moment.[38] A more recent study suggested that bracing decreases muscle cocontraction of the vastus medialis and medial hamstrings and thereby decreases medial joint forces.[39] The limitations of treating knee OA with bracing include patient noncompliance, brace durability, and cost.

Muscle Strengthening

Quadriceps weakness caused by unloading of the painful extremity is common among patients with knee OA. Quadriceps weakness may be present in patients with no knee pain who have radiographic OA changes and have greater lower extremity muscle mass than other individuals who are deconditioned and have an increased body mass index.[40] Quadriceps weakness may be a risk factor for the development of knee OA secondary to the decreased stability and shock-attenuating capacity of the weakened muscle groups.[41,42] Patients who participated in a muscle-strengthening program had decreased pain and disability.[43,44]

Other Treatments

Oral opioids are commonly used for treating OA pain. Topical treatments such as capsaicin (Zostrix; Hi-Tech Pharmacal, Amityville, NY), methylsalicylate, lidocaine (Lidoderm; Endo Pharmaceuticals, Chadds Ford, PA), and diclofenac (Flector; King Pharmaceuticals, Bristol, TN) have been promoted for the relief of pain. Capsaicin applied as a topical cream to the painful joint lowers the levels of substance P in the periarticular tissues within 2 to 3 days. In randomized double-blind studies, capsaicin was found to be more effective than a placebo in relieving pain.[45] Methylsalicylate is related to aspirin (acetylsalicylic acid), which has been shown to decrease the synthesis of proinflammatory prostaglandins. Lidocaine is a topical anesthetic that acts by blocking neurotransmission of local pain fibers. Topical diclofenac, a NSAID, was found to be effective in relieving OA knee pain as early as 1 hour after application.[46]

Prospective, double-blind studies found that acupuncture yields better results than a sham procedure.[47] Pulsed electrical stimulation increases chondrocyte proliferation; glycosaminoglycan and type II collagen synthesis in vitro enhances cartilage repair after OA-inducing trauma in animals and improves pain and function in humans with OA. Pulsed electrical stimulation delayed the need for TKA for as long as 4 years in more than 60% of patients with significant OA.[48-51]

Diacerein (Dycerin; Glenmark Pharmaceuticals, Mumbai, India) reduces interleukin-1β–induced metalloprotease-13 production in osteoarthritic subchondral bone.[52] A Cochrane review of randomized controlled studies of diacerein in patients with OA found a statistically significant decrease in pain compared with a placebo.[53] In a 3-year study of hip OA, the progression of joint space narrowing was less in patients treated with diacerein than in those treated with a placebo.[54] However, no similar decrease was found in a 1-year study of knee OA.[55]

Conclusions

The conservative treatment of knee OA comprises a wide range of pharmaceutical and other treatment modalities. Some treatments focus on the symptoms alone; others act by reducing the level of inflammatory mediators in the knee. There is ample evidence of efficacy but a paucity of validated, controlled comparison studies. The goal of a treatment regimen tailored to an individual patient may be to forestall surgical intervention or simply to manage the symptoms. Multiple modalities can be used together to achieve the desired effect.

Surgical Treatment of Small Focal Lesions

Several methods for surgically treating focal articular cartilage defects in the knee have been developed within the past decade, but there is no consensus on the best approach, and the treatment of these lesions continues to be challenging. Several of these surgical treatment methods are also discussed in chapter 18. The published studies vary in their definition of a clinically relevant lesion. Outerbridge used a diameter of 0.5 inch (1.3 cm) to distinguish between a grade II and a grade III lesion.[56] In subsequent studies, the threshold size ranged from 0.75 cm^2 to 3 cm^2. For treatment, a measurement of 2 cm^2 typically is used to differentiate a small lesion from a large lesion. An in vitro biomechanical study of the effect of defect size on cartilage rim stress found that the load distribution to the surrounding cartilage increased with a lesion diameter of approximately 10 mm, and that there was progressively more stress with a larger diameter lesion.[57] Although the concept of lesion size is important in the treatment algorithm, edge integrity, lesion depth, and location also have a role.

Fixation of OCD Lesions

OCD lesions are a unique subset of osteochondral defects. Unlike chronic degenerative lesions or lesions resulting from traumatic injury, OCD lesions are defined by a structure in which an intact unit of cartilage and subchondral bone detaches from its surrounding matrix. The process is not entirely understood. The patient's age and the interval before the pathophysiologic presentation of symptoms (the onset of pain, swelling, and catching or structural changes associated with detachment and resorption) are prognosticators of healing potential. It is important to distinguish between juvenile and adult OCD, although most adult lesions represent chronic juvenile OCD.[58]

Depending on the extent and viability of the associated bony tissue and subchondral bone base, fixation of unstable fragments often can preserve the native hyaline surface. The bony undersurface is thoroughly débrided to remove any apposed fibrous tissue, and an optimal compressive fixation is achieved through orthogonal application of hardware. Bone grafting may be needed to maintain the articular height. It remains unclear whether better results are obtained when resorbable or removable screws are used. The use of resorbable screws obviates the need for a second hardware removal procedure, but traditional hardware typically achieves better fixation.[59,60] Osteochondral plugs also have been used for the fixation of OCD lesions.[61,62]

Débridement

Surgical treatment traditionally has focused on limiting the progression of OA. In 1940, Haggert[63] described an open débridement of the knee that included synovectomy, shaving of fibrillated and degenerative cartilage, and total patellectomy; 19 of the 20 patients had subjective improvement at a mean 28-month follow-up (range, 19 months to 5 years). Magnuson[64] described similar results after open débridement. Arthroscopic techniques progressed during the 1970s, and several retrospective analyses reported successful results of débridement of more diffuse degenerative disease in the knee. Sprague[65] found that 52 of 62 patients (84%) who underwent arthroscopic débridement had a good or fair result at a mean 13.6-month follow-up (range, 6 to 19 months). In a prospective randomized study, Merchan and Galindo[66] found that 26 of 35 patients (75%) had improved at a mean 25-month follow-up (range, 12 to 36 months). However, more recent randomized

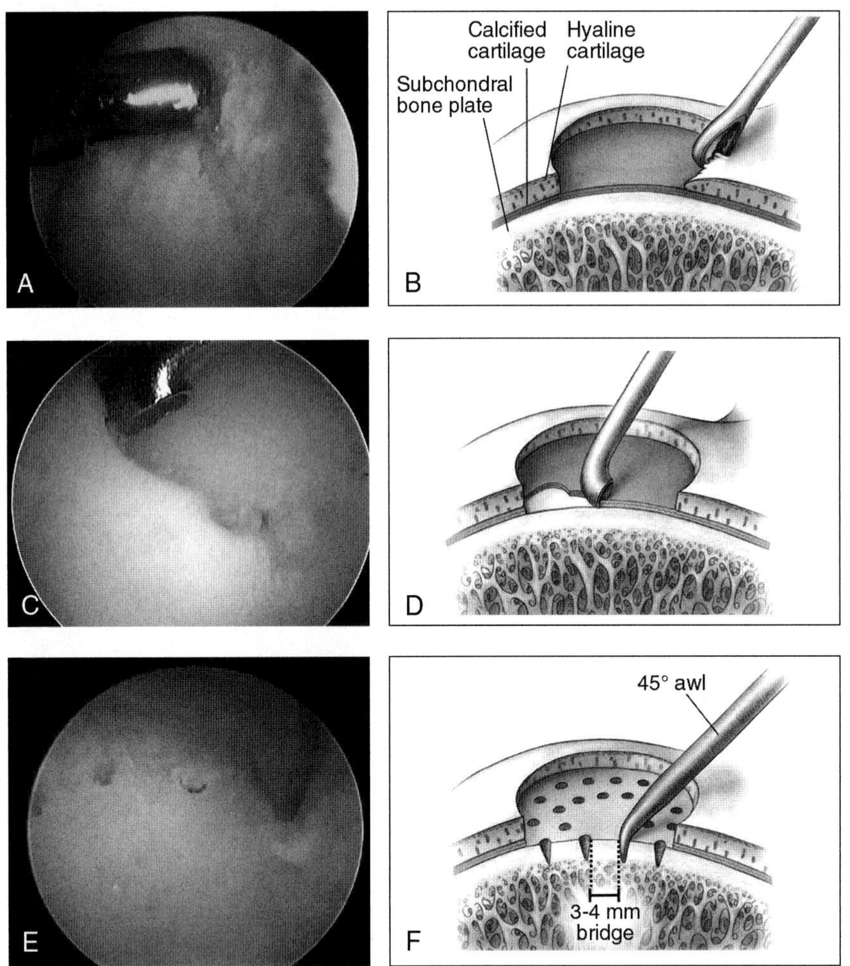

Figure 2 Intraoperative photographs (left) and schematic diagrams (right) showing microfracture technique. **A** and **B,** Preparation of the perpendicular edges. **C** and **D,** Débridement of the calcified cartilage base. **E** and **F,** Puncture of the subchondral bone with an awl. (Reproduced with permission from Mithoefer K, Williams RJ III, Warren RF, et al: Chondral resurfacing of articular cartilage defects in the knee with the microfracture technique: Surgical technique. *J Bone Joint Surg Am* 2006;88: S294 S304.)

controlled studies questioned the role of débridement in the management of OA. In a 2002 double-blind study, Moseley and associates[67] compared arthroscopic débridement and a sham surgical procedure in patients at a US Department of Veterans Affairs hospital, finding that arthroscopy had no clear benefit. Kirkley and associates[68] revisited this study in 2008 to include a more typical distribution of patients and seven experienced arthroscopic surgeons; the outcomes were assessed using validated subjective grading systems. Once again, the results suggested only a short-term benefit from arthroscopy, and this benefit was deemed a placebo effect. Patients with a suspected large meniscal tear or mechanical symptoms were excluded from these studies; the implication is that these patients would definitely benefit from surgery.

Several studies noted difficulty in predicting which patients can benefit from surgery. The best results were achieved in patients with early OA. The negative prognostic indicators included Outerbridge grade III or IV articular wear, gross malalignment (varus greater than 4° or valgus greater than 10°), obesity, tobacco use, and advanced age.[69,70] Most of the studies did not distinguish between chondral and meniscal pathology. It has not been determined whether removing articular cartilage fibrillation is beneficial; however, débriding flaps to prevent further delamination and débriding hypertrophic, severely inflamed synovium may be helpful.

Microfracture

Marrow Stimulation

Pridie[71] first documented the potential for chondral resurfacing, noting that patients who had undergone extensive débridement in the manner described by Magnuson[64] developed a layer of smooth fibrocartilage over areas of raw bone. Histologic analysis showed that the basis of this repair was subchondral bone. Drilling through sclerotic subchondral bone to expose the bony undersurface was found to reconstitute a fibrocartilaginous healing response. Abrasion arthroplasty was developed as a similar arthroscopic means of generating fibrocartilage repair. The superficial subchondral bone surface is arthroscopically abraded to uncover the vascular bone underneath.[72] However, the imprecise extent of the débridement and concern about thermal necrosis have limited the applicability of this technique.

Surgical Technique

Steadman and associates[73] described microfracture as an arthroscopic means of achieving the same effect as Pridie drilling (Figure 2). A sharp awl is used to perforate the subchondral bone, with the holes regularly spaced throughout the affected area to provide optimal coverage of the defect. The débridement establishes a discrete perimeter or shoulder with a perpendicular edge for the purpose of creating a contained defect and shielding it from contact forces. Débridement of the calcified cartilage layer also is critical for bonding between the repair tissue and the defect bed. The perforations of the subchondral bone are initiated at the rim and progress inward, with penetration 3 to 4 mm deep and spacing 3 to 4 mm apart. Adequate access to the subchondral marrow is ensured by turning off the arthroscopy pump while observing for bone bleeding; this technique is essential for the success of the procedure.

Postoperative Rehabilitation

A precise postoperative regimen has been described using continuous passive motion starting immediately, with only touch-down weight bearing allowed for 6 weeks after repair of a femoral condyle lesion.[74] After repair of a trochlear defect, weight bearing is allowed only in extension, with limited flexion loading and a flexion-limiting brace. In a case-control study of 43 patients, Marder and associates[75] compared the standard postoperative protocol (continuous passive motion with no weight bearing) to weight bearing as tolerated without continuous passive motion. Functional measures of activity revealed no difference between the two groups of patients at a mean 4.2-year follow-up (range, 2 to 9 years). However, no attempt was made to characterize the repair using imaging, repeat arthroscopy, or biopsy. A study of chondral defect healing after microfracture in a macaque model showed that healing continued during the period from 6 to 12 weeks after surgery; an extended period of protected weight bearing therefore may be beneficial.[76]

Results

Several studies found that marrow stimulation achieves good results. Steadman and associates[77] measured pain, activity level, and function after microfracture in 71 patients with no other concomitant knee pathology (associated ligament deficiency) requiring treatment. At a mean 11-year follow-up (range, 7 to 17 years), 80% of patients had subjective improvement. In a prospective study of 53 athletes, Gobbi and associates[78] found that approximately 60% had improved activity and function at a mean 72-month follow-up (range, 36 to 120 months). However, a study of high-demand athletes found that only 25% had regained full preinjury activity levels, although 66% reported a good or excellent result.[79] The prognostic indicators of good results include age younger than 35 to 40 years, good fill grade, low body mass, and short duration of preoperative symptoms.[80,81] The relative contraindications include a significant subchondral bone loss, poor joint alignment, and probable noncompliance with postoperative rehabilitation.

The nature of the repair tissue in microfracture has been an important concern. On second-look arthroscopy and MRI, a mixture of fibrous, fibrocartilaginous, and hyaline-like cartilage tissue was observed.[82] Differences between the stiffness, compressibility, and permeability of the repair tissue and the native hyaline cartilage suggest that repair tissue has inferior wear characteristics and function.[83] There is clinical evidence of the progressive deterioration of repair tissue after microfracture.[84]

Osteochondral Autograft Transplantation

OAT, mosaicplasty, chondral osseous replacement, and autogenous chondral transplantation all involve transferring viable full-thickness osteochondral units to extend from the articular cartilage to the subchondral bone, thereby directly restoring hyaline cartilage to areas of need. Osteochondral plugs typically are removed from the femoral trochlea at the intercondylar notch and along the superomedial and superolateral borders of the patellofemoral articulation, which are sites that have less contact pressure. Biomechanical mapping studies of cadaver knees found that contact pressures are lowest along the medial trochlea and the distal lateral trochlea,[85,86] but these areas have the thinnest articular cartilage. Topographic considerations also must be taken into account when transferring segments to the reverse saddle-shaped intercondylar notch or the convex medial and lateral condyles.[87] When reconstituting a larger defect, it is important to reapproximate the native contour of the articular surface, maintain smooth transitions across multiple plugs, and limit morbidity at the harvest site.

The results of the first procedures were poor, with graft subsidence and consequent fibrous overgrowth. However, the placement of grafts proud to the articular surface in sheep resulted in poor bony incorporation, and histologic findings were consistent with hypertrophic nonunion.[88] Biomechanical studies of grafts delivered proud, flush, or sunk found the lowest peak contact pressures when the plugs were placed flush to

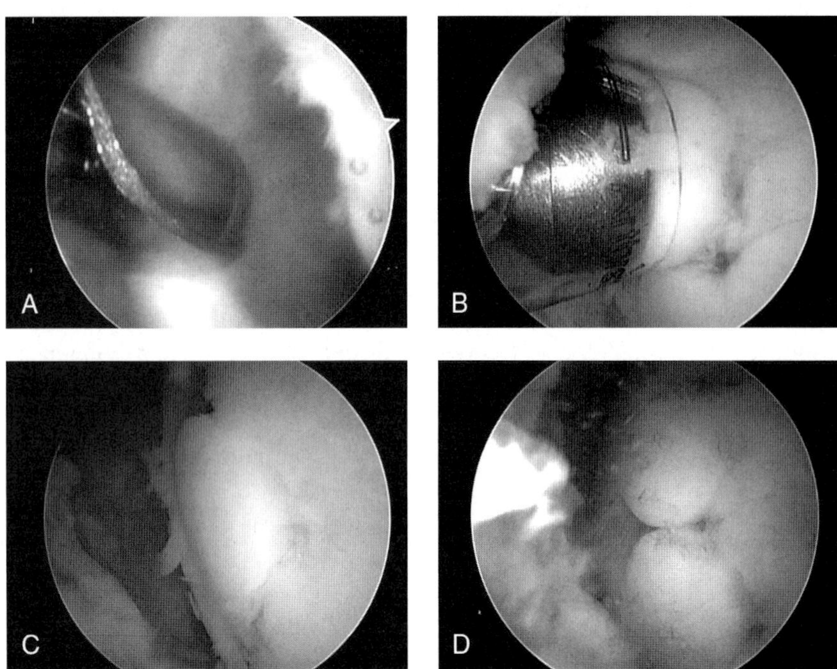

Figure 3 Intraoperative photographs showing arthroscopic OAT. **A,** Preparation of the defect bed. **B,** Placement of the osteochondral plugs into the prepared defect. The marking on the delivery device refers to the arthroscopic depth of insertion. **C,** Osteochondral plugs in the defect bed. **D,** Multiple osteochondral plugs filling the defect.

the intact cartilage surface; plugs placed sunk had lower pressures than those placed proud.[89] Similarly, cylindrical grafts placed into recipient sites cut at an angle had lower contact pressures when the donor-recipient mismatch resulted in a defect located below, rather than above, the articular surface.[90]

Surgical Technique

Depending on the size and location of the defect, OAT can be done arthroscopically, through a miniarthrotomy, or through an extended arthrotomy[91] (Figure 3). A template of the recipient lesion site is created, and the type of graft needed is assessed. The arrangement of plugs is determined, and graft harvesting is planned. It is preferable to remove the osteochondral plugs using a manual trephine, with care to harvest each plug at an angle perpendicular to the joint surface. The plugs can vary in diameter from 4.5 mm to more than 8 mm, but possible donor site morbidity should be taken into account. Holes are drilled into the lesion to correspond to the depth and diameter of each plug, again at a perpendicular angle. It is recommended that the implants be spaced 1 mm apart to allow better graft incorporation. Meticulous attention must be paid to restoring the normal articular surface contour. Minimal force should be used to seat the plugs because increased force is associated with decreased viability of surface chondrocytes.[92,93]

Postoperative Rehabilitation

A structured postoperative regimen is used, with early continuous passive motion and an emphasis on a full active or active-assisted range of motion during the first 3 weeks. The patient does not bear weight during this period.[94] Activity is advanced to short-arc quadriceps strengthening exercises and 50% weight bearing for the next 3 weeks. Full weight bearing is initiated at 6 weeks, with closed-chain and eccentric strengthening exercises. Open-chain exercises are permitted at 9 weeks, with sport-specific conditioning and a return to full sports participation at 12 weeks.

Results

Several studies found good clinical outcomes after OAT. In a case study of young, active patients (mean age, 29.5 years) with defects of 1.5 to 2.5 cm^2, Marcacci and associates[95] found that 77% had a good or excellent result at a 7-year follow-up, and 73% had returned to their earlier level of sports activity. Similarly, Chow and associates[96] reported that 25 of 30 patients (83%) with a defect between 1 and 2.5 cm^2 had a good or excellent outcome at a mean 45-month follow-up (range, 24 to 63 months). Of the 9 patients who underwent an elective second-look arthroscopy, 7 (78%) had complete healing; the other 2 patients had partial healing, with viable chondrocytes in all fully healed plugs. Postoperative MRI revealed congruency at the articular surface in 11 of 12 patients. In a prospective randomized study, Gudas and associates[97] compared OAT and microfracture in 60 athletes (mean age, 24.3 years) with an isolated 1- to 4-cm^2 defect in the weight-bearing surface of the medial or lateral femoral condyle. The patients were followed for a mean 37.1 months (range, 36 to 38 months), with MRI and clinical assessment at intervals. After OAT, 96% of the patients subjectively reported a good or excellent result, compared with 52% of patients after microfracture. Histologic analysis of tissue biopsies at 12 months identified hyaline cartilage in all patients in the OAT group. Of patients in the microfracture group, 57% had fibrocartilage repair; the remaining patients had a soft fibroelastic tissue different from the surrounding articular cartilage. MRI analysis revealed good plug incorporation in 84% of patients in the OAT group, with small cysts found in the remaining patients. The repair tissue thickness was similar to that of the adjacent tissue in 68% of the patients in the OAT group, compared with 18% of the patients in the microfracture group. Joint congruity was achieved in 96% of the patients in the OAT group, compared with 52% in the microfracture group. A return to preinjury levels of athletic activity was reported by 93% of the patients in the OAT group and 52% of those in the microfracture group. In second-look arthroscopies, all OAT donor sites were found to be covered with a firm fibrocartilage repair similar to that seen in microfracture.

The most important disadvantage of OAT is the potential for donor site morbidity. A study of osteochondral grafts taken from a previously asymptomatic distal femur to treat talar defects found significant donor site morbidity in 4 of 11 patients.[98] Similar OAT using distal femoral grafts to treat elbow defects resulted in transient knee pain in one of seven patients.[99] The suitability of a defect for OAT also is constrained by the size of the defect in relation to the availability of graft material and the potential pathophysiologic compromise of the patellofemoral joint.

Conclusions

The management of small articular cartilage defects (less than 2 cm^2) follows an algorithm that takes into account the size, location, and depth of the defect as well as patient factors such as age, body mass index, and functional expectations (Figure 4). Native hyaline cartilage should be preserved whenever possible, and therefore every attempt should be made to fix an OCD lesion. If fixation is unsuccessful, débridement can be used to manage a lesion smaller than 1 cm in diameter. Conservative débridement is favored, with resection of perceived pain generators only. In the absence of intrinsic cartilage or meniscal healing, the priority should be to retain as much native hyaline tissue as possible and thereby forestall the onset of OA. The stimulation of subchondral bone via microfracture is a reasonable first-line treatment of symptomatic articular cartilage defects. Microfracture is a relatively easy, completely arthroscopic procedure that requires minimal instrumentation, spares the bone and cartilage, and does not preclude any future procedures. The primary disadvantage of microfracture is that the repair material is fibrocartilage rather than hyaline cartilage. As with other restorative procedures, the patient may not tolerate the postoperative activity limitations.

Patient selection is the key to success in treating articular cartilage defects. The best candidate is a patient younger than 35 years who has a small, isolated lesion with good containment and who can be expected to comply with the postoperative rehabilitation protocol. An older patient with a larger degenerative lesion and signs of OA may have a less-than-optimal result. Low body mass index is associated with higher success rates.

OAT is an option for a patient who has a lesion that is unsuitable for microfracture (because of, for example, poor containment) or has had an unsuccessful microfracture. Although OAT is more invasive than microfracture and is limited by donor site availability and morbidity, it is associated with higher rates of full functional recovery. The technical limitations of OAT, as well as a paucity of research data, preclude the use of this technique for patellar or tibial lesions. Lower extremity axial alignment is essential for any reparative procedure.

Surgical Treatment of Large and Complex Lesions

The treatment of a large or complex lesion involving the articular cartilage is challenging and requires a carefully considered approach. A large or complex lesion generally is defined as a lesion having one or more of the following characteristics: size greater than 2 cm^2, subchondral bone involvement, multifocal or bipolar character, an unsuccessful earlier repair procedure, a patellofemoral or tibial location, an associated meniscal or ligamentous deficiency, or limb malalignment. The currently available techniques for treating a large or complex lesion include autologous chondrocyte implantation (ACI) and osteochondral allograft transplantation (OCA). Many patients have an abnormality of the joint or limb in addition to the articular cartilage lesion and may need concomitant ligament reconstruction, meniscus allografting, an osteotomy, or patellofemoral realignment. Stratification of patients into distinct categories can help define the appropriate treatment and predict the outcomes (Table 1).

The presence of OCD is one of the best indications for cartilage repair. Patients with OCD generally

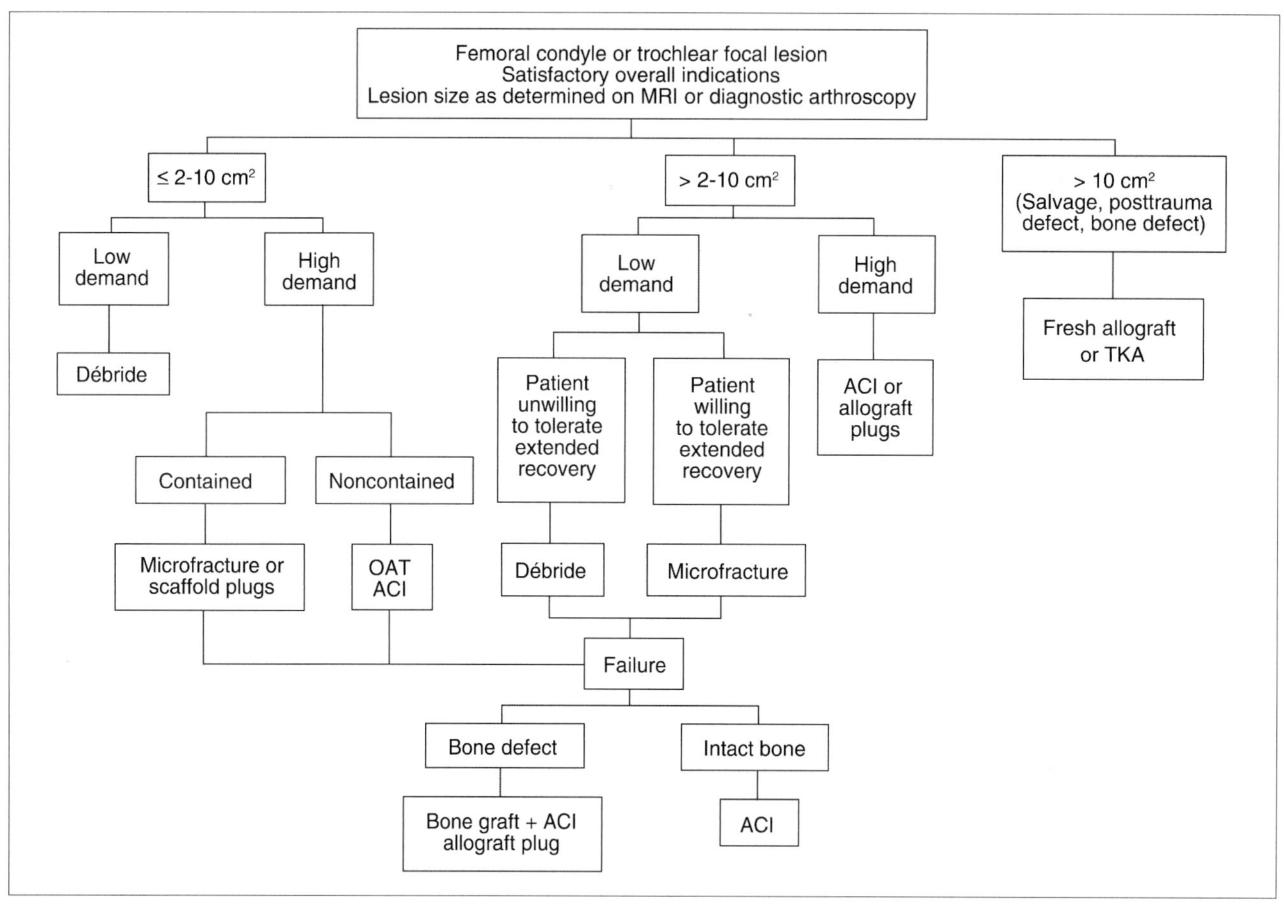

Figure 4 Clinical algorithm for the treatment of articular cartilage defects. Satisfactory overall indications = a knee that is symptomatic, unipolar, nonarthritic, and aligned, with no patholaxity and a meniscus that is two thirds intact in a patient who is younger than 55 years, has a body mass index below 30, does not have rheumatoid arthritis or cardiovascular disease, and will comply with the requirements of treatment. OAT = osteochondral autograft transplantation, ACI = autologous chondrocyte implantation. (Reproduced with permission from Sgaglione NA, Miniaci A, Gillogly SD, Carter TR: Update on advanced surgical techniques in the treatment of traumatic focal articular cartilage lesions in the knee. *Arthroscopy* 2002;18[2 suppl 1]:29. http://www.sciencedirect.com/science/journal/07498063.)

Table 1
Categorization of Complex Lesions

Size
> 2 cm²
Irregular shape
Location
Multiple foci
Tibial/patellar sites
Bipolar "kissing" lesions
Depth
Osteochondritis dissecans
Previous microfracture
Previous OAT
Load Characteristics
Joint malalignment
Ligamentous deficiency
Meniscal deficiency

are young (between ages 15 and 30 years); have a focal and often large lesion of the medial or lateral femoral condyle; and have no underlying pathology, with the occasional exception of malalignment. A type III or IV OCD fragment is not salvageable and is ideal for OCA, which is unique in restoring both the osseous and chondral deficit. ACI also is effective for an OCD lesion that is smaller or shallow (less than 8 mm deep).[100] Autologous bone grafting may be necessary for a very deep lesion. The treatment outcome in patients with OCD is excellent, with success rates of 80% to 90%.[101]

An articular cartilage defect can result from one of the two types of osteonecrosis. Spontaneous osteonecrosis of the knee generally is characterized by a focal osseous lesion or cyst, which in a patient age 35 to 60 years may be a prodrome of OA. True osteonecrosis is more diffuse and can be idiopathic or, in a younger patient, associated with corticosteroid treatment. Spontaneous osteonecrosis of the knee can be effectively treated with bone grafting of the cystic lesion, with or without ACI or OCA. Diffuse osteonecrosis is best treated with small- or large-fragment allografts, particularly in a young patient for whom it is desirable to avoid prosthetic arthroplasty. Osteochondral fracture or malunion may be a result of high-energy trauma such as a motor vehicle crash or a fall, but occasionally it occurs with patellar dislocation. Typically, there is joint incongruity resulting from malunion of a tibial plateau fracture or from a nonsalvageable fragment associated with a subacute or chronic osteochondral femoral injury. Anatomic bone restoration is the most critical component of treatment for these patients; OCA usually is the best option, and ACI is rarely indicated. Realignment osteotomies are commonly used, with meniscal transplantation if tibial plateau grafts are needed.

A degenerative chondral lesion usually occurs in a patient who is age 35 to 55 years, and it represents a chronic disease state resulting from trauma or surgery. Degenerative lesions and OA probably represent the same disease continuum, and the distinction between them is only in the extent and severity of disease. The knee is characterized by multiple lesions with meniscal and ligamentous compromise. Either ACI or OCA can be used. Multiple, technically challenging grafts may be necessary, and staged or combination realignment procedures are common. The results of treatment with either modality are fair to good, and patients must be willing to accept arthroplasty as a salvage option.

Autologous Chondrocyte Implantation

ACI is predicated on the potential for mesenchymal cells to differentiate into mature cartilage. Autologous chondrocytes are cultured in vitro and implanted into a cartilage defect. The procedure involves ex vivo cell manipulation and subsequent delivery of chondrocytes to the injury site, with coverage by a periosteal patch to contain the cells and provide them with growth factors. A so-called sandwich procedure, in which an underlying bone graft is covered by a second periosteal patch, can be used for a deeper osteochondral lesion. ACI requires two separate procedures: first, arthroscopy to harvest articular cartilage for chondrocyte expansion and culture; and second, arthrotomy to prepare the lesion, harvest and suture the periosteal patch, and inject the cells.

The ACI technique originally was developed in rabbits,[102] and its use in humans was first reported in 1994 by Brittberg and associates.[103] The complexity and morbidity of the staged procedure led to the development of second-generation ACI techniques that involve the culturing of cartilage-like tissue in a three-dimensional culture system.[104] Biodegradable polymers are used as temporary scaffolds for the in vitro growth of chondrocytes, which are directly transplanted into the defect site. Several synthetic and natural scaffolds have been developed to improve the relative proportion of chondrocytes compared with cells grown in a two-dimensional system.[105] These scaffolds obviate the need for periosteum harvest and suturing, thus allowing all-arthroscopic delivery to be considered. In matrix-associated ACI (MACI; Genzyme, Cambridge, MA), cells grown for 4 weeks in a culture medium are seeded onto a three-dimensional porcine collagen matrix for 3 days in a culture medium before being implanted. With Hyalograft C (Fidia Advanced Biopolymers; Abano Terme, Italy), cells are grown in a fibrous network composed of the benzylic ester of hyaluronic acid, and they are directly implanted into the defect. Neither product is available in the United States, pending approval by the US Food and Drug Administration.

Surgical Technique

ACI begins with an arthroscopic assessment of the joint and a systematic evaluation of all articular surfaces to document the presence and extent of cartilage lesions.[106,107] The quality and thickness of the surrounding cartilage is assessed to determine its role in periosteum suturing. It is critical to document a posterior extension of a lesion because of the technical difficulty of reaching it, even with arthrotomy. After a decision is made that the lesion is suitable for ACI, a biopsy site is selected for cartilage procurement. As with OAT donor sites, areas of decreased contact or load bearing are selected to minimize morbidity. Approximately 200 to 300 mg of cartilage are harvested; the yield is approximately 200,000 to 300,000 cells, which can be expanded to several million cells. Full-thickness cartilage should be harvested, with careful incision at the biopsy margins to prevent damage to other areas. Any factors creating a predisposition to chondral injury must be assessed so they can be corrected before or during the implantation procedure; corrective osteotomy or ligament repair-reconstruction may be required. The depth of the OCD lesion must be determined because a defect greater than 1 cm deep requires additional bone grafting before cartilage resurfacing.

The second ACI treatment stage involves arthrotomy, defect preparation, periosteum procurement, fixation, and chondrocyte implantation. To prepare the repair bed, all fissured and undermined articular cartilage at the lesions is débrided. An orthogonal incision with a blade down to subchondral bone can be used to define clear margins. The dimensions of the final prepared defect are used as a template for periosteum procurement. The proximal medial tibia is most commonly used as a periosteum harvest site. An elevator is used to gently remove the full-thickness patch. The periosteum is then fixed to the defect using a 6-0 suture in interrupted fashion, and watertight integrity is tested by injection with normal saline. Fibrin glue is used to augment the seal. The chondrocyte suspension is injected, and the injection portal is closed with sutures and fibrin sealant.

Postoperative Rehabilitation

The goals of the postoperative period are to prevent intra-articular adhesions by using aggressive range-of-motion exercises, protect the periosteum seal by limiting weight bearing, and maintain muscle tone by using isometric exercises. Continuous passive motion is initiated as early as 6 hours after surgery and is used 6 to 8 hours daily for 6 to 8 weeks. For femoral condyle lesions, full range of motion is allowed beginning 6 to 8 weeks after surgery; for trochlear lesions, maximal flexion is limited to 40° to minimize the patellofemoral forces. Only touch-down weight bearing is allowed after repair of a femoral condyle lesion during the first 6 weeks; full weight bearing begins at 12 weeks. After repair of a trochlear lesion, the patient is permitted full, immediate weight bearing while using a knee immobilizer locked in full extension.

Results

Several studies have reported on the clinical success of ACI. At a mean 39-month follow-up (range, 16 to 66 months), Brittberg and associates[103] in 1994 found that 14 of 16 patients with a femoral condylar transplant had a good or excellent result, but only 2 of 9 patients with a patellar transplant had a good or excellent result. Second-look arthroscopies at 3 months revealed a repair bed that was level with the surrounding tissue but had visible borders and was somewhat spongy; later probing revealed that the bed had become firmer. In a 2000 study of 101 patients, Petersen and associates[108] found that 92% of those with a single femoral condyle lesion and 89% of those with an OCD lesion had a good or excellent result at 2- to 9-year follow-up. The results were less favorable among patients with a patellar lesion or a concomitant ACL reconstruction; 62% or 75%, respectively, had a good or excellent result. A later report suggested that formation of a durable repair bed requires as long as 11 years.[109] Zaslav and associates[110] reported that 96 of 126 patients (76%) who were treated with ACI after an earlier unsuccessful articular cartilage treatment had a successful result at 48-month follow-up, as determined on the basis of knee pain, function, quality of life, and overall health.

The complications of ACI include cell leakage from the repair site, periosteal hypertrophy, dedifferentiation of chondrocytes into fibroblasts, and uneven distribution of cells. Although few studies have specifically examined mechanisms of failure, several case series have suggested that periosteal hypertrophy occurs in 2.4% to 20% of cases, delamination in 3.8%, and chondromalacia in 3.8% of ACIs, with combined reoperation rates ranging from 5.1% to 37%.[111,112]

Osteochondral Allograft Transplantation

OCA procedures are based on transplantation of intact osteochondral tissue with living chondrocytes and mature hyaline cartilage. OCA was first described in 1908 as a means of reconstituting articular defects.[113] In the first case study, Gross and associates[114] in 1975 reported on nine transplants in eight patients. Among the factors contributing to the success of OCA is the immunoprivileged character of hyaline cartilage, which receives its nutrition through diffusion from synovial fluid. In addition, the osseous component of the allograft allows for secure fixation to the host site. Osteochondral allografts are harvested within 24 hours of the donor's death. Implantation times vary from center to center. Cold storage in a liquid medium maintains the structural properties and durability of the allograft more optimally when compared to frozen tissue; chondrocyte viability and metabolic activity remain essentially unchanged for as long as 14 days.[115,116]

Surgical Technique

The OCA technique has been well described.[117,118] Allograft sizing is based on an AP radiograph. The acceptable margin is 2 mm, although there is substantial anatomic variability, particularly in condylar lesions. Most commonly, 15- to 30-mm dowels or plugs are used; shell or small-fragment grafts often are necessary for a lesion that is difficult to reach or exceptionally large. A standard midline arthrotomy incision is made from the center of the patella to the tip of the tibial tubercle and is elevated subcutaneously either medial or lateral to the patellar tendon, depending on the location of the lesion. Patellar eversion is not needed for most femoral lesions.

The press-fit plug (dowel) technique (Figure 5) and the shell graft technique are commonly used. The press-fit plug technique is best for contained condylar lesions 15 to 35 mm in diameter. Fixation is achieved by means of a press fit, and the considerations are similar to those for the OAT procedure. After determining the size of the cylinder to be transplanted, a guidewire is driven into the center of the lesion, perpendicular to the articular surface. A core reamer is used to remove the cylinder of affected bone and at least 3 to 4 mm of subchondral bone. Lesions that are deeper than 10 mm are packed with morcellized autologous bone graft, in lieu of an attempt to transplant a larger plug. A donor plug is harvested from the corresponding anatomic location on the graft, with care to match the articular contour and fit of the host site by marking the orientation of both the donor plug and recipient site. The plug is gently tamped into place and press fit until it is flush, while minimizing the mechanical insult to the native and graft tissue.

The shell graft technique is best used for a defect that is not entirely circular, such as a very posterior femoral, trochlear, or patellar lesion. After careful preparation of the repair bed, a graft of corresponding shape and size is hand crafted to fit into the defect margins. The fixation often is augmented by means of bioabsorbable pins or compression screws.

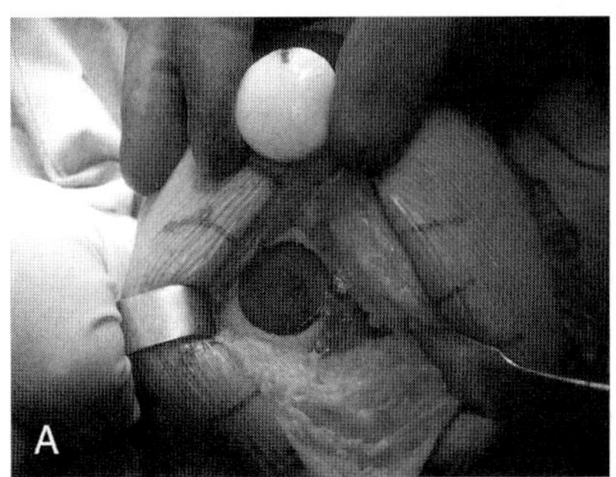

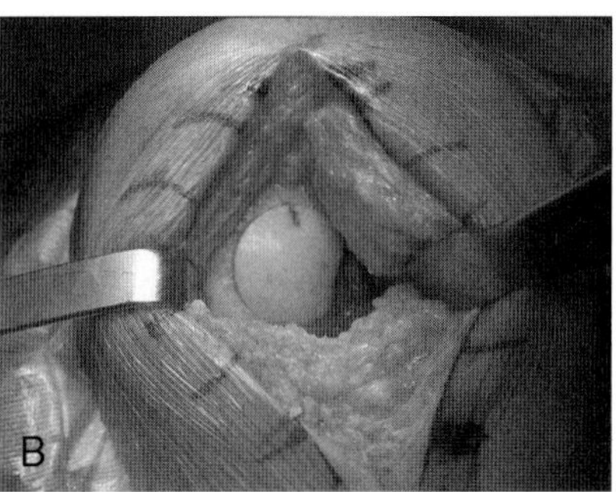

Figure 5 Clinical photographs showing implantation of a press-fit allograft plug. **A**, Preparation of the lesion site for implantation. **B,** The allograft in situ.

Postoperative Rehabilitation

The early postoperative rehabilitation includes continuous passive motion with full range of motion. Only touch-down weight bearing is permitted for at least the first 8 weeks and sometimes for as long as 12 weeks, depending on the transplant size, the type of fixation, and radiographic evidence of incorporation. Closed-chain exercises are permitted at 4 weeks, with progressive weight bearing at 3 months. Patients typically are advised to limit impact loading of the graft during the first year. After a complex concomitant reconstruction procedure or bipolar femoral and tibial graft placement, an unloader brace can be used to limit the stress applied to the grafted areas. Patients with a patellofemoral joint reconstruction are limited to approximately 45° of flexion during the first 4 to 6 weeks.

Results

Several studies reported good results after OCA. At a mean 7.5-year follow-up (range, 2 to 22 years, Ghazavi and associates[119] found that OCA had a subjectively successful outcome in 108 of 126 knees (86%) in 123 patients with a posttraumatic osteochondral defect. The transplant survivorship was 95% at 5 years, 71% at 10 years, and 66% at 20 years. Emmerson and associates[101] found that 47 of 65 knees (72%) in 63 patients with an OCD lesion treated using OCA had a subjectively rated good or excellent outcome at a mean 7.7-year follow-up (range, 2 to 22 years). The factors related to an unsuccessful outcome included age older than 50 years, a workers' compensation filing, a bipolar defect, and malalignment. Inflammatory conditions, diffuse arthrosis, and ligamentous instability also contributed to a relatively high failure rate.[120]

Conclusions

The treatment of a large or complex cartilage lesion requires a broader, more complex approach than the more common small focal lesion. The patient evaluation should include a comprehensive clinical assessment, with particular attention to the biomechanics of the limb and joint. The diagnostic category appears to be more useful in clinical decision making than the lesion size. ACI and OCA are typically done after an unsuccessful, less invasive salvage procedure such as OAT or microfracture. The indications include a lesion larger than 2 cm^2, bone involvement deeper than 1 cm, and bipolar disease (for OCA). The contraindications include limb malalignment, ligamentous instability, meniscal insufficiency, and advanced multicompartmental arthrosis. ACI, as an autologous repair, avoids issues of graft availability, possible disease transmission, or immunoreactivity. However, ACI requires a staged procedure and leads to the formation of a fibrocartilage mix rather than native cartilage. OCA involves direct reconstitution of a native hyaline cartilage bed, but the procedure is complicated by issues related to cost, graft procurement, disease transmission, and surgical arthrotomy.

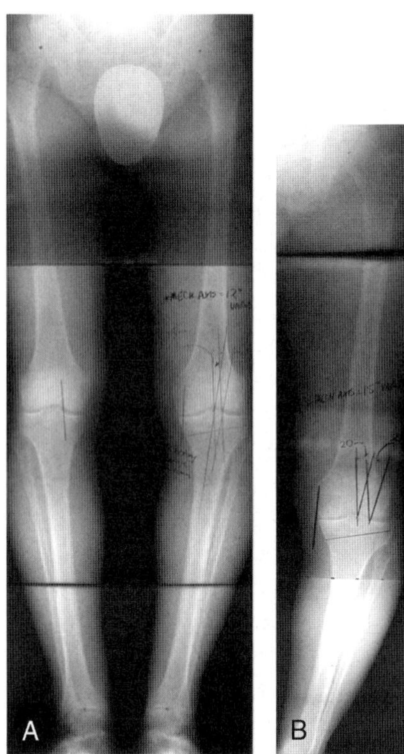

Figure 6 **A,** Double-leg standing AP radiograph. Lines drawn along the anatomic and mechanical axes of the left leg intersect at approximately 15°. **B,** Single-leg standing radiograph of the left leg of the same patient shows an increase in varus deformity. Anatomic and mechanical axes now intersect at approximately 20°. If the single-leg standing radiograph is used to determine the required correction rather than the double-leg standing radiograph, an overcorrection of the deformity may result.

Osteotomy for Correcting Malalignment

High tibial and distal femoral osteotomies are widely accepted treatments for relatively young, active patients with symptomatic medial or lateral compartment gonarthrosis associated with varus or valgus deformity. Knee alignment is a significant factor in arthritis progression.[121] Indications for realignment osteotomy include compartmental overload, as seen in unicompartmental OA or with prearthritic cartilage lesions. In addition, osteotomy can be used to improve the functional stability of the knee by reducing a lateral or hyperextension thrust resulting from posterolateral instability.[122] Osteotomies also are commonly used to realign the limb in association with articular resurfacing or meniscal transplantation.[123-126] The medial compartment typically is involved in primary OA, in association with a varus deformity; it also is involved in secondary OA resulting from OCD lesions, a meniscectomy, or a chronic ACL injury. Lateral compartment involvement is less common and usually is associated with a valgus deformity. The lateral compartment is dependent on meniscal integrity, and removal of the lateral meniscus can lead to lateral compartment overload and secondary OA.

Surgical Technique

Long standing radiographs of the leg are essential for determining the mechanical axis, which generally is found within the compartment exhibiting signs of overload. Single-leg standing radiographs may provide a dynamic evaluation of a thrust but overestimate the amount of correction needed. Lateral radiographs are important for assessing tibial slope, which may affect cruciate stability. Increasing the slope improves posterior cruciate ligament stability at the cost of ACL stability. Templating the desired mechanical axis through the center of the knee allows the angle of correction to be determined (Figure 6).

An osteotomy can be performed as an opening wedge or a closing wedge. Opening wedge osteotomies require only a single cut and therefore are easier to perform. Closing wedge osteotomies involve removal of a wedge of bone and therefore require greater precision. The correction can be done acutely or with gradual distraction. Usually the deformity is mild and can be easily treated with acute correction. Gradual distraction is reserved for more complex deformities and entails bone healing during the distraction process. An osteotomy can be done at the distal femur or the proximal tibia. Varus deformity often is caused by a proximal tibia vara and is best treated using high tibial osteotomy; valgus deformity of the knee generally is caused by a distal femoral deformity, and distal femoral osteotomy therefore is indicated.

For a medial opening wedge osteotomy, a medial incision is made midway between the anterior and posteromedial borders of the tibia. The incision is carried down to bone, a subperiosteal elevation is done to elevate the medial collateral ligament and, if necessary, the pes anserinus insertion. Under fluoroscopic guidance, a guidewire is inserted, and the cortex is cut in line with the guidewire, using a microsizeable saw (Figure 7). AO osteotomes are used to carry out the osteotomy, and larger osteotomes are inserted to create the opening wedge. It is important to leave a lateral hinge. The wedge is opened the desired amount. Fixation is done with an opening wedge plate (available in different patterns). Fixation and completion of the osteotomy are done under fluoroscopic guidance. Bone graft is used to fill the opening wedge defect. If the slope needs to be increased because of a posterior cruciate ligament deficiency, the plate can be placed slightly more anterior; doing so causes some increase in the anterior opening of the osteotomy. If the slope is not being changed, the plate must be placed posteriorly to close the wedge anteriorly. If the plate is very posterior and the slope needs to be decreased to correct an ACL deficiency, some anterior fixation may be necessary to make sure the slope is closed anteriorly.

A valgus closing wedge osteotomy is done with an anterolateral incision, as described by Coventry.[127] The incision is made longitudinally along the anterolateral aspect of the knee, just anterior to the fibular head. Dissection down to the fibular head is done, with subperiosteal dissection of a sleeve including the lateral collateral ligament and biceps femoris attachments. The fibula is transected at the level of the fibular neck, and the head and neck are excised. Posterior and anterior exposure of the proximal tibia is done by subperiosteal elevation, thus allowing visualization from the level of the articular cartilage to a few centimeters distally. The proximal osteotomy is done 2 cm distal to the joint line and parallel to the articular surface, and it is followed by an oblique osteotomy to create a closing wedge. Fixation is achieved by placing a staple across the osteotomy site. Billings and associates[128] described a similar technique that spares the fibular head by dividing the proximal tibiofibular joint capsule with proximal migration of the fibula. Osteotomies are done using a cutting guide and a sagittal saw, with fixation using an L-shaped plate.

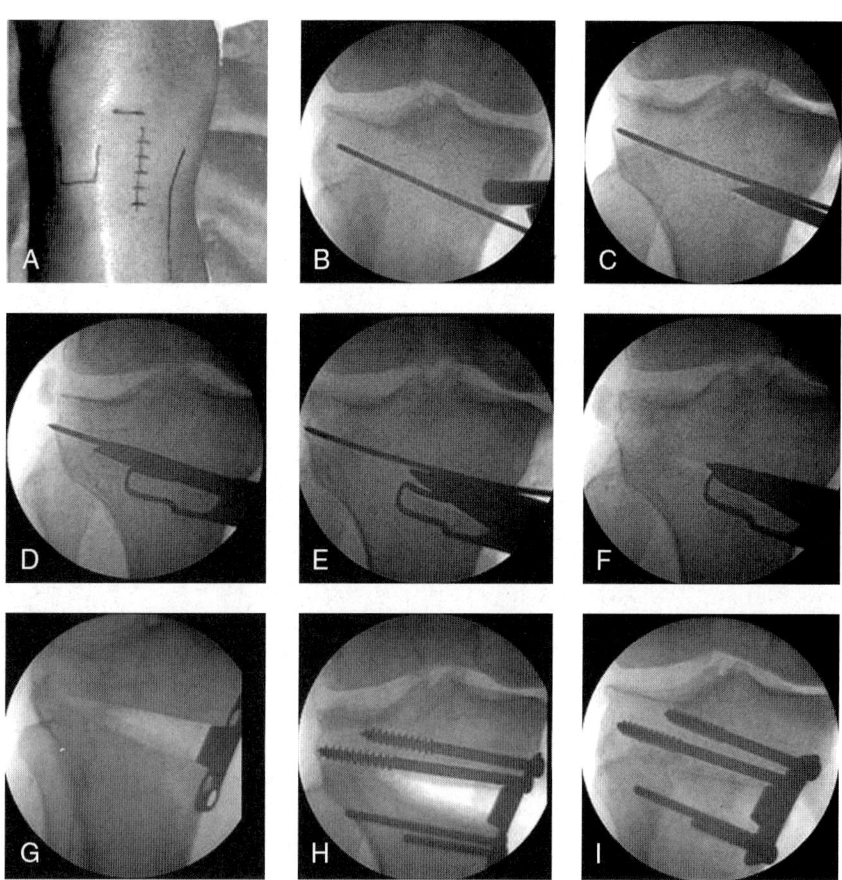

Figure 7 A medial opening wedge high tibial osteotomy. **A,** Intraoperative photograph showing skin markings: tibial tubercle, joint line and posterior margin of the tibia are marked, as well as the skin incision. **B,** Intraoperative fluoroscopic image showing a Kirschner wire inserted along the plane of the planned osteotomy. **C,** An osteotome is directed in line with the Kirschner wire. **D** and **E,** Expansion along the osteotome cut creates an opening wedge. **F,** The Kirschner wire is removed after the opening wedge has been completed. **G,** Placement of a spacer for fixation after the opening wedge. Final AP **(H)** and oblique **(I)** fluoroscopic images showing the completed medial opening wedge high tibial osteotomy. Note the maintenance of joint spaces throughout the correction of the mechanical axis.

A distal femoral opening wedge osteotomy involves a lateral approach to the distal femur, as described by Puddu and associates.[129] A longitudinal incision is made over the iliotibial band approximately 2 finger breadths distal to the lateral epicondyle and is extended proximally. The dissection is carried down to the vastus lateralis, which is retracted forward from the posterolateral intermuscular septum. Flexion of the knee allows exposure of the lateral cortex of the distal femur. An oblique osteotomy is done at approximately 20° to the joint surface, with care to leave a medial hinge. The osteotomy is wedged open, a tricorticocancellous graft is placed, and fixation is achieved using a lateral plate (Figure 8).

A medial closing wedge osteotomy can be used to achieve similar

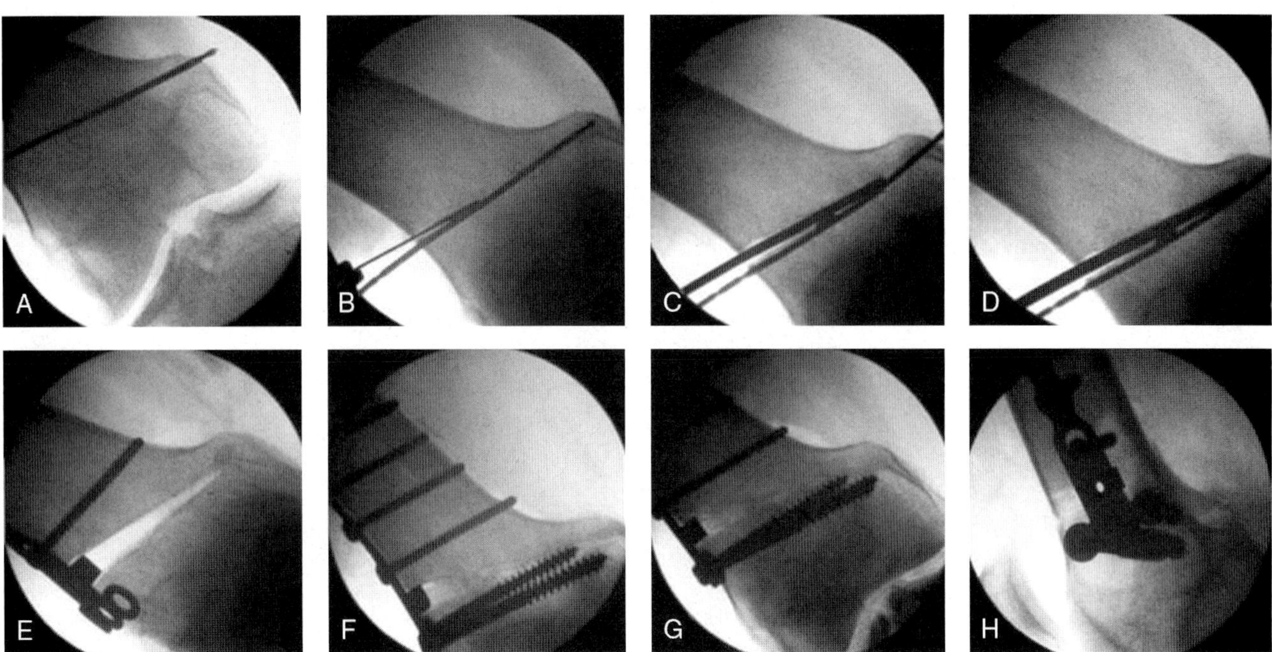

Figure 8 Intraoperative fluoroscopic images of a lateral opening wedge distal femoral osteotomy. **A,** A Kirschner wire is inserted along the plane of a planned osteotomy. **B** through **D,** The osteotome is directed in line with the Kirschner wire. **E,** Expansion along the osteotome cut to create the opening wedge and placement of the spacer for fixation after the opening wedge. Final radiographs show the completed lateral opening wedge distal femoral osteotomy: AP **(F)**, oblique **(G)**, and lateral **(H)**.

results.[130,131] A longitudinal incision is made medially and carried down to the vastus medialis, which is retracted anteriorly to expose the shaft of the femur. Care is taken to leave a small cuff of tissue with the medial intermuscular septum to protect the neurovascular bundle. Similar subperiosteal dissection is used to expose the posterior cortex of the femur. Guide pins are inserted proximally and distally in the templated direction of the osteotomies. Parallel cuts in the coronal plane ensure that the flexion-extension of the distal femur is not changed. Following excision of the wedge of bone and varus closure, fixation typically is achieved using a blade plate.

Postoperative Rehabilitation

It is important to allow a tibial or femoral osteotomy to heal before weight bearing is initiated. In the first week, the patient's knee is placed in a hinged brace with progressive continuous passive motion to 90°. Radiographs are taken at 6 weeks; if there is evidence of osteotomy healing, the patient is advanced to 50% weight bearing. The gradual progression to full weight bearing at 12 weeks is accompanied by physical therapy and quadriceps strengthening exercises. Interval radiographs are used to confirm healing of the osteotomy.

Results

The use of realignment osteotomy rather than other procedures for treating a young patient with early OA is controversial. The survivorship of an osteotomy is less predictable than that of unicompartmental or total knee replacement for these patients. Limb malalignment, instability, component fixation, or extensor mechanism maltracking can present a challenge if an osteotomy must be revised to TKA.[132-134] Nonetheless, osteotomy can be successful for a properly selected patient. Good results have been reported after high tibial osteotomy in several patient groups.[135] Holden and associates[136] found good or excellent results in 36 of 51 knees (70%) in 45 patients at a mean 10-year follow-up (range, 5 to 13 years). Similarly, Marti and associates[137] found that 30 of 34 patients (88%) had good or excellent results at a mean 11-year follow-up (range, 5 to 21 years). The complications included transient peroneal nerve palsy, thrombophlebitis, and wound infection. Earlier studies reported higher rates of failure and conversion to TKA;[138,139] however, these studies included patients with more significant deformity or OA progression.

Similar successes have been reported after distal femoral osteotomy. Aglietti and Menchetti[140] found that 14 of 18 patients (77%) had a good or excellent result at a mean 9-year follow-up (range, 5 to 16 years). McDermott and associates[131] reported subjective improvement in 22 of 24 knees (92%) at a mean 4-year follow-up. Healy and associates[130] reported a good or excellent result in 19 of 23 knees (83%) in 21 patients at a mean 4-year follow-up (range, 2 to 9 years). Miniaci and associates[141] reported a good or excellent result in 34 of 40 patients (86%) at a mean 5.5-year follow-up. The complications included subluxation at the osteotomy site (caused by inadequate retention of a hinge) and malunion.

Conclusions

Correcting mechanical alignment is essential in the biologic treatment of osteochondral lesions and early OA in a young, active patient; in any resurfacing procedure that involves articular cartilage; or in meniscal transplantation that involves mechanical axis deviation and overload of that involved compartment. Osteotomy of the proximal tibia or the distal femur is effective in correcting mechanical alignment and slowing the progression of OA. Preoperative planning is essential to determine the mechanical axis and plan the osteotomy sites and angles. The severity of the preexisting malalignment or OA is correlated with the likelihood of osteotomy failure, and the increased difficulty of revision to TKA should be considered before realignment is attempted in such patients. Nonetheless, osteotomy is a useful means of balancing or redistributing contact forces across the tibiofemoral articulation.

Unicompartmental Knee Arthroplasty

OA of the knee is restricted to one compartment in approximately 25% of patients. In another 10% of patients, OA of the knee is characterized as isolated patellofemoral arthritis, and in 5% the OA primarily is in the lateral compartment.[142] Unicompartmental knee arthroplasty (UKA) may be indicated to treat unicompartmental OA of the knee if nonsurgical treatment and arthroscopic and realignment procedures have been unsuccessful. Metallic spacers were used for knee hemiarthroplasty beginning in the mid 1950s,[143,144] and newer metallic interposition arthroplasty devices were introduced between 2000 and 2005. A properly done UKA preserves bone stock and thus greatly simplifies a revision procedure.[145] UKA allows for a more physiologic range of motion than TKA.[146] There is minimal blood loss during the procedure. The patient's hospital stay is shorter than with TKA, and UKA is less expensive than TKA.[147]

Patient selection is the most important factor leading to a successful UKA. The patient should have less than 10° of varus deformity, a range of motion of at least 90° without flexion contracture, intact cruciate and lateral collateral ligaments with only medial instability, OA or posttraumatic arthritis, and pain restricted to one compartment.[147,148] In addition, the patient should have an acceptable body mass index and not be employed in manual labor. The one-finger test confirms that the patient is suitable for a UKA. In a positive test, the patient indicates the location of the pain by pointing to the involved compartment with one finger; if the patient clasps the entire knee to indicate the location of the pain, TKA probably is required.

Improvements in the reported survivorship of UKAs suggest that UKA may be a satisfactory means of reducing pain and improving function in patients age 55 to 65 years, especially if TKA is precluded because of comorbidity. UKA also can be used to treat a younger patient (age 35 to 50 years) with unicompartmental OA to avoid a realignment osteotomy. Although reports of UKA in the early 1970s had a high revision rate (approximately 10% at 2-year follow-up), subsequent survivorship rates increase from 37% to 92% at 2- to 8-year follow-ups in the late 1970s, to 87% to 98% survival at 6- to 14-year follow-ups in the late 1990s.[147] This compares favorably to survival rates for TKA, cited as 97% at 10 years and 90% at 18 years.[149,150]

The design of the UKA prosthesis is important. Some designs that attempted to increase knee stability led to premature mechanical failure, and designs with high contact stresses have failed because of polyethylene wear.[148] The surgical approach is chosen based on the instrumentation; a medial, lateral parapatellar, or midvastus approach can be used. The exposure is similar to that used in TKA, except that minimally invasive instrumentation systems require far less dissection.

Surgical Technique

Several surgical technique suggestions can be helpful in obtaining a well-positioned, long-lasting UKA with minimal tibial and femoral bone removal (Figure 9). With a mini-incision technique, it is helpful to use a Steinmann pin in the intercondylar notch to retract the patella. Removing only the essential

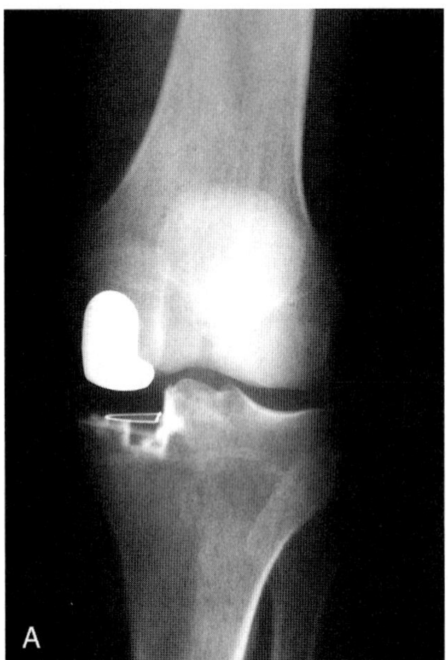

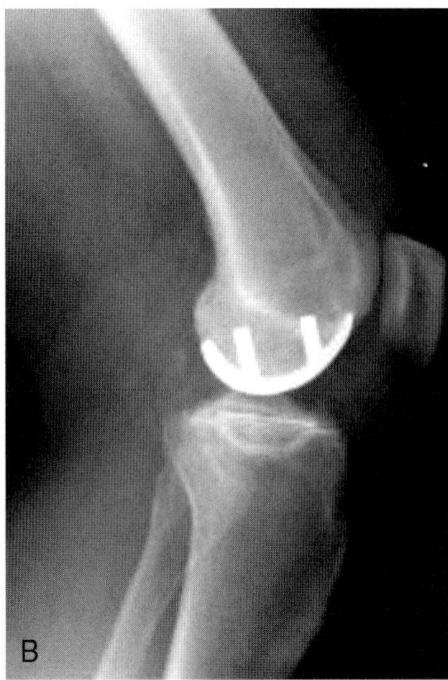

Figure 9 AP **(A)** and lateral **(B)** radiographs showing a well-aligned UKA with joint space maintenance and minimal tibial bone removal.

amount of tibial bone during tibial resection is critical for preventing a tibial plateau fracture during implantation and avoiding a difficult later TKA revision. The tibial component should be wide enough to cover the entire resected tibial surface, including the cortical rim if possible, and it should extend laterally to the ACL insertion. In general, the vertical cut for the tibia should not be rotated internally or externally. However, the vertical cut should be slightly internally rotated in a lateral compartment UKA because the tibia externally rotates during extension. Lateralizing the femoral component during a medial UKA helps avoid a medial-lateral mismatch caused by rotation during extension.[151] Overstuffing the medial compartment with a thick tibial component results in valgus alignment and premature wear of the lateral compartment. The use of multiple drill holes, pulse lavage, and drying of the surfaces before final cementing maximizes the cement fixation.[152] Care must be taken to avoid placing more cement than necessary on the posterior aspect of the tibial prosthesis; the use of too much cement can create a snowplow effect, leading to posterior cement retention that can fracture and create an intra-articular loose body.[153] Femoral tibial tracking throughout the full range of motion should be confirmed before closure.[154]

Postoperative Rehabilitation

The postoperative rehabilitation protocol used after UKA is similar to the TKA protocol. Full weight bearing is permitted immediately, and continuous passive motion is initiated soon after surgery to promote full range of motion. Gait and strength training are advanced as tolerated, with light sports activity as soon as 1 month after surgery.

Results

UKAs came into use in the 1970s. Success rates increased over subsequent years, with more recent success rates reported at 80% to 98% at 6- to 25-year follow-up.[155-166] In the United States, the use of UKA rather than TKA has quadrupled during the past 5 years because of improved instrumentation, components, and limited-incision techniques.[145] The improper choice of patients (especially of patients with a high body mass index), component failure, the development of OA in the contralateral compartment, poor surgical technique, and inappropriate postoperative alignment are most commonly responsible for the failure of a UKA.[167] Microscopic OA may be present even in the pristine articular surface of the lateral compartment, and it can lead to progression of lateral compartment OA despite appropriate surgical technique and postoperative alignment.[168]

Conclusions

UKA is an excellent procedure for carefully selected patients after unsuccessful nonsurgical treatment and arthroscopic articular surface procedures. However, a satisfactory clinical result requires strict adherence to the established indications and surgical technique. The continuing evolution of UKA implant designs promises to resolve concerns about implant wear and longevity. The use of a minimally invasive approach and a suitable implant design, as well as retention of bone stock, should limit the likelihood of a future revision. Computer-assisted navigation systems may be useful in aligning a prosthesis with minimal exposure.

Summary

The management of knee cartilage pathology encompasses a wide range of modalities. Pharmacologic and physiologic treatment strategies can be used, and improved dynamic stabilization through muscle strengthening and replacement of joint fluid constituents can forestall the progression of OA. It is important to limit the inflammatory response that leads to articular cartilage damage. Recent biosurgical developments have challenged the belief that articular cartilage damage is irreversible. The resurfacing of cartilage defects using marrow stimulation has had success, although the repair tissue poorly approximates the native hyaline cartilage. Nonetheless, meticulous surgical technique can lead to a successful clinical outcome in a properly selected patient.

The evolution of ex vivo manipulation of chondrocyte progenitors and improved delivery systems should lead to better repairs in the future. Currently, the articular surface can be reconstituted by transplanting viable segments of osteochondral tissue. Articular cartilage pathology caused by poor mechanical alignment can be treated by using osteotomy. Overload of a single compartment typically appears as early OA, and redistributing these contact forces can forestall the progression of OA without directly affecting the articular surface; this technique also is useful in conjunction with resurfacing or transplantation strategies.

UKA requires minimal exposure or bone resection and has improved the survival rates of implants. Patients retain more physiologic function and have far less morbidity after UKA than TKA. In a properly selected patient, it is reasonable to expect the implant to survive more than 10 years.

The armamentarium of treatments now available for knee cartilage pathology allows a patient-specific strategy to be chosen, particularly for a younger patient in whom TKA may not survive long-term use. A detailed conversation about the patient's goals and realistic expectations of each treatment can be useful in tailoring the treatment strategy to the patient. Each strategy can be seen as part of a sequential progression leading toward TKA, with the goal of maximizing function through the practical management of symptoms.

References

1. Lawrence RC, Felson DT, Helmick CG, et al: Estimates of the prevalence of arthritis and other rheumatic conditions in the United States: Part II. *Arthritis Rheum* 2008;58:26-35.
2. Yelin E, Cisternas MG, Pasta DJ, Trupin L, Murphy L, Helmick CG: Medical care expenditures and earnings losses of persons with arthritis and other rheumatic conditions in the United States in 1997: Total and incremental estimates. *Arthritis Rheum* 2004;50:2317-2326.
3. Murphy L, Schwartz TA, Helmick CG, et al: Lifetime risk of symptomatic knee osteoarthritis. *Arthritis Rheum* 2008;59:1207-1213.
4. Curl WW, Krome J, Gordon ES, Rushing J, Smith BP, Poehling GG: Cartilage injuries: A review of 31,516 knee arthroscopies. *Arthroscopy* 1997;13:456-460.
5. Hjelle K, Solheim E, Strand T, Muri R, Brittberg M: Articular cartilage defects in 1,000 knee arthroscopies. *Arthroscopy* 2002;18:730-734.
6. Potter HG, Foo LF: Magnetic resonance imaging of articular cartilage: Trauma, degeneration, and repair. *Am J Sports Med* 2006;34:661-677.
7. Poole A: Imbalances of anabolism and catabolism of cartilage matrix components in osteoarthritis, in Kuettner K, Goldger V, eds: *Osteoarthritic Disorders.* Rosemont, IL, American Academy of Orthopedic Surgeons, 1995, pp 247-260.
8. Bloom BS: Direct medical costs of disease and gastrointestinal side effects during treatment for arthritis. *Am J Med* 1988;84:20-24.
9. Dahners LE, Mullis BH: Effects of nonsteroidal anti-inflammatory drugs on bone formation and soft-tissue healing. *J Am Acad Orthop Surg* 2004; 12:139-143.
10. Goodman SB, Jiranek W, Petrow E, Yasko AW: The effects of medications on bone. *J Am Acad Orthop Surg* 2007; 15:450-460.
11. Mason L, Moore RA, Edwards JE, Derry S, McQuay HJ: Topical NSAIDs for chronic musculoskeletal pain: Systematic review and meta-analysis. *BMC Musculoskelet Disord* 2004;5:28.
12. Lane JM: Anti-inflammatory medications: Selective COX-2 inhibitors. *J Am Acad Orthop Surg* 2002;10:75-78.
13. Silverstein FE, Faich G, Goldstein JL, et al: Gastrointestinal toxicity with celecoxib vs nonsteroidal anti-inflammatory drugs for osteoarthritis and rheumatoid arthritis: The CLASS study. A randomized controlled trial: Celecoxib Long-term Arthritis Safety Study. *JAMA* 2000;284:1247-1255.
14. Rostom A, Muir K, Dubé C, et al: Gastrointestinal safety of cyclooxygenase-2 inhibitors: A Cochrane Collaboration systematic review. *Clin Gastroenterol Hepatol* 2007;5: 818-828.
15. Leese PT, Recker DP, Kent JD: The COX-2 selective inhibitor, valdecoxib, does not impair platelet function in the elderly: Results of a randomized controlled trial. *J Clin Pharmacol* 2003;43:504-513.
16. Forwood MR: Inducible cyclo-oxygenase (COX-2) mediates the induction of bone formation by mechanical loading in vivo. *J Bone Miner Res* 1996;11:1688-1693.
17. Cole BJ, Schumacher HR Jr: Injectable corticosteroids in modern practice. *J Am Acad Orthop Surg* 2005;13: 37-46.
18. Mankin HJ, Conger KA: The acute effects of intra-articular hydrocorti-

sone on articular cartilage in rabbits. *J Bone Joint Surg Am* 1966;48:1383-1388.

19. Ishikawa K, Ohira T, Sakata H: Effects of intraarticular injection of halopredone diacetate on the articular cartilage of rabbit knees: A comparison with methylprednisolone acetate. *Toxicol Appl Pharmacol* 1984;75:423-436.
20. Seshadri V, Coyle CH, Chu CR: Lidocaine potentiates the chondrotoxicity of methylprednisolone. *Arthroscopy* 2009;25:337-347.
21. Raynauld JP, Buckland-Wright C, Ward R, et al: Safety and efficacy of long-term intraarticular steroid injections in osteoarthritis of the knee: A randomized, double-blind, placebo-controlled trial. *Arthritis Rheum* 2003;48:370-377.
22. Bagga H, Burkhardt D, Sambrook P, March L: Longterm effects of intraarticular hyaluronan on synovial fluid in osteoarthritis of the knee. *J Rheumatol* 2006;33:946-950.
23. Wang CT, Lin J, Chang CJ, Lin YT, Hou SM: Therapeutic effects of hyaluronic acid on osteoarthritis of the knee: A meta-analysis of randomized controlled trials. *J Bone Joint Surg Am* 2004;86:538-545.
24. Waddell DD, Bricker DC: Hylan G-F 20 tolerability with repeat treatment in a large orthopedic practice: A retrospective review. *J Surg Orthop Adv* 2006;15:53-59.
25. Hempfling H: Intra-articular hyaluronic acid after knee arthroscopy: A two-year study. *Knee Surg Sports Traumatol Arthrosc* 2007;15:537-546.
26. Huang MH, Yang RC, Chou PH: Preliminary effects of hyaluronic acid on early rehabilitation of patients with isolated anterior cruciate ligament reconstruction. *Clin J Sport Med* 2007;17:242-250.
27. Tytherleigh-Strong G, Hurtig M, Miniaci A: Intra-articular hyaluronan following autogenous osteochondral grafting of the knee. *Arthroscopy* 2005;21:999-1005.
28. Waddell DD, Bricker DC: Total knee replacement delayed with hylan G-F 20 use in patients with grade IV osteoarthritis. *J Manag Care Pharm* 2007;13:113-121.
29. Goomer RS, Leslie K, Maris T, Amiel D: Native hyaluronan produces less hypersensitivity than cross-linked hyaluronan. *Clin Orthop Relat Res* 2005;434:239-245.
30. Frech TM, Clegg DO: The utility of nutraceuticals in the treatment of osteoarthritis. *Curr Rheumatol Rep* 2007;9:25-30.
31. Chan PS, Caron JP, Orth MW: Short-term gene expression changes in cartilage explants stimulated with interleukin beta plus glucosamine and chondroitin sulfate. *J Rheumatol* 2006;33:1329-1340.
32. McAlindon TE, LaValley MP, Gulin JP, Felson DT: Glucosamine and chondroitin for treatment of osteoarthritis: A systematic quality assessment and meta-analysis. *JAMA* 2000;283:1469-1475.
33. Towheed TE, Maxwell L, Anastassiades TP, et al: Glucosamine therapy for treating osteoarthritis. *Cochrane Database Syst Rev* 2005;2:CD002946.
34. Clegg DO, Reda DJ, Harris CL, et al: Glucosamine, chondroitin sulfate, and the two in combination for painful knee osteoarthritis. *N Engl J Med* 2006;354:795-808.
35. Goggs R, Vaughan-Thomas A, Clegg PD, et al: Nutraceutical therapies for degenerative joint diseases: A critical review. *Crit Rev Food Sci Nutr* 2005;45:145-164.
36. Dennis DA, Komistek RD, Nadaud MC, Mahfouz M: Evaluation of off-loading braces for treatment of unicompartmental knee arthrosis. *J Arthroplasty* 2006;21:2-8.
37. Giori NJ: Load-shifting brace treatment for osteoarthritis of the knee: A minimum 2½-year follow-up study. *J Rehabil Res Dev* 2004;41:187-194.
38. Pollo FE, Otis JC, Backus SI, Warren RF, Wickiewicz TL: Reduction of medial compartment loads with valgus bracing of the osteoarthritic knee. *Am J Sports Med* 2002;30:414-421.
39. Ramsey DK, Briem K, Axe MJ, Snyder-Mackler L: A mechanical theory for the effectiveness of bracing for medial compartment osteoarthritis of the knee. *J Bone Joint Surg Am* 2007;89:2398-2407.
40. Slemenda C, Brandt KD, Heilman DK, et al: Quadriceps weakness and osteoarthritis of the knee. *Ann Intern Med* 1997;127:97-104.
41. Slemenda C, Heilman DK, Brandt KD, et al: Reduced quadriceps strength relative to body weight: A risk factor for knee osteoarthritis in women? *Arthritis Rheum* 1998;41:1951-1959.
42. Hurley MV: The role of muscle weakness in the pathogenesis of osteoarthritis. *Rheum Dis Clin North Am* 1999;25:283-298.
43. Ettinger WH Jr, Burns R, Messier SP, et al: A randomized trial comparing aerobic exercise and resistance exercise with a health education program in older adults with knee osteoarthritis: The Fitness Arthritis and Seniors Trial (FAST). *JAMA* 1997;277:25-31.
44. Amin S, Baker K, Niu J, et al: Quadriceps strength and the risk of cartilage loss and symptom progression in knee osteoarthritis. *Arthritis Rheum* 2009;60:189-198.
45. Moore RA, Tramèr MR, Carroll D, Wiffen PJ, McQuay HJ: Quantitative systematic review of topically applied non-steroidal anti-inflammatory drugs. *BMJ* 1998;316:333-338.
46. Petersen B, Rovati S: Diclofenac epolamine (Flector) patch: Evidence for topical activity. *Clin Drug Investig* 2009;29:1-9.
47. Vas J, White A: Evidence from RCTs on optimal acupuncture treatment for knee osteoarthritis: An exploratory review. *Acupunct Med* 2007;25:29-35.
48. Ciombor DM, Aaron RK, Wang S, Simon B: Modification of osteoarthritis by pulsed electromagnetic field: A morphological study. *Osteoarthr Cartil* 2003;11:455-462.

49. Garland D, Holt P, Harrington JT, Caldwell J, Zizic T, Cholewczynski J: A 3-month, randomized, double-blind, placebo-controlled study to evaluate the safety and efficacy of a highly optimized, capacitively coupled, pulsed electrical stimulator in patients with osteoarthritis of the knee. *Osteoarthr Cartil* 2007;15: 630-637.

50. Hulme J, Robinson V, DeBie R, Wells G, Judd M, Tugwell P: Electromagnetic fields for the treatment of osteoarthritis. *Cochrane Database Syst Rev* 2002;1:CD003523.

51. Fary RE, Carroll GJ, Briffa TG, Gupta R, Briffa NK: The effectiveness of pulsed electrical stimulation (E-PES) in the management of osteoarthritis of the knee: A protocol for a randomised controlled trial. *BMC Musculoskelet Disord* 2008;9:18.

52. Boileau C, Tat SK, Pelletier JP, Cheng S, Martel-Pelletier J: Diacerein inhibits the synthesis of resorptive enzymes and reduces osteoclastic differentiation/survival in osteoarthritic subchondral bone: A possible mechanism for a protective effect against subchondral bone remodeling. *Arthritis Res Ther* 2008;10:R71.

53. Fidelix TS, Soares BG, Trevisani VF: Diacerein for osteoarthritis. *Cochrane Database Syst Rev* 2006;1:CD005117.

54. Dougados M, Nguyen M, Berdah L, et al: Evaluation of the structure-modifying effects of diacerein in hip osteoarthritis: ECHODIAH, a three-year, placebo-controlled trial. Evaluation of the Chondromodulating Effect of Diacerein in OA of the Hip. *Arthritis Rheum* 2001;44:2539-2547.

55. Pham T, Le Henanff A, Ravaud P, Dieppe P, Paolozzi L, Dougados M: Evaluation of the symptomatic and structural efficacy of a new hyaluronic acid compound, NRD101, in comparison with diacerein and placebo in a 1 year randomized controlled study in symptomatic knee osteoarthritis. *Ann Rheum Dis* 2004;63:1611-1617.

56. Outerbridge RE: The etiology of chondromalacia patellae: 1961. *Clin Orthop Relat Res* 2001;389:5-8.

57. Guettler JH, Demetropoulos CK, Yang KH, Jurist KA: Osteochondral defects in the human knee: Influence of defect size on cartilage rim stress and load redistribution to surrounding cartilage. *Am J Sports Med* 2004;32: 1451-1458.

58. Kocher MS, Tucker R, Ganley TJ, Flynn JM: Management of osteochondritis dissecans of the knee: Current concepts review. *Am J Sports Med* 2006;34:1181-1191.

59. Sgaglione NA, Abrutyn DA: Update on the treatment of osteochondral fractures and osteochondritis dissecans of the knee. *Sports Med Arthrosc Rev* 2003;11:222-235.

60. Dines JS, Fealy S, Potter HG, Warren RF: Outcomes of osteochondral lesions of the knee repaired with a bioabsorbable device. *Arthroscopy* 2008;24:62-68.

61. Kobayashi T, Fujikawa K, Oohashi M: Surgical fixation of massive osteochondritis dissecans lesion using cylindrical osteochondral plugs. *Arthroscopy* 2004;20:981-986.

62. Miura K, Ishibashi Y, Tsuda E, Sato H, Toh S: Results of arthroscopic fixation of osteochondritis dissecans lesion of the knee with cylindrical autogenous osteochondral plugs. *Am J Sports Med* 2007;35:216-222.

63. Haggert GE: The surgical treatment of degenerative arthritis of the knee joint. *J Bone Joint Surg Am* 1940;22: 717-729.

64. Magnuson PB: Joint debridement: Surgical treatment of degenerative arthritis. *Clin Orthop Relat Res* 1974; 101:4-12.

65. Sprague NF III: Arthroscopic debridement for degenerative knee joint disease. *Clin Orthop Relat Res* 1981; 160:118-123.

66. Merchan EC, Galindo E: Arthroscope-guided surgery versus nonoperative treatment for limited degenerative osteoarthritis of the femorotibial joint in patients over 50 years of age: A prospective comparative study. *Arthroscopy* 1993;9: 663-667.

67. Moseley JB, O'Malley K, Petersen NJ, et al: A controlled trial of arthroscopic surgery for osteoarthritis of the knee. *N Engl J Med* 2002;347: 81-88.

68. Kirkley A, Birmingham TB, Litchfield RB, et al: A randomized trial of arthroscopic surgery for osteoarthritis of the knee. *N Engl J Med* 2008;359: 1097-1107.

69. Aaron RK, Skolnick AH, Reinert SE, Ciombor DM: Arthroscopic débridement for osteoarthritis of the knee. *J Bone Joint Surg Am* 2006;88: 936-943.

70. Spahn G, Mückley T, Kahl E, Hofmann GO: Factors affecting the outcome of arthroscopy in medial-compartment osteoarthritis of the knee. *Arthroscopy* 2006;22:1233-1240.

71. Pridie AH: A method of resurfacing osteoarthritic knee joints. *J Bone Joint Surg Br* 1959;41:618.

72. Friedman MJ, Berasi CC, Fox JM, Del Pizzo W, Snyder SJ, Ferkel RD: Preliminary results with abrasion arthroplasty in the osteoarthritic knee. *Clin Orthop Relat Res* 1984;182: 200-205.

73. Steadman JR, Rodkey WG, Singleton SB, Briggs KK: Microfracture technique for full-thickness chondral defects: Technique and clinical results. *Oper Tech Orthop* 1997;7: 300-304.

74. Mithoefer K, Williams RJ III , Warren RF, et al: Chondral resurfacing of articular cartilage defects in the knee with the microfracture technique: Surgical technique. *J Bone Joint Surg Am* 2006;88:S294-S304.

75. Marder RA, Hopkins G Jr, Timmerman LA: Arthroscopic microfracture of chondral defects of the knee: A comparison of two postoperative treatments. *Arthroscopy* 2005;21: 152-158.

76. Gill TJ, McCulloch PC, Glasson SS, Blanchet T, Morris EA: Chondral defect repair after the microfracture procedure: A nonhuman primate model. *Am J Sports Med* 2005;33: 680-685.

77. Steadman JR, Briggs KK, Rodrigo JJ, Kocher MS, Gill TJ, Rodkey WG: Outcomes of microfracture for traumatic chondral defects of the knee: Average 11-year follow-up. *Arthroscopy* 2003;19:477-484.

78. Gobbi A, Nunag P, Malinowski K: Treatment of full thickness chondral lesions of the knee with microfracture in a group of athletes. *Knee Surg Sports Traumatol Arthrosc* 2005;13:213-221.

79. Mithoefer K, Williams RJ III, Warren RF, Wickiewicz TL, Marx RG: High-impact athletics after knee articular cartilage repair: A prospective evaluation of the microfracture technique. *Am J Sports Med* 2006;34: 1413-1418.

80. Kreuz PC, Erggelet C, Steinwachs MR, et al: Is microfracture of chondral defects in the knee associated with different results in patients aged 40 years or younger? *Arthroscopy* 2006; 22:1180-1186.

81. Mithoefer K, Williams RJ III, Warren RF, et al: The microfracture technique for the treatment of articular cartilage lesions in the knee: A prospective cohort study. *J Bone Joint Surg Am* 2005;87:1911-1920.

82. Buckwalter JA, Martin JA, Olmstead M, Athanasiou KA, Rosenwasser MP, Mow VC: Osteochondral repair of primate knee femoral and patellar articular surfaces: Implications for preventing post-traumatic osteoarthritis. *Iowa Orthop J* 2003;23:66-74.

83. Buckwalter JA, Mankin HJ: Articular cartilage: Degeneration and osteoarthritis, repair, regeneration, and transplantation. *Instr Course Lect* 1998;47: 487-504.

84. Kreuz PC, Steinwachs MR, Erggelet C, et al: Results after microfracture of full-thickness chondral defects in different compartments in the knee. *Osteoarthritis Cartilage* 2006;14: 1119-1125.

85. Garretson RB III, Katolik LI, Verma N, Beck PR, Bach BR, Cole BJ: Contact pressure at osteochondral donor sites in the patellofemoral joint. *Am J Sports Med* 2004;32:967-974.

86. Ahmad CS, Cohen ZA, Levine WN, Ateshian GA, Mow VC: Biomechanical and topographic considerations for autologous osteochondral grafting in the knee. *Am J Sports Med* 2001;29: 201-206.

87. Bartz RL, Kamaric E, Noble PC, Lintner D, Bocell J: Topographic matching of selected donor and recipient sites for osteochondral autografting of the articular surface of the femoral condyles. *Am J Sports Med* 2001;29:207-212.

88. Pearce SG, Hurtig MB, Clarnette R, Kalra M, Cowan B, Miniaci A: An investigation of 2 techniques for optimizing joint surface congruency using multiple cylindrical osteochondral autografts. *Arthroscopy* 2001;17:50-55.

89. Koh JL, Wirsing K, Lautenschlager E, Zhang LO: The effect of graft height mismatch on contact pressure following osteochondral grafting: A biomechanical study. *Am J Sports Med* 2004; 32:317-320.

90. Koh JL, Kowalski A, Lautenschlager E: The effect of angled osteochondral grafting on contact pressure: A biomechanical study. *Am J Sports Med* 2006; 34:116-119.

91. Hangody L, Ráthonyi GK, Duska Z, Vásárhelyi G, Füles P, Módis L: Autologous osteochondral mosaicplasty: Surgical technique. *J Bone Joint Surg Am* 2004;86:65-72.

92. Borazjani BH, Chen AC, Bae WC, et al: Effect of impact on chondrocyte viability during insertion of human osteochondral grafts. *J Bone Joint Surg Am* 2006;88:1934-1943.

93. Barber FA, Herbert MA, McGarry JE, Barber CA: Insertion force of articular cartilage transplantation systems. *J Knee Surg* 2008;21:200-204.

94. Levy AS: Osteochondral autograft for the treatment of focal cartilage lesions. *Oper Tech Orthop* 2001;11: 108-114.

95. Marcacci M, Kon E, Delcogliano M, Filardo G, Busacca M, Zaffagnini S: Arthroscopic autologous osteochondral grafting for cartilage defects of the knee: Prospective study results at a minimum 7-year follow-up. *Am J Sports Med* 2007;35:2014-2021.

96. Chow JC, Hantes ME, Houle JB, Zalavras CG: Arthroscopic autogenous osteochondral transplantation for treating knee cartilage defects: A 2- to 5-year follow-up study. *Arthroscopy* 2004;20:681-690.

97. Gudas R, Kalesinskas RJ, Kimtys V, et al: A prospective randomized clinical study of mosaic osteochondral autologous transplantation versus microfracture for the treatment of osteochondral defects in the knee joint in young athletes. *Arthroscopy* 2005;21:1066-1075.

98. Reddy S, Pedowitz DI, Parekh SG, Sennett BJ, Okereke E: The morbidity associated with osteochondral harvest from asymptomatic knees for the treatment of osteochondral lesions of the talus. *Am J Sports Med* 2007;35: 80-85.

99. Ansah P, Vogt S, Ueblacker P, Martinek V, Woertler K, Imhoff AB: Osteochondral transplantation to treat osteochondral lesions in the elbow. *J Bone Joint Surg Am* 2007;89:2188-2194.

100. Peterson L, Minas T, Brittberg M, Lindahl A: Treatment of osteochondritis dissecans of the knee with autologous chondrocyte transplantation: Results at two to ten years. *J Bone Joint Surg Am* 2003;85:17-24.

101. Emmerson BC, Görtz S, Jamali AA, Chung C, Amiel D, Bugbee WD: Fresh osteochondral allografting in the treatment of osteochondritis dissecans of the femoral condyle. *Am J Sports Med* 2007;35:907-914.

102. Grande DA, Pitman MI, Peterson L, Menche D, Klein M: The repair of experimentally produced defects in rabbit articular cartilage by autologous chondrocyte transplantation. *J Orthop Res* 1989;7:208-218.

103. Brittberg M, Lindahl A, Nilsson A, Ohlsson C, Isaksson O, Peterson L: Treatment of deep cartilage defects in the knee with autologous chondrocyte transplantation. *N Engl J Med* 1994;331:889-895.

104. Kon E, Delcogliano M, Filardo G, Montaperto C, Marcacci M: Second generation issues in cartilage repair. *Sports Med Arthrosc* 2008;16:221-229.

105. Kerker JT, Leo AJ, Sgaglione NA: Cartilage repair: Synthetics and scaffolds. Basic science, surgical techniques, and clinical outcomes. *Sports Med Arthrosc* 2008;16:208-216.

106. Minas T, Peterson L: Chondrocyte transplantation. *Oper Tech Orthop* 1997;7:323-333.

107. Brittberg M, Peterson L, Sjögren-Jansson E, Tallheden T, Lindahl A: Articular cartilage engineering with autologous chondrocyte transplantation: A review of recent developments. *J Bone Joint Surg Am* 2003;85: 109-115.

108. Peterson L, Minas T, Brittberg M, Nilsson A, Sjögren-Jansson E, Lindahl A: Two- to 9-year outcome after autologous chondrocyte transplantation of the knee. *Clin Orthop Relat Res* 2000;374:212-234.

109. Peterson L, Brittberg M, Kiviranta I, Akerlund EL, Lindahl A: Autologous chondrocyte transplantation: Biomechanics and long-term durability. *Am J Sports Med* 2002;30:2-12.

110. Zaslav K, Cole B, Brewster R, et al: A prospective study of autologous chondrocyte implantation in patients with failed prior treatment for articular cartilage defect of the knee: Results of the study of the treatment of articular repair (STAR) clinical trial. *Am J Sports Med* 2009;37:42-55.

111. Henderson I, Tuy B, Oakes B: Reoperation after autologous chondrocyte implantation: Indications and findings. *J Bone Joint Surg Br* 2004;86: 205-211.

112. Niemeyer P, Pestka JM, Kreuz PC, et al: Characteristic complications after autologous chondrocyte implantation for cartilage defects of the knee joint. *Am J Sports Med* 2008;36: 2091-2099.

113. Convery FR, Akeson WH, Meyers MH: The operative technique of fresh osteochondral allografting of the knee. *Oper Tech Orthop* 1997;7:340-344.

114. Gross AE, Silverstein EA, Falk J, Falk R, Langer F: The allotransplantation of partial joints in the treatment of osteoarthritis of the knee. *Clin Orthop Relat Res* 1975;108:7-14.

115. Williams SK, Amiel D, Ball ST, et al: Prolonged storage effects on the articular cartilage of fresh human osteochondral allografts. *J Bone Joint Surg Am* 2003;85:2111-2120.

116. Ball ST, Amiel D, Williams SK, et al: The effects of storage on fresh human osteochondral allografts. *Clin Orthop Relat Res* 2004;418:246-252.

117. Görtz S, Bugbee WD: Allografts in articular cartilage repair. *Instr Course Lect* 2007;56:469-480.

118. Gross AE: Fresh osteochondral allografts for post-traumatic knee defects: Surgical technique. *Oper Tech Orthop* 1997;7:334-339.

119. Ghazavi MT, Pritzker KP, Davis AM, Gross AE: Fresh osteochondral allografts for post-traumatic osteochondral defects of the knee. *J Bone Joint Surg Br* 1997;79:1008-1013.

120. Bugbee WD, Convery FR: Osteochondral allograft transplantation. *Clin Sports Med* 1999;18:67-75.

121. Sharma L, Song J, Felson DT, Cahue S, Shamiyeh E, Dunlop DD: The role of knee alignment in disease progression and functional decline in knee osteoarthritis. *JAMA* 2001;286: 188-195.

122. Naudie DD, Amendola A, Fowler PJ: Opening wedge high tibial osteotomy for symptomatic hyperextension-varus thrust. *Am J Sports Med* 2004;32: 60-70.

123. Aubin PP, Cheah HK, Davis AM, Gross AE: Long-term followup of fresh femoral osteochondral allografts for posttraumatic knee defects. *Clin Orthop Relat Res* 2001;391:S318-S327.

124. Jamali AA, Emmerson BC, Chung C, Convery FR, Bugbee WD: Fresh osteochondral allografts: Results in the patellofemoral joint. *Clin Orthop Relat Res* 2005;437:176-185.

125. McCulloch PC, Kang RW, Sobhy MH, Hayden JK, Cole BJ: Prospective evaluation of prolonged fresh osteochondral allograft transplantation of the femoral condyle: Minimum 2-year follow-up. *Am J Sports Med* 2007;35:411-420.

126. Amendola A: Knee osteotomy and meniscal transplantation: Indications, technical considerations, and results. *Sports Med Arthrosc* 2007;15:32-38.

127. Coventry MB: Valgus osteotomy of the upper tibia. *Tech Orthop* 1989;4: 35-40.

128. Billings A, Scott DF, Camargo MP, Hofmann AA: High tibial osteotomy with a calibrated osteotomy guide, rigid internal fixation, and early motion: Long-term follow-up. *J Bone Joint Surg Am* 2000;82:70-79.

129. Puddu G, Cipolla M, Cerullo G, Franco V, Giannì E: Osteotomies: The surgical treatment of the valgus knee. *Sports Med Arthrosc* 2007;15:15-22.

130. Healy WL, Anglen JO, Wasilewski SA, Krackow KA: Distal femoral varus osteotomy. *J Bone Joint Surg Am* 1988; 70:102-109.

131. McDermott AG, Finklestein JA, Farine I, Boynton EL, MacIntosh DL, Gross A: Distal femoral varus osteotomy for valgus deformity of the knee. *J Bone Joint Surg Am* 1988;70:110-116.

132. Parvizi J, Hanssen AD, Spangehl MJ: Total knee arthroplasty following proximal tibial osteotomy: Risk factors for failure. *J Bone Joint Surg Am* 2004;86:474-479.

133. Katz MM, Hungerford DS, Krackow KA, Lennox DW: Results of total knee arthroplasty after failed proximal tibial osteotomy for osteoarthritis. *J Bone Joint Surg Am* 1987;69:225-233.

134. Nelson CL, Saleh KJ, Kassim RA, et al: Total knee arthroplasty after varus osteotomy of the distal part of the femur. *J Bone Joint Surg Am* 2003; 85:1062-1065.

135. Wright JM, Crockett HC, Slawski DP, Madsen MW, Windsor RE: High tibial osteotomy. *J Am Acad Orthop Surg* 2005;13:279-289.

136. Holden DL, James SL, Larson RL, Slocum DB: Proximal tibial osteotomy in patients who are fifty years old or less: A long-term follow-up

study. *J Bone Joint Surg Am* 1988;70: 977-982.

137. Marti RK, Verhagen RA, Kerkhoffs GM, Moojen TM: Proximal tibial varus osteotomy: Indications, technique, and five to twenty-one-year results. *J Bone Joint Surg Am* 2001; 83:164-170.

138. Naudie D, Bourne RB, Rorabeck CH, Bourne TJ: Survivorship of the high tibial valgus osteotomy. A 10- to -22-year followup study. *Clin Orthop Relat Res* 1999;367:18-27.

139. Hernigou P, Medevielle D, Debeyre J, Goutallier D: Proximal tibial osteotomy for osteoarthritis with varus deformity: A ten to thirteen-year follow-up study. *J Bone Joint Surg Am* 1987;69:332-354.

140. Aglietti P, Menchetti PP: Distal femoral varus osteotomy in the valgus osteoarthritic knee. *Am J Knee Surg* 2000;13:89-95.

141. Miniaci A, Grossman SP, Jacob RP: Supracondylar femoral varus osteotomy in the treatment of valgus knee deformity. *Am J Knee Surg* 1990;3:65-73.

142. Felson DT, Zhang Y: An update on the epidemiology of knee and hip osteoarthritis with a view to prevention. *Arthritis Rheum* 1998;41:1343-1355.

143. McKeever DC: Tibial plateau prosthesis: 1960. *Clin Orthop Relat Res* 2005;440:4-8.

144. MacIntosh DL, Hunter GA: The use of the hemiarthroplasty prosthesis for advanced osteoarthritis and rheumatoid arthritis of the knee. *J Bone Joint Surg Br* 1972;54:244-255.

145. Riddle DL, Jiranek WA, McGlynn FJ: Yearly incidence of unicompartmental knee arthroplasty in the United States. *J Arthroplasty* 2008;23:408-412.

146. Laurencin CT, Zelicof SB, Scott RD, Ewald FC: Unicompartmental versus total knee arthroplasty in the same patient: A comparative study. *Clin Orthop Relat Res* 1991;273:151-156.

147. Bert JM: Unicompartmental knee replacement. *Orthop Clin North Am* 2005;36:513-522.

148. Borus T, Thornhill T: Unicompartmental knee arthroplasty. *J Am Acad Orthop Surg* 2008;16:9-18.

149. Diduch DR, Insall JN, Scott WN, Scuderi GR, Font-Rodriquez D: Total knee replacement in young, active patients: Long-term follow-up and functional outcome. *J Bone Joint Surg Am* 1997;79:575-582.

150. Dalury DF, Barrett WP, Mason JB, Goldstein WM, Murphy JA, Roche MW: Midterm survival of a contemporary modular total knee replacement: A multicentre study of 1970 knees. *J Bone Joint Surg Br* 2008; 90:1594-1596.

151. Bert JM, Smith R: Failures of metal-backed unicompartmental arthroplasty. *Knee* 1997;4:41-48.

152. Rosa RA, Bert JM, Bruce W, Gross M, Carroll M, Hartdegen V: An evaluation of all-ultra-high molecular weight polyethylene unicompartmental tibial component cement-fixation mechanisms. *J Bone Joint Surg Am* 2002;84: 102-104.

153. Hamilton WG, Collier MB, Tarabee E, McAuley JP, Engh CAJr , Engh GA: Incidence and reasons for reoperation after minimally invasive unicompartmental knee arthroplasty. *J Arthroplasty* 2006;21:98-107.

154. Bert JM: Unicompartmental arthroplasty for unicompartmental knee arthritis. *Tech Knee Surg* 2008;7:51-60.

155. Bae DK, Guhl JF, Keane SP: Unicompartmental knee arthroplasty for single compartment disease: Clinical experience with an average four-year follow-up study. *Clin Orthop Relat Res* 1983;176:233-238.

156. Insall J, Aglietti P: A five to seven-year follow-up of unicondylar arthroplasty. *J Bone Joint Surg Am* 1980;62: 1329-1337.

157. Marmor L: Unicompartmental arthroplasty of the knee with a minimum ten-year follow-up period. *Clin Orthop Relat Res* 1988;228:171-177.

158. Scott RD, Cobb AG, McQueary FG, Thornhill TS: Unicompartmental knee arthroplasty: Eight- to 12-year follow-up evaluation with survivorship analysis. *Clin Orthop Relat Res* 1991;271:96-100.

159. Heck DA, Marmor L, Gibson A, Rougraff BT: Unicompartmental knee arthroplasty: A multicenter investigation with long-term follow-up evaluation. *Clin Orthop Relat Res* 1993; 286:154-159.

160. Bert JM: 10-year survivorship of metal-backed, unicompartmental arthroplasty. *J Arthroplasty* 1998;13: 901-905.

161. Price AJ, Waite JC, Svard U: Long-term clinical results of the medial Oxford unicompartmental knee arthroplasty. *Clin Orthop Relat Res* 2005; 435:171-180.

162. Gioe TJ, Killeen KK, Hoeffel DP, et al: Analysis of unicompartmental knee arthroplasty in a community-based implant registry. *Clin Orthop Relat Res* 2003;416:111-119.

163. Pennington DW, Swienckowski JJ, Lutes WB, Drake GN: Unicompartmental knee arthroplasty in patients sixty years of age or younger. *J Bone Joint Surg Am* 2003;85:1968-1973.

164. Steele RG, Hutabarat S, Evans RL, Ackroyd CE, Newman JH: Survivorship of the St Georg Sled medial unicompartmental knee replacement beyond ten years. *J Bone Joint Surg Br* 2006;88:1164-1168.

165. Newman J, Pydisetty RV, Ackroyd C: Unicompartmental or total knee replacement: The 15-year results of a prospective randomized controlled trial. *J Bone Joint Surg Br* 2009;91:52 57.

166. O'Rourke MR, Gardner JJ, Callaghan JJ, et al: Unicompartmental knee replacement: A minimum twenty-one-year followup, end-result study. *Clin Orthop Relat Res* 2005;440:27-37.

167. Berger RA, Meneghini RM, Jacobs JJ, et al: Results of unicompartmental knee arthroplasty at a minimum of ten years of follow-up. *J Bone Joint Surg Am* 2005;87:999-1006.

168. Bert JM, Leverone J: Histologic appearance of "pristine" articular cartilage in knees with unicompartmental osteoarthritis. *J Knee Surg* 2007;20: 15-19.

Surgical Management of Articular Cartilage Defects in the Knee

Brian J. Cole, MD, MBA
Cecilia Pascual-Garrido, MD
Robert C. Grumet, MD

Abstract

The treatment of isolated cartilage lesions of the knee is based on several underlying principles, including a predictable reduction in the patient's symptoms, improvements in function and joint congruence, and prevention of progressive damage. Surgical options for cartilage restoration are described as palliative treatments, such as débridement and lavage; reparative, such as marrow stimulation techniques; or restorative, such as osteochondral grafting and autologous chondrocyte implantation. The choice of an appropriate treatment should be made on an individual basis, with consideration for the patient's specific goals (such as pain reduction or functional improvement), physical demand level, prior treatment history, lesion size and location, and a systematic evaluation of the knee that considers comorbidities, including alignment, meniscal status, and ligament integrity. It is important for the physician to be familiar with the indications, surgical techniques, and clinical outcomes of the available treatment options for chondral defects of the knee.

Instr Course Lect 2010;59:181-204.

Articular cartilage is vulnerable to traumatic injury and subsequent degeneration. These changes are likely related to the limited capacity for cartilage repair, poor vascular supply, and deficiency in terms of the ability of an undifferentiated cell population to respond to the insult. Although the natural history of isolated chondral and osteochondral defects is not predictable, clinical experience suggests that, when left untreated, these lesions do not heal and may progress to symptomatic degeneration of the joint.[1] Therefore, early surgical intervention for symptomatic lesions is often suggested in an effort to restore normal joint congruity and pressure distribution and prevent further injury. Treatment recommendations are made after an evaluation of symptomatic lesions and should be tailored to the specifics of each case.

The goals of surgical treatment are to provide pain relief and improve joint function, thus allowing patients to comfortably perform activities of daily living and potentially maintain or return to higher levels of activity. Multiple algorithms have been described in an effort to simplify the treatment of cartilage lesions. These are useful tools with which to organize thoughts. In general, surgical options can be grouped into three categories: palliative (arthroscopic débridement and lavage), reparative (marrow stimulation techniques), and restorative (osteochondral grafting and autologous chondrocyte implantation). All of these techniques have been reported to improve the clinical status compared with the preoperative state. Thus, the appropriate treatment of any given cartilage lesion is patient specific. The size and location of the lesion, the physical demands of the patient, and

Dr. Cole or an immediate family member has received royalties from Arthrex and Stryker; serves as a paid consultant to or is an employee of Genzyme, Zimmer, DePuy, Arthrex, Carticept, and Regentis; and has received research or institutional support from Arthrex, DePuy, and Zimmer. Neither of the following authors or members of their immediate families has received anything of value from or owns stock in a commercial company or institution related directly or indirectly to the subject of this chapter: Dr. Pascual-Garrido and Dr. Grumet.

the treatment history all are important preoperative considerations. In addition, the surgeon must consider what subsequent treatment options are available if the current treatment fails to relieve the symptoms. A realistic and comprehensive understanding of the patient's goals is critical to any decision regarding how to treat a symptomatic chondral defect. In keeping with these principles, the treatment algorithm consists of a graduated surgical plan. The least destructive and least invasive treatment option necessary to alleviate the symptoms and restore joint function is performed first. The more extensive treatments are reserved for potential salvage operations later. If the symptoms persist despite conservative treatment, subsequent treatments are not impeded by previous management.

Decision Making

When treating articular cartilage lesions in the knee, the surgeon should focus on patient-specific and defect-specific variables and avoid "linear thinking." The clinical presentation should correlate with the underlying pathoanatomy. For example, a patient with known classic osteochondritis dissecans of the medial femoral condyle who reports bilateral anterior knee pain with stair-climbing should be evaluated initially with a presumptive diagnosis of patellofemoral pain before ascribing the symptoms to the osteochondritis dissecans lesion. Because the natural history of cartilage lesions is not known and the surgical treatments are neither benign nor associated with a predictable outcome (particularly with regard to the prevention of arthritis), surgical decision making must be taken quite seriously.

Understanding and addressing the patient's specific concerns and goals are critical to achieving a successful outcome from the patient's perspective. More specifically, patients often express concerns about whether it is safe to remain active despite symptoms and whether a delay in surgical intervention precludes certain treatment options because of disease progression. Knowledge of the specific marginal improvements that a procedure should provide gives the patient a reasonable expectation regarding the outcome. Unfortunately, the lack of understanding of the natural history of these defects makes it difficult to advise patients, and it is best to carry out careful discussions on a case-by-case basis.

Patient age, body mass index, symptom type (weight-bearing pain, non–weight-bearing pain, swelling, mechanical symptoms, giving way, and aggravation of symptoms related to walking on level ground as opposed to stair-climbing), occupation and/or family commitments, risk aversion (desire to avoid subsequent surgical procedures), responsiveness and rehabilitation after previous surgical treatments, and the patient's specific concerns related to his or her disorder are all important preoperative considerations. Although chronologic age is often cited as a relative indication or contraindication to cartilage repair, it is really physiologic age that determines the patient's eligibility for a nonarthroplasty solution. Typically, patients who become symptomatic in the fourth or fifth decade of life have concomitant chondral and subchondral disease involving apposing articular surfaces that precludes a biologic treatment option. In addition, the results of partial and total knee arthroplasty are predictably gratifying and satisfy most patients, even those who are relatively young. One must carefully search for associated pathologic conditions, such as malalignment, ligament insufficiency, and concomitant meniscal deficiency that may contribute to treatment failure and should be corrected before or during the surgery to treat the chondral lesion.

Defect-specific variables include defect location, number, size, depth, and geometry; the condition of the subchondral bone and surrounding cartilage; and the degree of containment. The condition of the apposing surface, which is often overlooked, is also an important variable. Even minor areas of early degeneration make achieving a satisfactory clinical outcome challenging. Specific management of each of these defect-specific variables increases the likelihood of a good clinical outcome.

Treatment Algorithm

Malalignment, ligament insufficiency, and concomitant meniscal deficiency are assessed and, when necessary, are treated with a concomitant or staged osteotomy (high tibial, distal femoral, or tibial tuberosity), ligament reconstruction, and perhaps a meniscal allograft transplantation.[2] Patellofemoral lesions are often treated with a simultaneous realignment procedure such as anteromedialization of the tibial tuberosity. Anteromedialization is more successful for lateral patellofemoral lesions than it is for lesions located along the medial aspect of the patellofemoral joint.[3] Medial patellofemoral lesions are treated with a more vertically oriented anteromedialization.[2] The treatment algorithm for chondral lesions is guided by the lesion size and location and the patient activity level (Figure 1).

Primary repair is done for any chondral injury that is amenable to fixation. Any acute osteochondral

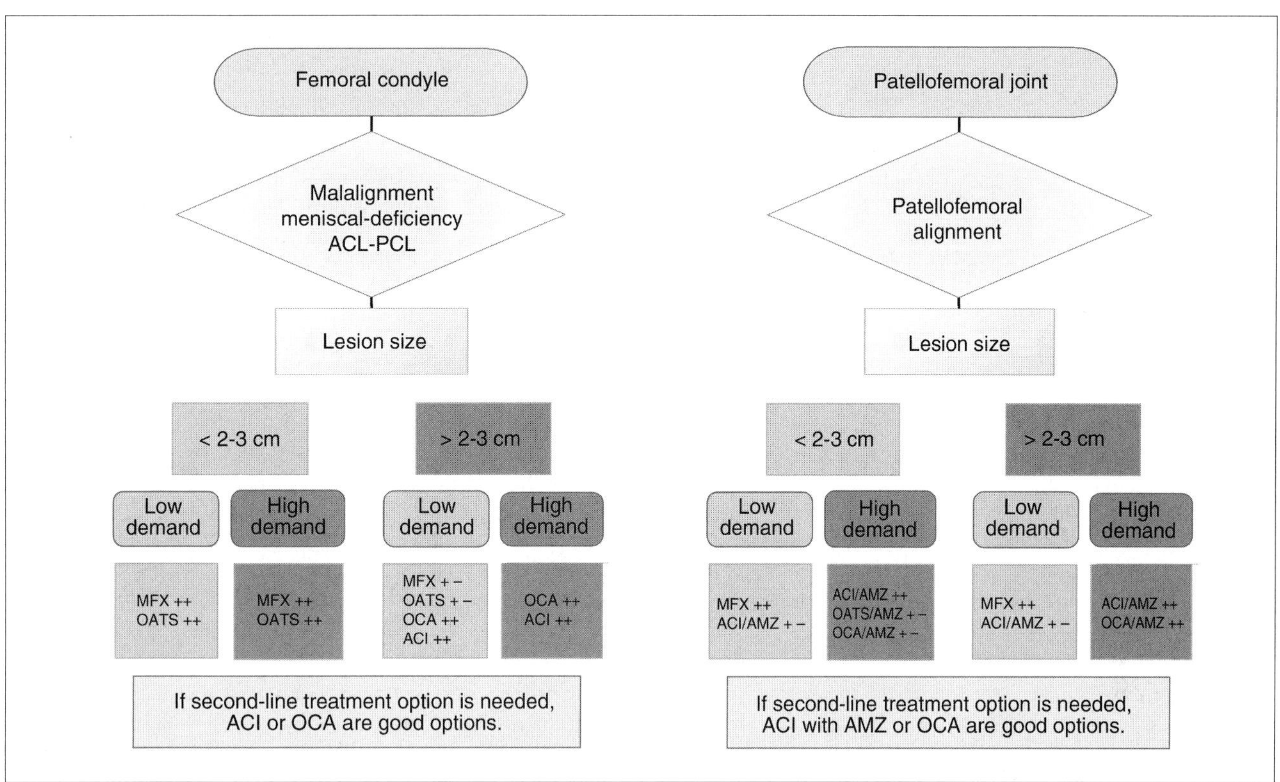

Figure 1 Treatment algorithm for focal chondral lesions. Before treatment, it is important to assess the presence of correctable lesions. Surgical treatment should be considered for trochlear and patellar lesions only after the use of rehabilitation programs has failed. The treatment decision is guided by the size and location of the defect, the patient's demands, and whether it is first or second-line treatment. ACL = anterior cruciate ligament, PCL = posterior cruciate ligament, MFX = microfracture, OATS = osteochondral autograft transplantation, ACI = autologous chondrocyte implantation, OCA = osteochondral allograft, AMZ = anteromedialization, ++ = best treatment option, and +– = possible option depending on patient's characteristics.

fragment or in situ and unstable osteochondritis dissecans lesion is repaired primarily. It is particularly critical to fix large fragments (> 1 cm^2) from the weight-bearing portion of the femoral condyles. The basic principles for primary repair include elevation of the unstable fragment, débridement of the fibrous base, microfracture if necessary to gain access to the subchondral blood supply to promote healing, bone grafting of areas of cystic changes or bone loss, and rigid fixation of the fragment under compression. Headless compression screw fixation, with subsequent screw removal in younger patients after 8 weeks of not bearing weight, is often used. Continuous passive motion for up to 6 hours each day is recommended. Because fragments can settle over time, even headless screws can become prominent and damage the apposing surface. Performing a second-look arthroscopy to evaluate the defect helps the surgeon to judge the success of the procedure and to provide accurate advice to the patient.

Patients with lesions that cannot be repaired primarily may benefit from another type of treatment (palliative, reparative, or regenerative). Marrow stimulation techniques are typically a first-line treatment. These techniques are often used for smaller lesions (< 2 cm^2), or in patients with larger lesions (> 3 cm^2) and modest physical or physiologic demand levels. Small lesions in high-demand patients or those for whom marrow stimulation has failed can be treated with one or two 10-mm osteochondral autografts harvested from the lateral femoral trochlea just proximal to the sulcus terminalis. Larger lesions (> 2.5 cm^2) are typically more amenable to osteochondral allografting or autologous chondrocyte implantation. Autologous chondrocyte implantation is advised for younger patients with shallow lesions, especially of the patellofemoral joint. This method does not violate the subchondral bone and minimizes the impact on future treatment such

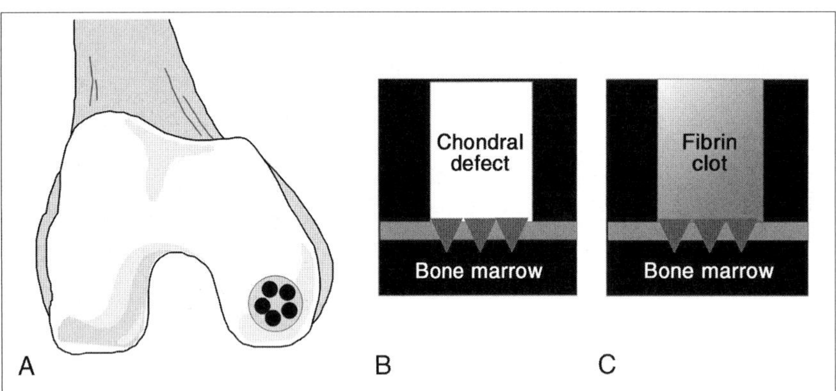

Figure 2 Microfracture. **A,** Holes should be created 2 to 3 mm apart, beginning at the periphery of the lesion. Great care should be taken to prevent confluence of the holes. **B,** A surgical awl is used to create the holes. The awl is kept perpendicular to the subchondral plate. **C,** The defect fills with fibrin clot, which is contained by the vertical walls of intact cartilage surrounding the lesion.

as osteochondral allograft transplantation. Larger, deeper lesions with bone loss typically require an osteochondral allograft.

Treatment is also guided by the location of the lesion. For example, osteochondral allografts are used for femoral condyle lesions because they allow accurate anatomic reconstruction. Lesions of the patellofemoral joint are often treated with autologous chondrocyte implantation because the lesions are small, and the varying anatomic concavity and convexity make structural grafts too difficult to fit in place. The tibia remains a difficult articular surface to treat. Small tibial lesions that are found when the femoral articular cartilage is being restored are commonly treated with marrow stimulation techniques. Other options include the use of osteochondral autografts placed in a retrograde manner with use of a cannulated reamer system such as the Arthrex cannulated reamer (Arthrex, Naples, FL). The use of osteochondral allografts with an intact meniscus and concomitant realignment has been reported for the treatment of larger lesions of the tibial plateau, especially after fracture and the development of secondary arthritis, with graft survival rates of up to 65% at 15 years.[4]

Surgical Options

Marrow Stimulation Technique (Microfracture)

The microfracture marrow stimulation technique is performed with a surgical awl to penetrate the subchondral bone. The violation of the subchondral plate promotes bleeding and the local migration of stem cells and other anabolic factors that support the formation of a "superclot." It is believed that the pluripotent nature of these stem cells allows the formation of reparative fibrocartilage tissue[5] (Figure 2).

Critical to the success of this technique is the creation of vertical walls of stable articular cartilage to create a "well-shouldered" lesion. This improves the local mechanical environment during healing by reducing shear and compression. All unstable cartilage is removed when the lesion site is prepared. The calcified cartilage layer is carefully débrided, and surgical awls are used to penetrate the subchondral bone (Figure 3). The holes are placed perpendicular to the bone surface, 2 to 3 mm apart, and confluence is avoided. Postoperative rehabilitation is guided by the location of the lesion, but typically it involves up to 6 weeks of not bearing weight and the use of a continuous passive motion machine for 6 hours per day. Patients with a lesion in the patellofemoral joint wear a brace with a flexion stop of 30° to limit patellofemoral contact; weight bearing is permitted.

The best outcomes of this technique are seen in younger patients with small traumatic lesions.[6] After 2 and 5 years of follow-up, Knutsen and associates[7] found no difference between the outcomes of microfracture and those of autologous chondrocyte implantation for femoral condyle lesions, but patients with smaller lesions treated with microfracture did better than those with larger lesions. Similarly, Gudas and associates[8] observed that, among patients with lesions exceeding 2 cm^2 in the central part of the medial femoral condyle, those treated with microfracture had lower clinical outcome scores than did those treated with an osteochondral autograft transplantation (Table 1). Location also plays a role in the success of marrow stimulation techniques, with better results seen after the treatment of femoral condyle lesions.[9]

Osteochondral Autograft Transplantation

Osteochondral autograft transplantation is the transfer of one or more cylindrical osteochondral autografts into the cartilage defect, providing a congruent hyaline cartilage-covered surface (Figure 4). The autografts

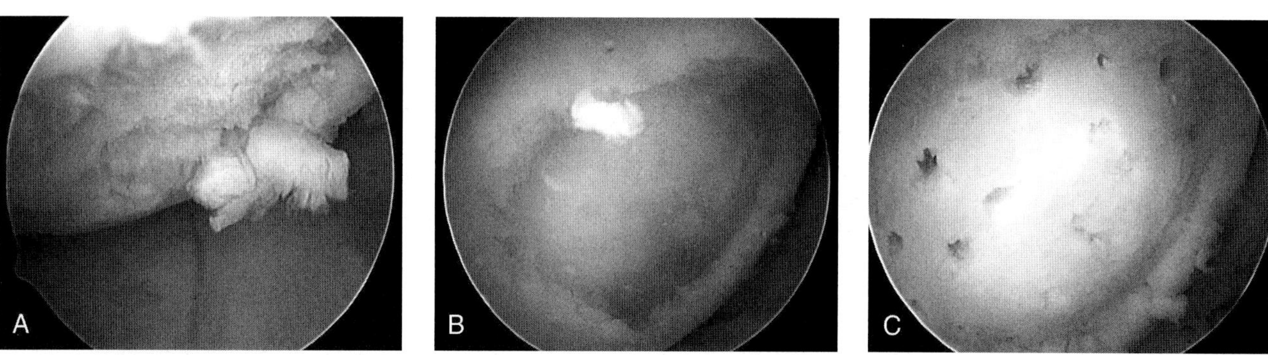

Figure 3 Microfracture. **A,** A chondral lesion in the femoral condyle. **B,** The lesion was carefully débrided, with the surgeon making sure that it had stable vertical borders. **C,** Microfracture holes were created in the subchondral bone, allowing a fibrin clot to fill the defect.

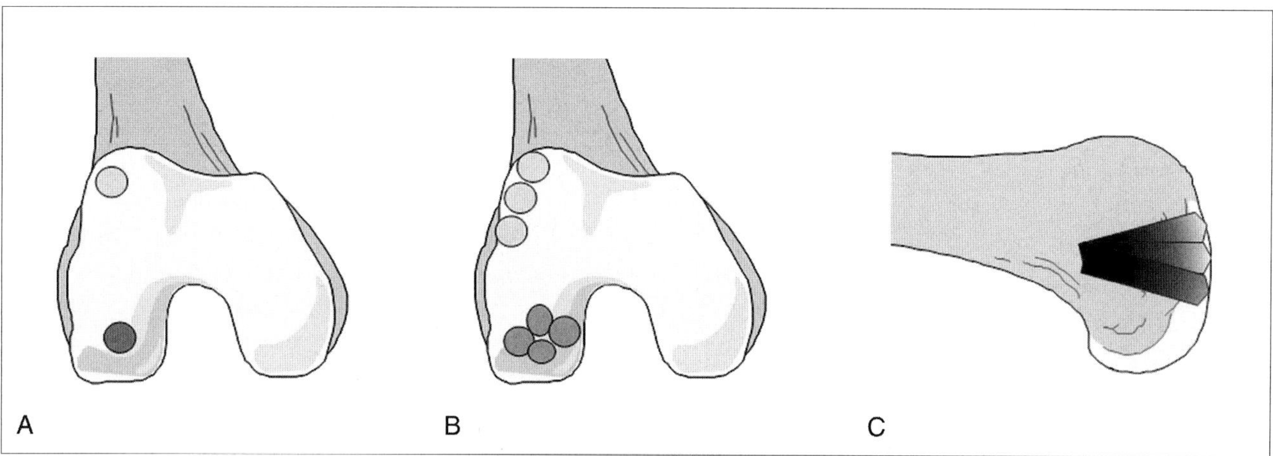

Figure 4 Illustration of osteochondral autograft transplantation. **A** and **B,** Depending on the defect size, one or multiple osteochondral plugs can be used to fill the defect. The plugs are often harvested from the intercondylar notch or from the margins of the lateral or medial condyles above the sulcus terminalis. **C,** This sagittal section shows how the osteochondral graft should be placed to fill the defect.

are harvested from the non–weight-bearing periphery of the femoral trochlea or the margin of the intercondylar notch. With a combination of different graft sizes, 90% to 100% of the defect can be filled.[10] This technique is limited by the amount of donor tissue available in the knee, and donor site morbidity increases as more tissue is harvested. Osteochondral autograft transplantation is best for small lesions (< 2 cm^2), but good clinical results have been reported[11] with lesions between 2 and 4 cm^2. The use of "mega" osteochondral autograft transplants ("megaOATS") from the posterior part of the femoral condyle for large osteochondral lesions (> 4 cm^2) has had good clinical results at 5.5 years postoperatively.[12]

Osteochondral autograft transplantation can be done through a small arthrotomy or entirely arthroscopically. To harvest donor grafts perpendicular to the surface, obtaining the donor plugs through a small lateral arthrotomy is preferable because the lateral edge of the patella can interfere with an arthroscopic harvest. The plugs are then implanted arthroscopically. There are many available commercial systems that provide a series of donor and recipient harvesting tubes to create a press-fit implant of up to 10 mm in diameter. A sizing guide is used to determine the number and size of grafts that are needed. A properly sized graft harvester with a collared pin is introduced perpendicular to the donor site to a depth of approximately 12 to 15 mm (Figure 5). The recipient socket is created to a depth that is 2 mm less than the length of the donor graft. It is important to maintain a perpendicular relationship between the donor graft and

Table 1
Demographic Data and Outcomes in Studies Comparing Microfracture With Other Cartilage Restoration Procedures

Author(s)	Group 1	Group 2	No. of Patients	Mean Age (yr)	Mean Lesion Size (cm^2)	Lesion Location
Saris et al[25]	Autologous chondrocyte implantation	Microfracture	118	33.9	Range, 2.4-2.6	Medial and lateral femoral condyles
Knutsen et al[7]	Autologous chondrocyte implantation	Microfracture	80	Not reported	Not reported	89% medial femoral condyle; 11% lateral femoral condyle
Gudas et al[8]	Osteochondral autograft transplantation	Microfracture	60	24.3	2.8	84% medial femoral condyle, 16% lateral femoral condyle
Knutsen et al[26]	Autologous chondrocyte implantation	Microfracture	80	32.2	4.8	89% medial femoral condyle; 11% lateral femoral condyle

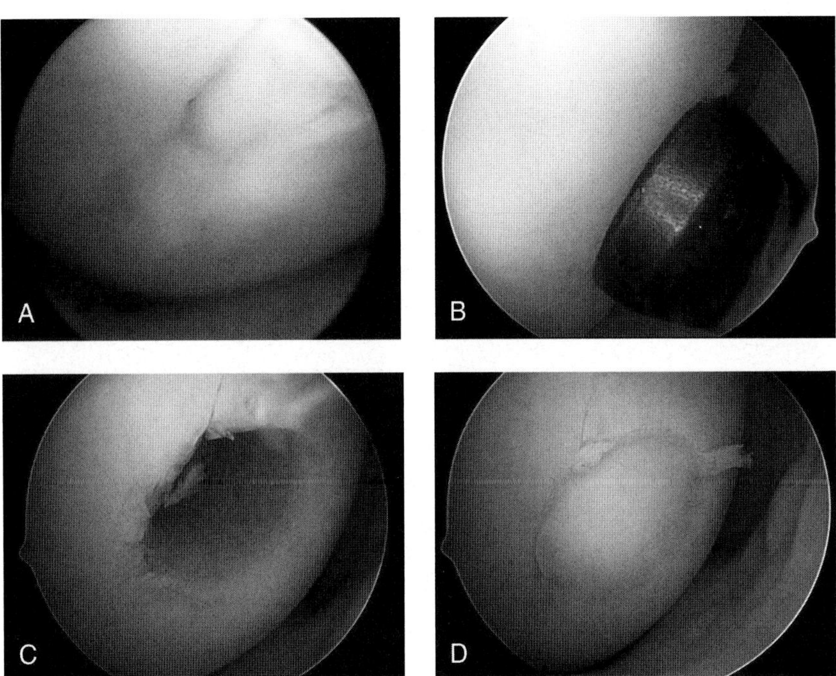

Figure 5 Osteochondral autograft transplantation. **A,** Identification of the lesion on the medial femoral condyle. **B,** A sizer is used to determine the number and size of the autografts. In this case, the lesion measured 8 mm in diameter. **C,** An 8-mm plug was harvested. **D,** The donor plug position should be flush with the surrounding articular cartilage.

the articular surface to create well-defined vertical walls in the recipient socket because this facilitates congruent plug placement (Figure 5, *C*). The donor plug is placed over the recipient site and gently advanced into the defect, where it is often left slightly proud. The chondrocytes can be damaged during impaction; therefore, it is critical to avoid high loads when inserting the graft.[13] The final plug position should be flush with the surrounding articular cartilage (Figure 5, *D*). Postoperatively, patients are protected from weight bearing for 6 weeks and use a continuous passive motion machine 6 hours per day.

Hangody and Kárpáti[14] evaluated the survival of the transplanted hyaline cartilage. The graft undergoes osseous incorporation to the subchondral bone while the transplanted cartilage integrates with the adjacent host articular cartilage with fibrocartilage. Recently, Hangody and associates[11] evaluated clinical outcomes at a mean of 14 years after 1,097 osteochondral autograft transplantation procedures. Encouraging results in this large multicenter series support the use of this technique for the treatment of small and medium focal chondral and osteochondral defects of the knee. The osteochondral autograft transplanta-

Table 1 *(continued)*
Demographic Data and Outcomes in Studies Comparing Microfracture With Other Cartilage Restoration Procedures

Mean Duration of Follow-up	Clinical Outcome	Histologic Findings	Additional Findings
18 months	Improvement in both groups; no significant difference	Better structural repair in autologous chondrocyte implantation group	
5 years	77% good clinical results in both groups; no significant difference	No significant difference	Younger patients did better in both groups
HSS score significantly superior in osteochondral autograft transplantation group ($P < 0.01$)	100% hyaline cartilage in osteochondral autograft transplantation group; 57% fibrocartilage, 43% fibroelastic tissue in microfracture group	Patients < 30 years old had better clinical scores; HSS scores better for traumatic lesions than osteochondritis dissecans lesions; HSS scores lower for lesions of > 2 cm^2 in microfracture group	
2 years	SF-36 score significantly superior in microfracture group	No significant difference in the percent of fibrocartilage tissue	Patients < 30 years old had better outcomes; SF-36 scores higher for lesions of < 4 cm^2 in microfracture group

HSS = Hospital for Special Surgery; SF-36 = Medical Outcomes Study 36-Item Short Form

tion procedure has been compared with other cartilage restoration procedures (Table 2).

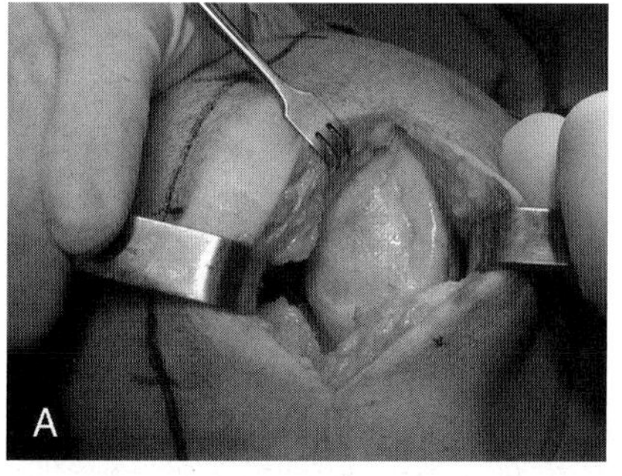

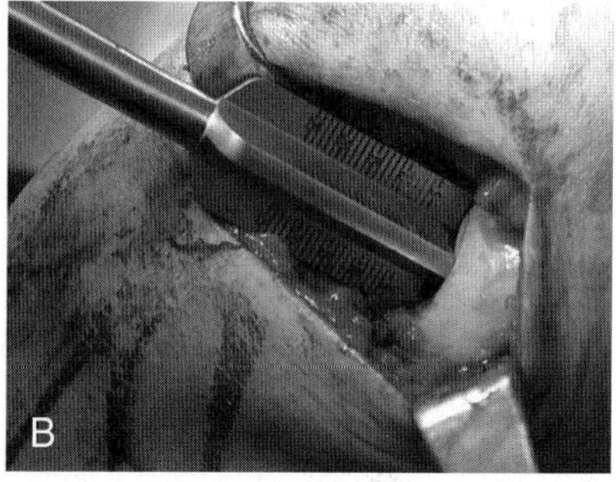

Figure 6 Osteochondral allograft transplantation. **A,** The procedure is typically performed through a small arthrotomy to expose the lesion. **B,** A reamer is used to convert the defect to a circular recipient socket with a uniform depth of 6 to 8 mm.

Osteochondral Allograft Transplantation

Osteochondral allograft transplantation provides an option for treatment of larger lesions (> 2.5 cm^2) or those with substantial bone loss. It is normally a second-line treatment option but can be a first-line treatment of high-demand patients with large lesions.

Osteochondral allograft transplantation can be used to resurface large, deep defects with mature hyaline articular cartilage while also filling any underlying osseous defect. Tissue matching and immunosuppression are not necessary because the transplanted chondrocytes are isolated by the cartilage matrix and not exposed to the host immune surveillance.[15] The allografts can be fresh or frozen. Fresh grafts are normally maintained at 4°C in standard or enriched culture medium for no more than 28 days, which allows chondrocytes to survive after transplantation. Frozen allografts are maintained at −40°C for years. The fresh allografts elicit a minimal immune response, the chondrocytes survive, and the bone is successfully revascularized.[16-18]

Allograft transplantation can be done arthroscopically; however, it is more often performed through a small arthrotomy. The allograft is slowly warmed from 4°C to 37°C by placing it in normal saline solution at room temperature. The slow warming minimizes damage to the graft.[19] The lesion is sized with a template, and a correspondingly sized reamer is used to convert the defect to a circular recipient socket with a uniform depth of 6 to 8 mm (Figure 6). This bone depth facilitates graft implantation and limits the amount of immunogenic donor bone that is implanted. A sterile marking pen is used to mark the 12 o'clock position of the lesion to orient the donor plug appropriately. An instrumentation system is used to size and harvest a cylindrical plug from the allograft (Figure 7). The donor graft is drilled through its entire depth with

Table 2
Demographic Data and Outcomes in Studies of Osteochondral Autograft Transplantation

Author(s)	Group 1	Group 2 (or 2 and 3)	No. of Patients	Mean Age (yr)	Mean Lesion Size (cm²)
Hangody et al[11]	Osteochondral autograft transplantation	—	1,097	36	Not reported
Marcacci et al[27]	Osteochondral autograft transplantation	—	30	29.3	< 2.5
Gobbi et al[6]	Osteochondral autograft transplantation	Microfracture; chondroplasty	32	Osteochondral autograft transplantation: 27; microfracture: 24; chondroplasty: 32	Osteochondral autograft transplantation: 4; microfracture: 4.5; chondroplasty: 3.7
Dozin et al[28]	Débride then autologous chondrocyte implantation	Débride then osteochondral autograft transplantation	47	Autologous chondrocyte implantation: 29; osteochondral autograft transplantation: 27	Autologous chondrocyte implantation: 1.97; osteochondral autograft transplantation: 1.88
Bentley et al[29]	Osteochondral autograft transplantation	Autologous chondrocyte implantation	100	31.3	4.66

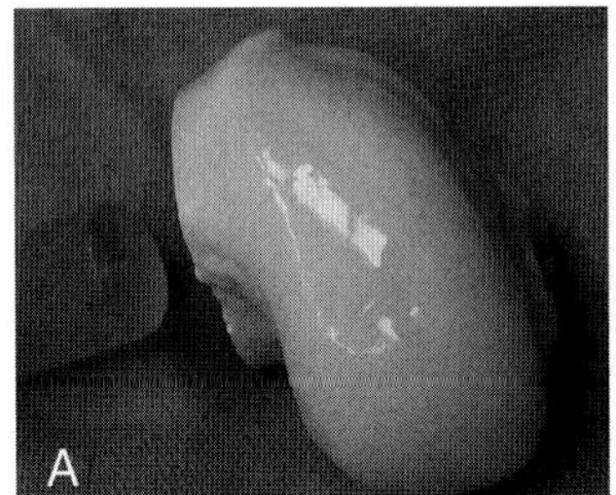

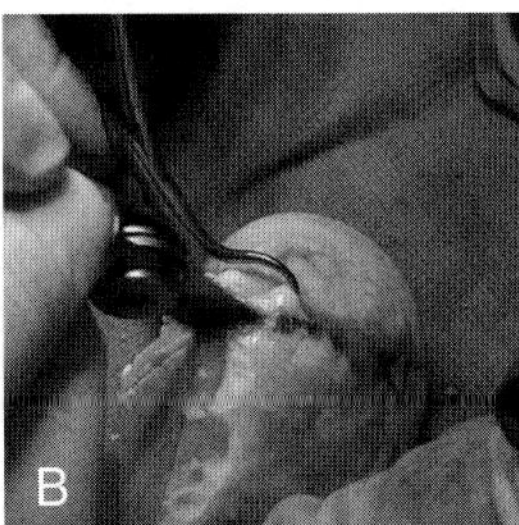

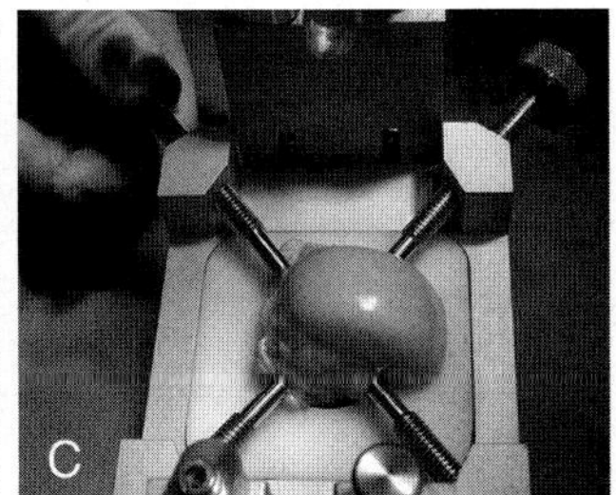

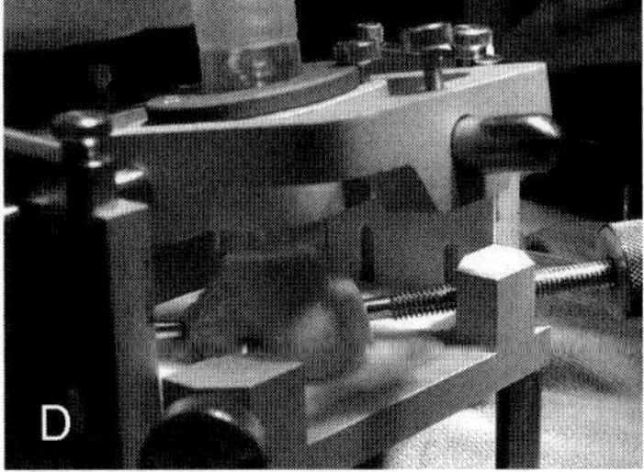

Figure 7 Osteochondral allograft transplantation. **A,** Fresh donor femoral condyle. **B,** The condyle is trimmed to create a flat surface to place on the workstation. This cut is made parallel to the potential harvest site. **C,** Condyle securely fixed to the workstation. **D,** Graft template placed on the condyle to match the bottom of the recipient site.

a harvester under irrigation with normal saline solution. The graft is extracted, and a ruler is used to measure and mark the four quadrants of the graft at the depth of the previously measured recipient sites. Before insertion, pulsatile lavage (approximately 2 L) is used to remove the residual blood and bone marrow elements from the allograft to reduce the risk of disease transmission and graft immunogenicity. The graft is then press-fit into the socket by hand after careful alignment of the four quadrants to the recipient site (Figure 8). If the implanted allograft is particularly large, fixation may be augmented with bioabsorbable or metal compression screws.

Postoperatively, weight bearing is limited to toe-touch for the first 6 weeks. Patients with a patellofemoral graft are allowed to bear weight as tolerated in extension and generally

Table 2 *(continued)*
Demographic Data and Outcomes in Studies of Osteochondral Autograft Transplantation

Lesion Location	Mean Duration of Follow- up	Clinical Outcome	Histologic Findings	Additional Findings
798 femoral condyle, 147 patellofemoral, 31 tibia, 98 talus, 8 capitellum, 3 humeral head, 11 femoral head	14 years	Rate of good-to-excellent. results: 92% for femoral condylar implantation, 87% for tibial resurfacings, 74% for patellar and/or trochlear mosaicplasties, 93% for talar procedures	Graft survival in 81 of 98	Comorbidities should be assessed; postoperative bleeding from donor site—prevention with donor site biodegradable plugs
Medial and lateral femoral condyles	Range, 2-7 years	77% good clinical results	Not performed	MRI showed good integration and survival of graft in 60%
Talus	54 months	No clinical difference among three treatment groups	Not performed	Results of microfracture and osteochondral autograft transplantation better for small lesions
Autologous chondrocyte implantation: 73% femoral condyle, 27% patella; osteochondral autograft transplantation: 68% femoral condyle; 32% patella		Complete recovery in 88% of mosaicplasty group and 68% of autologous chondrocyte implantation group ($P = 0.093$)	Not performed	14 patients improved significantly with débridement
53% medial femoral condyle; 18% lateral femoral condyle; 25% patella; 3% trochlea; 1% tibial plateau	19 months	Modified Cincinnati score > 55 for 88% of autologous chondrocyte implantation group and 74% of osteochondral autograft transplantation group	74% with hyaline-like or fibrocartilage tissue in autologous chondrocyte implantation group; not reported for osteochondral autograft transplantation group	Technique documented placing plugs slightly prominently

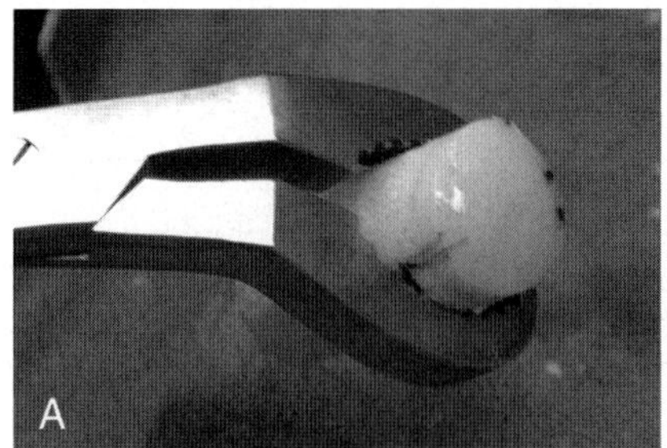

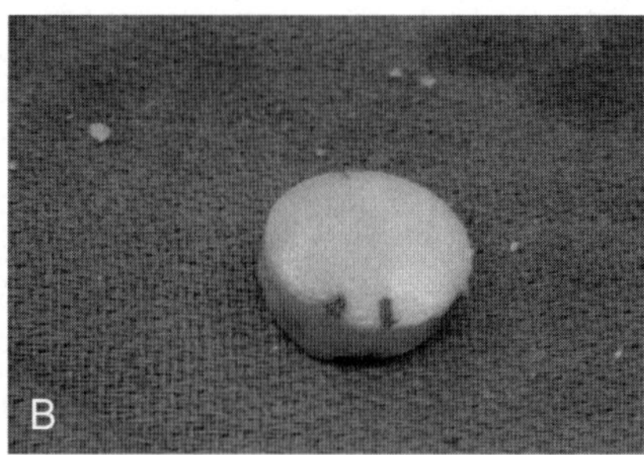

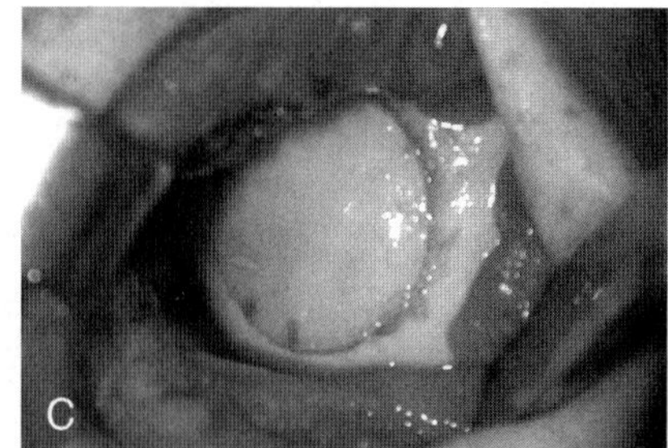

Figure 8 Osteochondral allograft transplantation. **A,** After removal of the plug, depth measurement markings are made on the graft to match the measurements of the recipient socket in four quadrants. **B,** Matching of the donor plug. The depth of bone should be limited to 8 to 10 mm to facilitate graft implantation and limit the amount of immunogenic donor bone that is implanted. **C,** The graft is press-fit into the socket by hand after careful alignment of the four quadrants to the recipient site. The graft is flush with the recipient articular surface.

are limited to 45° of flexion during the first 4 weeks. Continuous passive motion is used immediately after the surgery. A return to normal activities of daily living and light sports activity is considered at 8 to 12 months.

Video 18.1: Osteochondral Allograft Transplantation. Brian J. Cole, MD, MBA (13 min)

Subjective improvement can be expected in 75% to 85% of patients after osteochondral allograft implantation for properly selected chondral lesions[4,20] (Table 3).

Table 3
Demographic Data and Outcomes in Studies of Osteochondral Allograft Transplantation

Author(s)	Type of Osteochondral Allograft	Mean Age (yr)	Type of Study	No. of Patients	Lesion Location
Gross et al[30]	Failed fresh	47	Histologic	69	Knee (exact location not specified)
Davidson et al[31]	Fresh	32	Clinical, histologic, MRI	8 (10 knees)	6 medial femoral condyle, 2 trochlea, 2 medial femoral condyle and trochlea
McCulloch et al[32]	Fresh	35	Clinical, radiographic	25	Femoral condyle
Jamali et al[33]	Fresh patellofemoral	28	Clinical, radiographic	18	Patellofemoral
Gross et al[4]	Fresh	27	Clinical outcome	60	30 medial femoral condyle; 30 lateral femoral condyle

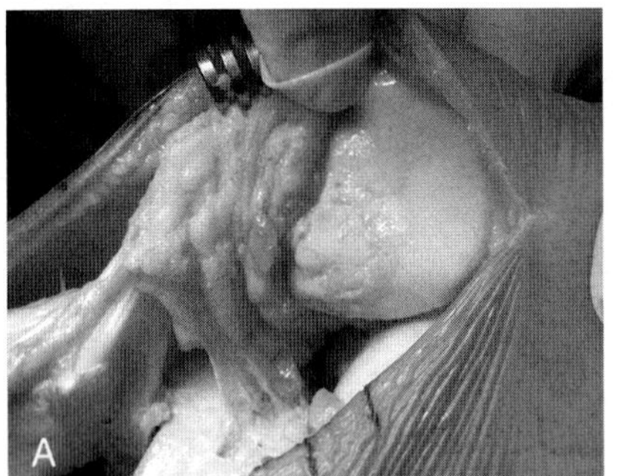

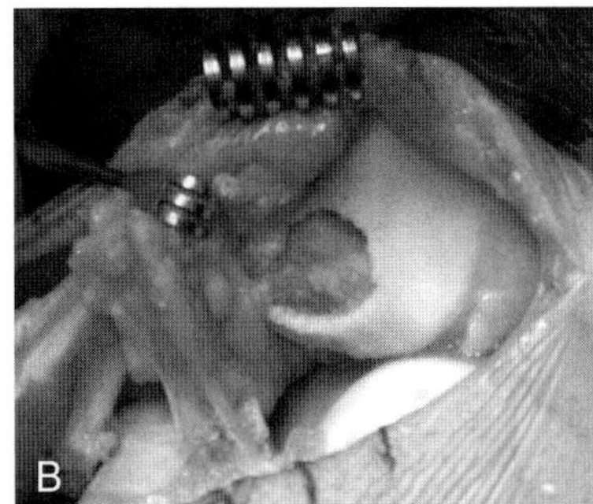

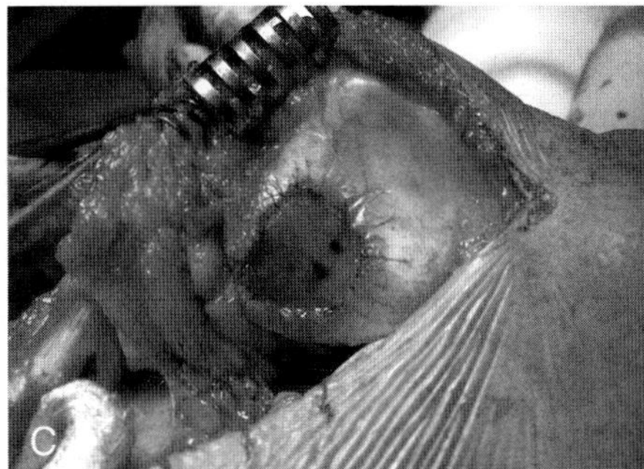

Figure 9 Autologous chondrocyte implantation. **A,** A chondral lesion in the patella. **B,** Preparation of the defect. **C,** After the chondrocytes are delivered, the gap is closed with suture and fibrin glue.

Autologous Chondrocyte Implantation

Autologous chondrocyte implantation is ideal for symptomatic, unipolar, well-contained chondral or osteochondral defects measuring between 2 and 10 cm^2 with bone loss of less than 6 to 8 mm. It is typically a second-line treatment after at least arthroscopic débridement has been performed.

The first stage of autologous chondrocyte implantation is an arthroscopic evaluation of the size and depth of the focal chondral lesion and a cartilage biopsy. The total volume of the biopsied material should be approximately 200 to 300 mg. The second stage is implantation of the cells. This is done usually no sooner than 6 weeks after the biopsy. At the time of implantation, the defect is prepared by removing any existing fibrocartilage down to the underlying calcified layer. Vertical walls are created at the periphery of the lesion with use of a combination of a No. 15 blade and sharp ring curets. After débridement, the tourniquet, if used, should be deflated, and complete hemostasis should be obtained. The use of cotton pledgets soaked with epinephrine may help to obtain hemostasis (Figure 9).

Next, a periosteal patch is harvested from the proximal-medial part of the tibia, just distal to the pes anserinus insertion, through a separate incision. The patch should be at least 2 mm larger than the defect. The patch edges are detached with a No. 15 scalpel blade and elevated with a sharp, curved periosteal elevator, beginning distally. Synthetic collagen-membrane substitutes are

Table 3 *(continued)*
Demographic Data and Outcomes in Studies of Osteochondral Allograft Transplantation

Mean Duration of Follow-up	Outcome	Additional Findings
< 1, 2-5, > 5 years	Cartilage: viable chondrocytes, normal matrix and structure in middle and deep layers Bone: creeping substitution	
40 months	Clinical: improvements in SF-36, IKDC, Tegner, Lysholm scores (*P* < 0.05) Histologic: cellular density and viability similar in host and donor cartilage MRI: improvement in Outerbridge score	Prevention of short-term degenerative changes
3 years	Clinical: improvements in Lysholm, IKDC, KOOS, SF-12 scores (*P* < 0.05); 84% of patients satisfied Radiographic: 88% had graft incorporation	Patients with uncorrected malalignment did worse; clinical results did not deteriorate with increasing age of graft
94 months	Clinical: 5 failures; good results in 60% Radiographic: no signs of patellofemoral arthrosis in 10 of 12	No patellofemoral bone alignment procedures performed
10 years	Survival: 95% at 5 years, 85% at 10 years, 65% at 15 years	Comorbidities should be assessed and corrected in same procedure

IKDC = International Knee Documentation Committee; KOOS = Knee Injury and Osteoarthritis Outcome Score; SF-12 = Medical Outcomes Study 12-Item Short Form; SF-36 = Medical Outcomes Study 36-Item Short Form

commercially available (Chondro-Gide; Geistlich Biomaterials, Wolhusen, Switzerland) and can be used as a substitute for the periosteal patch. The use of these scaffolds not only reduces operating time but also has been shown to avoid typical problems related to the periosteum.[21]

The patch or scaffold is then sewn to the cartilage. When periosteum is used, the cambium layer is placed toward the lesion. With the Chondro-Gide scaffold, the porous surface should be placed toward the lesion with the smooth side facing out. Sutures (6-0 polyglactin [Vicryl; Ethicon, Somerville, NJ]) are first passed into the patch approximately 2 mm from the edge and then passed through the cartilage at a depth of 2 to 3 mm below the cartilage surface. Sutures should be placed approximately 4 mm apart, and a gap should be maintained in the upper edge to allow chondrocyte implantation (Figure 10). The edges of the patch are sealed with fibrin glue, and a water tightness test is performed with an 18-gauge angiocatheter. The chondrocytes are then delivered through the opening with use of an angiocatheter. After the cells have been implanted, the opening gap is closed with suture and fibrin glue (Figure 9, *C*).

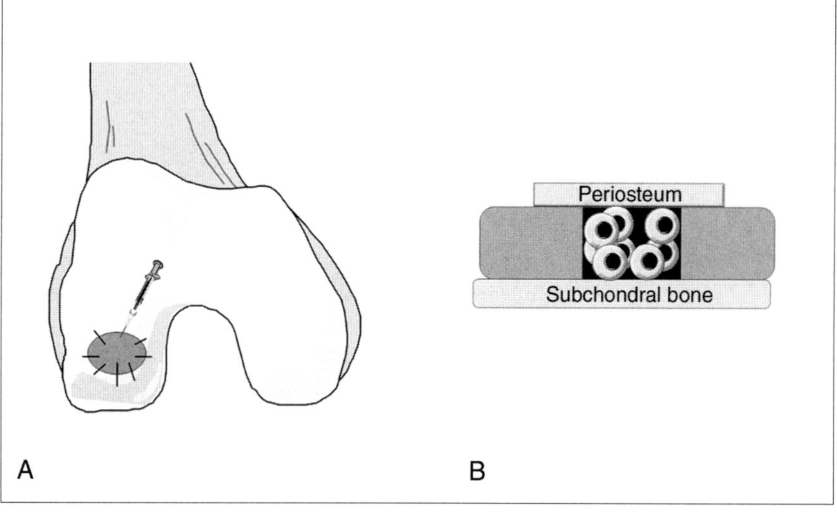

Figure 10 Illustration of autologous chondrocyte implantation. **A,** Injection of the chondrocytes under the upper edge of the patch. The cells should be injected slowly. **B,** A periosteal patch with the cambium layer facing down into the defect is carefully sutured onto the top of the defect. Chondrocytes are injected into the contained defect.

Postoperatively, patients with a femoral condyle lesion do not bear weight and use a continuous passive

Table 4
Demographic Data and Clinical Outcomes in Studies of Autologous Chondrocyte Implantation

Author(s)	No. of Patients	Mean Age (yr)	Mean Lesion Size (cm²)
Zaslav et al[34]	126 with autologous chondrocyte implantation after other failed cartilage procedures (multicenter study)	34.5	4.63
Rosenberger et al[35]	56; 50% with concomitant osteotomies	48.6 (range, 45-60); all > 45	4.7 (range, 1-15.0)
Mandelbaum et al[36]	40	Range, 16-48	4.5
Kreuz et al[37]	118 with isolated chondral lesion	35 (range, 18-50)	
Knutsen et al[7]	40 with autologous chondrocyte implantation, 40 with microfracture		
Steinwachs and Kreuz[38]	63	34	

motion machine. Patients with a patellofemoral lesion are permitted full weight bearing with the knee in extension. Continuous passive motion for 6 to 8 hours per day at one cycle per minute is used for 6 weeks after the surgery. A return to normal activities of daily living and sports activities is allowed 6 months after the surgery.

Video 18.2: Autologous Chondrocyte Implantation. Brian J. Cole, MD, MBA (8 min)

It is estimated that autologous chondrocyte implantation has been performed in more than 10,000 patients worldwide. The procedure has better results when it is done for lesions in the femoral condyle or in patients with a patellofemoral lesion who are undergoing a concomitant realignment procedure.[22-24] There have been several studies comparing autologous chondrocyte implantation with other biologic reconstructive procedures (Table 4).

Summary

Articular cartilage defects of the knee are common. Treatment options range from palliative (débridement) to reparative (marrow stimulation) to restorative (osteochondral grafting and autologous chondrocyte implantation). All of these techniques improve the clinical status compared with the preoperative state. Decision making is done case by case and is guided by the patient's physical and physiologic demand level, previous failed treatment, and the location and size of the defect. It is critical that the surgeon also consider what subsequent treatment options might be necessary should the first-line treatment fail to relieve the symptoms.

References

1. Maletius W, Messner K: The effect of partial meniscectomy on the long-term prognosis of knees with localized, severe chondral damage: A twelve- to fifteen-year followup. *Am J Sports Med* 1996;24:258-262.

2. Rue JP, Yanke AB, Busam ML, McNickle AG, Cole BJ: Prospective evaluation of concurrent meniscus transplantation and articular cartilage repair: Minimum 2-year follow-up. *Am J Sports Med* 2008;36:1770-1778.

3. Farr J: Autologous chondrocyte implantation improves patellofemoral cartilage treatment outcomes. *Clin Orthop Relat Res* 2007;463:187-194.

4. Gross AE, Shasha N, Aubin P: Long-term followup of the use of fresh osteochondral allografts for posttraumatic knee defects. *Clin Orthop Relat Res* 2005;435:79-87.

5. Shapiro F, Koide S, Glimcher MJ: Cell origin and differentiation in the repair of full-thickness defects of ar-

Table 4 *(continued)*
Demographic Data and Clinical Outcomes in Studies of Autologous Chondrocyte Implantation

Lesion Location	Mean Duration of Follow-up	Outcome
102 (67%) medial femoral condyle; 27 (18%) lateral femoral condyle; 24 (16%) trochlea	48 months	76% were treatment successes; no difference between results of marrow stimulating procedure and débridement at primary surgery; mean improvements in Cincinnati, VAS, and SF-36 scores from baseline to all time points ($P < 0.001$)
	4.7 years (range, 2-11 years)	8 failures (14%); additional arthroscopic procedures required in 24 patients (43%) for periosteal-related problems and adhesions; 88% of these patients had lasting improvement, 78% felt improved, 81% would again choose autologous chondrocyte implantation as a treatment option
Trochlea	59 ± 18 months	Significant improvement in Cincinnati score, overall condition (3.1 points preoperatively to 6.4 points postoperatively), pain (2.6 to 6.2 points), swelling (3.9 to 6.3 points); no failed implantations
78 femoral condyle; 17 trochlea; 23 patella	Clinical and MRI evaluation at 6, 18, and 36 months	Patients with regular (1-3 times/week) or competitive (4-7 times/week) sports involvement had significantly better ICRS and Cincinnati scores than patients with no or rare sports involvement ($P < 0.01$); correlation between sports activity levels and clinical scores significant (increasing from 6 to 18 months, 18 to 36 months postoperatively)
89% medial femoral condyle; 11% lateral femoral condyle	2 years	77% good clinical results in both groups; no significant difference between groups; younger patients did better in each group
Femoral condyle, trochlea, patella	6, 18, and 36 months	Evaluation of autologous chondrocyte implantation with type I/III collagen membrane; significant improvement in ICRS and modified Cincinnati scores ($P < 0.01$); graft hypertrophy can be avoided by using a collagen membrane

VAS = visual analog scale, SF-36 = Medical Outcomes Study 36-Item Short Form;, ICRS = International Cartilage Repair Society

ticular cartilage. *J Bone Joint Surg Am* 1993;75:532-553.

6. Gobbi A, Francisco RA, Lubowitz JH, Allegra F, Canata G: Osteochondral lesions of the talus: Randomized controlled trial comparing chondroplasty, microfracture, and osteochondral autograft transplantation. *Arthroscopy* 2006;22:1085-1092.
7. Knutsen G, Drogset JO, Engebretsen L, et al: A randomized trial comparing autologous chondrocyte implantation with microfracture: Findings at five years. *J Bone Joint Surg Am* 2007;89:2105-2112.
8. Gudas R, Kalesinskas RJ, Kimtys V, et al: A prospective randomized clinical study of mosaic osteochondral autologous transplantation versus microfracture for the treatment of osteochondral defects in the knee joint in young athletes. *Arthroscopy* 2005;21:1066-1075.
9. Kreuz PC, Steinwachs MR, Erggelet C, et al: Results after microfracture of full-thickness chondral defects in different compartments in the knee. *Osteoarthritis Cartilage* 2006;14:1119-1125.
10. Hangody L, Ráthonyi GK, Duska Z, Vásárhelyi G, Füles P, Módis L: Autologous osteochondral mosaicplasty: Surgical technique. *J Bone Joint Surg Am* 2004;86:65-72.
11. Hangody L, Vásárhelyi G, Hangody LR, et al: Autologous osteochondral grafting: Technique and long-term results. *Injury* 2008;39: S32-S39.
12. Braun S, Minzlaff P, Hollweck R, Wörtler K, Imhoff AB: The 5.5-year results of megaOATS: Autologous transfer of the posterior femoral condyle. A case-series study. *Arthritis Res Ther* 2008;10:R68.
13. Pylawka TK, Wimmer M, Cole BJ, Virdi AS, Williams JM: Impaction affects cell viability in osteochondral tissues during transplantation. *J Knee Surg* 2007;20:105-110.
14. Hangody L, Kárpáti Z: New possibilities in the management of severe circumscribed cartilage damage in the knee. *Magy Traumatol Ortop Kezseb Plasztikai Seb* 1994;37:237-243.
15. Czitrom AA, Keating S, Gross AE: The viability of articular cartilage in fresh osteochondral allografts after clinical transplantation. *J Bone Joint Surg Am* 1990;72:574-581.
16. Acosta CA, Izal I, Ripalda P, Forriol F: Cell viability and protein composition in cryopreserved cartilage. *Clin Orthop Relat Res* 2007;460:234-239.
17. Williams JM, Virdi AS, Pylawka TK, Edwards RB III , Markel MD, Cole BJ: Prolonged-fresh preservation of intact whole canine femoral condyles for the potential use as osteochondral allografts. *J Orthop Res* 2005;23:831-837.
18. Pearsall AW IV, Tucker JA, Hester RB, Heitman RJ: Chondrocyte viability in refrigerated osteochondral allografts used for transplantation within the knee. *Am J Sports Med* 2004;32:125-131.

19. Pylawka TK, Virdi AS, Cole BJ, Williams JM: Reversal of suppressed metabolism in prolonged cold preserved cartilage. *J Orthop Res* 2008;26: 247-254.

20. Muscolo DL, Ayerza MA, Aponte-Tinao LA, Abalo E, Farfalli G: Unicondylar osteoarticular allografts of the knee. *J Bone Joint Surg Am* 2007; 89:2137-2142.

21. Haddo O, Mahroof S, Higgs D, et al: The use of chondrogide membrane in autologous chondrocyte implantation. *Knee* 2004;11:51-55.

22. Brittberg M, Lindahl A, Nilsson A, Ohlsson C, Isaksson O, Peterson L: Treatment of deep cartilage defects in the knee with autologous chondrocyte transplantation. *N Engl J Med* 1994;331:889-895.

23. Peterson L, Minas T, Brittberg M, Nilsson A, Sjögren-Jansson E, Lindahl A: Two- to 9-year outcome after autologous chondrocyte transplantation of the knee. *Clin Orthop Relat Res* 2000;374:212-234.

24. Peterson L, Brittberg M, Kiviranta I, Akerlund EL, Lindahl A: Autologous chondrocyte transplantation: Biomechanics and long-term durability. *Am J Sports Med* 2002;30:2-12.

25. Saris DB, Vanlauwe J, Victor J, et al: Characterized chondrocyte implantation results in better structural repair when treating symptomatic cartilage defects of the knee in a randomized controlled trial versus microfracture. *Am J Sports Med* 2008;36:235-246.

26. Knutsen G, Engebretsen L, Ludvigsen TC, et al: Autologous chondrocyte implantation compared with microfracture in the knee: A randomized trial. *J Bone Joint Surg Am* 2004; 86:455-464.

27. Marcacci M, Kon E, Delcogliano M, Filardo G, Busacca M, Zaffagnini S: Arthroscopic autologous osteochondral grafting for cartilage defects of the knee: Prospective study results at a minimum 7-year follow-up. *Am J Sports Med* 2007;35:2014-2021.

28. Dozin B, Malpeli M, Cancedda R, et al: Comparative evaluation of autologous chondrocyte implantation and mosaicplasty: A multicentered randomized clinical trial. *Clin J Sport Med* 2005;15:220-226.

29. Bentley G, Biant LC, Carrington RW, et al: A prospective, randomised comparison of autologous chondrocyte implantation versus mosaicplasty for osteochondral defects in the knee. *J Bone Joint Surg Br* 2003;85: 223-230.

30. Gross AE, Kim W, Las Heras F, Backstein D, Safir O, Pritzker KP: Fresh osteochondral allografts for posttraumatic knee defects: Long-term followup. *Clin Orthop Relat Res* 2008; 466:1863-1870.

31. Davidson PA, Rivenburgh DW, Dawson PE, Rozin R: Clinical, histologic, and radiographic outcomes of distal femoral resurfacing with hypothermically stored osteoarticular allografts. *Am J Sports Med* 2007;35: 1082-1090.

32. McCulloch PC, Kang RW, Sobhy MH, Hayden JK, Cole BJ: Prospective evaluation of prolonged fresh osteochondral allograft transplantation of the femoral condyle: Minimum 2-year follow-up. *Am J Sports Med* 2007;35:411-420.

33. Jamali AA, Emmerson BC, Chung C, Convery FR, Bugbee WD: Fresh osteochondral allografts: Results in the patellofemoral joint. *Clin Orthop Relat Res* 2005;437:176-185.

34. Zaslav K, Cole B, Brewster R, et al: A prospective study of autologous chondrocyte implantation in patients with failed prior treatment for articular cartilage defect of the knee: Results of the Study of the Treatment of Articular Repair (STAR) clinical trial. *Am J Sports Med* 2009;37:42-55.

35. Rosenberger RE, Gomoll AH, Bryant T, Minas T: Repair of large chondral defects of the knee with autologous chondrocyte implantation in patients 45 years or older. *Am J Sports Med* 2008;36:2336-2344.

36. Mandelbaum B, Browne JE, Fu F, et al: Treatment outcomes of autologous chondrocyte implantation for full-thickness articular cartilage defects of the trochlea. *Am J Sports Med* 2007;35:915-921.

37. Kreuz PC, Steinwachs M, Erggelet C, et al: Importance of sports in cartilage regeneration after autologous chondrocyte implantation: A prospective study with a 3-year follow-up. *Am J Sports Med* 2007;35:1261-1268.

38. Steinwachs M, Kreuz PC: Autologous chondrocyte implantation in chondral defects of the knee with a type I/III collagen membrane: A prospective study with a 3-year follow-up. *Arthroscopy* 2007;23:381-387.

Video References

18.1: Cole BJ: Video. Osteochondral allograft transplantation, in Cole BJ, ed: *Surgical Techniques in Orthopaedics: Cartilage Restoration of the Knee.* DVD. Rosemont, IL, American Academy of Ortho paedic Surgeons, 2003.

18.2: Cole BJ: Video. Autologous chondrocyte implantation, in Cole BJ, ed: *Surgical Techniques in Orthopaedics: Cartilage Restoration of the Knee.* DVD. Rosemont, IL, American Academy of Orthopaedic Surgeons, 2003.

Patellar Instability

Daniel E. Redziniak, MD
David R. Diduch, MD
William M. Mihalko, MD, PhD
John P. Fulkerson, MD
Wendy M. Novicoff, PhD
Shahin Sheibani-Rad, MD
Khaled J. Saleh, MD, MSc, FRCSC

Abstract

Patellar instability is a generic term that is used to describe patellar dislocation, patellar subluxation, and general symptomatic instability. Patellofemoral instability is a relatively difficult condition to treat; accurate management of the condition should take into account the anatomy of the joint and its stabilizing structures. The goal of any treatment should be to restore the normal anatomy of the joint. It is important to understand the basic anatomy and biomechanics of this condition, the classification of different types of patellar instability, varying presentations, and diagnostic techniques and criteria, including the types of imaging studies that can be useful in determining the ultimate course of treatment.

Instr Course Lect 2010;59:195-206.

Dr. Diduch or an immediate family member has received royalties from Arthrocare; has received research or institutional support from Mitek and Zimmer; and has stock or stock options held in Arthrocare. Dr. Mihalko or an immediate family member has received royalties from Elsevier; is a member of a speakers' bureau or has made paid presentations on behalf of Ethicon and Aesculap/B. Braun; serves as a paid consultant to or is an employee of Aesculap/B. Braun, Ethicon, Johnson & Johnson, and Stryker; and has received research or institutional support from the Journal of Bone and Joint Surgery–American, *Smith & Nephew, and Aesculap/B. Braun. Dr. Fulkerson, or an immediate family member serves as a board member, owner, officer, or committee member of the American Board of Orthopaedic Surgery, the American Orthopaedic Association, the American Orthopaedic Society for Sports Medicine, the Arthroscopy Association of North America, the International Society of Arthroscopy, Knee Surgery, and Orthopaedic Sports Medicine, and the Orthopaedic Research and Education Foundation; has received royalties from Arthrex, DJ Orthopaedics, and Lippincott; serves as an unpaid consultant to DJ Orthopaedics and the Musculoskeletal Transplant Foundation; has received research or institutional support from Kinamed; has stock or stock options held in DJ Orthopaedics; and has received nonincome support (such as equipment or services), commercially derived honoraria, or other non–research-related funding (such as paid travel) from SLACK Incorporated. Dr. Novicoff or an immediate family member has received research or institutional support from Aesculap/B. Braun, DePuy, Smith & Nephew, Stryker, and Zimmer. Dr. Saleh or an immediate family member has received royalties from Smith & Nephew; is a member of a speakers' bureau or has made paid presentations on behalf of Aesculap/B. Braun, Stryker, OMNI, and Kimberly Clark; serves as a paid consultant to or is an employee of Aesculap/B. Braun, Stryker, and OMNI; has received research or institutional support from the* Journal of Bone and Joint Surgery–American, *Stryker, EKR Therapeutics, and Aesculap/B. Braun; and has received nonincome support (such as equipment or services), commercially derived honoraria, or other non–research-related funding (such as paid travel) from Blue Cross Blue Shield and Kimberly Clark. Neither of the following authors or a member of their immediate families has received anything of value from or owns stock in a commercial company or institution related directly or indirectly to the subject of this chapter: Dr. Redziniak, and Dr. Sheibani-Rad.*

Patellar instability is a generic term that describes patellar dislocation, patellar subluxation, and general symptomatic patellar instability.[1] It is estimated that patellar instability affects between 7 and 49 people per 100,000.[2,3] It accounts for 11% of the musculoskeletal symptoms seen in the office setting as well as 16% to 25% of all injuries in runners. There is a higher incidence in females.[4]

Anatomy and Biomechanics

Understanding the functional anatomy and basic mechanics of the patellofemoral joint will help the clinician to comprehend how instability occurs and how the described treatments can help stabilize the joint. In full extension, the patella is typically not engaged in the trochlear groove. Once motion is initiated in early flexion, only the distal part of the patellar articular surface is in contact with the superior aspect of the trochlear groove. Appropriate engagement of the trochlea is important for the stability of the patellofemoral joint. The quadriceps functions as a dy-

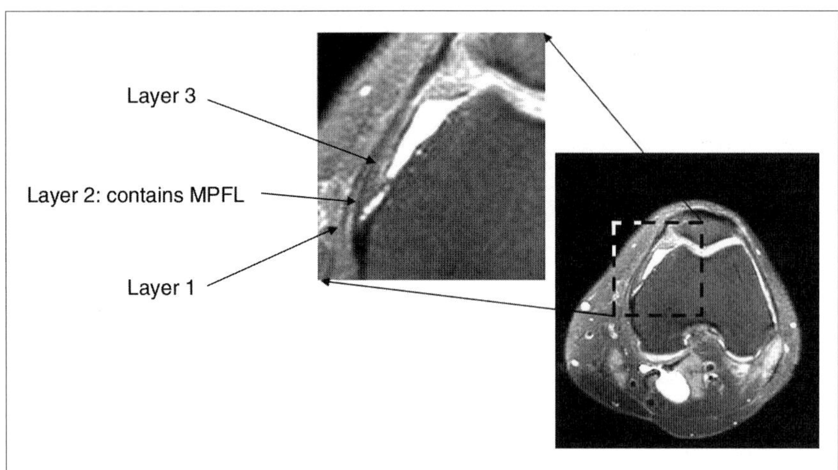

Figure 1 T2-weighted MRIs of the knee with the medial soft-tissue sleeve enhanced to reveal the three anatomic layers. MPFL = medial patellofemoral ligament.

namic stabilizer of the patella within the trochlear groove, and the medial patellofemoral ligament is the primary static soft-tissue restraint to lateral patellar translation. When engaged in the trochlear groove, the patella is held in place by both the soft-tissue tension of the medial soft-tissue sleeve of the knee and the lateral aspect of the trochlea. As flexion increases, the contact area of the patella moves proximally until 90° of flexion, at which point the proximal pole is in contact with the distal aspect of the trochlear groove. In this position of knee flexion, the patella is more deeply engaged in the trochlear groove, and increasing flexion further causes the medial facet to articulate with the lateral edge of the medial femoral condyle and the lateral facet to articulate with the medial edge of the lateral femoral condyle.[5,6] Most knees have a third patellar facet, which is a small area of the medial border of the patella that engages the lateral aspect of the medial femoral condyle past 90° of flexion. After flexion is initiated, the patella typically lags in flexion within the sagittal plane by 30° to 40° compared with the tibiofemoral flexion angle.

The medial patellofemoral ligament is an important structure for patellofemoral stability. Warren and Marshall[7] described the medial anatomy of the knee as being a three-layered system (Figure 1). The superficial layer includes the deep crural fascia, which also incorporates the fascia over the vastus medialis. The second layer includes the superficial fibers of the medial collateral ligament and blending of the fibers of the posterior oblique ligament on the medial side of the knee. It is in this layer that the medial patellofemoral ligament is located. The deepest layer includes the knee capsule and the deep fibers of the medial collateral ligament as well as the meniscotibial and meniscofemoral ligament structures. The medial patellofemoral ligament is a medial structure that inserts on the superomedial border of the patella approximately 6 mm below the superior pole. Its origin is along the entire height of the anterior aspect of the medial femoral epicondyle. The structure has been reported in numerous studies as having an average length of between 5 and 6 cm (53 to 57 mm on the average, with standard deviations of 4 to 5 mm).[8-10] The medial patellofemoral ligament has been reported to have connections to the undersurface of the vastus medialis obliquus on its superior border in the second layer of the medial aspect of the knee as well. Its patellar attachment is typically broader than its origin on the anterior aspect of the medial epicondyle. The medial patellofemoral ligament has been reported to provide more than 50% of the medial restraint forces to the patella during testing in cadaver models.[11-13] The anatomic and mechanical attributes of the medial patellofemoral ligament listed above have generated the attention that the ligament has been afforded in the literature over the past few years.

Classification of Patellar Instability

Patellar malalignment is a rotational or translational deviation of the patella. The movements of the patellofemoral joint are complex.[6] The traditional classification of patellar instability includes congenital, traumatic, habitual, obligatory, subluxation, and dislocation. The classification by Dejour and associates is based on clinical symptoms[14] (Table 1).

Etiology

The etiology of patellar instability is multifactorial (Table 2). Structural and functional imbalance of the patellofemoral joint leads to chronic instability and secondary flattening, or dysplasia, of the lateral part of the trochlea. This dysplasia and patella alta both reduce the containment of the patella within the femoral trochlea, a problem that is aggravated by underlying structural and functional imbalance. The consequence is that the patella is not securely engaged at the start of flexion, causing it to slip laterally. As flexion continues, it either dislocates completely or slips back medially to its correct position.

Imbalance and secondary osseous and retinacular adaptive dysplasia result in the lateral subluxation of the patella from the intercondylar groove. When the tibial tubercle is lateral to the long axis of the femur and the quadriceps muscle, the patella is subjected to laterally directed forces. Other aggravating factors, in some patients, are vastus medialis insufficiency and joint laxity.

Table 1
Classification of Patellar Instability as Described by Dejour and Associates

Major patellar instability	More than one documented dislocation
Objective patellar instability	One dislocation with associated anatomic abnormality
Potential patellar instability	Patellar pain with associated radiographic abnormalities

Presentation and History

Patients with patellar instability sometimes experience anterior knee pain, but episodes of collapsing or shifting in the knee are more prominent. A common clue is the feeling of the knee "giving way" or "going out." It should be determined whether symptoms began with a sudden traumatic event. Previous treatment and the patient's response to that treatment should be noted. If treatment was unsuccessful, it is essential to determine whether the failure was caused by an incorrect diagnosis, inappropriate treatment, poor patient compliance, or instability that exceeded the effectiveness of nonsurgical treatment.

Physical Examination

The patella is best examined with the patient flexing the knee to determine if the patella engages smoothly at the proximal end of the trochlea or more distally than normal. This also demonstrates whether knee flexion is restricted by tight structures or obstructed by an osteochondral fragment broken off during patellar dislocation. A thorough ligamentous examination is necessary to rule out concomitant cruciate or collateral ligament tears. It is not uncommon to confuse the symptoms of a torn anterior cruciate ligament with those of patellar instability. Medial collateral ligament injuries also commonly occur at the time of patellar dislocation. The examiner should identify the area of maximal tenderness along the course of the medial patellofemoral ligament, which usually identifies the location of the injury.

Patellar stability is assessed by the examiner pushing the patella laterally while flexing the knee. The medial patellofemoral ligament is palpated to establish if it is doing its normal job of pulling the patella into the trochlea during the first 20° of knee flexion. The examiner holds the relaxed knee in 20° to 30° of flexion while subluxating the patella laterally. If the patient is apprehensive during this maneuver, the test is considered to be positive. The patient will report pain and resist further lateral motion of the patella, and the examiner can assess the degree of medial patellofemoral ligament deficiency. If the patient continues to have symptoms following surgery, the examiner should repeat this maneuver by holding the patella medially while flexing the knee to re-create a medial subluxation (relocation from medial to lateral) and noting whether this elicits any apprehension. Patients with patellar instability experience medial to lateral shifting of the patella and have very sudden giving way, which may be mistaken for lateral subluxation.

Table 2
Etiology of Patellar Instability

Patella alta
Trochlear dysplasia
Dysplasia of lateral femoral condyle
Defective lateral trochlear margin
Shallow trochlear groove
Vastus medialis obliquus insufficiency
Joint laxity
Trauma
Previous surgery
Tight lateral structures (for example, lateral retinaculum and iliotibial band)

The quadriceps (Q) angle is defined as the angle between lines joining the anterior superior iliac spine, the center of the patella, and the tibial tubercle. It is normally between 8° and 10° in males and between 15° and 20° in females; however, some authors believe that there is no sex difference in the Q angle if the angle measurement is normalized for height. The factors that increase the Q angle are external tibial torsion, a laterally positioned tibial tuberosity, genu valgum, and increased femoral anteversion. Any factor increasing the Q angle increases the laterally directed force on the extensor mechanism, predisposing the patella to instability.

The patellar grind test is performed by directly applying pressure to the patella and manually displacing it medially, laterally, superiorly,

Table 3
Surgical Techniques for Patellar Instability

Proximal malalignment	Primary repair of medial patellofemoral ligament, medial imbrication and advancement of vastus medialis obliquus, lateral retinacular release, reconstruction of medial patellofemoral ligament
Distal malalignment	Anteromedial tibial tubercle transfer, tibial osteotomy

and inferiorly in the trochlear groove. When there is a pathologic patellofemoral condition, this test reproduces anterior knee pain.

The patellar tilt test is done with the patient lying supine and the knee in 20° of flexion. The examiner holds the patella between the thumb and index finger and pushes the patella down in an attempt to flip its lateral edge upward. Elevation of the lateral aspect of the patella to less than neutral suggests an abnormal result, whereas 0° to 20° of elevation is normal. Limited upward movements indicate an excessively tight lateral retinaculum.

Imaging

Radiographs

The AP radiograph is of limited use. Occasionally, an osteochondral fracture of the medial patellar edge or loose bodies can be seen. The patellar height can be measured on the lateral radiograph. The Blackburne-Peel index relates the length of the articular surface of the patella to the distance of its inferior margin from the tibial plateau; it ranges from 0.85 to 1.09 in men and from 0.79 to 1.09 in women.[15] The index provides a useful measure of the relationship of the patella to the trochlea. Alternatively, the Insall-Salvati index can be used.[16] This index compares the diagonal length of the patella with the length of the patellar tendon and ranges from 0.9 to 1.1 in men and from 0.94 to 1.18 in women. However, the measurement has limitations because the length of the patella is not always an indication of the length of its articular surface.

Computed Tomography Scans

Patellar tilt is measured on a CT scan obtained with the knee in full extension with use of a line drawn through the posterior femoral condyles as the reference line and the long axis of the patella as the measurement line. The normal angle is less than 20°.[17] Inoue and associates[18] found that, with the knee extended, the lateral tilt of the patella was more pronounced in patients who had patellar subluxation than it was in a control group.

The tibial tubercle-trochlear groove distance is also determined on the CT scan but with the knee flexed 90°. This is a measurement of the offset of the tubercle relative to the true trochlear groove and is more accurate than the Q angle. With the knee flexed 90°, the tibial tubercle should lie less than 20 mm lateral to the midline of the femur at the proximal edge of the femoral condyles. Values of 20 mm or greater are considered abnormal.[19]

Magnetic Resonance Imaging

MRI is also used to evaluate the patella. Sallay and associates[20] demonstrated that a rupture of the medial patellofemoral ligament is visible on both sagittal and axial T2-weighted images. The characteristic bone bruise on the medial facet of the patella and the lateral femoral condyle in patients who have recently sustained a patellar dislocation can be seen on MRI, and MRI is also very useful for detecting an osteochondral fracture, which is an indication for early surgical intervention.

Nonsurgical Management

Patellar instability can often be treated successfully without surgery. Ideal rehabilitation requires the avoidance of pain during exercise. Stretching and strengthening are used. Although strengthening of the quadriceps muscle and the vastus medialis obliquus is the initial management of many patients, stretching of the lateral retinaculum, hamstrings, quadriceps, Achilles tendon, and iliotibial band should also be performed. Physical therapy should include closed-chain exercises and strengthening of the vastus medialis obliquus (the main dynamic stabilizer of the knee). Establishing proper core stability and functional alignment of the lower extremity is important. Weight loss is another way to reduce patellofemoral loads. Other methods include the use of a patellar brace to modify the position of the patella, patellar taping to pull the patella away from a painful area, use of an orthotic device in the shoe when a patient has excessive foot pronation, and use of analgesic medications.

Surgical Management

If there is no clinical improvement with nonsurgical management, surgical treatment may be indicated. There are widely differing views regarding the correction of malalignment. The operation must be selected with respect to the patient's age and level of activity, as well as the condition of the joint. The traditional view has focused on two types of procedures: proximal realignment and distal realignment (Table 3). Trochleoplasty is rarely indicated, particularly in young patients, as the long-term consequences of this procedure are not known.

The purpose of proximal realignment procedures is to alter the medial-lateral position of the patella by manipulating the soft tissues—most importantly, the medial patellofemoral ligament—proximal to the inferior patellar pole. Distal realignment procedures modify the position of the patella by the transfer of the tibial tuberosity.

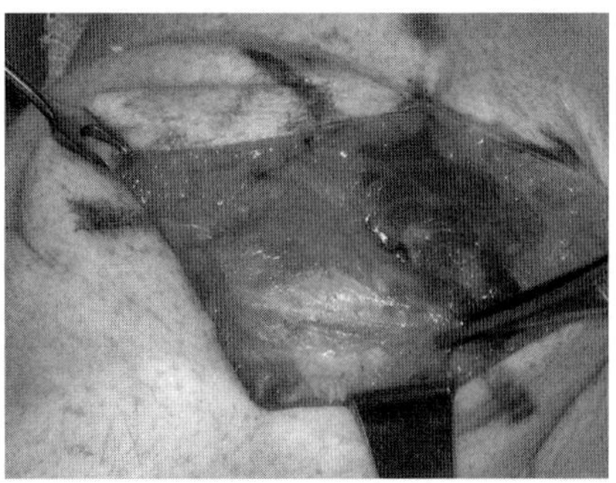

Figure 2 The medial patellofemoral ligament has been localized deep to the vastus medialis obliquus. Traction is applied to determine its point of disruption.

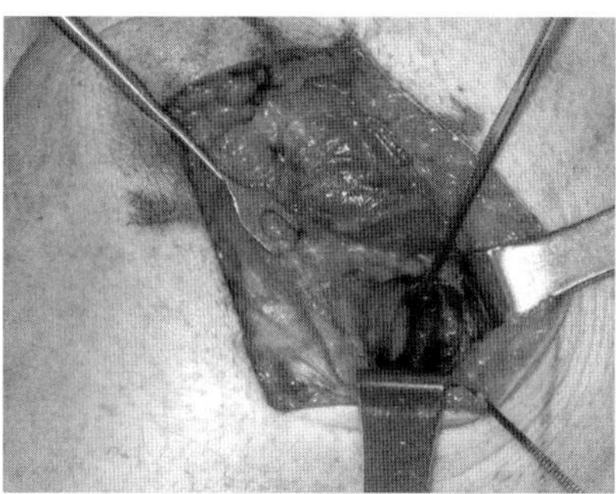

Figure 3 A longitudinal incision in the deep fascia and periosteum is used to expose the origin of the medial patellofemoral ligament for the placement of two suture anchors.

Proximal Repair and Realignment Procedures

To decide whether a proximal realignment is appropriate, it is important to determine whether the patellar instability is caused by a deficiency of the medial patellar stabilizers or whether the primary problem is abnormal alignment. Often the two problems coexist. If the patient has malalignment, then proximal realignment procedures alone may not be successful in restoring patellar stability. Myers and associates[21] pointed out that proximal realignment does not work well in patients with patellofemoral pain and should be reserved for patients who have sustained a dislocation and require stabilization. When proximal realignment is selected as a treatment option, the surgeon should assess the medial patellofemoral ligament and retinaculum and decide if a primary repair of the medial patellofemoral ligament is indicated, or medial imbrication is sufficient, or if a reconstruction of the medial patellofemoral ligament with use of a tendon graft should be undertaken. The surgical treatment of patellar instability should be individualized.

Primary Repair of the Medial Patellofemoral Ligament

For repair of the medial patellofemoral ligament, a horizontal incision is made parallel to the medial patellofemoral ligament, starting anterior to the medial epicondyle and extending toward the proximal-medial part of the patella. The vastus medialis obliquus-investing fascia is then incised parallel to the skin incision, and the edge of the vastus medialis obliquus is elevated to reveal the deep surface of the medial patellofemoral ligament in its anatomic orientation just distal to the vastus medialis obliquus (Figure 2). With use of this technique, the medial patellofemoral ligament can be palpated in its entirety, and its point of disruption can be identified.[22] To assist in identifying the medial patellofemoral ligament, traction is applied to the ligament and patellar stability is checked. This technique also allows determination of the location of the injury to the medial patellofemoral ligament. If the medial patellofemoral ligament is torn off of the patella, stability cannot be established with longitudinal traction parallel to the medial patellofemoral ligament. In these cases, which are limited in number, the medial patellofemoral ligament is repaired back to the patella with the use of nonabsorbable sutures placed through drill holes in the patella as needed.

Most commonly, the medial patellofemoral ligament is torn from its origin on the medial epicondyle. For primary repair, a longitudinal incision is made in the deep fascia and periosteum just anterior and superior to the medial epicondyle to expose the osseous origin. The medial patellofemoral ligament is generally more palpable than it is directly visible as a thickening in the medial retinaculum. Lateral patellar translation is checked as the forceps is used to stabilize the medial patellofemoral ligament to ensure that the appropriate tissue is incorporated in the repair. Two suture anchors are then placed into the femur at the origin of the medial patellofemoral ligament, and the repair is performed with the knee in 30° to 45° of flexion (Figure 3). Mattress sutures are used to advance and secure the medial patellofemoral ligament to its osseous origin in this position (Figure 4). In cases in which the tissue is attenuated, and the origin and insertion sites of the medial patellofemoral ligament are intact, an imbrication of the medial patellofemoral ligament is performed (Figure 5). The optimal physiometric position is confirmed by moving

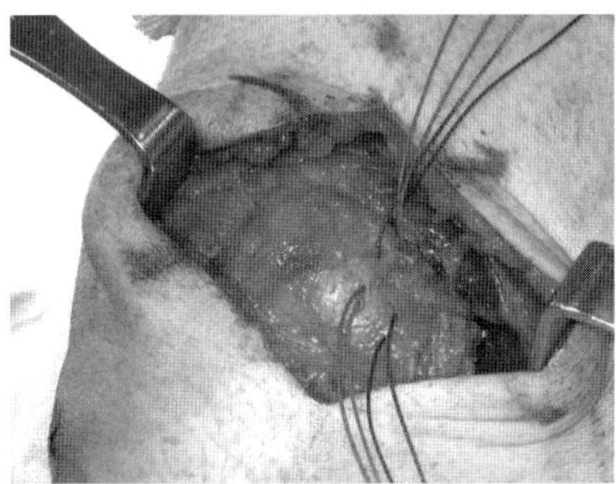

Figure 4 Horizontal mattress sutures are placed through the medial patellofemoral ligament and the medial retinaculum.

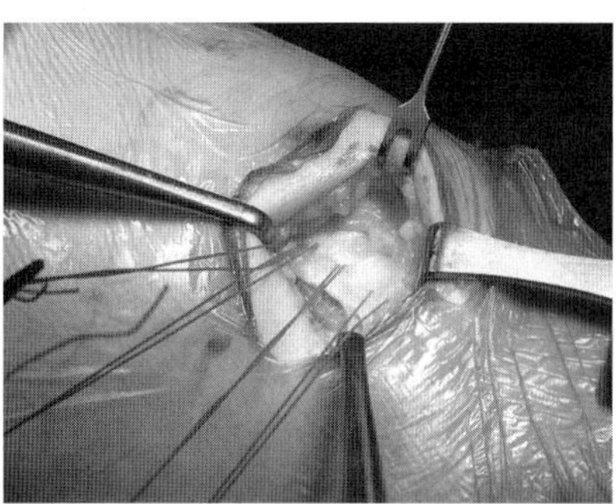

Figure 5 In cases in which the medial patellofemoral ligament and medial retinaculum are attenuated, imbricating sutures are used to tighten the medial structures.

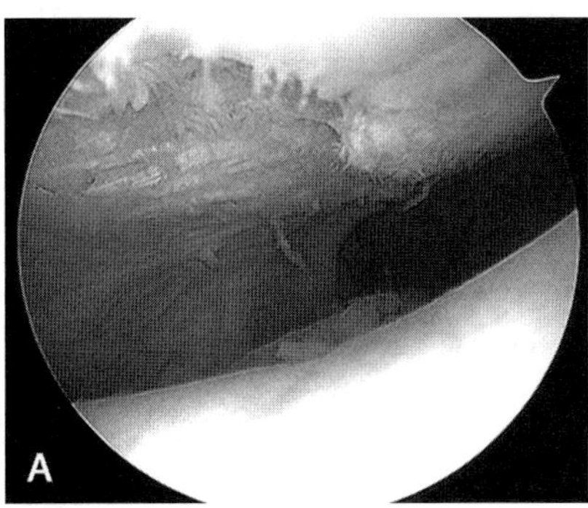

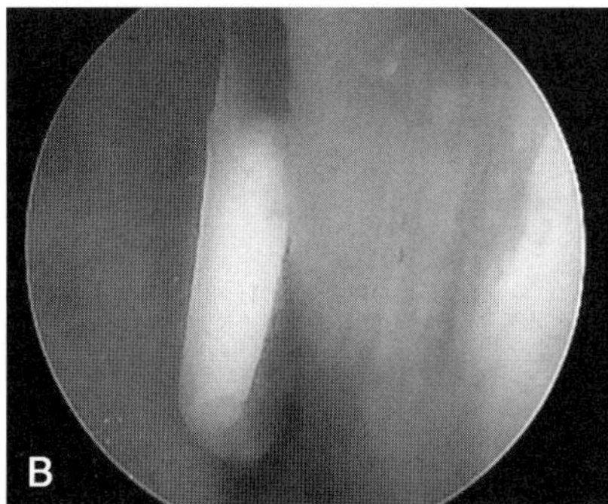

Figure 6 **A** and **B**, Arthroscopic images showing a primary patellar dislocation with a medial patellar facet injury and an associated osteochondral loose body.

the knee through a range of motion. The investing fascia is repaired before skin closure. After the repair has been performed, patellar tracking is assessed and a firm end point to lateral patellar displacement should be appreciated. Postoperatively, a hinged knee brace is applied to allow 50% weight bearing and a range of motion of 0° to 30°, which is advanced in 30° increments every 2 weeks. Use of the brace and crutches is discontinued by 6 weeks postoperatively. Progressive quadriceps-strengthening exercises are advanced, with a return to sports activities usually after 3 months.

In an ongoing study at one institution, 12 patients (14 knees) who had undergone repair of the medial patellofemoral ligament had an average International Knee Documentation Committee (IKDC) score of 75.1 points and a mean Kujala patellofemoral subjective evaluation score of 80 points (maximum, 100 points) at a mean of 45 months (range, 20 to 75 months) postoperatively.[23] The scores on the Tegner activity scale[24] were 6.0 points before the surgery and 6.9 points after the surgery, indicating that patients were able to resume activity at a level that was at least the same as their preoperative level. The visual analog score showed good pain relief, with an average score of 1.2 points (on a 10-point scale) after the procedure. Two patients had an episode of subluxation postoperatively, but there were no recurrent dislocations and no patient required revision surgery. Although the patients had completed the postoperative physical therapy program and had returned to sports activities, side-to-side comparison of quadriceps muscle function showed an average 35% deficit in the strength of the repaired knee during contraction in a more flexed position (at 60°). In addition, there was an average 63% reduction in quadriceps activity of the vastus medialis obliquus on electromyography.

Repair of the medial patellofemoral ligament currently is recommended for patients with chronic recurrent patellar instability following failed nonsurgical treatment or those with acute patellar instability and a loose osteochondral fragment following dislocation (Figure 6). Diagnostic arthroscopy is done first to address any associated intra-articular pathologic conditions and to visualize patellar tracking. Occasionally, the point of disruption of the medial patellofemoral ligament can be visualized arthroscopically (Figure 7). If a tibial tubercle osteotomy is to be performed, it is done before the repair of the medial patellofemoral ligament to allow the surgeon to obtain correct tensioning of that ligament after the transfer of the tuberosity.

Reconstruction of the Medial Patellofemoral Ligament

Indications for reconstruction of the medial patellofemoral ligament include lateral patellar instability secondary to laxity of the medial patellar stabilizers with or without trochlear dysplasia. As is the case with primary repair, this procedure should be done to treat patellar instability, not to correct malalignment or to treat patellofemoral arthritis. Overtightening of the graft

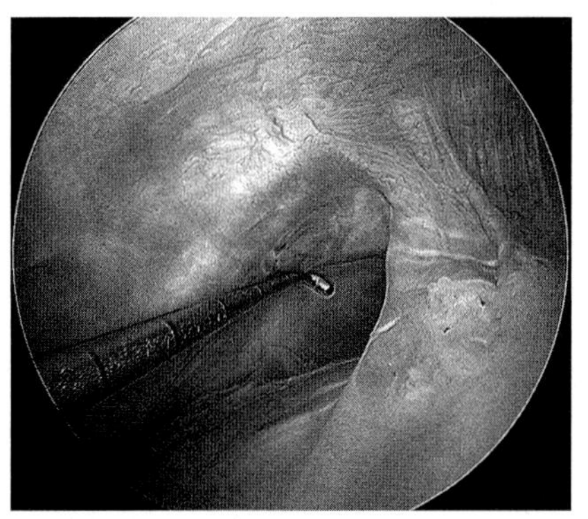

Figure 7 Intra-articular view of the medial patellofemoral ligament torn from its femoral origin.

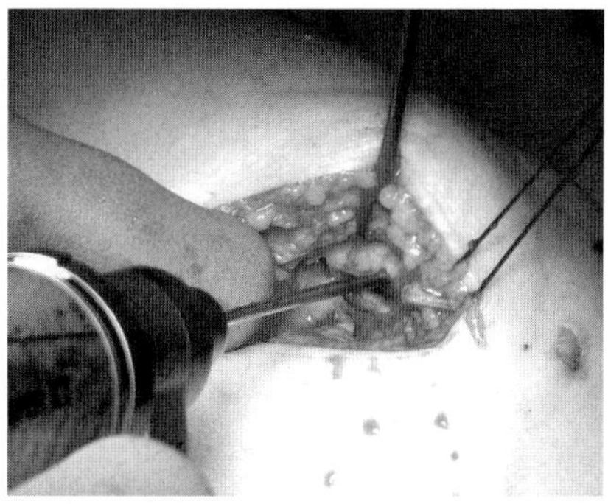

Figure 8 A Beath pin is drilled through the proximal third of the patella at the insertion of the medial patellofemoral ligament.

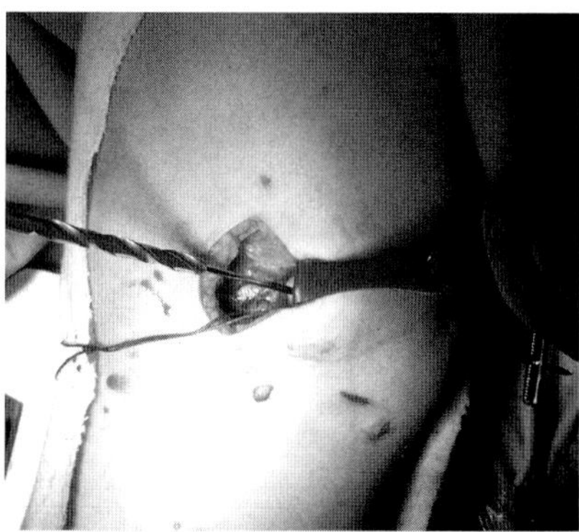

Figure 9 The patellar tunnel is drilled to a size sufficient to allow passage of the graft and the EndoButton.

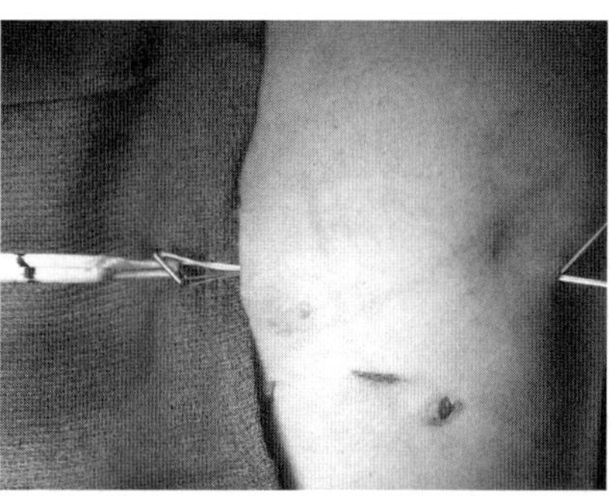

Figure 10 The Beath pin is used to pass the graft and the EndoButton through the patellar tunnel.

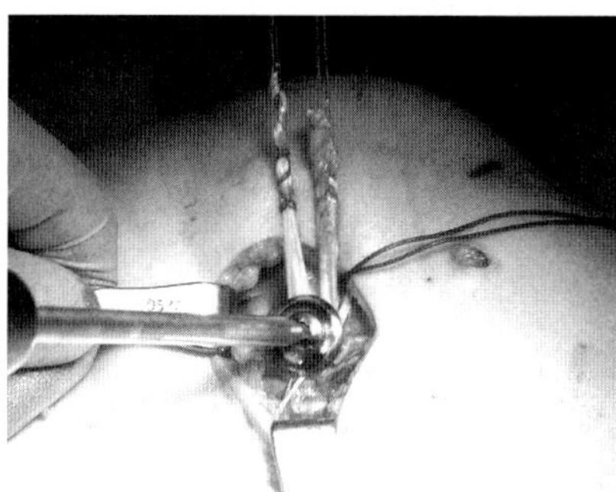

Figure 11 A 6.5-mm screw and washer are then applied for femoral fixation with the knee in 30° to 45° of flexion.

will result in an overconstrained patella that is painful, perhaps leading to arthritis caused by increased joint contact forces.[25]

Use of a soft-tissue graft such as an ipsilateral hamstring tendon is especially helpful when the medial patellofemoral ligament is deficient or attenuated, as it often is in patients with chronic instability, in revisions, and in association with a congenital dislocation. A variety of graft sources is available for reconstruction of the medial patellofemoral ligament. The semitendinosus tendon, which is near the reconstruction site and easy to harvest, is preferable to use. The tendon is doubled over and is measured with a tunnel sizer. A closed-loop EndoButton fixation device (Smith & Nephew Endoscopy, Andover, MA) is used for patellar fixation. The exposure of the medial patellofemoral ligament is the same as that described above. A Beath pin is drilled from medial to lateral in the midportion of the medial patellofemoral ligament insertion on the patella, which is located in the proximal third of the patella (Figure 8). The pin is then carefully advanced to the lateral edge of the patella without violating the anterior cortex or the articular surface. Lateral fluoroscopy is used to confirm appropriate positioning of the pin. The patellar tunnel is then drilled with the appropriately sized cannulated drill bit to the depth required to flip the EndoButton (Figure 9). The Beath pin is used to pull the graft through the patellar tunnel, and the previously placed sutures are used to flip the EndoButton so that it sits flush along the lateral side of the patella (Figure 10). The position of the EndoButton is confirmed fluoroscopically. The location of the medial patellofemoral ligament is identified, a Beath pin is drilled just anterior to the medial epicondyle, and its location is confirmed fluoroscopically. The graft is wrapped around the Beath pin, allowing an assessment of graft isometry as the knee is brought through a full range of motion. The pin is then overdrilled with a 4.5-mm cannulated drill bit to the appropriate depth, which is verified fluoroscopically. A 6.5-mm screw and washer are then used for femoral fixation with the knee in 30° to 45° of flexion (Figure 11).

Alternatively, to minimize the risk of patellar fracture caused by the transosseous graft tunnel, the graft can be placed into a shorter tunnel and fixed with a soft-tissue interference screw, such as the Biotenodesis screw (Arthrex, Naples, FL). Farr and Schepsis[26] used semitendinosus autograft or allograft with Biotenodesis screw fixation on the femur and either Biotenodesis screw fixation or suture-anchor fixation on the patella. Suture-anchor fixation on the patella eliminates the complication of a patellar fracture associated with the transosseous tunnel.

Multiple techniques have been described for reconstruction of the medial patellofemoral ligament, and they all differ with regard to graft choice and fixation method.[26-32] They are all designed to reestablish the checkrein against lateral patellar motion. The medial patellofemoral ligament is most important during the first 30° to 45° of knee flexion, during which it allows the patella to engage the trochlea properly. Increased flexion causes the medial patellofemoral ligament to relax as the trochlear anatomy provides stability to the patellofemoral joint. After graft fixation is obtained, the knee should be examined to ensure that there is a full range of motion with a good end point to lateral translation in full extension and at 30° of flexion. When the surgeon is tensioning the medial patellofemoral ligament graft, it should tighten only on lateral patellar translation.[25] Obtaining the appropriate amount of tension in the reconstruction guarantees that the patella is not overconstrained. It is extremely important to not overtighten the medial structures and constrain patellofemoral motion, regardless of the realignment procedure that is chosen. Elias and Cosgarea[33] showed that small errors in graft length and position in medial patellofemoral ligament reconstructions involving the use of a hamstring autograft can dramatically increase the force and pressure applied to the medial patellofemoral cartilage.

Another important step during a reconstruction of the medial patellofemoral ligament is placement of the femoral attachment. The origin of the medial patellofemoral ligament is located on the ridge between the adductor tubercle and the medial femoral epicondyle.[34] When the femoral fixation is too proximal, the medial patellar facet can become overloaded with increasing flexion. When the femoral fixation is too distal, the medial patellofemoral ligament can become inappropriately tight in extension and prevent the patella from engaging the trochlea correctly. The principle of isometry enables the graft and the trochlea to function in tandem to allow the patella to enter the trochlea smoothly at about 30° to 45° of knee flexion. Placement of guidewires to secure a length of suture as the knee is moved through a range of motion can help to determine isometry before drilling of the graft tunnels. In addition, fluoroscopic images can be helpful to confirm graft placement on the femur and to prevent violation of the patellar articular surface. When these principles have been strictly followed, reconstruction of the medial patellofemoral ligament has been found to have good results at up to 5 years postoperatively.[26,29,31,32,35-37] After surgery, a hinged knee brace is applied to allow 50% weight bearing and a range of motion of 0° to 30°, which is advanced in 30° increments every 2 weeks. Use of the brace and crutches is discontinued by 6 weeks after the surgery. Progressive quadriceps-strengthening exercises are advanced, with return to sports activities usually after 3 months.

Because of a high prevalence of medial articular lesions after dislocation, caution must be exercised when performing a reconstruction of the medial patellofemoral ligament, with a need to consider the location of the articular lesions in the design of the procedure. There is a risk that the reconstruction of the medial patellofemoral ligament will add a load to a medial articular lesion. According to Myers and associates,[21] this procedure should be reserved for patients who have sustained a dislocation and require stabilization. In the opinion of one of the authors (JPF), reconstruction of the medial patellofemoral ligament with a tendon graft should be reserved for patients with more severe dysplasia (in whom the procedure is often combined with tibial tubercle transfer), a grossly deficient medial structure with failure of the medial patellofemoral ligament to heal, or generalized laxity and for salvage following a failed imbrication of the medial patellofemoral ligament in patients with a normal tibial tubercle-trochlear groove index. One alternative for medial patellofemoral ligament reconstruction is to completely avoid drilling into the patella and pass the tendon graft deep to the vastus medialis obliquus tendon and through it at its patellar attachment site, suturing the patellar side of the graft to the vastus medialis obliquus tendon and also to the quadriceps tendon immediately above (Figure 12).

Medial Imbrication and Vastus Medialis Obliquus Advancement

Insall and associates[38] initially described an extensive medial imbrication procedure. After exposure of the quadriceps mechanism, two incisions are made. The first incision is a medial parapatellar arthrotomy that passes over the medial quarter of the patella. The second is a lateral release extending just distal to the fibers of the vastus lateralis. Realignment is performed by advancing the medial flap containing the vastus medialis obliquus laterally and distally in the line of the fibers of the vastus medialis. After suturing, the incision lies in a straight line across the front of the patella, and the lateral release should be left open. Insall and associates[39] reported a 91% rate of good or excellent results at 48 months following the performance of this procedure to treat symptoms of recurrent patellar subluxation in 53 knees. Hughston and Walsh[40] recommended isolated proximal realignment in patients with instability when the Q angle is less than 10° and the addition of medialization of the tibial tubercle when the angle is more than 10°. This strategy resulted in a 71% rate of good or excellent results. The extensive medial imbrication described by Insall and associates[39] is not used as frequently now because it is more likely to cause abnormal contact stresses in the patellofemoral joint and to be followed by postoperative stiffness. Nam and Karzel[41] described a less invasive surgical technique that included a mini-open medial reefing and an arthroscopic lateral release for the treatment of patellar dislocation. Of 23 knees that were treated with this procedure, 1 had recurrent dislocation and 1 had subluxation at a mean of 4.4 years postoperatively. The redislocation rate compared favorably with that following use of traditional, more extensile open approaches. The authors concluded that the mini-open technique provides anatomic restoration with limited morbidity and cosmetically appealing results.

Many methods of realigning the patella have been described. Most techniques for proximal realignment involve an open medial reefing or advancement of the vastus medialis obliquus. A less extensive imbrication of the medial retinaculum may also be accomplished arthroscopically. Ali and Bhatti[42] reported a 78% rate of good or excellent results at a mean of 51 months after arthroscopic proximal realignment. With this technique, spinal needles are used to pass a series of sutures medial to the patella; the sutures are subsequently retrieved under the skin and tied to plicate the medial retinaculum in a nonspecific fashion. Halbrecht[43] described a similar technique, in which the medial imbrication was performed by percutaneous passage of sutures followed by knot tying inside the joint, thus eliminating the need for extra incisions. All patients also had a lateral release. At 2 years postoperatively, 93% of their 26 patients reported substantial subjective improvement with no redislocations. Whether the imbrication is open or arthroscopic, the goal is to rebalance the patella within the trochlea without overtightening the medial structures, which ultimately would increase patellar contact pressures. The main feature of this surgery is reestablishing the proper length and tension of the medial patellofemoral ligament.

Lateral Retinacular Release

Historically, a lateral retinacular release was added to a medial stabilization procedure in the treatment of lateral patellar instability. The release was performed because it was believed that a tight lateral retinaculum was a predisposing factor for lateral patellar instability. More recently, indications have been refined, and a lateral release is considered to be appropriate only for patients with a tight retinaculum and patellar tilt.[42-46] This phenomenon is associated with lateral patellar compression syndrome, as originally described by Ficat and associates[47]

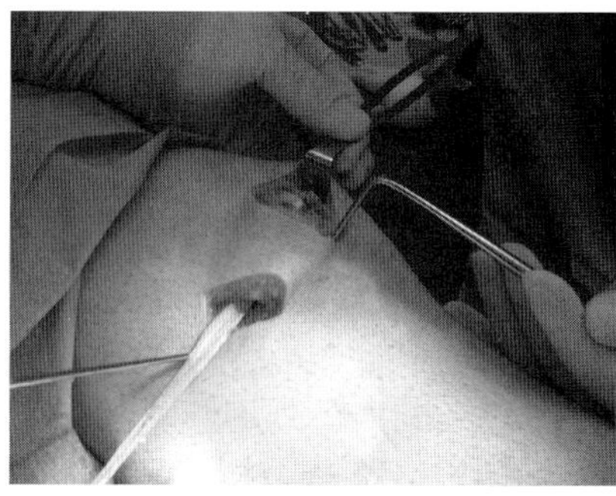

Figure 12 The medial patellofemoral ligament tendon graft has been passed under and through the vastus medialis obliquus tendon. It will be secured by sutures into the vastus medialis obliquus and quadriceps tendons without drilling into the patella.

Lateral release alone for the treatment of lateral patellar instability has yielded poor results and is not recommended. Jensen and Roosen[48] reported that a lateral release added no benefit in a study of 23 patients who underwent medial imbrication for treatment of acute dislocation of the patella. Dainer and associates[49] reported worse results when a lateral release was added to medial capsular repair, with a higher prevalence of redislocation and fewer good or excellent results. Kolowich and associates[50] found that the most predictable criterion for the success of a lateral release was a negative passive patellar tilt on physical examination. In this study, all 28 patients who received a lateral release alone for the treatment of patellar instability continued to have episodes of dislocation.

An improperly performed lateral release can cause medial patellar subluxation, a particularly debilitating condition.[40] In most cases, a lateral release extending just proximal to the proximal patellar pole is all that is needed. Maintaining an intact vastus lateralis helps to reduce medial patellar subluxation and pain.

Hemarthrosis is the most common postoperative complication.

Most surgeons recommend that a lateral release never be used in isolation for the treatment of patellar instability. However, it may be performed as an adjunct when there is residual patellar tilt caused by an excessively tight lateral retinaculum after the medial structures, specifically the medial patellofemoral ligament, have been addressed.

Distal Realignment

Distal realignment is the preferred treatment if there is an abnormal trochlea or a high patella. It is accomplished by the transfer of the tibial tubercle distally to allow the patella to engage correctly in the trochlea. As a result, the Blackburne-Peel index is lowered to the normal range.

Anteromedial Tibial Tubercle Transfer (Fulkerson Procedure)

Transferring the tibial tubercle has long proven to be effective for the treatment of patellar instability. This procedure is meant to correct the Q angle by medializing the tibial tubercle, and it should be used only when the patella does not track in the central part of the trochlea. Following the transfer, cortical screws are used to secure the transferred tubercle. The tubercle is anteriorized as well to unload the patellofemoral joint and produce a proximal shift of contact area for any given degree of flexion. The shift in contact area is attributed to a change in the angle between the patellar tendon and the quadriceps tendon and the distal shift of the patella in relation to the trochlea.

When an anteromedial tubercle transfer is being considered, it is helpful to consider the severity and pattern of articular degeneration. Some patients with patellofemoral instability may also have secondary dysplastic changes, and the trochlea may be flattened from long-standing lateral patellar tracking. As a result, any lateral tracking will be exacerbated by this secondary trochlear deficiency. This may produce continued strain on the medial patellofemoral ligament. As the medial patellofemoral ligament is stretched over time, it leads to a further predisposition of the patella to dislocate laterally. The hallmark reason for moving a tibial tubercle medially is an increased tibial tubercle-trochlear groove index. Imaging with either CT or MRI allows specific measurement of the distance in millimeters between the tibial tubercle and the center of the trochlear groove. Complications from this procedure include tibial fracture, a prominent tubercle, and skin necrosis. Patients should not bear weight for 6 to 8 weeks postoperatively. The rates of good results following the procedure range from 89% to 93%.[51]

Trochleoplasty

A trochleoplasty procedure was first described by Albee.[52] It is an elevating osteotomy of the lateral trochlear facet, and it is performed to correct trochlear dysplasia. A consistent complication of the procedure is disruption of the cartilage surface and changes in the contact pressure, potentially leading to patellofemoral arthritis. There are two types of trochleoplasty: the Dejour method and the Bereiter method.[53,54] With the Dejour method, a staple or screws are used to anchor a thicker osteochondral flap. It has had a success rate of 77%.[55] With the Bereiter method, a polyglactin tape is used to anchor a thinner flexible flap. The Bereiter method is best suited for patients with intact articular cartilage. Instability following trochleoplasty is uncommon, but articular damage is expected; therefore, this technique is rarely indicated.

Summary

Patellofemoral instability is a difficult condition to treat, and the anatomy of the joint and its stabilizing structures must be taken into account. The aim of the surgical technique should be to restore the normal anatomy of the joint. Restoring the balance of patellar tracking as a first step for the treatment of patellar instability is recommended. The restoration of normal restraints should then follow. Treatment of patellar instability with a repair or reconstruction of the medial patellofemoral ligament, in conjunction with a tibial tubercle osteotomy if indicated to correct the Q angle, provides acceptable results. When the medial patellofemoral ligament is intact but attenuated, an imbrication of that ligament and the medial retinaculum can be performed. Alternatively, when medial patellar stabilizers are attenuated, when the patient has congenital dislocation or severe generalized ligamentous laxity, or when a revision is being performed, reconstruction of the medial patellofemoral ligament with a tendon graft is a viable option to restore patellar stability. There is a need for future studies to compare repairs of the medial patellofemoral ligament with reconstructions of the medial patellofemoral ligament with use of a graft for the treatment of lateral patellar instability. A tibial tubercle osteotomy is an essential adjunct to repair of the medial patellofemoral ligament in patients with a large Q angle or severe trochlear dysplasia. Most surgeons recommend that a lateral release never be used in isolation for the treatment of patellar instability. However, it may be performed as an adjunct when there is residual patellar tilt after the medial retinacular structures, specifically the medial patellofemoral ligament, have been treated.

References

1. Aglietti P, Buzzi R, Insall JN: Disorders of the patellofemoral joint, in Insall JN, Scott WN, eds: *Surgery of the Knee*, ed 3. Philadelphia, PA, Churchill Livingstone, 2001, pp 913-1043.
2. Atkin DM, Fithian DC, Marangi KS, Stone ML, Dobson BE, Medelsohn C: Characteristics of patients with primary acute lateral patellar dislocation and their recovery within the first 6 months of injury. *Am J Sports Med* 2000;28:472-479.
3. Nietosvaara Y, Aalto K, Kallio PE: Acute patellar dislocation in children: Incidence and associated osteochondral fractures. *J Pediatr Orthop* 1994; 14:513-515.
4. Kasim NQ, Fulkerson JP: Acute and chronic injuries to the patellofemoral joint, in Garrett WE Jr, Speer KP, Kirkendall DT, eds: *Principles and Practice of Orthopaedic Sports Medicine*. Philadelphia, PA, Lippincott Williams and Wilkins, 2000, pp 709-742.
5. Grelsamer RP, Klein JR: The biomechanics of the patellofemoral joint. *J Orthop Sports Phys Ther* 1998;28: 286-298.
6. Goodfellow J, Hungerford DS, Zindel M: Patello-femoral joint mechanics and pathology: 1. Functional anatomy of the patello-femoral joint. *J Bone Joint Surg Br* 1976;58:287-290.
7. Warren LF, Marshall JL: The supporting structures and layers on the medial side of the knee: An anatomical analysis. *J Bone Joint Surg Am* 1979; 61:56-62.
8. Dopirak RM, Steensen RN, Maurus PB: The medial patellofemoral ligament. *Orthopedics* 2008;31: 331-338.
9. Smirk C, Morris H: The anatomy and reconstruction of the medial patellofemoral ligament. *Knee* 2003;10: 221-227.
10. Tuxøe JI, Teir M, Winge S, Nielsen PL: The medial patellofemoral ligament: A dissection study. *Knee Surg Sports Traumatol Arthrosc* 2002;10: 138-140.
11. Conlan T, Garth WP Jr, Lemons JE: Evaluation of the medial soft-tissue restraints of the extensor mechanism of the knee. *J Bone Joint Surg Am* 1993; 75:682-693.
12. Desio SM, Burks RT, Bachus KN: Soft tissue restraints to lateral patellar translation in the human knee. *Am J Sports Med* 1998;26:59-65.
13. Hautamaa PV, Fithian DC, Kaufman KR, Daniel DM, Pohlmeyer AM: Medial soft tissue restraints in lateral patellar instability and repair. *Clin Orthop Relat Res* 1998;349: 174-182.
14. Dejour H, Walch G, Nove-Josserand L, Guier C: Factors of patellar instability: An anatomic radiographic study. *Knee Surg Sports Traumatol Arthrosc* 1994;2:19-26.
15. Blackburne JS, Peel TE: A new method of measuring patellar height. *J Bone Joint Surg Br* 1977;59:241-242.
16. Insall J, Salvati E: Patella position in the normal knee joint. *Radiology* 1971; 101:101-104.
17. Lattermann C, Toth J, Bach BR Jr: The role of lateral retinacular release in the treatment of patellar instability. *Sports Med Arthrosc* 2007;15:57-60.
18. Inoue M, Shino K, Hirose H, Horibe S, Ono K: Subluxation of the patella: Computed tomography analysis of patellofemoral congruence. *J Bone Joint Surg Am* 1988;70:1331-1337.
19. Donell S: Patellofemoral dysfunction: Extensor mechanism malalignment. *Curr Orthop* 2006;20:103-111.
20. Sallay PI, Poggi J, Speer KP, Garrett WE: Acute dislocation of the patella: A correlative pathoanatomic study. *Am J Sports Med* 1996;24: 52-60.
21. Myers P, Williams A, Dodds R, Bülow J: The three-in-one proximal and distal soft tissue patellar realignment procedure: Results, and its place in the management of patellofemoral instability. *Am J Sports Med* 1999;27: 575-579.
22. Tom A, Fulkerson JP: Restoration of native medial patellofemoral ligament support after patella dislocation. *Sports Med Arthrosc* 2007;15:68-71.
23. Kujala UM, Jaakkola LH, Koskinen SK, Taimela S, Hurme M, Nelimarkka O: Scoring of patellofemoral disorders. *Arthroscopy* 1993;9:159-163.
24. Tegner Y, Lysholm J: Rating systems in the evaluation of knee ligament injuries. *Clin Orthop Relat Res* 1985; 198:43-49.
25. Beck P, Brown NA, Greis PE, Burks RT: Patellofemoral contact pressures and lateral patellar translation after medial patellofemoral ligament reconstruction. *Am J Sports Med* 2007;35:1557-1563.
26. Farr J, Schepsis AA: Reconstruction of the medial patellofemoral ligament for recurrent patellar instability. *J Knee Surg* 2006;19:307-316.
27. Davis DK, Fithian DC: Techniques of medial retinacular repair and reconstruction. *Clin Orthop Relat Res* 2002;402:38-52.
28. Deie M, Ochi M, Sumen Y, Yasumoto M, Kobayashi K, Kimura H: Reconstruction of the medial patellofemoral ligament for the treatment of habitual or recurrent dislocation of the patella in children. *J Bone Joint Surg Br* 2003;85:887-890.
29. Drez D Jr, Edwards TB, Wiliams CS: Results of medial patellofemoral ligament reconstruction in the treatment of patellar dislocation. *Arthroscopy* 2001;17:298-306.
30. Nomura E, Inoue M: Surgical technique and rationale for medial patellofemoral ligament reconstruction for recurrent patellar dislocation. *Arthroscopy* 2003;19:E47.
31. Steiner TM, Torga-Spak R, Teitge RA: Medial patellofemoral ligament reconstruction in patients with lateral patel-

lar instability and trochlear dysplasia. *Am J Sports Med* 2006;34:1254-1261.

32. Teitge RA, Torga-Spak R: Medial patellofemoral ligament reconstruction. *Orthopedics* 2004;27:1037-1040.

33. Elias JJ, Cosgarea AJ: Technical errors during medial patellofemoral ligament reconstruction could overload medial patellofemoral cartilage: A computational analysis. *Am J Sports Med* 2006;34:1478-1485.

34. Steensen RN, Dopirak RM, McDonald WG III: The anatomy and isometry of the medial patellofemoral ligament: Implications for reconstruction. *Am J Sports Med* 2004;32: 1509-1513.

35. Ellera Gomes JL, Stigler Marczyk LR, César de César P, Jungblut CF: Medial patellofemoral ligament reconstruction with semitendinosus autograft for chronic patellar instability: A follow-up study. *Arthroscopy* 2004; 20:147-151.

36. Nomura E, Horiuchi Y, Kihara M: A mid-term follow-up of medial patellofemoral ligament reconstruction using an artificial ligament for recurrent patellar dislocation. *Knee* 2000;7: 211-215.

37. Schöttle PB, Fucentese SF, Romero J: Clinical and radiological outcome of medial patellofemoral ligament reconstruction with a semitendinosus autograft for patella instability. *Knee Surg Sports Traumatol Arthrosc* 2005;13: 516-521.

38. Insall J, Bullough PG, Burstein AH: Proximal "tube" realignment of the patella for chondromalacia patellae. *Clin Orthop Relat Res* 1979;144:63-69.

39. Insall JN, Aglietti P, Tria AJ Jr: Patellar pain and incongruence: II. Clinical application. *Clin Orthop Relat Res* 1983;176:225-232.

40. Hughston JC, Walsh WM: Proximal and distal reconstruction of the extensor mechanism for patellar subluxation. *Clin Orthop Relat Res* 1979; 144:36-42.

41. Nam EK, Karzel RP: Mini-open medial reefing and arthroscopic lateral release for the treatment of recurrent patellar dislocation: A medium-term follow-up. *Am J Sports Med* 2005;33: 220-230.

42. Ali S, Bhatti A: Arthroscopic proximal realignment of the patella for recurrent instability: Report of a new surgical technique with 1 to 7 years of follow-up. *Arthroscopy* 2007;23: 305-311.

43. Halbrecht JL: Arthroscopic patella realignment: An all-inside technique. *Arthroscopy* 2001;17:940-945.

44. Ford DH, Post WR: Open or arthroscopic lateral release: Indications, techniques, and rehabilitation. *Clin Sports Med* 1997;16:29-49.

45. Fulkerson JP: Patellofemoral pain disorders: Evaluation and management. *J Am Acad Orthop Surg* 1994;2: 124-132.

46. Fulkerson JP, Schutzer SF, Ramsby GR, Bernstein RA: Computerized tomography of the patellofemoral joint before and after lateral release or realignment. *Arthroscopy* 1987;3:19-24.

47. Ficat P, Ficat C, Bailleux A: External hypertension syndrome of the patella: Its significance in the recognition of arthrosis. *Rev Chir Orthop Reparatrice Appar Mot* 1975;61:39-59.

48. Jensen CM, Roosen JU: Acute traumatic dislocations of the patella. *J Trauma* 1985;25:160-162.

49. Dainer RD, Barrack RL, Buckley SL, Alexander AH: Arthroscopic treatment of acute patellar dislocations. *Arthroscopy* 1988;4:267-271.

50. Kolowich PA, Paulos LE, Rosenberg TD, Farnsworth S: Lateral release of the patella: Indications and contraindications. *Am J Sports Med* 1990;18:359-365.

51. Fulkerson JP, Becker GJ, Meaney JA, Miranda M, Folcik MA: Anteromedial tibial tubercle transfer without bone graft. *Am J Sports Med* 1990;18: 490-497.

52. Albee FH: The bone graft wedge in the treatment of habitual dislocation of the patella. *Med Rec* 1915;88: 257-259.

53. Donell ST, Joseph G, Hing CB, Marshall TJ: Modified Dejour trochleoplasty for severe dysplasia: Operative technique and early clinical results. *Knee* 2006;13:266-273.

54. von Knoch F, Böhm T, Bürgi ML, von Knoch M, Bereiter H: Trochleaplasty for recurrent patellar dislocation in association with trochlear dysplasia: A 4- to 14-year follow-up study. *J Bone Joint Surg Br* 2006;88: 1331-1335.

55. Verdonk R, Jansegers E, Stuyts B: Trochleoplasty in dysplastic knee trochlea. *Knee Surg Sports Traumatol Arthrosc* 2005;13:529-533.

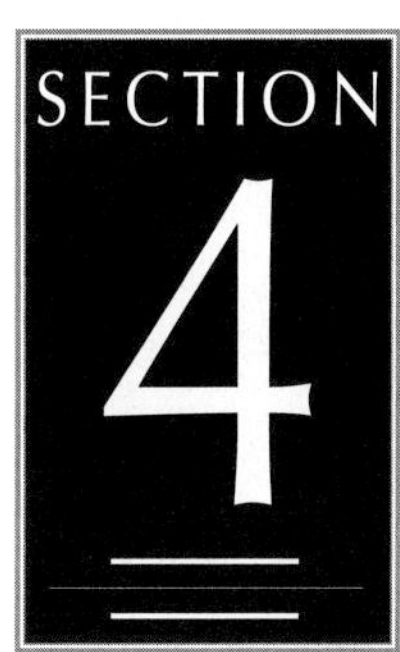

SECTION 4

Shoulder and Elbow

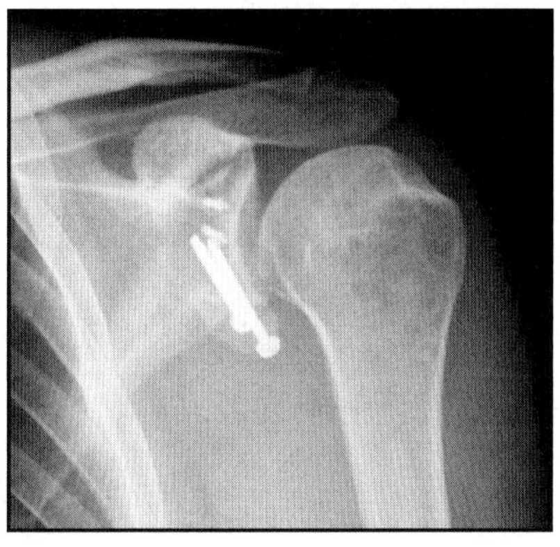

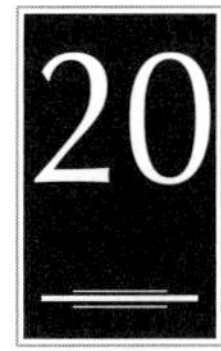

Acromioclavicular and Sternoclavicular Injuries and Clavicular, Glenoid, and Scapular Fractures

Michael S. Bahk, MD
John E. Kuhn, MD
Leesa M. Galatz, MD
Patrick M. Connor, MD
Gerald R. Williams Jr, MD

Abstract

Injuries to the acromioclavicular joint and the sternoclavicular joint and fractures of the clavicle, glenoid, and scapula vary widely in incidence, treatment, and prognosis. The treatment for acromioclavicular joint and clavicle injuries, which are relatively common, has significantly evolved. Controversy exists regarding the ideal treatment of type III acromioclavicular separations, whereas significant research has shown many potential benefits for surgically treating significantly displaced midshaft clavicle fractures that had traditionally been treated nonsurgically. Sternoclavicular injuries and scapula fractures are less common but are associated with high-energy mechanisms of injury and are potentially life threatening. Most of these injuries can be treated conservatively, although some injuries will benefit from surgical fixation. Identifying floating shoulders or unstable glenoid neck fractures without bony or ligamentous stabilization requires an understanding of the multiple anatomic stabilizers of the glenoid. Floating shoulders, glenoid neck fractures with 1 cm or 40° or more of displacement, and intra-articular glenoid fractures with associated glenohumeral instability or intra-articular displacement of 5 mm or more may require surgical repair.

Instr Course Lect 2010;59:209-226.

Dr. Bahk or an immediate family member owns stock or stock options in Stryker and Zimmer. Dr. Kuhn or an immediate family member has received research or institutional support from Arthrex and DJ Orthopedics and owns stock or stock options in Pfizer. Dr. Galatz or an immediate family member serves as an unpaid consultant to Tornier. Dr. Connor or an immediate family member has received royalties from Arthrotek and serves as a paid consultant to or is an employee of Arthrotek and Zimmer. Dr. Williams or an immediate family member serves as a board member, owner, officer, or committee member of the American Shoulder and Elbow Surgeons, the Pennsylvania Orthopaedic Society, the American Academy of Orthopaedic Surgeons, the Rothman Institute, and the Philadelphia Human Performance Laboratory; has received royalties from DePuy; is a member of a speaker's bureau or has made paid presentations on behalf of DePuy, Mitek, and Tornier; serves as a paid consultant to or is an employee of DePuy, Mitek, and Tornier; has received research or institutional support from Arthrex, National Institutes of Health, Stryker, and Synthes; owns stock or stock options in Invivo Therapeutics; and has received non-income support (such as equipment or servies), commercially derived honoraria, or other non–research-related funding (such as paid travel) from Wolters Kluwer Health-Lippincott Williams and Wilkins.

Acromioclavicular joint injuries—or separations, as they are commonly described—are common sports-related injuries resulting from falls or other direct forces on the superolateral aspect of the shoulder pushing the acromion in an inferior direction. Acromioclavicular joint injuries represent a spectrum of severity, ranging from a simple sprain of the acromioclavicular ligament with no displacement to widely displaced injuries associated with severe soft-tissue injury to the acromioclavicular ligament, the coracoclavicular ligament, and the deltotrapezial fascia. Treatment options vary according to the severity of the injury and logically reflect the associated soft-tissue involvement. A brief outline of the types of injuries and current recommendations for treatment are presented.

Classification

The modified Rockwood classification system is the most commonly used method of categorizing these injuries[1] (Table 1). A type I injury is a sprain (stretching) of the

Table 1
Modified Rockwood System for Classification of Acromioclavicular Separations

Type	Acromioclavicular Ligament	Coracoclavicular Ligament	Deltotrapezial Fascia
I	Sprained	Intact	—
II	Torn	Intact	—
III	Torn	Torn	Intact
IV	Torn	Torn	Torn
V	Torn	Torn	Torn

acromioclavicular ligament. Type II injuries tear the acromioclavicular ligament, leaving the coracoclavicular ligament intact. When the coracoclavicular and acromioclavicular ligaments are both torn and the acromioclavicular separation is reducible with gentle upward pressure under the elbow, the injury is classified as type III. A type IV acromioclavicular separation occurs when the coracoclavicular and acromioclavicular ligaments are torn and the scapula is displaced inferiorly and anteriorly, resulting in a relative posterior displacement of the distal part of the clavicle through a tear in the deltotrapezial fascia. The distal part of the clavicle lies directly subcutaneously in these injuries. A type V injury is characterized by a wide coracoclavicular separation. The distal part of the clavicle is herniated through a rent in the deltotrapezial fascia with the scapula displaced inferiorly. Type IV and V injuries are not reducible with upward pressure beneath the elbow, indicating interposition of soft tissue (deltotrapezial fascia) between the distal part of the clavicle and the acromioclavicular joint. Type VI is an exceedingly rare, high-energy injury characterized by inferior displacement of the clavicle beneath the coracoid. Most surgeons never encounter this injury, and it is not discussed in detail in this chapter.

Neviaser[2] developed a simpler classification system, also emphasizing the reducibility of the joint in determining the diagnosis and classification. Type I is a sprain of the acromioclavicular ligament, and type II is a tear of this ligament. Type III is subclassified as type IIIA if the injury is reducible and as type IIIB (corresponding to Rockwood types IV and V) if the injury is not reducible.

Diagnosis

Type I

Type I injuries, according to the Rockwood system, are sprains of the acromioclavicular ligament with no displacement. Radiographic findings are usually normal if the injury occurs in isolation. The diagnosis is based on the history and the findings of the physical examination. There is tenderness directly at the acromioclavicular joint. It is unusual for an inspection of the shoulder to reveal a deformity, with the exception of ecchymosis or abrasion on the superior aspect of the shoulder in the acute phase after the injury.

Type II

Type II injuries are tears of the acromioclavicular ligament with an intact coracoclavicular ligament. Physical examination reveals tenderness to palpation at the acromioclavicular joint. The acromion may be slightly displaced inferiorly relative to the distal part of the clavicle, but it continues to be at least partially in contact with the distal part of the clavicle. The joint is unstable in the anteroposterior plane. The distance between the coracoid and the clavicle remains normal, but the acromion is subluxated relative to the distal part of the clavicle.

Type III

When the acromioclavicular and coracoclavicular ligaments are both torn, the distal part of the clavicle is prominent as an obvious visible deformity. The distal part of the clavicle is usually tender to palpation, and the joint is reducible with upward pressure under the elbow. Chronic separations are less reducible because of scar formation around the joint. Nevertheless, the deltotrapezial aponeurosis is intact. The acromioclavicular joint is unstable in both the vertical and the horizontal plane. Complete separation of the acromioclavicular joint and an increase in the coracoclavicular distance are seen on radiographs.

Type IV

The clavicle is driven in a posterior direction in a type IV separation. This results in a distinct visible deformity with extreme prominence of the clavicle over the scapular spine. The clavicle is herniated through the trapezius and is subcutaneous. Although the acromioclavicular joint is unstable, because it is impaled over the scapula, it does not move on physical examination. Posterior displacement of the clavicle is seen on the axillary radiograph, whereas the dislocated acromioclavicular joint and a widened coracoclavicular distance are seen on the AP radiograph.

Type V

Displacement of the distal part of the clavicle occurs predominantly in the vertical plane. The injury results in obvious visible deformity of the distal part of the clavicle associated with downward and slightly anterior displacement of the scapula. The separation is not completely reducible because the distal part of the clavicle is herniated through the deltotrapezial fascia. There is usually substantial tenderness and swelling in the acute phase after the injury. An increase in the coracoclavicular distance (of up to 300%) and superior displacement of the distal part of the clavicle are seen on the AP radiograph.

Treatment

Treatment varies depending on the severity of the injury and the soft-tissue involvement. There is very little controversy regarding the treatment of type I and II injuries or type IV and V injuries. However, treatment of type III injuries is controversial, and there is no general consensus.[3-6]

Type I

Sling immobilization and symptomatic treatment of pain are usually all that are necessary for these injuries. Activities are resumed as tolerated.

Type II

These injuries are usually successfully managed with the methods used for type I. Occasionally, pain persists at the acromioclavicular joint, and additional treatment is indicated. Nonsurgical measures such as cortisone injections and nonsteroidal anti-inflammatory medication can be administered. An excision of the distal part of the clavicle alone is insufficient treatment; it results in a short, unstable distal part of the clavicle, continued pain, and disability. If surgery is selected because of the persistence of pain after nonsurgical treatment, the distal aspect of the clavicle should be removed, and a capsular plication with ligament reconstruction should be performed.

Type III

Type III injuries should initially be treated without surgery.[1,3,6] Most patients recover and regain normal shoulder function, although the visible deformity is permanent. Early surgical treatment can be considered for individuals with high sports or vocational demands, although this is controversial as many high-demand individuals do well with nonsurgical treatment.[4] Surgical treatment of patients with a high risk of recurrent injury, such as hockey or football players, is especially controversial as a surgical repair does not restore normal strength to the ligaments of the acromioclavicular joint and reinjury is common.

Surgical reconstruction of the ligaments is indicated for patients for whom nonsurgical treatment has failed.[1,3,7] Many different methods are available, and detailed descriptions are beyond the scope of this chapter.[1,5-8] There are common basic principles for all reconstructive methods. The coracoclavicular ligament is reconstructed with the use of sutures based in anchors at the base of the coracoid or around the coracoid. The sutures are usually brought through drill holes in the clavicle. Transfer of the coracoacromial ligament to the distal part of the clavicle augments the strength and biologic healing of the reconstruction and is advocated as part of the Weaver-Dunn procedure, the most common procedure performed for treatment of these injuries.[9] Autograft or allograft augmentation has been advocated for coracoclavicular ligament reconstruction, to improve the strength and facilitate healing, but long-term results are not yet available.[5,8]

Types IV and V

Surgical treatment of types IV and V is not controversial as early surgery improves the results following these injuries.[1] Ligament reconstruction is performed in the same way as it is for type III injuries. Careful attention is paid to the repair of the torn deltotrapezial aponeurosis because this is a critical aspect of the repair and reconstruction in patients with an acromioclavicular joint separation.

Arthroscopic Treatment

Arthroscopic treatment of type III injuries has been reported, but its role in the treatment of acromioclavicular separations has not been studied sufficiently for it to be recommended as an option.[10-12] The instrumentation has been developed but is still under investigation. Arthroscopy may be used as an adjunct to the treatment of type IV and V injuries, but the distal part of the clavicle must be exposed to reduce it through the torn deltotrapezial fascia, which is then repaired.

Fractures and Dislocations of the Medial Part of the Clavicle and the Sternoclavicular Joint

Anatomy and Clinical Assessment

The sternoclavicular joint is not commonly injured but, when it is, the injury is usually caused by high-energy trauma and may be associated with potentially life-threatening complications.

The sternoclavicular joint is saddle shaped with a very large

Table 2
Injuries Associated With Fracture of the Medial Aspect of the Clavicle

Associated Injury	Percent of Patients
Pneumothorax and/or hemothorax	42
Pulmonary contusion/respiratory failure	55
Rib fracture	73
Vascular injury	2
Facial fracture	31
Head injury	36
Cervical spine injury	25
Visceral injury	29
Upper extremity injury	45
Lower extremity injury	31

(Adapted with permission from Throckmorton T, Kuhn JE: Fractures of the medial end of the clavicle. *J Shoulder Elbow Surg* 2007;16: 49-54. http://www.sciencedirect.com/science/journal/10582746.)

clavicular head relative to the small fossa on the manubrium. This construct has little osseous constraint, and its stability is derived from the strong ligaments. The anterior and posterior aspects of the capsule provide the major stabilizing tissue.[13] The interclavicular ligament, which is important for the poise of the shoulder girdle, and the costoclavicular ligament have secondary roles.[14]

The subclavian vessels, esophagus, and trachea are behind the sternoclavicular joint and are at risk when this area is subjected to trauma. A thorough clinical and radiographic evaluation is recommended to assess these structures. Posterior displacement of the medial aspect of the clavicle relative to the sternum is associated with the greatest risk of associated injuries.[15]

Although a variety of radiographic views have been described to image the sternoclavicular joint and the medial aspect of the clavicle (the Hobbs view, Heinig lateral view, and serendipity view), CT and MRI increase the likelihood that a fracture will be diagnosed and help to determine whether the medial aspect of the clavicle is displaced anteriorly or posteriorly.[15,16]

Fractures of the Medial Aspect of the Clavicle

Fractures of the medial third of the clavicle are rare, accounting for between 2% and 9.3% of all clavicular fractures. These fractures are often sustained in high-speed motor vehicle collisions, and seat belt use, although lifesaving, may have a role in the production of these injuries.[16]

Typically, patients with a fracture of the medial third of the clavicle also have severe thoracic injuries, including pneumothorax and/or pulmonary contusion, with respiratory failure occurring in nearly half of the patients. Other injuries include rib fractures, head injuries, and cervical spine and other upper extremity injuries (Table 2). The mortality rate is as high as 19% for patients with these fractures.[16] The fractures are classified according to their configuration (Figure 1), with transverse and comminuted fractures presenting most commonly.[16]

Nonsurgical treatment is most often recommended, but an open fracture is an indication for surgical fixation.[16] Many patients have residual pain, and the nonunion rate may approach 15%.[16,17] Some authors have reported success with surgical reduction and internal fixation.[18]

Dislocations of the Sternoclavicular Joint

Dislocations of the sternoclavicular joint are rare, accounting for approximately 3% of all shoulder injuries, and they can be life threatening.[19] The epiphysis of the medial end of the clavicle does not close until a person is in his or her mid 20s.[15] As such, what is initially perceived as a dislocation in a young adult may in fact be a Salter-Harris type I or II physeal fracture; however, reduction and immobilization remain the treatment of choice. Anterior dislocations are two to three times more common than posterior dislocations, and fortunately they are less dangerous. Posterior dislocations have been associated with a variety of life- or limb-threatening injuries, including tracheal compression, injury to the great vessels, mediastinal compression, and compression of the innominate vein.[20-22] Untreated dislocations have been associated with late complications, including erosion into the great vessels, tracheoesophageal fistulas, compression of the subclavian artery, thoracic outlet syndrome, and compression of the brachial plexus.[23-26]

The mechanisms of injury for sternoclavicular dislocation include motor vehicle collisions, falls, and sports. Most dislocations occur as a result of an indirect force. As the shoulder girdle is pushed back, the clavicle pivots on the first rib and the medial aspect of the clavicle is pushed forward, producing an anterior dislocation. Conversely, when the shoulder girdle is pushed forward, a posterior dislocation may be produced.

These injuries are classified by the direction of the dislocation (anterior or posterior), by their chronicity (acute, subacute, or chronic), and by their severity (ranging from capsular sprains to subluxation events that reduce spontaneously to dislocations that require assistance with reduction).

Acute traumatic instability is usually treated with an acute reduction of the sternoclavicular joint. Closed

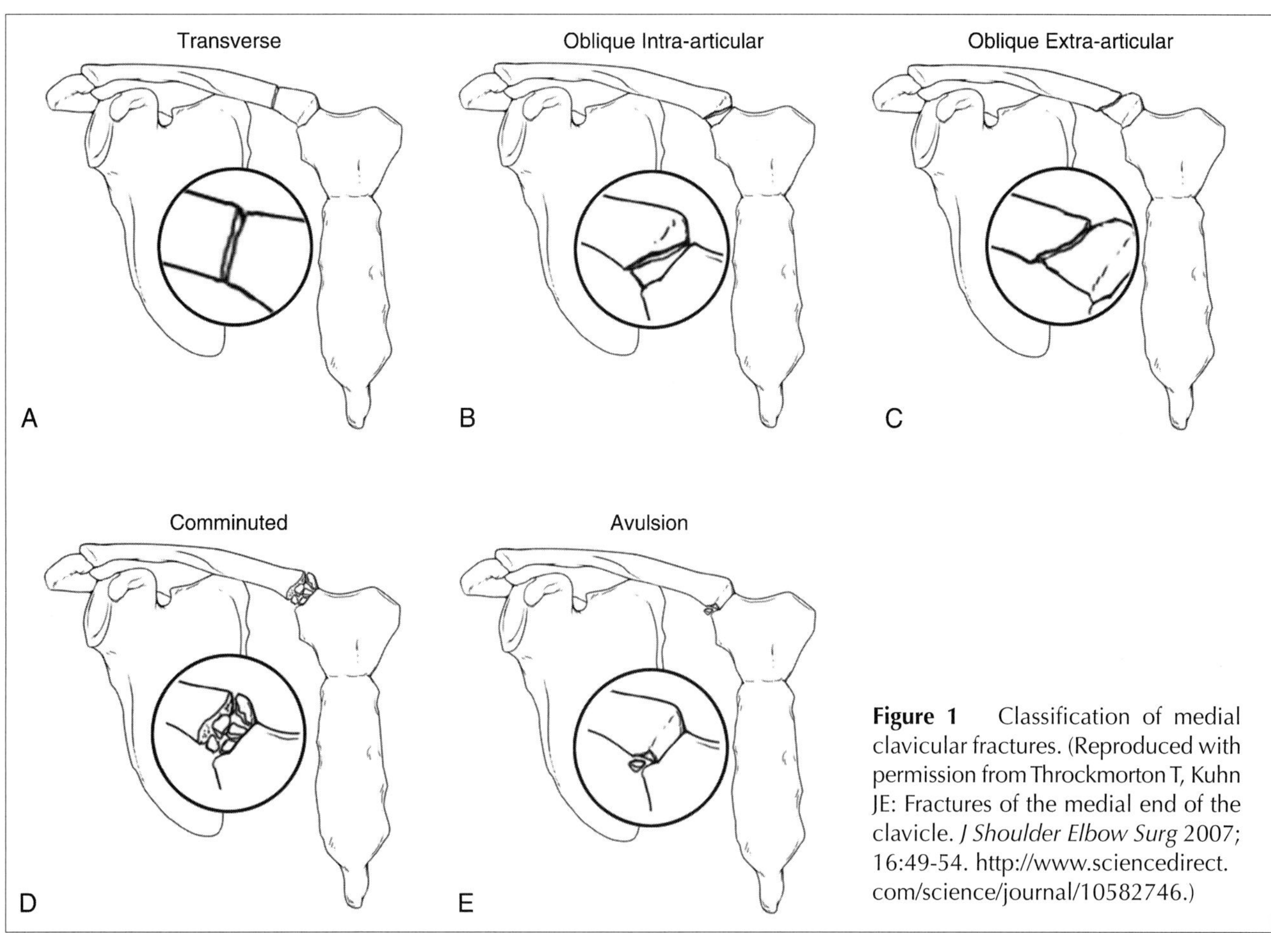

Figure 1 Classification of medial clavicular fractures. (Reproduced with permission from Throckmorton T, Kuhn JE: Fractures of the medial end of the clavicle. *J Shoulder Elbow Surg* 2007; 16:49-54. http://www.sciencedirect.com/science/journal/10582746.)

reduction is recommended for both acute anterior and acute posterior dislocations, and several techniques have been described. Closed reduction is generally successful if it is done early.[27] The reduction of a posterior dislocation of the sternoclavicular joint must be performed carefully as the sternal head could be providing a tamponade of a torn vessel.[28] It is advisable to reduce posterior dislocations of the sternoclavicular joint with the patient under general anesthesia, with thoracic surgery available as a backup.

Irreducible anterior dislocations are commonly left unreduced, and many patients do well without the need for further intervention.[29,30] Posterior dislocations should not be left unreduced as late sequelae such as erosion into the great vessels or tracheoesophageal fistulas can occur.[31] Open reduction and reconstruction of the sternoclavicular joint ligaments is indicated for both an acute irreducible posterior dislocation and a chronic posterior dislocation. Patients with a chronic anterior dislocation and sufficiently bothersome symptoms may benefit from reconstruction of the sternoclavicular joint.

Surgery is contraindicated for patients who have atraumatic, voluntary instability of the sternoclavicular joint. A connective tissue disorder such as Ehlers-Danlos syndrome is a relative contraindication.

A variety of surgical techniques have been described for treating an unstable sternoclavicular joint. Resection of the sternal head of the clavicle yields poor results.[32-34] Spencer and Kuhn[35] reviewed the biomechanical properties of three of the most popular procedures: transfer of the subclavius tendon, transfer of the intra-articular disk and ligament into the resected end of the clavicle, and reconstruction of the anterior and posterior aspects of the capsule with use of a figure-of-8 semitendinosus autograft.[34,36] The figure-of-8 reconstruction with the semitendinosus was found to have significantly better mechanical properties than the reconstructions performed with the other techniques[35] (Figure 2). Because of pin breakage and migration into vital structures with disastrous complications, the use of Steinmann pins,

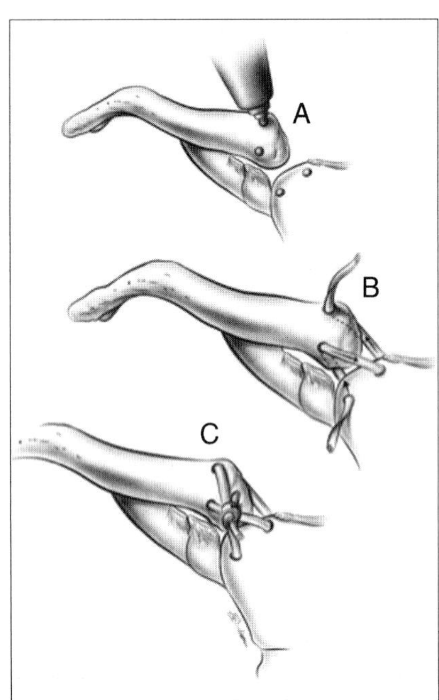

Figure 2 Figure-of-8 reconstruction of the sternoclavicular joint. (Reproduced from Spencer EE Jr, Kuhn JE: Biomechanical analysis of reconstructions for sternoclavicular joint instability. *J Bone Joint Surg Am* 2004;86:98-105.)

Kirschner wires, threaded pins with bent ends, and Hagie pins is contraindicated for the treatment of sternoclavicular joint instability.[37-42]

Midshaft Clavicular Fractures

Acute midshaft fractures of the clavicle have historically been treated with benign neglect, with the clinical perception that most of these fractures heal and patients have successful clinical outcomes. In addition, historic reviews showed the prevalence of nonunion after surgical management to be higher than that after nonsurgical treatment.[43] However, the current literature reveals that not all patients with this injury do well with nonsurgical treatment. In a recent review of 2,144 clavicular fractures, Zlowodzki and associates[44] reported a 15.1% prevalence of nonunion of fractures treated without surgery and a 2.2% rate of nonunion of fractures treated with plate fixation. In a study of 242 consecutive clavicular fractures, Hill and associates[45] found that 16 of 52 patients (31%) with a completely displaced middle-third clavicular fracture that had been treated with nonsurgical means had an unsatisfactory clinical result. In a similar study of 245 consecutive clavicular fractures, Nowak and associates[46] found that 46% of the patients continued to have clinical sequelae up to 9 years after the injury. In their study of 281 diaphyseal clavicular fractures, Robinson and associates[17] showed that the prevalence of clavicular nonunion following nonsurgical treatment increased with advancing age, female sex, complete displacement of the fracture ends, and the presence of comminution. Although the overall prevalence of clavicular fracture nonunion was found to be 4.5% in their series, the prevalence of nonunion following nonsurgical treatment of completely displaced and comminuted fractures ranged from 20% to 47% in patients between 25 and 65 years of age. McKee and associates[47,48] suggested that use of a patient-based outcome measurement (the Disabilities of the Arm, Shoulder and Hand [DASH] score)[49] may reveal more residual clinical impairment following nonsurgical management of displaced clavicular fractures than is demonstrated by surgeon-based or radiographic measures. Thus, the evolution of management of these injuries has included efforts to define which fractures are most likely to progress to symptomatic nonunion or malunion if they are treated initially without surgery and to determine whether primary surgical treatment of these specific fractures may improve the clinical results.

Indications for surgical treatment of acute midshaft clavicular fractures include open fractures, fractures with compromised skin caused by severe fracture displacement ("tented skin"), and fractures associated with a vascular or neurologic injury. On the basis of several studies that have defined the clinical outcome of the nonsurgical management of midshaft clavicular fractures,[17,44-47,50] evolving indications for acute surgical management include midshaft clavicular fractures with complete displacement (no osseous contact), initial clavicular shortening of 2 cm or more, and comminuted fractures with a displaced transverse "zed" (or z-shaped) fragment. As female sex and increasing patient age have been associated with increased rates of nonunion, these confounding variables should also be taken into consideration when choosing surgical or nonsurgical treatment.[17]

The Canadian Orthopaedic Trauma Society performed a multicenter, randomized clinical trial comparing nonsurgical treatment and plate fixation of displaced midshaft clavicular fractures in 132 patients.[50] Acute surgical fixation led to statistically better results with regard to Constant and DASH scores, return to activities, time to union, nonunions, symptomatic malunions, and patient satisfaction. Although hardware removal was the most common reason for repeat intervention in the surgically treated group, only 2 of 67 patients required removal of symptomatic hardware after the fracture had healed. Three patients with a postoperative infection were managed with antibiotics and local wound care and ultimately had the plate removed after bone

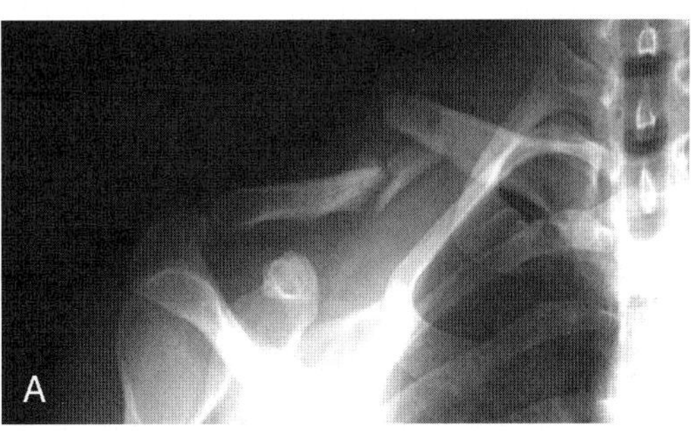

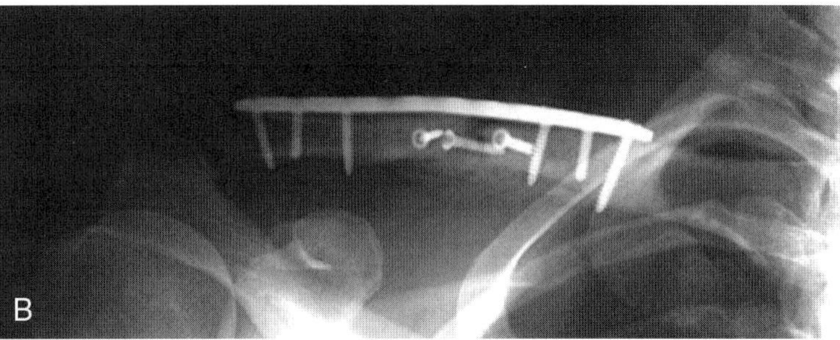

Figure 3 **A,** Markedly displaced midshaft clavicular fracture with comminution. **B,** Healed fracture after open reduction and internal fixation with use of a precontoured clavicular plate and supplemental interfragmentary fixation.

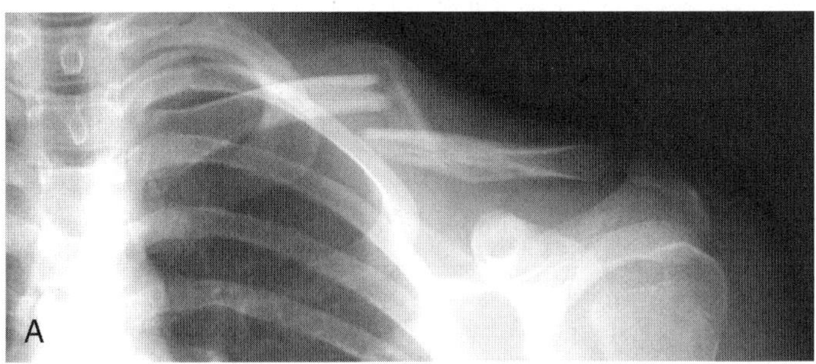

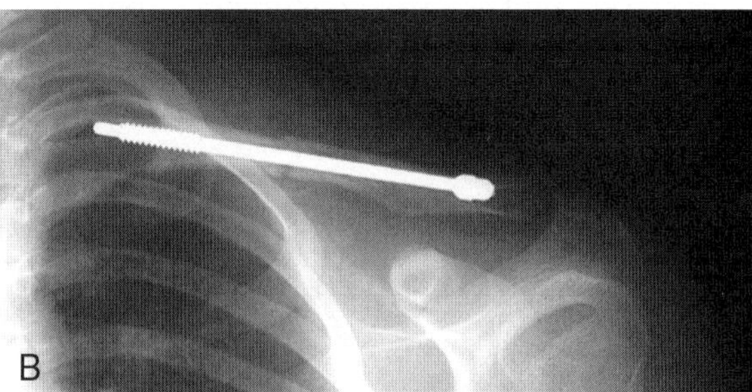

Figure 4 **A,** Markedly displaced midshaft clavicular fracture with a vertical comminuted fragment (a "zed" fracture). **B,** Immediate postoperative radiograph after intramedullary fixation.

healing, and one broken plate was removed after the patient was involved in an all-terrain-vehicle accident 6 weeks postoperatively. There were no catastrophic complications related to surgical management. In addition to this prospective randomized clinical trial, there have been multiple other cohort studies showing success with surgical management of displaced midshaft clavicular fractures.[51-56]

Although the literature contains anecdotal reports of many complications of plate fixation (hardware prominence requiring removal, nonunion, malunion, hardware failure, infection, supraclavicular neuroma, subclavian vein injury, and pneumothorax), these complications can be avoided through meticulous surgical technique (Figure 3). The supraclavicular nerves, which traverse the clavicle from a superomedial to an inferolateral direction, should be identified and protected throughout the procedure. It is important to be precise about creating a full-thickness deltotrapezial fascial approach that can be meticulously repaired at the conclusion of the procedure. This thick "watertight" deltotrapezial fascial repair will augment the vascular supply to the fracture; minimize dead space and the potential for a postoperative hematoma; and provide a physiologic barrier to the plate and screws, thereby playing an important role in avoiding hardware prominence. It is important to achieve anatomic reduction of the fracture fragments and stable, compressive fixation with the use of either a limited-contact dynamic compression plate (or its equivalent) or one of the newer anatomic plates. The use of a tubular plate is not recommended.[52,57,58] It has been shown that placing the plate on the superior (tension) side of the clavicle creates the most stable construct, and ensuring that the plate does not protrude off the medial aspect of the clavicle anteriorly will help to avoid painful hardware.[59] The periosteum and soft-tissue attachments of the fracture fragments should be saved, and bone grafting should be considered in acute cases with severe comminution and in all cases of nonunion.

Intramedullary fixation is another option for the surgical management of a displaced midshaft clavicular fracture (Figure 4). Use of this technique makes it possible to avoid the larger approach necessary for plate fixation, and, if the implant is later removed through a small posterior approach as is typically recommended, the issue of persistent or painful hardware is eliminated. The primary disadvantage of intramedullary fixation is that it does not provide axial or rotational stability when used for nontransverse and comminuted fractures.[60] In addition, smooth Kirschner wires and other nonstable intramedullary fixation methods have had an unacceptably variable complication rate (range, 5% to 50%), the most notable of which is hardware migration into the vital structures near the shoulder girdle.[39,61,62] Methods of intramedullary fixation that provide more stability while minimizing the complications of loss of fixation and hardware migration have been devised. Successful outcomes have been reported after use of these techniques,[61-64] although the authors of this chapter are not aware of any prospective randomized studies comparing intramedullary and plate fixation.

As is the case with plate fixation, complications following intramedullary fixation of displaced midshaft clavicular fractures can often be minimized through meticulous surgical technique. Only a minimal incision over the fracture site is necessary to reduce the fracture fragments; the soft-tissue and periosteal attachments to osseous fragments should be maintained. The largest-diameter device that will traverse the medullary canal is recommended to enhance fracture stability (particularly for nontransverse fractures and those with comminution), and the threads of the implant should not lie at the level of the fracture site. It is important to completely reduce the fracture before placement of the intramedullary device; this requires superior translation of the lateral part of the shoulder girdle, which prevents the creation of an "A-frame" malalignment of the clavicle. In addition, there is a tendency for the intramedullary device to exit the distal part of the clavicle too superiorly; care should be taken to ensure that the device exits the posterior part of the clavicle as far distally and inferiorly as possible. At the conclusion of the procedure, comminuted fragments are reapproximated with cerclage suture, and the deltotrapezial fascia is closed over the fracture site.

An important issue regarding recommendations for the treatment of displaced midshaft clavicular fractures is the timing of surgical treatment. In a study to address this issue, Potter and associates[65] compared 15 patients treated with immediate fixation of this injury with 15 who had undergone delayed fixation of a clavicular nonunion or symptomatic malunion after failure of nonsurgical care. Although no significant differences in fracture healing; in strength of shoulder flexion, abduction, or rotation; or in DASH scores were noted between the groups, the Constant scores and endurance strength were marginally better after the acute fracture repair. The authors pointed out that these data should not be used in isolation to recommend primary surgical fixation of this injury but rather could be used in counseling patients on the relative advantages and disadvantages of immediate surgical repair compared with potentially delayed reconstruction for the treatment of displaced midshaft fractures.[65]

Lateral Clavicular Fractures

There is general agreement that lateral clavicular fractures, which account for 10% to 15% of all clavicular fractures, with complete displacement are associated with a higher prevalence of nonunion than are midshaft clavicular fractures;[17,43,66] this is likely a result of a combination of bone and ligamentous injury. Nordqvist and associates[66] found that 25% of type II lateral clavicular fractures (fractures that occur between the conoid and trapezoid coracoclavicular ligaments) progressed to nonunion or caused chronic pain, and Robinson and associates[17] showed that 21% of patients with this injury required surgery. Although the proportion of lateral clavicular fractures that progress to nonunion, particularly in elderly patients, may be higher than the proportion of midshaft clavicular fractures that do so, many of the nonunions are asymptomatic and do not require further treatment.[17]

The authors of this chapter are not aware of any prospective studies comparing surgical and nonsurgical treatment of fractures of the lateral third of the clavicle. When these fractures are managed surgically, the remaining part of the clavicle that is lateral to the fracture site is often either substantially comminuted or of insufficient quantity to enable rigid fixation with traditional plates or intramedullary implants. An array of different technical procedures to address this problem, with the use of screws, pins, and plates, have been described in multiple small case series.[60,67-72] Newer, precontoured anatomic plates that enable locking screw fixation into the lateral fracture fragment have been created; however, even these may be of insufficient strength to withstand the traction forces of the lateral part of the shoulder girdle. Thus, it has been recommended that coracoclavicular fixation or reconstruction be used to supplement the osseous fixation.[73] This is typically provided through suture or allograft ligament sling fixation around the base of the coracoid and the reduced clavicle to augment or reconstruct the injured coracoclavicular ligament (Figure 5). Occasionally, if the lateral-

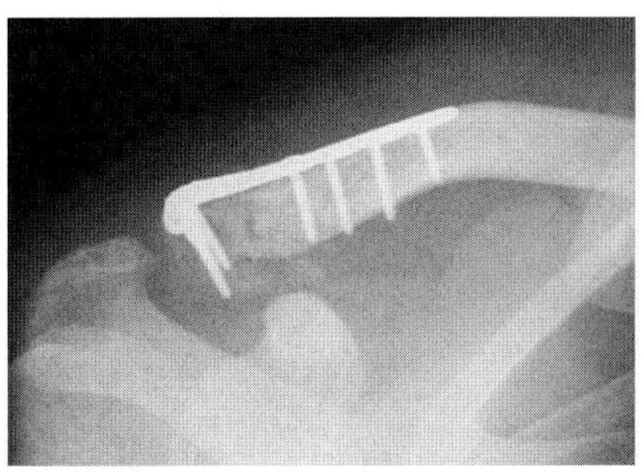

Figure 5 A distal clavicular plate was used to treat this type II distal clavicular fracture. The repair was augmented with coracoclavicular sling fixation.

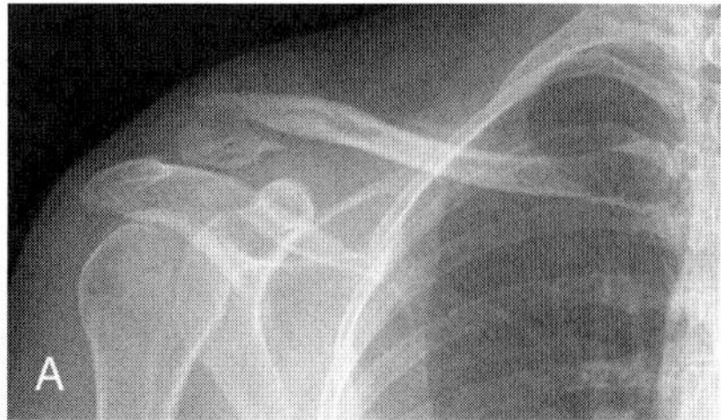

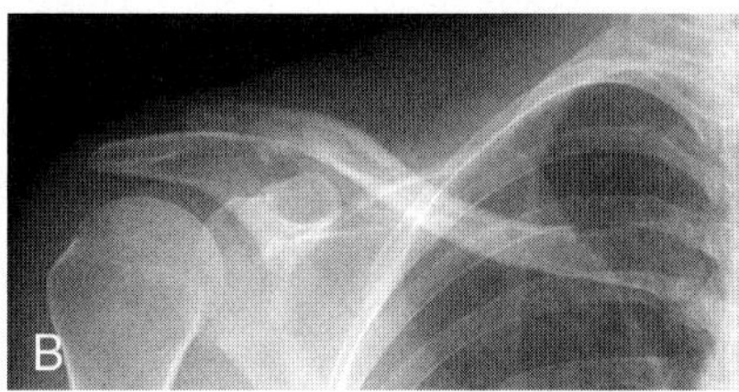

Figure 6 **A,** A displaced type II distal clavicular fracture with comminution of the distal fracture fragment. **B,** Isolated coracoclavicular fixation led to successful healing and an excellent clinical result.

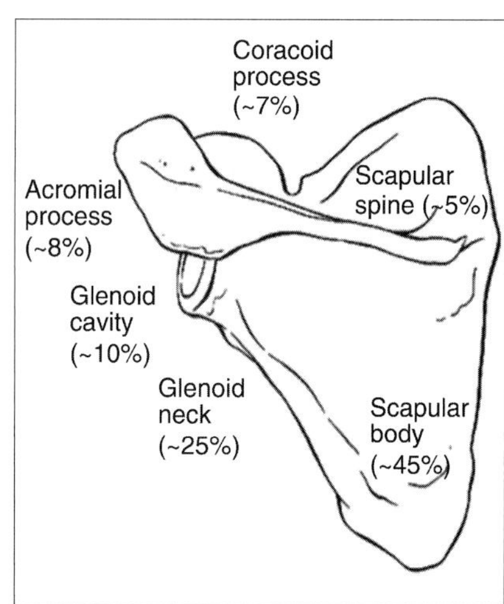

Figure 7 Frequency of scapular fractures. (Reproduced with permission from Goss TP: Fractures of the scapula, in Rockwood CA, Matsen FA, Wirth MA, Lippitt SB, eds: *The Shoulder*, ed 3. Philadelphia, PA, Saunders, 2004, pp 413-454.)

distal part of the clavicular bone has been determined, qualitatively or quantitatively, to be unable to accept osseous fixation, isolated coracoclavicular fixation can be used successfully to treat these injuries (Figure 6). The use of a hook plate has also been described for this particular injury.[69,70,74] Although isolated studies have shown successful results with this implant, the prevalence and magnitude of complications preclude its universal recommendation. If it is used, it should always be removed approximately 3 months postoperatively because of the high prevalence of acromial erosion and rotator cuff damage from the hook.

Glenoid and Scapular Fractures

Fractures of the glenoid and scapula account for 1% of all fractures and 5% of all shoulder fractures.[75-78] These fractures most commonly involve the scapular body (45%), the glenoid neck (25%), and the glenoid cavity (10%). Fractures affecting the acromion process (8%), coracoid process (7%), and scapular spine (5%) are less common[75,79] (Figure 7). Management varies according to the fracture location and displacement.

Scapular Body Fractures

Fractures of the scapular body are often associated with concomitant injuries, which are sometimes life threatening.[75-77,80,81] These injuries include rib fractures, hemothorax or pneumothorax, a ruptured viscus, closed head injury, and long-bone fracture. Management of a scapular body fracture may be deferred because of these other injuries, especially in patients who have sustained polytrauma. In 90% of cases, the scapular body fracture is treated nonsurgically with a sling for comfort for 7 to 10 days, followed by pendulum exercises and passive range-of-motion exercises for 4 to 6 weeks. An overhead pulley exercise program can usually be added by 6 weeks postinjury. Rotator cuff and scapular muscle strengthening is initiated at 6 to 8 weeks and is continued for 2 to 3 months. Improvement occurs for 9 to 12 months. Successful fracture union, minimal pain, and good function are expected in most cases.[75,80,81] However, nonunion and symptomatic malunion have been reported.[75,82-84]

Glenoid Neck Fractures

Glenoid neck fractures exit the superior part of the scapula either medial or lateral to the base of the coracoid[75,85] (Figure 8). Those that exit laterally are inherently unstable and often require surgical stabilization. However, they are very uncommon. Glenoid neck fractures that exit medial to the base of the coracoid divide the scapula into a medial fragment (consisting of the scapular body, scapular spine, and acromion) and a lateral fragment (the glenoid and the coracoid process). The lateral fragment is attached to the medial fragment by the coracoacromial ligament and to the axial skeleton by the coracoclavicular and acromioclavicular ligaments and the clavicle.[86]

Goss[75,81,85,87] described the superior shoulder suspensory complex as a lateral osseous and soft-tissue ring (glenoid process, coracoid process,

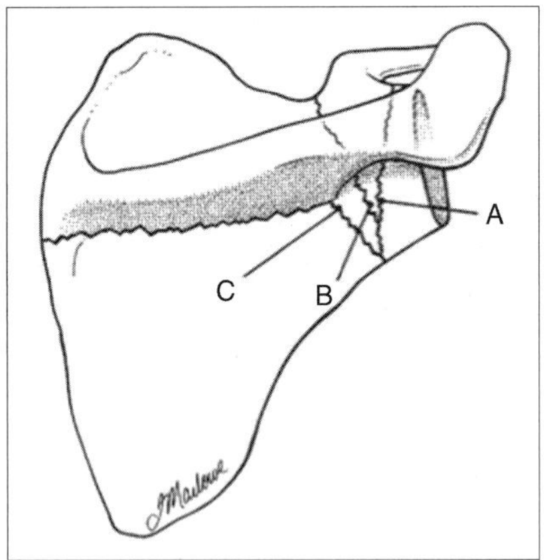

Figure 8 Scapular neck fractures most commonly occur medial to the coracoid (line B) and uncommonly lateral to the coracoid (line A). (Reproduced with permission from Goss TP: Fractures of the glenoid neck. *J Shoulder Elbow Surg* 1994;3: 42-52. http://www.sciencedirect.com/science/journal/10582746.)

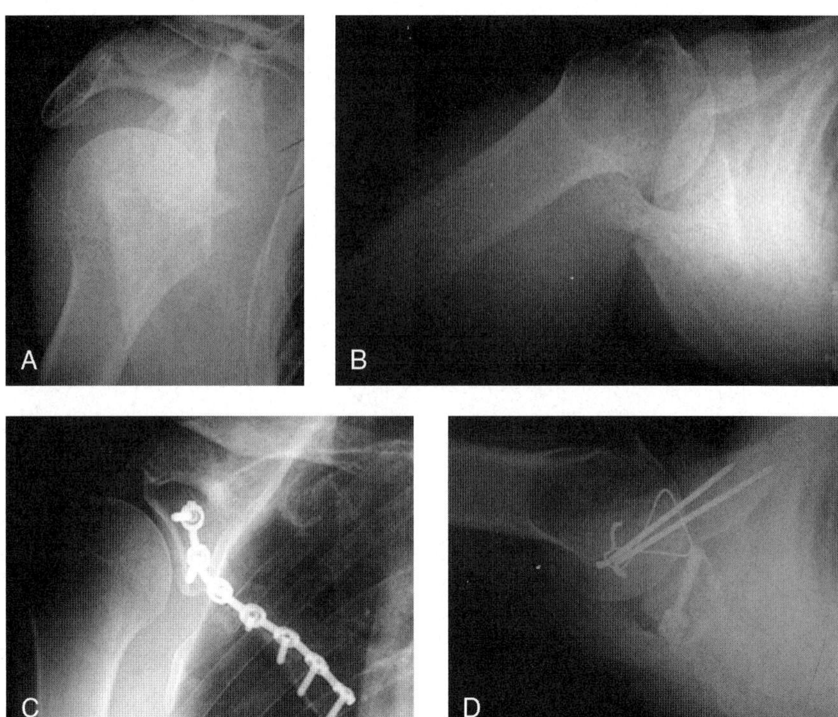

Figure 9 **A** and **B,** Radiographs of a distal clavicular fracture and a displaced scapular neck fracture. The displaced scapular neck fracture has been reduced and fixed posteriorly with a plate that curves inferiorly along the lateral border **(C)**, and the distal clavicular fracture has been reduced and fixed with tension-band and Kirschner wires **(D)**. (Reproduced with permission from Getz C, Deutsch A, Williams GR Jr: Scapular and glenoid fractures, in Warner JJP, Iannotti JP, Flatow EL, eds: *Complex and Revision Problems in Shoulder Surgery*, ed 2. Philadelphia, PA, Lippincott Williams and Wilkins, 2005, pp 365-394.)

coracoclavicular ligament, distal part of the clavicle, acromioclavicular joint, and acromion process) supported by superior and inferior osseous struts (the clavicular shaft and the lateral scapular body and spine). Together with the coracoacromial ligament, the remaining intact portions of the superior shoulder suspensory complex resist displacement and angulation of glenoid neck fractures.

Glenoid neck fractures can be classified according to the amount of displacement and angulation.[85] Type I glenoid neck fractures are displaced less than 1 cm, are angulated less than 40°, and account for 90% of cases. Type II fractures are displaced more than 1 cm, are angulated more than 40°, and represent only 10% of glenoid neck fractures.[75,88-90] In the absence of an additional fracture or ligamentous injury, most glenoid neck fractures are inherently stable and can be managed nonsurgically with a protocol similar to the one described above for scapular body fractures.[86]

Displaced or angulated fractures in young, active patients are treated surgically.[75,90] The type of surgical treatment depends on the associated injuries to the superior shoulder suspensory complex and the time from the injury. For example, an acute (less than 7 days old) displaced glenoid neck fracture combined with an ipsilateral clavicular shaft fracture and disruption of the coracoacromial and acromioclavicular ligaments can be managed with open reduction and internal fixation of the clavicle. The glenoid neck will be reduced by the intact coracoclavicular ligament (by ligamentotaxis). Likewise, an acute displaced glenoid neck fracture combined with displaced ipsilateral clavicular shaft and scapular spine fractures can be treated with open reduction and internal fixation of the clavicular shaft and the scapular spine. The glenoid neck will be reduced by ligamentotaxis through the intact coracoclavicular and/or coracoacromial ligaments. In patients with a subacute fracture, or a fracture pattern that is not amenable to ligamentotaxis, the glenoid neck must be reduced and stabilized directly through a posterior approach deep to the posterior border of the posterior part of the deltoid through the internervous plane between the teres minor and the infraspinatus. A plate is placed along the posterior aspect of the glenoid and curves down the lateral angle of the scapula (Figure 9).

Table 3
Results of Treatment of Glenoid Neck Fractures*

Author(s)	Year	No. of Patients	Mean Duration of Follow-up (Range)	Treatment	Results
Herscovici et al[91]	1992	7	Not available	Clavicle surgically fixed	All excellent
Nordqvist and Petersson[80]	1992	68	14 years	Nonsurgical	51 good, 15 fair, 2 poor; residual deformity associated with pain
Leung and Lam[92]	1993	15	25 months (14-47)	Surgical fixation	14 good to excellent, 1 fair; no stratification by displacement
Edwards et al[93]	2000	20	28 months (9-79)	Nonsurgical	17 excellent, 3 good; less displacement associated with better results
Low and Lam[94]	2000	4	3.3 years (2-4)	Clavicle surgically fixed	3 excellent, 1 good; no stratification by displacement
Egol et al[95]	2001	19	Not available	7 surgical, 12 nonsurgical	More flexion in surgical group; no difference in shoulder outcome scores
van Noort et al[96]	2001	35	35 months	31 nonsurgical, 4 surgical	3 late reconstructions; no difference between groups except that severe displacement resulted in caudal dislocation
Hashiguchi and Ito[97]	2003	5	57.4 months	Clavicle surgically fixed	5 good; average UCLA score, 34.2 points
Labler et al[98]	2004	17	Not available	8 nonsurgical, 9 surgical	5 good to excellent in each group; associated injures affected outcome; displacement was poor prognostic indicator

UCLA = University of California at Los Angeles
*Although the patient groups and treatment methods are variable, patient satisfaction seemed to be related to residual displacement or angulation in nonsurgically treated patients, and surgical management was most successful when anatomic reduction and healing were achieved.

Reported results of the treatment of glenoid neck fractures are sparse and difficult to interpret. Patients with and without combined injuries to the superior shoulder suspensory complex have been included in studies of the treatment of glenoid neck fractures, and results have been rarely stratified according to displacement or angulation. However, patient satisfaction after nonsurgical treatment seems to be related to residual displacement or angulation, and surgical management is most successful when anatomic reduction and healing are achieved. The results of several reported studies[80,91-98] are summarized in Table 3.

Glenoid Cavity Fractures

Glenoid cavity fractures involve the glenoid rim and are usually associated with instability or are fractures of the glenoid fossa causing incongruity of the articular surface. They are classified, according to their location and severity, into six types[75,87,99,100] (Figure 10).

Type I fractures involve the anterior (Ia) or posterior (Ib) aspect of the glenoid rim. Type II through IV fractures start with a transverse fracture between the superior and inferior halves of the glenoid and exit inferiorly through the lateral scapular border (II), superiorly through or near the superior scapular notch (III), or medially through the medial scapular border (IV). Type V fractures are more complex and are a combination of type II through IV fractures. Type VI fractures are severely comminuted and often not reconstructible.

Most glenoid fractures can be treated nonsurgically in a manner similar to what is used for scapular body fractures. Nonsurgical treatment is also indicated for type VI fractures that are too comminuted to support stable fixation. Surgical treatment is reserved for type I fractures associated with an unstable glenohumeral joint or any fracture (other than type VI) with intra-articular displacement exceeding 5 mm.[101]

Surgery for type I fractures is often done arthroscopically, especially if it is performed acutely.[102] When the rim fragment contains the labrum, which it often does, it can be used for fixation. In many cases, the most inferior portion of the osseous fragment is still attached to the native glenoid through an intact labral connection. The superior part of the

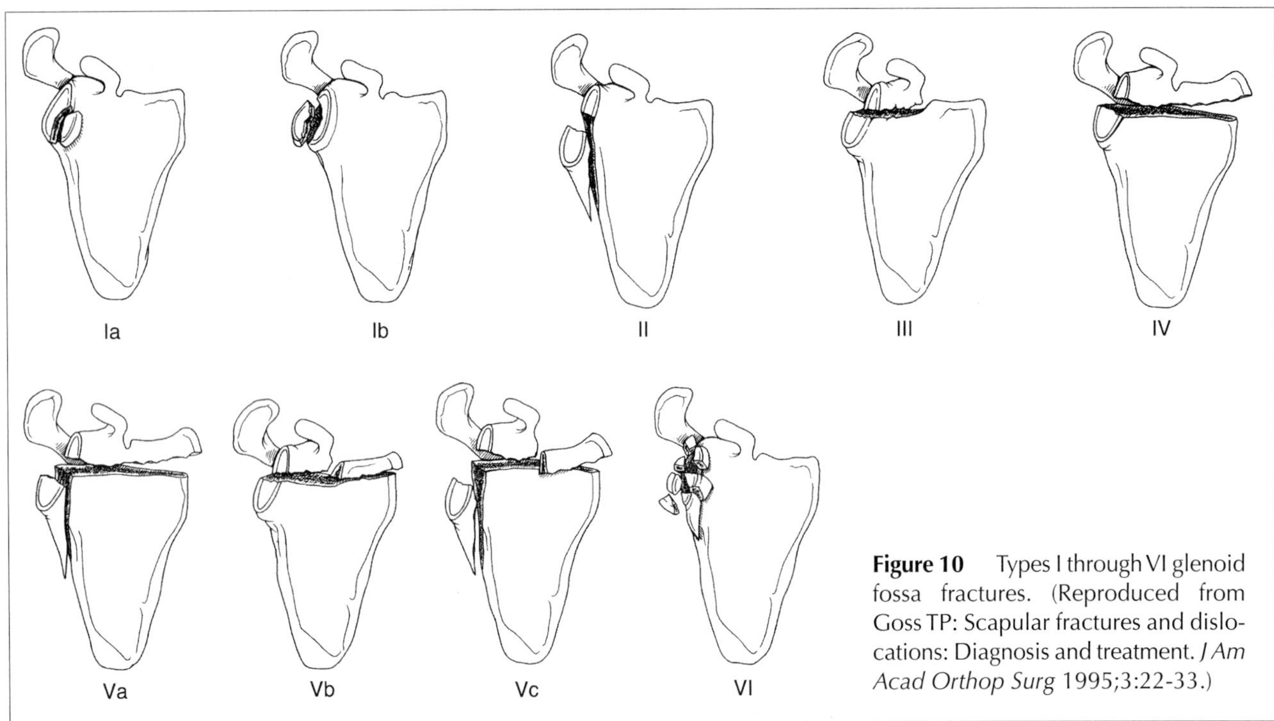

Figure 10 Types I through VI glenoid fossa fractures. (Reproduced from Goss TP: Scapular fractures and dislocations: Diagnosis and treatment. *J Am Acad Orthop Surg* 1995;3:22-33.)

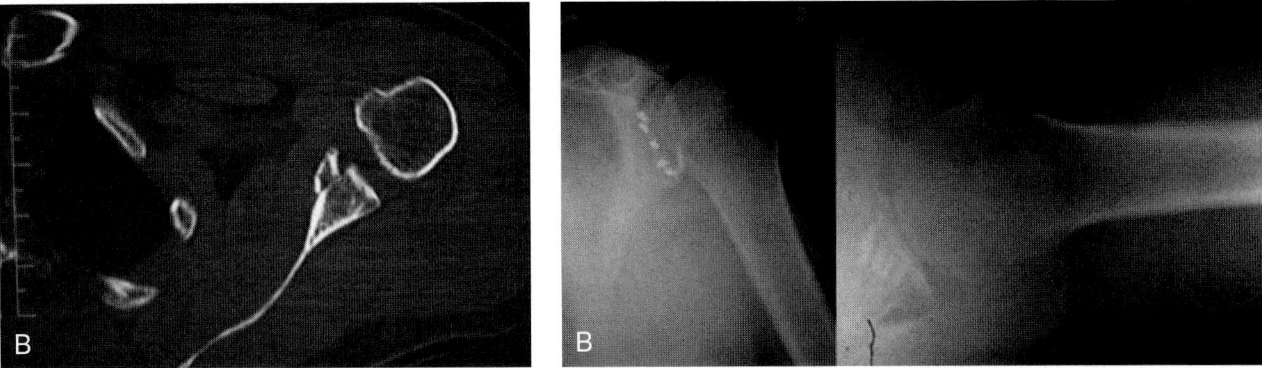

Figure 11 **A,** A type Ia glenoid rim fracture. **B,** Suture anchors have been placed in the fracture bed, and sutures have been passed through the fragment and tied extra-articularly. (Reproduced with permission from Getz C, Deutsch A, Williams GR Jr: Scapular and glenoid fractures, in Warner JP, Iannotti JP, Flatow EL, eds: *Complex and Revision Problems in Shoulder Surgery*, ed 2. Philadelphia, PA, Lippincott Williams and Wilkins, 2005, pp 365-394.)

fragment usually contains a portion of the labrum superior to it that can be reattached to the glenoid with suture anchors.

Open treatment of type Ia fractures is performed through a standard deltopectoral or anterior axillary approach. The displaced fragment is stabilized with interfragmentary screws (if it is large enough) or suture anchors. The anchors are placed in the native glenoid inferior and superior to the fragment, with the labrum used for fixation. Alternatively, the anchors are placed in the fracture bed, and the sutures are passed through the fragment and tied extra-articularly (Figure 11).

Type Ib fractures that are associated with an unstable glenohumeral joint are usually fixed with interfragmentary screws through a limited posterior axillary approach. With the patient in the lateral decubitus position and the arm abducted, the posterior part of the deltoid is retracted superolaterally without detaching any of its origin or insertion. The interval between the infraspinatus and the teres minor is split, and the infraspinatus is retracted superiorly while the teres minor is retracted inferiorly. The infraspinatus insertion does not require detachment in most cases. The capsule is incised to visualize the articular surface. The fragment is then reduced and fixed with two screws (Figure 12).

Type II fractures are also approached through a posterior axillary incision, through the same interval without detachment of the infraspinatus. If a plate is required to obtain adequate fixation, the inferior limb of the posterior axillary incision is extended inferiorly and medially over the lateral scapular margin. The infraspinatus origin and the dorsal portions of the origins of the teres minor and teres major are reflected off the scapula to expose the lateral border and the fracture line. The fracture is reduced, held provisionally with pins, and stabilized with a plate that starts below the fracture line on the lateral scapular border and extends superiorly onto the posterior surface of the glenoid. Care must be taken to avoid damage to the suprascapular nerve by the plate and to avoid placing screws into the joint.

Type III fractures are often best approached anteriorly. The strongest deforming force is the conjoined tendon of the short head of the biceps and the coracobrachialis. Control of the fragment is easiest when the coracoid can be used to lever the fragment. A neutralization plate can be placed anteriorly and supplemented with a lag screw placed percutaneously from superior to inferior, between the clavicle and the scapular spine or acromion.

The treatment of type IV fractures is similar to that of type II fractures. In some cases, even after a plate has been applied laterally, the fracture is rotationally unstable. Under these circumstances, the medial border of the scapula is exposed, and a plate is placed across the medial extent of the fracture.

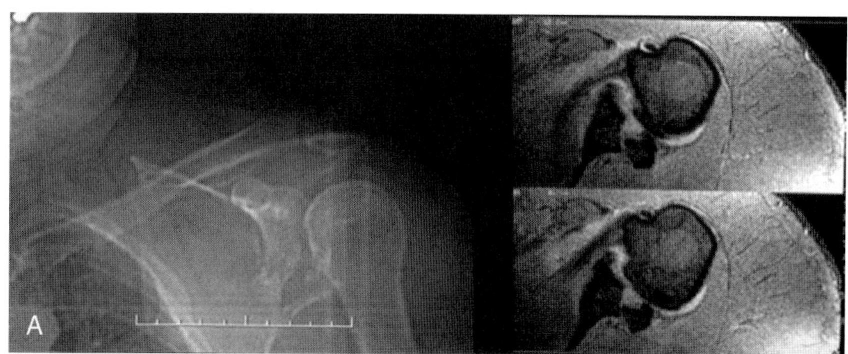

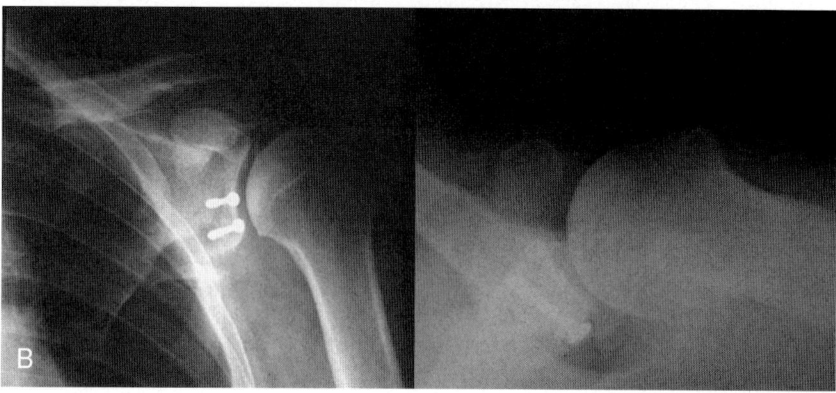

Figure 12 **A,** A type Ib glenoid rim fracture. **B,** The posterior fragment has been fixed with two screws. (Reproduced with permission from Getz C, Deutsch A, Williams GR Jr: Scapular and glenoid fractures, in Warner JP, Iannotti JP, Flatow EL, eds: *Complex and Revision Problems in Shoulder Surgery*, ed 2. Philadelphia, PA, Lippincott Williams and Wilkins, 2005, pp 365-394.)

The most important aspect of surgical management of type V fractures is to be sure that there are enough large fragments for stable and anatomic fixation of the articular surface. An extensile posterior approach is used in most cases.[78,103] Combining anterior and posterior approaches is rarely required but may be necessary for type Vb and Vc fractures when the superior glenoid fragment is severely rotated by the conjoined tendon.

The extensile posterior approach is performed with the patient lying in the lateral decubitus position. The skin incision starts at the medial extent of the scapular spine, courses laterally to the posterior corner of the acromion, and then curves inferiorly and medially to follow the lateral scapular border (Figure 13). The posterior deltoid origin is released from the scapular spine and retracted laterally. The interval between the infraspinatus and the teres minor is split, and the infraspinatus is detached from the humerus and reflected medially. Care is taken to prevent traction on the suprascapular nerve. The capsule is then incised to expose the joint surface. The teres minor and teres major origins are partially reflected off the lateral scapular margin, and the fracture is reduced. The articular surface is reconstructed and is fixed provisionally with pins. The remaining fractures are reduced, and a plate is placed from the lateral scap-

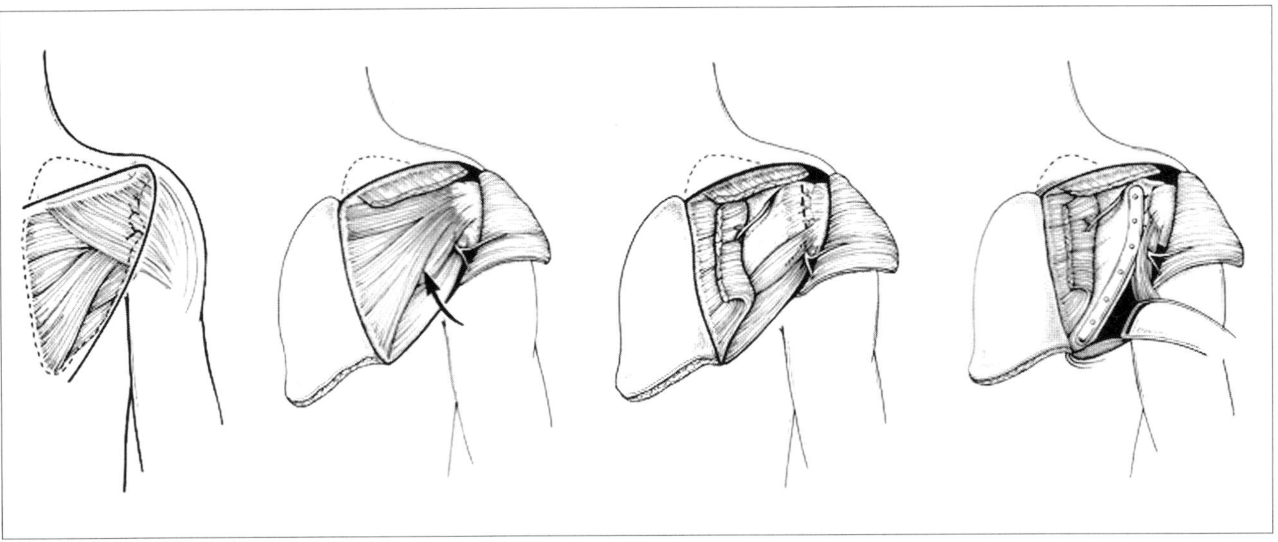

Figure 13 An extended posterior approach is used to expose the glenoid, glenoid neck, and lateral border of the scapula. (Reproduced with permission from Getz C, Deutsch A, Williams GR Jr: Scapular and glenoid fractures, in Warner JP, Iannotti JP, Flatow EL, eds: *Complex and Revision Problems in Shoulder Surgery*, ed 2. Philadelphia, PA, Lippincott Williams and Wilkins, 2005, pp 365-394.)

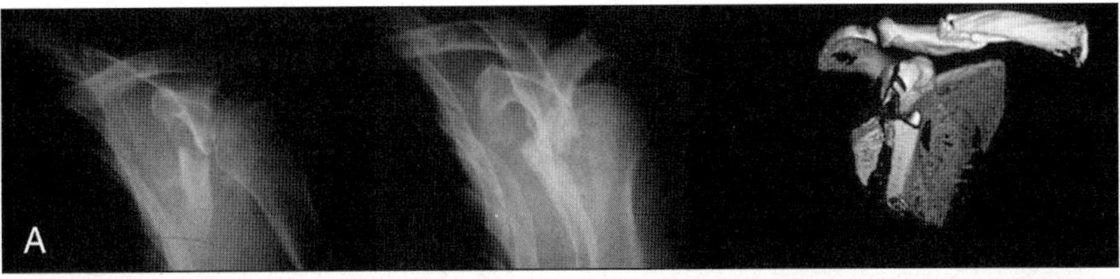

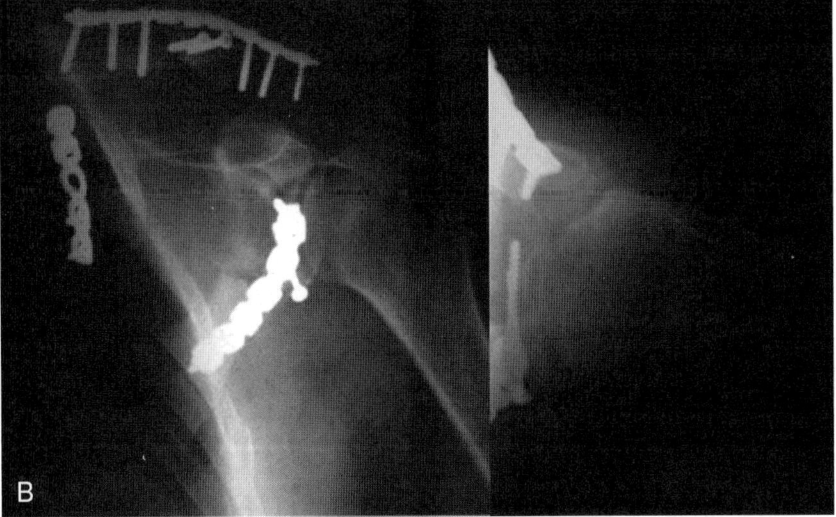

Figure 14 **A,** A type Va glenoid fossa fracture with an associated midshaft clavicular fracture. **B,** An extended posterior approach was used to fix the glenoid with supplementation by a medial border plate. (Reproduced with permission from Getz C, Deutsch A, Williams GR Jr: Scapular and glenoid fractures, in Warner JP, Iannotti JP, Flatow EL, eds: *Complex and Revision Problems in Shoulder Surgery*, ed 2. Philadelphia, PA, Lippincott Williams and Wilkins, 2005, pp 365-394.)

ular border to the posterior surface of the glenoid. Cannulated screws can be passed over the pins that were used for provisional fixation. After the plate has been secured, fracture stability is assessed. In some cases, a medial plate may also be required (Figure 14).

The results of surgical management of glenoid cavity fractures depend on the quality of the reduction. When residual joint incongruity is less than 2 mm, results are good or excellent in 80% to 90% of cases, and posttraumatic arthritis is minimal after 4 years of follow-up.[78,101]

Summary

Collectively, fractures and dislocations of the acromioclavicular joint, sternoclavicular joint, clavicle, and scapula account for a large percentage of shoulder girdle injuries. Treatment recommendations vary according to the severity and location of the injury. Most acromioclavicular injuries are treated nonsurgically unless the displacement is severe or irreducible. Sternoclavicular dislocations are treated with closed reduction. Anterior dislocations often are unstable after reduction and are subsequently treated nonsurgically. Unstable or irreducible posterior dislocations are reduced and stabilized with open means because of the potential for mediastinal injury. Markedly displaced medial and lateral clavicular fractures are associated with a high prevalence of symptomatic nonunion; therefore, surgical reduction and fixation are often recommended. Traditionally, midshaft clavicular fractures have been treated nonsurgically in most cases. Recently, high prevalences of symptomatic nonunion and malunion have been identified. Hence, surgical management with a plate or intramedullary pin has been advocated for displaced fractures. Scapular fractures are most often treated nonsurgically. Surgical reduction and internal fixation is reserved for displaced or angulated glenoid neck fractures, glenoid rim fractures associated with instability, and glenoid fossa fractures with articular displacement of more than 5 mm.

References

1. Rockwood CA, Williams GR, Young DC: Disorders of the acromioclavicular joint, in Rockwood CA, Matsen FA, Wirth MA, Lippitt SB, eds: *The Shoulder*, ed 3. Philadelphia, PA, Saunders, 2004, pp 521-595.
2. Neviaser RJ: Injuries to the clavicle and acromioclavicular joint. *Orthop Clin North Am* 1987;18:433-438.
3. Trainer G, Arciero RA, Mazzocca AD: Practical management of grade III acromioclavicular separations. *Clin J Sport Med* 2008;18:162-166.
4. Gstettner C, Tauber M, Hitzl W, Resch H: Rockwood type III acromioclavicular dislocation: Surgical versus conservative treatment. *J Shoulder Elbow Surg* 2008;17:220-225.
5. Nicholas SJ, Lee SJ, Mullaney MJ, Tyler TF, McHugh MP: Clinical outcomes of coracoclavicular ligament reconstructions using tendon grafts. *Am J Sports Med* 2007;35:1912-1917.
6. Nissen CW, Chatterjee A: Type III acromioclavicular separation: Results of a recent survey on its management. *Am J Orthop* 2007;36:89-93.
7. Guy DK, Wirth MA, Griffin JL, Rockwood CA Jr: Reconstruction of chronic and complete dislocations of the acromioclavicular joint. *Clin Orthop Relat Res* 1998;347:138-149.
8. Mazzocca AD, Santangelo SA, Johnson ST, Rios CG, Dumonski ML, Arciero RA: A biomechanical evaluation of an anatomical coracoclavicular ligament reconstruction. *Am J Sports Med* 2006;34:236-246.
9. Weaver JK, Dunn HK: Treatment of acromioclavicular injuries, especially complete acromioclavicular separation. *J Bone Joint Surg Am* 1972;54:1187-1194.
10. Salzmann GM, Walz L, Schoettle PB, Imhoff AB: Arthroscopic anatomical reconstruction of the acromioclavicular joint. *Acta Orthop Belg* 2008;74:397-400.
11. Tomlinson DP, Altchek DW, Davila J, Cordasco FA: A modified technique of arthroscopically assisted AC joint reconstruction and preliminary results. *Clin Orthop Relat Res* 2008;466:639-645.
12. Baumgarten KM, Altchek DW, Cordasco FA: Arthroscopically assisted acromioclavicular joint reconstruction. *Arthroscopy* 2006;22:228e1-228e6.
13. Spencer EE, Kuhn JE, Huston LJ, Carpenter JE, Hughes RE: Ligamentous restraints to anterior and posterior translation of the sternoclavicular joint. *J Shoulder Elbow Surg* 2002;11:43-47.
14. Bearn JG: Direct observations on the function of the capsule of the sternoclavicular joint in clavicular support. *J Anat* 1967;101(pt 1):159-170.
15. Rockwood CA, Wirth MA: Disorders of the sternoclavicular joint, in Rockwood CA, Matsen FA, Wirth MA, Lippitt SB, eds: *The Shoulder*, ed 3. Philadelphia, PA, Saunders, 2004, pp 597-653.
16. Throckmorton T, Kuhn JE: Fractures of the medial end of the clavicle. *J Shoulder Elbow Surg* 2007;16:49-54.
17. Robinson CM, Court-Brown CM, McQueen MM, Wakefield AE: Estimating the risk of nonunion following nonoperative treatment of a clavicular fracture. *J Bone Joint Surg Am* 2004;86:1359-1365.
18. Low AK, Duckworth DG, Bokor DJ: Operative outcome of displaced medial-end clavicle fractures in adults. *J Shoulder Elbow Surg* 2008;17:751-754.
19. Cave EF: Shoulder girdle injuries, in Cave EF, ed: *Fractures and Other Injuries*. Chicago, IL, Year Book Publishers, 1958, pp 258-259.
20. Gardner MA, Bidstrup BP: Intrathoracic great vessel injury resulting from blunt chest trauma associated with posterior dislocation of the sternoclavicular joint. *Aust N Z J Surg* 1983;53:427-430.
21. Jougon JB, Lepront DJ, Dromer CE: Posterior dislocation of the sternoclavicular joint leading to mediastinal compression. *Ann Thorac Surg* 1996;61:711-713.
22. Ono K, Inagawa H, Kiyota K, Terada T, Suzuki S, Maekawa K: Posterior dislocation of the sternoclavicular joint with obstruction of the innominate vein: Case report. *J Trauma* 1998;44:381-383.
23. Ecke H: Late lesions following luxation of the sternoclavicular joint. *Hefte Unfallheilkd* 1984;170:52-55.
24. Noda M, Shiraishi H, Mizuno K: Chronic posterior sternoclavicular dislocation causing compression of a subclavian artery. *J Shoulder Elbow Surg* 1997;6:564-569.
25. Gangahar DM, Flogaites T: Retrosternal dislocation of the clavicle producing thoracic outlet syndrome. *J Trauma* 1978;18:369-372.

26. Rayan GM: Compression brachial plexopathy caused by chronic posterior dislocation of the sternoclavicular joint. *J Okla State Med Assoc* 1994;87:7-9.

27. Bicos J, Nicholson GP: Treatment and results of sternoclavicular joint injuries. *Clin Sports Med* 2003;22:359-370.

28. Southworth SR, Merritt TR: Asymptomatic innominate vein tamponade with retromanubrial clavicular dislocation: A case report. *Orthop Rev* 1988;17:789-791.

29. de Jong KP, Sukul DM: Anterior sternoclavicular dislocation: A long-term follow-up study. *J Orthop Trauma* 1990;4:420-423.

30. Wirth MA, Rockwood CA Jr: Acute and chronic traumatic injuries of the sternoclavicular joint. *J Am Acad Orthop Surg* 1996;4:268-278.

31. Wasylenko MJ, Busse EF: Posterior dislocation of the clavicle causing fatal tracheoesophageal fistula. *Can J Surg* 1981;24:626-627.

32. Acus RW III, Bell RH, Fisher DL: Proximal clavicle excision: An analysis of results. *J Shoulder Elbow Surg* 1995;4:182-187.

33. Eskola A, Vainionpää S, Vastamäki M, Slätis P, Rokkanen P: Operation for old sternoclavicular dislocation: Results in 12 cases. *J Bone Joint Surg Br* 1989;71:63-65.

34. Rockwood CA Jr, Groh GI, Wirth MA, Grassi FA: Resection arthroplasty of the sternoclavicular joint. *J Bone Joint Surg Am* 1997;79:387-393.

35. Spencer EE Jr, Kuhn JE: Biomechanical analysis of reconstructions for sternoclavicular joint instability. *J Bone Joint Surg Am* 2004;86:98-105.

36. Burrows HJ: Tenodesis of the subclavius in the treatment of recurrent dislocation of the sterno-clavicular joint. *J Bone Joint Surg Br* 1951;33:240-243.

37. Smolle-Juettner FM, Hofer PH, Pinter H, Friehs G, Szyskowitz R: Intracardiac malpositioning of a sternoclavicular fixation wire. *J Orthop Trauma* 1992;6:102-105.

38. Pate JW, Wilhite JL: Migration of a foreign body from the sternoclavicular joint to the heart: A case report. *Am Surg* 1969;35:448-449.

39. Lyons FA, Rockwood CA Jr: Migration of pins used in operations on the shoulder. *J Bone Joint Surg Am* 1990;72:1262-1267.

40. Clark RL, Milgram JW, Yawn DH: Fatal aortic perforation and cardiac tamponade due to a Kirschner wire migrating from the right sternoclavicular joint. *South Med J* 1974;67:316-318.

41. Ferrández L, Usabiaga J, Ramos L, Yubero J, No L: Migration of Kirschner wires into the mediastinum after stabilization of sterno-clavicular lesions: A report of two cases. *Chir Organi Mov* 1991;76:301-304.

42. Janssens de Varebeke B, Van Osselaer G: Migration of Kirschner's pin from the right sternoclavicular joint resulting in perforation of the pulmonary artery main trunk. *Acta Chir Belg* 1993;93:287-291.

43. Neer CS II: Nonunion of the clavicle. *J Am Med Assoc* 1960;172:1006-1011.

44. Zlowodzki M, Zelle BA, Cole PA, Jeray K, McKee MD: Treatment of acute midshaft clavicle fractures: Systematic review of 2144 fractures. On behalf of the Evidence-Based Orthopaedic Trauma Working Group. *J Orthop Trauma* 2005;19:504-507.

45. Hill JM, McGuire MH, Crosby LA: Closed treatment of displaced middle-third fractures of the clavicle gives poor results. *J Bone Joint Surg Br* 1997;79:537-539.

46. Nowak J, Mallmin H, Larsson S: The aetiology and epidemiology of clavicular fractures: A prospective study during a two-year period in Uppsala, Sweden. *Injury* 2000;31:353-358.

47. McKee MD, Schemitsch EH, Stephen DJ, Kreder HJ, Yoo D, Harrington J: Functional outcome following clavicle fractures in polytrauma patients. *J Trauma* 1999;47:616.

48. McKee MD, Pedersen EM, Jones C, et al: Deficits following nonoperative treatment of displaced midshaft clavicular fractures. *J Bone Joint Surg Am* 2006;88:35-40.

49. Hudak PL, Amadio PC, Bombardier C, The Upper Extremity Collaborative Group (UECG): Development of an upper extremity outcome measure: The DASH (disabilities of the arm, shoulder and hand). *Am J Ind Med* 1996;29:602-608.

50. Canadian Orthopaedic Trauma Society: Nonoperative treatment compared with plate fixation of displaced midshaft clavicular fractures: A multicenter, randomized clinical trial. *J Bone Joint Surg Am* 2007;89:1-10.

51. Ali Khan MA, Lucas HK: Plating of fractures of the middle third of the clavicle. *Injury* 1978;9:263-267.

52. Poigenfürst J, Rappold G, Fischer W: Plating of fresh clavicular fractures: Results of 122 operations. *Injury* 1992;23:237-241.

53. Shen WJ, Liu TJ, Shen YS: Plate fixation of fresh displaced midshaft clavicle fractures. *Injury* 1999;30:497-500.

54. Shahid R, Mushtaq A, Maqsood M: Plate fixation of clavicle fractures: A comparative study between reconstruction plate and dynamic compression plate. *Acta Orthop Belg* 2007;73:170-174.

55. McKee MD, Seiler JG, Jupiter JB: The application of the limited contact dynamic compression plate in the upper extremity: An analysis of 114 consecutive cases. *Injury* 1995;26:661-666.

56. Collinge C, Devinney S, Herscovici D, DiPasquale T, Sanders R: Anterior-inferior plate fixation of middle-third fractures and nonunions of the clavicle. *J Orthop Trauma* 2006;20:680-686.

57. Böstman O, Manninen M, Pihlajamäki H: Complications of plate fixation in fresh displaced midclavicular fractures. *J Trauma* 1997;43:778-783.

58. Schwarz N, Höcker K: Osteosynthesis of irreducible fractures of the clavicle with 2.7-mm ASIF plates. *J Trauma* 1992;33:179-183.

59. Iannotti MR, Crosby LA, Stafford P, Grayson G, Goulet R: Effects of plate location and selection on the stability of midshaft clavicle osteotomies: A biomechanical study. *J Shoulder Elbow Surg* 2002;11:457-462.

60. Kim W, McKee MD: Management of acute clavicle fractures. *Orthop Clin North Am* 2008;39:491-505.

61. Chu CM, Wang SJ, Lin LC: Fixation of mid-third clavicular fractures with Knowles pins: 78 patients followed for 2-7 years. *Acta Orthop Scand* 2002;73:134-139.

62. Strauss EJ, Egol KA, France MA, Koval KJ, Zuckerman JD: Complications of intramedullary Hagie pin fixation for acute midshaft clavicle fractures. *J Shoulder Elbow Surg* 2007;16:280-284.

63. Jubel A, Andermahr J, Schiffer G, Tsironis K, Rehm KE: Elastic stable intramedullary nailing of midclavicular fractures with a titanium nail. *Clin Orthop Relat Res* 2003;408:279-285.

64. Chuang TY, Ho WP, Hsieh PH, Lee PC, Chen CH, Chen YJ: Closed reduction and internal fixation for acute midshaft clavicular fractures using cannulated screws. *J Trauma* 2006;60:1315-1321.

65. Potter JM, Jones C, Wild LM, Schemitsch EH, McKee MD: Does delay matter? The restoration of objectively measured shoulder strength and patient-oriented outcome after immediate fixation versus delayed reconstruction of displaced midshaft fractures of the clavicle. *J Shoulder Elbow Surg* 2007;16:514-518.

66. Nordqvist A, Petersson C, Redlund-Johnell I: The natural course of lateral clavicle fracture: 15 (11-21) year follow-up of 110 cases. *Acta Orthop Scand* 1993;64:87-91.

67. Rockwood CA: Fractures of the outer clavicle in children and adults. *J Bone Joint Surg Br* 1982;64:642-647.

68. Ballmer FT, Gerber C: Coracoclavicular screw fixation for unstable fractures of the distal clavicle: A report of five cases. *J Bone Joint Surg Br* 1991;73:291-294.

69. Meda PV, Machani B, Sinopidis C, Braithwaite I, Brownson P, Frostick SP: Clavicular hook plate for lateral end fractures: A prospective study. *Injury* 2006;37:277-283.

70. Flinkkilä T, Ristiniemi J, Hyvönen P, Hämäläinen M: Surgical treatment of unstable fractures of the distal clavicle: A comparative study of Kirschner wire and clavicular hook plate fixation. *Acta Orthop Scand* 2002;73:50-53.

71. Nourissat G, Kakuda C, Dumontier C, Sautet A, Doursounian L: Arthroscopic stabilization of Neer type 2 fracture of the distal part of the clavicle. *Arthroscopy* 2007;23:674.e1-674.e4.

72. Jin CZ, Kim HK, Min BH: Surgical treatment for distal clavicle fracture associated with coracoclavicular ligament rupture using a cannulated screw fixation technique. *J Trauma* 2006;60:1358-1361.

73. Bezer M, Aydin N, Guven O: The treatment of distal clavicle fractures with coracoclavicular ligament disruption: A report of 10 cases. *J Orthop Trauma* 2005;19:524-528.

74. Kashii M, Inui H, Yamamoto K: Surgical treatment of distal clavicle fractures using the clavicular hook plate. *Clin Orthop Relat Res* 2006;447:158-164.

75. Goss TP: Fractures of the scapula, in Rockwood CA, Matsen FA, Wirth MA, Lippitt SB, eds: *The Shoulder*, ed 3. Philadelphia, PA, Saunders, 2004, pp 413-354.

76. Imatani RJ: Fractures of the scapula: A review of 53 fractures. *J Trauma* 1975;15:473-478.

77. Thompson DA, Flynn TC, Miller PW, Fischer RP: The significance of scapular fractures. *J Trauma* 1985;25:974-977.

78. Mayo KA, Benirschke SK, Mast JW: Displaced fractures of the glenoid fossa: Results of open reduction and internal fixation. *Clin Orthop Relat Res* 1998;347:122-130.

79. McGahan JP, Rab GT, Dublin A: Fractures of the scapula. *J Trauma* 1980;20:880-883.

80. Nordqvist A, Petersson C: Fracture of the body, neck, or spine of the scapula: A long-term follow-up study. *Clin Orthop Relat Res* 1992;283:139-144.

81. Goss TP: Scapular fractures and dislocations: Diagnosis and treatment. *J Am Acad Orthop Surg* 1995;3:22-33.

82. Ferraz IC, Papadimitriou NG, Sotereanos DG: Scapular body nonunion: A case report. *J Shoulder Elbow Surg* 2002;11:98-100.

83. Martin SD, Weiland AJ: Missed scapular fracture after trauma: A case report and a 23-year follow-up report. *Clin Orthop Relat Res* 1994;299:259-262.

84. Michael D, Fazal MA, Cohen B: Nonunion of a fracture of the body of the scapula: Case report and literature review. *J Shoulder Elbow Surg* 2001;10:385-386.

85. Goss TP: Fractures of the glenoid neck. *J Shoulder Elbow Surg* 1994;3:42-52.

86. Williams GR Jr, Naranja J, Klimkiewicz J, Karduna A, Iannotti JP, Ramsey M: The floating shoulder: A biomechanical basis for classification and management. *J Bone Joint Surg Am* 2001;83:1182-1187.

87. Goss TP: Double disruptions of the superior shoulder suspensory complex. *J Orthop Trauma* 1993;7:99-106.

88. Goss TP: Fractures of the glenoid cavity: Operative principles and techniques. *Tech Orthop* 1994;8:199-204.

89. Zdravkovic D, Damholt VV: Comminuted and severely displaced fractures of the scapula. *Acta Orthop Scand* 1974;45:60-65.

90. Ada JR, Miller ME: Scapular fractures: Analysis of 113 cases. *Clin Orthop Relat Res* 1991;269:174-180.

91. Herscovici D Jr, Fiennes AG, Allgöwer M, Rüedi TP: The floating

shoulder: Ipsilateral clavicle and scapular neck fractures. *J Bone Joint Surg Br* 1992;74:362-364.

92. Leung KS, Lam TP: Open reduction and internal fixation of ipsilateral fractures of the scapular neck and clavicle. *J Bone Joint Surg Am* 1993;75: 1015-1018.

93. Edwards SG, Whittle AP, Wood GW II: Nonoperative treatment of ipsilateral fractures of the scapula and clavicle. *J Bone Joint Surg Am* 2000;82:774-780.

94. Low CK, Lam AW: Results of fixation of clavicle alone in managing floating shoulder. *Singapore Med J* 2000;41: 452-453.

95. Egol KA, Connor PM, Karunakar MA, Sims SH, Bosse MJ, Kellam JF: The floating shoulder: Clinical and functional results. *J Bone Joint Surg Am* 2001;83-A:1188-1194.

96. van Noort A, te Slaa RL, Marti RK, van der Werken C: The floating shoulder: A multicentre study. *J Bone Joint Surg Br* 2001;83:795-798.

97. Hashiguchi H, Ito H: Clinical outcome of the treatment of floating shoulder by osteosynthesis for clavicular fracture alone. *J Shoulder Elbow Surg* 2003;12:589-591.

98. Labler L, Platz A, Weishaupt D, Trentz O: Clinical and functional results after floating shoulder injuries. *J Trauma* 2004;57:595-602.

99. Ideberg R, Grevsten S, Larsson S: Epidemiology of scapular fractures: Incidence and classification of 338 fractures. *Acta Orthop Scand* 1995; 66:395-397.

100. Goss TP: Fractures of the glenoid cavity. *J Bone Joint Surg Am* 1992;74: 299-305.

101. Kavanagh BF, Bradway JK, Cofield RH: Open reduction and internal fixation of displaced intra-articular fractures of the glenoid fossa. *J Bone Joint Surg Am* 1993;75:479-484.

102. Sugaya H, Kon Y, Tsuchiya A: Arthroscopic repair of glenoid fractures using suture anchors. *Arthroscopy* 2005;21:635.

103. Judet R: Surgical treatment of scapular fractures. *Acta Orthop Belg* 1964;30:673-678.

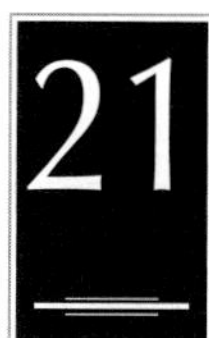

Key Factors in Primary and Revision Surgery for Shoulder Instability

CDR Matthew T. Provencher, MD, MC, USN
Robert A. Arciero, MD
Stephen S. Burkhart, MD
William N. Levine, MD
Andrew W. Ritting, MD
Anthony A. Romeo, MD

Abstract

The diagnosis and treatment of shoulder instability are predicated on a sound understanding of the patient's history and injury pattern as well as the examination and radiographic findings. The arthroscopic repair of instability is increasingly successful. However, glenohumeral bone loss, capsular injuries, and associated injury patterns have been linked to unsuccessful outcomes after either surgical or nonsurgical treatment. A comprehensive approach, from patient history to surgical technique, can increase the likelihood of a successful primary or secondary instability repair.

Instr Course Lect 2010;59:227-244.

Dr. Provencher or an immediate family member serves as a board member, owner, officer, or committee member of the American Orthopaedic Society for Sports Medicine; the International Society of Arthroscopy, Knee Surgery, and Orthopaedic Sports Medicine; the Society of Military Orthopaedic Surgeons; the American Academy of Orthopaedic Surgeons; and the Arthroscopy Association of North America; and has received research or institutional support from the Arthroscopy Association of North America; the American Orthopaedic Society for Sports Medicine, and the Orthopaedic Research and Education Foundation. Dr. Arciero or an immediate family member is a member of a speakers' bureau or has made paid presentations on behalf of Arthrex and has received research or institutional support from Arthrex. Dr. Burkhart or an immediate family member serves as a board member, owner, officer, or committee member of the San Antonio Orthopaedic Surgery Center; has received royalties from Arthrex; is a member of a speakers' bureau or has made paid presentations on behalf of Arthrex; serves as a paid consultant to or is an employee of Arthrex; and has received nonincome support (such as equipment or services), commercially derived honoraria, or other non–research-related funding (such as paid travel) from Wolters Kluwer Health–Lippincott Williams & Wilkins. Dr. Levine or an immediate family member serves as a board member, owner, officer, or committee member of the American Orthopaedic Association, the American Orthopaedic Society for Sports Medicine, and the American Shoulder and Elbow Surgeons and has received research or institutional support from Arthrex, Zimmer, and Smith & Nephew. Dr. Ritting or an immediate family member has received research or institutional support from Arthrex and has stock or stock options held in KCI. Dr. Romeo or an immediate family member has received royalties from Arthrex; is a member of a speakers' bureau or has made paid presentations on behalf of Arthrex; serves as a paid consultant to or is an employee of Arthrex; has received research or institutional support from Arthrex; has stock or stock options held in Arthrex; and has received nonincome support (such as equipment or services), commercially derived honoraria, or other non–research-related funding (such as paid travel) from Arthrex.

The surgical management of shoulder instability has dramatically changed during the past 20 years. Although open Bankart repair and capsular shift historically have been the gold standard for surgical treatment of an unstable shoulder, arthroscopic treatment increasingly is preferred. The choice of open or arthroscopic repair has become controversial.[1-4] Some early arthroscopic repairs had disappointingly high rates of failure,[5] but increased awareness of shoulder anatomy and pathology as well as technologic improvements have led to success rates comparable to those of open repair.[6]

The debate on the relative merits of arthroscopic and open repair has been accompanied by a trend toward identifying patients who may not be a candidate for any soft-tissue surgery, whether arthroscopic or open. Some bony defects of the glenoid or humeral head lead to failure of any soft-tissue procedure. The patient's age and functional demands must be considered, as well as capsular integrity and associated conditions such as a collagen disorder, rotator cuff tear, or biceps injury. The instability must be correctly diagnosed as anterior, posterior, or multidirectional.

Primary Surgery for Shoulder Instability

The factors that allow the surgeon to maximize the success of primary surgery to correct shoulder instability fall into three categories: selecting the patient, selecting the procedure, and selecting the rehabilitation program.

Selecting the Patient

History

Understanding the source and type of instability is critical to the success of any intervention. A thorough patient history must include hand dominance, type of instability (dislocation or subluxation), direction of instability (anterior, posterior, or multidirectional), age at first dislocation, activity level (including contact and noncontact sports), and any earlier treatment (including medically assisted reduction). The severity of trauma required for an instability episode to occur has obvious treatment implications; a patient whose shoulder slips into instability during sleep or a simple movement such as reaching overhead may require a different surgical plan than a patient with instability from severe trauma. The possibility of voluntary instability should be assessed because the instability pattern may have a psychological component that is relatively unlikely to be corrected by surgical repair.

Physical Examination

In addition to a patient history, a complete physical examination is integral to making the correct diagnosis and implementing the appropriate treatment plan. Most patients have normal range of motion, neurovascular status, and overall strength in the shoulder girdle and periscapular muscles. The apprehension, relocation, and anterior release tests are used to assess anterior shoulder instability. It is especially important to investigate the ease with which the humerus begins to dislocate and engage the glenoid. For example, humeral dislocation with glenoid engagement occurring at 30° of external rotation with the arm at the side probably indicates a significant engaging Hill-Sachs lesion with glenoid bone loss.[7] This condition usually is preceded by a history of shoulder instability in the mid ranges of shoulder abduction and external rotation.

It is important to distinguish between laxity and instability. Laxity is normal in the glenohumeral joint; for normal shoulder function, the humerus must have a minimal amount of obligate translation on the glenoid.[8,9] Instability generally is defined as symptomatic laxity, and its presence is determined by the perception of the patient. The extent of laxity is assessed through testing for anterior, posterior, and inferior sulcus translation. A finding of symptomatic directional laxity is called instability. The presence of a positive sulcus sign that does not decrease with external rotation with the arm at the side indicates a pathologic rotator cuff interval[10,11] (Figure 1). General ligamentous laxity also should be assessed by testing for thumb-to-forearm laxity, elbow recurvatum, metacarpophalangeal hyperextension, and increased external rotation with the arm in the abducted position.

Radiographic Evaluation

The AP, true AP, axillary lateral, and scapular lateral radiographic views are routinely obtained. The apical oblique, West Point, or Didiee view is used for close evaluation of the glenoid.[12-15] A Hill-Sachs defect is best seen on the true AP view in internal rotation or the Stryker notch view.[15] MRI is best used for identifying soft-tissue injury in an unstable shoulder, but the use of CT is recommended if bony injuries are suspected (Figure 2). Three-dimensional CT reconstruction may be beneficial for delineating the severity of the bony lesion, especially on the glenoid side.[16,17]

Bone Loss Evaluation

Certain patient history and examination factors are associated with glenoid and humeral head bone loss (Table 1). Patients with instability after a high-energy injury may have a glenoid fracture. More commonly, a patient with recurrent instability has had numerous instability events, some of which required reduction, and can describe a progression in the ease with which instability occurs. The shoulder position in which the patient becomes aware of instability should be carefully assessed to determine whether the instability is present in the mid ranges of motion (suggesting bone loss) and whether the humeral head is capable of engaging the glenoid anteriorly. Although an axillary lateral radiograph can provide some information, West Point and apical oblique radiographs are preferred.[12,14] However, plain radiographs probably are insufficient for a thorough evaluation of bone loss.

The extent of bone loss can be assessed using the most lateral glenoid image in a sagittal oblique MRI or magnetic resonance arthrography series. However, CT is more accurate for determining bone loss, particularly a three-dimensional CT re-

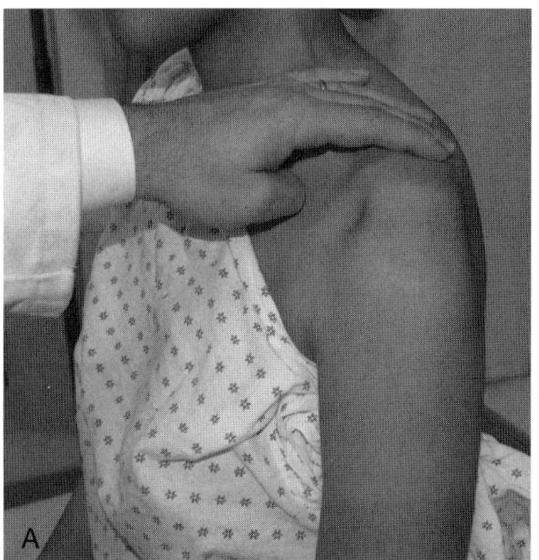

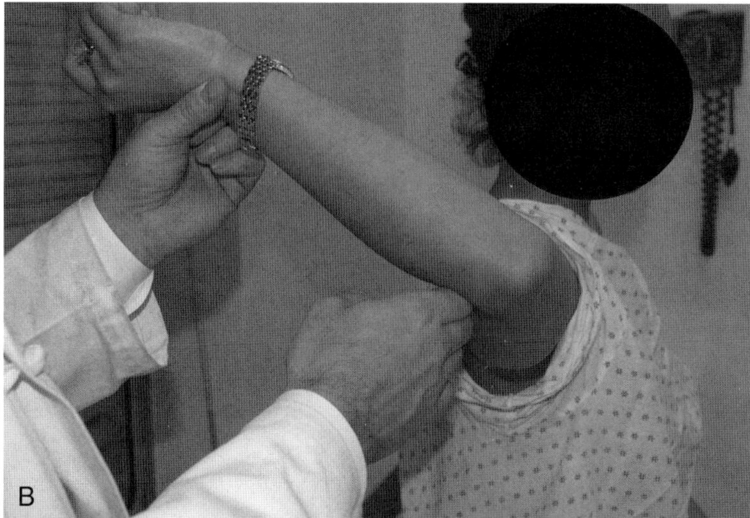

Figure 1 Clinical photographs showing left shoulder instability in a right-handed 24-year-old woman. **A,** A sulcus maneuver with external rotation of the arm and longitudinal traction is applied by the examiner. Placing the arm in external rotation has not decreased the positive sulcus sign, and therefore the rotator cuff interval is believed to be incompetent and may require closure if surgery is done. **B,** Maximal external rotation of the asymptomatic right shoulder, showing greater-than-normal ligamentous laxity.

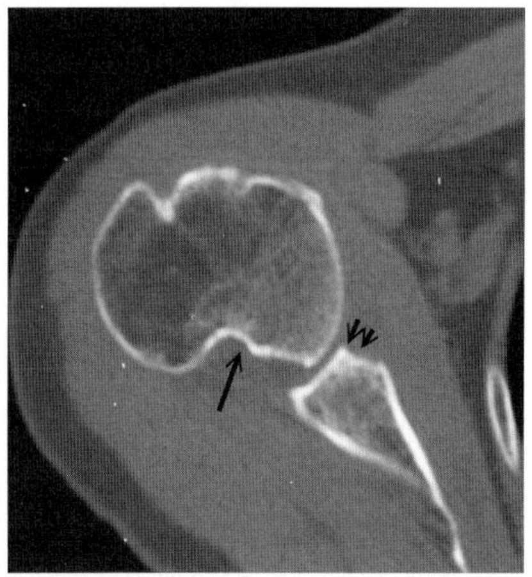

Figure 2 Axial CT of the right shoulder in a right-handed 45-year-old man with multiple traumatic anterior dislocations. A Hill-Sachs defect (*large arrow*) and anteroinferior glenoid deficiency (*small arrows*) can be seen.

Table 1
Factors Suggesting the Presence of Glenoid or Humeral Head Bone Loss

Patient History and Examination
Initial shoulder dislocation caused by a high-energy traumatic event
Multiple instability events
Recurrent anterior instability extending over several years or occurring as a single event several years after the initial instability
Progressive ease of instability (decreasing level of activity required)
Instability in the mid ranges of motion (45° to 60° abduction, with 45° of external rotation)
Imaging
Anteroinferior glenoid loss (on cortical rim or outline) seen on AP or true AP radiograph
Bone loss seen on axillary lateral radiograph
Bone loss seen on sagittal oblique MRI or magnetic resonance arthrogram
Bone loss seen on CT, especially three-dimensional reconstruction with the humeral head digitally subtracted
Anterior glenoid erosion seen on axial CT (the amount of anterior glenoid bone loss is underestimated on axial CT)

construction with the humeral head digitally subtracted from the sagittal view (Figure 3). The inferior two thirds of the glenoid forms a circle, and a deficiency within this circle indicates bone loss.[18] A circle is drawn onto the image to fill the inferior two thirds of the en face sagittal image,[18] and the missing bone is quantified by assessing surface area loss in the anteroinferior part of the circle (Figure 3, *B*). Bone loss must be precisely measured. The normal glenoid bone stock measurement from anterior to posterior is approximately 24 to 28 mm,[19] and a 6- to 8-mm loss of anterior glenoid bone therefore is a loss of 25% of the width of the glenoid. Such a loss may necessitate a change in strategy to include open bone augmentation in the primary repair. Bone loss usually occurs along a line parallel to the long axis of the glenoid[16,20] (Figures 3, *B* and 4).

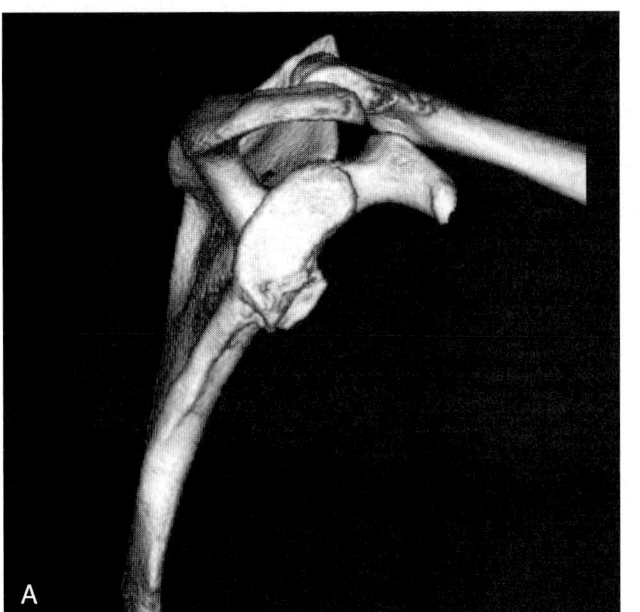

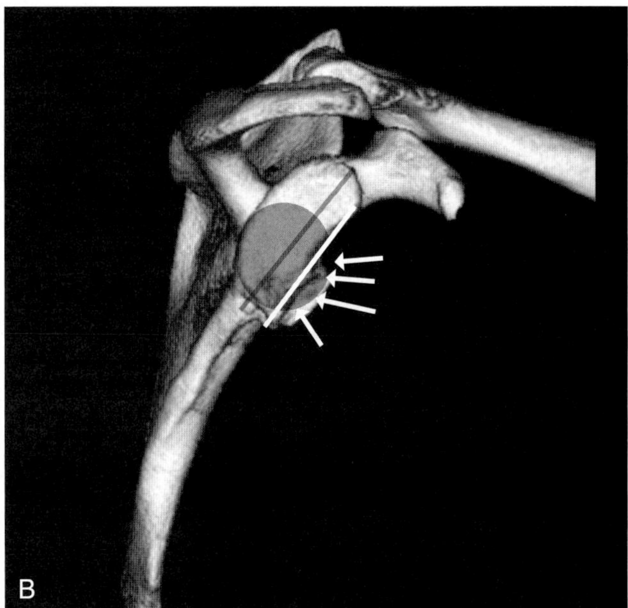

Figure 3 Three-dimensional CT reconstruction with the humeral head digitally subtracted, shown in the sagittal plane for determining glenoid bone loss. **A,** An anterior glenoid bone fragment with bone loss has healed medially. **B,** A circle is superimposed onto the inferior two thirds of the glenoid for quantifying bone loss (*arrows*); bone loss almost always occurs along a line parallel to the long axis of the glenoid (light and dark lines, respectively).

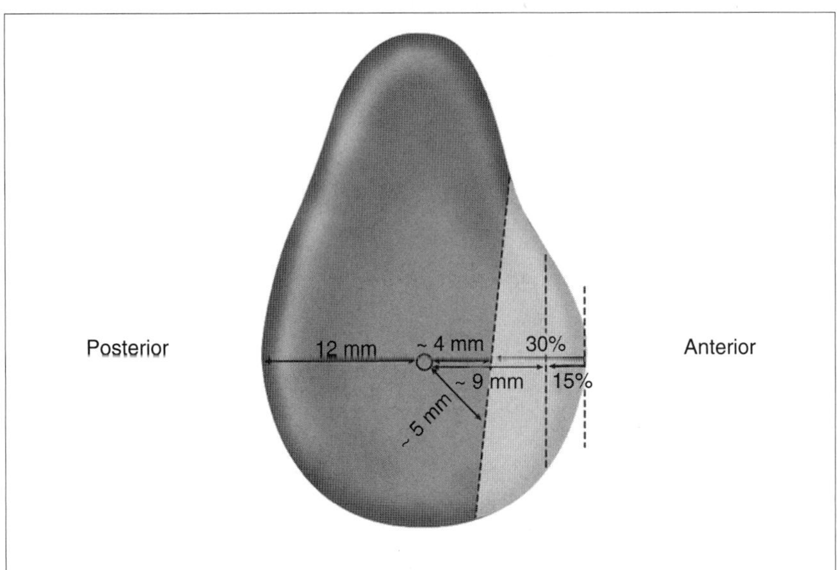

Figure 4 Schematic diagram depicting the quantification of bone loss. The center circle represents the bare spot of the glenoid. (Reproduced from Piasecki DP, Verma NN, Romeo AA, Levine WN, Bach BR, Provencher MT: Glenoid bone deficiency in recurrent anterior shoulder instability: Diagnosis and management. *J Am Acad Orthop Surg* 2009:17:487.)

If bone loss is not assessed preoperatively, it should be determined arthroscopically to confirm the appropriateness of the anterior stabilization procedure. The arthroscopic technique for determining glenoid bone loss has been validated in clinical and research studies.[19-21] As described by Lo and associates,[19] glenoid bone loss can be quantified by measuring the anterior-to-posterior width of the defect at the level of the bare spot. With the arthroscope in the anterosuperior portal, a calibrated probe is inserted from the posterior portal to measure the distance from the anterior and posterior rims to the bare spot (Figure 5). The difference between the anterior and posterior radii is used to calculate the bone loss, as follows: percentage of glenoid bone loss = (distance from the bare spot to the posterior rim − distance from the bare spot to the anterior rim) ÷ 2 × distance from the bare spot to the posterior rim. The result is expressed as a percentage.

The percentage of glenoid bone loss that should be considered critical in treating recurrent anterior shoulder instability is controversial.

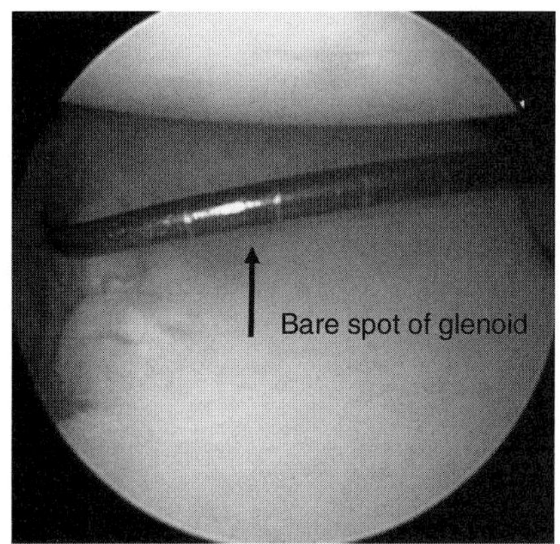

Figure 5 Arthroscopic view from the anterosuperior portal showing the measurement of glenoid bone loss using a calibrated probe inserted from the posterior portal. (Reproduced from Piasecki DP, Verma NN, Romeo AA, Levine WN, Bach BR, Provencher MT: Glenoid bone deficiency in recurrent anterior shoulder instability: Diagnosis and management. *J Am Acad Orthop Surg* 2009:17:485.)

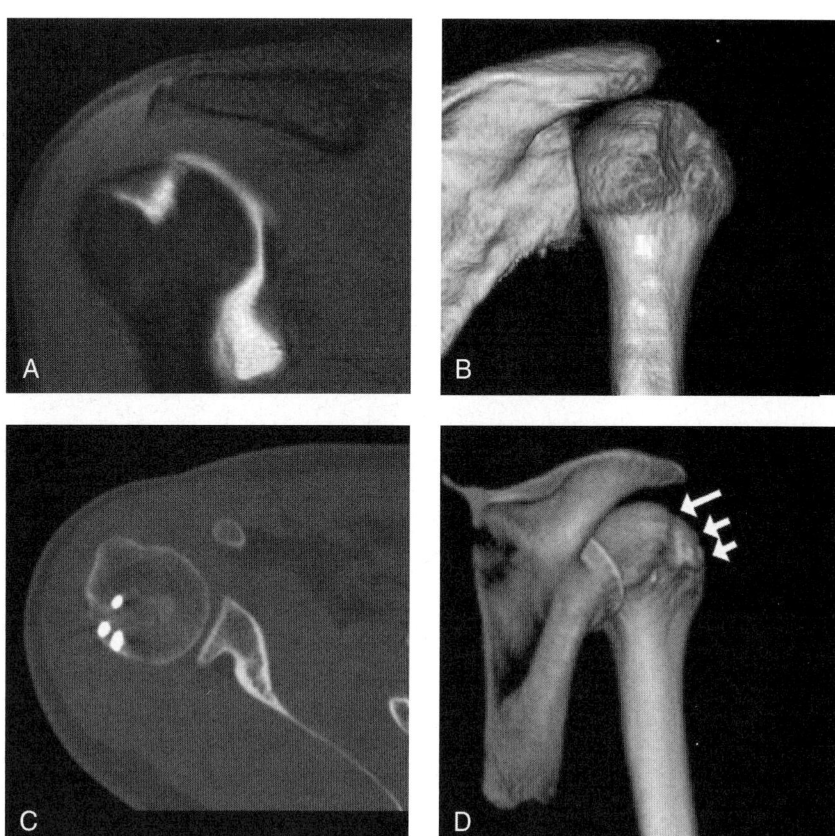

Figure 6 A large Hill-Sachs lesion as seen on a coronal magnetic resonance arthrogram **(A)** and a three-dimensional CT reconstruction **(B)**. There is no glenoid bone loss, and the Hill-Sachs lesion is isolated, with an anterior labral tear. The lesion was treated with an open procedure using a fresh osteochondral allograft to the humeral head. Full incorporation of the graft at 1-year follow-up can be seen on CT **(C)** and three-dimensional CT reconstruction (*arrows*) **(D)**.

Itoi and associates[22,23] found that the stability of the glenohumeral joint is adversely affected by glenoid bone loss of 21% or more. However, repaired capsular structures were found to provide sufficient stability. Other researchers[24] suggested that even 6 to 8 mm of anterior glenoid bone loss may require bony augmentation or a robust arthroscopic repair.

The reported recurrence rates after arthroscopic repair of a glenoid bone defect are as high as 67%.[7] However, Mologne and associates[25] reported a 14% recurrence rate after arthroscopic treatment of patients with a mean glenoid bone loss of 25%. All of the recurrences occurred in patients who had so-called attritional bone loss and erosion of the glenoid bone loss fragment. Although none of the patients with a bony fragment developed recurrent instability, the 14% overall recurrence rate was considered unsatisfactory. Sugaya and associates[26] reported an 8% recurrence rate after arthroscopic treatment in patients with a mean 25% bone loss. A bony fragment was incorporated into all of the repairs. These studies highlight the importance of glenoid bone stock for the success of the initial instability repair.

The preferred treatment of patients with humeral bone loss is less well defined because of the difficulty of determining whether a Hill-Sachs lesion is clinically important. In an engaging Hill-Sachs lesion, as described by Burkhart and De Beer,[7] the anterior glenoid is engaged by a posterolateral humeral head with an impression injury (the Hill-Sachs lesion) when the arm is abducted and externally rotated. Cadaver studies established that the humeral head more easily engages the glenoid if the anterior glenoid has a bone deficiency.[27] A Hill-Sachs injury may be present in 80% to 95% of patients with recurrent shoulder instability,[28,29] but most such injuries can safely be ignored.[7] However, a sizable Hill-Sachs defect (usually deeper than 5 to 7 mm) or instability with humeral head engagement can be surgically treated with soft-tissue augmentation,

Table 2
Surgical Procedures for a Hill-Sachs Lesion

Procedure	Description
Soft tissue	Capsulolabral repair to the native glenoid with suture anchors
Remplissage	Tenodesis of the infraspinatus tendon into the defect with suture anchors
Anterior capsulolabral repair	Limits external rotation to prevent engagement
Posterior capsular plication	Recenters the humeral head in conjunction with anterior instability repair and prevents engagement
Glenoid	Lengthens the articular arc of the glenoid and effectively prevents engagement; commonly used for a humeral-sided lesion
Latarjet	Transfers the coracoid to the anterior glenoid to lengthen the glenoid functional arc
Iliac crest graft	Transfers the iliac crest inner table (tricortical) to the anterior glenoid to lengthen the glenoid functional arc
Humeral head	Rarely necessary, except for a severe defect or a reverse or isolated Hill-Sachs lesion
Fresh osteochondral humeral head allograft	A size-matched humeral head allograft is placed into the defect.
Cylindrical synthetic plugs	Synthetic plugs are placed into the defect.
Partial metal resurfacing	A partial metal resurfacing implant is placed into the defect.
Remplissage	Tenodesis of the infraspinatus tendon into the defect with suture anchors
Combined glenoid and humeral head	Rarely necessary, except for severe glenoid and humeral head bone loss (in, for example, a patient with seizures)

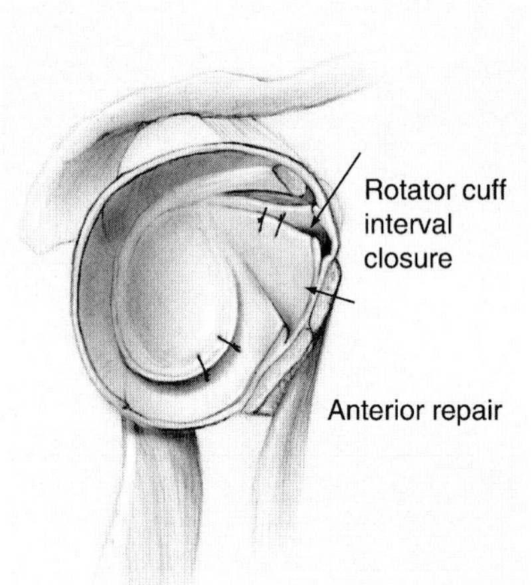

Figure 7 Schematic diagram showing a typical arthroscopic closure of the rotator cuff interval after an anterior instability repair. The superior glenohumeral ligament (*long arrow*) is imbricated to the middle glenohumeral ligament (*short arrow*); this closure biomechanically improves the anterior stability of the glenohumeral joint.

glenoid-based bone augmentation, a humeral head procedure (Figure 6), or occasionally a combined glenoid–humeral head procedure (Table 2).

Video 21.1: Glenoid Bone Loss: Evaluation and Management. LCDR Matthew T. Provencher, MD, MC, USN; Daniel J. Solomon, MD (12 min)

Rotator Cuff Interval Closure

The rotator cuff interval is the tissue that occupies the space between the supraspinatus and subscapularis tendons, including the superior and middle glenohumeral ligaments, long head of the biceps, coracohumeral ligament, and capsule. Arthroscopic rotator cuff interval closure in the setting of shoulder instability remains controversial. Most patients with primary anterior instability do not require rotator cuff interval closure. However, recent biomechanical evidence suggests that arthroscopic closure of the rotator cuff interval may improve anterior stability after an anterior instability repair, predominantly because of the bumper effect and tensioning of the middle glenohumeral ligament.[30-32] Thus, rotator interval closure may be considered, particularly if the patient is undergoing revision surgery or has hyperlaxity (especially inferior). However, closure should be used judiciously because of possible loss of motion, especially external rotation at the side.[31-33] Closure should be done with the arm in maximal external rotation (Figure 7).

For patients with posterior instability, arthroscopic rotator cuff interval closure has been recommended to supplement the construct and repair damaged rotator cuff interval structures.[34] Some authors believe that rotator cuff interval closure should be a routine part of all posterior instability repairs.[35] However, recent clinical studies reported excellent results without closure.[36-40]

The use of rotator cuff interval closure in patients with multidirectional instability is controversial. Closure has been recommended to decrease inferior translation of the glenohumeral joint, which is a key component of multidirectional instability.[31,33] However, the inferior capsule and associated stretch, not the rotator cuff interval structures, were found to be the most impor-

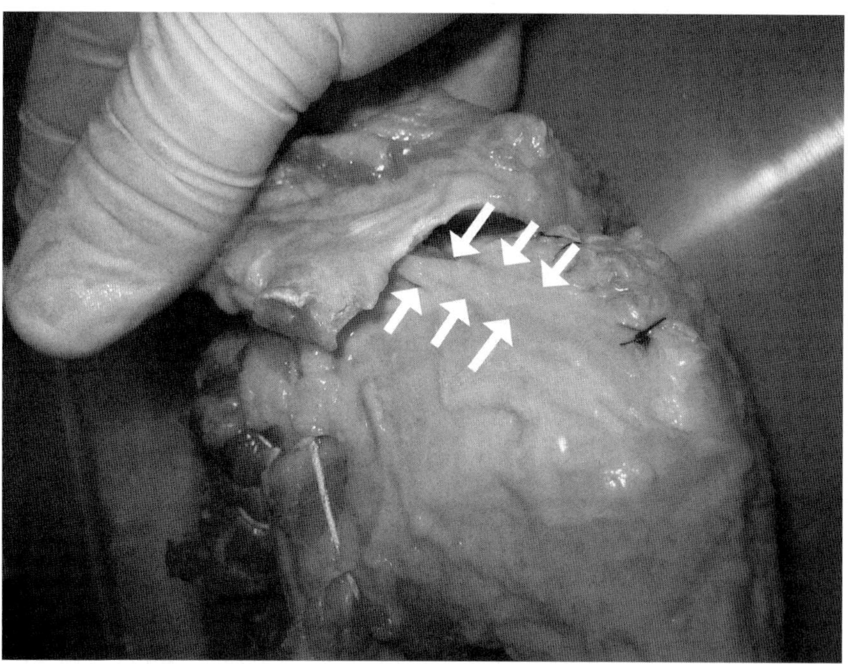

Figure 8 Photograph showing the coracohumeral ligament (arrows), which originates at the base of the coracoid and inserts on the lesser tuberosity; it contributes to the inferior stability of the glenohumeral joint.

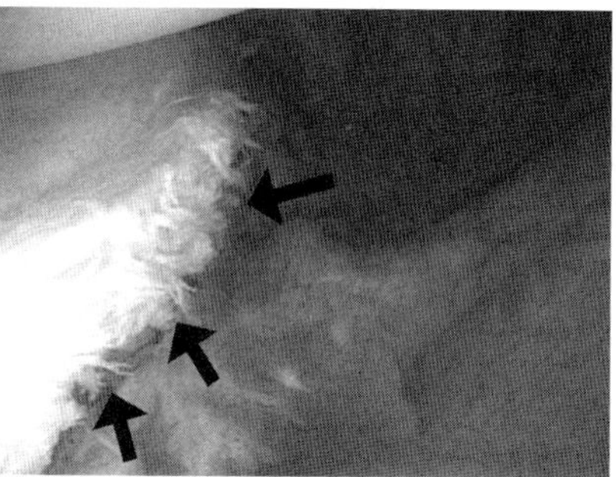

Figure 9 Arthroscopic photograph showing an anterior labral periosteal sleeve avulsion after a shoulder dislocation. The labral tissue, attached capsule, and inferior glenohumeral ligament have healed medially down the glenoid neck (arrows).

tant aspects of maintaining inferior stability of the shoulder.[41-44] The coracohumeral ligament is important to the inferior stability of the shoulder, especially when the arm is positioned at the side (Figure 8); however, arthroscopic imbrication of this structure is unreliable.[45,46] Nonetheless, supplementing the repair with rotator cuff interval closure has been recommended to obtain a robust multidirectional instability repair construct while preserving range of motion.[47]

Selecting the Procedure

Appropriate patient selection makes it easier to choose the appropriate surgical treatment. A soft-tissue procedure should be chosen if the primary defect involves the labrum and capsule. Both open and arthroscopic Bankart procedures have successful outcomes, and the choice is a matter of surgeon preference. If an arthroscopic repair is chosen, the surgeon should be mindful of several considerations that can enhance healing and improve the outcome. An evaluation under anesthesia should be done to confirm the preoperative plan. Although patient positioning is a matter of surgeon preference, the lateral decubitus position is recommended for global access to the superior, posterior, inferior, and anterior labrum and capsule. The defect always should be viewed from the anterosuperior portal to avoid missing an anterior labral periosteal sleeve avulsion (ALPSA) tear in which the labrum and capsule are healed medially on the glenoid neck, which is associated with a relatively poor outcome.[48] (Figure 9). The soft tissue should be removed from the glenoid repair site, and there should be a bleeding bone bed to enhance healing. Suture anchors should be placed at the margins of the articular cartilage and scapular neck to avoid a nonanatomic medial scapular neck placement. For most anteroinferior labral tears, at least three suture anchors should be used (from the 3 o'clock to 6 o'clock positions on a right shoulder and from the 6 o'clock to 9 o'clock positions on a left shoulder). If increased capsular laxity is indicated by preoperative examination and arthroscopic evaluation, a capsular plication may be necessary. The capsule should be abraded to enhance healing to the labrum. The plication can be to intact labral tissue if it is robust, but a suture anchor is preferred if there is any question.

A bony procedure should be considered if significant bony defects of the glenoid or humeral head are present. A Latarjet coracoid transfer is recommended for a glenoid deficiency of more than 20% to 25%. For a large Hill-Sachs deformity, the options include humeral head osteochondral allograft with screw fixation, synthetic plugs, arthroscopic reduction and bone grafting, and arthroscopic remplissage (in which the Hill-Sachs defect is filled with the infraspinatus tendon).[49-52]

Selecting the Rehabilitation Program

The rehabilitation program should be preceded by thorough preoperative counseling of the patient. As determined intraoperatively, the factors to be considered include the type of instability (traumatic or atraumatic), the direction of instability (anterior, posterior, or multidirectional), the integrity of the tissue, any associated findings (such as a biceps tendon or rotator cuff tear) and required treatment, and the surgeon's confidence in the quality of the repair. The type of postoperative immobilization varies with the procedure. The use of a commercially available sling with abduction abdominal pillow support is recommended after most anterior instability repairs because this type of sling keeps the shoulder in a neutral position. A similar sling that keeps the arm in 30° of external rotation is recommended after a posterior instability repair. The sling typically is used for 4 to 6 weeks after an anterior or posterior instability repair or a Latarjet or humeral head allograft procedure. A gunslinger-style brace often is used for 4 to 6 weeks after a multidirectional instability repair, especially if the patient had an unsuccessful earlier instability repair. Physical therapy is not recommended during the first 4 to 6 weeks after a multidirectional instability repair.

Physical therapy typically begins 7 to 10 days after a routine anterior or posterior instability repair, with progression through passive and active-assisted range-of-motion exercises during the first 4 weeks until forward elevation to 130° and external rotation to 30° is achieved. Forward elevation is increased to 180°, and external rotation is increased to 60° during the next 2 weeks. Active range-of-motion exercises are followed by resistance strengthening from 8 to 12 weeks after the repair and by a return to full participation in sports and other activities usually 4 to 6 months after the repair. After a complex repair or a revision repair, 9 to 12 months may be required before a return to full activity.

Revision Surgery for Shoulder Instability

Failure of a shoulder stabilization procedure can be categorized as postoperative recurrence, stiffness, or pain. Some failures involve bone loss, an untreated preexisting injury (superior labrum anterior and posterior [SLAP] tear, rotator cuff tear, humeral avulsion of the glenohumeral ligament [HAGL] lesion, or extensive labral tearing), an improper diagnosis of the type of instability, a neurologic injury, subscapularis insufficiency (after open stabilization), chondrolysis, hardware failure and impingement, or posttraumatic arthritis (Table 3).

The most common mode of failure is recurrence, which can result from recurrent trauma, compromised surgical technique, or failure to address bone loss.[7,53] Failure to diagnose a HAGL lesion can lead to recurrent instability after an arthroscopic repair (Figure 10). Treatment that reflects an incorrect diagnosis (such as an anterior instability repair for a patient who has multidirectional or posterior instability) also can lead to repair failure, as can complications directly related to the procedure. Loss of motion can occur after an open or arthroscopic instability repair; severe loss of motion may require further treatment. Subscapularis rupture after an open Bankart repair can cause failure that requires further treatment.[54,55] Hardware impingement from metal or bioabsorbable anchors can cause devastating articular cartilage injury. Chondrolysis can occur with the use of anchors, thermal ablation, or an intra-articular pain pump, but it is rare.[56-58] Capsular deficiency can occur after multiple shoulder procedures, especially if the procedures were open or involved thermal capsulorrhaphy. Systematic evaluation of all possible causes is the key to successfully treating a patient with a failed instability repair.

Evaluating the Patient

Patient History, Examination, and Imaging

A thorough history, physical examination, and radiographic evaluation are necessary to determine the cause of failure after an instability repair. The primary symptom may be pain, recurrent instability, loss of motion, weakness, apprehension, or inability to return to sports or other activity. If recurrent instability is the primary symptom, the examiner should determine the mode of recurrence as well as its cause. Dislocation requiring a reduction after a major trauma suggests a disruption of the index repair and is likely to involve a recurrent labral tear and capsular injury, possibly with glenoid or humeral head bone loss. Recurrent subluxation occurring after trivial trauma or unrelated to trauma probably involves capsular laxity or deficiency, bone loss, or improper surgical technique. Instability that occurs during sleep suggests significant capsular laxity or bone loss. The presence of dead arm syndrome suggests recurrent subluxation. Patients with hyperlaxity or inadequate bone or soft tissue are especially at risk of recurrence. Contact athletes, particularly male athletes younger than 20 years, are at an inherent risk of recurrence.[53] Balg and Boileau[59]

Table 3
Etiology of Failed Instability Shoulder Surgery

Reason for Failure	Diagnostic Considerations
Improper diagnosis	Posterior and multidirectional instability must be ruled out.
	Thorough history and physical examination are required.
Inadequate imaging	Advanced imaging should be obtained if bone loss is suspected on plain radiographs. Glenoid bone loss must be detected on three-dimensional CT or sagittal oblique MRI.
	A HAGL lesion is difficult to diagnose without a magnetic resonance arthrogram.
	Hill-Sachs injury is detected using a Stryker notch radiograph, MRI, or CT.
	Concomitant pathology (SLAP tear, rotator cuff tear) is detected on MRI or magnetic resonance arthrogram.
Preexisting condition	Rotator cuff tear (especially in a patient older than 40 years who has a dislocation)
	Glenoid bone loss
	Humeral bone loss
Capsular integrity	Earlier surgery involving thermal treatment; open or arthroscopic shift
Technical issues	Inability to correct underlying instability; the anchor position is important (especially from the 6 o'clock to 3 o'clock position)
	Poor retensioning of the capsulolabral structures
	Poor knot, loop, or suture anchor integrity during the repair
	Inadequate restoration of the glenoid labrum to the native location
	Inadequate preparation of the anterior glenoid neck for repair
	Inadequate capsular shift for treating the nearly ubiquitous capsular stretch
	Hardware failure; failure to avoid proud anchors
Bone loss	A leading cause of shoulder stabilization failure
	An adequate radiographic workup is required, with advanced imaging (MRI, CT), especially after a failed stabilization procedure.
Rehabilitation	The postoperative protocol should balance limitations and stiffness against capsulolabral healing.
Persistent weakness	Axillary and suprascapular nerve palsy must be ruled out if there is associated muscle atrophy.
	Postoperative subscapularis dysfunction may be present.
Persistent pain	Associated pathology, other diagnoses, chondral injuries, and capsulitis must be investigated.
	Differential joint and subacromial injections can provide diagnostic and therapeutic benefit.
Postoperative stiffness	The earlier repair location must be investigated. With loss of external rotation at the side, repair should be considered for the anterosuperior aspect of the shoulder.
	Existing or new subscapularis deficiency may be present, especially with loss of external rotation at the side.

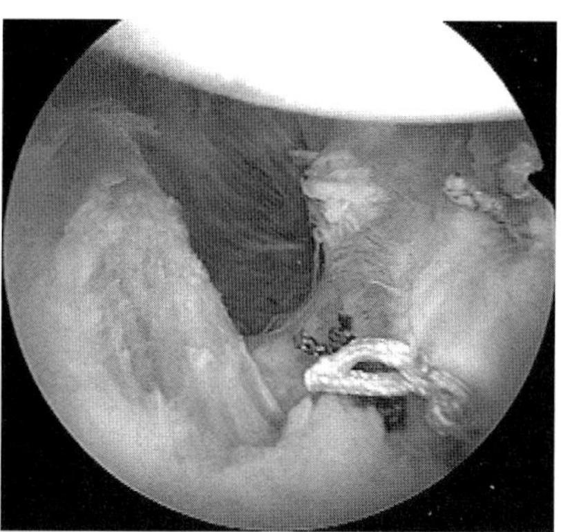

Figure 10 Arthroscopic photograph from the posterior portal, showing a HAGL lesion in a left shoulder after a failed arthroscopic labral instability repair with suture anchors.

described the Instability Severity Index Score, which can be used to determine whether the patient should receive arthroscopic or open treatment for an optimal outcome; patients with both bone loss and hyperlaxity were found to have a 75% recurrence rate after an arthroscopic repair. In another study, contact athletes with no bone loss had a recurrence rate of 6.5% after arthroscopic stabilization, but contact athletes with significant bone loss had an 89% recurrence rate.[7]

Capsular contracture with loss of motion can cause pain after stabilization surgery. Severe pain should alert the physician to the possibility of infection, chondrolysis, or exposed suture anchors with articular cartilage injury. Weakness suggests the presence of a neurologic injury; a subscapularis rupture (after an open repair); or a torn rotator cuff, particularly if the patient is older than 40 years. Paresthesias, especially along the ulnar nerve distribution, suggests the presence of hyperlaxity and multidirectional instability.

The examination should begin with an evaluation of active and passive motion, which can reveal range-of-motion deficits and neuromuscular weakness and injury. Increased external rotation after an open instability repair suggests a subscapularis deficiency. The presence of a squeaking sound suggests prominent suture knots or hardware. The pertinent neurovascular and soft-tissue structures should be thor-

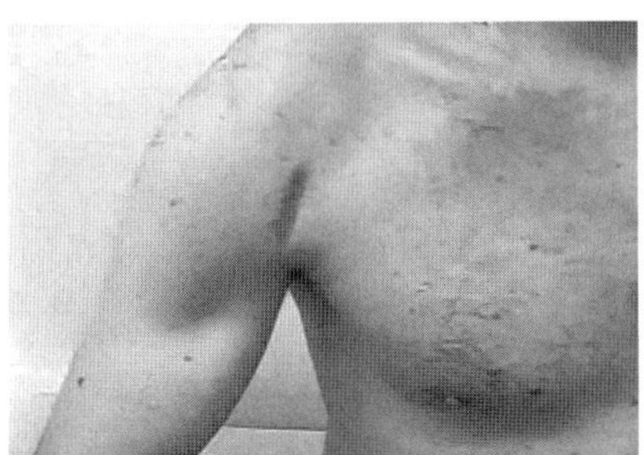

Figure 11 Photograph showing a positive belly press test, which indicates a subscapularis tear. The incision scar from an earlier open stabilization procedure can be seen.

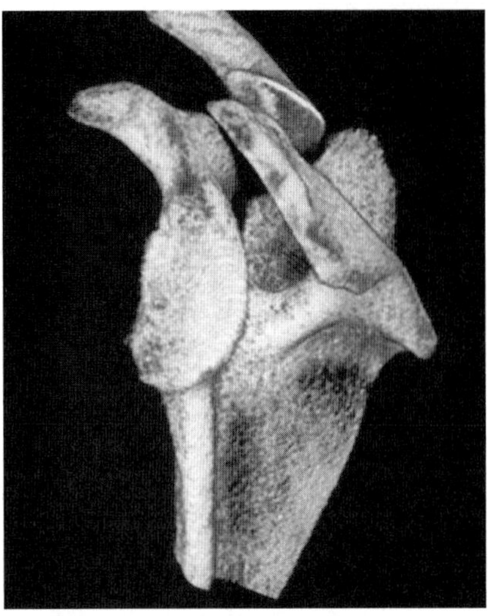

Figure 12 Glenoid bone loss as seen on a three-dimensional CT reconstruction.

oughly examined, with attention to the musculocutaneous and axillary nerves and strength testing of all major muscle groups about the shoulder girdle. The strength of each component of the rotator cuff should be tested, with particular attention to the belly press and lift-off tests for subscapularis integrity (Figure 11). Apprehension testing can then be used for the position that elicited a positive result. A positive relocation test result suggests the presence of an undiagnosed SLAP tear or recurrent subluxation. Apprehension with the arm in abduction and external rotation suggests a recurrence of anterior instability; apprehension in forward flexion and relative adduction suggests posterior instability. The shoulder also should be evaluated for capsular laxity and glenohumeral translation. A sulcus sign that reproduces pain or instability suggests inferior laxity or redundancy with multidirectional instability.[10,59] The load-and-shift test is primarily used to detect anterior-posterior translation; the result always should be compared with the asymptomatic shoulder. Crepitus during this maneuver suggests a recurrent Bankart lesion or articular cartilage injury. The posterior jerk maneuver should be done to detect or rule out posterior instability or a posterior labral tear.

Imaging is important for determining the reason for failure of an instability repair. Bone loss, as seen on the West Point radiographic view, was shown to be correlated with bone loss observed on CT.[22] In general, CT, especially with three-dimensional reconstruction, should be obtained to precisely assess bone loss (Figure 12). CT arthrography permits detection of a recurrent Bankart lesion, capsular redundancy, improper anchor placement, anchor impingement, or rotator cuff defects. MRI is the standard method of evaluating the soft tissue, but it is less useful than CT for assessing bone loss. MRI, particularly with a glenohumeral gadolinium injection, is extremely useful for detecting a recurrent Bankart lesion, a HAGL lesion, a SLAP tear, a posterior labral tear, capsular redundancy or deficiency, chondrolysis, or rotator cuff defects.

The evaluation should allow the cause of failure to be determined and a surgical strategy to be developed that will lead to optimal results. It is important to discuss with the patient and family the rationale for the surgical strategy. Contingency plans should be developed because the examination under anesthesia and arthroscopic evaluation occasionally reveal an additional defect that requires treatment. However, usually a thorough history, the physical examination, and appropriate imaging allow the surgeon to fully determine the cause of failure and establish a definitive treatment plan before the revision surgery.

Examination Under Anesthesia and Arthroscopic Evaluation

An examination under anesthesia should be considered part of the overall evaluation, although usually its primary purpose is to confirm the mode of failure and the prevailing instability direction and pattern. A severe loss of rotation, as verified under anesthesia, can indicate the presence of capsular contracture or overtightening, adhesive capsulitis, glenohumeral arthrosis, or chondrolysis. The examiner should listen for crepitus and brisement, which suggest hardware impingement. The treatment can include arthroscopic capsular release, débridement, hardware removal, or, rarely, cartilage resurfacing.

Glenohumeral translation is assessed using a sulcus test with the arm at the side and in external rotation. If the sulcus sign remains with external rotation, increased inferior capsular redundancy and incompetence of the rotator cuff interval may be present.[10,60] The anterior-posterior load-and-shift test is done with the arm in abduction and neutral rotation, in the plane of the scapula. The presence of an engaging Hill-Sachs defect is suggested if the humeral head catches or becomes locked on the edge of the glenoid, requiring reduction under anesthesia. An engaging Hill-Sachs lesion may be managed with remplissage (tenodesis of the infraspinatus into the defect)[52] or glenoid bone augmentation to prevent engagement and lengthen the articular arc of the glenoid.[7,61,62]

The placement of the arthroscopic portal should allow complete visualization of all aspects of the glenohumeral joint. From the posterior viewing portal, all components of the rotator cuff, biceps tendon, superior labrum, rotator cuff interval, inferior capsule, lateral capsular attachment, humeral head, and glenohumeral articular surfaces can be examined. The arm is placed out of traction and into forward elevation, abduction, and external rotation to determine whether a humeral head defect is engaging the glenoid rim. The arthroscope is moved to an anterosuperior portal for evaluation of the anterior and posterior capsulolabral attachments, earlier anchor placement, and, perhaps most important, glenoid bone loss. Inferior glenoid bone loss appears as the so-called inverted pear glenoid.[19]

The selection of surgical technique for the primary repair and the anatomic precision of the repair are related to the risk of a recurrence of instability. Other than bone loss, the most common causes of failure after an instability repair are unaddressed capsular laxity, improper anchor positioning, and recurrent trauma. In an arthroscopic repair, the labrum must be completely mobilized, and the subscapularis muscle fibers must be exposed to allow correct capsulolabral retensioning. Accurately positioning the suture anchors on the glenoid with penetration at the margin of the articular surface allows the glenoid concavity to be re-created and avoids medialization of the repair (Figure 13). Boileau and associates[53] recommended that at least four suture anchors be used; using only one or two suture anchors was associated with recurrent instability. Asymmetric tensioning during open or arthroscopic capsulorrhaphy is rare but can create instability in the opposite direction.

Significant bone loss in the glenoid or humeral head has been considered the primary reason for failure after arthroscopic repair. In cadaver studies, a glenoid osseous defect involving 21% of the glenoid diameter was correlated with increased translation and decreased force for dislocation after a standard Bankart repair.[63] Hyperlaxity also creates a predisposition to recurrence; Boileau and associates[53] found a significant correlation between recurrence of anteroinferior shoulder laxity and arthroscopic Bankart repair. On multivariate analysis, the combination of inferior hyperlaxity with glenoid bone loss of more than 25% resulted in a 75% recurrence rate after arthroscopic stabilization. The average time to failure of arthroscopic Bankart surgery was 17.6 months.

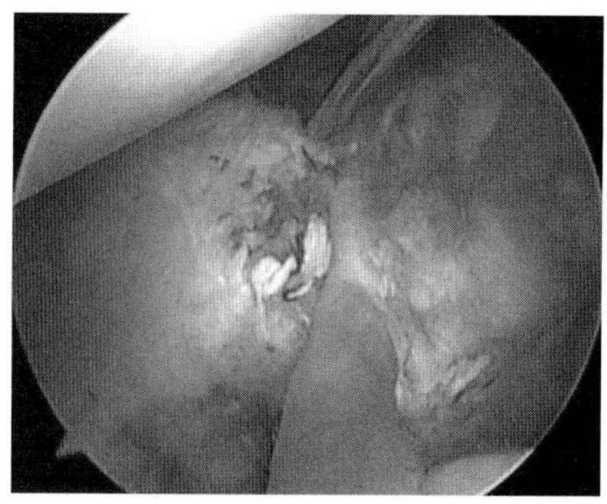

Figure 13 Arthroscopic view of a left shoulder from the anterosuperior portal, showing a medialized anchor and labrum after a failed repair.

Selecting the Procedure

The treatment of a failed anterior instability repair can be challenging. Although both arthroscopic and open procedures have been described, open procedures have gained favor; the Latarjet procedure, which augments the anterior glenoid, is an especially good option. Arthroscopic repair generally is considered if the instability was insufficiently treated during the index procedure because of a technical issue (for example, the anchors were not placed in an optimal position) or a missed diagnosis (for example, true posterior instability treated as if it were anterior instability with continued posterior instability).[64,65] The most common cause of failure after an instability repair is the inadequate treatment of significant bone deficiency during the index procedure. An open revision should be done if either the glenoid bone deficiency or the humeral head deficiency is considered significant. A significant glenoid bone deficiency is defined as a loss of more than 25% of the inferior glenoid diameter, which creates the inverted pear glenoid.[7,61] A significant humeral head deficiency is defined as a Hill-Sachs lesion that is deeper than 3 to 5 mm and engages the anterior glenoid rim in a position of 90° abduction and 90° of external rotation. Bone loss on either the glenoid or humeral side can be adequately treated using a Latarjet reconstruction, in which coracoid bone is grafted to the anterior glenoid, leaving the conjoined tendon attached to the coracoid[62,66] (Figure 14). The Latarjet procedure establishes three stabilizing mechanisms: extension of the articular arc of the glenoid by means of the coracoid graft; the sling effect of the conjoined tendon; and tensioning of the

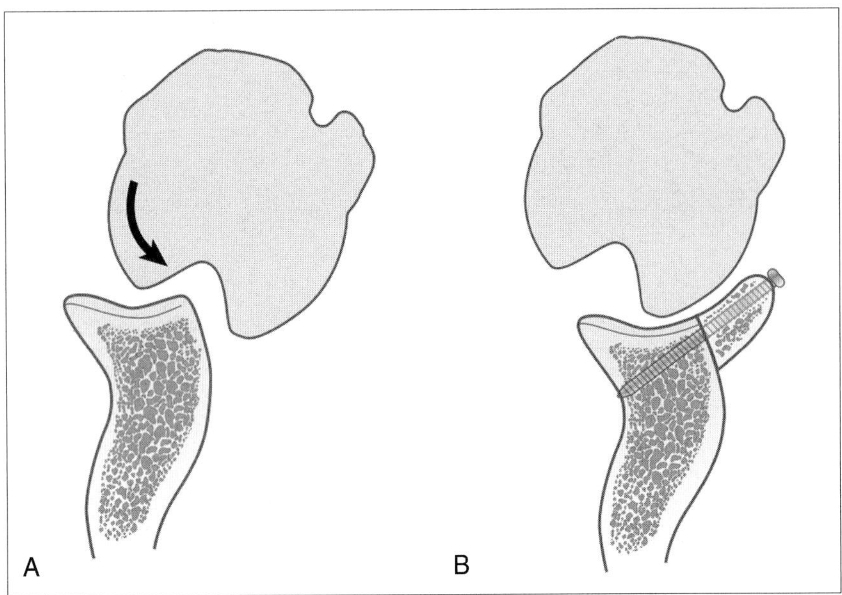

Figure 14 Schematic diagrams showing an engaging Hill-Sachs lesion **(A)** and surgical prevention of engagement by lengthening the glenoid arc **(B)**.

lower subscapularis by the conjoined tendon. The Latarjet procedure can include intra-articular or extra-articular coracoid placement (with capsular repair to the intact glenoid rather than the anterior aspect of the bone graft); coracoid and conjoined tendon placement through a split in the subscapularis tendon rather than a full subscapularis takedown (to create a sling effect); dissection of the conjoined tendon from the coracoid, with the coracoid used as free bone graft; and orientation of the coracoid graft so that the inferior or lateral edge becomes the glenoid face.

Ghodadra and associates[67] found that the optimal orientation of the coracoid for restoring the glenoid contact forces is for the inferior surface of the coracoid to become the glenoid face (Figure 15). This method also provides the most bone stock for the anterior glenoid. The bone graft extends the articular arc far enough that the Hill-Sachs lesion is unable to engage, even in full external rotation. Biomechanical testing has established that the sling effect of the conjoined tendon is a significant anterior restraint after a Latarjet procedure.[68]

The Latarjet procedure can be very effective for stabilizing a capsular deficiency, which can be caused by multiple failed surgical procedures or thermal capsular necrosis (Figure 16). The stabilizing mechanisms achieved by the Latarjet procedure are so effective that a shoulder with a completely absent anterior capsule can be completely stabilized without additional soft-tissue grafting.[62] If there is severe bone loss, an iliac crest autograft can be considered[70] (Figure 17).

Some instability repairs fail because all pathologic structures were not recognized and treated; these may include a concomitant subscapularis tear, a SLAP lesion, a partial articular-surface rotator cuff tear, loose bodies, localized grade IV chondromalacia, or a posterior Bankart lesion. Arrigoni and associates[70] reported that arthroscopic evaluation before an open Latarjet reconstruction revealed an additional significant defect in 73% of patients. Because of the high incidence of associated defects, diagnostic arthroscopy is recommended in all instability surgery, including open instability repair.

Symptomatic stiffness after instability surgery is uncommon but challenging. The capsule can be as thick as 1 cm; a capsule of such thickness is completely resistant to manipulation under anesthesia and is best treated with arthroscopic capsular release. The use of a monopolar pencil-tip electrode is recommended to cut the capsule approximately 1 cm lateral to the labrum, avoiding destruction of the labral bumper and the suction cup effect of an intact labrum. The rotator cuff interval must be divided anteriorly, and any subcoracoid adhesions must be excised to eliminate subcoracoid capture. Range-of-motion exercises are begun immediately after surgery to prevent recurrent stiffness.

Postoperative chondrolysis, although rare, is extremely debilitating. Arthroscopic glenoid resurfacing with acellular allograft dermis is successful in 50% to 70% of patients with chondrolysis (A Romeo, MD, Chicago, IL, unpublished data, 2009). However, it is unknown whether the dramatic improvement in some patients will be long lasting. For a young patient who does not improve with biologic resurfacing, humeral head allograft, total shoulder arthroplasty, or arthrodesis of the shoulder may be necessary as a last resort[57] (Figure 18).

Postoperative rupture of the subscapularis after an open repair is extremely disabling[54,55] (Figure 19). Patients have weakness and pain with most activities and may de-

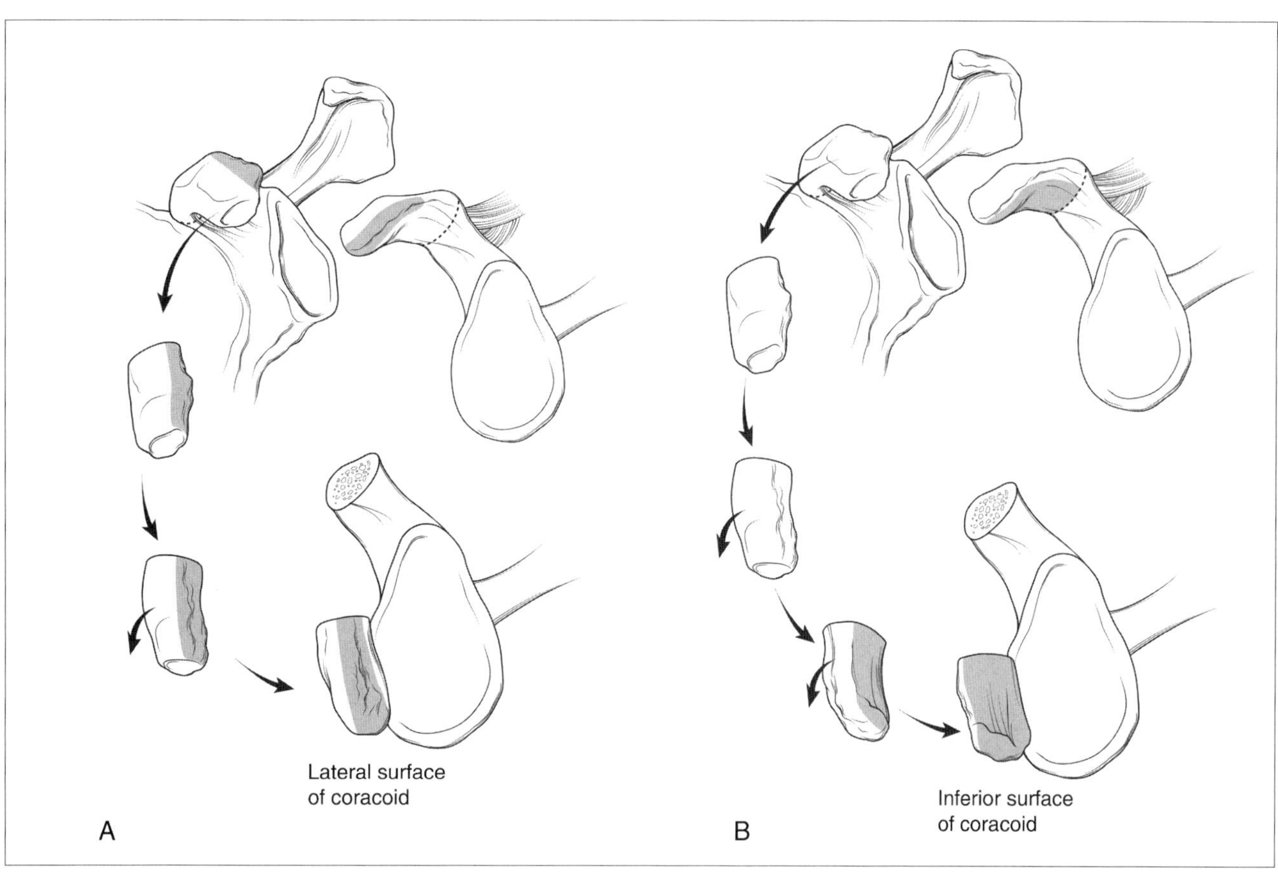

Figure 15 Schematic diagrams showing two methods of orienting a coracoid bone graft for a Latarjet procedure. **A,** The lateral edge of the coracoid used as the glenoid face; this is the traditional method. **B,** The inferior aspect of the coracoid used as the glenoid face; this method can improve joint congruity and provide more glenoid bone stock for reconstruction.

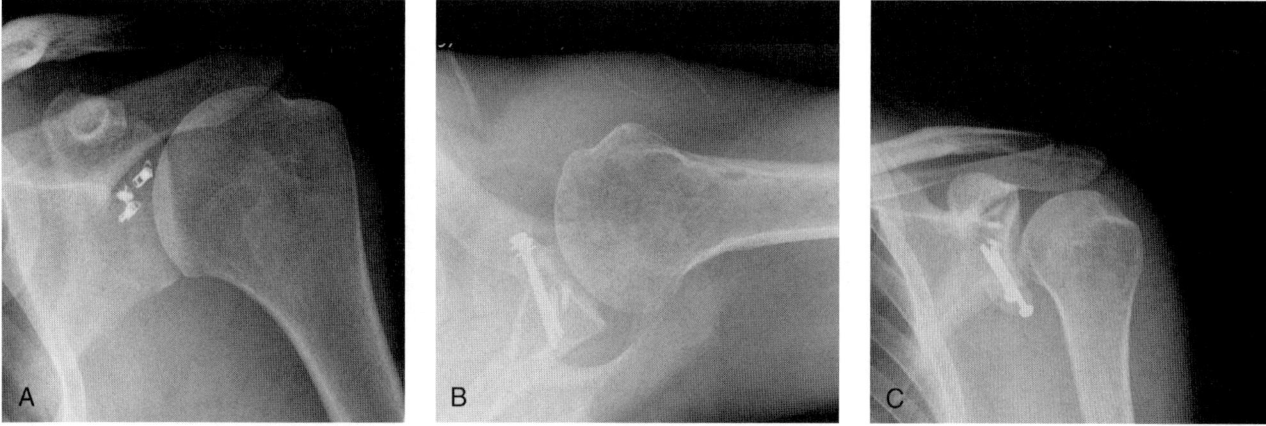

Figure 16 **A,** AP radiograph showing a failed anterior instability repair; suboptimal placement of three glenoid anchors can be seen above the 3 o'clock position. The Latarjet procedure was used for revision repair. **B,** Axillary lateral radiograph showing incorporation of the Latarjet graft. **C,** AP radiograph showing the healed repair.

velop disabling fixed anterior subluxation. If the disruption occurs in the tendinous portion of the subscapularis, arthroscopic repair can be achieved using suture anchors. If the tendon length is insufficient to reach the anatomic footprint, the bone bed for repair can be medialized as much as 5 mm.[71] A three-

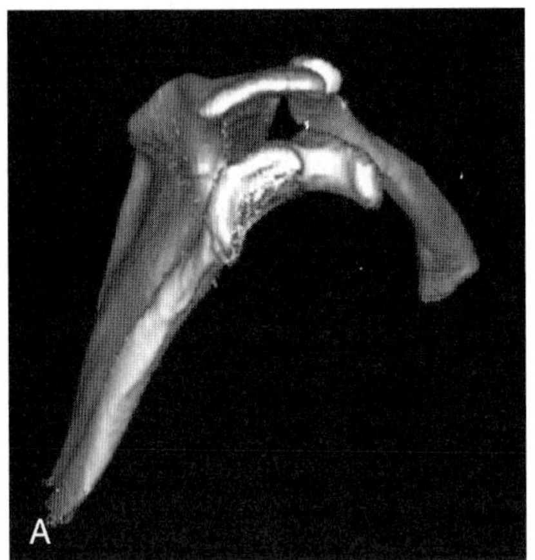

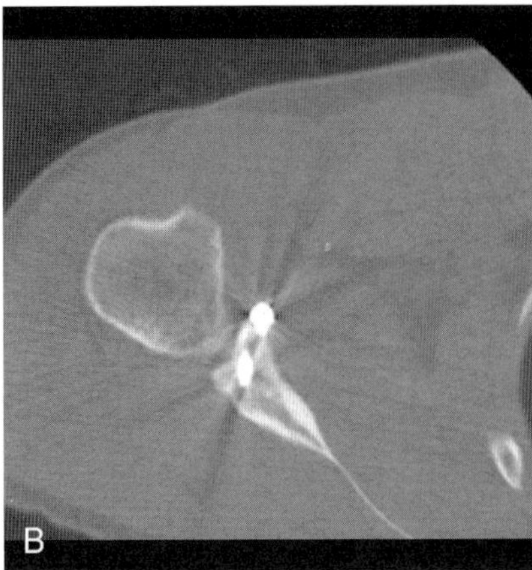

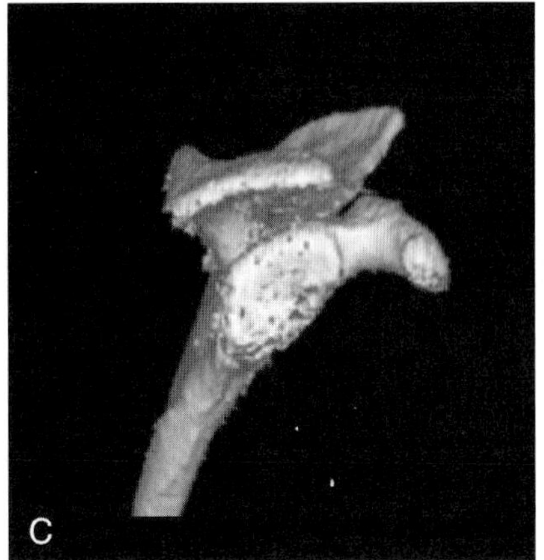

Figure 17 **A,** Three-dimensional CT reconstruction showing a large glenoid defect (40% to 50%). **B,** CT scan showing full incorporation of iliac crest autograft 6 months after surgery. **C,** Three-dimensional CT reconstruction showing reconstitution of the glenoid bone stock 6 months after surgery.

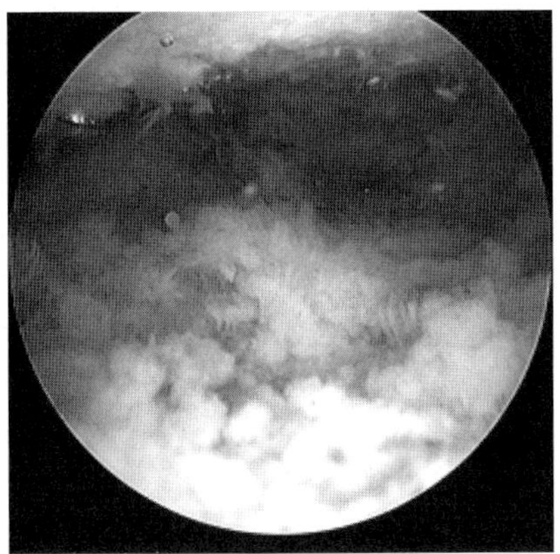

Figure 18 Glenohumeral arthroscopic view showing extensive bipolar chondrolysis in a 19-year-old patient 6 months after repair of a SLAP lesion.

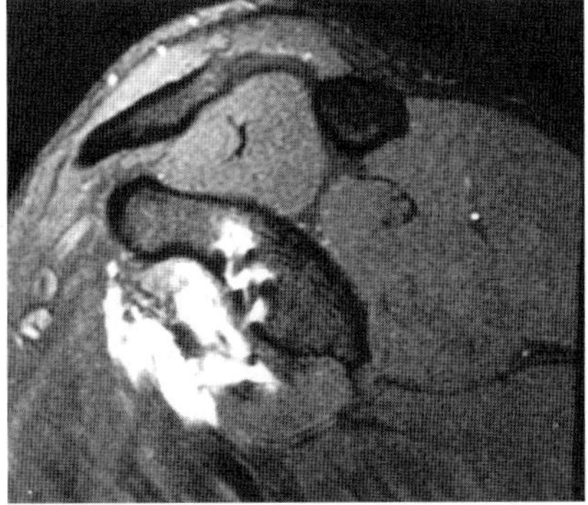

Figure 19 Sagittal oblique MRI showing a subscapularis deficiency in a 34-year-old man 3 years after open anterior instability repair. The belly press and lift-off tests were positive. The Latarjet procedure was used for the revision repair.

sided release is recommended for mobilizing a retracted subscapularis while avoiding injury to the musculocutaneous and axillary nerves.[71] Postoperative rupture of the subscapularis through the muscle or at the musculotendinous junction presumably occurs because of a medialized takedown of the subscapularis during the index surgery. A repair is not possible because no tendon is available for reattachment. Particularly if there is fixed anterior subluxation, a Latarjet reconstruction can be used to add enough length to the glenoid articular arc to contain the humeral head and prevent subluxation. The sling effect of the conjoined tendon enhances anterior stability, even though there is no capsule, and function can be greatly improved. However, it may be impossible to treat the internal rotation strength deficit. A subcoracoid transfer of the pectoralis minor (the Resch technique)[72] is not possible because the coracoid would have been moved inferolaterally to its new location as a bone graft. A standard, non–subcoracoid pectoralis major transfer is not recommended because the force vector is directed anteromedially and could exacerbate any tendency toward anterior-inferior subluxation. Because postoperative rupture of the subscapularis occurs only after an open repair and is extremely disabling, the surgeon should consider taking down only the upper half of the subscapularis or splitting the subscapularis during an open instability repair. Only 57% of patients who had subscapularis dysfunction after open Bankart surgery were satisfied with the surgical result, and only 57% would have the surgery again.[54]

Revision arthroscopic and open repairs are equally successful if skillfully done, there is no loss of bone stock, and the recurrence was caused by a true traumatic episode that disrupted an intact, skillful initial repair.[64,73] Good results have been achieved arthroscopically for overhead throwing athletes with a traumatic recurrence, a deficient initial repair, good remaining tissue for repair, and minimal bone loss (less than 15%). An arthroscopic revision stabilization procedure may require a thorough mobilization of the capsulolabral complex, additional fixation points, and additional capsular plication (including posteroinferior capsular plication sutures). Capsular tears, redundancy, and even lateral humeral ligament avulsions can be treated with an arthroscopic revision procedure. Scant literature is available to document the results of revision arthroscopic stabilization after a failed open instability repair. However, arthroscopic revision stabilization may be effective for a traumatic disruption of an intact repair with good capsulolabral tissue, minimal bone loss, and no hyperlaxity.[64]

The results of open or arthroscopic revision surgery for shoulder instability are likely to be inferior to those of the primary intervention.[64,65,73,74] Range-of-motion limitations, pain, stiffness, and subscapularis dysfunction are more likely to occur after revision surgery. The number of earlier stabilizing procedures is correlated with a poor functional outcome. In a study of 28 patients, Meehan and Petersen[66] identified glenohumeral arthritis, age younger than 30 years, two or more earlier instability procedures, a bony Bankart lesion, multidirectional instability, and involvement of the nondominant extremity as the key factors associated with poor patient satisfaction.

Selecting the Rehabilitation Program

The correct postoperative care is essential after a revision instability procedure. Rapid mobilization can lead to failure of the repair. After an open revision procedure with exposure through a subscapularis tendon incision, external rotation and active subscapularis contraction must be avoided for the first 6 weeks to allow complete healing and avoid subscapularis deficiency. Most rehabilitation programs allow a protected range of motion during a 4- to 6-week period of immobilization, with sling removal for pendulum exercises within a few days of the surgery. Strengthening should start within 8 to 12 weeks, with a return to sport no earlier than 6 months after surgery.

Summary

A successful primary instability repair requires a careful patient history and physical examination, with preoperative imaging studies to identify pitfalls associated with failure. Multiple surgical and postoperative strategies can lead to a reliable repair with a predictable return to full function. However, it is important to note the common reasons for instability failure, especially unrecognized glenoid and humeral head bone loss, hyperlaxity or residual capsular redundancy, poor surgical technique, and failure to address the correct direction of instability. A patient with recurrent instability after surgery must be carefully evaluated for bone loss to determine the optimal strategy for revision repair. Arthroscopic revision stabilization may be appropriate for overhead throwing athletes and other patients who have excellent tissue, little bone loss, and traumatic failure of an otherwise well-done initial repair. Open revision surgery should be considered in the presence of glenoid bone loss or an engaging Hill-Sachs lesion. A spectrum of pathology may be involved in the failure of an instability repair, and an individual shoulder may have multiple components. The surgical approach must be customized to the pathology.[69]

References

1. Bottoni CR, Smith EL, Berkowitz MJ, Towle RB, Moore JH: Arthroscopic versus open shoulder stabilization for recurrent anterior instability: A prospective randomized clinical trial. *Am J Sports Med* 2006;34: 1730-1737.

2. Freedman KB, Smith AP, Romeo AA, Cole BJ, Bach BR Jr: Open Bankart repair versus arthroscopic repair with transglenoid sutures or bioabsorbable tacks for recurrent anterior instability of the shoulder: A meta-analysis. *Am J Sports Med* 2004;32:1520-1527.

3. Guanche CA, Quick DC, Sodergren KM, Buss DD: Arthroscopic versus open reconstruction of the shoulder in patients with isolated Bankart lesions. *Am J Sports Med* 1996; 24: 144-148.

4. Kailes SB, Richmond JC: Arthroscopic vs. open Bankart reconstruction: A comparison using expected value decision analysis. *Knee Surg Sports Traumatol Arthrosc* 2001;9: 379-385.

5. Grana WA, Buckley PD, Yates CK: Arthroscopic Bankart suture repair. *Am J Sports Med* 1993;21:348-353.

6. Kim SH, Ha KI, Cho YB, Ryu BD, Oh I: Arthroscopic anterior stabilization of the shoulder: Two to six-year follow-up. *J Bone Joint Surg Am* 2003; 85:1511-1518.

7. Burkhart SS, De Beer JF: Traumatic glenohumeral bone defects and their relationship to failure of arthroscopic Bankart repairs: Significance of the inverted-pear glenoid and the humeral engaging Hill-Sachs lesion. *Arthroscopy* 2000;16:677-694.

8. Arciero RA, Taylor DC: Primary anterior dislocation of the shoulder in young patients: A ten-year prospective study. *J Bone Joint Surg Am* 1998; 80:299-300.

9. Bigliani LU, Kelkar R, Flatow EL, Pollock RG, Mow VC: Glenohumeral stability: Biomechanical properties of passive and active stabilizers. *Clin Orthop Relat Res* 1996;330:13-30.

10. Ikeda H: "Rotator interval" lesion: Part 1. Clinical study. *Nippon Seikeigeka Gakkai Zasshi* 1986;60:1261-1273.

11. Ovesen J, Nielsen S: Stability of the shoulder joint: Cadaver study of stabilizing structures. *Acta Orthop Scand* 1985;56:149-151.

12. Garth WP Jr, Slappey CE, Ochs CW: Roentgenographic demonstration of instability of the shoulder: The apical oblique projection. A technical note. *J Bone Joint Surg Am* 1984;66:1450-1453.

13. Kornguth PJ, Salazar AM: The apical oblique view of the shoulder: Its usefulness in acute trauma. *AJR Am J Roentgenol* 1987;149:113-116.

14. Roukos JR, Feagin JA, Abbott HG: Modified axillary roentgenogram: A useful adjunct in the diagnosis of recurrent instability of the shoulder. *Clin Orthop Relat Res* 1972;82:84-86.

15. Pavlov H, Warren RF, Weiss CB Jr, Dines DM: The roentgenographic evaluation of anterior shoulder instability. *Clin Orthop Relat Res* 1985;194:153-158.

16. Saito H, Itoi E, Sugaya H, Minagawa H, Yamamoto N, Tuoheti Y: Location of the glenoid defect in shoulders with recurrent anterior dislocation. *Am J Sports Med* 2005;33:889-893.

17. Sugaya H, Moriishi J, Dohi M, Kon Y, Tsuchiya A: Glenoid rim morphology in recurrent anterior glenohumeral instability. *J Bone Joint Surg Am* 2003;85:878-884.

18. Huysmans PE, Haen PS, Kidd M, Dhert WJ, Willems JW: The shape of the inferior part of the glenoid: A cadaveric study. *J Shoulder Elbow Surg* 2006;15:759-763.

19. Lo IK, Parten PM, Burkhart SS: The inverted pear glenoid: An indicator of significant glenoid bone loss. *Arthroscopy* 2004;20:169-174.

20. Provencher MT, Detterline AJ, Ghodadra N, et al: Measurement of glenoid bone loss: A comparison of measurement error between 45 degrees and 0 degrees bone loss models and with different posterior arthroscopy portal locations. *Am J Sports Med* 2008;36:1132-1138.

21. Burkhart SS, De Beer JF, Tehrany AM, Parten PM: Quantifying glenoid bone loss arthroscopically in shoulder instability. *Arthroscopy* 2002;18:488-491.

22. Itoi E, Lee SB, Amrami KK, Wenger DE, An KN: Quantitative assessment of classic anteroinferior bony Bankart lesions by radiography and computed tomography. *Am J Sports Med* 2003;31:112-118.

23. Itoi E, Lee SB, Berglund LJ, Berge LL, An KN: The effect of a glenoid defect on anteroinferior stability of the shoulder after Bankart repair: A cadaveric study. *J Bone Joint Surg Am* 2000;82:35-46.

24. Greis PE, Scuderi MG, Mohr A, Bachus KN, Burks RT: Glenohumeral articular contact areas and pressures following labral and osseous injury to the anteroinferior quadrant of the glenoid. *J Shoulder Elbow Surg* 2002;11:442-451.

25. Mologne TS, Provencher MT, Menzel KA, Vachon TA, Dewing CB: Arthroscopic stabilization in patients with an inverted pear glenoid: Results in patients with bone loss of the anterior glenoid. *Am J Sports Med* 2007;35:1276-1283.

26. Sugaya H, Moriishi J, Kanisawa I, Tsuchiya A: Arthroscopic osseous Bankart repair for chronic recurrent traumatic anterior glenohumeral instability: Surgical technique. *J Bone Joint Surg Am* 2006;88:159-169.

27. Yamamoto N, Itoi E, Abe H, et al: Contact between the glenoid and the humeral head in abduction, external rotation, and horizontal extension: A new concept of glenoid track. *J Shoulder Elbow Surg* 2007;16:649-656.

28. Calandra JJ, Baker CL, Uribe J: The incidence of Hill-Sachs lesions in initial anterior shoulder dislocations. *Arthroscopy* 1989;5:254-257.

29. Cetik O, Uslu M, Ozsar BK: The relationship between Hill-Sachs lesion and recurrent anterior shoulder dislocation. *Acta Orthop Belg* 2007;73:175-178.

30. Mologne TS, Zhao K, Hongo M, Romeo AA, An KN, Provencher MT: The addition of rotator interval closure after arthroscopic repair of either anterior or posterior shoulder instability: Effect on glenohumeral translation and range of motion. *Am J Sports Med* 2008;36:1123-1131.

31. Provencher MT, Mologne TS, Hongo M, Zhao K, Tasto JP, An KN: Arthroscopic versus open rotator interval closure: Biomechanical evaluation of stability and motion. *Arthroscopy* 2007;23:583-592.

32. Yamamoto N, Itoi E, Tuoheti Y, et al: Effect of rotator interval closure on glenohumeral stability and motion: A cadaveric study. *J Shoulder Elbow Surg* 2006;15:750-758.

33. Gerber C, Werner CM, Macy JC, Jacob HA, Nyffeler RW: Effect of selective capsulorrhaphy on the passive range of motion of the glenohumeral joint. *J Bone Joint Surg Am* 2003;85:48-55.

34. Harryman DT II, Sidles JA, Harris SL, Matsen FA III: The role of the rotator interval capsule in passive motion and stability of the shoulder. *J Bone Joint Surg Am* 1992;74:53-66.

35. Savoie FH III, Holt MS, Field LD, Ramsey JR: Arthroscopic management of posterior instability: Evolution of technique and results. *Arthroscopy* 2008;24:389-396.

36. Weber SC, Caspari RB: A biomechanical evaluation of the restraints to posterior shoulder dislocation. *Arthroscopy* 1989;5:115-121.

37. Bradley JP, Baker CL III, Kline AJ, Armfield DR, Chhabra A: Arthroscopic capsulolabral reconstruction for posterior instability of the shoulder: A prospective study of 100 shoulders. *Am J Sports Med* 2006;34:1061-1071.

38. Kim SH, Kim HK, Sun JI, Park JS, Oh I: Arthroscopic capsulolabroplasty for posteroinferior multidirectional instability of the shoulder. *Am J Sports Med* 2004;32:594-607.

39. Provencher MT, Bell SJ, Menzel KA, Mologne TS: Arthroscopic treatment of posterior shoulder instability: Results in 33 patients. *Am J Sports Med* 2005;33:1463-1471.

40. Williams RJ III, Strickland S, Cohen M, Altchek DW, Warren RF: Arthroscopic repair for traumatic posterior shoulder instability. *Am J Sports Med* 2003;31:203-209.

41. Soslowsky LJ, Malicky DM, Blasier RB: Active and passive factors in inferior glenohumeral stabilization: A biomechanical model. *J Shoulder Elbow Surg* 1997;6:371-379.

42. Blasier RB, Soslowsky LJ, Malicky DM, Palmer ML: Posterior glenohumeral subluxation: Active and passive stabilization in a biomechanical model. *J Bone Joint Surg Am* 1997; 79:433-440.

43. Boardman ND, Debski RE, Warner JJ, et al: Tensile properties of the superior glenohumeral and coracohumeral ligaments. *J Shoulder Elbow Surg* 1996;5:249-254.

44. Warner JJ, Deng XH, Warren RF, Torzilli PA: Static capsuloligamentous restraints to superior-inferior translation of the glenohumeral joint. *Am J Sports Med* 1992;20:675-685.

45. Cooper DE, O'Brien SJ, Arnoczky SP, Warren RF: The structure and function of the coracohumeral ligament: An anatomic and microscopic study. *J Shoulder Elbow Surg* 1993;2:70-77.

46. Harryman DT II, Sidles JA, Harris SL, Matsen FA III: Laxity of the normal glenohumeral joint: A quantitative in vivo assessment. *J Shoulder Elbow Surg* 1992;1:66-67.

47. Taverna E, Sansone V, Battistella F: Arthroscopic rotator interval repair: The three-step all-inside technique. *Arthroscopy* 2004;20:105-109.

48. Ozbaydar M, Elhassan B, Diller D, Massimini D, Higgins LD, Warner JJ: Results of arthroscopic capsulolabral repair: Bankart lesion versus anterior labroligamentous periosteal sleeve avulsion lesion. *Arthroscopy* 2008;24: 1277-1283.

49. Kropf EJ, Sekiya JK: Osteoarticular allograft transplantation for large humeral head defects in glenohumeral instability. *Arthroscopy* 2007;23:322.e1-322.e5.

50. Kelly J, Ogunro S: Arthroscopic "filling" of Hill-Sachs lesions. *Arthroscopy* 2007;23:e2.

51. Re P, Gallo RA, Richmond JC: Transhumeral head plasty for large Hill-Sachs lesions. *Arthroscopy* 2006; 22:798.e1-798.e4.

52. Purchase RJ, Wolf EM, Hobgood ER, Pollock ME, Smalley CC: Hill-Sachs "remplissage": An arthroscopic solution for the engaging Hill-Sachs lesion. *Arthroscopy* 2008;24:723-726.

53. Boileau P, Villalba M, Héry JY, Balg F, Ahrens P, Neyton L: Risk factors for recurrence of shoulder instability after arthroscopic Bankart repair. *J Bone Joint Surg Am* 2006;88: 1755-1763.

54. Sachs RA, Williams B, Stone ML, Paxton L, Kuney M: Open Bankart repair: Correlation of results with postoperative subscapularis function. *Am J Sports Med* 2005;33:1458-1462.

55. Scheibel M, Nikulka C, Dick A, Schroeder RJ, Popp AG, Haas NP: Structural integrity and clinical function of the subscapularis musculotendinous unit after arthroscopic and open shoulder stabilization. *Am J Sports Med* 2007;35:1153-1161.

56. Hansen BP, Beck CL, Beck EP, Townsley RW: Postarthroscopic glenohumeral chondrolysis. *Am J Sports Med* 2007;35:1628-1634.

57. McNickle AG, L'Heureux DR, Provencher MT, Romeo AA, Cole BJ: Postsurgical glenohumeral arthritis in young adults. *Am J Sports Med* 2009; 37:1784-1791.

58. Petty DH, Jazrawi LM, Estrada LS, Andrews JR: Glenohumeral chondrolysis after shoulder arthroscopy: Case reports and review of the literature. *Am J Sports Med* 2004;32: 509-515.

59. Balg F, Boileau P: The instability severity index score: A simple preoperative score to select patients for arthroscopic or open shoulder stabilisation. *J Bone Joint Surg Br* 2007;89: 1470-1477.

60. Ovesen J, Nielsen S: Experimental distal subluxation in the glenohumeral joint. *Arch Orthop Trauma Surg* 1985;104:78-81.

61. Burkhart SS, Danaceau SM: Articular arc length mismatch as a cause of failed Bankart repair. *Arthroscopy* 2000; 16:740-744.

62. Burkhart SS, De Beer JF, Barth JR, Cresswell T, Roberts C, Richards DP: Results of modified Latarjet reconstruction in patients with anteroinferior instability and significant bone loss. *Arthroscopy* 2007;23:1033-1041.

63. Itoi E, Lee SB, Berglund LJ, Berge LL, An KN: The effect of a glenoid defect on anteroinferior stability of the shoulder after Bankart repair: A cadaveric study. *J Bone Joint Surg Am* 2000;82:35-46.

64. Marquardt B, Garmann S, Schulte T, Witt KA, Steinbeck J, Pötzl W: Outcome after failed traumatic anterior shoulder instability repair with and without surgical revision. *J Shoulder Elbow Surg* 2007;16:742-747.

65. Meehan RE, Petersen SA: Results and factors affecting outcome of revision surgery for shoulder instability. *J Shoulder Elbow Surg* 2005;14:31-37.

66. Latarjet M: Surgical technics in the treatment of recurrent dislocation of the shoulder (antero-internal). *Lyon Chir* 1965;61:313-318.

67. Ghodadra N, Gupta A, Romeo AA, et al: Normalization of glenohumeral articular contact pressures after either Latarjet or iliac crest bone grafting procedure: Impact of graft type and position. *J Bone Joint Surg Am*, in press.

68. Yamamoto N, Itoi E, Abe H, et al: Effect of an anterior glenoid defect on anterior shoulder stability: A cadaveric study. *Am J Sports Med* 2009;37: 949-954.

69. Warner JJ, Gill TJ, O'Hollerhan JD, Pathare N, Millett PJ: Anatomical glenoid reconstruction for recurrent

anterior glenohumeral instability with glenoid deficiency using an autogenous tricortical iliac crest bone graft. *Am J Sports Med* 2006;34: 205-212.

70. Arrigoni P, Huberty D, Brady PC, Weber IC, Burkhart SS: The value of arthroscopy before an open modified Latarjet reconstruction. *Arthroscopy* 2008;24:514-519.

71. Burkhart SS, Brady PC: Arthroscopic subscapularis repair: Surgical tips and pearls A to Z. *Arthroscopy* 2006;22: 1014-1027.

72. Resch H, Povacz P, Ritter E, Matschi W: Transfer of the pectoralis major muscle for the treatment of irreparable rupture of the subscapularis tendon. *J Bone Joint Surg Am* 2000;82: 372-382.

73. Barnes CJ, Getelman MH, Snyder SJ: Results of arthroscopic revision anterior shoulder reconstruction. *Am J Sports Med* 2009;37:715-719.

74. Kim SH, Ha KI, Kim YM: Arthroscopic revision Bankart repair: A prospective outcome study. *Arthroscopy* 2002;18:469-482.

Video Reference

21.1 Provencher MT, Solomon DJ: Video. *Glenoid Bone Loss: Evaluation and Management*. San Diego, CA, 2008.

Surgical Management of Traumatic Anterior Glenohumeral Instability: An International Perspective

Bradford O. Parsons, MD
Pascal Boileau, MD
Yong Girl Rhee, MD
David A. Sonnabend, MD, BSc (Med), FRACS
Sergio L. Checchia, MD
Alessandro Castagna, MD
Evan L. Flatow, MD

Abstract

The treatment of traumatic anterior glenohumeral instability has evolved considerably in recent years. The results of arthroscopic repair have considerably improved, and, for many surgeons, arthroscopic techniques have supplanted traditional open techniques. Although a scoring system and other assessment tools can be useful, the choice of a surgical treatment for glenohumeral stabilization requires a careful assimilation of the patient's expectations and the surgeon's experience as well as an understanding of the relevant individual pathoanatomy. Pathoanatomy, nonsurgical and surgical treatment of shoulder instability, bone loss, unsuccessful stabilization treatment, and review of recent literature are important factors.

Instr Course Lect 2010;59:245-253.

Dr. Parsons or an immediate family member serves as a paid consultant to or is an employee of Zimmer and has received research or institutional support from Zimmer. Dr. Boileau or an immediate family member serves as a board member, owner, officer, or committee member of the European Society for Surgery of the Shoulder and Elbow and the Nice University Hospital Center; has received royalties from Tornier; and serves as a paid consultant to or is an employee of DePuy and Smith & Nephew. Dr. Sonnabend or an immediate family member serves as a paid consultant to or is an employee of DePuy and has received research or institutional support from DePuy and Zimmer. Dr. Checchia or an immediate family member is a board member, owner, officer, or committee member of the International Board of Shoulder and Elbow Surgeons; has received royalties from Arthrex; and is a paid consultant for or is an employee of Arthrex. Dr. Castagna or an immediate family member serves as a paid consultant to or is an employee of CONMED Linvatec and Tornier. Dr. Flatow or an immediate family member serves as a board member, owner, officer, or committee member of the American Shoulder and Elbow Surgeons, the Arthroscopy Association of North America, and the Mount Sinai Medical Center; has received royalties from Innomed and Zimmer; serves as a paid consultant to or is an employee of Wyeth; serves as an unpaid consultant to Zimmer; has received research or institutional support from Zimmer; and has received nonincome support (such as equipment or services), commercially derived honoraria, or other non–research-related funding (such as paid travel) from Springer and Wolters Kluwer Health–Lippincott Williams & Wilkins. Neither Dr. Rhee nor any immediate family members have received anything of value from or own stock in a commercial company or institution related directly or indirectly to the subject of this chapter.

Management of traumatic anterior glenohumeral instability has evolved considerably in recent years. Although open labral repair and capsulorrhaphy often are considered the gold standard, many surgeons now prefer arthroscopic techniques, and some consider arthroscopic repair to be the new gold standard. The early reports of arthroscopic techniques included unacceptably high rates of recurrence,[1-7] but a better understanding of pathoanatomy, instrumentation, and technique has led to improved rates of recurrence, and the current rates are similar after open and arthroscopic anatomic repairs.[8-13] Not all patients or unstable shoulders should be treated arthroscopically; for some, open techniques, including soft-tissue and bony procedures such as the Bristow-Latarjet procedure, may be preferred.

Pathoanatomy

Traumatic anterior dislocation often causes injuries involving the capsulolabral structures, the glenoid, and the humeral head. Of 247 shoulders undergoing anterior shoulder stabilization, 180 (73%) had a classic Bankart lesion, 30 (12%) had a bony Bankart lesion, 20 (8%) had an anterior labroligamentous periosteal sleeve avulsion (ALPSA) lesion, 5 (2%) had a humeral avulsion of the glenohumeral ligament (HAGL) lesion, and 12 (5%) had a midsubstance tear of the anteroinferior capsule (YG Rhee, MD, unpublished data, 2009). In general, a pathoanatomic lesion contributing to anterior shoulder instability can be classified as a soft-tissue (capsulolabral) or bony (glenoid or humeral head) lesion.

Soft-Tissue Lesions

The inferior glenohumeral ligament (IGHL) is the primary restraint to anteroinferior instability, with contributions from the labrum, the osseous glenoid dish, and the rotator cuff, which provides dynamic muscular restraint. A detachment of the anterior labrum, middle glenohumeral ligament, and IGHL from the anteroinferior glenoid rim, called a Bankart lesion, often is the primary lesion resulting from traumatic anterior shoulder instability.[14] However, cadaver sectioning has revealed that an isolated labral deficiency generally is insufficient to cause glenohumeral dislocation[15] and that the IGHL complex also must be deficient.[16]

Recurrent trauma and instability often lead to attenuation of the anteroinferior capsule and increased laxity of the IGHL, even after the labrum is anatomically repaired.[17] An anteroinferior capsulolabral lesion sometimes extends into the medial glenoid neck periosteum. This ALPSA lesion most frequently is observed in shoulders with recurrent instability and may be associated with an increased risk of recurrence after repair.[18,19] Extension of the labral lesion into the superior labral complex, called a superior labrum anterior and posterior lesion, sometimes occurs. A HAGL lesion is rare.[20,21] Nevertheless, care should be taken to determine whether a HAGL lesion is present, as it often requires surgical management, and an open repair may be preferable to the conventional arthroscopic Bankart lesion repair.

Osseous Lesions

Traumatic anterior dislocation rarely results in a bony avulsion of the anteroinferior glenoid and IGHL complex, which is called a bony Bankart lesion.[22] Conversely, recurrent instability may lead to resorption of osseous fragments or compression of the glenoid rim, creating a glenoid deficiency. Boileau and associates[23] classified a glenoid rim lesion as either a separation fracture, in which an avulsion of a bony fragment can be seen radiographically, or a compression fracture, in which there is a glenoid rim deficiency but no visible free bony fragment. Glenoid bone loss, especially in a compression lesion, is a factor in the failure of both arthroscopic and open stabilization procedures.[23-26] The management of glenoid bone loss is controversial, especially with respect to the critical threshold of bone loss that can safely be managed with a soft-tissue Bankart repair.

A humeral lesion can affect the treatment of a recurrently unstable shoulder. Most commonly, the posterosuperior humeral head has a depression fracture from recurrent impaction onto the anteroinferior glenoid rim. This Hill-Sachs lesion is extremely common, occurring in almost all shoulders with recurrent instability.[27] If a Hill-Sachs lesion is large (more than 30% of the articular surface) or associated with glenoid rim deficiency, it can engage the edge of the glenoid rim during abduction and external rotation and thus lead to recurrent instability.[28] Balg and Boileau[29] found that Hill-Sachs lesions, as seen on an AP scapular radiograph with the arm in external rotation, are associated with a higher risk of failure after arthroscopic stabilization. A large Hill-Sachs lesion (more than 40% of the humeral head) often requires bone grafting or other direct treatment, whereas a smaller lesion (less than 20% of the humeral head) often does not engage the glenoid rim after anterior capsulorrhaphy.

Patient Evaluation

A routine patient evaluation includes a detailed history of instability episodes, with attention to the patient's age at the first traumatic dislocation; the number of recurrent instability episodes, including true dislocations requiring physician reduction, subluxations, and patient-reduced dislocations; any atraumatic instability after the initial traumatic primary dislocation (for example, instability at night or during activities of daily living); and earlier nonsurgical and surgical treatment. Patients with multiple instability episodes often have an attenuated capsuloligamentous complex and are relatively likely to have associated bone loss. A history of manual labor, sports activity (especially in a contact sport such as football), or seizure disorder should be identified, as these factors can have an impact on surgical decision making.

The physical examination should identify objective signs of instability through testing for apprehension and relocation, assessment for multidirectional instability or rotator cuff interval lesions, and identification of associated conditions such as rotator cuff deficiency (in particular, a subscapularis tear) or nerve palsy. The assessment also should identify any signs of ligamentous laxity such as elbow or metacarpal-phalangeal hyperextension.

Orthogonal plain radiographs in the true AP, AP with the arm in external rotation, outlet, and axillary lateral views are used, with attention to identifying any glenoid or humeral bone loss. Patients with recurrent instability often are evaluated using MRI and magnetic resonance arthrography to assess the severity of soft-tissue capsulolabral lesions. Careful MRI assessment should identify an ALPSA lesion with an attenuated anterior capsule (Figure 1), a HAGL lesion, or an associated superior labrum anterior and posterior lesion or rotator cuff tear. Bony lesions often can be identified and quantified using MRI but can be better delineated using CT, especially if three-dimensional reconstruction is used.

Nonsurgical Management

Recurrence rates as high as 92% to 95% have been reported in younger, high-demand patients after acute traumatic anterior shoulder dislocation.[8,30-32] Nonsurgical treatment is intended to restore stability and function while decreasing the likelihood of a recurrence. Several studies examined the effect of external rotation after acute traumatic anterior shoulder instability.[33-35] Itoi and associates[34] found that better anatomic apposition of the Bankart lesion to the glenoid rim can be seen on MRI when the arm is positioned in external rotation (approximately 35°) rather than internal rotation (using a sling). Miller and associates[35] reported similar findings in a cadaver study. Itoi and associates[33,36] also found lower recurrence rates in patients treated with external rotation bracing after traumatic anterior dislocation. Scheibel and associates[37] recommended 3 weeks of immobilization with bracing rather than the 5 to 6 weeks used by Itoi and associates.[33,36] After the period of immobilization, most patients participate in a program of physical therapy for controlled stretching and improving dynamic stability by strengthening the rotator cuff and periscapular muscles.

If symptomatic recurrent instability recurs despite nonsurgical treatment, surgical stabilization may be indicated. There is a trend toward the use of arthroscopic stabilization for most patients.

Arthroscopic Stabilization

The goal of an anatomic stabilization, whether open or arthroscopic, is to reestablish the normal orientation of the Bankart labral lesion and restore appropriate tension to the attenuated capsulolabral structures. Decreases in the rate of recurrence after arthroscopic stabilization often have been associated with the use of better instrumentation and fixation techniques, including suture anchors (rather than arthroscopically placed tacks or staples)[1-3,9,30,31,38] and capsular management with arthroscopic plication rather than thermal capsular shrinkage.[39-43] Thermal capsular shrinkage is associated with adverse effects, including axillary nerve injury, chondrolysis, and capsular attenuation,[44-46] and it has been abandoned by most surgeons.

Because of the advances in instrumentation and techniques, most patients who have anteroinferior glenohumeral instability without a significant glenoid or humeral bony lesion can be treated arthroscopically after unsuccessful nonsurgical management. The reported rates of recurrence are 10% or lower.[9,10,13,47] More significant capsular lesions, such as an ALPSA lesion, are amenable to arthroscopic treatment, but they require a more extensive release of the medially scarred capsulolabral complex from the glenoid neck and more extensive capsulorrhaphy to minimize the risk of recurrence.[19] Arthroscopic stabilization is believed to lead to less morbidity than open stabilization, with a lower incidence of stiffness or subscapularis weakness.[8,10,48] Some recent studies found better results after arthroscopic treatment than after open treatment in certain groups of patients historically managed with open stabilization, including contact or collision athletes, patients undergoing revision stabilization surgery, and patients with select small bony Bankart (separation) fractures.[49-54]

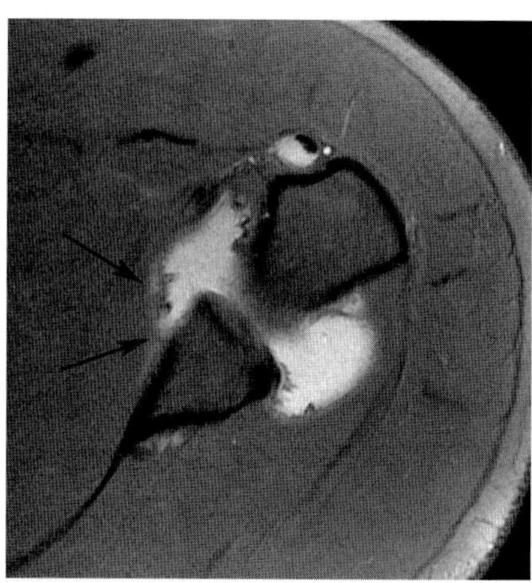

Figure 1 An axial MRI showing an ALPSA lesion and attenuated anterior capsule in a patient with recurrent instability.

Bone Deficiency

Several conditions are not amenable to arthroscopic stabilization.

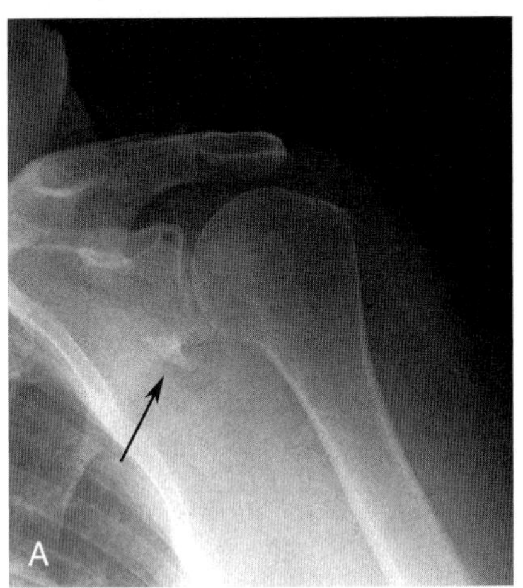

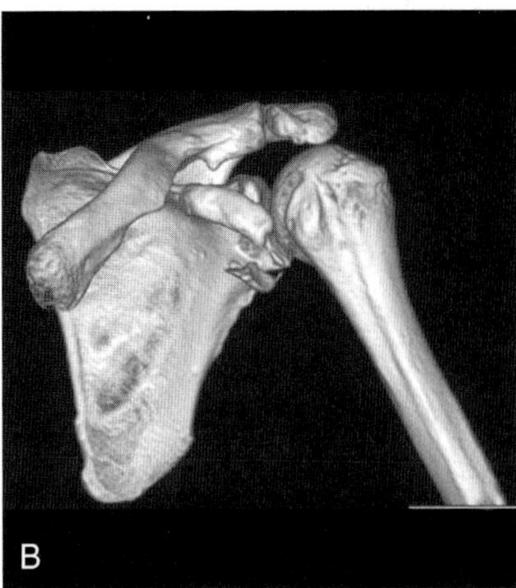

Figure 2 A bony Bankart lesion (*arrow*) is shown in an AP scapular radiograph **(A)** and three-dimensional CT reconstruction **(B)**.

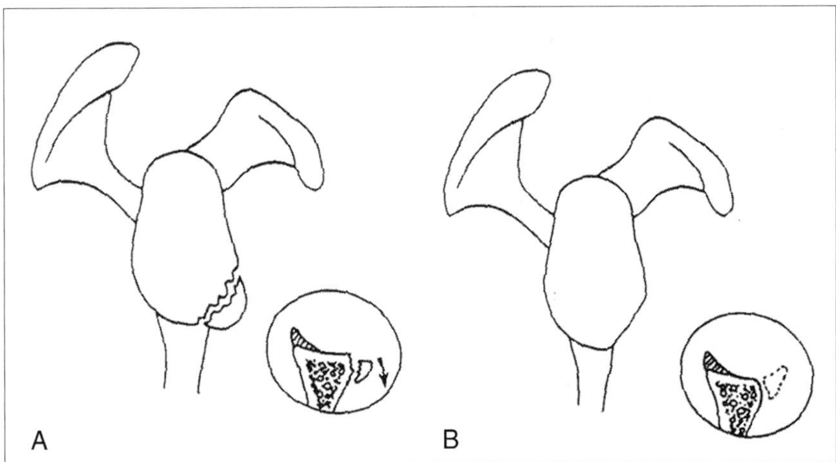

Figure 3 Schematic diagram of the glenoid face showing two patterns of glenoid rim lesions. **A,** A typical bony Bankart lesion. **B,** A compression lesion with associated bone loss of the anteroinferior glenoid. (Reproduced with permission from Boileau P, Villalba M, Héry JY, Balg F, Ahrens P, Neyton L: Risk factors for recurrence of shoulder instability after arthroscopic Bankart repair. *J Bone Joint Surg Am* 2006; 88(8):1755-1763.)

Significant bone deficiency, most commonly in the glenoid, is the primary indication for open stabilization, which often is done using a bone graft. Controversy remains as to the critical amount of bone deficiency that can be managed with an arthroscopic soft-tissue repair rather than an open stabilization or bone-grafting procedure.

Rowe and Sakellarides[55] found that the presence of a glenoid bone deficiency greatly increased the likelihood of recurrent instability. In their study, the recurrence rate after open stabilization was 62%. Even with the use of improved arthroscopic techniques, glenoid insufficiency remains a primary cause of failure. Glenoid lesions may be quite common, especially in patients with a history of multiple dislocations. Sugaya and associates[26] evaluated 100 unstable shoulders using CT and found a 40% incidence of glenoid rim insufficiency; this rate was confirmed arthroscopically.

Bone augmentation is not always required for a glenoid deficiency, and glenoid deficiency does not always preclude an arthroscopic repair. Glenoid bone loss of less than 20% is the traditional threshold for repairing a lesion with a soft-tissue procedure, but little evidence is available to validate this demarcation. Many patients with a glenoid lesion have a corresponding Hill-Sachs lesion that may affect the success of a soft-tissue repair.[27] Therefore, identifying and quantifying a glenoid bone lesion is key to managing an unstable shoulder with glenoid insufficiency.

The bony Bankart lesion represents an avulsion of the anteroinferior glenoid from the glenoid rim along the capsulolabral complex, and often it is amenable to arthroscopic or open repair[22] (Figure 2). The bony Bankart lesion is not equivalent to the compression fracture, as described by Boileau and associates,[23] in which the glenoid has been whittled away by recurrent instability and little or no bone exists for repair (Figure 3). A compression lesion often is missed or underappreciated on radiographs, but it can have a significant impact on the success of a stabilization procedure.

Plain radiographs can yield clues to the presence of a glenoid deficiency. Using the Bernageau axillary view, Edwards and associates[56] described three forms of glenoid bone loss: the bony Bankart lesion, in which there is a visible fragment; the cliff sign, in which anteroinferior bone loss is present, with no visible fragment; and the blunted angle, in which rounding and compression of the glenoid rim are present. Three-dimensional CT can be helpful if

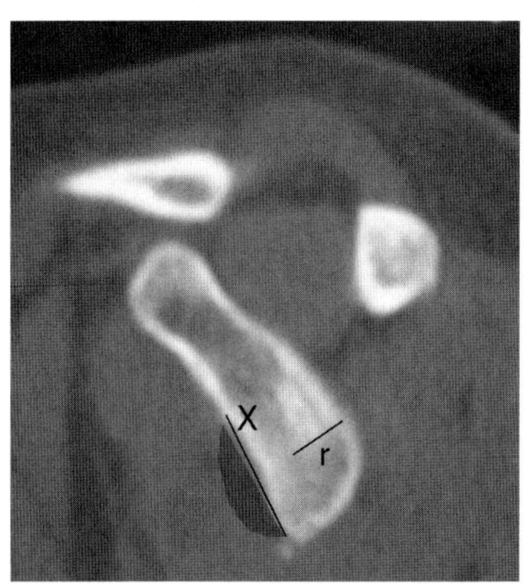

Figure 4 The assessment of glenoid bone loss, as described by Gerber and Nyffeler.[25] The radius (r) of the glenoid face is compared to the length of the defect (X); the dislocation resistance is less than 70% of the value of an intact joint if the defect is longer than the radius. This quantitive assessment is shown on a sagittal CT scan of a glenoid face with significant anteroinferior bone loss (shaded area). Bone grafting may be necessary for the glenoid defect.

Table 1
The Instability Severity Index Score

Prognostic Factor	Categories	Points
Age at surgery	Younger than age 20 years	2
	Older than age 20 years	0
Sports participation before injury	Competitive	2
	Recreational or none	0
Type of sports participation before injury	Contact sport or sport involving forced abduction–external rotation	1
	Other	0
Shoulder laxity	Hyperlaxity	1
	Normal laxity	0
Hill-Sachs lesion in external rotation (on AP radiograph)	Visible	2
	Not visible	0
Glenoid contour (on AP radiograph)	Loss of contour	2
	No loss of contour	0

(Adapted with permission from Balg F, Boileau P: The instability severity index score: A simple preoperative score to select patients for arthroscopic or open shoulder stabilisation. *J Bone Joint Surg Br* 2007;89:1470-1477.)

Table 2
Recurrence Rates Associated With the Instability Severity Index Score

Total Score	Recurrence Rate ($P < 0.001$)	Preferred Treatment
0 to 3	4.8%	Soft-tissue stabilization
3 to 6	9.9%	Bristow-Latarjet procedure
6 or higher	70.0%	Bristow-Latarjet procedure

(Adapted with permission from Balg F, Boileau P: The instability severity index score: A simple preoperative score to select patients for arthroscopic or open shoulder stabilisation. *J Bone Joint Surg Br* 2007;89:1470-1477.)

the presence or type of glenoid deficiency is in doubt. Gerber and Nyffeler[25] developed a method of quantifying glenoid bone defects on CT by comparing the radius of the inferior glenoid to the length of the defect. If the length of the defect is greater than the radius of the maximum width of the glenoid, the force required to dislocate the glenohumeral joint is reduced by 30% (Figure 4). Other, similar formulaic assessments on CT or MRI have been developed in an effort to quantify glenoid bone loss.[26,57] Although helpful, none of the available studies determined the critical threshold for bone augmentation, and therefore the entire spectrum of the patient's condition, including any humeral lesion or soft-tissue attenuation, is important in surgical decision making.

The preoperative Instability Severity Index Score of Balg and Boileau[29] incorporates the patient history, examination, and radiographic imaging (Tables 1 and 2). Factors associated with the failure of arthroscopic repair include age younger than 20 years; involvement in overhead throwing or a collision sport; and hyperlax joints, as indicated by glenohumeral external rotation of more than 85° with the arm adducted or hyperabduction of 20° more than the contralateral shoulder. Patients with a score of 3 or lower can successfully be treated with arthroscopic stabilization; those with a score higher than 3 should be treated with a Bristow-Latarjet coracoid transfer because of their higher risk of recurrence after arthroscopic stabilization.[29]

Glenoid Bone Grafting

If the patient has both a glenoid deficiency and a corresponding engaging humeral deficiency, many surgeons recommend osseous reconstruction to minimize the risk of recurrence. Although in rare circumstances a Hill-Sachs lesion of more than 25% to 40% of the humeral head requires humeral bone grafting with reconstruction, most smaller Hill-Sachs lesions can be successfully managed with glenoid bone augmentation. Warner and associates[58] described successful

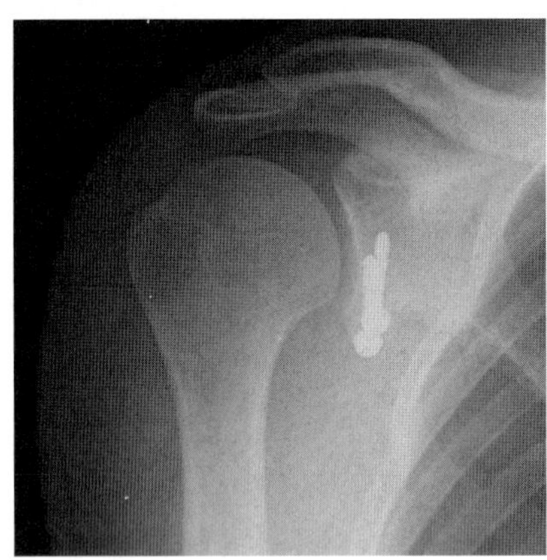

Figure 5 AP radiograph showing a Bristow-Latarjet reconstruction with anteroinferior placement of the transferred coracoid process along the glenoid rim.

iliac crest bone grafting for glenoid lesions, in which the harvested tricortical crest is contoured and placed intra-articularly along the deficient glenoid neck and the anterior capsule-labrum is repaired along the native glenoid rim. At 33-month follow-up of 11 patients after treatment for recurrent instability and associated significant glenoid bone loss (quantified using Gerber's method), the average American Shoulder and Elbow Surgeons Shoulder Index and Rowe scores were 94. None of the patients had recurrent instability, and all had complete graft union on CT.[58]

The Bristow-Latarjet coracoid transfer procedure recently has achieved renewed popularity for managing recurrent instability with associated bone loss (Figure 5). The transferred coracoid increases the glenoid width in a manner similar to that of Warner's method for iliac crest grafting. The result is improved static stability without the morbidity associated with iliac crest tricortical harvest. When the arm is abducted and externally rotated, the attached conjoined tendon adds dynamic stability by acting as an internal sling along the axillary pouch. Burkhart and associates[59] reported a 4.9% recurrence rate and an average Constant Shoulder Score of 94 in 102 shoulders with recurrent instability and glenoid bone loss of more than 25%. Similarly, Hovelius and associates[60] reported patient satisfaction for 98% of 116 shoulders at 15-year follow-up after a Bristow-Latarjet repair; 4 patients had recurrent dislocation. Although the Bristow-Latarjet procedure traditionally is done in an open fashion, Boileau and associates[61] and Lafosse and associates[62] recently described an arthroscopic Bristow-Latarjet procedure, with promising early results.

Complications and Revision Surgery

Complications are rare after surgical stabilization of the shoulder. The risk of complications inherent in nearly all orthopaedic procedures, such as those related to infection or hardware, is extremely low. As arthroscopic techniques and instrumentation have evolved, most surgeons have adopted the use of bioabsorbable anchors around the glenoid because of concerns about metal anchor prominence in the joint and the potential for arthrosis. Many surgeons have discontinued the use of capsular shrinkage with thermal capsulorrhaphy because of reports of degrading and chondrolysis.[42-46]

Stiffness is rare after shoulder stabilization, especially when the procedure is done arthroscopically,[8,10] but it is more common after revision surgery. Historically, in the Putti-Platt procedure and other procedures involving subscapularis tightening, the anterior tissues were deliberately overtightened, often leading to a loss of external rotation or early arthritis.[63] Excessive stiffness can lead to early arthrosis, and careful attention to proper capsular tightening is critical during open or arthroscopic stabilization.[63,64]

Arthritis can be a consequence of instability. At 25-year radiographic follow-up, Hovelius and Saeboe[65] reported 26% incidence of moderate or severe arthropathy in patients treated nonsurgically for traumatic anterior instability. Postcapsulorrhaphy arthritis has been observed after open and arthroscopic soft-tissue stabilization procedures as well as bony reconstructive procedures.[59,60,63,64,66] However, it is difficult to delineate the risk of arthritic changes following any particular surgical or nonsurgical treatment for instability. Excessive overtensioning of the joint capsule resulting in a significant loss of external rotation (more than 30% compared with the contralateral shoulder) is recognized as a risk factor for arthrosis. The positioning of the glenoid bone graft can have an impact; a lateral overhang of the coracoid or iliac bone graft anterior to the joint has been associated with an increased rate of early arthrosis and should be avoided.[67]

The primary complication of surgical stabilization is recurrent instability. Although early reports of unacceptably high recurrence rates after arthroscopic shoulder stabilization have been superseded by more recent reports of similar recurrence rates after open and arthroscopic stabilization, recurrence remains a concern. A careful assessment of the cause of recurrence is critical whenever revision surgery is considered. Bone deficiency is a common cause, and careful preoperative assessment of bony lesions can help in the selection of the most appropriate stabilization procedure. No consensus exists as to the threshold at which a bone deficiency must be treated with grafting, but most experts agree that an isolated glenoid bone deficiency of less than 20% often can be managed with soft-tissue repair. However, as reflected in the Balg and Boileau[29] scoring system for instability, all contributors to shoulder instability, including patient activity level, must be considered in surgical decision making.

The Bristow-Latarjet procedure is recommended for treating a patient with anteroinferior glenoid deficiency after an unsuccessful arthroscopic stabilization procedure. An arthroscopic procedure often is appropriate for treating a traumatic recurrence without bone loss or a recurrence caused by poorly stabilized soft tissues, provided that the quality of the capsulolabral tissue is adequate for such a repair.

Summary

The surgical stabilization of recurrent anterior shoulder instability has evolved in recent years with improvements in arthroscopic instrumentation, techniques, and results. However, an open stabilization or a bone graft procedure sometimes is warranted. An understanding of the indications for using an arthroscopic or open technique, especially with a bone deficiency, leads to optimal patient outcomes and avoids a recurrence.

References

1. Freedman KB, Smith AP, Romeo AA, Cole BJ, Bach BR Jr: Open Bankart repair versus arthroscopic repair with transglenoid sutures or bioabsorbable tacks for recurrent anterior instability of the shoulder: A meta-analysis. *Am J Sports Med* 2004;32:1520-1527.
2. Gross RM: Arthroscopic shoulder capsulorrhaphy: Does it work? *Am J Sports Med* 1989;17:495-500.
3. Hawkins RB: Arthroscopic stapling repair for shoulder instability: A retrospective study of 50 cases. *Arthroscopy* 1989;5:122-128.
4. Hayashida K, Yoneda M, Nakagawa S, Okamura K, Fukushima S: Arthroscopic Bankart suture repair for traumatic anterior shoulder instability: Analysis of the causes of a recurrence. *Arthroscopy* 1998;14:295-301.
5. Magnusson L, Kartus J, Ejerhed L, Hultenheim I, Sernert N, Karlsson J: Revisiting the open Bankart experience: A four- to nine-year follow-up. *Am J Sports Med* 2002;30:778-782.
6. Mohtadi NG, Bitar IJ, Sasyniuk TM, Hollinshead RM, Harper WP: Arthroscopic versus open repair for traumatic anterior shoulder instability: A meta-analysis. *Arthroscopy* 2005; 21:652-658.
7. Mologne TS, McBride MT, Lapoint JM: Assessment of failed arthroscopic anterior labral repairs: Findings at open surgery. *Am J Sports Med* 1997; 25:813-817.
8. Bottoni CR, Smith EL, Berkowitz MJ, Towle RB, Moore JH: Arthroscopic versus open shoulder stabilization for recurrent anterior instability: A prospective randomized clinical trial. *Am J Sports Med* 2006;34:1730-1737.
9. Carreira DS, Mazzocca AD, Oryhon J, Brown FM, Hayden JK, Romeo AA: A prospective outcome evaluation of arthroscopic Bankart repairs: Minimum 2-year follow-up. *Am J Sports Med* 2006;34:771-777.
10. Fabbriciani C, Milano G, Demontis A, Fadda S, Ziranu F, Mulas PD: Arthroscopic versus open treatment of Bankart lesion of the shoulder: A prospective randomized study. *Arthroscopy* 2004;20:456-462.
11. Kim SH, Ha KI, Cho YB, Ryu BD, Oh I: Arthroscopic anterior stabilization of the shoulder: Two to six-year follow-up. *J Bone Joint Surg Am* 2003; 85:1511-1518.
12. Tjoumakaris FP, Abboud JA, Hasan SA, Ramsey ML, Williams GR: Arthroscopic and open Bankart repairs provide similar outcomes. *Clin Orthop Relat Res* 2006;446:227-232.
13. Westerheide KJ, Dopirak RM, Snyder SJ: Arthroscopic anterior stabilization and posterior capsular plication for anterior glenohumeral instability: A report of 71 cases. *Arthroscopy* 2006; 22:539-547.
14. Bankart A: Pathology and treatment of recurrent dislocation of shoulder-joint. *Br J Surg* 1938;26:23-29.
15. Pouliart N, Marmor S, Gagey O: Simulated capsulolabral lesion in cadavers: Dislocation does not result from a bankart lesion only. *Arthroscopy* 2006;22:748-754.
16. Itoi E, Hsu HC, An KN: Biomechanical investigation of the glenohumeral joint. *J Shoulder Elbow Surg* 1996;5:407-424.
17. Speer KP, Deng X, Borrero S, Torzilli PA, Altchek DA, Warren RF: Biomechanical evaluation of a simulated Bankart lesion. *J Bone Joint Surg Am* 1994;76:1819-1826.
18. Neviaser TJ: The anterior labroligamentous periosteal sleeve avulsion lesion: A cause of anterior instability of the shoulder. *Arthroscopy* 1993;9: 17-21.
19. Ozbaydar M, Elhassan B, Diller D, Massimini D, Higgins LD, Warner JJ: Results of arthroscopic capsulolabral repair: Bankart lesion versus anterior labroligamentous periosteal sleeve avulsion lesion. *Arthroscopy* 2008;24: 1277-1283.
20. Nicola T: Recurrent dislocation of the shoulder. *Am J Surg* 1953;86: 85-91.
21. Wolf EM, Cheng JC, Dickson K: Humeral avulsion of glenohumeral ligaments as a cause of anterior shoulder instability. *Arthroscopy* 1995;11:600-607.
22. Bigliani LU, Newton PM, Steinmann SP, Connor PM, McIlveen SJ: Glenoid rim lesions associated with recurrent anterior dislocation of the

shoulder. *Am J Sports Med* 1998;26: 41-45.

23. Boileau P, Villalba M, Héry JY, Balg F, Ahrens P, Neyton L: Risk factors for recurrence of shoulder instability after arthroscopic Bankart repair. *J Bone Joint Surg Am* 2006;88: 1755-1763.
24. Burkhart SS, De Beer JF: Traumatic glenohumeral bone defects and their relationship to failure of arthroscopic Bankart repairs: Significance of the inverted-pear glenoid and the humeral engaging Hill-Sachs lesion. *Arthroscopy* 2000;16:677-694.
25. Gerber C, Nyffeler RW: Classification of glenohumeral joint instability. *Clin Orthop Relat Res* 2002;400:65-76.
26. Sugaya H, Moriishi J, Dohi M, Kon Y, Tsuchiya A: Glenoid rim morphology in recurrent anterior glenohumeral instability. *J Bone Joint Surg Am* 2003;85:878-884.
27. Calandra JJ, Baker CL, Uribe J: The incidence of Hill-Sachs lesions in initial anterior shoulder dislocations. *Arthroscopy* 1989;5:254-257.
28. Gerber C, Lambert SM: Allograft reconstruction of segmental defects of the humeral head for the treatment of chronic locked posterior dislocation of the shoulder. *J Bone Joint Surg Am* 1996;78:376-382.
29. Balg F, Boileau P: The instability severity index score: A simple preoperative score to select patients for arthroscopic or open shoulder stabilisation. *J Bone Joint Surg Br* 2007;89: 1470-1477.
30. Kirkley A, Werstine R, Ratjek A, Griffin S: Prospective randomized clinical trial comparing the effectiveness of immediate arthroscopic stabilization versus immobilization and rehabilitation in first traumatic anterior dislocations of the shoulder: Long-term evaluation. *Arthroscopy* 2005;21:55-63.
31. Larrain MV, Botto GJ, Montenegro HJ, Mauas DM: Arthroscopic repair of acute traumatic anterior shoulder dislocation in young athletes. *Arthroscopy* 2001;17:373-377.
32. Wheeler JH, Ryan JB, Arciero RA, Molinari RN: Arthroscopic versus nonoperative treatment of acute shoulder dislocations in young athletes. *Arthroscopy* 1989;5:213-217.
33. Itoi E, Hatakeyama Y, Kido T, et al: A new method of immobilization after traumatic anterior dislocation of the shoulder: A preliminary study. *J Shoulder Elbow Surg* 2003;12:413-415.
34. Itoi E, Sashi R, Minagawa H, Shimizu T, Wakabayashi I, Sato K: Position of immobilization after dislocation of the glenohumeral joint: A study with use of magnetic resonance imaging. *J Bone Joint Surg Am* 2001;83:661-667.
35. Miller BS, Sonnabend DH, Hatrick C, et al: Should acute anterior dislocations of the shoulder be immobilized in external rotation? A cadaveric study. *J Shoulder Elbow Surg* 2004;13: 589-592.
36. Itoi E, Hatakeyama Y, Sato T, et al: Immobilization in external rotation after shoulder dislocation reduces the risk of recurrence: A randomized controlled trial. *J Bone Joint Surg Am* 2007;89:2124-2131.
37. Scheibel M, Kuke A, Nikulka C, Magosch P, Ziesler O, Schroeder RJ: How long should acute anterior dislocations of the shoulder be immobilized in external rotation? *Am J Sports Med* 2009;37:1309-1316.
38. Marquardt B, Witt KA, Liem D, Steinbeck J, Pötzl W: Arthroscopic Bankart repair in traumatic anterior shoulder instability using a suture anchor technique. *Arthroscopy* 2006;22: 931-936.
39. Alberta FG, ElAttrache NS, Mihata T, McGarry MH, Tibone JE, Lee TQ: Arthroscopic anteroinferior suture plication resulting in decreased glenohumeral translation and external rotation: Study of a cadaver model. *J Bone Joint Surg Am* 2006;88:179-187.
40. Cohen SB, Wiley W, Goradia VK, Pearson S, Miller MD: Anterior capsulorrhaphy: An in vitro comparison of volume reduction. Arthroscopic plication versus open capsular shift. *Arthroscopy* 2005;21:659-664.
41. Gerber C, Werner CM, Macy JC, Jacob HA, Nyffeler RW: Effect of selective capsulorrhaphy on the passive range of motion of the glenohumeral joint. *J Bone Joint Surg Am* 2003;85: 48-55.
42. Chen S, Haen PS, Walton J, Murrell GA: The effects of thermal capsular shrinkage on the outcomes of arthroscopic stabilization for primary anterior shoulder instability. *Am J Sports Med* 2005;33:705-711.
43. D'Alessandro DF, Bradley JP, Fleischli JE, Connor PM: Prospective evaluation of thermal capsulorrhaphy for shoulder instability: Indications and results. Two- to five-year follow-up. *Am J Sports Med* 2004;32:21-33.
44. Greis PE, Burks RT, Schickendantz MS, Sandmeier R: Axillary nerve injury after thermal capsular shrinkage of the shoulder. *J Shoulder Elbow Surg* 2001;10:231-235.
45. Good CR, Shindle MK, Kelly BT, Wanich T, Warren RF: Glenohumeral chondrolysis after shoulder arthroscopy with thermal capsulorrhaphy. *Arthroscopy* 2007;23:797.e1-5.
46. McFarland EG, Kim TK, Banchasuek P, McCarthy EF: Histologic evaluation of the shoulder capsule in normal shoulders, unstable shoulders, and after failed thermal capsulorrhaphy. *Am J Sports Med* 2002;30:636-642.
47. Brophy RH, Marx RG: The treatment of traumatic anterior instability of the shoulder: Nonoperative and surgical treatment. *Arthroscopy* 2009; 25:298-304.
48. Sachs RA, Williams B, Stone ML, Paxton L, Kuney M: Open Bankart repair: Correlation of results with postoperative subscapularis function. *Am J Sports Med* 2005;33:1458-1462.
49. Mazzocca AD, Brown FM Jr, Carreira DS, Hayden J, Romeo AA: Arthroscopic anterior shoulder stabilization of collision and contact athletes. *Am J Sports Med* 2005;33:52-60.
50. Barnes CJ, Getelman MH, Snyder SJ: Results of arthroscopic revision anterior shoulder reconstruction. *Am J Sports Med* 2009;37:715-719.

51. Creighton RA, Romeo AA, Brown FM Jr, Hayden JK, Verma NN: Revision arthroscopic shoulder instability repair. *Arthroscopy* 2007;23:703-709.

52. Neri BR, Tuckman DV, Bravman JT, Yim D, Sahajpal DT, Rokito AS: Arthroscopic revision of Bankart repair. *J Shoulder Elbow Surg* 2007;16:419-424.

53. Porcellini G, Campi F, Paladini P: Arthroscopic approach to acute bony Bankart lesion. *Arthroscopy* 2002;18:764-769.

54. Sugaya H, Moriishi J, Kanisawa I, Tsuchiya A: Arthroscopic osseous Bankart repair for chronic recurrent traumatic anterior glenohumeral instability. *J Bone Joint Surg Am* 2005;87:1752-1760.

55. Rowe CR, Sakellarides HT: Factors related to recurrences of anterior dislocations of the shoulder. *Clin Orthop* 1961;20:40-48.

56. Edwards TB, Boulahia A, Walch G: Radiographic analysis of bone defects in chronic anterior shoulder instability. *Arthroscopy* 2003;19:732-739.

57. Griffith JF, Antonio GE, Tong CW, Ming CK: Anterior shoulder dislocation: Quantification of glenoid bone loss with CT. *AJR Am J Roentgenol* 2003;180:1423-1430.

58. Warner JJ, Gill TJ, O'Hollerhan JD, Pathare N, Millett PJ: Anatomical glenoid reconstruction for recurrent anterior glenohumeral instability with glenoid deficiency using an autogenous tricortical iliac crest bone graft. *Am J Sports Med* 2006;34:205-212.

59. Burkhart SS, De Beer JF, Barth JR, Cresswell T, Roberts C, Richards DP: Results of modified Latarjet reconstruction in patients with anteroinferior instability and significant bone loss. *Arthroscopy* 2007;23:1033-1041.

60. Hovelius L, Sandström B, Saebö M: One hundred eighteen Bristow-Latarjet repairs for recurrent anterior dislocation of the shoulder prospectively followed for fifteen years: Study II. The evolution of dislocation arthropathy. *J Shoulder Elbow Surg* 2006;15:279-289.

61. Boileau P, Bicknell RT, El Fegoun AB, Chuinard C: Arthroscopic Bristow procedure for anterior instability in shoulders with a stretched or deficient capsule: The "belt-and-suspenders" operative technique and preliminary results. *Arthroscopy* 2007;23:593-601.

62. Lafosse L, Lejeune E, Bouchard A, Kakuda C, Gobezie R, Kochhar T: The arthroscopic Latarjet procedure for the treatment of anterior shoulder instability. *Arthroscopy* 2007;23:1242.e1-5.

63. Hawkins RJ, Angelo RL: Glenohumeral osteoarthrosis: A late complication of the Putti-Platt repair. *J Bone Joint Surg Am* 1990;72:1193-1197.

64. Walch G, Ascani C, Boulahia A, Nové-Josserand L, Edwards TB: Static posterior subluxation of the humeral head: An unrecognized entity responsible for glenohumeral osteoarthritis in the young adult. *J Shoulder Elbow Surg* 2002;11:309-314.

65. Hovelius L, Saeboe M: Arthropathy after primary anterior shoulder dislocation: 223 shoulders prospectively followed up for twenty-five years. *J Shoulder Elbow Surg* 2009;18:339-347.

66. Pelet S, Jolles BM, Farron A: Bankart repair for recurrent anterior glenohumeral instability: Results at twenty-nine years' follow-up. *J Shoulder Elbow Surg* 2006;15:203-207.

67. Allain J, Goutallier D, Glorion C: Long-term results of the Bristow-Latarjet procedure for the treatment of anterior instability of the shoulder. *J Bone Joint Surg Am* 1998;80:841-852.

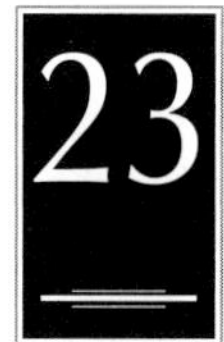

Massive Rotator Cuff Tears: Arthroscopy to Arthroplasty

Anshu Singh, MD
Andrew Jawa, MD
Monica Morman, MD
Benjamin Sanofsky, BA
Laurence Higgins, MD

Abstract

The understanding of rotator cuff disease has increased exponentially since Codman drew attention to this pathology in the early 1900s. Although challenging, the surgical treatment of massive rotator cuff tears is rational, with treatment decisions based on physical examination, imaging, biologic, and patient factors. Arthroscopy can be used to treat ancillary pain generators, débride necrotic tissue, and possibly restore balance to the force couples about the shoulder. Tendon transfers may be effective in restoring functional strength to irreparable, ineffectual muscle units. Arthroplasty is both a primary treatment and a salvage option.

Instr Course Lect 2010;59:255-267.

Since Codman[1] drew attention to rotator cuff disease in the early 1900s, the understanding of this pathology has increased exponentially. The surgical treatment of massive rotator cuff tears is challenging but rational and is based on physical examination, imaging, biologic, and patient factors. The three broad treatment categories for this disease include arthroscopy, tendon transfers, and arthroplasty. Arthroscopy can be used to manage ancillary pain generators, débride degenerative tissue, and possibly restore balance to the force couples about the shoulder. The functional strength of irreparable, ineffectual muscle units may be effectively restored with tendon transfers. Arthroplasty can be used as a primary treatment and a salvage option. This chapter will present findings from the current literature regarding the indications and outcomes for treating rotator cuff disease, with the goals of providing effective pain relief and restoring functional range of motion.

Arthroscopy

The evolution in the arthroscopic surgical treatment of rotator cuff disease has accelerated over the past 20 years, with a transition from open repair to mini open repair to complete arthroscopic repair.[2] In the early period of arthroscopic rotator cuff repair, techniques, implants, and instruments quickly evolved. As expected, initial failure rates were high. Massive rotator cuff tears, the most difficult to visualize and mobilize arthroscopically, were the last tears to be treated arthroscopically. As techniques improved, failure rates decreased; surgeons are now routinely treating complex tears with a fully arthroscopic approach.[3]

None of the following authors nor any immediate family members have received anything of value from or own stock in a commercial company or institution related directly or indirectly to the subject of this chapter: Dr. Singh, Dr. Jawa, Dr. Morman, and Mr. Sanofsky. Dr. Higgins or an immediate family member has received royalties from Zimmer; is a member of a speakers' bureau or has made paid presentations on behalf of DePuy; serves as a paid consultant to or is an employee of DePuy; and has received research or institutional support from Zimmer, DePuy, and DJ Orthopaedics.

Goals

Not all massive rotator cuff tears are irreparable, and all irreparable tears are not necessarily massive.[4] "Massive" describes the size of the tear, whereas "reparability" describes the sum of the multiple factors that determine the healing potential of a torn rotator cuff.[5] Such factors include patient age, activity level, chronicity of the tear, acromiohumeral distance, and fatty infiltration of the rotator cuff muscles.[6] Massive rotator cuff tears may be classified as posterosuperior (involving the supraspinatus and infraspinatus) or less commonly anterosuperior (involving the subscapularis and supraspinatus).

The accepted teaching for surgical repair has been to restore the native anatomy of the rotator cuff in a watertight fashion. Although the literature reports higher failure rates in large arthroscopically repaired tears, the statistics do not necessarily correlate with patient satisfaction.[3,7-10] Factors previously considered contraindicative to arthroscopic repair (such as arthroscopic rotator cuff repair in the presence of proximal humeral head migration, grade 3 fatty infiltration, and massive tear size) may now be treated arthroscopically with the patient's acceptance of limited goals.

In 1944, Inman and associates[11] described the coronal plane force couple of the deltoid opposing the inferior rotator cuff. The transverse plane force couple involves the infraspinatus and teres minor posteriorly balancing the subscapularis anteriorly.[12] Restoration of the coronal and transverse force couples forms the basis of partial repair, which reestablishes balance about the shoulder, allowing conversion of a massive rotator cuff tear to a more functional pathology.[13] For patients who want to remain active, partial repair is a potential alternative to early arthroplasty and avoids many of the complications of open procedures.

History and Examination

A comprehensive patient history should include the duration of symptoms, mechanism of injury, comorbidities, and information on the quality, quantity, and location of pain. A routine physical examination is performed to assess range of motion, rotator cuff strength, and concomitant pathology, such as biceps tenosynovitis, acromioclavicular disease, and osteoarthritis. With the elbow at the side (to evaluate infraspinatus function) and with the shoulder in 90° abduction (to assess the teres minor), the patient should be examined for the presence or absence of an external rotation lag sign. The subscapularis is assessed by the belly-press, bear-hug, and/or lift-off tests. Electromyography has shown that the bear-hug test is the most sensitive test for subscapularis tears involving the upper 30% of the tendon at 45° of forward flexion and is sensitive for inferior subscapularis dysfunction at 90° of forward flexion.[14]

Imaging

Imaging studies to assess the rotator cuff should include plain radiographs with a true AP view of the glenohumeral joint, axillary lateral view, and a transcapular outlet or Y view. These studies can be used to assess the congruency of the glenohumeral joint, proximal migration of the humeral head, arthritic changes in the glenohumeral joint, and other bony pathology about the shoulder. MRI and CT arthrograms may be used to further evaluate the rotator cuff, especially for fatty infiltration in the rotator cuff musculature, and assess the status of the glenohumeral articulation. Ultrasound is used in some centers to evaluate the presence or extent of a rotator cuff tear preoperatively or assess the postoperative integrity of a rotator cuff repair.[4]

Treatment

A variety of surgical treatments of massive, irreparable rotator cuff tears have been advocated in the orthopaedic literature. Although arthroscopic débridement has yielded variable outcomes, other more definitive treatments include transposition of intact portions of the rotator cuff musculature and formal tendon transfers.[15-18] Transfer of the pectoralis major has been used for isolated, irreparable subscapularis tendon tears but is not believed to be sufficiently effective in recentering the humeral head in the context of static anterosuperior subluxation.[8,18-20] Hemiarthroplasty may provide pain relief in patients with massive irreparable rotator cuff tears but probably will not improve function because of the absence of kinematic restoration. More recently, reverse total shoulder arthroplasty has become popular in the treatment of rotator cuff arthropathy, but it has narrow indications and a higher complication rate than that of conventional arthroplasty.

Partial repair of massive, irreparable rotator cuff tears may be performed arthroscopically to restore balance to force couples in the shoulder while avoiding the potential complications of open procedures and postponing the need for arthroplasty.[11] This repair usually mobilizes the posterior cuff anteriorly and fixates the posterior cuff to the greater tuberosity with suture anchors. Other advantages of arthroscopy compared with open procedures include decreased postoperative pain, decreased stiffness, and the ability to better visualize the specific tear pattern.

Subscapularis Tears

The largest rotator cuff muscle, the subscapularis, functions as both an internal rotator and key stabilizer of the glenohumeral joint, especially in the anteroinferior direction.[21] Using electromyographic analysis, Kelly and associates[22] showed a difference in the firing patterns of muscles about the shoulder in symptomatic and asymptomatic tears. In this study, all patients with cuff tears showed increased muscle firing with certain actions compared with their normal counterparts; those with asymptomatic tears showed increased function of the intact subscapularis, whereas symptomatic patients showed increased activity in the torn rotator cuff tendons and perimuscular substitution, which resulted in suboptimal function.

The less frequent subscapularis tendon tear usually occurs after trauma but is most often associated with a superior rotator cuff tear.[23,24] Given its essential function and the impossibility of spontaneous healing, conservative treatment is not recommended. Even if complete repair is not possible, partial repair can restore the balance of the transverse plane force couple.

Subscapularis tendon tears are often repaired through an open approach; however, some authors have reported residual weakness or stiffness caused by adhesions or by failure of the repair.[24,25] Lafosse and associates[23] reported the results of arthroscopic repair of 17 isolated subscapularis tears in a larger study of 342 arthroscopic rotator cuff tears. Biceps tenodesis was performed in 9 of 15 intact, long head, biceps tendons. At a mean follow-up of 29 months, the authors reported improvement in the Constant score from 58% to 96% and improvement in the University of California Los Angeles score from 16 points to 32 points. Improvements in subscapularis strength and function with a diminution in pain also were observed without postoperative stiffness. Postoperative CT arthrography confirmed an intact repair in 15 patients and partial rerupture (of the subscapularis/cuff) in 2 patients.

Secondary Pain Generators

In massive, irreparable rotator cuff tears, function is enhanced not only by restoring balanced force couples in the shoulder but also by treating other pain generators. Impingement-related pain is diminished by débridement of the unstable edges and partial tears. Chen and associates[25] showed that 93 of 122 (76%) of surgically treated complete cuff tears had obvious pathology of the biceps tendon ranging from tendinitis to complete rupture. All chronic rotator cuff tears (> 3 months duration) were associated with biceps pathology, and tears greater than 5 cm had a strong relationship with severe lesions of the long head biceps tendon (Figure 1). Boileau and associates[26] reported that in 72 shoulder patients treated with isolated biceps tenotomy or tenodesis for a massive irreparable rotator cuff tear, 78% of patients were subjectively satisfied with their treatment and had an average 20-point improvement in the Constant score at 35 months after surgery. Although biceps tenotomy or tenodesis does not restore muscle strength and balance, a significant improvement in pain often results in an overall improvement in function, range of motion, and activity level. Szabó and associates[27] recently confirmed the findings of Boileau and associates[26] and recommended biceps tenotomy or tenodesis as a valid palliative treatment.

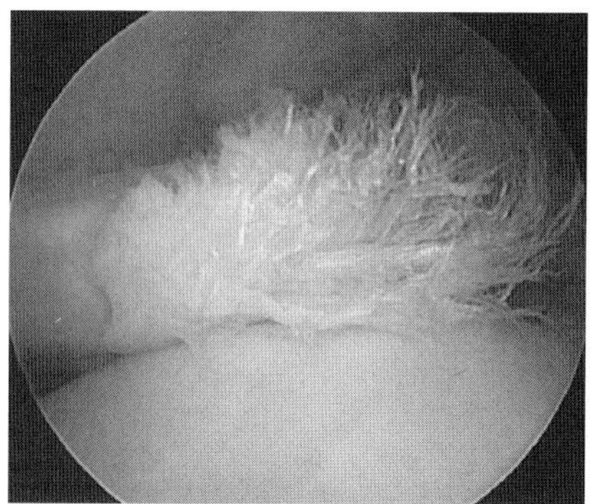

Figure 1 Arthroscopic view of biceps tenosynovitis leading to a frank tear.

Suprascapular nerve entrapment also has been reported as a source of chronic, diffuse, shoulder pain.[28-32] Compression has been described at the level of the suprascapular notch and the spinoglenoid notch.[33] The causes of suprascapular nerve entrapment include idiopathic neuritis, trauma, repetitive overuse, traction, and compression from an adjacent mass or ganglion cyst. The anatomy of the suprascapular notch is well defined and may contribute to nerve compression.[33] More recently, the association between massive rotator cuff tears and tethering of the suprascapular nerve has been described.[34] Based on follow-up electromyographic and nerve conduction velocity studies, Costouros and associates[30] showed reversal of suprascapular neuropathy in patients treated with either complete or partial repair of a massive rotator cuff tear. They also reported improvement in pain and function. There was no statistical difference between the groups treated with partial and complete rotator cuff repair.

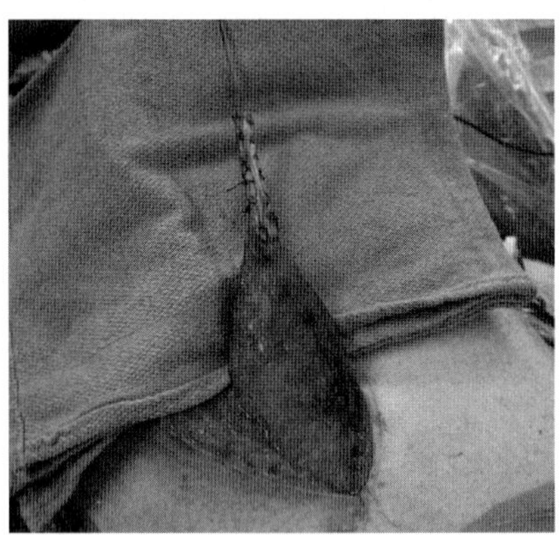

Figure 2 Photograph showing isolation of latissimus dorsi musculotendinous pedicle for transfer.

Clinical suspicion of suprascapular neuropathy may be confirmed with neurodiagnostic evaluation. Antoniou and associates[29] showed that compressive lesions at the level of the suprascapular notch had the greatest improvement with surgical decompression. Arthroscopic decompression offers better cosmesis, minimal trauma, better visualization, and the ability to concomitantly treat intra-articular pathology. Lafosse and Tomasi[31] showed clinical improvement in 14 of 15 patients with decompression at the level of the spinoglenoid notch and in 2 of 3 patients at the level of the suprascapular notch. In another study of 10 patients treated with suprascapular nerve release at the suprascapular notch through a posterior approach, Post and Mayer[28] reported four excellent and four good results; two patients had a decrease in symptoms.

Conclusion

Partial or complete arthroscopic repair of massive rotator cuff tendon tears facilitates evaluation and treatment of concomitant painful pathology, such as biceps tendinitis, impingement, and acromioclavicular disease. Decompression of the suprascapular nerve is helpful when indicated. This broad approach to complex pathology results in functional improvement, decreased pain, and reliable patient satisfaction.

Tendon Transfers

Patients with massive rotator cuff tears that cannot be repaired by conventional means may be candidates for tendon transfers. Many intrinsic and extrinsic tendon transfers have been described, including transfers of the subscapularis, triceps, and deltoid tendons.[35-38] However, latissimus dorsi and pectoralis major tendon transfers have gained favor among many surgeons for treating massive irreparable posterosuperior and anterosuperior tears, respectively.

Indications

The primary indication for a tendon transfer is a massive irreparable rotator cuff tear in a patient with pain and weakness.[17] The feasibility of repairing the rotator cuff can be determined by evaluating prior surgeries, the fatty infiltration on CT scans or MRI, and physical examination findings showing significant weakness in external rotation, lag signs, and atrophy.[18] Open or arthroscopic débridement may be appropriate for patients with pain and minimal loss of strength and function.[15]

Several factors are relevant for successful tendon transfers. Stiffness, arthritic changes, loss of the coracoacromial arch, nerve injury, and deltoid insufficiency are all contraindications to a tendon transfer. In latissimus dorsi transfers for treating posterosuperior tears, subscapularis dysfunction may be a relative contraindication to surgery because the humeral head will not remain centered on the glenoid.[39] Patients with multiple failed rotator cuff repairs have worse outcomes.

Other important factors to consider in preoperative planning are nicotine dependence and the ability of the patient to comply with a long and demanding course of postoperative rehabilitation and participation in physical therapy.

Latissimus Dorsi Transfers

Patients with disruption of the supraspinatus and infraspinatus tendons may lose abduction and external rotation strength. The latissimus dorsi transfer has gained favor for treating these patients because of the width of the tendon and the length of its excursion, as well as its length and the predictable location of the neurovascular pedicle (Figure 2). However, it is important to note that the direction of pull and function of the latissimus dorsi are not similar to those of the tendons it is replacing. Furthermore, the tendon crosses two articulations (scapulothoracic and glenohumeral), which decreases the effectiveness of the transfer.

It is critical to understand the limitations of the procedure; most patients will gain one grade of muscle power, which is not sufficient to overcome true pseudoparesis. The additional power provided by the latissimus dorsi transfer can be preoperatively estimated with the "one finger test," in which the patient's ability to flex the shoulder is evaluated by the examiner assisting with the index finger.

Many authors have reported favorable results with the procedure.[17,40,41] In a study of 14 patients, Gerber and associates,[17] who popularized the transfer in 1988, reported no complications. Four patients, with more than 1 year follow-up, had improved function. Aoki and associates[40] reported fair to excellent results in 9 of 12 patients after latissimus dorsi transfer and concluded that the procedure was effective in restoring function. Warner and Parsons[41] reported that 70% of patients with no prior surgeries had improved function, compared with 55% of patients with previous repairs. Additionally, 44% of patients in the salvage group had late ruptures compared with 17% in the primary group.

In 2006, Pearle and associates[42] performed an anatomic study that showed three important findings relevant to safe dissection and mobilization of a latissimus dorsi-teres major transfer: (1) The neurovascular pedicles for the latissimus dorsi and teres major are, on average, 13.1 cm and 7.4 cm medial to the respective humeral insertions. (2) The radial nerve runs 2.9 cm medial to the top of the latissimus and 2.3 cm medial to the bottom of the teres major insertion on the humerus. (3) The axillary nerve runs an average of 1.4 cm proximal to the superior edge of the teres major. These findings were confirmed by Morrelli and associates[43] in a 2008 study. They reported that the neurovascular pedicle insertion into the latissimus dorsi is 11.0 cm.

In a 2006 study, Gervasi and associates[44] described a technique of open latissimus dorsi harvest with arthroscopic reattachment through standard arthroscopic portals. Habermeyer and associates[45] also described a technique using one dorsal incision, moving the point of fixation further posteriorly and inferiorly. They reported an increase in the mean Constant score from 46.5 to 74.6 points and increased range of motion. Electromyographic analysis showed activity in the tendon transfers of all of the patients. The authors concluded that the results were comparable to those achieved with a two-incision technique. In 2009, a technique was described in which the latissimus dorsi tendon is harvested and secured with a bony fleck, providing secure bone-to-bone healing. (H Resch, MD, Las Vegas, NV, unpublished data presented at the American Academy of Orthopaedic Surgeons annual meeting, 2009.)

Several recent studies examined the factors that predict patient outcome. In 2006, Iannotti and associates[46] evaluated the anatomic and patient factors that affected the clinical result of latissimus dorsi transfers for posterosuperior tears. They reported that preoperative shoulder function and strength were predictive of postoperative function; synchronous in-phase contraction of the transfer was variable but associated with better results; and females may have worse clinical outcomes. Costouros and associates[47] used MRI studies to help predict outcomes after transfer and reported that fatty atrophy of the teres minor of Goutallier stage 2 or less was associated with better postoperative Constant scores and better active external rotation and active flexion. Interestingly, the presence of a teres minor tear did not have an effect on outcome.

In a 2008 study, Werner and associates[48] examined the correlation between psychomotor skills and latissimus dorsi tendon transfer outcomes. Patients with the 10 best and 10 worst results after transfer were tested with a battery of psychomotor tests and electromyographic assessment. Although there were no preoperative differences in other factors known to effect outcome, there was a significant difference in the activity pattern and innervation between the two groups. These tests may offer a method of preoperatively predicting success before tendon transfers.

With the use of electromyographic analysis, Irlenbusch and associates[49] showed that functional improvement after tendon transfer is not simply related to a tenodesis effect, as had been previously speculated, but is caused by active muscle contraction.

Pectoralis Major Transfers

Massive anterosuperior rotator cuff tears involving both the subscapularis and supraspinatus are less common than posterosuperior tears.[9] The subscapularis plays an important role in centering the humeral head in the joint and also functions as a powerful internal rotator. Unlike the treatment for posterosuperior tears, there are few available tendon transfer options for restoring subscapularis function. The trapezius has been suggested, but there are no data regarding its successful use.[15] Pectoralis major transfers have been used with success in treating subscapularis tears; however, because the line of pull is anterior to the center of rotation, it cannot function as a humeral head stabilizer. The force vector is improved if the transfer is performed in a retrocoracoid fashion.

Wirth and Rockwood[20] reported satisfactory results in regaining stability of the humeral head in 10 of 13 patients, all of whom had multiple previous surgeries and irreparable subscapularis tears. Using pectoralis major transfer to treat irreparable subscapularis tears, Jost and associates[50] reported satisfactory results in 25 of 30 patients with improvement in active forward flexion, abduction strength, range of motion, and Constant and subjective shoulder value scores. Importantly, they found pectoralis transfers to have less favorable results for patients with both subscapularis tears

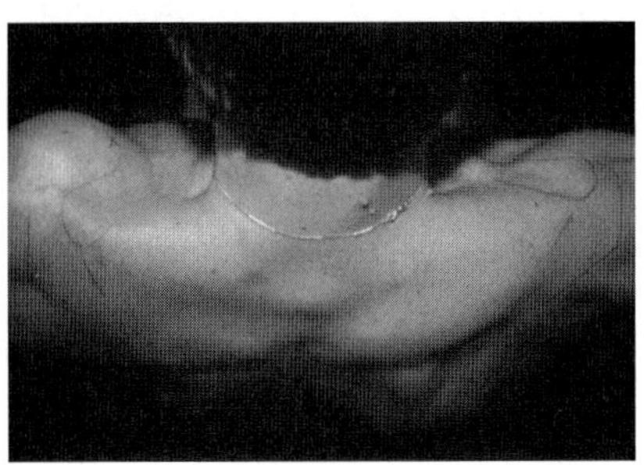

Figure 3 Photograph of the left shoulder of a patient with dynamic anterosuperior subluxation caused by incompetence of the coracoacromial arch. (Reproduced with permission from Gerber C: Massive rotator cuff repairs, in Ianotti JP, Williams GR Jr, eds: *Disorders of the Shoulder: Diagnosis and Management.* Philadelphia, PA, Lippincott Williams & Wilkins, 1999, pp 57-90.)

and associated irreparable supraspinatus tears.

The number of studies evaluating the effectiveness of pectoralis transfers is small in comparison with the interest in latissimus dorsi transfers. Nonetheless, two recent studies have provided greater insight into the technique and outcomes of pectoralis major transfers. In 2007, Konrad and associates[51] performed a biomechanical analysis evaluating pectoralis major transfers for treating irreparable subscapularis tears that were either routed superficially (the standard technique) or deep to the conjoined tendon, which potentially increased the stabilizing effect to the humeral head by decreasing the anterior force vector. Using six cadaver shoulders, the group found that routing the pectoralis major underneath the conjoined tendon partially restored the glenohumeral kinematics, probably because of its greater degree of alignment with subscapularis pull. It is unclear whether this finding will have clinical relevance.

In 2008, Elhassan and associates[52] compared the use of pectoralis major transfer in three groups of patients—group 1: those with irreparable subscapularis tears who had previous unsuccessful instability surgery; group 2: those with previous unsuccessful shoulder arthroplasty; and group 3: those with massive subscapularis tears. The mean Constant score improved for patients in groups 1 and 3 but did not improve for those in group 2. Failure of the pectoralis major transfer in all groups was correlated with preoperative anterior subluxation of the humeral head (Figure 3). Restoration of normal glenohumeral joint position was never restored after subluxation.

Discussion

Tendon transfers for massive irreparable posterosuperior and anterosuperior tears are a good treatment option in patients with both pain and significant weakness. Latissimus dorsi tendon transfer is supported by a strong, growing body of literature that has reported good outcomes. However, it is important to recognize that the failure of previous surgeries, significant fatty infiltration causing atrophy of the supraspinatus and infraspinatus muscles, profound weakness, and poor findings on psychomotor testing may preclude good outcomes. Pectoralis major transfers for subscapularis tears may improve function and stability but will likely fail in patients previously treated with arthroplasty or in those with preoperative humeral head subluxation. Routing the transfer under the conjoined tendon is biomechanically advantageous, but clinical outcome data are lacking.

Arthroplasty

Pathophysiology

Large, chronic tears of the rotator cuff decrease the depressive and compressive forces at the glenohumeral joint, producing several stepwise ramifications. The decrease in forces leads to a loss of concavity-compression, which is the key stabilizer in mid and upper ranges of abduction. Uncoupling of the superoinferior force couple allows unopposed action of the deltoid during active elevation of the arm. This deviant motion leads to increased shear forces on the glenoid and concomitant superior migration of the humeral head.

During the initial stages of rotator cuff tear arthropathy (RCTA), anterosuperior migration is an active phenomenon, placing excessive strain on secondary static stabilizers such as the coracoacromial arch, the glenoid labrum, the joint capsule, and the glenohumeral and coracohumeral ligaments. This migration manifests on plain radiographs as "acetabularization" of the acromion and "femoralization" of the humeral head. Eventually these secondary mechanisms fail, resulting in pseudoparesis of the shoulder, or painful anterosuperior escape of the humeral head with attempted elevation. The Hamada classification organizes this process, which ranges from a massive rotator cuff tear without arthritis to end-stage RCTA[53] (Figure 4).

Historic Implant Designs

RCTA represents the crossroads of rotator cuff disease (which in its incipient stages continues to be approached as a soft-tissue disease) and shoulder arthritis (which has traditionally been treated with joint arthroplasty procedures). By definition, RCTA is the final stage of irreparable rotator cuff tears. To treat RCTA, shoulder surgeons abandoned soft-tissue procedures and attempted to adapt conventional arthroplasty to treat the secondary arthrosis. Neer

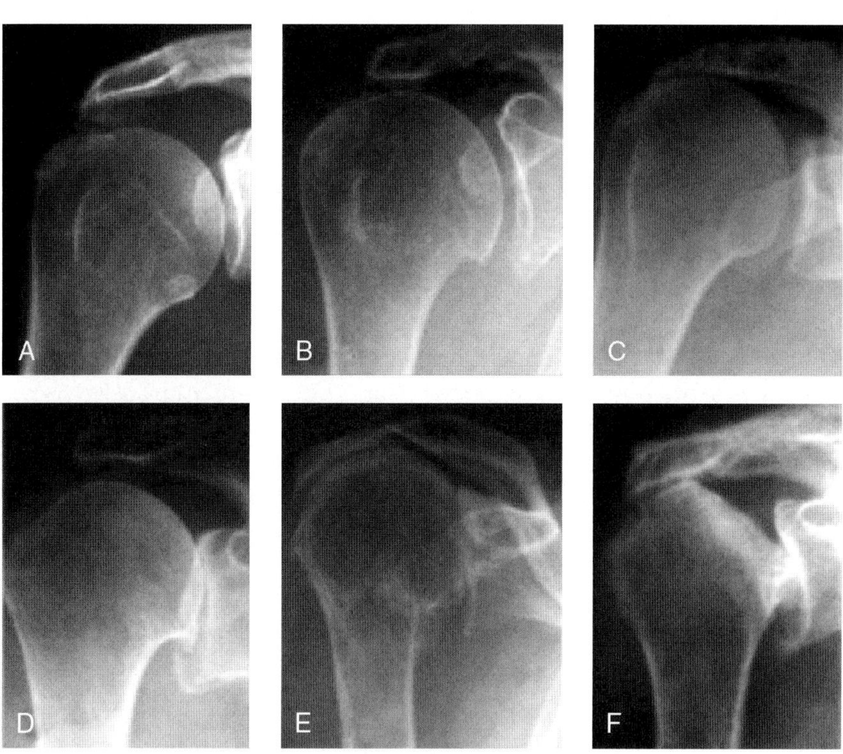

Figure 4 Radiographs of the stages of RCTA based on the Hamada classification system. **A,** Stage 1, well-balanced force couples. **B,** Stage 2, superior migration caused by loss of depressive forces of the inferior cuff. **C,** Stage 3, arthrosis in glenoacromial interval. **D,** Stage 4a, glenohumeral arthritis. **E,** Stage 4b, static superior subluxation. **F,** Stage 5, end-stage RCTA. (Reproduced with permission from Wall B, Nové-Josserand, O'Connor DP, Edwards TB, Walch G: Reverse total shoulder arthroplasty: A review of results according to etiology. *J Bone Joint Surg Am* 2007;89:1476-1485.)

and associates[54] proposed using a conventional total shoulder arthroplasty to treat RCTA; however, a subsequent investigation showed that the implant could not control the superoinferior migration of the center of rotation, which led to a "rocking horse" phenomenon on the face of the glenoid, with resultant early component loosening.[55]

A constrained total shoulder arthroplasty was one of the first designs and was intended to counteract the inherent instability of RCTA using an implant with a high degree of conformity and constraint. The center of rotation was a "fixed fulcrum," meaning that the humeral head could move within the glenoid component but could not disengage from it. This design, which led to unacceptably high rates of hardware failure, instability, and revision, is no longer used.[56]

Designs for total shoulder arthroplasty evolved to semiconstrained implants with hooded glenoid components to mechanically limit superior excursion of the humeral head only.[57] This design was more effective at centering the humeral head in the glenoid, but range of motion tended to be unsatisfactory. Semiconstrained implants also allowed the rocking horse phenomenon because the humeral head engaged with the hooded component, creating compressive forces on the top of the glenoid and tensile forces at the bottom.[58] Radiolucent lines became prevalent at the glenoid bone–implant interface, heralding ultimate implant failure.

Bipolar hip arthroplasty was designed for situations in which instability was a concern, and a bipolar shoulder hemiarthroplasty was designed for similar reasons.[59] Short-term follow-up of patients with RCTA treated with bipolar shoulder hemiarthroplasty showed good results based on Neer's limited goals (20° external rotation and 90° forward elevation) as an end point.[60,61] However, these prostheses overstuffed the glenohumeral joint, lateralized the center of rotation, created significant polyethylene debris, and caused superior medial wear of the glenoid. A recent fluoroscopic study showed that most of the motion occurs at the outer bone-implant interface.[62] Clinical studies have failed to show an advantage of bipolar shoulder hemiarthroplasty over traditional unipolar hemiarthroplasty.

Current Treatments

There are three types of arthroplasty for rotator cuff disease: unconstrained total shoulder arthroplasty, hemiarthroplasty, and reverse total shoulder arthroplasty. The choice of treatment requires consideration of the patient's physiologic age, physical demands, migration of the humeral head, and the condition of the rotator cuff itself. Patients with burdensome pain refractory to nonsurgical measures, such as activity modification, physical therapy, and oral anti-inflammatory medications, may be candidates for surgical treatment.

Unconstrained Total Shoulder Arthroplasty

The use of traditional unconstrained total shoulder arthroplasty is based

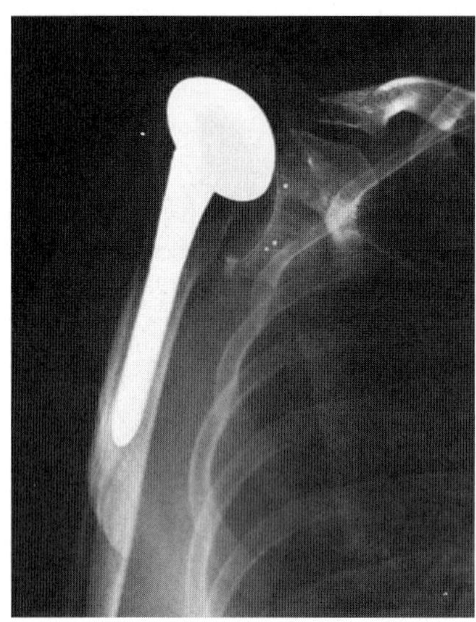

Figure 5 Radiograph of the shoulder of a patient with a rotator cuff and coracoacromial arch failure after conventional total shoulder arthroplasty.

on the condition of the rotator cuff and other factors. For patients with glenohumeral degenerative joint disease and isolated supraspinatus tendon dysfunction without proximal migration, traditional total shoulder arthroplasty is indicated. In a 2002 study, Edwards and associates[63] found that 8% of patients treated with total shoulder arthroplasty for primary osteoarthritis had concomitant rotator cuff pathology. Patients with tears of the supraspinatus, documented at the time of surgery, had identical performance statistics to those with an intact rotator cuff. Extension of the tear into the infraspinatus produced poorer results.

One caveat to treating patients with small cuff tears with unconstrained arthroplasty is that if tears progress to massive tears, such that the superoinferior force couple is lost, glenoid failure can be expected because of the rocking horse phenomenon. These small tears may indicate poor quality rotator cuff tissue, which is more likely to fail in a stepwise manner (Figure 5). Long-term follow-up of the outcomes of unconstrained total shoulder arthroplasty to treat patients with and without isolated supraspinatus tears have not been reported. Cemented stems have been shown to provide higher initial stability compared with press-fit humeral stems;[64] however, they lack the remodeling potential of press-fit stems in good bone stock. Therefore, cementation should be reserved for patients with osteopenic bone, which is commonly associated with fracture and RCTA.

Hemiarthroplasty

Hemiarthroplasty has historically been viewed as a salvage procedure for advanced RCTA and still has a role in treating younger patients (in whom the longevity of an inverse arthroplasty is a concern) and elderly patients with pain and forward flexion in excess of 90°. The competence of the coracoacromial arch is of paramount importance in all patients, regardless of age.

Recent studies show successful outcomes when judged by the limited goals criteria proposed by Neer.[61,65,66] In 2000, Zuckerman and associates[65] reported on 15 hemiarthroplasties performed in elderly patients with advanced RCTA. They found a significant decrease in pain, increased active flexion from 69° to 86°, and improved active external rotation from 15° to 29° at 28-month follow-up. Sanchez-Sotelo and associates[66] reviewed midterm (5-year) results of 33 shoulders treated at the Mayo Clinic with hemiarthroplasty for RCTA. They found similar improvements in pain and range of motion. The authors reported anterosuperior instability in seven shoulders that had previous subacromial decompressions, ostensibly caused by resection of the coracoacromial ligament.

It is important to inform patients treated with hemiarthroplasty that pain resolution may not be complete, range of motion will improve slightly, the ability to perform strenuous labor will be limited, and results may not be durable because of glenoid wear or instability. Conversion to a reverse arthroplasty is the salvage procedure for instability or continued pain and is facilitated by a prosthesis that is convertible to an inverse prosthesis without stem removal.

Reverse Total Shoulder Arthroplasty

For elderly patients with a massive irreparable rotator cuff tear, RCTA, pseudoparalysis, or fractures with rotator cuff incompetence, reverse total shoulder arthroplasty is indicated. A functioning deltoid muscle is vital to a satisfactory outcome. The reverse ball and socket geometry compensates for both the weakness and instability inherent in RCTA (Figure 6).

From a biomechanical standpoint, the reverse arthroplasty improves strength by increasing the lever arm of the deltoid, therefore increasing the amount of torque it generates for a given contractile force. The deltoid then can substitute for a weak or absent rotator cuff in abduction and elevation. The original Grammont Delta prosthesis (Medinov, Roanne, France) designed in 1985, as well as all subsequent designs, accomplished this by moving the center of rotation inferiorly and medially. The only exception to this design is the Encore reverse shoulder prosthesis (Encore Medical/Danjoy Orthopedics, Austin, TX), which moves the center of rotation inferiorly and laterally. Instability is countered by the semicon-

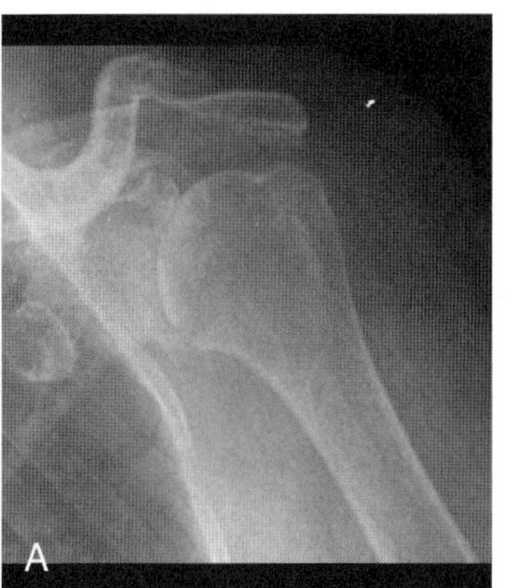

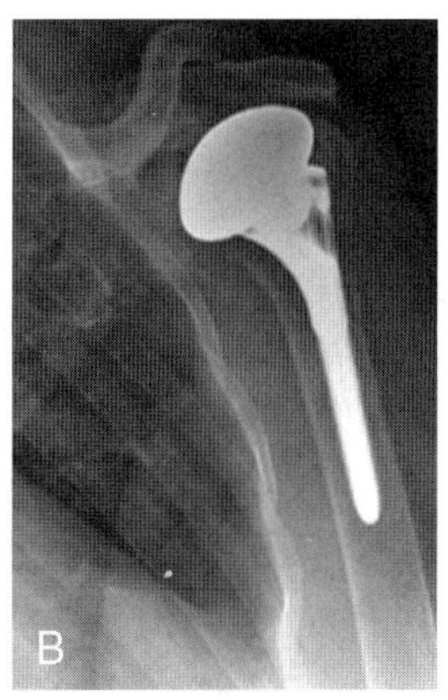

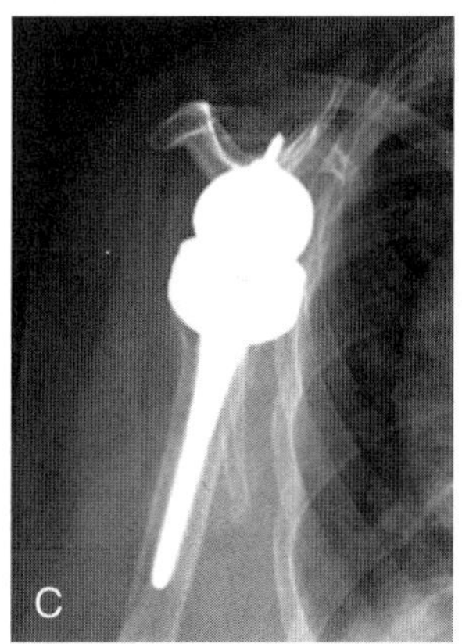

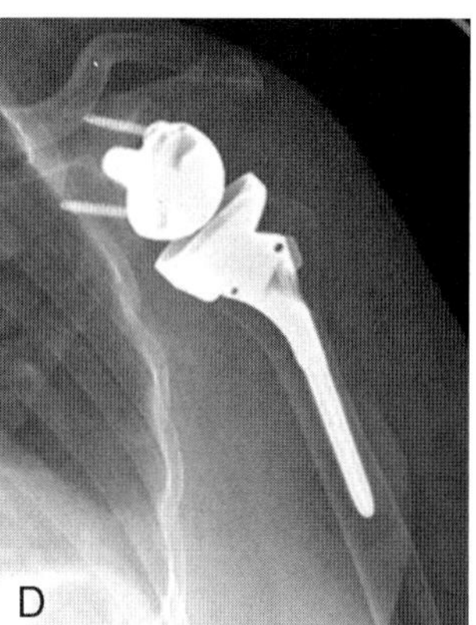

Figure 6 Preoperative **(A)** and postoperative **(B)** radiographs of the shoulder of a patient treated with reverse geometry shoulder arthroplasty, which increases stability and compensates for rotator cuff insufficiency. Scapular Y **(C)** and AP **(D)** postoperative radiographs after revision to an inverse prosthesis with well-placed components.

strained nature of the implant that prevents anterior and superior escape. This stability is accomplished by a large, stable glenosphere and the high degree of conformity of the implant compared with standard shoulder arthroplasty implants.

Early results of reverse arthroplasty were encouraging in terms of restoring elevation but not external rotation. Given that hemiarthroplasty was the traditional procedure of choice, Sirveaux and associates[67] conducted a multicenter study comparing age-matched control subjects treated with hemiarthroplasty and the Grammont Delta total shoulder prosthesis. They found that patients with classic RCTA treated with reverse arthroplasty had a significant improvement in Constant score (20 points), elevation (40°), and pain compared with those treated with hemiarthroplasty.

Both the traditional deltopectoral and deltoid-splitting superior approaches may be used for primary surgery. The choice is usually based on the surgeon's training and experience because no comparative studies of the approaches have been published. The superior approach does not violate the subscapularis and may be more stable, whereas the deltopectoral approach is more extensile and does not violate the deltoid, which powers the shoulder after reverse arthroplasty. Although the superior approach may have a lower rate of instability, inferior positioning of the glenoid component is difficult to achieve, possibly contributing to prosthetic impingement and notching.

In a 2005 study, Frankle and associates[68] reviewed the 2-year results of 60 patients with RCTA treated with reverse arthroplasty. These patients were generally older and more functionally limited than patients in prior studies who had been treated with hemiarthroplasty;[65,66] however, short-term results were better in terms of flexion (improved from 55 to 105.1) and pain on the visual analog scale (improved from 6.3 to 2.2) than those reported in earlier studies, and patients were generally satisfied with the procedure. Seven patients (12%) required revision to another arthroplasty at 2-year follow-up, which raises concern regarding the midterm and long-term durability of the technique.

Many early studies of reverse arthroplasty were affected by inclusion bias. Patients were not stratified by diagnoses or comorbidity, so it was difficult to draw conclusions regarding a specific indication. Currently, the best midterm data are from the database of a French multicenter study in which 672 shoulder arthroplasties for RCTA have been followed since 1991.[69] A 2007 study used etiologic factors to analyze the results of Grammont reverse arthroplasty in 240 patients.[53] Patients with rotator cuff pathology, including massive irreparable tears, RCTA, and osteoarthritis with cuff tears, performed well in terms of Constant scores and function in comparison with other indications. Revision surgery had a significantly higher rate of complications (37% compared with 13%) at a minimum 2-year follow-up.

Reverse shoulder arthroplasty provides pain relief and restores active elevation and abduction but fails to restore active external rotation. Often, this leads to frustration and poor functional outcome caused by the inability to position the hand in space despite adequate active eleva-

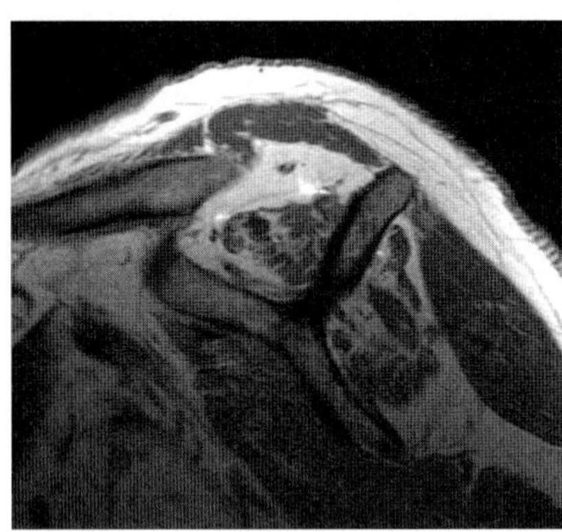

Figure 7 Sagittal MRI scan showing fatty degeneration of the supraspinatus, the infraspinatus, and the teres minor.

tion. In a 2007 study, Simovitch and associates[70] used MRI to show that preoperative fatty infiltration of the teres minor in patients treated with reverse arthroplasty for rotator cuff tears resulted in a loss of external rotation (7°) and modest improvement of the subjective shoulder score (25%) relative to their intact counterparts (Figure 7). It was postulated that posteroinferior rotator cuff function could not be adequately compensated by the deltoid alone.

Given the importance of the posteroinferior rotator cuff, it is critically important to clinically and radiographically evaluate its function before contemplating reverse arthroplasty. In patients with a positive hornblower sign or significant external rotation lag with the arm adducted (which is indicative of teres minor dysfunction), a concomitant latissimus dorsi transfer at the time of reverse arthroplasty is preferred. The use of latissimus dorsi transfer to restore active external rotation has been validated clinically and biomechanically.[39,48,71] Recently, a cadaver model showed that the transfer to the posterior aspect of the greater tuberosity produced the greatest external rotation moment arm.[72]

Complications from reverse arthroplasty are multiple, and there is a significant learning curve for surgeons. Reported revision rates are as high as 40%, and the complications rate is reported to be as high as 50% in procedures performed by experienced surgeons.[53] Complications include infection, glenoid notching, instability, dislocation, implant loosening, and acromial stress fractures. A 2006 review of 80 reverse shoulder arthroplasty prostheses in a multicenter trial provided some of the first midterm data.[73] Implant survivorship was more than 90%, and glenoid loosening was present in fewer than 15% of implants at 5 years. However, two interesting observations were reported. At 1 to 3 years, a break occurred in the survivorship curve, which represented early loosening of the prostheses that was believed to be caused by poor placement, rheumatoid arthritis, and infection. This break in the survivorship curve did not affect prostheses used to treat patients with RCTA. At 6 years, some patients had declines in their functional results. This decline did not occur in aged-matched control subjects, and there is no clear explanation for this observation. The decline in function has not been well studied and is of unknown significance.

Because of concerns about implant durability, reverse arthroplasty prosthesis implantation is not recommended in patients younger than 65 years. If this prothesis is used in younger patients, the surgeon should advise the patient of the high likelihood of revision surgery and should be capable of performing complicated revision surgery. Although the complication rate for revisions is high in terms of instability and infection, good functional results and pain control are possible. Reverse arthroplasty should be considered for the benefits it represents for patients with no acceptable alternative; however, these must be balanced with the disadvantages of its high complication rate and long learning curve.

Summary

Multiple surgical options are available to the surgeon when treating patients with a massive rotator cuff tear. Arthroscopy is the least invasive method and should be considered in patients who have achieved good pain relief and improved function with subacromial injection. Ancillary pain generators, such as the biceps tendon and suprascapular nerve, should be evaluated and treated to maximize results. Latissimus dorsi transfer restores one grade of functional strength to patients with irreparable tears without profound weakness. Pectoralis major transfer may restore the anteroposterior couple by substituting for an incompetent subscapularis. Hemiarthroplasty provides satisfactory results by Neer's limited goals criteria in patients with an intact coracoacromial arch. Reverse geometry shoulder arthroplasty is a salvage option for restoring active flexion and providing pain relief to elderly patients with pseudoparalysis. Reverse arthroplasty may be combined with latissimus dorsi transfer in shoulders with external rotation lag caused by teres minor deficiency. With proper treatment, most patients with massive rotator cuff tears can expect pain relief and functional range of motion.

References

1. Codman EA: *The Shoulder-Rupture of the Supraspinatus Tendon and Other Lesions in or About the Subacromial Bursa.* Malabar, Florida, Krieger Publishing Company, 1934.

2. Yamaguchi K. Levine WN, Marra G, Galatz LM, Klepps F, Flatow EL: Transitioning to arthroscopic rotator cuff repair: The pros and cons. *Instr Course Lect* 2003;52:81-92.

3. Burkhart SS: Arthroscopic treatment of massive rotator cuff tears: Clinical results and biomechanical rationale. *Clin Orthop Relat Res* 1991;267:45-56.

4. Elhassen B, Endres NK, Higgins W, Warner JJ: Massive irreparable tendon tears of the rotator cuff: Salvage options. *Instr Course Lect* 2008;57: 153-166.

5. Galatz LM, Silva MJ, Rothermich SY, Zaegel MA, Havlioglu N, Thomopoulos S: Nicotine delays tendon-to-bone healing in a rat shoulder model. *J Bone Joint Surg Am* 2006;88: 2027-2034.

6. Goutallier D, Postel JM, Bernageau J, Lavau L, Voisin MC: Fatty muscle degeneration in cuff ruptures: Pre- and postoperative evaluation by CT scan. *Clin Orthop Relat Res*1994;304:78-83.

7. Bishop J, Klepps S, Lo IK, Bird J, Gladstone JN, Flatow EL: Cuff integrity after arthroscopic versus open rotator cuff repair: A prospective study. *J Shoulder Elbow Surg* 2006;15: 290-299.

8. Galatz LM, Ball CM, Teefey SA, Middleton WD, Yamaguchi K: The outcome and repair integrity of completely arthroscopically repaired large and massive rotator cuff tears. *J Bone Joint Surg Am* 2004;86:219-224.

9. Harryman DT II, Mack LA, Wang KY, Jackins SE, Richardson ML, Matsen FA III: Repairs of the rotator cuff: Correlation of functional results with integrity of the cuff. *J Bone Joint Surg Am* 1991;73:982-989.

10. Calvert PT, Packer NP, Stoker DJ, Bayley JI, Kessel L: Arthrography of the shoulder after operative repair of the torn rotator cuff. *J Bone Joint Surg Br* 1986;68:147-150.

11. Inman VT, Saunders JB, Abbott LC: Observations on the function of the shoulder joint. *J Bone Joint Surg Am* 1944;26:1-30.

12. Burkhart SS: Reconciling the paradox of rotator cuff repair versus debridement: A unified biomechanical rationale for the treatment of rotator cuff tears. *Arthroscopy* 1994;10:4-19.

13. Burkhart SS, Nottage WM, Ogilvie-Harris DJ, Kohn HS, Pachelli A: Partial repair of irreparable rotator cuff tears. *Arthroscopy* 1994;10:363-370.

14. Barth JR, Burkhart SS, De Beer JF: The bear-hug test: A new and sensitive test for diagnosing a subscapularis tear. *Arthroscopy* 2006;22:1076-1084.

15. Rockwood CA Jr, Williams GR Jr, Burkhead WZ Jr: Débridement of degenerative, irreparable lesions of the rotator cuff. *J Bone Joint Surg Am* 1995; 77:857-866.

16. Gartsman GM: Massive, irreparable tears of the rotator cuff: Results of operative debridement and subacromial decompression. *J Bone Joint Surg Am* 1997;79:715-721.

17. Gerber C, Vinh TS, Hertel R, Hess CW: Latissimus dorsi transfer for the treatment of massive tears of the rotator cuff: A preliminary report. *Clin Orthop Relat Res* 1988;232:51-61.

18. Warner JJ: Management of massive irreparable rotator cuff tears: The role of tendon transfer. *Instr Course Lect* 2001;50:63-71.

19. Kreuz PC, Remiger A, Erggelet C, Hinterwimmer S, Niemeyer P, Gächter A: Isolated and combined tears of the subscapularis tendon. *Am J Sports Med* 2005;33:1831-1837.

20. Wirth MA, Rockwood CA Jr: Operative treatment of irreparable rupture of the subscapularis. *J Bone Joint Surg Am* 1997;79:722-731.

21. Burkhart SS, Ochoa E Jr: Subscapularis tendon tears: Diagnosis and treatment strategies. *Curr Orthop Pract* 2008;19:542-547.

22. Kelly BT, Williams RJ, Cordasco FA, et al: Differential patterns of muscle activation in patients with symptomatic and asymptomatic rotator cuff tears. *J Shoulder Elbow Surg* 2005;14: 165-171.

23. Lafosse L, Jost B, Reiland Y, Audebert S, Toussaint B, Gobezie R: Structural integrity and clinical outcomes after arthroscopic repair of isolated subscapularis tears. *J Bone Joint Surg Am* 2007;89:1184-1193.

24. Scheibel M, Nikulka C, Dick A, Schroeder RJ, Popp AG, Haas NP: Structural integrity and clinical function of the subscapularis musculotendinous unit after arthroscopic and open shoulder stabilization. *Am J Sports Med* 2007;35:1153-1161.

25. Chen CH, Hsu KY, Chen WJ, Shih CH: Incidence and severity of biceps long head tendon lesion in patients with complete rotator cuff tears. *J Trauma* 2005;58:1189-1193.

26. Boileau P, Baqué F, Valerio L, Ahrens P, Chuinard C, Trojani C: Isolated arthroscopic biceps tenotomy or tenodesis improves symptoms in patients with massive irreparable rotator cuff tears. *J Bone Joint Surg Am* 2007; 89:747-757.

27. Szabó I, Boileau P, Walch G: The proximal biceps as a pain generator and results of tenotomy. *Sports Med Arthrosc* 2008;16:180-186.

28. Post M, Mayer J: Suprascapular nerve entrapment: Diagnosis and treatment. *Clin Orthop Relat Res* 1987;223: 126-136.

29. Antoniou J, Tae SK, Williams GR, Bird S, Ramsey ML, Iannotti JP: Suprascapular neuropathy: Variability in diagnosis, treatment, and outcome. *Clin Orthop Relat Res* 2001;386: 131-138.

30. Costouros JG, Porramatikul M, Lie DT, Warner JJ: Reversal of suprascapular neuropathy following arthroscopic repair of massive supraspinatus and infraspinatus rotator cuff tears. *Arthroscopy* 2007;23:1152-1161.

31. Lafosse L, Tomasi A: Technique for endoscopic release of suprascapular nerve entrapment at the suprascapular notch. *Tech Shoulder Elbow Surg* 2006;7:1-6.

32. Millett PJ, Barton RS, Pacheco IH, Gobezie R: Suprascapular nerve entrapment: Technique for arthroscopic release. *Tech Shoulder Elbow Surg* 2006;7:89-94.

33. Albritton MJ, Graham RD, Richards RS II, Basamania CJ: An anatomic study of the effects on the suprascapular nerve due to retraction of the supraspinatus muscle after rotator cuff tear. *J Shoulder Elbow Surg* 2003; 12:497-500.

34. Mallon WJ, Wilson RJ, Basamania CJ: The association of suprascapular neuropathy with massive rotator cuff tears: A preliminary report. *J Shoulder Elbow Surg* 2006;15:395-398.

35. Karas SE, Giachello TL: Subscapularis transfer for reconstruction of massive tears of the rotator cuff. *J Bone Joint Surg Am* 1996;78:239-245.

36. Malkani AL, Sundine MJ, Tillett ED, Baker DL, Rogers RA, Morton TA: Transfer of the long head of the triceps tendon for irreparable rotator cuff tears. *Clin Orthop Relat Res* 2004; 428:228-236.

37. Sundine MJ, Malkani AL: The use of the long head of triceps interposition muscle flap for treatment of massive rotator cuff tears. *Plast Reconstr Surg* 2002;110:1266-1274.

38. Apoil A, Augereau B: Deltoid flap repair of large losses of substance of the shoulder rotator cuff. *Chirurgie* 1985; 111:287-290.

39. Gerber C, Maquieira G, Espinosa N: Latissimus dorsi transfer for the treatment of irreparable rotator cuff tears. *J Bone Joint Surg Am* 2006;88:113-120.

40. Aoki M, Okamura K, Fukushima S, Takahashi T, Ogino T: Transfer of latissimus dorsi for irreparable rotator-cuff tears. *J Bone Joint Surg Br* 1996;78:761-766.

41. Warner JJ, Parsons IM IV: Latissimus dorsi tendon transfer: A comparative analysis of primary and salvage reconstruction of massive, irreparable rotator cuff tears. *J Shoulder Elbow Surg* 2001;10:514-521.

42. Pearle AD, Kelly BT, Voos JE, Chehab EL, Warren RF: Surgical technique and anatomic study of latissimus dorsi and teres major transfers. *J Bone Joint Surg Am* 2006;88:1524-1531.

43. Morelli M, Nagamori J, Gilbart M, Miniaci A: Latissimus dorsi tendon transfer for massive irreparable cuff tears: An anatomic study. *J Shoulder Elbow Surg* 2008;17:139-143.

44. Gervasi E, Causero A, Parodi PC, Raimondo D, Tancredi G: Arthroscopic latissimus dorsi transfer. *Arthroscopy* 2007;23:1243.e1-4.

45. Habermeyer P, Magosch P, Rudolph T, Lichtenberg S, Liem D: Transfer of the tendon of latissimus dorsi for the treatment of massive tears of the rotator cuff: A new single-incision technique. *J Bone Joint Surg Br* 2006;88:208-212.

46. Iannotti JP, Hennigan S, Herzog R, et al: Latissimus dorsi tendon transfer for irreparable posterosuperior rotator cuff tears: Factors affecting outcome. *J Bone Joint Surg Am* 2006;88: 342-348.

47. Costouros JG, Espinosa N, Schmid MR, Gerber C: Teres minor integrity predicts outcome of latissimus dorsi tendon transfer for irreparable rotator cuff tears. *J Shoulder Elbow Surg* 2007;16:727-734.

48. Werner CM, Ruckstuhl T, Müller R, Zanetti M, Gerber C: Influence of psychomotor skills and innervation patterns on results of latissimus dorsi tendon transfer for irreparable rotator cuff tears. *J Shoulder Elbow Surg* 2008; 17:22S-28S.

49. Irlenbusch U, Bernsdorf M, Born S, Gansen HK, Lorenz U: Electromyographic analysis of muscle function after latissimus dorsi tendon transfer. *J Shoulder Elbow Surg* 2008;17: 492-499.

50. Jost B, Puskas GJ, Lustenberger A, Gerber C: Outcome of pectoralis major transfer for the treatment of irreparable subscapularis tears. *J Bone Joint Surg Am* 2003;85:1944-1951.

51. Konrad GG, Sudkamp NP, Kreuz PC, Jolly JT, McMahon PJ, Debski RE: Pectoralis major tendon transfers above or underneath the conjoint tendon in subscapularis-deficient shoulders: An in vitro biomechanical analysis. *J Bone Joint Surg Am* 2007;89: 2477-2484.

52. Elhassan B, Ozbaydar M, Massimini D, Diller D, Higgins L, Warner JJ: Transfer of pectoralis major for the treatment of irreparable tears of subscapularis: Does it work? *J Bone Joint Surg Br* 2008;90:1059-1065.

53. Wall B, Nové-Josserand L, O'Connor T, Edwards TB, Walch G: Reverse total shoulder arthroplasty: A review of results according to etiology. *J Bone Joint Surg Am* 2007;89: 1476-1485.

54. Neer CS III, Craig EV, Fukuda H: Cuff-tear arthropathy. *J Bone Joint Surg Am* 1983;65:1232-1244.

55. Franklin JL, Barrett WP, Jackins SE, Matsen FA III: Glenoid loosening in total shoulder arthroplasty: Association with rotator cuff deficiency. *J Arthroplasty* 1988;3:39-46.

56. Post M, Jablon M: Constrained total shoulder arthroplasty: Long-term follow-up observations. *Clin Orthop Relat Res* 1983;173:109-116.

57. Amstutz HC, Thomas BJ, Kabo JM, Jinnah RH, Dorey FJ: The Dana total shoulder arthroplasty. *J Bone Joint Surg Am* 1988;70:1174-1182.

58. Orr TE, Carter DR, Schurman DJ: Stress analyses of glenoid component designs. *Clin Orthop Relat Res* 1988; 232:217-224.

59. Swanson AB, de Groot Swanson G, Sattel AB, Cendo RD, Hynes D, Jar-Ning W: Bipolar implant shoulder arthroplasty: Long-term results. *Clin Orthop Relat Res* 1989;249:227-247.

60. Worland RL, Jessup DE, Arredando J, Warburton KJ: Bipolar shoulder arthroplasty for rotator cuff arthropathy. *J Shoulder Elbow Surg* 1997;6: 512-515.

61. Neer CS II, Watson KC, Stanton FJ: Recent experience in total shoulder replacement. *J Bone Joint Surg Am* 1982;64:319-337.

62. Stavrou P, Slavotinek J, Krishnan J: A radiographic evaluation of birotational head motion in the bipolar

shoulder hemiarthroplasty. *J Shoulder Elbow Surg* 2006;15:399-401.

63. Edwards TB, Boulahia A, Kempf JF, Boileau P, Nemoz C, Walch G: The influence of rotator cuff disease on the results of shoulder arthroplasty for primary osteoarthritis: Results of a multicenter study. *J Bone Joint Surg Am* 2002;84:2240-2248.

64. Ooms EM, Verdonschot N, Wolke JG, et al: Enhancement of initial stability of press-fit femoral stems using injectable calcium phosphate cement: An in vitro study in dog bones. *Biomaterials* 2004;25:3887-3894.

65. Zuckerman JD, Scott AJ, Gallagher MA: Hemiarthroplasty for cuff tear arthropathy. *J Shoulder Elbow Surg* 2000;9:169-172.

66. Sanchez-Sotelo J, Cofield RH, Rowland CM: Shoulder hemiarthroplasty for glenohumeral arthritis associated with severe rotator cuff deficiency. *J Bone Joint Surg Am* 2001;83:1814-1822.

67. Sirveaux F, Favard L, Oudet D, Huquet D, Walch G, Molé D: Grammont inverted total shoulder arthroplasty in the treatment of glenohumeral osteoarthritis with massive rupture of the cuff: Results of a multicentre study of 80 shoulders. *J Bone Joint Surg Br* 2004;86:388-395.

68. Frankle M, Siegal S, Pupello D, Saleem A, Mighell M, Vasey M: The Reverse Shoulder Prosthesis for glenohumeral arthritis associated with severe rotator cuff deficiency: A minimum two-year follow-up of sixty patients. *J Bone Joint Surg Am* 2005;87:1697-1705.

69. Middernacht B, De Wilde L, Molé D, Favard L, Debeer P. Glenosphere disengagement: A potentially serious default in reverse shoulder surgery. *Clin Orthop Relat Res* 2008;466:892-898.

70. Simovitch RW, Helmy N, Zumstein MA, Gerber C: Impact of fatty infiltration of the teres minor muscle on the outcome of reverse total shoulder arthroplasty. *J Bone Joint Surg Am* 2007;89:934-939.

71. Gerber C, Pennington SD, Lingenfelter EJ, Sukthankar A: Reverse Delta-III total shoulder replacement combined with latissimus dorsi transfer: A preliminary report. *J Bone Joint Surg Am* 2007;89:940-947.

72. Favre P, Loeb MD, Helmy N, Gerber C: Latissimus dorsi transfer to restore external rotation with reverse shoulder arthroplasty: A biomechanical study. *J Shoulder Elbow Surg* 2008;17:650-658.

73. Guery J, Favard L, Sirveaux F, Oudet D, Mole D, Walch G: Reverse total shoulder arthroplasty: Survivorship analysis of eighty replacements followed five to ten years. *J Bone Joint Surg Am* 2006;88:1742-1747.

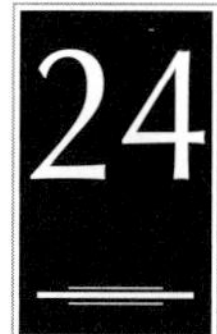

Principles of Arthroscopic Repair of Large and Massive Rotator Cuff Tears

Peter B. MacDonald, MD, FRCS
Sahal Altamimi, MD, FRCSC

Abstract

Minimally invasive arthroscopic techniques for rotator cuff tears have been greatly advanced during the past decade. It is important to review the clinical presentation and common physical findings of a large or massive rotator cuff tear, essential preoperative imaging, and the principles and technical aspects of all-arthroscopic repair. An anatomic repair of the footprint must begin with an understanding of the three-dimensional morphology of the rotator cuff tear and an accurate reduction of the tear. A contracted, immobile massive rotator cuff tear is challenging. Advanced arthroscopic mobilization techniques and margin convergence principles may allow repair of an otherwise irreparable tear. Failure of tendon healing is common but can be minimized by using dual-row, transosseous-equivalent techniques. A relatively slow rehabilitation program is paramount to protect the repair. The result of using arthroscopic techniques for a large or massive rotator cuff tear is comparable to that of a traditional open repair. Pain relief has been a far more reliable result than gains in function or strength.

Instr Course Lect 2010;59:269-280.

The effect of the force couple between the rotator cuff and the deltoid muscle has been investigated in several studies.[1-3] Inman and associates[4] initially described the concept of force couple in the coronal plane, which consists of the superiorly directed force vector of the deltoid muscle balanced against the inferiorly directed force couple of the inferior aspect of the rotator cuff (the subscapularis, infraspinatus, and teres minor) and the weight of the arm. Burkhart[5] emphasized the importance of the transverse plane force couple, in which the anterior rotator cuff (the subscapularis) is balanced against the posterior cuff (the infraspinatus and teres minor). The inferiorly directed force serves as a stable fulcrum for the force of the deltoid in the coronal plane. If a posterior massive rotator cuff tear is present, the force couple is imbalanced, an unstable fulcrum is created by the unopposed pull of the subscapularis anteriorly and the deltoid muscle superiorly, and anterosuperior escape of the humeral head results.

Preoperative Clinical Assessment

A detailed history and thorough physical examination of the upper extremity and cervical spine often provide sufficient information for establishing a diagnosis and estimating the size of the rotator cuff tear. Useful information about symptoms often can be obtained by asking the patient to fill out a standardized history form during the first clinical assessment. A gradual onset of pain is typical of a rotator cuff tear, and the dominant extremity is most commonly affected. The pain characteristically interferes with sleep and intensifies with overhead activity. Pain usually is localized at the anterolateral aspect of the shoulder and radiates to the midarm along

Dr. MacDonald or an immediate family member is a member of a speakers' bureau or has made paid presentations on behalf of Linvatec; serves as an unpaid consultant to Linvatec; and has received research or institutional support from Linvatec and Biosysntech. Neither Dr. Altamimi nor an immediate family member has received anything of value from or owns stock in a commercial company or institution related directly or indirectly to the subject of this chapter.

the deltoid muscle. Gerber and associates[6] found that pain radiated into the deltoid region when normal saline was injected into the subacromial space. Pain and numbness distal to the elbow usually are related to the cervical spine rather than rotator cuff pathology.

Most patients report insidious shoulder pain with no history of trauma. Younger patients with a massive rotator cuff tear are likely to have a history of traumatic insult. Occasionally, patients have painless shoulder weakness. A gradual onset of weakness suggests a chronic tear, and an acute onset after years of shoulder pain suggests an acute-on-chronic tear.

A shoulder lesion is common with a rotator cuff tear. A biceps tendon rupture or instability may accompany rotator cuff tear; a history of a "pop" may suggest a rupture of the long head of the biceps tendon. Acromioclavicular arthritis is a common source of shoulder pain centered at the superior aspect of the shoulder.

Physical Examination

The examiner should be able to estimate the size of the tear based on the clinical assessment. The shoulder evaluation should include a careful examination of the cervical spine and a thorough neurologic assessment. Visually scanning the shoulders and scapulae is important. Supraspinatus and infraspinatus muscle atrophy and rupture of the long head of the biceps tendon are common in massive rotator cuff tears. The supraspinatus and infraspinatus are best viewed from behind and from the side. The supraspinatus is covered by the trapezius; infraspinatus atrophy therefore is easier to detect.

Palpation can elicit tenderness at the rotator cuff insertion site on the greater tuberosity, and palpation of the adjacent biceps groove can suggest biceps pathology. Subacromial crepitus can be detected by palpation with the arm actively or passively rotated. The acromioclavicular joint is palpated for tenderness and compared with palpation of the opposite side with equivalent pressure.

After palpation, active and passive internal rotation, external rotation, and overhead forward elevation and abduction are observed. Active range of motion is measured with the patient sitting or standing. Observing range of motion from the patient's back can provide an estimation of scapulothoracic rhythm. Inferior capsular tightness can cause premature abduction of the scapula. A patient with complete rupture of the subscapularis has excessive passive external rotation. The patient's symptoms can be elicited with impingement. Neer[7] first described the painful arc in rotator cuff pathology. The test finding is positive if the patient has pain with abduction of the arm between 70° and 120°. A painful arc in more than 120° of abduction may indicate acromioclavicular joint pathology.[8] A positive Hawkins sign occurs when the patient has pain with passive internal rotation and forward elevation of 90°.[9]

Rotator cuff strength is assessed with resisted maneuvers. Supraspinatus muscle strength is tested with the arm in internal rotation and at 90° of elevation in the scapular plane. If supraspinatus strength is almost normal during this Jobe or empty can test, the tear may be relatively small.[10] The optimal position for testing the strength of the infraspinatus muscle is resisted external rotation with the arm at the side and the elbow flexed at 90°. Profound weakness of external rotation is characteristic of a large or massive rotator cuff tear. Gerber and Krushell[11] described the lift-off and belly-press signs for assessment of subscapularis muscle strength.

The drop arm, external rotation lag, and hornblower signs are characteristic of a massive rotator cuff tear. Codman[12] defined the drop arm sign as an inability to hold the arm above the shoulder against gravity. The external rotation lag sign, as described by Hertel and associates,[13] is used to determine the integrity of the supraspinatus and the infraspinatus. In a positive test, the patient cannot maintain an external rotation position or falls into a position of internal rotation with the arm examined at the side. Walch and associates,[14] who first described the hornblower sign, found a sensitivity of 100% and a specificity of 93% for the presence of Goutallier stage III or IV fatty degeneration of the teres minor. In a positive test, the patient cannot hold the arm in the externally rotated position when the arm is placed at 90° of abduction in the scapular plane with the elbow flexed at 90°. Combinations of these tests can provide information as to the number of involved tendons and the size of the rotator cuff tear. Surgical repair should be considered after unsuccessful nonsurgical treatment using physical therapy, nonsteroidal anti-inflammatory drugs, and steroid injections.

Imaging

Conventional radiography is an important part of the preoperative evaluation of rotator cuff pathology. The AP view allows assessment of the position of the humeral head relative to the glenoid and acromion, arthritis of the glenohumeral joint, cystic changes of the greater tuberosity, sclerosis of the undersurface of the acromion, and the acromio-

Table 1
The Goutallier Staging System for Fatty Degeneration of the Rotator Cuff Muscles

Stage	Description
0	Normal muscle
1	Some fatty streaks
2	Fat < muscle
3	Fat = muscle
4	Fat > muscle

Data from Goutallier D, Postel JM, BernageauJ, Lavau L, Voisin MC: Fatty muscle degeneration in cuff ruptures: Pre- and postoperative evaluation by CT scan. *Clin Orthop Relat Res* 1994;304: 78-83.

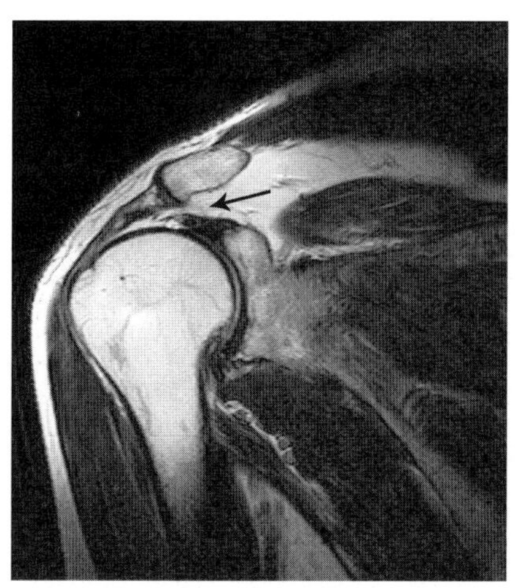

Figure 1 Coronal MRI scan showing a large rotator cuff tear (*arrow*).

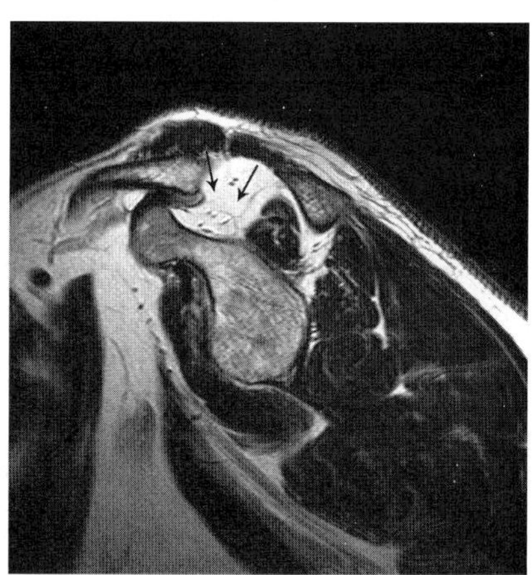

Figure 2 Sagittal MRI scan showing a large rotator cuff tear *(arrows)* with fatty atrophy of the supraspinatus.

humeral distance. Arthrosis of the acromioclavicular joint can be seen on an AP view; however, this joint has a variable orientation, and visualization is enhanced by a 15° cephalic tilt of the x-ray beam.[15] A narrowing of the subacromial space of less than 7 mm is consistent with a large rotator cuff tear[16] (Figure 1). Anterosuperior escape of the humeral head and evidence of rotator cuff tear arthropathy can be seen in patients with massive rotator cuff tears. The supraspinatus outlet view is used to outline the acromion morphology and may reveal evidence of acromial spurs. The axillary view provides excellent visualization of the glenoid and humeral head; it also can be used to rule out the presence of os acromiale, which often is associated with rotator cuff tears.[17,18]

Conventional radiographs show the osseous structure of the shoulder girdle but little soft-tissue anatomy, such as that of the rotator cuff or biceps tendon. MRI is the modality of choice for evaluating rotator cuff pathology, followed by ultrasonography. Soft-tissue structures, including the tendons and muscles of the rotator cuff and the long head of the biceps tendon, can be well displayed using MRI or ultrasonography. A full-thickness rotator cuff tear always creates a communication between the joint cavity and the subacromial space. Fatty replacement and a substantial loss in mass can be seen with a long-standing muscle tear. Balich and associates[19] reported MRI sensitivity of 84% to 96%, specificity of 94% to 98%, and accuracy of 92% to 97% for complete rotator cuff tears. MRI provides important information about tear size, location, chronicity, degree of medial retraction, extent of fatty infiltration, and quality of remaining tissue. Compared with conventional spin-echo technique, fat-saturation techniques can improve the detection of both complete and partial tears.[20,21] The coronal oblique, sagittal oblique, and axial planes are standard for an MRI protocol. The typical slice is 3 to 4 mm thick. Coronal oblique images are most useful for detecting a supraspinatus tear, medial tendon retraction, or acromioclavicular joint abnormality. T2-weighted sagittal oblique images are used to identify the anteroposterior extent of the rotator cuff tear. Subscapularis and infraspinatus tendon tears are evaluated on both axial and sagittal images. Biceps tendon pathology is best seen on axial images. Goutallier[22] first described the extent of fatty infiltration seen on CT scans (Table 1). Fatty infiltration can be easily detected on axial or sagittal T1-weighted MRI studies (Figure 2).

Ultrasonography of the shoulder has recently increased in popularity, and technical advances continue to improve its usefulness as a diagnostic tool for rotator cuff pathology. The advantage of ultrasonography is its ability to examine the shoulder both statically and dynamically. Ultrasonography does not have the contraindications of MRI, and it is relatively inexpensive, well tolerated by the patient, and less time consuming than MRI. On the other hand, the accuracy of ultrasonography is operator dependent, and there is a long learning curve. Information about fatty infiltration of the muscle and articular cartilage defect is imprecise.[23] Ultrasonography has had conflicting results in detecting partial thickness tears.[24,25] In the absence of well-defined local expertise, ultrasonography has not been

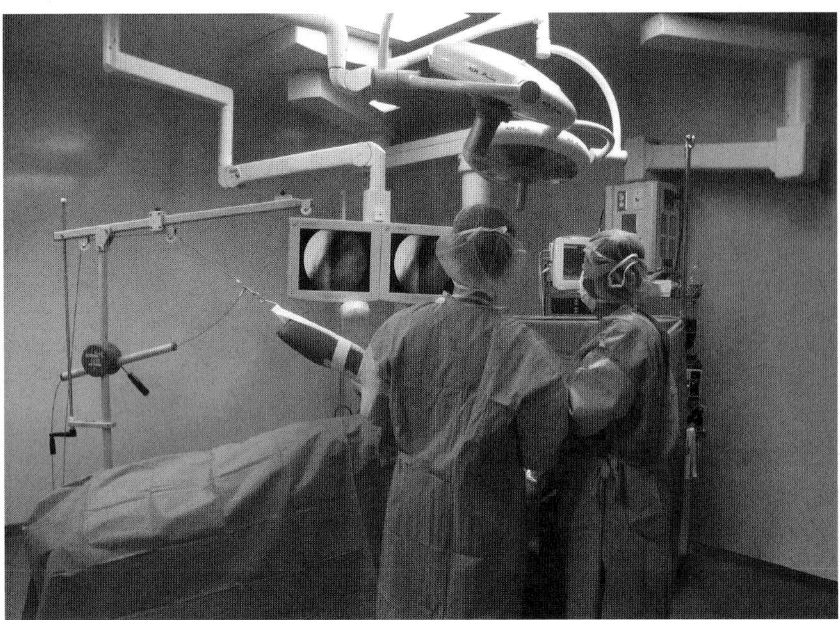

Figure 3 Photograph showing the operating room setup for arthroscopic repair of a rotator cuff tear. The patient is placed in the lateral decubitus position with the arm attached to a shoulder traction system.

Table 2
Surgical Steps in an All-Arthroscopic Rotator Cuff Repair

1. Establish accurate portals.
2. Perform diagnostic arthroscopy.
3. Examine the biceps tendon and decide whether tenodesis or tenotomy is required.
4. Define the tear pattern and prepare the tendons.
5. Perform a bursectomy and decide whether acromioplasty is needed.
6. Mobilize the rotator cuff tendons.
7. Prepare the footprint on the greater tuberosity.
8. Place a margin convergence suture for an L- or U-shaped tear.
9. Insert the anchors percutaneously and test their seating.
10. Pass the sutures and retrieve their limbs.
11. Determine the post limb, and tie a secure knot.
12. Assess the integrity of the repair.

universally accepted by radiologists and orthopaedic surgeons for the preoperative evaluation of rotator cuff tears.

The Arthroscopic Repair Procedure

The use of a stepwise approach to learning rotator cuff repair is suggested, beginning with repair of a small tear using a miniopen deltoid split to perfect the art of subacromial decompression and treat intra-articular pathology, such as a partial biceps tear or a superior labrum anterior and posterior tear. Complete arthroscopic repair of a small tear then can be mastered. The transition to the repair of large and massive tears should be accomplished by perfecting rotator cuff tear mobilization techniques and margin convergence. The most difficult tears require an interval slide, which is the most advanced and time-consuming skill. It must be remembered that surgical repair time exceeding 120 minutes with traction is undesirable because of the complications of swelling and fluid extravasation.

The Surgical Setup

A standard 4.5-mm, 30° angle arthroscope, a light source, a camera, a television monitor, and a recorder are used in all-arthroscopic shoulder procedures (Figure 3). A versatile traction system with easy attachment can enhance shoulder access and visualization. Shavers and burrs most commonly are used in sizes from 4.5 to 6.5 mm. A rotary shaver with variable speeds and a suction attachment is necessary. Disposable plastic cannulas are required to minimize fluid leakage and extravasation. To allow passage of the arthroscopic instruments, two cannulas (6 and 8 mm) are commonly used. The cannula should be clear to allow visualization of the suture and the knots. The procedure for an all-arthroscopic repair of a large or massive rotator cuff tear is summarized in Table 2.

Anesthesia, Positioning, and Examination Under Anesthesia

An interscalene regional block is routinely done while the patient is awake to provide long-lasting postoperative pain relief. The intraoperative pain relief provided by the regional block significantly reduces the general anesthesia requirement. A light general anesthesia is administered as a means of ensuring muscle relaxation and instituting controlled hypotension.

The procedure can be performed with the patient in the lateral decubitus or beach chair position. The lateral decubitus position provides better access to the entire shoulder region and therefore is preferred by the authors. All bony prominences are carefully padded, especially the fibular head and lateral malleolus of the lower leg, and the patient's position is stabilized using a beanbag and safety strap. The affected shoulder is prepared and draped in standard sterile fashion. The arm is placed on a shoulder traction device attached to the end of the table. Axial traction of 10 to 15 lb is applied, depending on the size of the arm and the patient's weight. The arm is held in 30° to 40° of abduction with 15° of forward flexion and slight internal rotation.

When the anesthesiologist confirms that the airway is secure, the shoulder is examined under anesthesia and compared with the opposite side. The range of motion is assessed in all planes, with careful attention to passive external and internal rotation.

Surface Landmarks and Portals

Accurate, safe portals are created as the first important step toward an adequate visual field. The bony anatomic landmarks are palpated and outlined with a sterile pen. The posterolateral corner of the acromion is marked first because it is the most easily identifiable landmark,[26] and the scapular spine, anterolateral border of the acromion, distal clavicle, and acromioclavicular joint also are marked. The final location of the key portals is determined by marking the tip of the coracoid process. The humeral head and glenohumeral joint are palpated by placing the fingers anteriorly and the thumb posteriorly, then moving the humeral head in an anteroposterior direction to identify the soft spot in the triangular region between acromion, glenoid, and humeral head. A standard posterior viewing portal is established in the soft spot, typically 2 cm distal (along the axis of the arm) and 2 cm medial to the posterolateral corner of the acromion. The axillary nerve is relatively safe in this location. The anterosuperior portal is created using the outside-in technique; an 18-gauge spinal needle is directed into the triangle formed by the biceps tendon superiorly, the subscapularis tendon inferiorly, and the glenoid medially. It is important to place all anterior portals lateral to the coracoid process to avoid injury to the neurovascular structures. The arthroscope is repositioned into the subacromial space, and the midlateral portal is established 2 to 3 cm distal to the acromion. The superolateral portal is created by passing the spinal needle percutaneously anywhere along the lateral acromion border; the exact location depends on the location of the rotator cuff tear and the rotation of the arm.

Principle of Fluid Management and Visualization

The most critical aspect of an all-arthroscopic procedure is to maintain a clear visual field. A good understanding of the arthroscopic flow dynamic and maintenance of adequate inflow pressure is necessary to control hemostasis. Several factors can improve arthroscopic visualization, including the use of hypotensive anesthesia, electrocautery, increased pump pressure or fluid height, a cold irrigation fluid, and epinephrine added to the irrigation fluid. In a randomized, controlled study, Jensen and associates[27] found that adding epinephrine to the irrigation fluid reduced bleeding and improved visual clarity. Although hypotensive anesthesia is quite helpful, it should be used carefully in a patient with atherosclerotic cardiovascular disease; cerebral ischemia can occur if the beach chair position is used.

Diagnostic Arthroscopy

The glenohumeral joint is completely and systematically evaluated through a standard posterior viewing portal. Diagnostic arthroscopy typically begins with identification of the long head of the biceps tendon and its origin at the superior glenoid.[28] Pathologic processes involving the biceps tendon include tendinitis, partial or complete rupture, and subluxation or dislocation. The biceps tendon and its origin are palpated with a probe through the anterior portal, and its stability is tested. The articular cartilage of the humeral head and glenoid are carefully assessed. Superior glenoid erosion is noted if the rotator cuff is massively torn. The axillary pouch is examined for the presence of any loose bodies. The quality and integrity of the rotator cuff is determined. Special attention is paid to the insertion of the supraspinatus tendon; the midtendon insertion typically is 1.5 mm from the articular margin of the humeral head.[29,30]

Biceps Pathology

Possible biceps tendon pathology is assessed by a careful examination of the biceps anchor and proximal long head, and the results are correlated with those of the clinical examination. If there is any suggestion of biceps-related pain or biceps pathology, particularly in the presence of a large or massive rotator cuff tear, a biceps tenotomy or tenodesis is done. The choice of tenotomy or tenodesis depends on the age and functional demands of the patient. For a sedentary patient who is older

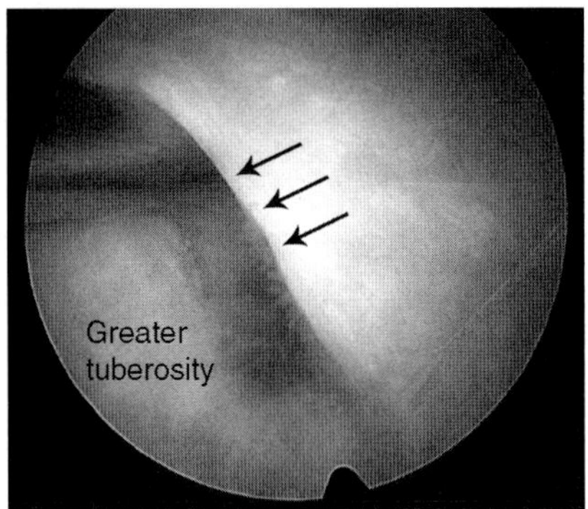

Figure 4 Intraoperative photograph showing a crescent-shaped rotator cuff tear from the posterior portal. Arrows show the edges of the rotator cuff tear.

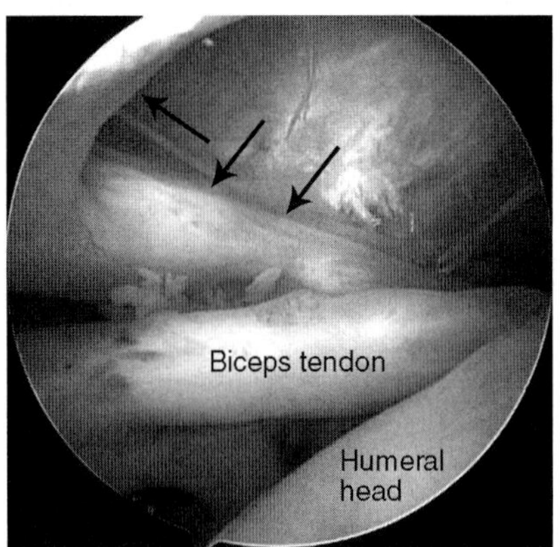

Figure 5 Intraoperative photograph showing a U-shaped rotator cuff tear from the posterior portal. Arrows show the edges of the rotator cuff tear.

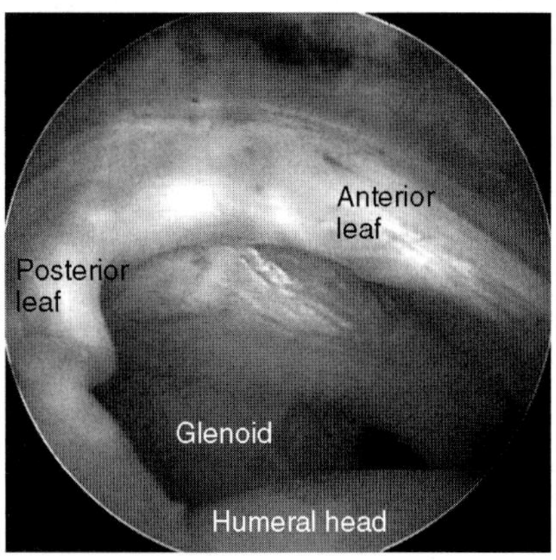

Figure 6 Intraoperative photograph showing a U-shaped rotator cuff tear from the lateral portal.

than 60 years, the authors prefer tenotomy, especially if the tear is on the nondominant side. Tenodesis is preferred for other patients to avoid the complications of biceps cramping and weakness as well as the cosmetic deformity. Many different techniques can be used for tenodesis; the authors prefer a biodegradable screw with humeral head tunnel fixation at the proximal part of the biceps groove. Although groove-related pain is a possibility, this complication appears to be uncommon.

Tear Pattern

A three-dimensional understanding of the morphology of a large or massive cuff tear is essential for the repair. The tear is viewed from multiple portals, and the tear edges are grasped from multiple trajectories to allow the shape of the tear (crescent, U, L, or reverse L) to become more apparent and to establish a plan for the repair and a position for the convergence sutures.[31] Débridement of the anterior and posterior bursa is helpful for identifying the rotator cuff margin. As in fracture management, it is critical to determine the direction of reduction before any stabilization attempt.[32] However, frequently it is difficult to determine the direction of a rotator cuff tear reduction. The size and shape of the rotator cuff tear may appear different when assessed from the lateral and posterior viewing portals. To determine tear morphology, reduction is tried from medial to lateral, anterior to posterior, and posterior to anterior, using an atraumatic tendon grasper. The width of the tear at its insertion on the greater tuberosity can be measured with a probe inserted through the lateral portal. Crescent-shaped tears are the most common, and they have excellent medial-to-lateral mobility[5,33] (Figure 4). U-shaped tears extend much further medially, with the apex of the tear adjacent to the glenoid rim (Figures 5 and 6). A U-shaped tear typically has mobile anterior and posterior leaves, but medial to lateral mobility is restricted. Although L-shaped and reverse L-shaped tears may appear to be U shaped because of the physiologic pull of the rotator cuff, one leaf is more mobile than the other leaf.[31] A massive, contracted tear has no mobility from medial to lateral or from anterior to posterior.

When the tear pattern has been determined, the planned locations of the margin convergence sutures and bone anchors are planed to ensure a tension-free anatomic repair.

Subacromial Decompression

The preoperative assessment of clinical impingement, radiographic acromial morphology, and intraoperative findings are crucial to determining the size of the acromioplasty or the amount of bone removed. Subacromial decompression can improve visualization of the rotator cuff tear, facilitate the technical aspect of the repair, and eliminate extrinsic pressure from the repair. However, excessive acromioplasty and coracoacromial ligament resection should be avoided in the presence of a massive rotator cuff tear. If the repair fails and the coracoacromial arch is disrupted, an anterosuperior escape may develop. Subacromial smoothing is recommended for a massive rotator cuff tear, rather than a formal decompression that removes a significant portion of the acromion and releases the coracoacromial ligament. The smoothing includes débridement of soft tissue on the undersurface of the acromion and the removal of small bony prominences. The integrity of the coracoacromial arch is preserved as a last restraint against anterosuperior humeral head migration. The anterolateral edge of the acromion must be clearly delineated. An os acromiale can be mistaken intraoperatively for the acromioclavicular joint if it is not identified by preoperative imaging.

Rotator Cuff Mobilization

Repair of a large rotator cuff tear without adequate cuff mobilization can lead to tension overload and ultimately cause the repair to fail. The adhesions that tend to form on both the bursal and the articular sides of the tear must be removed. Posterolateral adhesion between the rotator cuff and the deltoid fascia in the lateral gutter also should be removed. An articular side release, with an elevator passed between the glenoid rim and the supraspinatus, is used to free the contracted superior capsule. Rotator cuff mobility is reassessed following this release. For satisfactory repair of a crescent-shaped tear, the tendon edges should be reduced to their footprint in the greater tuberosity, with minimal tension; a longitudinal tear should be reduced side to side.

If the tear remains irreducible or immobile, the advanced interval slide arthroscopic mobilization technique is used. An anterior interval slide provides 1 to 2 cm lateral excursion of the supraspinatus tendon.[34] Arthroscopic scissors are introduced from the lateral portal while being viewed from the posterior portal, to separate the anterior supraspinatus tendon from the rotator cuff interval along the course of the biceps toward the base of the coracoid. The division effectively releases the contracted coracohumeral ligament. If supraspinatus and infraspinatus excursion is still poor, a double interval slide (anterior and posterior) can provide as much as 5 cm of additional lateral excursion of the posterior rotator cuff, as described by Lo and Burkhart.[35] The posterior rotator cuff interval lies between the supraspinatus and the infraspinatus tendons. The scapular spine, which serves as a landmark between the supraspinatus and infraspinatus tendons, is identified first through the lateral working portal. A radiofrequency device or arthroscopic scissor is used to divide the tissue between the supraspinatus and infraspinatus. A posterior rotator cuff interval slide places the suprascapular nerve at risk if the release is carried more than 2 cm medial to the glenoid rim in the suprascapular notch.[36] Some of the pain from a large retracted rotator cuff tear results from traction on the suprascapular nerve, which can be relieved through a partial or complete repair.[37,38]

Footprint Preparation

The anatomic footprint is reestablished after the rotator cuff tendon is successfully mobilized. A shaver or light burr is used to prepare the greater tuberosity bed down to a bleeding bone without decortication. Decortication of the greater tuberosity should be avoided to ensure secure anchor fixation. Patients with osteoporotic bone often require larger suture anchors, and particular caution must be used to avoid weakening the tuberosity during preparation.

Margin Convergence

The margin convergence repair principle typically is used for a U-shaped tear or the longitudinal limb of an L-shaped or reverse L-shaped tear.[39] Sutures are placed in a side-to-side fashion through the anterior and posterior leaves of the tear (Figure 7). This technique distributes forces to the anterior and posterior tear leaves, minimizes overall tension on the tendon-bone repair, and allows repair of an otherwise irreparable tear. Side-to-side suture placement is repeated as necessary, moving laterally with each suture. As the side-to-side sutures are sequentially tied, the free margin of the rotator cuff converges laterally toward the bone bed. Care must be taken with a side-to-side repair to minimize a dog ear formation of the tendon. Despite using the best mobilization techniques, some large or massive tears may not be completely repairable because of tissue loss and retraction. A margin convergence partial repair of such a tear can improve function and decrease pain, although the longevity of this type of repair is questionable.[40]

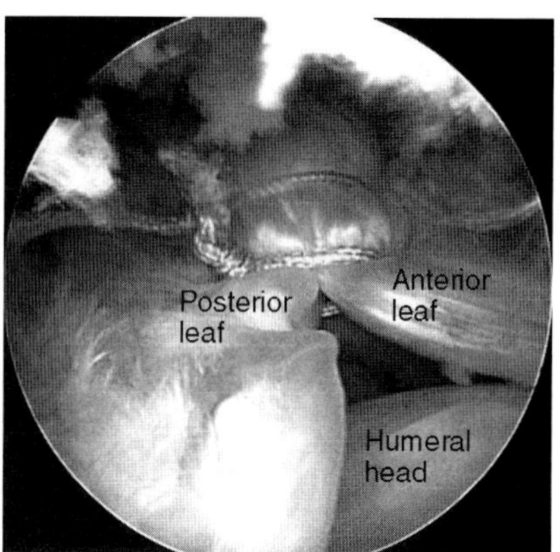

Figure 7 Intraoperative photograph showing margin convergence from the lateral portal. Sutures are placed in a side-to-side fashion through the anterior and posterior leaves. The sutures are sequentially tied from medial to lateral.

Anchor Placement

After the rotator cuff tear is approximated on the tuberosity, suture anchors are placed on the prepared bone bed. The trajectory of a suture anchor is critical to maximizing its pullout

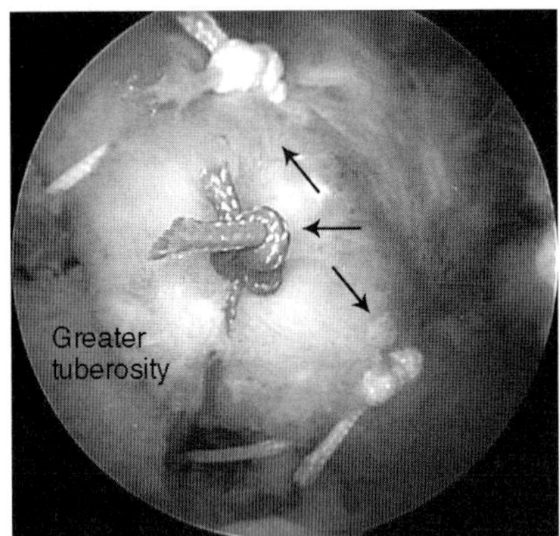

Figure 8 Intraoperative photograph showing a post single-row repair. Arrows point to the reattached rotator cuff tendons.

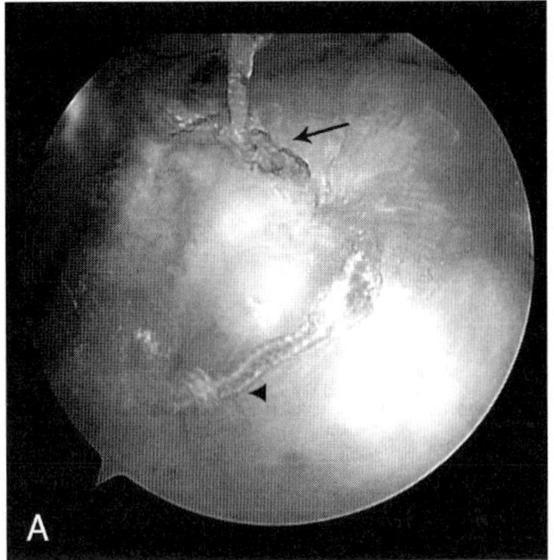

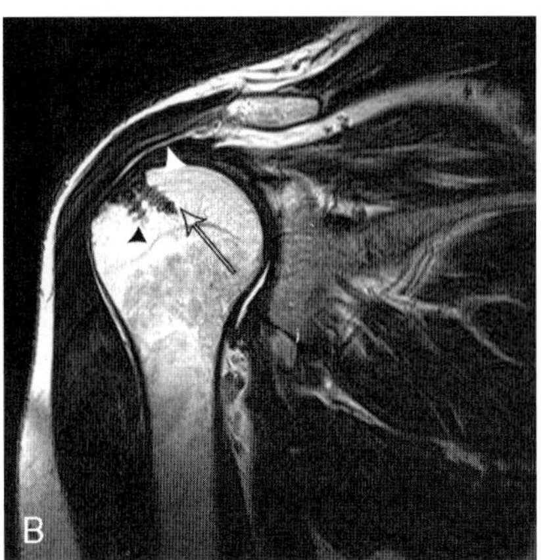

Figure 9 **A,** Intraoperative photograph showing a post dual-row repair. Medial row repair (*arrow*) and lateral row repair (*arrowhead*). **B,** Coronal MRI scan showing postoperative healing of a dual-row repair. The reattached rotator cuff (*white arrowhead*), medial row anchor (*open arrow*), and the lateral row anchor (*black arrowhead*) are shown.

strength. The anchor should be placed at a 45° angle to the vector of rotator cuff tension (the so-called deadman's angle) to improve pullout strength.[41] The suture anchors are passed percutaneously through a small stab incision and seated adjacent to the articular margin (Figure 8).

The number of anchors used is determined by the size of the tear and the configuration of the repair. In general, one suture anchor is used for every 1 cm of rotator cuff tear. A spinal needle is inserted percutaneously adjacent to the lateral margin of the acromion to ensure that the location and angle of the anchors is accurate. The suture anchor is seated, and gentle traction is applied through the suture limb to ensure adequate holding power. Large, 6.5-mm suture anchors are placed if the bone is osteoporotic. Double- or triple-loaded anchors are recommended to achieve an adequate fixation while minimizing the load on the suture.

The fixation strength of the bone-anchor-suture-tendon construct depends on bone quality, fatty degeneration of the rotator cuff, suture material, and configuration. Failure most commonly occurs at the suture-tendon junction rather than the bone-suture junction.[42] For a screw-in biodegradable anchor, a tap is routinely used after a pilot hole is created using a punch. A biodegradable anchor has the advantage of being more visible than other types of anchors on any postsurgical MRI studies.

Dual-row fixation is preferable for a massive tear, unless the tuberosity surface area is small (Figure 9). The medial anchor is placed first on the edge of the articular surface. A 1.5-cm bone bridge is preferred between the medial and lateral row. The dual row can be modified to a transosseous equivalent using a lateral PushLock (Arthrex, Naples, FL) knotless anchor system.[43] These configurations increase the rotator cuff footprint, contact pressure, and pullout strength but may immediately decrease tendon blood flow.

Suture Passing and Knot Tying

Following anchor placement, one suture strand is retrieved through the lateral working portal, an appropriate suture-passing device is selected, and the retrieved suture limb is loaded into the device. An arthroscopic surgeon should be familiar with a variety of suture-passing instruments.

Despite recent advances in knotless technology, surgeons should be familiar with arthroscopic knot-tying techniques.[44] Several suture configurations can be used to maximize suture-holding power in the tendon. To avoid unloading the suture, an assistant holds one limb of the suture during retrieval. The suture limb that passes through the rotator cuff tissue is the post, and the knot is routinely placed on the top of the rotator cuff. The suture should be tied from the cannula that permits the most direct route for tying. An extra cannula through the anterior deltoid just lateral to the acromioclavicular joint can serve as a waiting room portal to avoid suture tangling. A sliding locking knot backed with three alternating half-hitch knots is routinely used. Only the suture limbs that are actively being tied should be in the working cannula. The suture limbs are cut close to the knot using an arthroscopic suture scissor. This sequence can be performed repeatedly. The security of the final repair is assessed while the arm is gently rotated.[28]

Postoperative Course

Arthroscopic repair of a large or massive rotator cuff tear is an outpatient procedure. At the conclusion of surgery, the shoulder is immobilized in a sling to protect the repair. Postoperative rehabilitation is as important as the surgery itself, and patient noncompliance can lead to early repair failure. A cold therapy device is applied in the recovery room, and its use is encouraged for the first 2 weeks after surgery.[45] Most authors agree that a small rotator cuff repair must be protected from active exercises for approximately 4 to 6 weeks. Repair of a large or massive tear should be protected for 6 to 8 weeks. The patient is allowed to remove the sling only while bathing or performing elbow exercises. An abduction splint reduces the tension in the repaired cuff tear and therefore could maximize the healing process and decrease pain; it should be used for a large or massive cuff tear.[46] Handgrip strength and elbow supination-pronation exercises are encouraged beginning on the first postoperative day.

After 4 weeks for a small tear and 8 weeks for a large or massive tear, active forward elevation is initiated. It is easier to perform most of the exercises in the supine position to eliminate the need to work against gravity. Formal physical therapy is a supplement, not a replacement, for home exercises. Home therapy exercises should be performed three to five times per day. A resistance and strengthening program for the deltoid and rotator cuff is initiated after 3 months. To avoid retearing the rotator cuff, patients are cautioned against lifting weights or heavy objects. A return to manual work and overhead activity is discouraged until sufficient range of motion and strength have been gained, usually 6 to 9 months after surgery. The patient should be aware that maximal improvement may not be reached until 12 to 18 months after surgery.

Complications

Arthroscopic rotator cuff repair has high rates of success and favorable outcomes. The reported rates of complications range from 0% to 10.6%;[47-49] complications often are attributed to the surgeon's learning curve or the duration of surgery. The complications of arthroscopic rotator cuff repair include postoperative stiffness, infection, fluid extravasation and local swelling, failure of healing, deep venous thrombosis, regional pain syndrome, transient neurapraxias, direct nerve injury, loose anchors, and articular cartilage scuffing.

The reported incidence of stiffness ranges from 2.7% to 10.6%.[47,50] The contributing factors include diabetes mellitus, preoperative stiffness, an overly tight repair, inadequate postoperative pain control, and inappropriate rehabilitation. Preoperative stiffness should be treated before the associated rotator cuff tear is repaired. Intra-articular capsular contracture and extra-articular subacromial adhesions are the most important pathologic features. The first line of treatment is a physical therapy program accompanied by steroid injections; recalcitrant stiffness is effectively managed with manipulation and arthroscopic release.

Infection after arthroscopic rotator cuff repair is relatively rare and much less common than after open repair. The pathogen most commonly isolated from rotator cuff infections is *Propionibacterium acnes*, which is commonly found in moist skin such as that of the axilla.[51] *P acnes* is a slow-growing, gram-positive, anaerobic bacterium. Cultures should be monitored for a minimum of 7 days. A high index of suspicion and early recognition of infection are crucial for optimal treatment results.

Shoulder edema and fluid extravasation are relatively common following subacromial arthroscopy because the subacromial area is not encapsulated. Surgical time of more than 2 hours is directly correlated with the development of fluid overload and, more severely, airway edema.[52] Lo and Burkhart[53] reported an average weight gain of 8.7 lb immediately after shoulder arthroscopy. Careful monitoring of fluid pressure and procedure length are important to avoid these complications.

Results

Arthroscopic repair of large and massive cuff tears has a high level of success, with significant pain relief and improvement in shoulder function.[28] The reported results are comparable to the results of traditional open repair.[54] Pain relief often is substantial, and it is the most predictable outcome following arthroscopic repair. Jones and Savoie[55] reported the results of arthroscopic repair of 37 large and 13 massive rotator cuff tears at an average 32-month follow-up. Forty-four patients (88%) had a good or excellent outcome based on the University of California Los Angeles Shoulder Scale, with significant improvement in function, strength, and pain relief. There was no significant difference in the outcome scores of patients with a large or massive rotator cuff tear. Forty-nine patients (98%) were satisfied with the result; only 1 patient (2%) required revision arthroscopic repair. Bennett[56] reported that 35 of 37 patients (95%) were satisfied at 2- to 4-year follow-up after arthroscopic repair of a massive rotator cuff tear. Complete coverage was achieved during surgery in 29 (78%) of the patients. No significant difference was found after repair of anterosuperior or posterosuperior tears. This finding emphasizes that many patients have a successful outcome despite incomplete coverage or postoperative persistence of a rotator cuff defect.

The discrepancy between the success of anatomic repairs and clinical outcomes has been investigated.[57-59] Galatz and associates[59] analyzed the relationship between repair integrity and the outcome of arthroscopically repaired large and massive rotator cuff tears. Based on ultrasonographic images, 17 of 18 patients had a recurrent tear at 12-month follow-up. Despite failure of healing, 16 of the patients had decreased pain, and the average functional outcome score improved from 48.3 to 84.6 points. Range of motion increased substantially; average forward flexion was 92° preoperatively, 152° at 12-month follow-up, and 142° at 24-month follow-up. The relatively high tendon-healing failure rate may be attributed to the aggressive rehabilitation protocol, which included immediate use of active-assisted pulley exercise.

In a recent multicenter study of 576 patients who had undergone arthroscopic repair of a small or medium-sized rotator cuff tear, Flurin and associates[60] found no significant correlation between pain relief and anatomic repair or cuff integrity. At an average 18.5-month follow-up, 541 patients (94%) had a good or excellent result, although 25.3% of the repaired rotator cuffs had leakage of contrast on CT or magnetic resonance arthrogram. Although overall outcomes are good regardless of whether tendon healing is achieved, an intact rotator cuff is associated with significantly better shoulder function, particularly in terms of strength. Lee and associates[49] reported significant clinical improvement regardless of tear size following arthroscopic rotator cuff repair. Pain scores were significantly improved in 21 patients with a massive cuff tear; overall function improved, but the gains in strength and motion were less dramatic than after the repair of smaller tears.

Vad and associates,[61] in a retrospective study of 108 patients with a massive rotator cuff tear, identified five negative prognostic factors: superior migration of the humeral head, external rotation and abduction strength less than grade III, decreased passive range of motion, muscle atrophy, and glenohumeral arthritis. The presence of three or more of these factors was correlated with a poor treatment outcome. Similarly, Ellman and associates[62] identified four factors that may lead to a poor outcome of surgical repair: acromiohumeral distance of 7 mm or less, inability to abduct the arm actively to 100°, low abduction and external rotation strength, and relatively long duration of symptoms. Burkhart and associates[63] reported the results of arthroscopic repair of a massive rotator cuff tear in 22 patients; 17 patients had 52% to 75% fatty degeneration, and 5 had more than 75% fatty degeneration. Three (60%) of the 5 patients with more than 75% fatty degeneration had a poor outcome. Overall clinical improvement was observed in 19 (86.4%) of the patients, with modest gains in function. The best results were obtained when the patient had less than 75% fatty degeneration. Lafosse[64] reported that healing rates after dual-row repair were higher than those of historical control subjects.

Summary

Arthroscopic repair of a large or massive rotator cuff tear is technically demanding. Considerable experience with shoulder arthroscopy is required to achieve success with a minimal risk of complications. Future advances in technology and innovative techniques will continue to simplify the arthroscopic approach to rotator cuff repair.

References

1. Howell SM, Galinat BJ, Renzi AJ, Marone PJ: Normal and abnormal mechanics of the glenohumeral joint in the horizontal plane. *J Bone Joint Surg Am* 1988;70:227-232.
2. Hansen ML, Otis JC, Johnson JS, Cordasco FA, Craig EV, Warren RF: Biomechanics of massive rotator cuff tears: Implications for treatment. *J Bone Joint Surg Am* 2008;90:316-325.
3. Bechtol CO: Biomechanics of the shoulder. *Clin Orthop Relat Res* 1980; 146:37-41.
4. Inman VT, Saunders JB, Abbot LC: Observations on the function of the shoulder joint: 1944. *Clin Orthop Relat Res* 1996;330:3-12.
5. Burkhart SS: Arthroscopic treatment of massive rotator cuff tears: Clinical results and biomechanical rationale. *Clin Orthop Relat Res* 1991;267:45-56.
6. Gerber C, Galantay RV, Hersche O: The pattern of pain produced by irritation of the acromioclavicular joint and the subacromial space. *J Shoulder Elbow Surg* 1998;7:352-355.

7. Neer CS II: Anterior acromioplasty for the chronic impingement syndrome in the shoulder: 1972. *J Bone Joint Surg Am* 2005;87:1399.

8. Kessel L, Watson M: The painful arc syndrome: Clinical classification as a guide to management. *J Bone Joint Surg Br* 1977;59:166-172.

9. Hawkins RJ, Kennedy JC: Impingement syndrome in athletes. *Am J Sports Med* 1980;8:151-158.

10. Jobe FW, Jobe CM: Painful athletic injuries of the shoulder. *Clin Orthop Relat Res* 1983;173:117-124.

11. Gerber C, Krushell RJ: Isolated rupture of the tendon of the subscapularis muscle: Clinical features in 16 cases. *J Bone Joint Surg Br* 1991;73: 389-394.

12. Codman E: *The Shoulder: Rupture of the Supraspinatus Tendon and Other Lesions in or About the Subacromial Bursa*. Boston, MA, Thomas Todd Company, 1934.

13. Hertel R, Ballmer FT, Lombert SM, Gerber C: Lag signs in the diagnosis of rotator cuff rupture. *J Shoulder Elbow Surg* 1996;5:307-313.

14. Walch G, Boulahia A, Calderone S, Robinson AH: The 'dropping' and 'hornblower's' signs in evaluation of rotator-cuff tears. *J Bone Joint Surg Br* 1998;80:624-628.

15. Zanca P: Shoulder pain: Involvement of the acromioclavicular joint (Analysis of 1,000 cases). *Am J Roentgenol Radium Ther Nucl Med* 1971;112: 493-506.

16. Weiner DS, Macnab I: Superior migration of the humeral head: A radiological aid in the diagnosis of tears of the rotator cuff. *J Bone Joint Surg Br* 1970;52:524-527.

17. Mudge MK, Wood VE, Frykman GK: Rotator cuff tears associated with os acromiale. *J Bone Joint Surg Am* 1984; 66:427-429.

18. Bigliani L, Norris T, Fischer J, Neer CS II: The relationship between the unfused acromial epiphysis and subacromial impingement lesions. *Orthop Trans* 1983;7:138.

19. Balich SM, Sheley RC, Brown TR, Sauser DD, Quinn SF: MR imaging of the rotator cuff tendon: Interobserver agreement and analysis of interpretive errors. *Radiology* 1997;204: 191-194.

20. Quinn SF, Sheley RC, Demlow TA, Szumowski J: Rotator cuff tendon tears: Evaluation with fat-suppressed MR imaging with arthroscopic correlation in 100 patients. *Radiology* 1995; 195:497-500.

21. Stanwood W, Marra G: Massive rotator cuff tears. *Curr Opinion Ortho* 2001;12:319-324.

22. Goutallier D, Postel JM, Bernageau J, Lavau L, Voisin MC: Fatty muscle degeneration in cuff ruptures: Pre- and postoperative evaluation by CT scan. *Clin Orthop Relat Res* 1994;304:78-83.

23. Beggs I: Ultrasound of the shoulder and elbow. *Orthop Clin North Am* 2006;37:277-285.

24. Iannotti JP, Ciccone J, Buss DD, et al: Accuracy of office-based ultrasonography of the shoulder for the diagnosis of rotator cuff tears. *J Bone Joint Surg Am* 2005;87:1305-1311.

25. Martin-Hervás C, Romero J, Navas-Acién A, Reboiras JJ, Munuera L: Ultrasonographic and magnetic resonance images of rotator cuff lesions compared with arthroscopy or open surgery findings. *J Shoulder Elbow Surg* 2001;10:410-415.

26. Gramstad G, Galatz LM, Yamaguchi K: Arthroscopic shoulder anatomy, in Blaine T, ed: *Shoulder Arthroscopy*. Rosemont, IL, American Academy of Orthopaedic Surgeons, 2006, pp 1-22.

27. Jensen KH, Werther K, Stryger V, Schultz K, Falkenberg B: Arthroscopic shoulder surgery with epinephrine saline irrigation. *Arthroscopy* 2001;17:578-581.

28. Abrams J: Arthroscopic techniques for massive rotator cuff repairs. *Tech Should Elbow Surg* 2007;8:126-134.

29. Ruotolo C, Fow JE, Nottage WM: The supraspinatus footprint: An anatomic study of the supraspinatus insertion. *Arthroscopy* 2004;20:246-249.

30. DeFranco M, Cole B: Current perspectives on rotator cuff anatomy. *Arthroscopy* 2009;25:305-320.

31. Lo IK, Burkhart SS: Current concepts in arthroscopic rotator cuff repair. *Am J Sports Med* 2003;31:308-324.

32. Fouse M, Nottage WM: All-arthroscopic rotator cuff repair. *Sports Med Arthrosc* 2007;15:208-215.

33. Burkhart SS: A stepwise approach to arthroscopic rotator cuff repair based on biomechanical principles. *Arthroscopy* 2000;16:82-90.

34. Tauro JC: Arthroscopic repair of large rotator cuff tears using the interval slide technique. *Arthroscopy* 2004;20: 13-21.

35. Lo IK, Burkhart SS: Arthroscopic repair of massive, contracted, immobile rotator cuff tears using single and double interval slides: Technique and preliminary results. *Arthroscopy* 2004; 20:22-33.

36. Warner JP, Krushell RJ, Masquelet A, Gerber C: Anatomy and relationships of the suprascapular nerve: Anatomical constraints to mobilization of the supraspinatus and infraspinatus muscles in the management of massive rotator-cuff tears. *J Bone Joint Surg Am* 1992;74:36-45.

37. Costouros JG, Porramatikul M, Lie DT, Warner JJ: Reversal of suprascapular neuropathy following arthroscopic repair of massive supraspinatus and infraspinatus rotator cuff tears. *Arthroscopy* 2007;23:1152-1161.

38. Mallon WJ, Wilson RJ, Basamania CJ: The association of suprascapular neuropathy with massive rotator cuff tears: A preliminary report. *J Shoulder Elbow Surg* 2006;15:395-398.

39. Burkhart SS, Athanasiou KA, Wirth MA: Margin convergence: A method of reducing strain in massive rotator cuff tears. *Arthroscopy* 1996;12: 335-338.

40. Burkhart SS, Nottage WM, Ogilvie-Harris DJ, Kohn HS, Pachelli A: Partial repair of irreparable rotator cuff tears. *Arthroscopy* 1994;10:363-370.

41. Burkhart SS: The deadman theory of suture anchors: Observations along a south Texas fence line. *Arthroscopy* 1995;11:119-123.

42. Cummins CA, Murrell GA: Mode of failure for rotator cuff repair with suture anchors identified at revision surgery. *J Shoulder Elbow Surg* 2003; 12:128-133.

43. Park MC, ElAttrache NS, Tibone JE, Ahmad CS, Jun BJ, Lee TQ: Part I: Footprint contact characteristics for a transosseous-equivalent rotator cuff repair technique compared with a double-row repair technique. *J Shoulder Elbow Surg* 2007;16:461-468.

44. Lo IK, Burkhart SS, Chan KC, Athanasiou K: Arthroscopic knots: Determining the optimal balance of loop security and knot security. *Arthroscopy* 2004;20:489-502.

45. Speer KP, Warren RF, Horowitz L: The efficacy of cryotherapy in the postoperative shoulder. *J Shoulder Elbow Surg* 1996;5:62-68.

46. Millett PJ, Wilcox RB III, O'Holleran JD, Warner JJ: Rehabilitation of the rotator cuff: An evaluation-based approach. *J Am Acad Orthop Surg* 2006; 14:599-609.

47. Brislin KJ, Field LD, Savoie FH III: Complications after arthroscopic rotator cuff repair. *Arthroscopy* 2007;23: 124-128.

48. Berjano P, González BG, Olmedo JF, Perez-España LA, Munilla MG: Complications in arthroscopic shoulder surgery. *Arthroscopy* 1998;14: 785-788.

49. Lee E, Bishop JY, Braman JP, Langford J, Gelber J, Flatow EL: Outcomes after arthroscopic rotator cuff repairs. *J Shoulder Elbow Surg* 2007;16: 1-5.

50. Curtis A, Snyder S, Del Pizzo W, Friedman M, Ferkel R, Karzel R: Complications of shoulder arthroscopy. *Arthroscopy* 1992;8:395.

51. Athwal GS, Sperling JW, Rispoli DM, Cofield RH: Deep infection after rotator cuff repair. *J Shoulder Elbow Surg* 2007;16:306-311.

52. Orebaugh SL: Life-threatening airway edema resulting from prolonged shoulder arthroscopy. *Anesthesiology* 2003;99:1456-1458.

53. Lo IK, Burkhart SS: Immediate postoperative fluid retention and weight gain after shoulder arthroscopy. *Arthroscopy* 2005;21:605-610.

54. Nho SJ, Shindle MK, Sherman SL, Freedman KB, Lyman S, MacGillivray JD: Systematic review of arthroscopic rotator cuff repair and mini-open rotator cuff repair. *J Bone Joint Surg Am* 2007;89:127-136.

55. Jones CK, Savoie FH III: Arthroscopic repair of large and massive rotator cuff tears. *Arthroscopy* 2003;19: 564-571.

56. Bennett WF: Arthroscopic repair of massive rotator cuff tears: A prospective cohort with 2- to 4-year follow-up. *Arthroscopy* 2003;19:380-390.

57. Boileau P, Brassart N, Watkinson DJ, Carles M, Hatzidakis AM, Krishnan SG: Arthroscopic repair of full-thickness tears of the supraspinatus: Does the tendon really heal? *J Bone Joint Surg Am* 2005;87:1229-1240.

58. Favard L, Bacle G, Berhouet J: Rotator cuff repair. *Joint Bone Spine* 2007; 74:551-557.

59. Galatz LM, Ball CM, Teefey SA, Middleton WD, Yamaguchi K: The outcome and repair integrity of completely arthroscopically repaired large and massive rotator cuff tears. *J Bone Joint Surg Am* 2004;86:219-224.

60. Flurin PH, Landreau P, Gregory T, et al: Arthroscopic repair of full-thickness cuff tears: A multicentric retrospective study of 576 cases with anatomical assessment. *Rev Chir Orthop Reparatrice Appar Mot* 2005;91: 31-42.

61. Vad VB, Warren RF, Altchek DW, O'Brien SJ, Rose HA, Wickiewicz TL: Negative prognostic factors in managing massive rotator cuff tears. *Clin J Sport Med* 2002;12:151-157.

62. Ellman H, Hanker G, Bayer M: Repair of the rotator cuff: End-result study of factors influencing reconstruction. *J Bone Joint Surg Am* 1986; 68:1136-1144.

63. Burkhart SS, Barth JR, Richards DP, Zlatkin MB, Larsen M: Arthroscopic repair of massive rotator cuff tears with stage 3 and 4 fatty degeneration. *Arthroscopy* 2007;23:347-354.

64. Lafosse L, Brozska R, Toussaint B, Gobezie R: The outcome and structural integrity of arthroscopic rotator cuff repair with use of the double-row suture anchor technique. *J Bone Joint Surg Am* 2007;89:1533-1541.

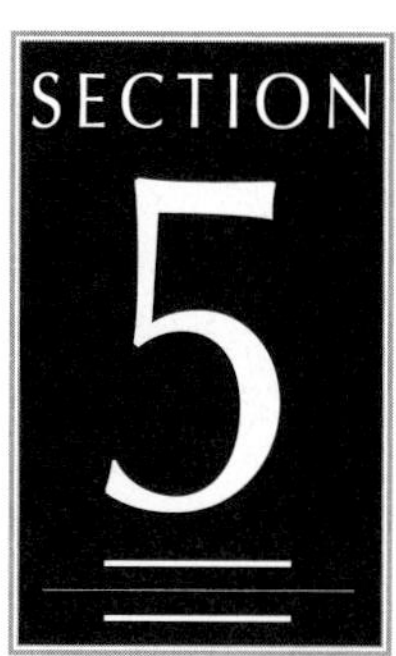

Hand and Wrist

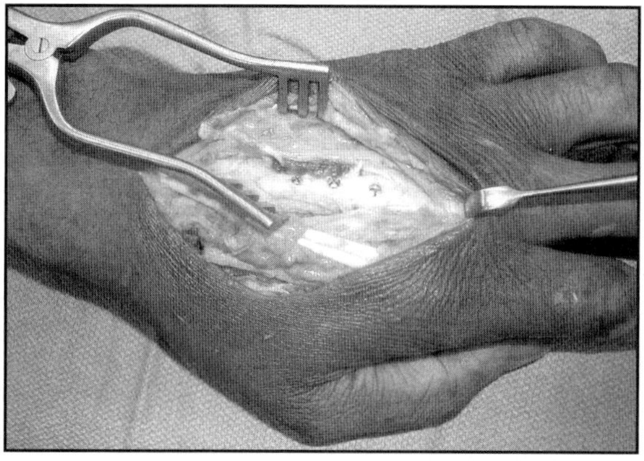

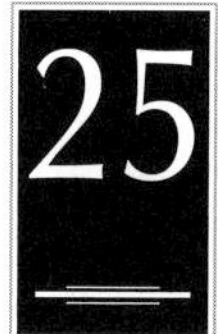

Reconstruction of Posttraumatic Disorders of the Forearm

Jesse B. Jupiter, MD
Diego L. Fernandez, MD
L. Scott Levin, MD, FACS
Robert W. Wysocki, MD

Abstract

Forearm rotation is crucial for full upper extremity mobility. The two-bone unit with its proximal and distal radioulnar joints should be considered as a single bicondylar articulation. After a traumatic bony forearm injury, surgical treatment for complications, such as deformity, bone loss, or failed fracture healing is challenging because complete return of forearm rotation can be difficult to achieve.

It is important to be aware of methods for assessing and managing posttraumatic forearm bony complications, including preoperative assessment and osteotomy techniques for malunited fractures. The vascularized fibular transplant also has been proven as an effective treatment method. Although nonunion of forearm fractures is uncommon, it can prove problematic; therefore, it is beneficial to review options for surgical management.

Instr Course Lect 2010;59:283-293.

Forearm Kinesiology

Forearm rotation is the most important contribution to the rotational mobility of the upper limb.[1] The two-bone unit with its proximal and distal radioulnar joints, and its rotational axis connecting the centers of the two, have been viewed as a single bicondylar joint. When combined with rotational motion of the shoulder, forearm rotation allows the hand to be positioned through an entire 360° arc of motion. With the shoulder fully abducted, nearly all of the rotational motion of the upper limb occurs through the forearm.[1] Activities such as accepting objects in the palm of the hand require nearly full forearm supination, whereas many other functional tasks require some degree of pronation. It has been suggested that, in addition to rotation along the axis of the forearm articulation, the distal aspect of the ulna moves in both adduction and abduction planes with forearm rotation, although some believe that this perceived motion may be caused by axial rotation of the humerus.[2,3]

The interosseous membrane, which is considered to be better described as a ligament, also contributes to the longitudinal stability of the forearm.[4-7] The central band contributes to the axial stability of the forearm, whereas the dorsal oblique band adds to the stability of the proximal radioulnar joint, and the distal membranous portion functions as a secondary stabilizer of the distal radioulnar joint.[7]

Malunion

When the forearm is considered to be a joint, diaphyseal fractures constitute intra-articular lesions and therefore require accurate anatomic reduction to ensure full function.

Dr. Jupiter or an immediate family member serves as an unpaid consultant to Synthes; has received research or institutional support from Aircast (DJ Orthopedics), Biomet, Hand Innovations, Linvatec, Mitek, SBI, Synthes, and Wright Medical Technology; owns stock or stock options in Hemaclear; and has received nonincome support (such as equipment or services), commercially derived honoraria, or other non–research-related funding (such as paid travel) from Saunders/Mosby-Elsevier and Wolters Kluwer Health. None of the following authors nor any immediate family members have received anything of value from or own stock in a commercial company or institution related directly or indirectly to the subject of this chapter: Dr. Fernandez, Dr. Levin, and Dr. Wysocki.

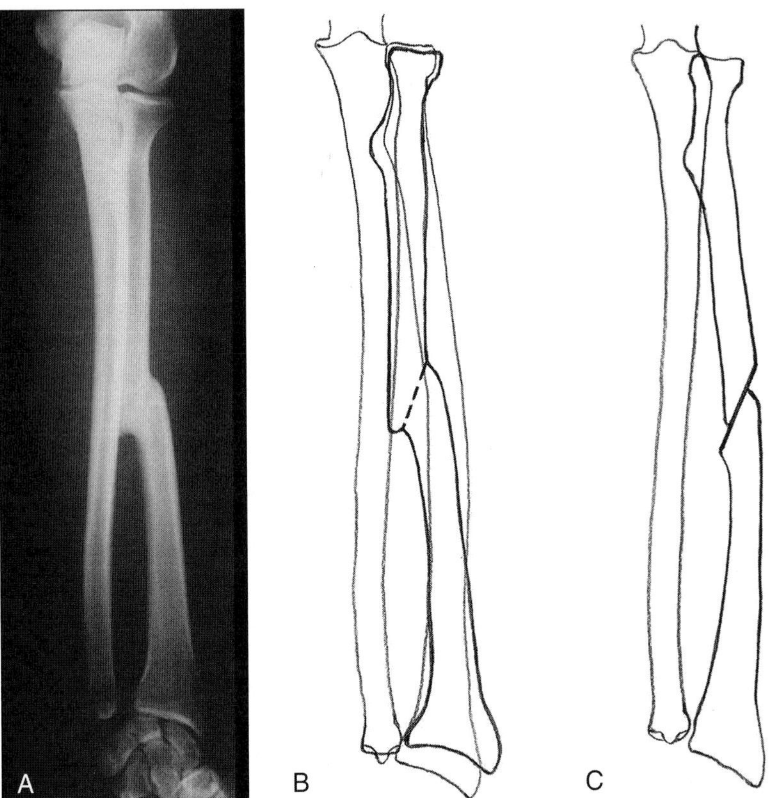

Figure 1 **A,** A radiograph of a malunited midshaft left radial fracture after closed treatment. There is reduction of the interosseous space, radial shortening resulting in a positive ulnar variance of 4 mm, and dissociation of the distal radioulnar joint. The patient had complete loss of pronation, unrestricted supination, and pain at the distal radioulnar joint. He also had a negative ulnar variance of 4 mm in the normal forearm. Tracings of the AP radiographs of the two forearms have been superimposed **(B)**, and an oblique osteotomy **(C)** was chosen to permit a lengthening of 8 mm, which was necessary to restore congruency of the distal radioulnar joint. The amount of lateral displacement of the proximal fragment indicates that a formal release of the interosseous membrane will be necessary.

The same principle applies to surgical reconstruction of malunited forearm fractures.

Surgical management of a diaphyseal malunion is a challenge because, despite the achievement of osseous union, correction of deformity, and relief of pain, complete and symmetric restoration of forearm rotation is difficult to obtain.[8] This results from the associated derangement of the proximal and distal radioulnar joints and the interosseous membrane.[9,10] Shortening of a single forearm bone with or without angular deformity automatically affects the articular anatomic relationships of either the proximal or the distal radioulnar joint. Loss of the physiologic bow of the radius limits pronation, and reduction of the interosseous space associated with angular or translational deformity can lead to osseous impingement and secondary contracture of the interosseous membrane, further reducing forearm rotation[10] (Figure 1, *A*).

Diaphyseal malunion in adults may be caused by insufficient reduction, usually with nonsurgical treatment, or may be an iatrogenic deformity after an attempted osteotomy. The deformity may include one or both bones of the forearm. The clinical scenario presents as restriction of forearm rotation, pain and instability of the radioulnar joints during pronation and supination, and often a cosmetic problem. Symptoms may be decreased by correcting all components of the deformity, including length discrepancy, angulation, rotation, and the bow of the radius.[9]

In children older than 10 years and in adults, restoration of normal anatomy and neighboring joint relationships following posttraumatic deformity can be achieved only with corrective osteotomies. This, together with the appropriate soft-tissue release, improves forearm rotation, while realignment of the radioulnar joints provides stability. Because there are no generally valid normal values, the contralateral, healthy forearm is used for preoperative planning. Fluoroscopy, CT scans, and cross-sectional MRIs are used to assess rotational malalignment, whereas three-dimensional plastic models based on the CT scans are used to assess complex deformities.[11-13]

Pathomechanics of Forearm Malunions and Clinical Correlation With Forearm Rotation

The influence of ulnar and radial malalignment on rotational motion has been demonstrated experimentally on cadaver forearms.[14-17] The amount of angulation directly correlates with the restriction of pronation and supination. Deformities in the distal third of the forearm, but not those in the middle or proximal third, decrease pronation.[14] Angulations of up to 10° in the middle third of the radius or ulna, or both, do not limit rotation, but deformities of 20° restrict forearm rotation by at least 30%, and angulations of more than 20° result in even greater restrictions.[14,15] Rotational deformities may also displace and decrease the pronation-supination arc of motion.[18,19]

Diaphyseal Deformity and Instability of the Distal Radioulnar Joint

Instability of the distal radioulnar joint can occur with angulation, malrotation, and length discrepancy of one or both forearm bones.[19] The loss of the normal spatial orientation of the joint surfaces prevents anatomic healing of acutely torn ligament restraints. This is true for fractures localized to the distal third of the radius.[20,21] If the fracture heals with a skeletal deformity, instability, subluxation, or complete dislocation, incompetence of the triangular fibrocartilage complex may occur.[21] Palmar subluxation of the distal part of the ulna is associated with dorsally angulated diaphyseal malunion. Conversely, malreduced Galeazzi fractures with persistent palmar angulation and pronated rotational malalignment are associated with dorsal displacement of the distal part of the ulna and complete loss of active supination.

Associated Disorders of the Proximal Radioulnar Joint

Chronic dislocation of the radial head can result from an unreduced Monteggia fracture with persistent angulation of the ulna or be associated with a forearm malunion with a discrepancy between the lengths of the radius and the ulna. An angulated metaphyseal malunion of the proximal part of the radius leads to incongruity of the radial head in the sigmoid notch and results in severe limitation of pronation. In general, valgus malalignment of the proximal part of the radius results in lateral subluxation of the radial head, creating substantial incongruity of both the proximal radioulnar joint and the radiocapitellar joint.

Surgical Techniques

Types of Osteotomies

A transverse osteotomy is preferred to treat a "simple" rotational or translational deformity. Moderate lengthening with angular correction in the plane of the osteotomy can be achieved with oblique osteotomies.[22,23] Rotational correction with oblique osteotomies is limited because rotation automatically induces a change in angular alignment and opens the osteotomy on one side, reducing the contact surface. For complex diaphyseal malunions, for which angular, rotational, and length adjustments are to be made, the single-cut osteotomy oriented in the combined oblique plane of deformity based on a mathematical analysis of the malalignment has been proposed.[24] Further refinements for planning and performing the single-cut osteotomy by applying a geometrical methodology were reported by Meyer and associates.[25] For an exact calculation of the true angle of deformity, Nagy[26] recommended the use of tables that readily provide these values on the basis of projected angles of the deformity on AP and lateral radiographs. During the performance of a single-cut osteotomy, the decision to create a closing or opening wedge osteotomy depends on the amount of length discrepancy of the involved bone. In patients with extreme bowing of the radius or a malunited segmental fracture, a double-level osteotomy may be required to restore alignment of the anatomic axis. Classically, step-cut osteotomies, although technically more demanding, have been used to lengthen long bones, thereby avoiding the need for bone grafting. An isolated rotational deformity is corrected with a transverse osteotomy.[27] Osseous defects created by lengthening require bone grafting except in children, in whom rapid periosteal bone healing readily fills the bone gap.

Deformity characterized by more than 4 cm of shortening of one forearm bone, such as occurs following physeal trauma, is better treated with progressive distraction/osteogenesis techniques that use external fixation.

Preoperative Planning

The contralateral, normal forearm is used as a guide for preoperative planning, as the correctional osteotomy should reproduce the osseous geometry of the normal side. Exact AP and lateral radiographs of both the radius and the ulna, including the proximal and distal joints, should be obtained. This may be difficult, especially when limited forearm rotation prevents the patient from placing the forearm in neutral rotation. In these cases, the correct position for exposure must be determined under an image intensifier. The distal epiphysis is used as the reference for the radius, and the humeroulnar joint is used for the ulna.

The contours of the healthy and deformed bones in both projections are drawn on separate sheets of tracing paper (Figure 1, *B* and *C*). The location of maximal deformity is determined by simple superimposition of the drawings. The angular deformity in both planes is measured with use of the values of these projected angles; the true angle of deformity and the orientation of the deformity in space are calculated with use of established tables.[19] In contrast, rotational deformity is determined by inspecting the relationship of the bicipital tuberosity to the radial styloid and the relationship of the coronoid process to the ulnar styloid. The exact degree of radial and ulnar torsion is measured by comparing the CT or MRI scans of the two forearms. The bicipital tuberosity and the square section of the radius at the level of the Lister tubercle are used to determine radial torsion, whereas the trochlea and the ulnar styloid are most commonly used for the ulna.[12,28] Rotational malalignment of the radius of more than 30° and rotational malalignment of the ulna of more than 20° should be corrected because these values exceed the physiologic limits of individual variations.[6]

To decide whether an opening-wedge or a closing-wedge osteotomy is suitable, the ulnar variances of the malunited and healthy sides are compared. If a single-cut closing-wedge osteotomy is performed, the wedge should include the true angle of correction. The base of the wedge is measured in millimeters and is included in the preoperative drawing. In an opening-wedge osteotomy, a variable amount of lengthening can be achieved with an interpositional bone graft, preferably a compression-resistant corticocancellous graft from the iliac crest. This graft, which may be triangular or trapezoidal in shape, should also include the true angle of deformity.

Techniques for Diaphyseal Osteotomies

The authors of this chapter prefer the Henry approach for exposure of the entire radius.[29] Proximal extension of this approach allows the surgeon to perform an anterior elbow joint arthrotomy to treat associated pathological conditions of the proximal radioulnar joint. Subperiosteal detachment of the supinator muscle and protection of the motor branch of the radial nerve are necessary for proximal osteotomies, whereas temporary release of the pronator teres may be needed for a midshaft malunion. The interval between the flexor and extensor carpi ulnaris is used to expose the ulna.

When both the radius and the ulna are malunited, the ulna should be realigned first. The radial realignment can then be "fine-tuned" to correct length and angular discrepancies to obtain accurate congruency of the radioulnar joints.

The site of the osteotomy (the apex of maximal deformity) is determined in the operating room on the basis of the distance from the distal or proximal end of the bone as measured on preoperative radiographic images. Before the osteotomy is performed, two Kirschner wires are placed to mark the exact anteroposterior and lateral planes proximal and distal to the osteotomy. A plate (usually a six- or eight-hole 3.5-mm compression plate) is temporarily fixed to the proximal fragment and is contoured to achieve the desired correction. In the middle third of the radius, shaping the plate to reconstruct the physiologic radial bow is of paramount importance.

The plate is then removed, and the base of the wedge is marked. If the angular deformity has markedly reduced the interosseous space, the scarred interosseous membrane should be released and partially resected before the osteotomy to facilitate reduction of the osteotomy. If a closing-wedge osteotomy is planned, the converging cuts are oriented in the plane of the true deformity. The osteotomy is closed with an intact periosteal hinge, and the plate is reapplied and is fixed to the distal fragment with one screw. The quality of the reduction is checked with fluoroscopy, and the amount of passive rotation is determined. If there is no substantial increase compared with the preoperative range of motion, a release of the interosseous membrane is performed. If, despite these measures, a reasonable improvement in rotation is not obtained, the radius should be derotated to achieve a balanced arc of rotation with at least 50° of pronation and 50° of supination. If bone graft is needed, interpositional corticocancellous bone blocks are preferred. If additional morcellized grafts are used, they should not be placed adjacent to the interosseous membrane because doing so increases the risk of creating a radioulnar synostosis. Associated subluxation of the distal radioulnar joint with malunion of the radial shaft (a healed Galeazzi fracture) usually does not require open reduction of the joint. Restoration of radial length and angular deformity should result in adequate congruity and stability of the joint.

Early active and passive assisted range-of-motion therapy is started on the second postoperative day. If passive motion does not reach 60% of that on the contralateral side by 4 weeks postoperatively, dynamic splinting for pronation and/or supination is started. Strengthening is started at 6 to 8 weeks after the surgery, and full weight bearing and sports are allowed once solid bone healing has been confirmed.

Techniques for Posttraumatic Chronic Radial Head Dislocations

Chronic radial head dislocations are less common in adults than they are in children, but they may be seen in a patient with a neglected initial subluxation associated with a complex high-energy forearm injury or in one with bipolar fracture-dislocations.[30-33] The most important factor responsible for chronic dislocation is insufficient reduction leading to posttraumatic ulnar shortening (Figure 2, *A*), not the loss of ligamentous restraints such as the anular ligament and the proximal part of the interosseous membrane. The discrepancy between the lengths of the radius and ulna is readily assessed by comparing radiographs of the affected and contralateral forearms. Open reduction of the radial head with simultaneous radial shortening is performed through a proximally extended Henry approach. The elongated capsule of the lateral elbow compartment is exposed between the brachioradialis and brachialis muscles after isolating and protecting the radial nerve. The proximal part of the radial shaft is exposed through subperiosteal detachment of the supinator muscle while the posterior interosseous nerve is visualized. The radius is shortened by the difference between the lengths of the ulnae on the affected and healthy sides (Figure 2, *B*). The plate is temporarily fixed with two screws into the proximal fragment. The predetermined transverse segment of bone is removed, and the plate is reapplied under compression. After the radius is shortened, the radial head usually reduces without tension against the capitellum. The elbow should be examined in full flexion, extension, and rotation to prove that the radial head is stable. Then, the capsule is closed, with resection of any excessive capsular tissue. Reconstruction of an anular ligament is not necessary if spontaneous reduction is maintained through passive range of motion.

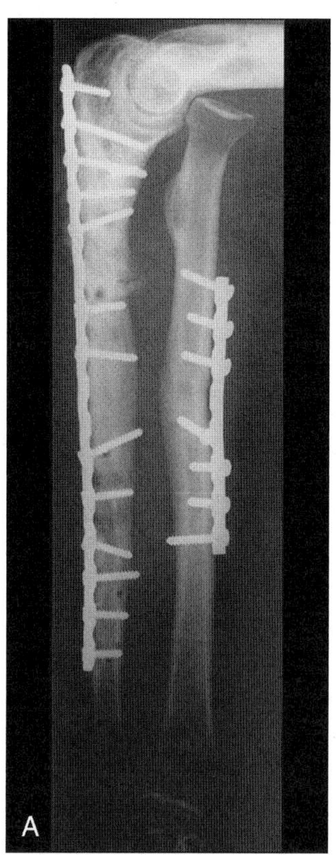

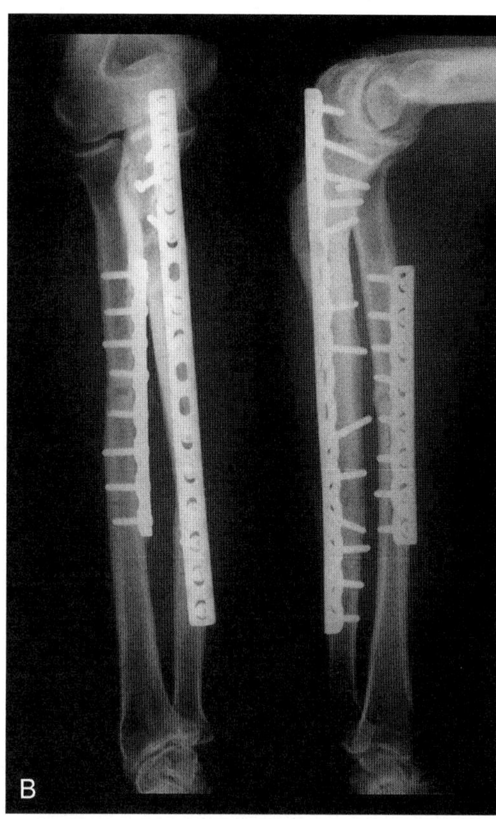

Figure 2 **A,** A radiograph of a forearm with a chronic radial head dislocation after an open both-bone forearm fracture. The ulna became infected and required multiple reoperations, which resulted in ulnar shortening. A tracing of a radiograph of the contralateral, normal forearm was used to plan an angular correction together with open reduction of the radial head. **B,** Radiographs made at 2 years show maintenance of radial head stability and uneventful healing of the radial osteotomy site.

Discussion

Several outcome studies have shown that satisfactory functional improvement can be expected after surgical correction of forearm malunions sustained in childhood.[34-37] Trousdale and Linscheid[38] reported that the results in adult patients treated within a year after the initial injury were substantially better than those in adults who were treated later. In a recent report by Nagy and associates,[19] 17 patients with a malunited forearm fracture were divided into three groups according to the clinical problem and the presentation of the deformity: (1) limitation of pronation, (2) limitation of supination, and (3) distal radioulnar joint instability. Ten patients had osteotomies of both the radius and the ulna, and seven had an osteotomy of the radius alone. The interosseous membrane was released in nine patients. Bone healing was uneventful in all cases, and no complications, infections, refractures, or synostoses occurred. Sixteen of the 17 patients reported subjective improvement, whereas 1 patient needed a repeat osteotomy to treat a residual symptomatic deformity and then had improvement as well. Patients with limited supination had better functional improvement after the osteotomy than did those with limited pronation. Stability of the distal radioulnar joint was restored after skeletal realignment of the radius without adjuvant ligament reconstruction, and release of the interosseous membrane did not impair function, including strength and stability.

Free Vascularized Fibular Grafting for Reconstruction of the Forearm Axis

General Reconstructive Options

The management of diaphyseal skeletal defects of the forearm is a complex, often multistage process, and vascularized fibular transfer has proven to be an effective reconstructive procedure in this setting.[39-44] Defects of less than 6 cm can be successfully treated with cancellous autograft or allograft, although this approach is less predictable in the presence of infection or following radiation therapy.[44,45] Alternatively, external fixation with bone transport works well and can be used to treat gaps of up to 3 cm, but the external fixation usually must be in place for several months and is fraught with complications such as infection and stiffness.[46,47] An additional reconstructive option for segmental bone loss is the creation of a one-bone forearm, but this eliminates all fore arm rotation and should be considered a final salvage option.[48,49]

Free bone transfer with microsurgical anastomoses is technically challenging and is associated with some donor site morbidity but has several distinct advantages.[50-52] Vascularized grafts heal rapidly, and periosteal new bone formation begins early irrespective of graft length. In contrast, nonvascularized grafts must undergo revascularization and creeping substitution before they are fully consolidated.[53,54] Because of its size and cortical nature, a free vascularized fibular graft is the treatment of choice for large segmental defects of the forearm.[50,55,56] Up to 26 cm of the fibula on a single vascular pedicle is available for reconstruction.[57]

In the presence of associated soft-tissue defects in the forearm, a skin paddle of up to 10 × 20 cm can be transferred with the fibula. This skin pedicle is based on the peroneal artery, and a 6 × 7-cm graft based on each septal perforator can be transferred with the fibula as an osteoseptocutaneous flap for single-stage reconstruction of combined skeletal and soft-tissue defects in the forearm.[44,50,55,58-61] The skin paddle also serves as a means of monitoring the vascular status of the graft.[60]

Osteoseptocutaneous Free Vascularized Fibular Flaps

The vascular pedicle of the vascularized fibular osteoseptocutaneous flap is the peroneal artery.[55,56] The artery has two venae comitantes and lies in the posterior compartment of the leg between the tibialis posterior and flexor hallucis longus muscles.

Clinical and cadaver evidence suggests that the best location for the skin paddle is at the junction of the middle and distal thirds of the fibula, 8 to 12 cm proximal to the ankle mortise, where the most consistent supramalleolar septocutaneous perforator is located.[62]

Preoperative angiography of the lower limb is not recommended routinely but is recommended for patients with atherosclerosis or symptoms of vascular insufficiency. Angiography of the recipient upper extremity, especially when there has been trauma or previous surgery, is indicated to establish the pedicle length that will be needed. An abnormal result of the Allen test should also prompt angiography. When planning the length of the fibular graft, one should err on the side of a longer graft. Achieving an appropriate final length is critical for alignment of the distal radioulnar joint, and it is much easier to trim excess bone than to make up for a residual deficit in length.

The procedure is preferably done with the patient under general anesthesia because of its anticipated duration, but the use of a supplementary regional blockade of the donor or recipient limb can assist with postoperative pain control. The patient is placed in the lateral decubitus position, with the involved upper limb lying on a hand table and the contralateral donor leg up. The arm should be prepared to the axilla, and a sterile tourniquet is used. The donor leg should be prepared to the groin, with sufficient space left for a skin-graft harvest from the proximal part of the thigh, if necessary.

A two-team approach with simultaneous preparation of the recipient site and harvest at the donor site is recommended. The radial artery should be used when possible, as it is usually not the primary source of blood flow to the hand. Two recipient veins should be identified and prepared as well.

Although up to 26 cm of viable fibular bone can be harvested, it is preferable to leave 8 to 10 cm of the fibula distally to maintain ankle stability, and 7 cm is left proximally for protection of the peroneal nerve. The specific surgical techniques of harvesting the osteocutaneous fibular transfer have been thoroughly described.[50,58-61]

Before the vascular anastomoses in the forearm are performed, the fibular graft should be placed in its expected final position and a PA radiograph of the wrist in neutral rotation should be made to verify anatomic restoration of the forearm axis, ulnar variance, and congruity of the distal radioulnar joint. Stable fixation is then achieved with small-fragment compression plates. This can be done by either direct fixation with a compression plate of the site of a transverse osteotomy or conversion to a step-cut osteotomy. Standard microvascular anastomoses of one artery and two veins are done.

The patients are encouraged to move their toes and ankle and are permitted partial weight bearing when comfortable up to 6 weeks after surgery. Passive stretching of the great toe is important because it is prone to the development of flexion contractures. The forearm and elbow are immobilized in a sugar tong splint or long arm cast until there is radiographic evidence of union.

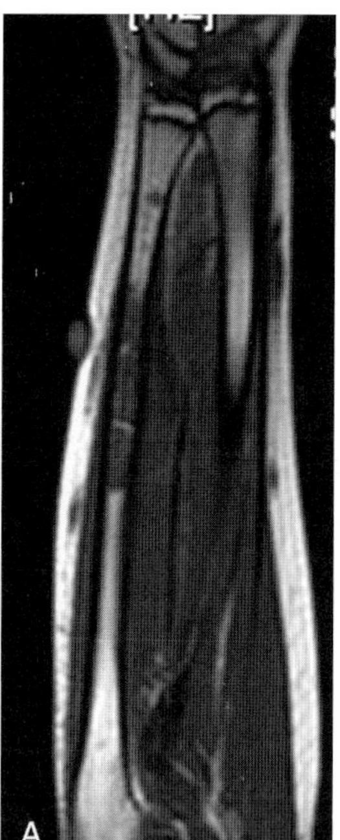

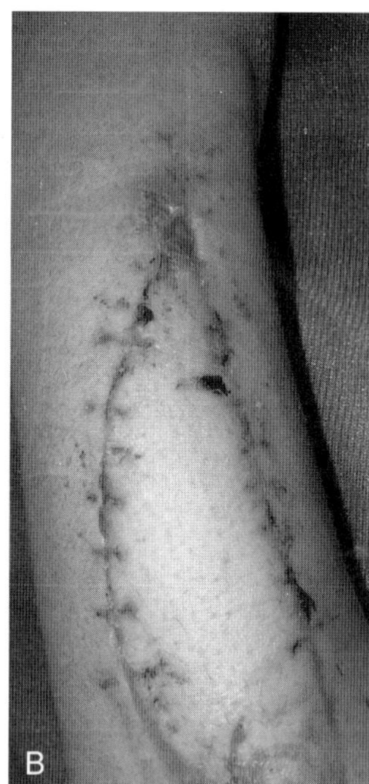

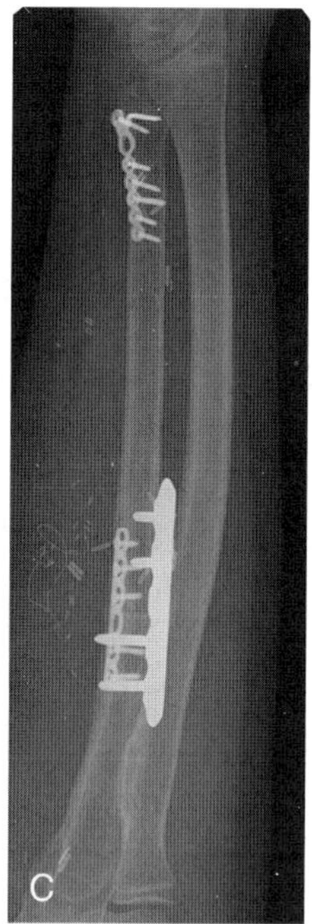

Figure 3 **A,** A coronal T1-weighted non–fat-suppression magnetic resonance scan of a 15-year-old boy with Ewing sarcoma of the ulna who underwent a wide resection that resulted in a 14-cm ulnar defect and a 4 × 6-cm soft-tissue defect. **B,** An osteoseptocutaneous fibular flap (including the fibula, soft tissue, and skin) was used to reconstruct the defect. **C,** A radiograph of the forearm after the vascularized fibular graft had healed.

Results

The reconstruction of defects caused by trauma, infection, and tumor have been reported to have encouraging results, with times to union of approximately 4 months.[63-66] Adani and associates[39] reported that 11 of 12 patients with a posttraumatic forearm defect, ranging from 6 to 13 cm in length, had successful union at a mean of 4.8 months. Two patients required additional bone grafting to achieve consolidation, and an osteoseptocutaneous flap was used in four patients. Jupiter and associates[50] used an osteoseptocutaneous fibular flap to treat nine patients with a large defect of the radius and an associated soft-tissue defect (Figure 3). The mean radial defect was 7.9 cm, and the soft-tissue defect averaged 11.8 × 5.9 cm. All cutaneous flaps survived, and all but one patient obtained osseous union at both host-graft junctions. There were no donor site complications. Kumar and associates[67] treated seven patients (five with a tumor and two with an infection) with application of a free vascularized fibular flap to the forearm. The mean time to union was 3.8 months. There were two nonunions, one of which was converted to a one-bone forearm and the other of which was not treated. Safoury[68] treated 18 patients with application of a free vascularized fibular graft to the forearm to bridge a posttraumatic segmental defect (mean, 17 cm) and reported a 100% rate of union at a mean of 4 months.

Donor site morbidity is not frequent after treatment with a fibular flap, but gait analysis has shown decreased walking velocity in comparison with control values.[68,69] Ankle valgus is a potential problem in children, and screw stabilization of the distal tibiofibular syndesmosis has been recommended.[43,70] Ankle malalignment or instability has not been a problem in adults.[71] Decreased motion and strength of the great toe have also been observed. The chapter authors believe that avoiding tight closure of the flexor hallucis and peroneal muscles and the skin interval helps to prevent this problem. Complications at the recipient site include nonunion, fracture of the graft, and thrombosis of the vascular pedicle.[41,50]

Diaphyseal Nonunions of the Forearm

Contemporary treatment of diaphyseal fractures of the radius and ulna with stable plate and screw fixation

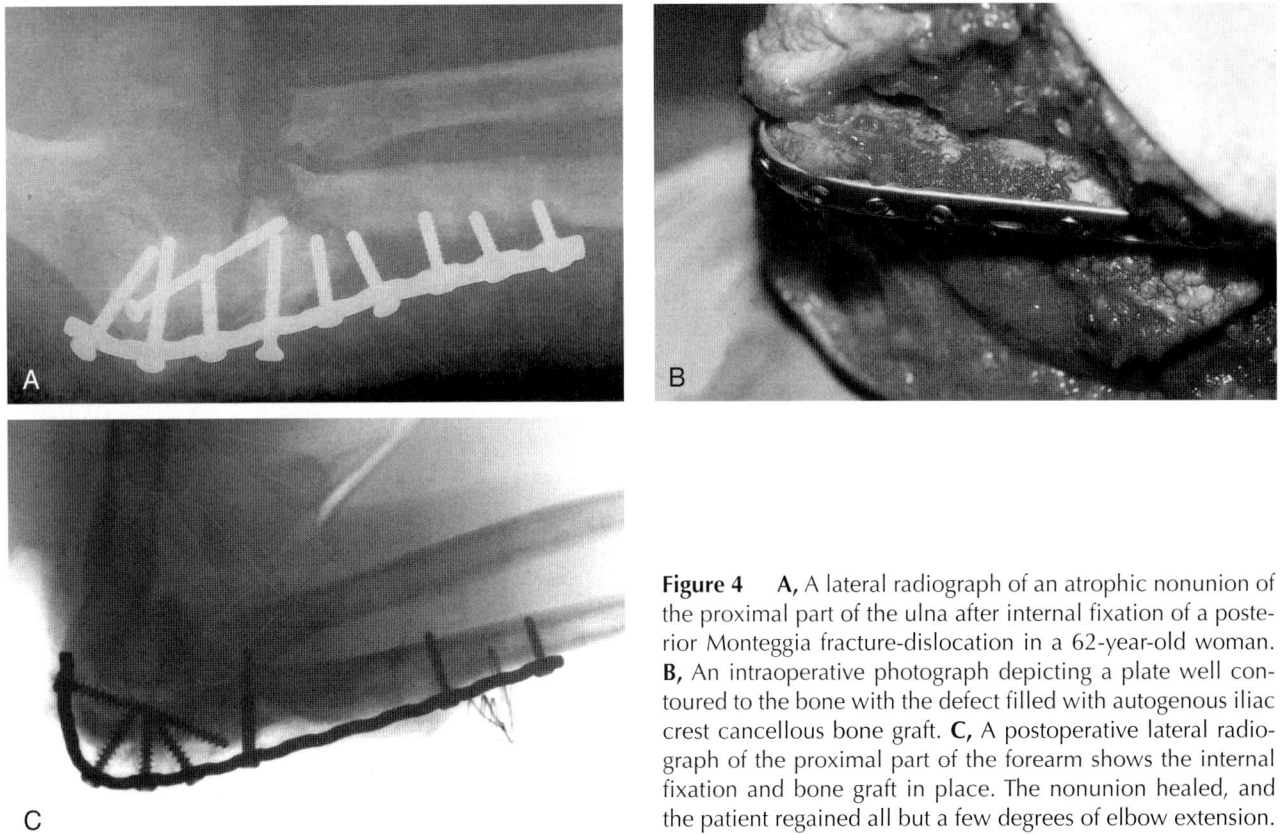

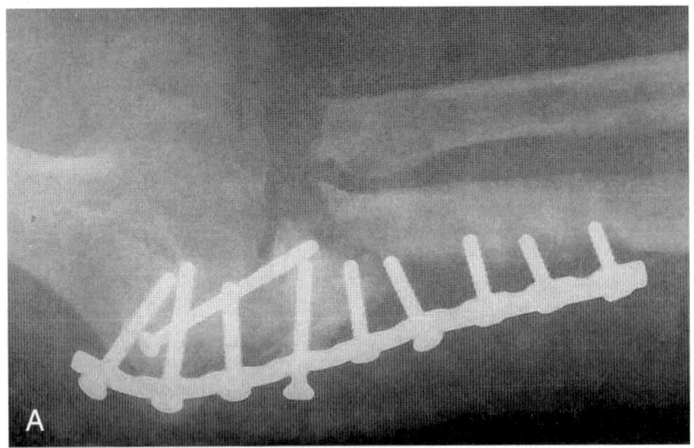

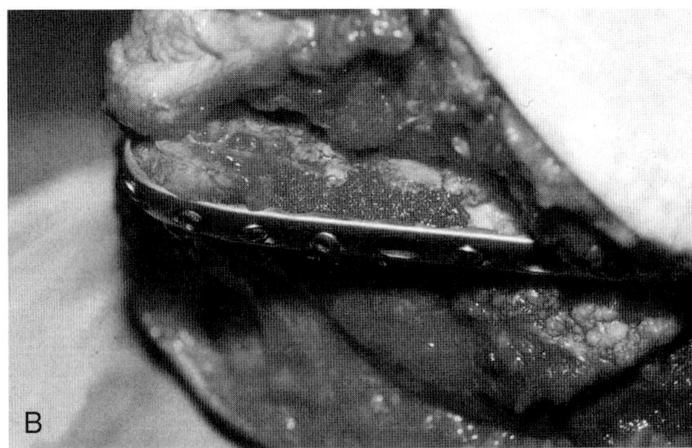

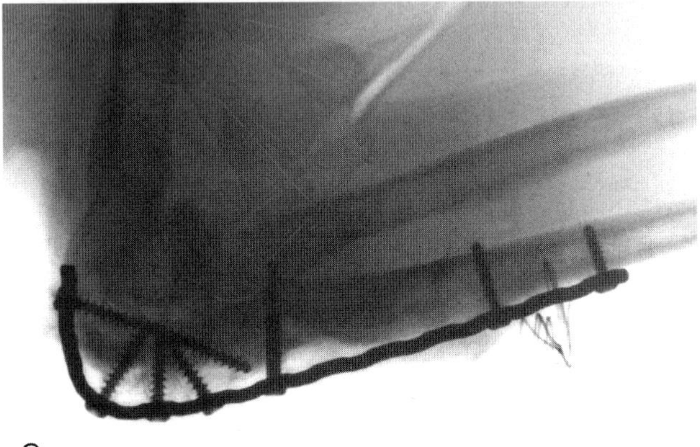

Figure 4 **A,** A lateral radiograph of an atrophic nonunion of the proximal part of the ulna after internal fixation of a posterior Monteggia fracture-dislocation in a 62-year-old woman. **B,** An intraoperative photograph depicting a plate well contoured to the bone with the defect filled with autogenous iliac crest cancellous bone graft. **C,** A postoperative lateral radiograph of the proximal part of the forearm shows the internal fixation and bone graft in place. The nonunion healed, and the patient regained all but a few degrees of elbow extension.

has led to nonunion rates of less than 5%.[72-75] When nonunion occurs, it is generally the result of a complex injury, a complication such as infection, or inadequate internal fixation.[72,73,76-78] Hypertrophic nonunions, characterized radiographically by abundant callus formation, are the result of inadequate mechanical stability of the fracture, usually after nonsurgical treatment or treatment with an intramedullary device.[79] Atrophic nonunions, characterized radiographically by tapering of the bones at the fracture without callus formation, lack both the biologic capacity to heal and adequate mechanical stability. These nonunions are related to loss of bone at the time of débridement of an open fracture, an infection, or an unexplained lack of healing capacity by the patient (Figure 4).

The treatment should restore the length and alignment of the diaphyseal segment, which in turn restores the radioulnar articulations and forearm rotation.[9] Successful treatment is based on stable plate fixation combined with the use of intercalary structural grafts, autogenous cancellous grafts, or a vascularized fibular graft.[50,80-85]

Ring and associates[78] reviewed the experience with 35 diaphyseal atrophic nonunions treated over a 15-year period by two surgeons using 3.5-mm compression plates and autogenous cancellous bone grafting. A segmental osseous defect, averaging 2 cm (range, 1 to 6 cm) in length, was present in each case. Twenty of the original fractures had been open injuries, and a deep infection had developed in association with 11 of them. The nonunion involved the radius alone in 16 patients, the ulna alone in 11, and both bones in 8. The 3.5-mm plates had an average of nine holes, and autogenous cancellous bone graft was used to fill the defect in each patient. All fractures healed within 6 months without additional intervention. Two patients required a subsequent resection of the distal end of the ulna for the treatment of arthritis of the distal radioulnar joint. After an average of 43 months, the average final arc of forearm rotation was 121°, and the average grip strength was 83% of that on the contralateral side. According to the criteria of Anderson and associates,[73] 5 patients had an excellent result; 18, a satisfactory result; 11, an unsatisfactory result (3 because of associated elbow injuries and 8 because of wrist stiffness); and 1, a poor result (cause by residual deformity).

Summary

The assessment and management of adverse sequelae of traumatic injury to the forearm can be exceedingly complex. The loss of forearm rotation has a substantial impact on effective function of the entire upper limb. The problems can include diaphyseal deformity, bone or soft-tissue loss, or a failure to heal—either alone or often in combination. Careful preoperative planning is essential to accurately define the extent and location of the clinical problem, establish a precise surgical plan, and better inform the patient regarding the risks and goals of the procedure.

References

1. Kapandji IA: Physiologie articulaire: Schémas commentés de mécanique humaine. *La Prono-Supination*, ed 6. Paris, France, Maloine, 2005, pp 104-115.
2. Rose-Innes AP: Anterior dislocation of the ulna at the inferior radio-ulnar joint: Case report, with a discussion of the anatomy of rotation of the forearm. *J Bone Joint Surg Br* 1960;42-B: 515-521.
3. Djbay HC: L'humerus dans la pronosupination. *Rev Med Limoges* 1972;3: 147-150.
4. Hotchkiss RN, An KN, Sowa DT, Basta S, Weiland AJ: An anatomic and mechanical study of the interosseous membrane of the forearm: Pathomechanics of proximal migration of the radius. *J Hand Surg Am* 1989;14 (2 Pt 1):256-261.
5. Rabinowitz RS, Light TR, Havey RM, et al: The role of the interosseous membrane and triangular fibrocartilage complex in forearm stability. *J Hand Surg Am* 1994;19:385-393.
6. Poitevin LA: Anatomy and biomechanics of the interosseous membrane: Its importance in the longitudinal stability of the forearm. *Hand Clin* 2001;17:97-110, vii.
7. Ofuchi S, Takahashi K, Yamagata M, Rokkaku T, Moriya H, Hara T: Pressure distribution in the humeroradial joint and force transmission to the capitellum during rotation of the forearm: Effects of the Sauvé-Kapandji procedure and incision of the interosseous membrane. *J Orthop Sci* 2001;6:33-38.
8. Stern PJ, Drury WJ: Complications of plate fixation of forearm fractures. *Clin Orthop Relat Res* 1983;175:25-29.
9. Schemitsch EH, Richards RR: The effect of malunion on functional outcome after plate fixation of fractures of both bones of the forearm in adults. *J Bone Joint Surg Am* 1992;74: 1068-1078.
10. Graham TJ, Fischer TJ, Hotchkiss RN, Kleinman WB: Disorders of the forearm axis. *Hand Clin* 1998;14: 305-316.
11. Dumont CE, Nagy L, Ziegler D, Pfirrmann CW: Fluoroscopic and magnetic resonance cross-sectional imaging assessments of radial and ulnar torsion profiles in volunteers. *J Hand Surg Am* 2007;32:501-509.
12. Dumont CE, Pfirrmann CW, Ziegler D, Nagy L: Assessment of radial and ulnar torsion profiles with cross-sectional magnetic resonance imaging: A study of volunteers. *J Bone Joint Surg Am* 2006;88:1582-1588.
13. Jupiter JB, Ruder J, Roth DA: Computer-generated bone models in the planning of osteotomy of multidirectional distal radius malunions. *J Hand Surg Am* 1992;17:406-415.
14. Sarmiento A, Ebramzadeh E, Brys D, Tarr R: Angular deformities and forearm function. *J Orthop Res* 1992;10: 121-133.
15. Matthews LS, Kaufer H, Garver DF, Sonstegard DA: The effect on supination-pronation of angular malalignment of fractures of both bones of the forearm. *J Bone Joint Surg Am* 1982;64:14-17.
16. Tynan MC, Fornalski S, McMahon PJ, Utkan A, Green SA, Lee TQ: The effects of ulnar axial malalignment on supination and pronation. *J Bone Joint Surg Am* 2000;82:1726-1731.
17. Tarr RR, Garfinkel AI, Sarmiento A: The effects of angular and rotational deformities of both bones of the forearm: An in vitro study. *J Bone Joint Surg Am* 1984;66:65-70.
18. Dumont CE, Thalmann R, Macy JC: The effect of rotational malunion of the radius and the ulna on supination and pronation. *J Bone Joint Surg Br* 2002;84:1070-1074.
19. Nagy L, Jankauskas L, Dumont CE: Correction of forearm malunion guided by the preoperative complaint. *Clin Orthop Relat Res* 2008;466:1419-1428.
20. Hughston JC: Fracture of the distal radial shaft: Mistakes in management. *J Bone Joint Surg Am* 1957;39:249-264.
21. Bowers WH: Instability of the distal radioulnar articulation. *Hand Clin* 1991;7:311-327.
22. Merle R, Descamps L: Plane oblique osteotomy in correction of deformities of the extremities. *Mem Adac Chir (Paris)* 1952;78:271-276.
23. Saffar P: Ulna oblique osteotomy for radius and ulna length inequality: Technique and applications. *Tech Hand Up Extrem Surg* 2006;10:47-53.
24. Sangeorzan BP, Judd RP, Sangeorzan BJ: Mathematical analysis of single-cut osteotomy for complex long bone deformity. *J Biomech* 1989; 22:1271-1278.
25. Meyer DC, Siebenrock KA, Schiele B, Gerber C: A new methodology for the planning of single-cut corrective osteotomies of mal-aligned long bones. *Clin Biomech (Bristol, Avon)* 2005;20:223-227.
26. Nagy L: Malunion of the distal end of the radius, in Fernandez DL, Jupiter JB, eds: *Fractures of the Distal Radius: A Practical Approach to Management*, ed 2. New York, NY, Springer, 2002, pp 289-344.
27. McNamara M, Munoz A: Alaskan three-dimensional osteotomy: Surgical correction for long bone malunions. *J Hand Surg Am* 2008;33: 776-779.

28. Bindra RR, Cole RJ, Yamaguchi K, et al: Quantification of the radial torsion angle with computerized tomography in cadaver specimens. *J Bone Joint Surg Am* 1997;79:833-837.

29. Henry AK: *Extensile Exposure Applied to Limb Surgery*. Edinburgh, United Kingdom, Livingstone, 1945, pp 59-65.

30. Bouyala JM, Bollini G, Jacquemier M, et al: The treatment of old dislocations of the radial head in children by osteotomy of the upper end of the ulna: Apropos of 15 cases. *Rev Chir Orthop Reparatrice Appar Mot* 1988;74:173-182.

31. Inoue G, Shionoya K: Corrective ulnar osteotomy for malunited anterior Monteggia lesions in children: 12 patients followed for 1-12 years. *Acta Orthop Scand* 1998;69:73-76.

32. Hasler CC, Von Laer L, Hell AK: Open reduction, ulnar osteotomy and external fixation for chronic anterior dislocation of the head of the radius. *J Bone Joint Surg Br* 2005;87:88-94.

33. Freedman L, Luk K, Leong JC: Radial head reduction after a missed Monteggia fracture: Brief report. *J Bone Joint Surg Br* 1988;70:846-847.

34. Blackburn N, Ziv I, Rang M: Correction of the malunited forearm fracture. *Clin Orthop Relat Res* 1984;188:54-57.

35. Meier R, Prommersberger KJ, Lanz U: Surgical correction of malunited fractures of the forearm in children. *Z Orthop Ihre Grenzgeb* 2003;141:328-335.

36. Price CT, Knapp DR: Osteotomy for malunited forearm shaft fractures in children. *J Pediatr Orthop* 2006;26:193-196.

37. van Geenen RC, Besselaar PP: Outcome after corrective osteotomy for malunited fractures of the forearm sustained in childhood. *J Bone Joint Surg Br* 2007;89:236-239.

38. Trousdale RT, Linscheid RL: Operative treatment of malunited fractures of the forearm. *J Bone Joint Surg Am* 1995;77:894-902.

39. Adani R, Delcroix L, Innocenti M, et al: Reconstruction of large posttraumatic skeletal defects of the forearm by vascularized free fibular graft. *Microsurgery* 2004;24:423-429.

40. Olekas J, Guobys A: Vascularised bone transfer for defects and pseudarthroses of forearm bones. *J Hand Surg Br* 1991;16:406-408.

41. Heitmann C, Levin LS: Applications of the vascularized fibula for upper extremity reconstruction. *Tech Hand Up Extrem Surg* 2003;7:12-17.

42. Giessler GA, Bickert B, Sauerbier M, Germann G: Free microvascular fibula graft for skeletal reconstruction after tumor resections in the forearm: Experience with five cases. *Handchir Mikrochir Plast Chir* 2004;36:301-307.

43. Bae DS, Waters PM, Sampson CE: Use of free vascularized fibular graft for congenital ulnar pseudarthrosis: Surgical decision making in the growing child. *J Pediatr Orthop* 2005;25:755-762.

44. Kremer T, Bickert B, Germann G, Heitmann C, Sauerbier M: Outcome assessment after reconstruction of complex defects of the forearm and hand with osteocutaneous free flaps. *Plast Reconstr Surg* 2006;118:443-456.

45. Hurst LC, Mirza MA, Spellman W: Vascularized fibular graft for infected loss of the ulna: Case report. *J Hand Surg Am* 1982;7:498-501.

46. Emara KM: Ilizarov technique in management of nonunited fracture of both bones of the forearm. *J Orthop Traumatol* 2002;3:177-180.

47. Grishin IG, Golubev VG, Goncharenko IV, Evgrafov AV, Kafarov FM: Transfer of free vascularized bone and skin-bone autografts: Experiences in the application of external fixation apparatus. *J Reconstr Microsurg* 1990;6:1-11.

48. Peterson CA II, Maki S, Wood MB: Clinical results of the one-bone forearm. *J Hand Surg Am* 1995;20:609-618.

49. Castle ME: One-bone forearm. *J Bone Joint Surg Am* 1974;56:1223-1227.

50. Jupiter JB, Gerhard HJ, Guerrero J, Nunley JA, Levin LS: Treatment of segmental defects of the radius with use of the vascularized osteoseptocutaneous fibular autogenous graft. *J Bone Joint Surg Am* 1997;79:542-550.

51. Brown KL: Limb reconstruction with vascularized fibular grafts after bone tumor resection. *Clin Orthop Relat Res* 1991;262:64-73.

52. Doi K, Tominaga S, Shibata T: Bone grafts with microvascular anastomoses of vascular pedicles: An experimental study in dogs. *J Bone Joint Surg Am* 1977;59:809-815.

53. Moore JB, Mazur JM, Zehr D, Davis PK, Zook EG: A biomechanical comparison of vascularized and conventional autogenous bone grafts. *Plast Reconstr Surg* 1984;73:382-386.

54. Enneking WF, Eady JL, Burchardt H: Autogenous cortical bone grafts in the reconstruction of segmental skeletal defects. *J Bone Joint Surg Am* 1980;62:1039-1058.

55. Stevanovic M, Gutow AP, Sharpe F: The management of bone defects of the forearm after trauma. *Hand Clin* 1999;15:299-318.

56. del Piñal F, Innocenti M: Evolving concepts in the management of the bone gap in the upper limb: Long and small defects. *J Plast Reconstr Aesthet Surg* 2007;60:776-792.

57. Jones NF, Swartz WM, Mears DC, Jupiter JB, Grossman A: The "double barrel" free vascularized fibular bone graft. *Plast Reconstr Surg* 1988;81:378-385.

58. Minami A, Usui M, Ogino T, Minami M: Simultaneous reconstruction of bone and skin defects by free fibular graft with a skin flap. *Microsurgery* 1986;7:38-45.

59. Chen ZW, Yan W: The study and clinical application of the osteocutaneous flap of fibula. *Microsurgery* 1983;4:11-16.

60. Yoshimura M, Shimamura K, Iwai Y, Yamauchi S, Ueno T: Free vascularized fibular transplant: A new method for monitoring circulation of the grafted fibula. *J Bone Joint Surg Am* 1983;65:1295-1301.

61. Harrison DH: The osteocutaneous free fibular graft. *J Bone Joint Surg Br* 1986;68:804-807.

62. Beppu M, Hanel DP, Johnston GH, Carmo JM, Tsai TM: The osteocutaneous fibula flap: An anatomic study. *J Reconstr Microsurg* 1992;8:215-223.

63. Sellers DS, Sowa DT, Moore JR, Weiland AJ: Congenital pseudarthrosis of the forearm. *J Hand Surg Am* 1988;13:89-93.

64. Witoonchart K, Uerpairojkit C, Leechavengvongs S, Thuvasethakul P: Congenital pseudarthrosis of the forearm treated by free vascularized fibular graft: A report of three cases and a review of the literature. *J Hand Surg Am* 1999;24:1045-1055.

65. Zaretski A, Amir A, Meller I, et al: Free fibula long bone reconstruction in orthopedic oncology: A surgical algorithm for reconstructive options. *Plast Reconstr Surg* 2004;113:1989-2000.

66. Minami A, Kasashima T, Iwasaki N, Kato H, Kaneda K: Vascularised fibular grafts: An experience of 102 patients. *J Bone Joint Surg Br* 2000;82:1022-1025.

67. Kumar VP, Satku K, Helm R, Pho RW: Radial reconstruction in segmental defects of both forearm bones. *J Bone Joint Surg Br* 1988;70:815-817.

68. Safoury Y: Free vascularized fibula for the treatment of traumatic bone defects and nonunion of the forearm bones. *J Hand Surg Br* 2005;30:67-72.

69. Bodde EW, de Visser E, Duysens JE, Hartman EH: Donor-site morbidity after free vascularized autogenous fibular transfer: Subjective and quantitative analyses. *Plast Reconstr Surg* 2003;111:2237-2242.

70. Germain MA, Mascard E, Dubousset J, Nguefack M: Free vascularized fibula and reconstruction of long bones in the child: Our evolution. *Microsurgery* 2007;27:415-419.

71. Lee EH, Goh JC, Helm R, Pho RW: Donor site morbidity following resection of the fibula. *J Bone Joint Surg Br* 1990;72:129-131.

72. Chapman MW, Gordon JE, Zissimos AG: Compression-plate fixation of acute fractures of the diaphyses of the radius and ulna. *J Bone Joint Surg Am* 1989;71:159-169.

73. Anderson LD, Sisk D, Tooms RE, Park WI III: Compression-plate fixation in acute diaphyseal fractures of the radius and ulna. *J Bone Joint Surg Am* 1975;57:287.

74. Wright RR, Schmeling GJ, Schwab JP: The necessity of acute bone grafting in diaphyseal forearm fractures: A retrospective review. *J Orthop Trauma* 1997;11:288-294.

75. Wei SY, Born CT, Abene A, Ong A, Hayda R, DeLong WG Jr: Diaphyseal forearm fractures treated with and without bone graft. *J Trauma* 1999;46:1045-1048.

76. Langkamer VG, Ackroyd CE: Internal fixation of forearm fractures in the 1980s: Lessons to be learnt. *Injury* 1991;22:97-102.

77. Jupiter JB, Rüedi T: Intraoperative distraction in the treatment of complex nonunions of the radius. *J Hand Surg Am* 1992;17:416-422.

78. Ring D, Allende C, Jafarnia K, Allende BT, Jupiter JB: Ununited diaphyseal forearm fractures with segmental defects: Plate fixation and autogenous cancellous bone-grafting. *J Bone Joint Surg Am* 2004;86:2440-2445.

79. Sage FP: Medullary fixation of fractures of the forearm: A study of the medullary canal of the radius and a report of fifty fractures of the radius treated with a prebent triangular nail. *J Bone Joint Surg Am* 1959;41:1489-1516.

80. Barbieri CH, Mazzer N, Aranda CA, Pinto MM: Use of a bone block graft from the iliac crest with rigid fixation to correct diaphyseal defects of the radius and ulna. *J Hand Surg Br* 1997;22:395-401.

81. Dabezies EJ, Stewart WE, Goodman FG, Deffer PA: Management of segmental defects of the radius and ulna. *J Trauma* 1971;11:778-788.

82. Grace TG, Eversmann WW Jr: The management of segmental bone loss associated with forearm fractures. *J Bone Joint Surg Am* 1980;62:1150-1155.

83. Miller RC, Phalen GS: The repair of defects of the radius with fibular bone grafts. *J Bone Joint Surg Am* 1947;29:629-636.

84. Nicoll EA: The treatment of gaps in long bones by cancellous insert grafts. *J Bone Joint Surg Br* 1956;38:70-82.

85. Dell PC, Sheppard JE: Vascularized bone grafts in the treatment of infected forearm nonunions. *J Hand Surg Am* 1984;9:653-658.

Disorders of the Distal Radioulnar Joint

Peter M. Murray, MD
Julie E. Adams, MD
Jonathan Lam, MD, PhD
A. Lee Osterman, MD
Scott Wolfe, MD

Abstract

Disorders of the distal radioulnar joint (DRUJ) are relatively common and often associated with the triangular fibrocartilage complex. Anatomically and biomechanically, the DRUJ should be considered in the broader context of the forearm joint, which has both distal and proximal articulations. Clinical examination is the best method of evaluating trauma to the DRUJ or DRUJ instability, although the clinical appearance of disorders may be subtle and imaging studies may be difficult to interpret. Arthroscopy is the best tool for evaluating the integrity of the triangular fibrocartilage complex. Although acute and chronic disorders of the triangular fibrocartilage complex can be treated arthroscopically, chronic DRUJ instability may require tenodesis reconstruction. Salvage of a DRUJ with degenerative arthritis generally requires resection arthrodesis. Implant arthroplasty has recently received attention, but further scrutiny of mid- and long-term results is needed.

Instr Course Lect 2010;59:295-311.

The higher order primates and hominids are distinguished by three evolutionary traits: a large brain, a prehensile thumb, and forearm rotation. Two of these traits are found in the upper extremity. Forearm and wrist function can be severely affected by dysfunction of the distal radioulnar joint (DRUJ), which is relatively common as the result of a developmental condition, trauma, or degenerative arthritis. Historically, treatment largely has been limited to resection of part or all of the ulnar head, which places the forearm at risk for instability, weakness, and pain.[1,2] Soft-tissue stabilization has been unreliable, although recent procedures are promising.[3,4] A salvage conversion to a one-bone forearm may be necessary for some patients.[5]

Dr. Murray or an immediate family member is a member of a speakers' bureau or has made paid presentations on behalf of SBI. Dr. Wolfe or an immediate family member is a member of a speakers' bureau or has made paid presentations on behalf of Trimed and Small Bone Innovations; serves as a paid consultant to or is an employee of Extremity Medical; and serves as an unpaid consultant to Trimed. Dr. Osterman or an immediate family member serves as a board member, owner, officer, or committee member of the American Society for Surgery of the Hand and the American Association for Hand Surgery; is a member of a speakers' bureau or has made paid presentations on behalf of SBI and Auxilium; serves as an unpaid consultant to Biomet, Medartis, and Trimed; and has received research or institutuional support from Synthes. Neither of the following authors nor any immediate family members have received anything of value from or own stock in a commercial company or institution related directly or indirectly to the subject of this chapter: Dr. Adams and Dr. Lam.

Anatomy and Biomechanics of the DRUJ

Anatomy

The radius and ulna articulate through the proximal and distal radioulnar joints, which together are called the forearm joint. The DRUJ is composed of the sigmoid notch of the distal radius and the ulnar head, which has an inherent ability to provide stability from the bony dorsal and cartilaginous volar rims of its notch.[6] Approximately 30% of DRUJ constraint is created by the articular contact of the ulnar head with the sigmoid notch.

The sigmoid notch is a shallow, concave articular surface at the ulnar surface of the radial epiphysis. Tolat and associates[7] described four possible configurations of the sigmoid

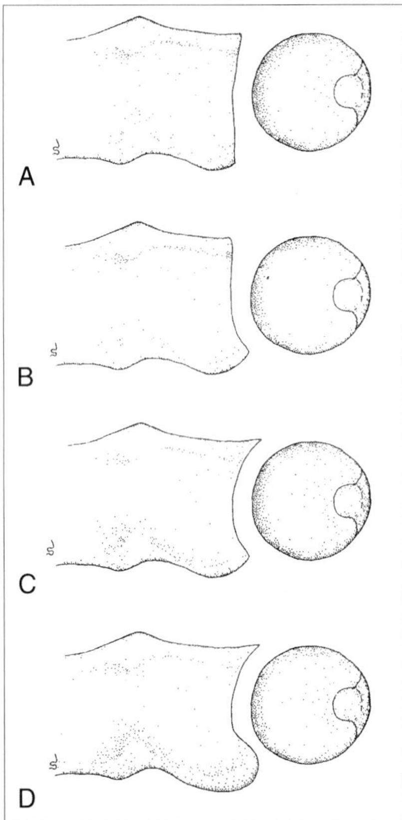

Figure 1 Schematic diagram showing the four possible shapes of the sigmoid notch: flat face **(A)**, ski slope **(B)**, C type **(C)**, and S type **(D)**. The configuration of the sigmoid notch can affect DRUJ stability. (Adapted with permission from Tolat AR, Stanley JK, Trail IA: A cadaveric study of the anatomy and stability of the distal radioulnar joint in the coronal and transverse planes. *J Hand Surg Br* 1996;21:592.)

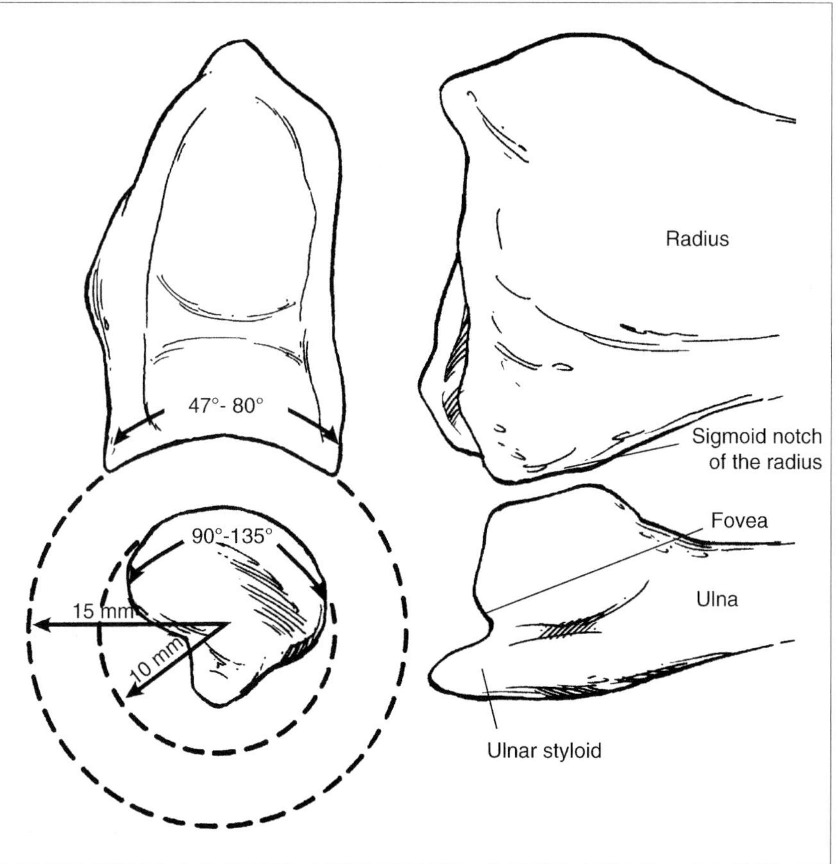

Figure 2 **A,** Axial view of the distal radius and ulna. The radius of the circle subtended by the sigmoid notch is greater than the radius of the circle subtended by the ulnar head articular surface, creating an incongruent joint. **B,** The distal radius and the distal ulna shown from the posterior perspective.

notch: flat face, ski slope, C type, and S type. The configuration can influence the stability of the DRUJ (Figure 1). The ulnar head is a cylindrical expansion of the distal ulna, and three quarters of its surface is covered in articular cartilage. The distal projection of the ulnar head is called the ulnar styloid process; the depression at the base of the styloid process is the fovea, which is nonarticular. The radius of curvature of the sigmoid notch is considerably greater than the radius of curvature of the ulnar head (Figure 2).

The triangular fibrocartilage complex (TFCC) is the primary soft-tissue stabilizer of the DRUJ. The TFCC is composed of the dorsal and volar radioulnar ligaments, the articular disk, the ulnotriquetral and ulnolunate ligaments, and the extensor carpi ulnaris subsheath (Figure 3). The dorsal radioulnar ligament originates from the dorsal articular margin of the sigmoid notch and tracks at a 45° angle, inserting at the fovea. The volar radioulnar ligament originates from the volar edge of the sigmoid notch and tracks at a 45° angle to converge with the dorsal radioulnar ligament at the fovea. The volar radioulnar ligament and the dorsal radioulnar ligament form a conjoined ligament that inserts into the fovea. The fibrocartilaginous articular disk lies between and in discontinuity with the dorsal and volar radioulnar ligaments. The thickness of the articular disk is directly proportional to the amount of ulnar minus variance.[8] The dorsal and volar DRUJ capsule is redundant, permitting the natural translation of the radius relative to the ulna during pronation and supination, which occurs because of the incongruent articular surfaces of the DRUJ. The extensor carpi ulnaris subsheath provides another constraint to separation of the ulna and radius at the DRUJ.

The anterior interosseous artery and the ulnar artery supply blood to the TFCC.[9] The dorsal and palmar branches of the anterior interosseous artery supply the dorsal and volar aspects, respectively, of the radial portion of the TFCC articular disk, as well as the dorsal and volar radioulnar ligaments. The ulnar portion of the articular disk and the foveal insertion of the dorsal and volar radioulnar ligaments are supplied by branches of the ulnar artery.[6] This vascularity provides the peripheral portion of the TFCC with an intrinsic healing ability but leaves the central 15% to 20% of the articular disk avascular and devoid of healing potential. The attachments of the dorsal and volar radioulnar ligaments at the base of the ulnar styloid are separated by richly vascularized tissue known as the ligamentum subcruentum.

The interosseous membrane, another soft tissue stabilizer of the DRUJ,[10] consists of a thin membranous portion and a thick ligamentous portion, called the central band. The central band is two to three times thicker than the membranous portion; it makes up the middle third of the structure and provides most of the strength of the interosseous membrane[10] (Figure 4). The origin of the interosseous membrane is relatively proximal on the radius, and its insertion is relatively distal on the ulna.[11]

The pronator quadratus, a dynamic stabilizer of the DRUJ, arises from the radial border of the distal radius and inserts along the ulnar border of the distal ulna just proximal to the DRUJ.[12] The pronator quadratus has deep and superficial heads; it both initiates pronation and maintains the convergence of the DRUJ.

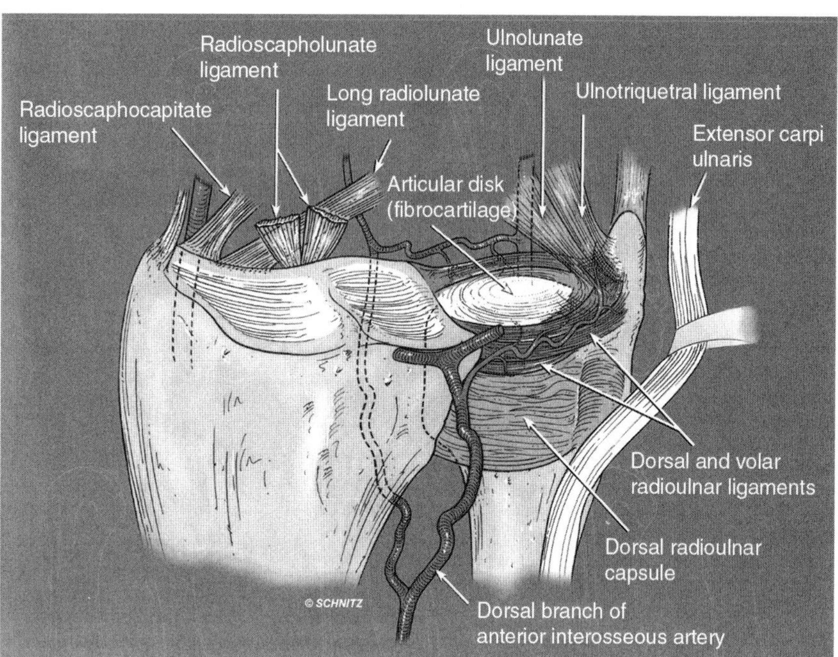

Figure 3 Schematic diagram showing the components of the TFCC. (Reproduced with permission from Kleinmann WB: Stability of the distal radioulna joint: Biomechanics, pathophysiology, physical diagnosis, and restoration of function. *J Hand Surg Am* 2007;32:1086-1087.)

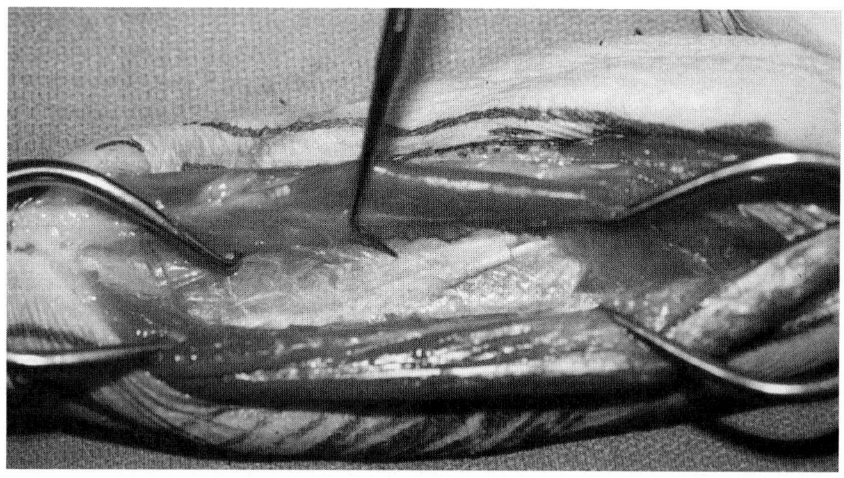

Figure 4 Photograph showing the thick central third of the interosseous membrane, which provides most of the structure's strength.

Biomechanics

The forearm essentially is a bicondylar joint articulating through the proximal and distal radioulnar joints. The axis of rotation passes obliquely from the radial head to the ulnar head, and the normal range of motion is between 150° and 180°.[6,13] The difference in the radii of curvature of the sigmoid notch and the ulnar head permits 4 to 6 mm of translation during forearm pronation and supination.[6,12,14] In pronation, the radius is translated volarly with respect to the ulnar head; in supination, the radius translates dorsally. Moore and associates[15] determined that this translation is caused by a shift in the helical axis or motion. Translation also affects the articular congruity of the joint, so that the greatest articular contact occurs with the forearm in neutral position, and the least articular contact occurs at the extremes of supination or pronation.[6] Instability of the DRUJ is conventionally described by the position of the ulna relative to the radial sigmoid notch. For example, a dorsal position of the ulna relative to the sigmoid notch is called dorsal subluxation of the DRUJ, even though the radius actually has migrated volar to the fixed ulna.

A cadaver study found that approximately 20% of the axial load across the wrist is transmitted through the ulna, and the remaining 80% is transmitted through the radius.[16] The interosseous membrane redistributes the load so that the radius and ulna share the load more equally in the proximal forearm.[11,17-20] The central band of the interosseous membrane is under peak strain with forearm pronation.[21,22] The material properties of the interosseous membrane are similar to those of the patellar tendon, and its stiffness is comparable to that of the anterior cruciate ligament.[23] As the dorsal angulation of the distal radius approaches 20°, the load transfer across the ulna reaches 67%. With increasing dorsal angulation, the incongruity of the DRUJ also increases.[24]

Although it is well accepted that the dorsal and volar radioulnar ligaments are the primary soft-tissue stabilizers of the DRUJ, debate continues as to which of these ligaments provides the primary constraint to translation during pronation or supination.[6,25-27] Biomechanical studies have used constraint testing, load-to-failure testing, and ligament tension testing. Schuind and associates[26] found that the dorsal radioulnar ligament constrains dorsal translation of the ulnar head during pronation, and the volar radioulnar ligament constrains volar translation of the ulnar head during supination. In contrast, Stuart and associates[27] found that volar radioulnar ligament tension peaks first during pronation and thereby prevents dorsal translation of the ulna; in supination, dorsal radioulnar ligament tension prevents volar translation of the ulna in a similar fashion. In patients with instability caused by incompetence of the palmar radioulnar ligament, the joint typically is unstable in pronation; with isolated disruption of the dorsal radioulnar ligament, the joint is unstable in supination.[26]

The biomechanics of the DRUJ can be summarized by three key points. Dorsal translation of the ulna is constrained by the palmar radioulnar ligament, regardless of forearm position. When the forearm is in the pronated position, volar translation of the ulna (dorsal translation of the radius) is constrained by the dorsal radioulnar ligament. When the forearm is in the supinated or neutral position, volar translation of the ulna (dorsal translation of the radius) is evenly constrained by the palmar radioulnar ligament, the dorsal radioulnar ligament, and the interosseous membrane.[26-28]

The dynamic stability of the DRUJ is provided by the pronator quadratus and the extensor carpi ulnaris tendon.[12,29] The deep and superficial heads of the pronator quadratus provide the convergence stability of the DRUJ, and the contraction of the extensor carpi ulnaris tendon and its subsheath depress the ulna palmarly. Although the interosseous membrane also provides convergence stability, it is not considered a dynamic stabilizer.

Mechanism of Injury and Diagnosis

Most DRUJ injuries result from a fall onto a hyperpronated extended wrist. The dorsal or volar radioulnar ligament fails, causing dorsal or volar dislocation or instability. DRUJ instability usually is related to a fracture of the distal radius. The fracture extends into the sigmoid notch of the distal radius, with concomitant injury to the dorsal or volar radioulnar ligament. A deformity of the distal radius also can lead to DRUJ instability. More than 20° of dorsal angulation or 7 to 10 mm of shortening can cause the TFCC to fail.[8] A fall or other high-energy mechanism of injury can cause an avulsion with detachment at the ulnar styloid base, leaving the wrist vulnerable in extension and the forearm vulnerable in pronation.

Clinical Examination

Instability of the DRUJ is more likely to appear as a dynamic, rather than fixed, deformity. If DRUJ instability is suspected, the wrist and forearm range of motion should be assessed, with attention to identifying the limits of motion, reproducing the patient's symptoms, and eliciting crepitus. Dynamic instability or a dislocation of the DRUJ can be subtle after an injury to the TFCC. Pain over the ulnar side of the wrist is worse at the extremes of forearm rotation, particularly supination. The range of motion generally is limited and painful, with weak rotational and grip strength in comparison with the normal contralateral side. There may be ulnar head asymmetry (compared with the contralateral side) as well as ulnar carpal or DRUJ tenderness. Pain can be elicited with DRUJ compression. A prominent, unstable distal ulnar head that can be reduced with ballottement of the ulna from a subluxated or dislocated position (in a manner similar to depressing the keys on a piano) represents the piano key sign. A DRUJ with the piano key sign should be compared with the contralateral side. Ulnar nerve injury may accompany a volar DRUJ dislocation. An acute dorsal dislocation may cause an obvious prominence of the distal ulna. In a patient with recurrent acute DRUJ dislocation or chronic instability appearing as a dislocating DRUJ, a characteristic clunking sound may be heard on physical examination. In dorsal dislocation, the forearm typically is fixed in pronation; in volar dislocation, the forearm is fixed in supination.[30]

In the shuck test to provoke DRUJ instability, the radius and ulna are stabilized in the examiner's hands, then stressed relative to each other in a dorsal-palmar motion. Laxity should be assessed in maximum supination, maximum pronation, and neutral position, and it should be compared with motion on the contralateral side.[31] In the push-up test, the patient rises from a seated position by supporting the body with the affected forearm. Pain suggests the presence of a TFCC tear or DRUJ instability. To rule out longitudinal instability of the forearm (the Essex-Lopresti lesion), a complete elbow examination should be done after an acute injury to the wrist in which a TFCC injury is suspected.

The clinical symptoms of chronic DRUJ instability include pain, decreased grip strength, limited mobility, and mechanical symptoms such as clicking or snapping with rotational movement of the forearm. Symptoms of mild instability may appear only with activities involving rotation of the forearm against resistance, such as using a screwdriver. Instability may appear as subluxation or recurrent dislocation of the joint during forearm rotation; these conditions are manifested by pain, loss of strength, and restricted range of motion. The examination should include identification of swelling, tenderness, and limitations on active and passive range of motion. A comparative examination of the contralateral forearm, wrist, and elbow should be done. Injury to the TFCC is suggested by the ulnar fovea sign, in which tenderness appears when pressure is applied in the depression subtended by the flexor carpi ulnaris tendon, the ulnar styloid, and the triquetrum[32] (Figure 5). Tay and associates[32] found that the ulnar fovea sign is more than 95% specific for detecting foveal or ulnotriquetral ligament disruption. Increased anteroposterior translation of the ulna within the sigmoid notch during passive manipulation (compared with the contralateral side) suggests chronic DRUJ instability or acute DRUJ injury, particularly if there is no firm end point. In a normal wrist, laxity typically is more pronounced in neutral rotation than in supination or pronation because the radioulnar ligaments are tensioned in pronation and supination.

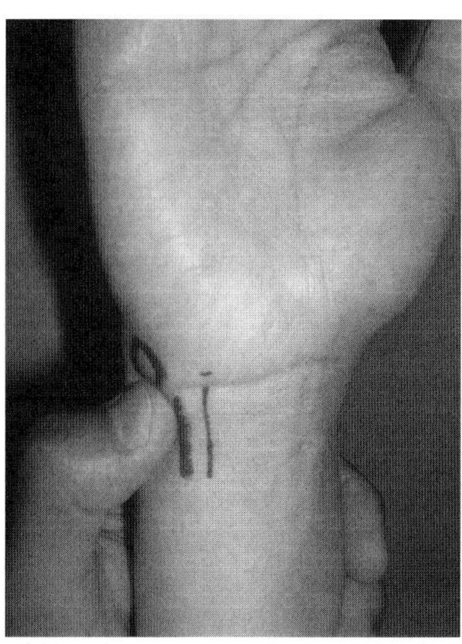

Figure 5 Clinical photograph showing a depression subtending the flexor carpi ulnaris tendon (two straight lines). Palpation of the ulnar styloid and pisiform (oval marking) will elicit tenderness in a patient with a TFCC tear or ulnotriquetral ligament pathology. Tenderness at this location is a positive ulnar fovea sign.

Imaging

A true lateral wrist radiograph may show subluxation or dislocation of the DRUJ. In a normal wrist, the true lateral view should show a superimposed lunate, scaphoid, and triquetrum; the ulna should be contained between the volar and dorsal borders of the radius. Ulnar head prominence dorsal or palmar to the long axis of the radius on a true lateral radiograph should raise concern about the stability of the DRUJ, particularly if there is recent or latent wrist trauma. PA views may show a gap between the distal radius and ulna in a dorsal dislocation or subluxation; in a volar dislocation, the two bones may overlap (Figure 6). A PA clenched fist radiograph in pronation is useful for assessing variance. Oblique radiographs in the semipronated and semisupinated positions show the dorsal and palmar ulnar articular aspects of the sigmoid notch, respectively. A stress view with a subluxating force applied to the ulna may reveal instability. Forearm grip or pronation may exacerbate symptoms of ulnocarpal impaction syndrome and increase the ulnar variance seen on radiographs[33] (Figure 7). Other radiographic findings that may suggest DRUJ insta-

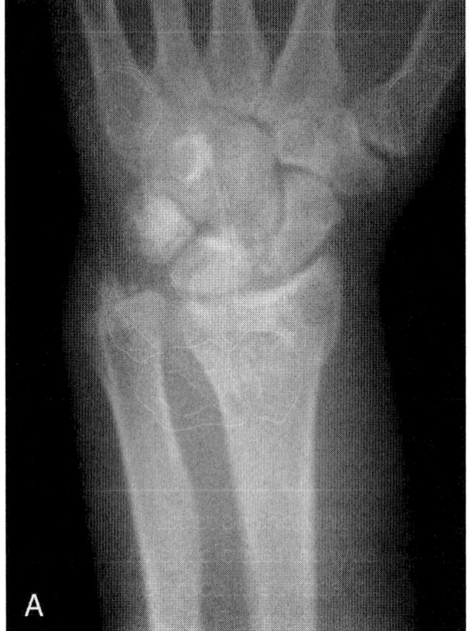

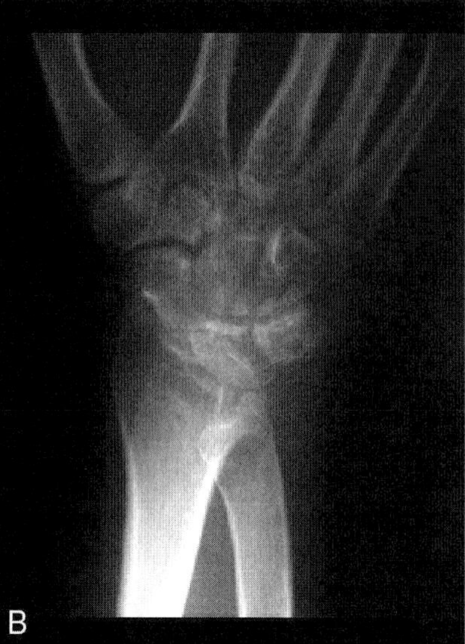

Figure 6 PA wrist radiographs showing dorsal **(A)** and volar **(B)** dislocation of the DRUJ.

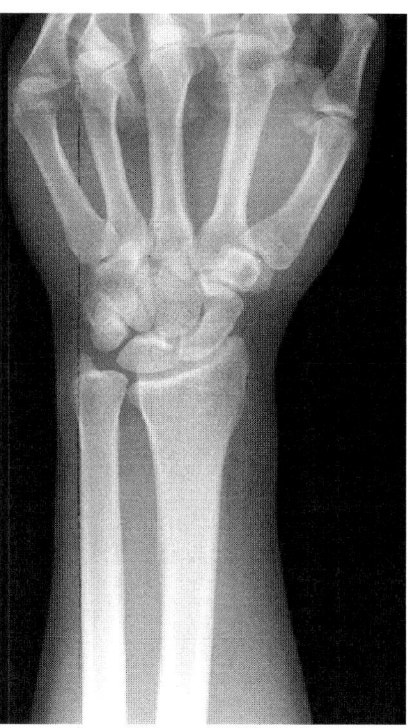

Figure 7 PA radiograph showing distal migration of the ulna relative to the radius with a clenched fist and pronation, which suggests DRUJ instability.

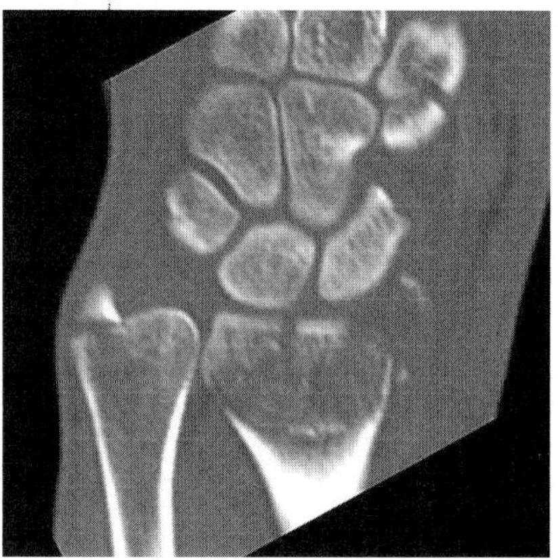

Figure 8 Coronal CT scan showing a displaced ulnar styloid base fracture suggestive of DRUJ instability.

bility include malunion of the distal radius, deformity of the distal radius or ulna, a displaced basilar fracture of the ulnar styloid (Figure 8), and more than 5 mm of radial shortening relative to the ulna.[34]

Some subtle findings can easily be overlooked on plain radiographs.[35,36] CT is the most accurate imaging modality for assessing DRUJ articular congruity. The patient should be positioned prone, with both arms extended overhead to permit simultaneous axial imaging through both radioulnar joints. The forearms should be parallel for comparison in the neutral, fully pronated, and fully supinated positions.[35] The positions of the ulnar head are compared side to side to assess for instability. Several assessment criteria have been described for determining DRUJ reduction with axial CT scanning.[37-39]

Although CT scans are useful in evaluating the DRUJ, they may appear normal even if there is significant soft-tissue disruption.[40] A magnetic resonance arthrogram is useful for evaluating the presence or absence of a TFCC tear or other soft-tissue injury. Images from higher resolution MRI equipment with a dedicated wrist coil have more than 90% accuracy in detecting traumatic tears or degenerative changes of the ligamentous and cartilaginous structures of the DRUJ and wrist.[41,42] Cartilage-sensitive MRI sequences allow a thorough evaluation of the articular surfaces of the ulnar head and sigmoid notch for degenerative arthritis, which can strongly influence treatment. Although diagnostic arthroscopy of the wrist and TFCC is the gold standard for diagnosing TFCC tears,[12] neither the foveal insertion of the radioulnar ligaments nor the sigmoid notch can be adequately evaluated with standard ulnocarpal diagnostic arthroscopy.

Acute Disorders of the DRUJ

A fracture of the distal forearm can affect the congruity and motion of the DRUJ, and a TFCC tear can cause pain and loss of function. A bony injury, a soft-tissue stabilizer disruption, or a combination injury can lead to acute DRUJ instability.

Acute Instability

Although the radius dislocates with respect to the stationary ulna, by convention DRUJ dislocations are classified on the basis of the position of the ulna relative to the radius. In a dorsal dislocation, the ulna is positioned dorsal to the radius; in a volar dislocation, the ulna is positioned volar to the radius. Multidirectional instability and an axial injury in which the radius shifts proximal to the ulna also are possible.

DRUJ dislocation frequently is caused by a fall onto an outstretched hand with a supination moment (leading to volar dislocation) or a pronation moment (leading to dorsal dislocation).[43,44] The presumed mechanism is injury to the dorsal radioulnar ligament in a palmar dislocation or injury to the volar radioulnar ligament in a dorsal dislocation.[30]

A dorsal dislocation should be reduced acutely by applying volarly directed pressure over the ulnar head and supinating the forearm. The forearm then is examined for stability of the reduction. If the DRUJ is stable after reduction, the forearm and elbow should be splinted for 6 weeks. Some authors recommend splinting in the position of full supination, and others prefer a neutral position.[45] Further treatment is needed if the dislocation cannot be reduced or is unstable after reduction.[43]

A volar dislocation is unusual and may be missed. If the dislocation is diagnosed acutely, a closed reduction usually is possible. However, a chronic volar dislocation frequently requires open treatment.[43,44] An acute dislocation can be reduced using dorsally directed pressure over the distal ulna with concomitant pronation. Long arm immobilization in neutral or slight pronation is recommended for 6 weeks.[45]

If closed reduction is unsuccessful, open reduction and extraction of the interposed tissue is required through a dorsal approach.[30] A dislocation that is unstable after open or closed reduction can be stabilized by placing a 0.062-inch Kirschner wire from the ulna into the radius just proximal to the DRUJ. The wrist is immobilized for 6 weeks, with the wires removed after 3 to 4 weeks to allow a controlled passive range of motion.

Although DRUJ dislocation or injury can occur in isolation, more frequently it is associated with a forearm fracture such as a distal radius fracture, an Essex-Lopresti lesion, or a Galeazzi fracture-dislocation.[46] The Galeazzi fracture is a diaphyseal radius fracture with a DRUJ dislocation.[45,47,48] Although formerly considered rare, this injury pattern now is believed to be underrecognized; in one study, it was found in almost 7% of forearm fractures.[34] The Galeazzi fracture is first treated with open reduction and internal fixation of the radius, which typically results in reduction of the DRUJ. If the DRUJ is stable, early motion can be initiated. If the DRUJ is reduced but unstable, immobilization in semisupination for 4 to 6 weeks is preferred. If a large ulnar styloid base fracture is present, open reduction and internal fixation of the styloid may improve stability. Open inspection may be needed if the DRUJ cannot be reduced. Repair of the TFCC or the ulnar styloid is followed by 6 weeks of immobilization in supination or neutral position.[45]

Rikli and associates[49] classified fractures of the distal forearm by delineating the radial, intermediate, and ulnar columns. With this three-column classification, treatment involves anatomically stabilizing the radius and then assessing the stability of the DRUJ. Even with a severe wrist injury in which a displaced distal radius fracture is accompanied by DRUJ disruption, restoration of the radial and intermediate columns can generate a stable DRUJ.

A fracture distal to the midulnar styloid generally is innocuous, regardless of whether there is a TFCC injury. An ulnar styloid base fracture frequently suggests the presence of DRUJ instability.[50] A fracture of the ulnar styloid occurs concomitantly in an estimated 51% to 65% of distal radius fractures,[51] and the implication of an ulnar styloid fracture for the stability of the DRUJ remains controversial. In one study, 8% of the patients required stabilization of the DRUJ.[51] Other studies found no association between instability and the presence of an ulnar styloid fracture.[51,52] It is generally believed that the presence of an ulnar styloid base fracture with displacement of more than 2 mm may be a risk factor for instability.[51] A displaced distal radius fracture, with or without a displaced ulnar styloid base fracture, should be regarded as having DRUJ instability until proved otherwise.[46] Reduction of the distal radius usually results in reduction of the ulnar styloid fracture and a stable DRUJ. If stability cannot be restored by positioning in supination alone, open reduction and internal fixation of the styloid fragment should be considered. Tension band wiring, Kirschner wires, screws, suture anchors, or fragment-specific fixation can be used; or the ulna can be stabilized to the radius with Kirschner wires proximal to the DRUJ. However, open reduction and internal fixation of the styloid fracture can lead to complications, including nonunion, malunion, and DRUJ capsule contracture. Prominent hardware may require later removal.

TFCC Tears

Types of TFCC Tears

Palmer[53] described patterns of injury to the TFCC as traumatic (type I) or degenerative (type II). A type I

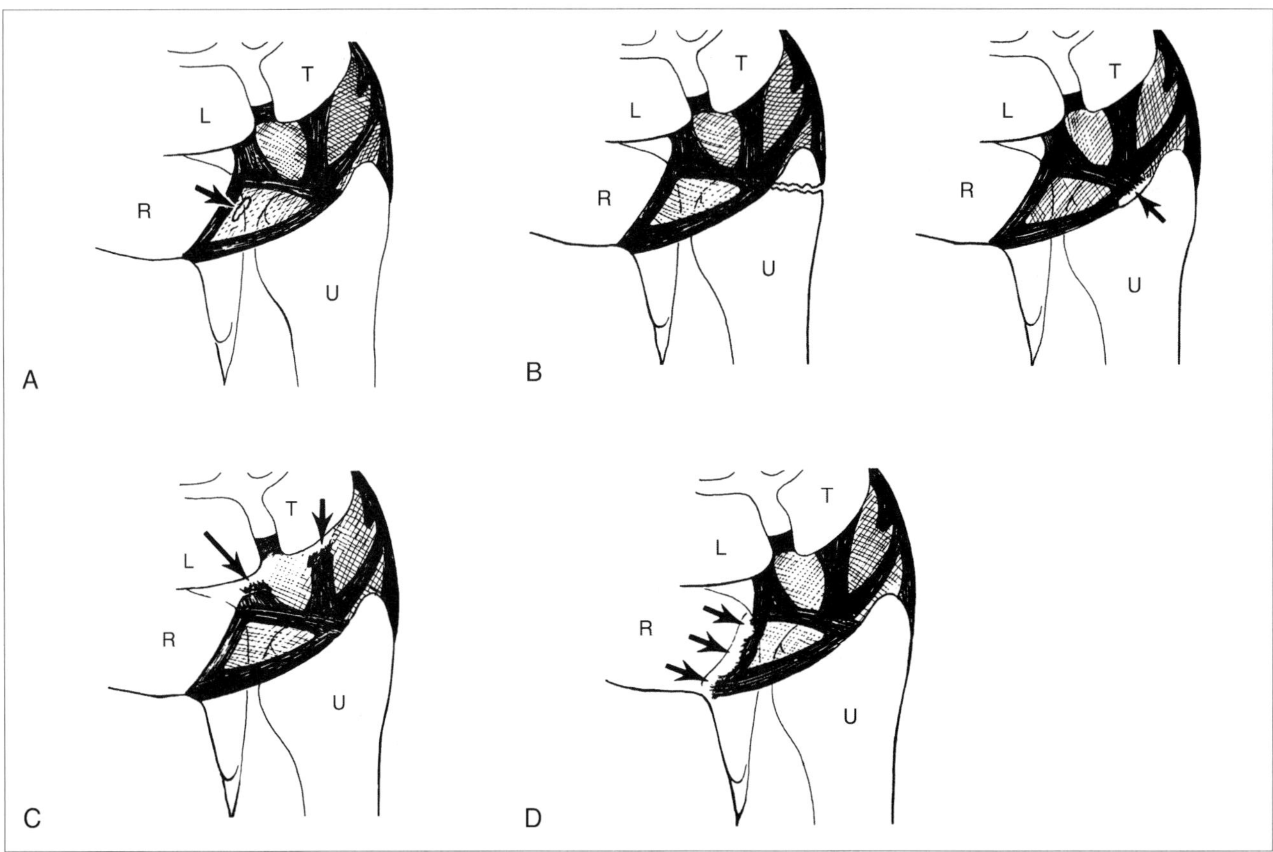

Figure 9 Schematic diagrams showing the Palmer classification of TFCC injuries. R = radius, L = lunate, T = triquetral, U = ulna. **A,** Type IA, a tear of the articular disk (*arrow*). **B,** Type IB, ulnar styloid avulsion fracture (left) and an avulsion from the fovea (right). **C,** Type IC, a tear of the ulnolunate ligament (*long arrow*) and a tear of the triquetral ligament (*short arrow*). **D,** Type ID, an avulsion of the TFCC from the ulnar margin of the distal radius (*arrows*).

tear is further classified as type IA, which is a central perforation; IB, an ulnar-sided avulsion with or without an ulnar styloid fracture; IC, a distal avulsion of the ulnocarpal ligament; or ID, a radial avulsion with or without a sigmoid notch fracture[53] (Figure 9).

Because of the vascular architecture of the TFCC, the location of the tear has implications for its healing potential. The peripheral 20% to 40% of the TFCC has a rich vascular supply and the capacity for healing, but the central portion is avascular with poor healing potential.[54] It is useful to consider DRUJ stability and the TFCC injury together when deciding on treatment. If the DRUJ is stable, the TFCC tear can be treated nonsurgically. However, if the DRUJ is unstable, the TFCC tear may require open or arthroscopic repair. Some tear patterns are correlated with instability (although not all TFCC tears occur in conjunction with or as a part of DRUJ instability). Lindau and associates[52] investigated the effect of an untreated TFCC tear on DRUJ stability in the setting of a distal radius fracture. The tear was diagnosed arthroscopically in 43 of the 51 relatively young patients (median age, 41 years) but was not treated. Ten of the 11 patients with complete peripheral tears had instability at 1-year follow-up. In patients without malunion whose instability was considered a function of tear type, none of those with a type IA tear had instability. However, 45% of those with a type IB tear, all of those with a type IC tear, and 54% of those with a type ID tear had instability. In this study, ulnar styloid fracture or nonunion was not correlated with DRUJ stability.[52]

Treatment of TFCC Tears

A type IA lesion is a central, slitlike tear or perforation of the TFCC. This type of injury is not destabilizing to the DRUJ, but the tear itself may become symptomatic and require treatment (Figure 10, *A*). A type IA lesion may become asymptomatic, even though it has poor healing potential. Nonsurgical treatment, such as immobilization in a long arm splint, therefore should be tried. If nonsurgical treatment is unsuccessful, arthroscopic débridement of the central portion of the tear is associated with good outcomes. As much as two thirds of the central TFCC may be débrided if the dorsal and palmar radioulnar ligaments and the ulnocarpal ligaments remain intact.[55] A 2-mm rim should be maintained to prevent alterations in load bearing and stability.[56]

A type IB tear is an avulsion of the TFCC from its ulnar attachment; another lesion with similar clinical consequences is an ulnar styloid fracture in which the dorsal and palmar distal radioulnar ligaments are injured[57] (Figure 10, *B*). Because of the loss of the integrity of these structures, DRUJ instability may occur as part of a type IB tear. In the setting of a IB tear and a stable DRUJ, this TFCC lesion may be treated nonsurgically with immobilization for 6 weeks. The vascular supply provides healing potential.[57,58] An unstable IB tear should be treated with open repair of the ulnar styloid fracture or open or arthroscopic reattachment of the TFCC avulsion.

A type IC lesion can be treated with immobilization, débridement, or open repair. A symptomatic tear may respond to tightening of the ligaments by an ulna-shortening osteotomy. Shortening the ulna increases the tension on the ulnocarpal ligaments and enhances the stability of the ulnar carpus.[57,58]

A type ID lesion represents a radial-sided tear. Although this type of tear can be repaired, surgical fixation is associated with a high complication rate. Débridement alone has a better result.

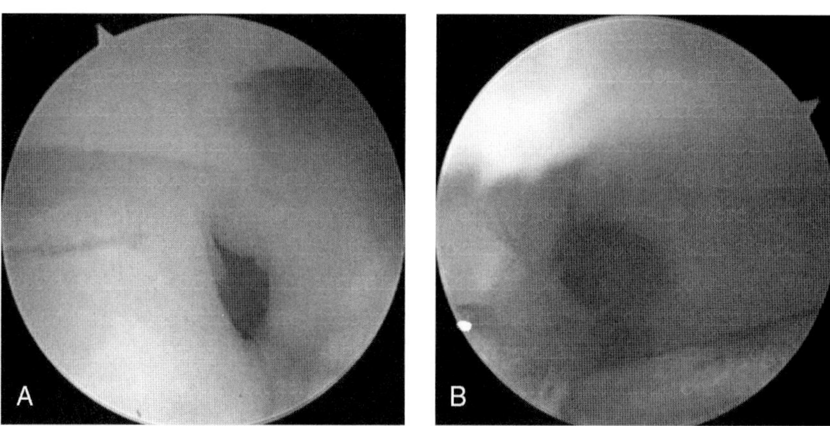

Figure 10 Arthroscopic views of Palmer TFCC tears. **A,** A type IA articular disk tear. **B,** A type IB tear.

Chronic Disorders of the DRUJ

Chronic instability can develop after injury to the osseous elements of the DRUJ or the soft-tissue structures that confer the joint's stability. Variability in the depth and contour of the sigmoid notch in the axial plane influences the stability of the native DRUJ. Malunion of the distal radius with more than 20° of dorsal angulation can be associated with radioulnar incongruity at the sigmoid notch, TFCC distortion, and DRUJ instability. Loss of radial length induces a relative increase in ulnar load and the symptoms of ulnocarpal impaction. Incompetent soft-issue stabilization of the DRUJ can lead to chronic instability after trauma or iatrogenic injury.[59]

Treatment

The factors to consider when devising a treatment plan for chronic DRUJ instability include the direction of instability (dorsal, palmar, multidirectional), the osseous anatomy of the sigmoid notch (dorsal or palmar rim deficit, depth, DRUJ congruity), the osseous anatomy and alignment of the forearm and wrist (malunion of the distal radius or ulna, ulnocarpal impaction, basilar fracture of the ulnar styloid), articular cartilage integrity (DRUJ arthritis), and attenuation of the soft-tissue stabilizing structures (TFCC, dorsal and palmar radioulnar ligaments, ulnocarpal ligaments, extensor carpi ulnaris, interosseous membrane).

Nonsurgical treatment involves restricting forearm rotation by splinting or casting in neutral rotation for 4 to 6 weeks to promote the healing or contracture of attenuated or lax soft-tissue stabilizing structures. Full immobilization of the DRUJ requires a cast extending above the elbow. A strengthening program of physical therapy for the dynamic stabilizers of the wrist can be beneficial. The program should include isometric strengthening of the extensor carpi ulnaris, the flexor carpi ulnaris, and the pronator quadratus. The nonsurgical approach is most appropriate for an acute injury, a subacute or chronic injury in a patient with low functional demands, an injury in a patient for whom surgery is contraindicated because of comorbidities, or a patient who is skeletally immature and would be susceptible to iatrogenic physeal injury.

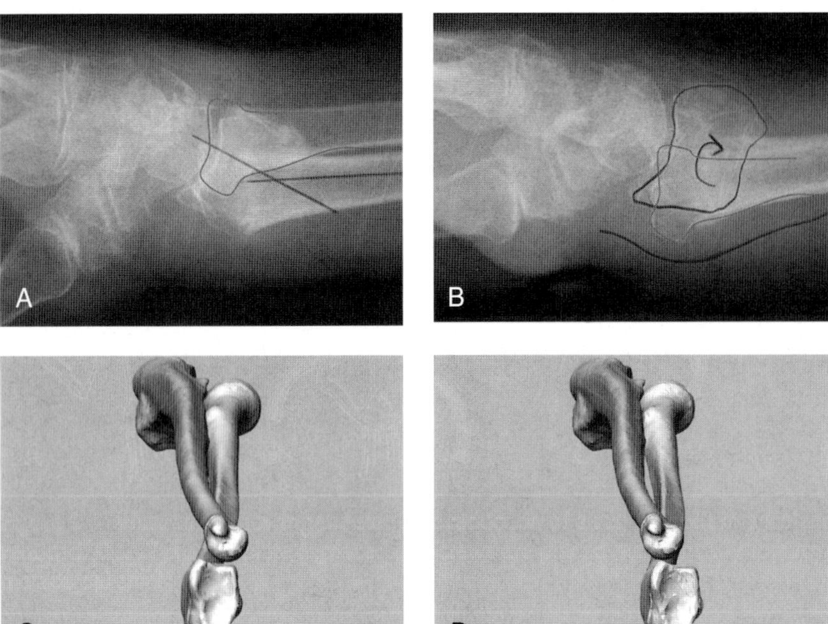

Figure 11 Lateral radiographs of a type I nondissociative malunion of the radius **(A)** and a type II dissociative malunion of the distal radius **(B)**. The superimposed lines show the outlines of the radius and ulna. The arrow in part B shows the direction of the distal radius fracture. Three-dimensional CT scans showing a type I nondissociative malunion of the radius **(C)** and a type II dissociative malunion of the distal radius **(D)**.

In a patient with no degenerative changes, the stability and motion of a chronically unstable DRUJ usually can be restored by surgically repairing or reconstructing the osseous alignment and soft-tissue integrity. A salvage procedure may be necessary if the instability has progressed to degenerative arthritis.

Bony Malalignment Procedures

Dynamic instability of the DRUJ may be classified as type I or II. An angular deformity of the distal radius can change the DRUJ kinematics and create painful and diminished forearm rotation or ulnocarpal impaction, even if the soft-tissue stabilizing structures are not disrupted. This condition is referred to as a type I or nondissociative radial malunion, in which the relationship of the radius, ulna, and carpus is maintained despite increased dorsal angulation of the distal fragment and the associated radial articular surface (Figure 11, *A* and *C*). A true lateral radiograph is necessary to properly evaluate the radioulnocarpal relationship.[60] In a type I radial malunion, the critical dorsal and palmar radioulnar ligaments remain intact so that the forearm rotational axis at the fovea is retained. Corrective osteotomy of a type I radial malunion restores anatomic alignment of the sigmoid notch, and it is both necessary and sufficient to restore normal DRUJ stability and kinematics. Fixation of a distal radius osteotomy most commonly is achieved using a volar plate, although some techniques involve a dorsal plate, Kirschner wire, or fragment-specific plate. The osteotomy void can be filled with allograft or a wedge-shaped autograft to correct the angulation or with a trapezoidal osseous graft to correct both the angulation and length discrepancy.[61,62] In addition to the angular deformity, the radioulnar length relationship must be assessed and restored to avoid an increased ulnar load and simultaneously treat any component of ulnocarpal impaction syndrome. The joint can be leveled by concomitant radius lengthening, an ulna-shortening osteotomy, or, for some patients, a combination procedure. An oblique cut typically is used for an ulna-shortening osteotomy; interfragmentary lag screw and compression plate fixation are used to maximize healing. The kinematics and stability of the DRUJ throughout the arc of forearm rotation should be assessed intraoperatively after the provisional fixation of the corrective osteotomy and before the final instrumentation.

In a type II dissociative radial malunion, the soft-tissue relationship between the angulated distal radial fragment and the ulna is disrupted, resulting in abnormal alignment of the radial articular fragment, the carpus, and the ulna on the lateral radiograph (Figure 11, *B* and *D*). The primary DRUJ ligaments and the secondary constraints, including the radioulnar capsule, the interosseous membrane, and the pronator quadratus, all may be disrupted. The rotational axis of the radius about the ulna is shifted away from the fovea, and radioulnar joint abutment occurs during rotation, especially if there are soft-tissue contractures caused by traumatic scarring. A mechanical block to supination usually is present. Restoration of osseous anatomy is the primary concern because isolated soft-tissue repair or reconstruction fails in the presence of marked bony deformity, joint incongruity, or arthritis. However, a type II malunion differs from a type I malunion in that a simple restoration of bony alignment, although necessary, may not be sufficient to restore rotational stability. Soft-tissue contracture release and/or repair or reconstruction of the radioulnar ligaments may be required.

Basilar fractures of the ulnar styloid compromise the stability of the DRUJ by disrupting the insertion of the deep fibers of the distal radioulnar and ulnocarpal ligaments at the ulnar fovea. Fixation of the styloid can restore DRUJ stability in the acute or subacute phase, if the TFCC is not otherwise injured or attenuated. The fracture is exposed along the subcutaneous border of the ulna, with care to avoid injury to the dorsal sensory branch of the ulnar nerve and the extensor carpi ulnaris tendon sheath. The method of fixation is determined by the fragment size and should avoid fragmentation of the styloid. The available implants include Kirschner wires (used alone or in a tension band construct), cannulated screws, variable-pitch compression screws, pin plates, minifragment plates, and suture anchors (tied over or through the fragment or in figure-of-8 fashion). The subcutaneous position of the implant can cause symptoms necessitating implant removal. Although a simple repair of an ulnar styloid base fracture generally is effective in restoring the stability of the dorsal radioulnar ligament in the acute or subacute stage of detachment, it may be insufficient for chronic detachment because of greater soft-tissue contracture or ligament attenuation.

Patients who have a flat or shallow sigmoid notch respond less predictably to soft-tissue reconstructive procedures for DRUJ instability. Stability of the DRUJ during forearm rotation relies on tension in the corresponding radioulnar ligament and coupled joint reactive forces of the ulnar head against a concentric and constraining sigmoid rim. Corrective osteoplasty for sigmoid notch deficiency can be done either as an isolated procedure to improve the mechanical constraint on the distal ulna or together with a soft-tissue reconstruction to augment ligamentous stability. As originally described by Wallwork and Bain,[63] transverse parallel osteotomies are done just proximal to the lunate fossa and at the proximal margin of the sigmoid notch, with a third longitudinal cut between the two transverse cuts to generate a hinged opening wedge osteocartilaginous flap that is elevated ulnarly to deepen the sigmoid notch. The defect is filled with osseous graft and fixed with a plate, Kirschner wires, or sutures.

Soft-Tissue Procedures

The ideal surgical treatment of chronic DRUJ instability without osseous malunion or cartilage degeneration (such as arthritis) is restoration of the mechanical integrity of the radioulnar ligaments of the TFCC. A delayed TFCC repair can reattach the radioulnar ligaments by suture fixation through drill holes to the ulnar fovea or, less commonly, the distal radius.[64] If a primary repair of the TFCC is not feasible because of chronic attenuation or the extent of injury, a reconstructive procedure can be done. The soft tissue can be extrinsically reconstructed using a radioulnar tether (direct link) or an ulnocarpal sling tenodesis (indirect link), or the dorsal and palmar radioulnar ligaments can be directly reconstructed. Numerous extrinsic soft-tissue stabilization procedures have been described, including those of Fulkerson and Watson,[65] Hui and Linscheid,[66] Tsai and Stilwell,[67] and the Boyes and Bunnell procedure.[4] Although an extra-articular tethering of the distal radius and ulna may improve clinical symptoms, it is nonanatomic and fails to restore normal joint stability or kinematics.[4] The Boyes-Bunnell and Hui-Linscheid procedures use a distally based strip of the flexor carpi ulnaris tendon to reconstruct the palmar ulnocarpal ligaments, and they may be the most appropriate techniques for combined ulnocarpal and DRUJ instability.

Anatomic, intrinsic radioulnar ligament reconstructive procedures have been described by Scheker and associates,[68] Johnston Jones and Sanders,[69] and Adams and Divelbiss.[70] Scheker and associates[68] used tendon graft woven through drill holes in the distal radius and ulna to reconstruct the dorsal radioulnar ligament. Johnston Jones and Sanders[69] used a palmaris tendon graft to reconstruct the radioulnar ligaments. The procedure described by Adams and Divelbiss[70] is recommended for anatomic reconstruction of both dorsal and palmar radioulnar ligaments. In this procedure, the DRUJ is exposed using a dorsal approach between the fifth and sixth extensor compartments. The TFCC remnant, the ulnar styloid, and the articular surfaces of the DRUJ are examined. If the TFCC remnant is attenuated and irreparable, the radioulnar ligament is reconstructed. Functional elements of the TFCC are retained; to preserve the stabilizing function of the extensor carpi ulnaris tendon sheath, care is taken to avoid opening it or disturbing its position within the ulnar groove. Any basilar styloid nonunion fragment is resected. The radioulnar lig-

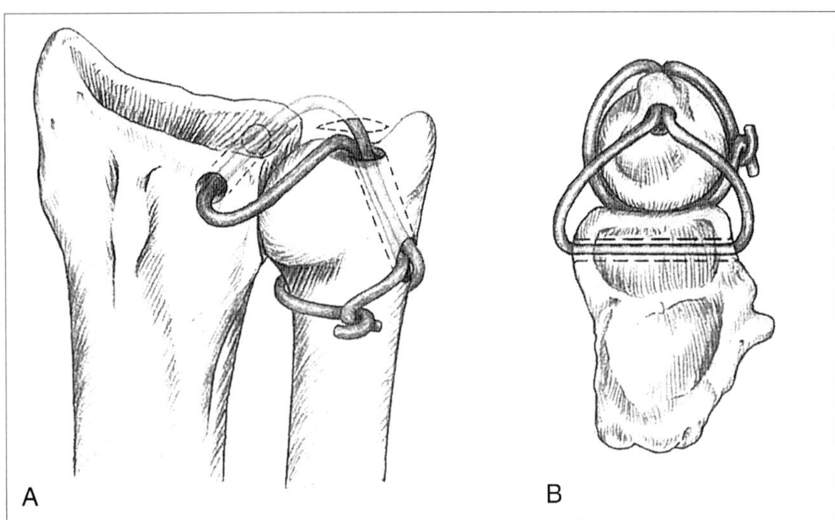

Figure 12 Schematic diagrams showing DRUJ reconstruction using a palmaris longus tendon graft, as described by Adams and Berger.[3] The tendon graft is passed from dorsal to palmar through a tunnel in the ulnar margin of the distal radius **(A)**, then tensioned through the ulnar neck **(B)**.

ament is reconstructed by passing a palmaris or plantaris tendon graft though a dorsal-palmar tunnel in the distal radius at the level of the sigmoid notch, with both ends merging in an ulnar tunnel from the fovea to the ulnar neck. Tensioning of the graft around the ulnar neck tightens both limbs of the dorsal and palmar radioulnar ligaments and their attachment at the fovea (Figure 12). Adams and Berger[3] used this technique for restoration of DRUJ stability in 12 of 14 patients (10 with bidirectional instability and 4 with unidirectional stability). Two patients required concomitant ulnar osteotomy. At a minimum 1-year follow-up, all patients in the study had recovered an average of 80% of supination, 84% of pronation, and 85% of grip strength compared with the contralateral unaffected side.

Salvage Procedures

Both chronic DRUJ instability and posttraumatic arthritis can lead to degenerative arthritis of the DRUJ. The success of bony and soft-tissue reconstructive procedures to address chronic DRUJ instability can be compromised by persistent pain or weakness caused by arthritis. A salvage procedure is indicated for DRUJ instability in the setting of advanced DRUJ arthritis, with the goal of eliminating the painful articulation between the distal radius and the ulna. These ablative treatments include the Darrach procedure,[1] the Bowers hemiresection-interposition arthroplasty,[71] the Sauvé-Kapandji procedure,[72] wide distal ulna resection, creation of a one-bone forearm by radioulnar arthrodesis, and implant arthroplasty.

The Darrach procedure, originally described in 1912, is best used for patients with low functional demands. Younger, more active patients generally have a poor result. The procedure entails resection of the distal ulna, with the osteotomy approximately 1 to 2 cm proximal to the most proximal extent of the sigmoid notch of the distal radius. This level of resection may help avoid convergence instability because it typically is proximal to the insertion of the pronator quadratus. A useful technical modification preserves the TFCC. The possible complications of the Darrach procedure include distal ulnar stump instability, particularly in a patient with preoperative joint instability. Therefore, the Darrach procedure is best reserved for patients with degenerative arthritis of the DRUJ. Dingman[73] observed that the Darrach procedure has the best clinical result in a patient with minimal distal ulnar resection and subsequent regeneration within the retained periosteal sleeve.

Several stabilization procedures have been described for the distal ulnar stump.[74] Breen and Jupiter[75] described a combined tenodesis of the distal ulnar stump using the extensor carpi ulnaris and the flexor carpi ulnaris, both of which are woven through the distal ulnar stump (Figure 13). Ruby and associates[76] described a procedure using the pronator quadratus. Sotereanos and associates[77] reported a salvage procedure using a large portion of allograft material for the treatment of complications arising from convergence instability of the distal ulnar stump.

The hemiresection-interposition arthroplasty was developed by Bowers[71] in response to the instability associated with the Darrach procedure. Hemiresection of the radial side of the arthritic ulnar head preserves the foveal attachments of the TFCC and the ulnar styloid. Capsular flaps and the pronator quadratus can be used for interposition, with suture fixation of the dorsal DRUJ capsule to the palmar capsule. The procedure is effective for the relief of arthritis pain, but the results are less predictable if the patient has

DRUJ instability, ulnar impaction syndrome, or ulnocarpal translation. A similar matched distal ulnar resection described by Watson and Gabuzda[78] requires sacrifice of the native insertions of the TFCC and ulnocarpal ligaments. Stability is derived from the healing of the exposed cancellous bone to the surrounding periosteal soft-tissue sleeve.

The Sauvé-Kapandji procedure[72] is an alternative to resection of the distal ulna. The symptoms of DRUJ degeneration are treated by arthrodesis. Forearm rotation is retained through a pseudarthrosis created proximal to the DRUJ. The advantage of this procedure over distal ulnar resection is the maintenance of bony support of the ulnar carpus. The débridement of eburnated bone from the articular surfaces of the DRUJ creates matched cancellous surfaces for arthrodesis. The ulnar head should be positioned in slight negative variance to minimize the development of ulnar impaction. Fixation typically is with cannulated compression screws or Kirschner wires positioned across the DRUJ. A 1-cm resection of the ulnar shaft just proximal to the level of the sigmoid notch enables forearm rotation. Instability of the proximal ulnar stump can become symptomatic; stabilization can be achieved by tenodesis with the extensor carpi ulnaris tendon, the flexor carpi ulnaris tendon, or both.[79,80] In a study of 22 patients, Gonçalves[81] found that the Sauvé-Kapandji procedure had consistently better results than the Darrach procedure. Taleisnik[82] described the elimination of pain and restoration of forearm rotation, with few complications, in 37 patients. The procedure typically is contraindicated in patients with DRUJ instability.

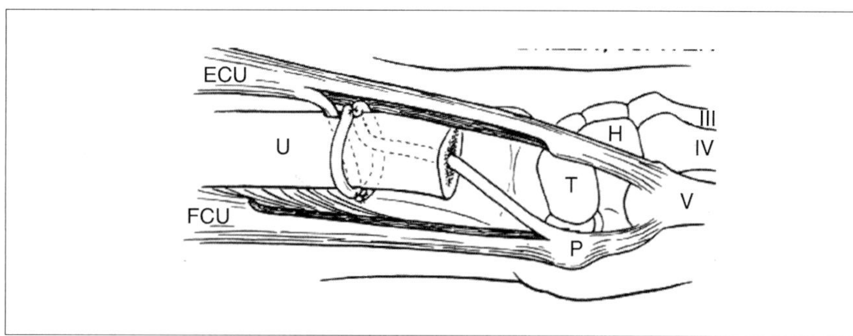

Figure 13 Schematic diagram showing tenodesis of the distal ulnar stump, as described by Breen and Jupiter.[75] This procedure is designed to prevent instability of the distal ulnar stump by using the extensor carpi ulnaris tendon. ECU = extensor carpi ulnaris, FCU = flexor carpi ulnaris, U = ulna, H = hamate, T = triquetrum, P = pisiform, III = third metacarpal, IV = fourth metacarpal, V = fifth metacarpal.

Wide resection of the distal ulna traditionally was reserved for the treatment of a tumor. However, Wolfe and associates[83] found that as much as one third of the ulnar length can be resected subperiosteally without sacrificing stability. Ulnocarpal translation is rare but can result from instability and radioulnar convergence. Earlier disruption of the integrity of the interosseous membrane is an absolute contraindication to wide resection because stability after a wide resection depends on this structure. In a combined series of 12 patients, Wolfe and associates[83] reported average range of motion and grip strength of 75% to 90%, with treatment failures caused by convergence or instability in 2 patients.

Creation of a one-bone forearm through radioulnar arthrodesis is the ultimate salvage procedure for chronic DRUJ instability and arthritis. It is indicated for chronic, end-stage DRUJ instability that has persisted despite surgical stabilization. Motion at the DRUJ is sacrificed to obtain stability and alleviate pain. The radius and ulna can be fixed together with autogenous osseous graft and a bridging plate, or the radius can be transposed onto the ulna by osteotomies and discarding of the proximal radius and distal ulna. The preferred position of arthrodesis typically is in neutral to slight pronation to facilitate activities of daily living and hygiene. Peterson and associates[5] reported a nonunion rate approaching 32% and a 50% rate of significant complications.

Degenerative Arthritis

Degenerative arthritis of the DRUJ occasionally develops after years of chronic DRUJ instability or as a result of posttraumatic arthritis caused by a distal radius fracture. This condition can cause debilitating pain and limit forearm and wrist function so that occupational, recreational, and ordinary daily activities are compromised. Most patients with severe degenerative arthritis of the DRUJ can achieve some temporary relief through nonsurgical measures. Nonsteroidal anti-inflammatory drugs, immobilization, and activity modification may help in reducing the discomfort. Occupational therapy modalities, such as ultrasonography, phonophoresis, and heat, also can be used. A fluoroscopically directed corticosteroid injection can be temporarily effective; it is best done with contrast enhancement to ensure correct needle placement in the joint.

Several surgical procedures can be used for resection or arthrodesis of a DRUJ with severe degenerative arthritis, including the Darrach procedure, an ulna-shortening osteotomy, the Sauvé-Kapandji procedure, hemiresection-interposition arthroplasty, one-bone forearm procedure, and prosthetic replacement of the DRUJ. An ulna-shortening osteotomy can be used to alter the contact surfaces in patients with degenerative arthritis of the DRUJ; Scheker and Severo[84] reported excellent results in 18 of 32 patients. The Darrach procedure should be considered only for an older, sedentary patient with degenerative arthritis of the DRUJ. A tenodesis stabilizing procedure, such as the extensor carpi ulnaris tenodesis described by Breen and Jupiter,[75] should be done with the Darrach procedure. The ultimate salvage procedure is conversion to a one-bone forearm, which is necessary only in extreme circumstances.

Implant arthroplasty of the distal ulna or DRUJ holds promise for the treatment of symptomatic DRUJ arthritis. Its role in the treatment of distal ulnar instability is not yet well understood, and alternatives to this procedure should be carefully considered. A metallic distal ulna implant can be used to restore mechanical integrity and load transmission across the distal forearm. Newer endoprostheses facilitate soft-tissue repair by allowing suture fixation of the TFCC and extensor carpi ulnaris subsheath to the implant. Sigmoid notch implants also have been developed. Long-term outcomes have not yet been reported to establish the durability of the fixation or any advantages over the use of an ulnar implant and soft-tissue reconstruction alone. An ulnar head endoprosthesis was used in 19 DRUJ arthroplasties in 17 patients; at 2-year follow-up, the average overall pain score decreased 50%, grip strength improved 16% (4 kg), forearm rotation was unchanged, and all wrists were clinically stable.[85] Two treatment failures occurred, at 7 and 14 months after surgery. Scheker and associates[86] used a ball-and-socket total DRUJ prosthesis that allows translation between the radius and the ulna. At a mean 15-month follow-up, all 23 patients reported complete pain relief, and normal forearm rotation was observed. The results were similar at 5.9-year follow-up of 31 patients.[87] Larger studies are necessary to determine the long-term durability of distal ulna implant arthroplasty.

Summary

Disorders of the DRUJ are common and may be underrecognized. The DRUJ is unique in that the radius of curvature of the sigmoid notch of the distal radius is greater than the radius of curvature of the distal ulnar head. The result is an inherently unstable joint that translates during pronation and supination. The biomechanics of the DRUJ are complex and have been understood only recently. It is now generally recognized that the volar radioulnar ligament provides a constraining force to dorsal translation of the DRUJ in any position, and the dorsal radioulnar ligament constrains volar translation of the DRUJ when the forearm is pronated. Clinical examination generally identifies DRUJ instability. Imaging of the joint has been enhanced by more powerful MRI technology. An acute injury of the DRUJ is a result of disruption of the TFCC and requires surgical repair. Successful repair may not be feasible for a chronic condition, and reconstruction of the dorsal and volar radioulnar ligaments may be necessary. Degenerative arthritis of the DRUJ can be disabling, but several surgical procedures have proved efficacious. The early results of prosthetic arthroplasty are encouraging, but the long-term success of the procedure remains unknown. The ultimate salvage procedure for disorders of the DRUJ is to create a one-bone forearm, thus converting the forearm to an immobile structure.

References

1. Bieber EJ, Linscheid RL, Dobyns JH, Beckenbaugh RD: Failed distal ulna resections. *J Hand Surg Am* 1988;13: 193-200.

2. Hartz CR, Beckenbaugh RD: Long-term results of resection of the distal ulna for post-traumatic conditions. *J Trauma* 1979;19:219-226.

3. Adams BD, Berger RA: An anatomic reconstruction of the distal radioulnar ligaments for posttraumatic distal radioulnar joint instability. *J Hand Surg Am* 2002;27:243-251.

4. Petersen MS, Adams BD: Biomechanical evaluation of distal radioulnar reconstructions. *J Hand Surg Am* 1993;18:328-334.

5. Peterson CA II, Maki S, Wood MB: Clinical results of the one-bone forearm. *J Hand Surg Am* 1995;20: 609-618.

6. Adams B: Distal radioulnar joint instability, in Green D, Hotchkiss R, Pederson W, Wolfe S, eds: *Green's Operative Hand Surgery*, ed 5. Amsterdam, The Netherlands, Elsevier, 2005, pp 605-644.

7. Tolat AR, Stanley JK, Trail IA: A cadaveric study of the anatomy and stability of the distal radioulnar joint in the coronal and transverse planes. *J Hand Surg Br* 1996;21:587-594.

8. Werner FW, Palmer AK, Fortino MD, Short WH: Force transmission

through the distal ulna: Effect of ulnar variance, lunate fossa angulation, and radial and palmar tilt of the distal radius. *J Hand Surg Am* 1992;17: 423-428.

9. Bednar MS, Arnoczky SP, Weiland AJ: The microvasculature of the triangular fibrocartilage complex: Its clinical significance. *J Hand Surg Am* 1991;16:1101-1105.

10. Hotchkiss RN: Injuries to the interosseous ligament of the forearm. *Hand Clin* 1994;10:391-398.

11. McGinley JC, Kozin SH: Interosseous membrane anatomy and functional mechanics. *Clin Orthop Relat Res* 2001;383:108-122.

12. Szabo RM: Distal radioulnar joint instability. *Instr Course Lect* 2007;56: 79-89.

13. Tay SC, Berger RA, Tomita K, Tan ET, Amrami KK, An KN: In vivo three-dimensional displacement of the distal radioulnar joint during resisted forearm rotation. *J Hand Surg Am* 2007;32:450-458.

14. Pirela-Cruz MA, Goll SR, Klug M, Windler D: Stress computed tomography analysis of the distal radioulnar joint: A diagnostic tool for determining translational motion. *J Hand Surg Am* 1991;16:75-82.

15. Moore DC, Hogan KA, Crisco JJ III, Akelman E, Dasilva MF, Weiss AP: Three-dimensional in vivo kinematics of the distal radioulnar joint in malunited distal radius fractures. *J Hand Surg Am* 2002;27:233-242.

16. Short WH, Palmer AK, Werner FW, Murphy DJ: A biomechanical study of distal radial fractures. *J Hand Surg Am* 1987;12:529-534.

17. Markolf KL, Dunbar AM, Hannani K: Mechanisms of load transfer in the cadaver forearm: Role of the interosseous membrane. *J Hand Surg Am* 2000;25:674-682.

18. Markolf KL, Lamey D, Yang S, Meals R, Hotchkiss R: Radioulnar load-sharing in the forearm: A study in cadavera. *J Bone Joint Surg Am* 1998; 80:879-888.

19. Pfaeffle HJ, Fischer KJ, Manson TT, Tomaino MM, Woo SL, Herndon JH: Role of the forearm interosseous ligament: Is it more than just longitudinal load transfer? *J Hand Surg Am* 2000;25:683-688.

20. Birkbeck DP, Failla JM, Hoshaw SJ, Fyhrie DP, Schaffler M: The interosseous membrane affects load distribution in the forearm. *J Hand Surg Am* 1997;22:975-980.

21. Manson TT, Pfaeffle HJ, Herdon JH, Tomaino MM, Fischer KJ: Forearm rotation alters interosseous ligament strain distribution. *J Hand Surg Am* 2000;25:1058-1063.

22. Nakamura T, Yabe Y, Horiuchi Y: In vivo MR studies of dynamic changes in the interosseous membrane of the forearm during rotation. *J Hand Surg Br* 1999;24:245-248.

23. Pfaeffle HJ, Tomaino MM, Grewal R, et al: Tensile properties of the interosseous membrane of the human forearm. *J Orthop Res* 1996;14: 842-845.

24. Kihara H, Palmer AK, Werner FW, Short WH, Fortino MD: The effect of dorsally angulated distal radius fractures on distal radioulnar joint congruency and forearm rotation. *J Hand Surg Am* 1996;21:40-47.

25. af Ekenstam F, Hagert CG: Anatomical studies on the geometry and stability of the distal radio ulnar joint. *Scand J Plast Reconstr Surg* 1985;19: 17-25.

26. Schuind F, An KN, Berglund L, et al: The distal radioulnar ligaments: A biomechanical study. *J Hand Surg Am* 1991;16:1106-1114.

27. Stuart PR, Berger RA, Linscheid RL, An KN: The dorsopalmar stability of the distal radioulnar joint. *J Hand Surg Am* 2000;25:689-699.

28. Ekenstam F: Osseous anatomy and articular relationships about the distal ulna. *Hand Clin* 1998;14:161-164.

29. Stuart PR: Pronator quadratus revisited. *J Hand Surg Br* 1996;21:714-722.

30. Nicolaidis SC, Hildreth DH, Lichtman DM: Acute injuries of the distal radioulnar joint. *Hand Clin* 2000;16: 449-459.

31. Chidgey LK: The distal radioulnar joint: Problems and solutions. *J Am Acad Orthop Surg* 1995;3:95-109.

32. Tay SC, Tomita K, Berger RA: The "ulnar fovea sign" for defining ulnar wrist pain: An analysis of sensitivity and specificity. *J Hand Surg Am* 2007; 32:438-444.

33. Tomaino MM: The importance of the pronated grip x-ray view in evaluating ulnar variance. *J Hand Surg Am* 2000; 25:352-357.

34. Moore TM, Lester DK, Sarmiento A: The stabilizing effect of soft-tissue constraints in artificial Galeazzi fractures. *Clin Orthop Relat Res* 1985; 194:189-194.

35. Mino DE, Palmer AK, Levinsohn EM: The role of radiography and computerized tomography in the diagnosis of subluxation and dislocation of the distal radioulnar joint. *J Hand Surg Am* 1983;8:23-31.

36. Morrissy RT, Nalebuff EA: Dislocation of the distal radioulnar joint: Anatomy and clues to prompt diagnosis. *Clin Orthop Relat Res* 1979; 144:154-158.

37. Mino DE, Palmer AK, Levinsohn EM: Radiography and computerized tomography in the diagnosis of incongruity of the distal radio-ulnar joint: A prospective study. *J Bone Joint Surg Am* 1985;67:247-252.

38. Wechsler RJ, Wehbe MA, Rifkin MD, Edeiken J, Branch HM: Computed tomography diagnosis of distal radioulnar subluxation. *Skeletal Radiol* 1987;16:1-5.

39. Lo IK, MacDermid JC, Bennett JD, Bogoch E, King GJ: The radioulnar ratio: A new method of quantifying distal radioulnar joint subluxation. *J Hand Surg Am* 2001;26:236-243.

40. King GJ, McMurtry RY, Rubenstein JD, Gertzbein SD: Kinematics of the distal radioulnar joint. *J Hand Surg Am* 1986;11:798-804.

41. Anderson ML, Skinner JA, Felmlee JP, Berger RA, Amrami KK: Diagnostic

comparison of 1.5 Tesla and 3.0 Tesla preoperative MRI of the wrist in patients with ulnar-sided wrist pain. *J Hand Surg Am* 2008;33:1153-1159.

42. Potter HG, Asnis-Ernberg L, Weiland AJ, Hotchkiss RN, Peterson MG, McCormack RR Jr: The utility of high-resolution magnetic resonance imaging in the evaluation of the triangular fibrocartilage complex of the wrist. *J Bone Joint Surg Am* 1997; 79:1675-1684.

43. Mulford JS, Axelrod TS: Traumatic injuries of the distal radioulnar joint. *Orthop Clin North Am* 2007;38: 289-297.

44. Schiller MG, af Ekenstam F, Kirsch PT: Volar dislocation of the distal radio-ulnar joint: A case report. *J Bone Joint Surg Am* 1991;73:617-619.

45. Szabo RM: Distal radioulnar joint instability. *J Bone Joint Surg Am* 2006;88: 884-894.

46. Mikic ZD: Treatment of acute injuries of the triangular fibrocartilage complex associated with distal radioulnar joint instability. *J Hand Surg Am* 1995;20:319-323.

47. Galeazzi R: Uber ein besondereres syndrom bei verletzungen im bereich der unterarmknochen. *Arch Orthop Unfallchir* 1935;35:557-562.

48. Rettig ME, Raskin KB: Galeazzi fracture-dislocation: A new treatment-oriented classification. *J Hand Surg Am* 2001;26:228-235.

49. Rikli DA, Regazzoni P: Fractures of the distal end of the radius treated by internal fixation and early function: A preliminary report of 20 cases. *J Bone Joint Surg Br* 1996;78:588-592.

50. Ruch DS, Lumsden BC, Papadonikolakis A: Distal radius fractures: A comparison of tension band wiring versus ulnar outrigger external fixation for the management of distal radioulnar instability. *J Hand Surg Am* 2005;30:969-977.

51. May MM, Lawton JN, Blazar PE: Ulnar styloid fractures associated with distal radius fractures: Incidence and implications for distal radioulnar joint instability. *J Hand Surg Am* 2002;27: 965-971.

52. Lindau T, Adlercreutz C, Aspenberg P: Peripheral tears of the triangular fibrocartilage complex cause distal radioulnar joint instability after distal radial fractures. *J Hand Surg Am* 2000;25:464-468.

53. Palmer AK: Triangular fibrocartilage complex lesions: A classification. *J Hand Surg Am* 1989;14:594-606.

54. Palmer AK: Triangular fibrocartilage disorders: Injury patterns and treatment. *Arthroscopy* 1990;6:125-132.

55. Palmer AK, Werner FW, Glisson RR, Murphy DJ: Partial excision of the triangular fibrocartilage complex. *J Hand Surg Am* 1988;13:391-394.

56. Adams BD: Partial excision of the triangular fibrocartilage complex articular disk: A biomechanical study. *J Hand Surg Am* 1993;18:334-340.

57. Osterman AL, Terrill RG: Arthroscopic treatment of TFCC lesions. *Hand Clin* 1991;7:277-281.

58. Bednar JM: Arthroscopic treatment of triangular fibrocartilage tears. *Hand Clin* 1999;15:479-488.

59. Kihara H, Short WH, Werner FW, Fortino MD, Palmer AK: The stabilizing mechanism of the distal radioulnar joint during pronation and supination. *J Hand Surg Am* 1995;20: 930-936.

60. Yang Z, Mann FA, Gilula LA, Haerr C, Larsen CF: Scaphopisocapitate alignment: Criterion to establish a neutral lateral view of the wrist. *Radiology* 1997;205:865-869.

61. Fingado B, Wolfe S: Reconstruction of secondary carpal problems following distal radius fractures, in Watson HK, Weinzweig J, eds: *The Wrist.* Philadelphia, PA, Lippincott Williams & Wilkins, 2001, pp 341-368.

62. Watson HK, Castle TH Jr: Trapezoidal osteotomy of the distal radius for unacceptable articular angulation after Colles' fracture. *J Hand Surg Am* 1988;13:837-843.

63. Wallwork NA, Bain GI: Sigmoid notch osteoplasty for chronic volar instability of the distal radioulnar joint: A case report. *J Hand Surg Am* 2001;26:454-459.

64. Hermansdorfer JD, Kleinman WB: Management of chronic peripheral tears of the triangular fibrocartilage complex. *J Hand Surg Am* 1991;16: 340-346.

65. Fulkerson JP, Watson HK: Congenital anterior subluxation of the distal ulna: A case report. *Clin Orthop Relat Res* 1978;131:179-182.

66. Hui FC, Linscheid RL: Ulnotriquetral augmentation tenodesis: A reconstructive procedure for dorsal subluxation of the distal radioulnar joint. *J Hand Surg Am* 1982;7:230-236.

67. Tsai TM, Stilwell JH: Repair of chronic subluxation of the distal radioulnar joint (ulnar dorsal) using flexor carpi ulnaris tendon. *J Hand Surg Br* 1984;9:289-294.

68. Scheker LR, Belliappa PP, Acosta R, German DS: Reconstruction of the dorsal ligament of the triangular fibrocartilage complex. *J Hand Surg Br* 1994;19:310-318.

69. Johnston Jones K, Sanders WE: Posttraumatic radioulnar instability: Treatment by anatomic reconstruction of the volar and dorsal radioulnar ligaments. *Orthop Trans* 1995-1996; 19:832.

70. Adams BD, Divelbiss BJ: Reconstruction of the posttraumatic unstable distal radioulnar joint. *Orthop Clin North Am* 2001;32:353-363.

71. Bowers WH: Distal radioulnar joint arthroplasty: The hemiresection-interposition technique. *J Hand Surg Am* 1985;10:169-178.

72. Sauvé L, Kapandji M: Nouvelle technique de traitement chirurgical des luxations récidivantes isolées de l'extrémité inferieure du cubitus. *J Chir (Paris)* 1936;47:589-594.

73. Dingman PV: Resection of the distal end of the ulna (Darrach operation): An end result study of twenty four cases. *J Bone Joint Surg Am* 1952;34: 893-900.

74. Leslie BM, Carlson G, Ruby LK: Results of extensor carpi ulnaris tenodesis in the rheumatoid wrist undergoing a distal ulnar excision. *J Hand Surg Am* 1990;15:547-551.

75. Breen TF, Jupiter JB: Extensor carpi ulnaris and flexor carpi ulnaris tenodesis of the unstable distal ulna. *J Hand Surg Am* 1989;14:612-617.

76. Ruby LK, Ferenz CC, Dell PC: The pronator quadratus interposition transfer: An adjunct to resection arthroplasty of the distal radioulnar joint. *J Hand Surg Am* 1996;21:60-65.

77. Sotereanos DG, Göbel F, Vardakas DG, Sarris I: An allograft salvage technique for failure of the Darrach procedure: A report of four cases. *J Hand Surg Br* 2002;27:317-321.

78. Watson HK, Gabuzda GM: Matched distal ulna resection for posttraumatic disorders of the distal radioulnar joint. *J Hand Surg Am* 1992;17:724-730.

79. Minami A, Suzuki K, Suenaga N, Ishikawa J: The Sauvé-Kapandji procedure for osteoarthritis of the distal radioulnar joint. *J Hand Surg Am* 1995;20:602-608.

80. Lamey DM, Fernandez DL: Results of the modified Sauvé-Kapandji procedure in the treatment of chronic posttraumatic derangement of the distal radioulnar joint. *J Bone Joint Surg Am* 1998;80:1758-1769.

81. Gonçalves D: Correction of disorders of the distal radio-ulnar joint by artificial pseudarthrosis of the ulna. *J Bone Joint Surg Br* 1974;56:462-464.

82. Taleisnik J: The Sauvé-Kapandji procedure. *Clin Orthop Relat Res* 1992;275:110-123.

83. Wolfe SW, Mih AD, Hotchkiss RN, Culp RW, Keifhaber TR, Nagle DJ: Wide excision of the distal ulna: A multicenter case study. *J Hand Surg Am* 1998;23:222-228.

84. Scheker LR, Severo A: Ulnar shortening for the treatment of early posttraumatic osteoarthritis at the distal radioulnar joint. *J Hand Surg Br* 2001;26:41-44.

85. Willis AA, Berger RA, Cooney WP III: Arthroplasty of the distal radioulnar joint using a new ulnar head endoprosthesis: Preliminary report. *J Hand Surg Am* 2007;32:177-189.

86. Scheker LR, Babb BA, Killion PE: Distal ulnar prosthetic replacement. *Orthop Clin North Am* 2001;32:365-376.

87. Laurentin-Pérez LA, Goodwin AN, Babb BA, Scheker LR: A study of functional outcomes following implantation of a total distal radioulnar joint prosthesis. *J Hand Surg Eur Vol* 2008;33:18-28.

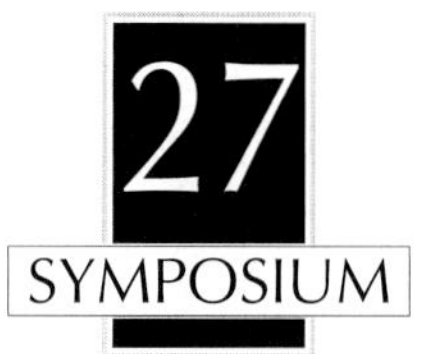

New Concepts in the Treatment of Distal Radius Fractures

John S. Taras, MD
Amy L. Ladd, MD
David M. Kalainov, MD
David S. Ruch, MD
David C. Ring, MD

Abstract

Fracture of the distal radius is the type of fracture most commonly seen in emergency departments. The understanding of nonsurgical and surgical care of distal radius fractures is evolving with recently developed methods of fixation. It is worthwhile to review some new methods of treatment, the role of bone grafting and synthetic substitutes, the principles of complex fracture management, and the treatment of common complications of distal radius fractures.

Instr Course Lect 2010;59:313-332.

Fracture alignment and the age of the patient are the most important factors determining the recovery of function after a distal radius fracture. There is no definitive rule for acceptable fracture alignment, but studies of patients who had a less-than-optimal outcome after healing with malalignment have helped to establish general guidelines. Malalignment and poor outcome are most highly correlated with an intra-articular incongruity exceeding 2 mm.[1-4] Dorsal angulation of more than 20° is associated with loss of wrist flexion and function.[1,5,6] Radial shortening of more than 4 mm is associated with loss of forearm rotation, and radial shortening of more than 5 mm is associated with ulnar wrist pain.[5,7] The relative risk of having a poor outcome was found to be 50% for patients younger than 65 years who had fracture healing with dorsal angulation of more than 10°, radial inclination of less than 15°, or radial shortening of more than 3 mm.[8] Therefore, reasonable treatment goals for an

Dr. Taras or an immediate family member is a board member, owner, officer, or committee member of Union Surgical; is a member of a speakers' bureau or has made paid presentations on behalf of Integra Life Sciences; and has received research or institutional support from Axogen. Dr. Ladd or an immediate family member is a board member, owner, officer, or committee member of the American Association for Hand Surgery, the American Society for Surgery of the Hand, the California Orthopaedic Association, the American Board of Orthopaedic Surgery, the American Orthopaedic Association, the Association of Bone and Joint Surgeons, and the Ruth Jackson Orthopaedic Society; has received royalties from the American Society for Surgery of the Hand and Orthohelix; is a member of a speakers' bureau or has made paid presentations on behalf of Medartis; serves as a paid consultant to or is an employee of Acumed; has stock or stock options in Orthovita; and has received nonincome support (such as equipment or services), commercially derived honoraria, or other non–research-related funding (such as paid travel) from the National Institutes of Health (National Institute of Arthritis and Musculoskeletal and Skin Diseases, National Institute of Child Health and Human Development). Dr. Kalainov or an immediate family member is a board member, owner, officer, or committee member of the American Society for Surgery of the Hand and Northwestern Memorial Hospital. Dr. Ruch or an immediate family member serves as a paid consultant to or is an employee of Zimmer and Synthes. Dr. Ring or an immediate family member has received royalties from DePuy and Wright Medical Technology; is a member of a speakers' bureau or has made paid presentations on behalf of Acumed, DePuy, and Synthes; serves as a paid consultant to or is an employee of Acumed and Wright Medical Technology; has received research or institutional support from Acumed, Biomet, Stryker, Tornier, and Joint Active Systems; has stock or stock options in Mimedex and Illuminoss; and has received nonincome support (such as equipment or services), commercially derived honoraria, or other non–research-related funding (such as paid travel) from the Journal of Hand Surgery–American.

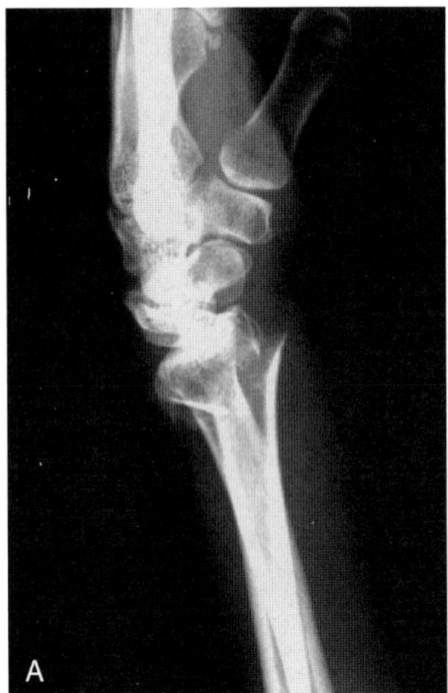

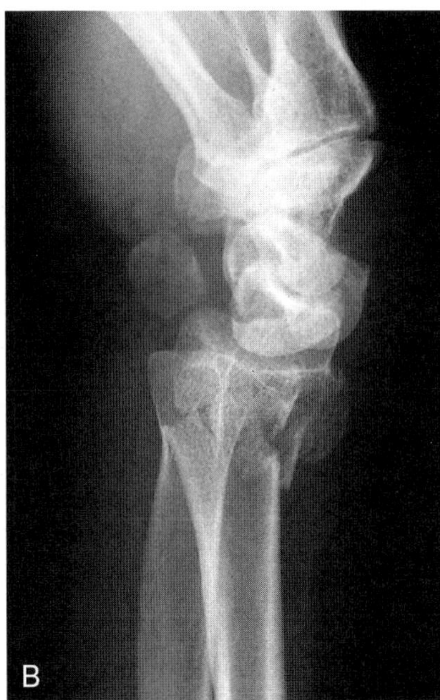

Figure 1 **A** and **B,** Lateral radiographs showing two comminuted distal radius fractures susceptible to redisplacement after closed treatment.

active person include a sustained reduction with less than 1 to 2 mm of articular displacement, 10° of dorsal angulation, and 2 to 3 mm of radial shortening.[9]

The optimal evidence-based treatment of distal radius fractures has not yet been clearly defined.[10] A wide array of methods and techniques is available for maintaining fracture alignment, including cast or splint immobilization, percutaneous pinning with casting, bridging or nonbridging external fixation, and internal fixation. The clinician can choose a treatment method based on experience and published research studies.

Pinning Techniques for the Treatment of Extra-articular Distal Radius Fractures

The factors that have been considered in developing procedures to treat extra-articular distal radius fractures include patient age, bone quality, ability to tolerate the procedure, and fracture type.[11] Treatment modalities have progressed from immobilization to percutaneous pinning, pins and plaster, external fixation, and internal fixation. The observed pitfalls of each technique have driven the evolution of treatment modalities. Fractures treated in plaster have a tendency to become redisplaced over time;[12] Mackenney and associates[13] reported that 60% of initially displaced fractures became redisplaced to a position of malunion when treated in a cast. Lafontaine and associates[14] identified the risk factors for redisplacement after an initial satisfactory reduction of a distal radius fracture as dorsal angulation of more than 20°, comminution, intra-articular involvement, associated fracture of the distal ulna, and patient age older than 60 years; if three or more risk factors were present, the likelihood of fracture collapse was high (Figure 1). Dias and associates[15] found that osteoporosis is a factor leading to progression of deformity after cast treatment.

The frequent failure of cast immobilization treatment of a displaced distal radius fracture led to attempts at stabilization using hardware fixation. The first widely used method was percutaneous pinning of the reduced fracture, usually with smooth straight wires and occasionally with threaded wires. Most techniques complement the use of pinning with cast immobilization for a period of 4 to 6 weeks. The reported pinning techniques include two pins placed through the radial styloid, two crossed pins, three or four intrafocal pins within the fracture site, transulnar oblique pinning with a threaded wire, a radial styloid pin with a second pin across the distal radioulnar joint, and multiple transulnar to radius pins that included the distal radioulnar joint.[16-25]

Several studies reported good or excellent results after pinning.[20,21,25-28] Other studies reported redisplacement rates of 25% to 33% despite pinning and casting.[16-18,23,24,29] The limitations of standard pinning techniques include a risk of infection if pins are left outside the skin for an extended time, irritation and skin breakdown if a pin cuts beneath the skin, tendon rupture if a pin is in close proximity to extensor tendons, and the necessity of a procedure to remove pins cut beneath the skin.

A purpose-designed threaded pin for distal radius fracture fixation (T-Pin, Union Surgical, Philadelphia, PA) recently has been introduced. This cannulated, threaded pin is designed to hold fracture fragments more securely than the commonly used smooth pins[11] (Figure 2). The technique for applying this

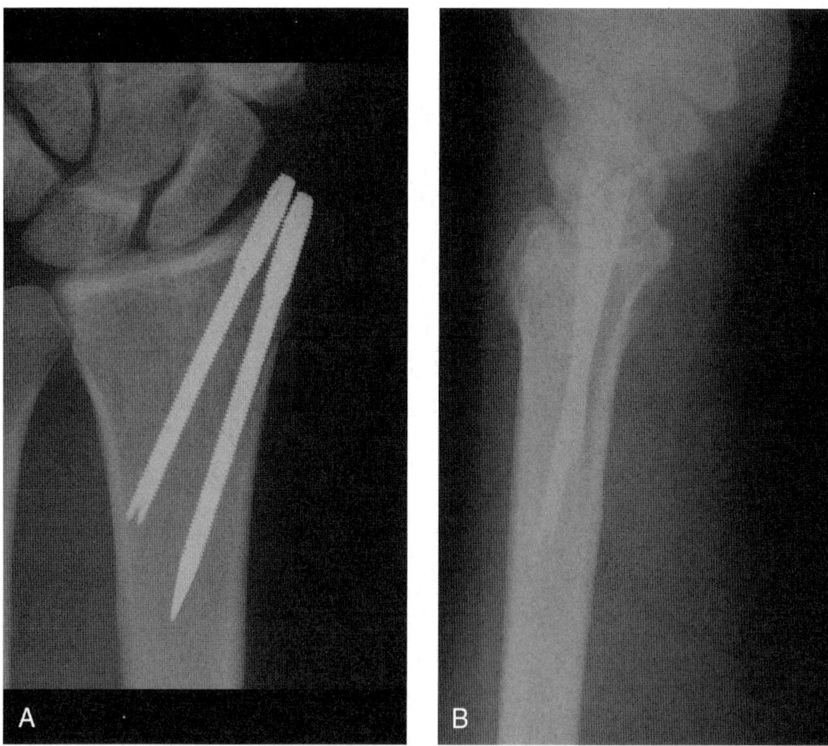

Figure 2 Postfixation PA **(A)** and lateral **(B)** radiographs of a distal radius fracture secured with two purpose-designed threaded pins inserted from the radial styloid.

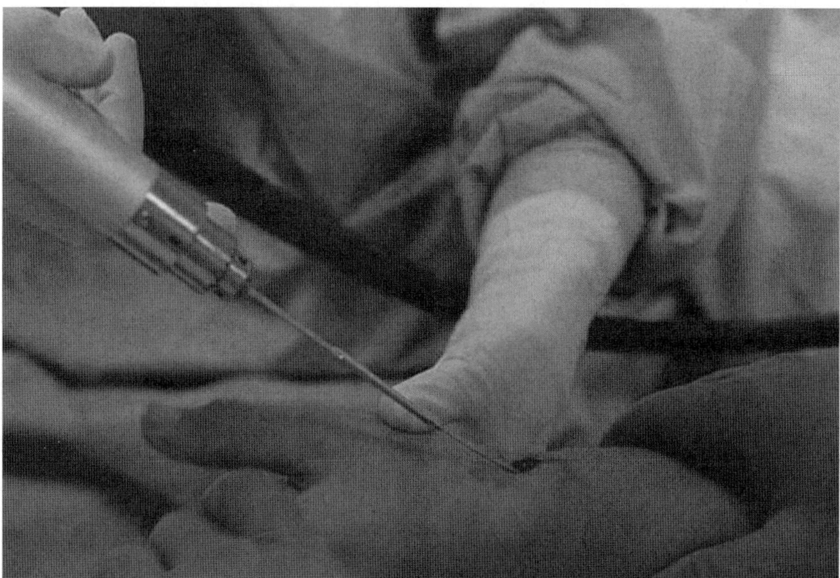

Figure 3 Intraoperative photograph showing the tip of the cannulated purpose-designed pin being placed over guidewire.

fixation device is similar to common pinning techniques. A break-off driver section allows the device to be placed entirely within the distal radius, thereby eliminating the possibility of tendon or skin irritation. The primary indication for using the purpose-designed threaded pin is the presence of an unstable, extra-articular, dorsally displaced distal radius fracture.

The purpose-designed threaded pin is placed over a guidewire through a small incision exposing the insertion site (Figure 3). In a typical fixation, two purpose-designed pins are inserted from the radial styloid. Other fixation configurations also can be used. The purpose-designed threaded pin creates a more secure purchase of the fracture fragments than smooth wires and thereby facilitates early wrist range of motion and recovery of function [11] (Table 1).

External fixation and internal fixation with plates are widely used alternatives to pinning for an unstable extra-articular distal radius fracture.[30] External fixation can bridge the fracture by distal fixation in the metacarpals, thereby indirectly reducing the fracture through ligamentotaxis or by direct distal fixation in the fracture fragment. Bridging external fixation is particularly useful for the initial treatment of an open fracture with soft-tissue loss, as a temporary measure in a patient with polytrauma, and for a distal shear fracture in which the distal fragment cannot be internally fixed. The current trend is to prefer internal fixation over percutaneous and external fixation.[30]

Nonbridging external fixation has been successfully used for treating unstable extra-articular fractures. At least 1 cm of intact volar cortex is required for pin purchase. In a comparison of bridging and nonbridging external fixation, McQueen[31] reported that nonbridging fixation led to better radiologic and functional indices during both early and late healing phases. The com-

Table 1
The Average Range of Motion 12 Months After Surgical Treatment of a Distal Radius Fracture Using Purpose-Designed Threaded Pins

Motion	Measurement
Flexion	54°
Extension	65°
Flexion-extension arc	119° (83% of the contralateral side)
Pronation	83°
Supination	65°
Pronation-supination arc	159° (94% of the contralateral side)

mon complications of external fixation include superficial radial nerve injury and pin tract infection. Stiffness and median nerve dysfunction can result from bridging external fixation because of excessive distraction, although the widespread recognition of this complication has led to greater diligence in avoiding it. The effectiveness of bridging external fixation is somewhat limited by the viscoelastic behavior of ligaments. There is a gradual loss of the initial distraction force applied through stress relaxation, which leads to some loss of initial fracture reduction during the healing phase.[32,33]

Formal open reduction and internal fixation requires surgical exposure of the fracture components. Plates specifically designed for common distal radius fracture patterns are most useful for fixing a displaced intra-articular fracture,[34] although they also are commonly used for unstable extra-articular fractures. Plates can be applied on the volar, dorsal, or radial cortices of the radius to maintain fracture reduction. Some implants incorporate screws that lock into the plate to enhance fracture stability; these designs are particularly useful for fractures with metaphyseal comminution.[35] Tendon rupture from chronic irritation over the plate or screws can occur after internal fixation with plates, although this complication is less likely to occur if a newer, low-profile plate design is used.[29,36] Because of the risk of tendon rupture, care must be taken when applying distal radius plates to ensure that the screws do not penetrate past the far cortex.

Bone Graft Substitutes

An extensive variety of bone graft substitutes is available for use in filling voids and restoring structural integrity during fracture fixation.[37-39] During the 1980s and 1990s, autogenous bone grafting was developed for use in both external and internal fixation of distal radius fractures, and it now is an important adjunct in the treatment of complex distal radius fractures.[40-42] The benefits of autogenous grafting include decreased time required for healing and removal of external fixation, as well as improvements in anatomic and functional outcome. However, autogenous grafting is associated with donor-site morbidity and increased surgical and hospital costs, especially with graft harvesting from the iliac crest[43] (Table 2). These disadvantages have influenced both surgeons and entrepreneurs to seek alternatives. Bone graft substitutes have been developed and used throughout the musculoskeletal system, including metaphyseal voids and fractures about the wrist.

Table 2
The Advantages and Disadvantages of Autologous Bone Graft

Advantages
Osteoinductivity and osteoconductivity
Osteogenesis
Cortical and cancellous forms
Structural support
Biocompatibility
Host site incorporation
Remodeling into normal bone
Disadvantages
Limited supply
Variable quality
Difficulty of harvesting
Harvest-related increases in surgical time, hospital stay, and cost
Harvest-related blood loss, postoperative pain, risk of infection, risk of fracture
Potential nidus for infection (avascular bone)

The use of graft substitutes can be considered for a comminuted distal radius fracture with a substantial metaphyseal void. In one respect, choosing a bone graft substitute is no different from choosing an autogenous or allograft bone graft. There is no absolute indication for using graft in the fracture setting, but it may be a useful adjunct.

Recommendations for Fixation of the Wrist Using Bone Graft Substitutes

It is difficult to compare bone graft substitutes of similar composition. These recommendations do not reflect the full range of available substitutes, and they do not constitute an endorsement for using a substitute rather than autogenous or allograft bone. The recommended methods for treating fractures, malunions, and other defects of the distal radius, including the use of bone grafts, are listed in Table 3. These recommendations for the

Table 3
Recommended Treatments of Fractures and Related Defects of the Radius

Fracture and/or Other Defect	Recommended Treatment
Simple distal radius fracture with significant metaphyseal defect	Calcium phosphate cement + pins
Significant cortical and metaphyseal defect	Calcium phosphate cement + plate and screws in osteoporotic bone *or* tricalcium phosphate in good-quality bone
Distal radius malunion (metaphyseal)	Plate and screws + calcium phosphate cement *or* iliac crest bone graft
Radius, ulna, humerus nonunion (metaphyseal or diaphyseal)	Iliac crest bone graft *or* tricalcium phosphate + bone marrow aspirate +/– BMP + electrical stimulation

BMP = bone morphogenetic protein

long bones can be extrapolated to defects elsewhere in the upper limb, including the metacarpals and phalanges. Calcium phosphate cement is recommended for metaphyseal defects typically associated with subchondral bone, which primarily resists compressive forces. Autogenous bone graft is preferred for areas known to heal poorly, such as the scaphoid. Calcium sulfate alone cannot be recommended for distal radius fractures because of its rapid dissolution characteristics and the lack of structural support.

Indications

Metaphyseal defects are ideally suited for using a calcium phosphate–based bone substitute as an osteoconductive material. The choice of porous, granular tricalcium phosphate or calcium phosphate cement depends on the stability of the fracture or void. Tricalcium phosphate can be used if sufficient cortical integrity exists, as in a simple fracture or defect, or if cortical strength is reestablished with plates, pins, or an external fixator. Calcium phosphate cement is chosen if the defect is larger than 1 cm and the primary purpose of reconstituting the metaphysis is to resist compressive forces.

Contraindications

Cement should not be used in the diaphysis because it has little ability to resist the shear and torsion forces normally borne by the diaphysis. Instead, tricalcium phosphate can be used in diaphyseal defects with adequate cortical reconstitution. Neither tricalcium phosphate nor calcium phosphate cement should be used if infection is present. The porosity of tricalcium phosphate may be an advantage in a nonunited fracture if the environment is optimized for healing by using bone marrow aspirate or another organic compound.

Calcium phosphate cement usually should not be used for a comminuted intra-articular fracture of the radius. A comminuted fracture with multiple unstable articular fragments creates local shear stresses that exceed the compressive strength capabilities of calcium phosphate cement. However, calcium phosphate cement can be used if the fracture construct can be adequately reduced, the articular pieces can be internally fixed without significant defects, and the void left after fixation of the primary metaphyseal fracture mimics an extra-articular fracture.

Technique

Tricalcium phosphate and calcium phosphate cement have different handling characteristics. Tricalcium phosphate bone graft substitutes are porous, with a texture resembling crumbly chalk. Most require reconstitution or softening with venous blood or bone marrow aspirate before being packed into the void with as much compression as possible. Tricalcium phosphate requires cortical integrity because it has poor strength. Therefore, it is best used in fractures with a well-defined and homogenous defect, in which the cortex already has been treated with an external fixator, pins, or a plate. Tricalcium phosphate may be preferred over autogenous graft for filling a diaphyseal defect if the healing environment is adequate and there is a desire to avoid the comorbidity associated with autograft harvest. Tricalcium phosphate also is ideal for a void such as that found in enchondroma, in which the cortex typically is intact and no additional hardware is needed. When used to fill a defect such as that created by benign tumor or implant removal, synthetic graft does not have the inherent strength afforded by intact cortices. Instead, the remodeling is similar to that of a metaphyseal fracture void. Figure 4 shows tricalcium phosphate filling a large defect after removal of a silicone implant used to treat a remote physeal bar of the distal radius; remodeling was gradual. Figure 5 shows a complex delayed union or nonunion of an unstable metaphyseal-diaphyseal fracture; the fracture was treated with hardware placed in 90° of opposition to provide cortical stability, and the nonunion was treated with tricalcium phosphate grafting in conjunction with bone morphogenetic protein (BMP)–7. It is unknown

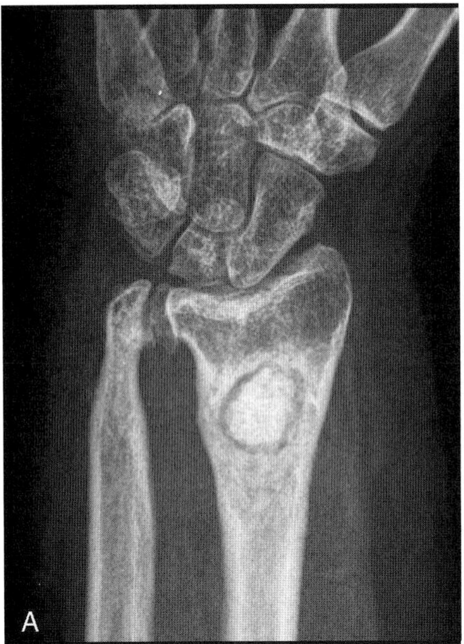

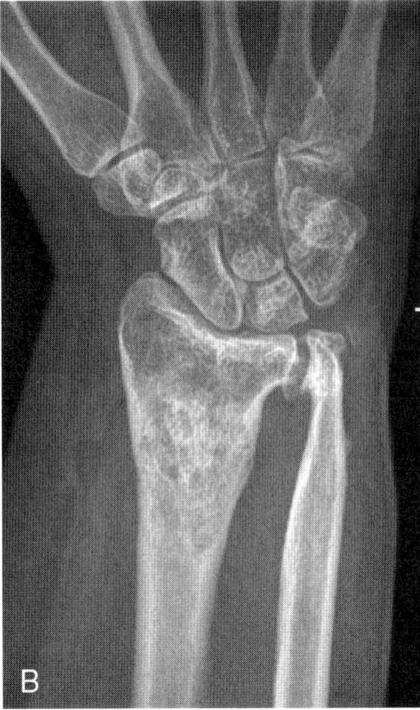

Figure 4 PA radiographs showing the remodeling of a large metaphyseal defect of the distal radius with a rim of osteoid after 4 months **(A)** and after 4 years **(B)**.

whether the BMP contributed to the subsequent healing. Such a complex fracture often is treated by using a variety of methods simultaneously, and the contribution of an individual treatment to the overall healing can be difficult to ascertain.

Calcium phosphate cement is ideally suited to a fracture with a large metaphyseal void and relatively intact cortices (Figure 6) or cortices that have been stabilized with pins, an external fixator (Figure 7), or a plate (Figure 8). Calcium phosphate cement should not be used for fractures involving the diaphysis because it poorly resists shear and torsion, which are critical to the role of the diaphysis. Similarly, calcium phosphate cement is contraindicated for a comminuted intra-articular fracture with oblique components unless articular alignment can be restored with no gap.

Extrusion of calcium phosphate cement into the soft tissues or joint can be minimized by banking the 12- or 14-gauge needle of the cement injection apparatus against the opposite cortex above or below the fracture line before the cement is injected. Banking the needle creates a high-pressure backfill and minimizes the flow of cement to the far cortex void, leaving a smooth, homogenous cement contour (Figures 6 and 8). The cement reaches half of its ultimate strength within the first 5 to 10 minutes of injection, and it is completely set within 24 hours. The cement hardens more rapidly if the tourniquet is released.

Pearls and Pitfalls

It is important to remove as much as possible of the tricalcium phosphate or calcium phosphate cement from the soft tissues before closing the wound because residual calcium substances are an irritant that can cause chemical cellulitis. Any calcium phosphate should be removed from the interface between the cortices and soft tissue before the cement hardens because it can solidify into a spike that can fray a tendon. Graft material should not be injected into the joint.

The surgeon must understand the material properties of the specific calcium phosphate cement to be used for fracture fixation and void filling. The handling characteristics of calcium phosphate cement differ greatly from those of polymethylmethacrylate cement. Calcium phosphate cement is only minimally exothermic, and it lacks the tensile properties of epoxy. In other words, it handles like grout rather than glue. Thorough mixing is required to ensure consistent setting. The variety of mixing and delivery techniques pertaining to different calcium phosphate cements can be confusing. Some, but not all, calcium phosphate cement formulations permit drilling through the material during or after setting. In general, manipulating the cement during the setting time, which is a critical period for crystallization and lattice formation, causes the material to crumble, rather than harden, more rapidly.

Calcium phosphate cement performs well as a homogenous construct in metaphyseal bone but should not be used as the primary means of fixing diaphyseal bone. Given their primarily osteoconductive nature and slow rate of bone remodeling, diaphyseal defects probably are better suited to the use of the more porous tricalcium phosphate or to autogenous or allograft bone graft. These materials can be used in combination with bone marrow aspirate or another type of harvested cell if healing is a concern, as with a delayed union or nonunion.

Evolving Techniques for Bone Graft Substitutes

In general, osteoconductive materials are used for metaphyseal defects

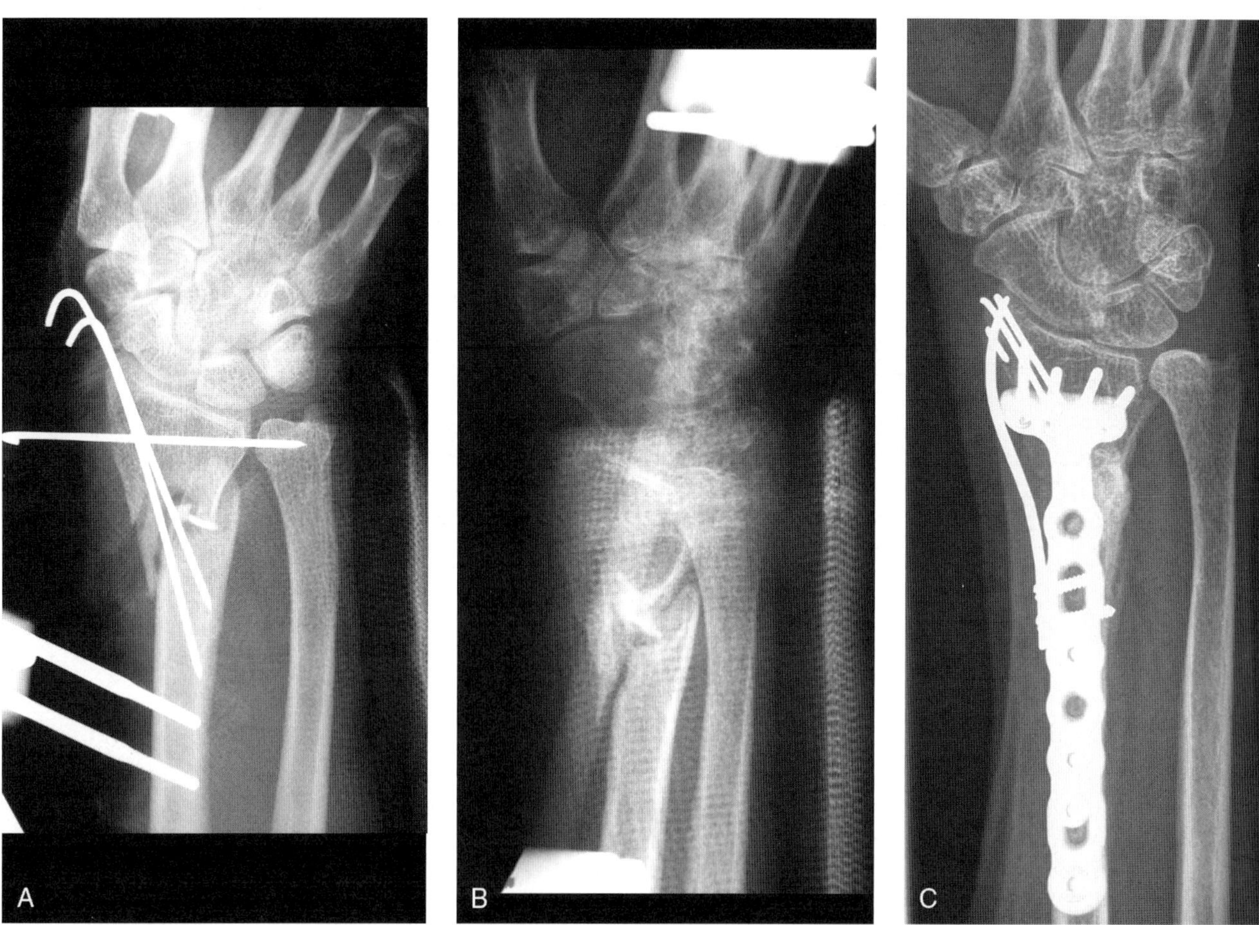

Figure 5 Radiographs showing treatment of an oblique (and, consequently, unstable) metaphyseal-diaphyseal fracture of the distal radius. **A,** The fracture was initially treated using external fixation with pins. **B,** After 4 months, a complex nonunion can be seen. **C,** A construct with 90° plating was used on the radial and volar column, with tricalcium phosphate and BMP-7; healing and remodeling can be seen after 1.5 years. Although iliac crest bone grafting is the graft of choice, the patient instead chose synthetic graft and BMP-7.

in conjunction with augmented fixation. Osteoinductive materials, including autograft, are used alone or as a graft extender if healing may be deterred, as in diaphyseal fractures or defects, osteoporotic bone, or nonunions. Composites of osteoinductive and osteoconductive materials may be useful for both periarticular metaphyseal defects and diaphyseal defects. In the future, proteins and growth factors may be used to promote healing in any common fracture. Calcium phosphate cement is the recommended graft substitute, with pin fixation, for a simple fracture with a significant distal radius defect. A more complex intra-articular fracture with a significant metaphyseal defect (typically larger than 1 cm) can be treated with internal fixation and calcium phosphate cement as an alternative to autogenous grafting. For the rare nonunion of the distal radius, internal fixation with iliac crest bone graft is preferred. For a distal radius malunion, an osteotomy with internal fixation is used, with calcium phosphate as a reasonable alternative to iliac crest bone graft. These recommendations are neither clear-cut nor backed by scientific evidence but are influenced by experience and practice patterns.

During the past 10 years, many types of graft substitutes have been developed, ranging from versatile demineralized bone graft products to mineral substitutes and growth factors. These products have been refined, and carrier substances have been developed. A new generation of substitutes allows tailoring to fit the specific patient needs, in much the way an internal fixation device is chosen. Although clinical need fuels the development and marketing of

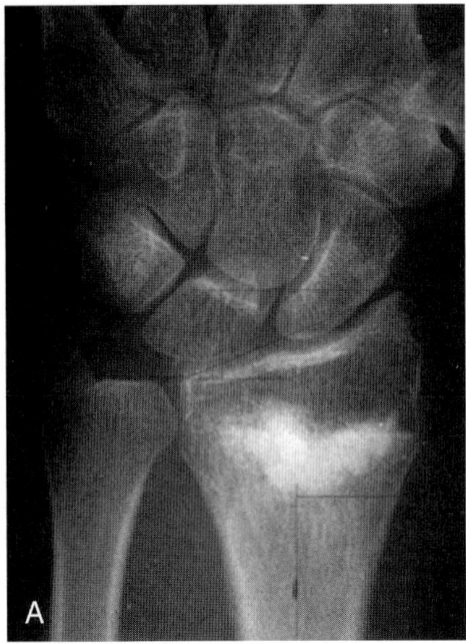

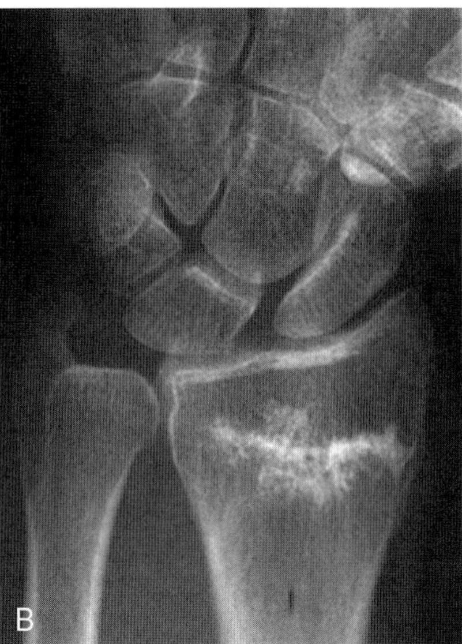

Figure 6 PA radiographs showing the appearance of calcium phosphate cement 2 weeks **(A)** and 2 years **(B)** after injection. (Courtesy of Norian Corporation, Cupertino, CA.)

bone graft substitutes, much of the clinical science is obscured by competitive marketing. The US Food and Drug Administration regulates products for safety and efficacy, but the standards are subject to interpretation. Each type of product raises unique concerns, with regulation overseen by several Food and Drug Administration centers. No biomechanical or other in vitro studies, animal studies, or clinical human studies are available to use for objective, quantitative comparison of the different substitutes. Clinical studies purporting to show equivalence between substitutes and autograft suggest either that the ability to assay bone healing is insufficiently sensitive or that osteoinduction, osteoconduction, and osteogenesis have negligible significance; the latter is highly unlikely.

Outcome studies and basic science analysis may prove helpful for assessing bone graft substitutes, and controlled comparisons of different products could provide useful information. Unfortunately, multicenter prospective studies are prohibitively expensive. In the absence of comparative information, sound clinical judgment must be the determining factor in decisions concerning the use of graft substitute.

Concomitant Injuries

Ligament Injuries and Carpal Malalignment

Tears of the intrinsic scapholunate and lunotriquetral interosseous ligaments are common in association with fractures of the distal radius. Scapholunate ligament defects have been observed in 18% to 64% of distal radius fractures by arthroscopy; approximately half of these defects represented partial tears.[44-47] Lunotriquetral tears have been detected in 12% to 16% of distal radius fractures, and combined defects of the scapholunate and lunotriquetral ligaments have been noted in as many as 22% of fractures by arthroscopy.[44-47]

Scapholunate or lunotriquetral ligament damage is more common with an intra-articular distal radius fracture, a displaced ulnar styloid fracture, a high-velocity injury, an increase in ulnar variance of more than 2 mm compared with the uninjured wrist, lunate hyperextension before fracture reduction, and in patients age 55 years or older.[44-50] Attritional tears of the scapholunate and lunotriquetral ligaments are common in patients near the seventh decade of life, and they may be difficult to differentiate from a traumatic defect.[44,51,52] Only sparse literature is available on other ligament injuries associated with distal radius fracture.

Carpal stability depends on intrinsic carpal ligaments, extrinsic ligaments that join the carpal bones to the forearm and hand, and skeletal anatomy.[53-55] Dynamic carpal instability may develop after a limited ligament injury and will escape detection in the absence of stress radiographic views. Static carpal instability is diagnosed on standard radiographs and can occur as a result of damage to more than one ligamentous structure or excessive displacement of a distal radius fracture. Delays have been reported in both the development and diagnosis of carpal malalignment,[56,57] and the true prevalence and natural history of carpal instability associated with distal radius fractures is not known.

The most commonly recognized pattern of carpal instability after a distal radius fracture is static scapholunate joint dissociation, which is denoted by a widened scapholunate interval. Scapholunate interval separation has been recognized in as many as 60% of distal radius fractures, often in association with increased scaphoid flexion and lunate hyperextension (known as dorsal intercalated segment instability).[49,51] Less commonly reported instability patterns include static

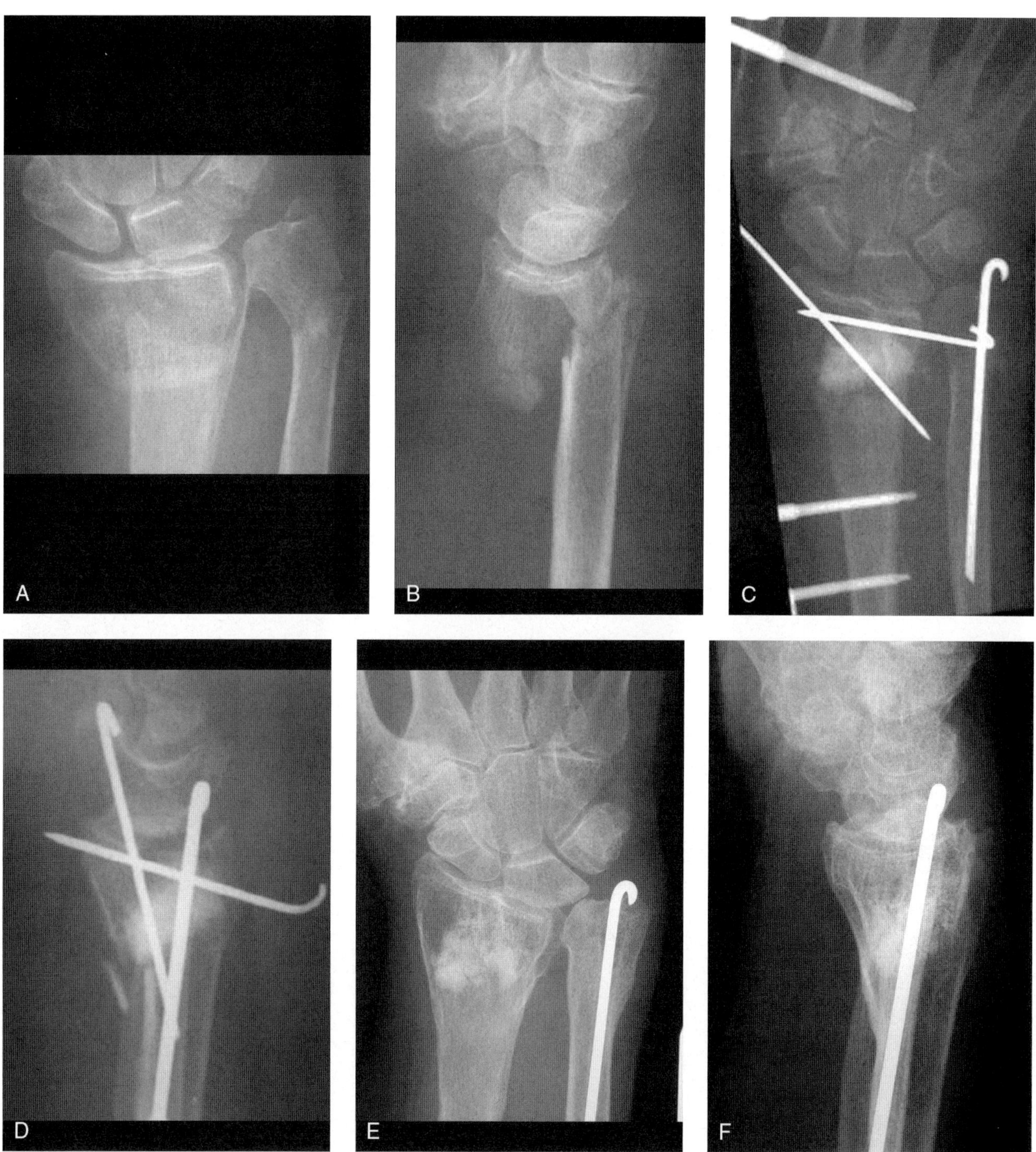

Figure 7 AP **(A)** and lateral **(B)** radiographs showing an unstable fracture of the distal radius and ulna in a 91-year-old woman with severe osteoporosis. AP **(C)** and lateral **(D)** radiographs showing treatment with an external fixator, percutaneous pins, and calcium phosphate cement. AP **(E)** and lateral **(F)** radiographs showing remodeling at 1 year with relative stress shielding of the central bone, in accordance with Wolff's law.

dorsal and palmar radiocarpal subluxation, static ulnar translocation of the carpus, and static midcarpal instability.[50,51,58-61]

In the absence of a destabilizing ligamentous injury, reduction of a distal radius fracture may effectively treat carpal malalignment. For example, dorsal intercalated segment instability may be resolved by correcting a dorsally angulated distal radius fracture.[62] Persistent carpal

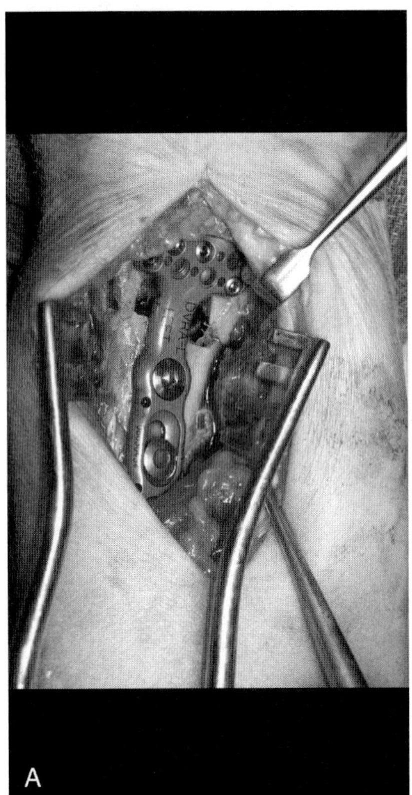

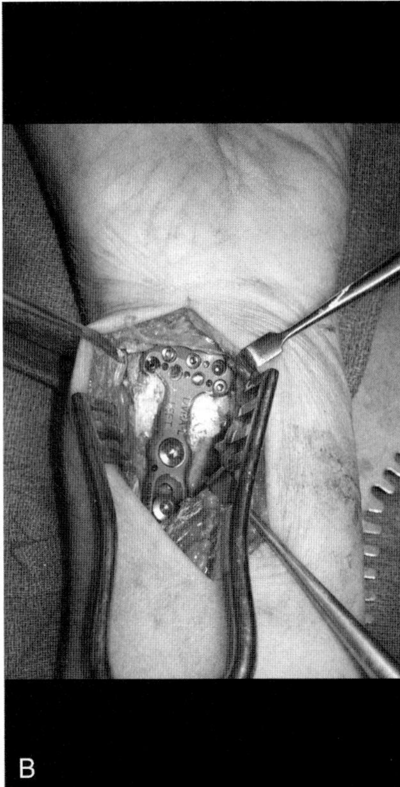

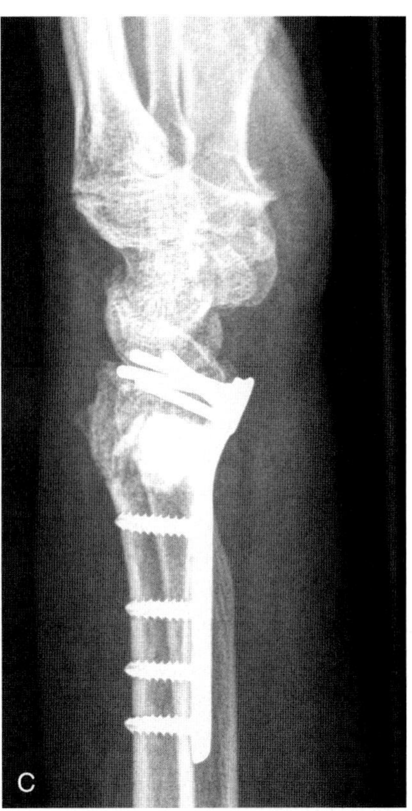

Figure 8 Treatment of a comminuted distal radius fracture with a void sufficiently large to warrant grafting. **A,** Intraoperative photograph showing plate fixation and the large fracture defect. **B,** Intraoperative photograph taken after injection of approximately 1.5 mL of calcium phosphate cement. **C,** Lateral radiograph showing homogenous filling of the void without extrusion through the dorsal cortex.

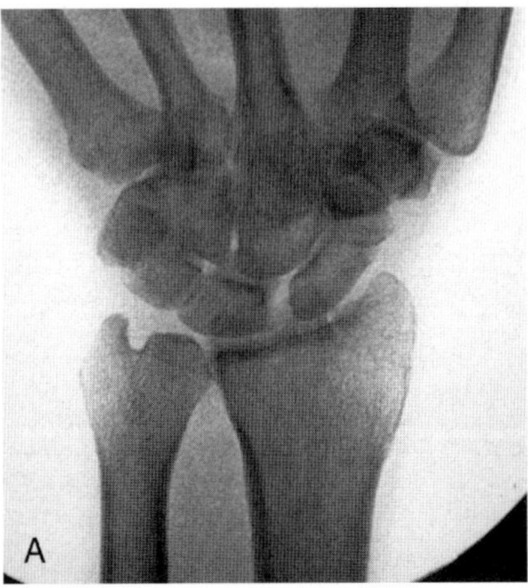

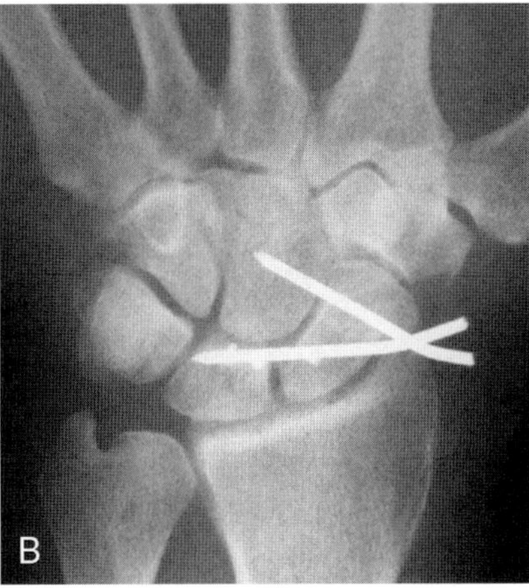

Figure 9 PA radiographs showing traumatic scapholunate joint dissociation. **A,** The dissociation was symptomatic 4 months after cast treatment of an intra-articular distal radius fracture. **B,** Treatment with open joint reduction, intercarpal pinning, and ligament reconstruction using a tendon graft.

instability after fracture reduction can be treated by intercarpal pinning, either alone or in combination with arthroscopic débridement, capsulodesis, ligament repair, or ligament reconstruction.[63,64] Carpal malalignment with late symptoms often is more difficult to manage. The treatment options range from benign neglect to total wrist arthrodesis, depending on the flexibility of the malaligned carpus, the presence of arthritis, the training and judgment of the surgeon, and, ultimately, the patient's choice (Figure 9).

Retrospective studies have found that the treatment of a distal radius fracture may be adversely affected if carpal ligament injury and carpal malalignment are not concurrently managed.[49,65-67] A recent prognostic level I arthroscopic study compared patients who had an untreated partial or complete scapholunate ligament tear with patients who had an intact or minimally damaged scapholunate ligament 1 year after distal radius fracture treatment. The patients with an untreated tear were found to have more pain and greater scapholunate interval gapping.[47] However, carpal ligament damage, carpal malalignment, or distal radius malunion does not always portend a suboptimal functional result. A scapholunate ligament injury may potentially allow the proximal carpal row to better conform to the altered geometry of the fractured distal radius;[55] consequently, repair or reconstruction of the ligament defect may conceivably lead to greater pain and progressive carpal arthrosis.[55,68]

Tendon Injuries

Spontaneous rupturing of the extensor pollicis longus tendon has been reported in as many as 8.6% of patients with a distal radius fracture.[69,70] Rupture of the extensor pollicis longus tendon usually occurs during the first 4 to 10 weeks after injury, in association with a nondisplaced or minimally displaced fracture. Proposed etiologies of tendon disruption include direct crushing of the tendon, excursion of the tendon over sharp bone or callus, increased thickness of the enveloping retinaculum, and vascular insufficiency.

Internal plate fixation of distal radius fractures has been associated with injury to the digital extensor and flexor tendons.[71-86] The extensor digitorum communis and extensor indicis proprius tendons are at greatest risk of injury from dorsal plate application, with reported rates of tenosynovitis or tendon rupture ranging from 0% to 32%.[71-76] Extensor tenosynovitis or tendon rupture related to the placement of screws and pegs through volar plates has been detected in up to 5% of cases.[79-83,85] The flexor pollicis longus tendon is particularly prone to injury from volar plate fixation;[77-86] disruption of this tendon was reported in 12% of patients in one study.[79]

The risk of tendon injury with plate fixation is affected by surgical exposure, implant design (in particular, a thick dorsal plate or a wide volar plate), implant modification that leaves a sharp edge, excessive screw or peg length, or loss of fracture reduction with secondary plate prominence.[74,78,82-88] Placement of a volar plate distal to the transverse ridge, or watershed line, of the distal radius is believed to create a specific risk for injury to the flexor pollicis longus and flexor digitorum profundus tendons.[86] The metallic composition of the implant may be a source of tendon damage; in animal studies, inflammatory changes have been attributed to both stainless steel and titanium plates.[89,90]

The prevention of tendon injury is of paramount importance in plate fixation of a distal radius fracture. There is considerable variation in the height of the Lister tubercle and the depth of the extensor pollicis longus tendon groove.[91] A minifluoroscopy unit can be used intraoperatively to obtain multiple tilt views for detecting inadvertent articular penetration and past-pointing of distal pegs and screws through cortical bone.[92-94] Tendon irritation after surgery can be managed with temporary wrist splint immobilization, anti-inflammatory medication, and physical therapy. Persistent pain attributable to an implant may require hardware removal. Tendon grafting and tendon transfers are the preferred surgical treatments for tendon rupture because the torn ends of the tendon may not be amenable to primary repair without débridement and extensive shortening.

Acute Carpal Tunnel Syndrome

Acute carpal tunnel syndrome (acute median neuropathy) occasionally occurs in association with distal radius fractures; one study found a 5.4% incidence after fracture repair.[95] Acute carpal tunnel syndrome is caused by elevated pressures within the carpal canal and is characterized by pain and dysesthesias in the median nerve distribution. Failure to recognize and treat this condition can lead to permanent median nerve dysfunction or complex regional pain syndrome.

Acute carpal tunnel syndrome is differentiated from a contusion of the median nerve by the course of symptom development after fracture.[96] Acute carpal tunnel syndrome develops over hours or days and progressively worsens. In contrast, the symptoms of a median nerve contusion appear at the time of fracture, often improve after manipulative reduction, and tend to dissipate within days or weeks. Acute carpal tunnel syndrome and contusion of the median nerve may occur in conjunction with chronic carpal tunnel syndrome, which should be suspected if the patient reports preexisting hand dysesthesias.

Risk factors for acute carpal tunnel syndrome include high-energy trauma in a young patient, translation of the distal radius epiphysis, tight casting, excess carpal traction, and extreme angulation of the wrist.[96] The treatment may include loosening or removal of the cast, fracture reduction, release of excessive wrist distraction, and surgical decompression of the carpal canal. Surgical decompression should be performed expediently if nonsurgical measures do not lead to immediate symptom improvement.

Prophylactic carpal tunnel decompression can be done in conjunction

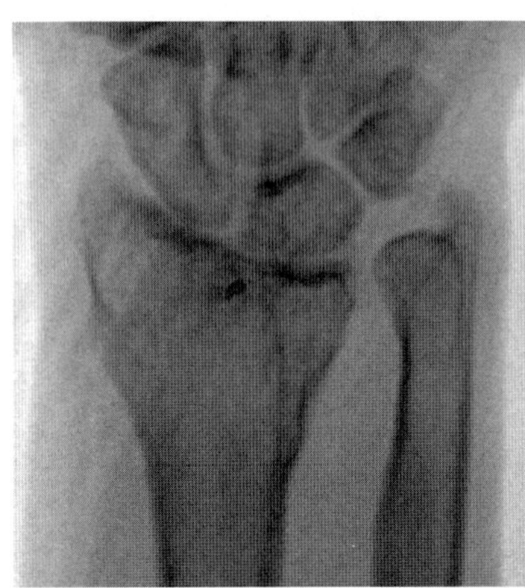

Figure 10 AP radiograph showing residual depression of the lunate facet of the radius. Eventually this condition will lead to loss of radiocarpal congruity caused by step-off in the articular surface, radiographically apparent arthrosis, radioulnar incongruity, and functional loss of rotation caused by ulnar positive variance.

with distal radius fracture repair, but the criteria are not well defined. In a retrospective case-control study, Dyer and associates[95] concluded that prophylactic surgical decompression may be appropriate for women younger than 48 years with more than 35% translation of the distal radius epiphysis. To prevent inadvertent injury to the palmar cutaneous branch of the median nerve, a separate incision is recommended when surgical release of the carpal canal is combined with a Henry approach to the distal radius fracture.

Distal Radioulnar Joint Injuries

The Role of the Intermediate Column

Treating the distal radioulnar joint in conjunction with a distal radius fracture is critical to the patient's short-term functional advance and the long-term prevention of arthrosis. The distal radioulnar joint is the most common source of persistent discomfort after treatment of a distal radius fracture.[97,98] The most common functional complaint after a distal radius fracture is the loss of supination of the forearm.[99-101] A classic article by Knirk and Jupiter[3] established that a 2-mm or greater residual depression of the lunate facet leads to articular incongruity and radiographically apparent arthrosis 5 to 7 years after the injury (Figure 10). Thus, the focus of treatment for distal radius fracture should be the intermediate column, which primarily consists of the lunate facet of the radius, the triangular fibrocartilage complex (TFCC), and the insertion of the TFCC on the ulnar styloid.

Radial Deformity

Loss of Radial Length

Loss of radial length, as measured by comparison to the intact ulna, can occur in a metaphyseal bending fracture or a lunate impaction fracture with residual depression of the lunate facet. A metaphyseal bending fracture typically results in both a loss of radial length and an increase in palmar tilt. The loss of radial length can lead to traumatic ulnocarpal impaction syndrome, which is characterized by pain with wrist extension and loss of rotation as the carpus encounters the fixed axis of the ulna. As little as 2 to 3 mm of ulnar positive variance can cause symptomatic ulnocarpal impaction, although the amount of shortening required to cause symptoms varies from patient to patient.

The best treatment of posttraumatic ulnocarpal impaction can be determined by examining other radiographic parameters for distal radius healing. With a neutral palmar tilt and no intra-articular incongruity, treatment using ulna-shortening osteotomy has a good overall outcome. With an isolated loss of radial length with at least neutral palmar tilt and no depression of the palmar lunate facet, the treatment can focus on the ulnocarpal impaction. An ulna-shortening osteotomy usually is sufficient, but a radial osteotomy can be used. Care must be taken to make certain the slope of the sigmoid notch is parallel to the slope of the ulnar head, so as to avoid the increased forces that may be seen after a ulna-shortening osteotomy. Posttraumatic degenerative changes at the distal radioulnar joint can cause an increase in pain over time.[102]

Loss of Radial Length and Palmar Tilt

The loss of palmar tilt in conjunction with a loss of radial length leads to both ulnocarpal impaction syndrome and increasing strain on the distal radioulnar joint ligaments, which causes loss of forearm rotation. A recent laboratory study found that a loss of 20° of palmar tilt with intact distal radioulnar joint ligaments requires increased work for forearm rotation and can explain the loss of supination in some patients.[101] In an elderly patient with a comminuted metaphyseal bending fracture, this deformity may be so severe that the distal radioulnar joint ligaments are completely stripped from the distal ulna. The result is an actual dislocation of the distal radioulnar joint, with overall restoration of freedom of motion. In a younger patient with less deformity and intact ligaments, the loss of palmar tilt in conjunction with a loss of radial length causes functional impairment in forearm supination. The management of this deformity should focus on restoring radial anatomy with a radial osteotomy.

An increase in palmar tilt may be of more concern than a loss of palmar

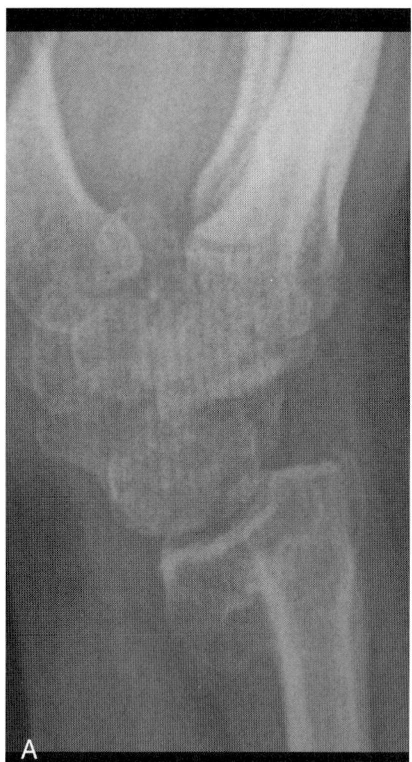

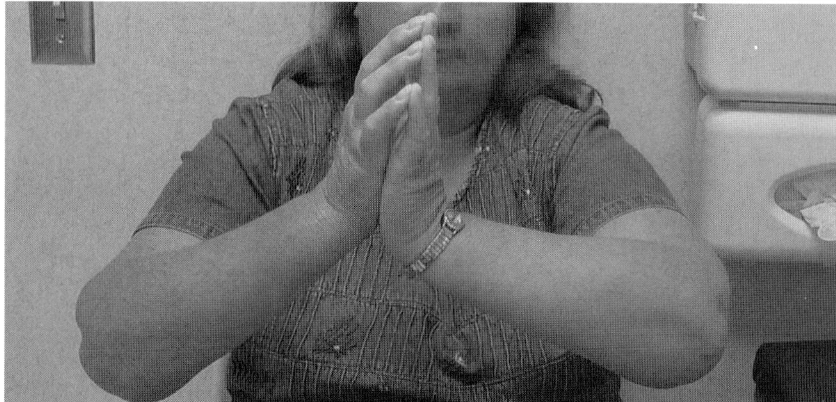

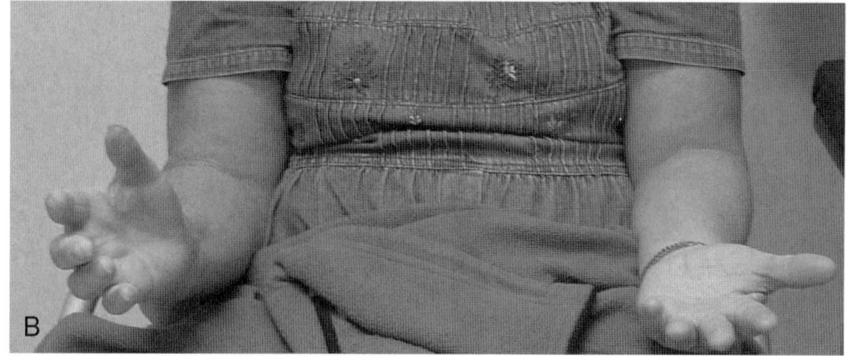

Figure 11 **A,** Lateral radiograph showing overreduction of a dorsally displaced fracture, resulting in an increased palmar tilt. The effect is to palmarly displace the radius relative to the ulna and cause relative subluxation of the distal radioulnar joint. **B,** Clinical photographs showing the significant loss of forearm rotation.

tilt (Figure 11). An increase from 12° to 17° after overreduction of a distal radius fracture was found to alter distal radioulnar joint mechanics and result in the loss of forearm rotation.[102-104] The exact indications for corrective osteotomy are unknown, but patients with functional loss of rotation have an excellent reported outcome after a palmar opening wedge osteotomy. An adjunctive carpal tunnel release may be appropriate to avoid traction injury to the median nerve as the radius is effectively lengthened by the osteotomy.

Residual Depression of the Palmar Lunate Facet

A lunate impaction fracture resulting in depression of the lunate facet may lead to ulnocarpal impaction or residual depression of the palmar lunate facet of the radius. Residual depression of the palmar lunate facet causes ulnocarpal incongruity, as well as radioulnar joint incongruity, as the carpus follows the palmar lunate–impacted segment. The result is a characteristic deformity with loss of wrist extension and forearm rotation. This deformity is best identified using CT with three-dimensional reconstruction. Corrective osteotomy of the palmar lunate facet restores the hand to the reduced position and restores forearm rotation without ligament reconstruction.

Ulnar Column Injury

The literature on treating ligamentous injuries and ulnar styloid fractures is conflicting. In a cadaver study, Adams[105] found that shortening the radius more than 5 mm results in disrupting the TFCC or fracturing the base of the ulnar styloid. Clinical observation suggests that ulnar-sided pain and loss of rotation are common after the radius is shortened. There is a current emphasis on improving outcomes by repairing the TFCC and the ulnar styloid. Studies have been published on repair of the TFCC in conjunction with external fixation and repair of ulnar styloid fractures in conjunction with external fixation of the distal radius.[105-107] A comparison of simple immobilization of the forearm in 60° of supination with direct repair of the ulnar styloid found that immobilization resulted in better outcomes than direct repair.[108] Most of the studies were conducted on the assumption that external fixation usually is the preferred primary fixation for a high-

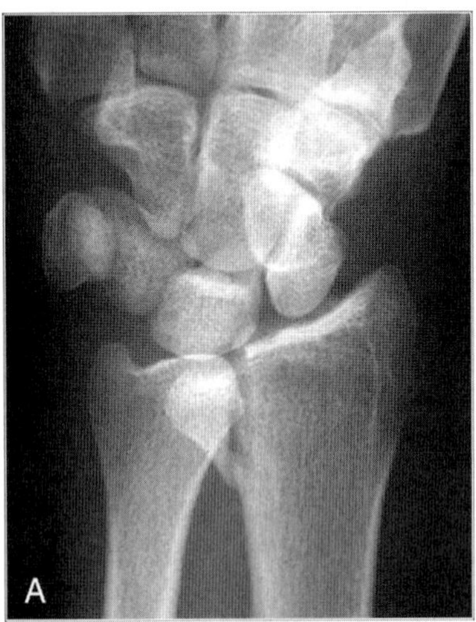

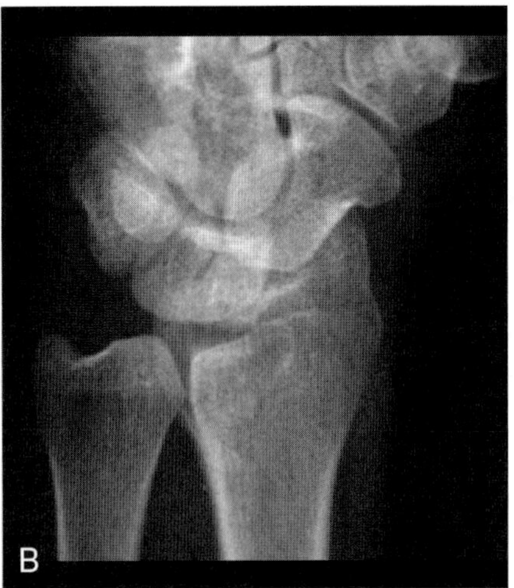

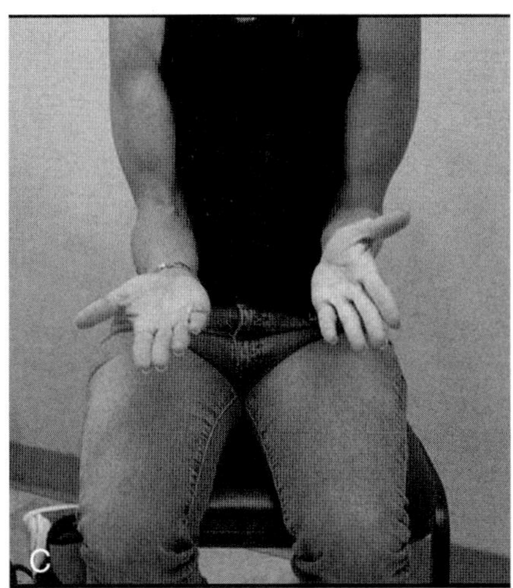

Figure 12 The effect of loss of the critical corner of the palmar lunate facet. **A,** AP radiograph showing a characteristic fracture of the critical ulnar corner of the lunate facet. **B,** AP radiograph showing the healed fracture, with articular incongruity and distal radioulnar joint malalignment. **C,** Clinical photograph showing the loss of extension and rotation resulting from healing in this position.

energy wrist fracture. The exact indications for repairing the TFCC or the ulnar styloid in conjunction with external fixation have not been determined.[44]

Repair of the ulnar styloid has been examined in conjunction with internal fixation of distal radius fracture. Study findings suggest that repair of the ulnar styloid does not improve the outcome when the radius heals anatomically.[109] In a study of displaced fractures involving at least three quarters of the height of the ulnar styloid, the fracture was fixed in 76 patients and not treated in another 76 patients. Although styloid fracture is predictive of a worse overall outcome, no difference was found in the outcomes of the treated and untreated patients.[110] This study emphasized the importance of restoring the critical corner consisting of the palmar lunate facet and the palmar distal radioulnar joint ligament (Figure 12).

It is apparent that injury to the distal radioulnar joint frequently is the source of residual symptoms after treatment of a distal radius fracture. These injuries appear to be related to high-energy trauma. There is a trend away from surgical repair, provided that the distal radius is anatomically reduced.

Distal Radius Malunion

A distal radius malunion is best defined as a malalignment associated with dysfunction. Malalignment does not always result in dysfunction; in particular, most low-demand older patients function very well with the deformity.[111] Dysfunction can take the form of loss of motion, loss of strength, or pain.[112-114] Pain can be the most difficult-to-treat symptom directly associated with the deformity. An osteotomy to relieve pain, like any surgery for this purpose, has relatively unpredictable results and should be undertaken with caution. Pain can be caused by articular malalignment, arthrosis, carpal malalignment, or distal radioulnar joint malalignment. These conditions can be treated using a salvage or reconstructive procedure. The relationship between distal radius malunion and carpal tunnel syndrome is disputed; some surgeons believe there is a direct causal relationship and that carpal tunnel syndrome can be alleviated with osteotomy alone.

Malunion is much less common than radiographic malalignment. Mackenney and associates[13] defined malalignment as a dorsal tilt of more than 10° or a positive ulnar variance of more than 3 mm. These radiographic parameters were used in finding that 744 of 1,296 initially displaced fractures (57%) later became redisplaced or malaligned. The factors associated with malalignment, as proposed by Lafontaine and associates,[115] include age older than 60 years; more than 20° of dorsal angulation, as seen on the initial postinjury lateral radiograph; dorsal metaphyseal comminution; comminution extending to the volar metaphyseal cortex; associated fracture of the ulna; and displaced articular fracture. Mackenney and associates[13] identified several predictors of loss of alignment in an initially displaced fracture: patient age, metaphyseal comminution, initial dorsal tilt, initial ulnar variance, and lack of functional independence. It is not worthwhile to remanipulate a reduced fracture that has become redisplaced in a cast or splint.[115,116] Patients having one or more of the predictive factors should be advised of the potential for fracture malalignment after nonsurgical treatment; however, they also should be informed that the relationship between malalignment and dysfunction (malunion) is incompletely defined. Optimal wrist alignment and function are important to many older patients, and treatment decisions should not be made solely on the basis of patient age.[117]

A surgically treated fracture can become malaligned. Percutaneous pins alone may not be sufficient to maintain the alignment if there is substantial metaphyseal comminution,[118] and external fixation alone (without ancillary percutaneous pin fixation of the fracture) may not be sufficient to maintain the reduction.[40,119,120] The fracture may settle after removal of the implant more than 6 weeks after injury, especially with substantial metaphyseal comminution.[3] A nonlocking plate can loosen in osteopenic metaphyseal bone;[121,122] a locking plate also can loosen, but the risk is much lower and incompletely defined.

Extra-articular malalignment is a combination of dorsovolar and radioulnar malalignment, shortening, and malrotation.[104,123] Articular malalignment can appear as subluxation or as a step-off in the subchondral line on an AP radiograph.[124-126] The diagnosis of malunion requires that the radiographic malalignment be correlated with the patient's symptoms. Caution is warranted. In particular, ulnar-sided wrist pain after a distal radius fracture can continue to improve for 1 year or longer. A lack of forearm rotation may be related to capsular contracture, which usually improves over time and responds to exercises, or bony malalignment. Pain is complex and multifactorial, and it can be difficult to relate directly to malalignment.

The patient's symptoms must be focused into a goal (for example, improved flexion or supination), and it must be determined whether the goal can be achieved with surgery. Distal radial osteotomy should be considered if the surgeon has confidence that it will achieve the goal, the patient has good understanding and compliance, and the potential benefits of surgical intervention outweigh the risks.

A malunited fracture of the distal radius can be treated with an osteotomy or salvage procedure (such as ulnar shortening or arthrodesis) if the patient has symptomatic ulnocarpal impaction syndrome, dysfunction of the distal radioulnar joint (such as limited forearm motion, instability, or arthrosis), a weak grip or restriction of motion related to extra-articular deformity, or simple articular incongruity sufficient to cause correctable arthrosis or subluxation. A malunion should not be surgically treated if the patient has a low functional activity level, an infection, a stiff hand, unrealistic expectations, or unclear goals. These surgical procedures are elective and should not be done if the indications do not clearly favor treatment. After the patient and the surgeon decide that the malalignment carries an unacceptable risk of dysfunction, the decision to proceed with osteotomy can be based on radiographic findings alone (for a so-called nascent malunion), without attempting to improve function over time and with exercises. A patient who has a limited deformity or is not highly motivated should consider postponing the surgical decision because motion can continue to improve for more than 1 year after injury with the use of active-assisted exercises and a dynamic or static splint.

Distal radial osteotomy traditionally has been done through a dorsal exposure with the use of a structural corticocancellous bone graft.[127] With the advent of angular stable (locking) plates, the use of adjunctive cancellous graft alone has proved adequate.[127] A nascent malunion or incompletely healed dorsally malaligned fracture can be treated from an extended volar exposure, during which the brachioradialis is lengthened or released and the dorsal periosteum is released as the fracture site is taken down. This extended flexor carpi radialis exposure restores mobility to the distal fracture fragment, allowing reduction to the metaphysis without undue force.[128-130] This extensile approach may also be useful for mature malunions. Several small case studies have established the safety and efficacy of volar osteotomy for a dorsally displaced fracture.[131-134] Intra-articular osteotomy, a technically challenging procedure, should be considered only for a simple, easily correctable articular malunion, preferably in the nascent stage; it should be done within 3 months of injury so that the original fracture line can be identified.[124-126] If there is established arthrosis of the distal radioulnar or radiocarpal joints, a salvage procedure may be preferable, such as a resection of the distal ulna, a Sauvé-Kapandji procedure (distal radioulnar arthrodesis with intentional ulnar pseudarthrosis), or a partial or total radiocarpal arthrodesis.

References

1. Forward DP, Davis TR, Sithole JS: Do young patients with malunited fractures of the distal radius inevitably develop symptomatic post-traumatic osteoarthritis? *J Bone Joint Surg Br* 2008;90:629-637.
2. Kreder HJ, Hanel DP, Agel J, et al: Indirect reduction and percutaneous fixation versus open reduction and internal fixation for displaced intra-articular fractures of the distal radius: A randomised, controlled trial. *J Bone Joint Surg Br* 2005;87:829-836.
3. Knirk JL, Jupiter JB: Intra-articular fractures of the distal end of the radius in young adults. *J Bone Joint Surg Am* 1986;68:647-659.
4. Catalano LW III, Cole RJ, Gelberman RH, Evanoff BA, Gilula LA, Borrelli J Jr: Displaced intra-articular fractures of the distal aspect of the radius: Long-term results in young adults after open reduction and internal fixation. *J Bone Joint Surg Am* 1997; 79:1290-1302.
5. Altissimi M, Antenucci R, Fiacca C, Mancini GB: Long-term results of conservative treatment of fractures of the distal radius. *Clin Orthop Relat Res* 1986;206:202-210.
6. Porter M, Stockley I: Fractures of the distal radius: Intermediate and end results in relation to radiologic parameters. *Clin Orthop Relat Res* 1987; 220:241-252.
7. Fernandez DL, Geissler WB: Treatment of displaced articular fractures of the radius. *J Hand Surg Am* 1991; 16:375-384.
8. Grewal R, MacDermid JC: The risk of adverse outcomes in extra-articular distal radius fractures is increased with malalignment in patients of all ages but mitigated in older patients. *J Hand Surg Am* 2007;32:962-970.
9. Abramo A, Kopylov P, Tagil M: Evaluation of a treatment protocol in distal radius fractures: A prospective study in 581 patients using DASH as outcome. *Acta Orthop* 2008;79: 376-385.
10. Handoll HH, Madhok R: Surgical interventions for treating distal radius fractures in adults. *Cochrane Database Syst Rev* 2003;3:CD003209.
11. Taras JS, Zambito KL, Abzug JM: T-Pin for distal radius fracture. *Tech Hand Up Extrem Surg* 2006;10:2-7.
12. Fernandez DL, Palmer AK: Fractures of the distal radius, in Green D, Hotchkiss R, Pederson W, eds: *Green's Operative Hand Surgery,* ed 4. New York, NY, Churchill Livingstone, 1999, pp 929-985.
13. Mackenney PJ, McQueen MM, Elton R: Prediction of instability in distal radial fractures. *J Bone Joint Surg Am* 2006;88:1944-1951.
14. Lafontaine MJ, Delince P, Hardy D, Simons M: Instability of fractures of the lower end of the radius: Apropos of a series of 167 cases. *Acta Orthop Belg* 1989;55:203-216.
15. Dias JJ, Wray CC, Jones JM: Osteoporosis and Colles' fractures in the elderly. *J Hand Surg Br* 1987;12:57-59.
16. Lenoble E, Dumontier C, Goutallier D, et al: Fracture of the distal radius: A prospective comparison between trans-styloid and Kapandji fixations. *J Bone Joint Surg Br* 1995;77: 562-567.
17. Clancey GJ: Percutaneous Kirschner-wire fixation of Colles fractures: A prospective study of thirty cases. *J Bone Joint Surg Am* 1984;66:1008-1014.
18. Stein AH Jr, Katz SF: Stabilization of comminuted fractures of the distal inch of the radius: Percutaneous pinning. *Clin Orthop Relat Res* 1975;108: 174-181.
19. Kapandji A: Treatment of non-articular distal radius fractures by intrafocal pinning with arum pins, in Saffer P, Cooney WP, eds: *Fractures of the Distal Radius.* Philadelphia, PA, Lippincott Williams & Wilkins, 1995, pp 71-83.
20. Kapandji A: Intra-focal pinning of fractures of the distal end of the radius 10 years later. *Ann Chir Main* 1987;6:57-63.
21. Kapandji A: L'osteosynthese par double enbrochage intrafocal: Traitement fonctionnel des fractures non-articulaires de l'extrémitié inferieure du radius. *Ann Chir* 1976;30:903-908.
22. Greatting MD, Bishop AT: Intrafocal (Kapandji) pinning of unstable fractures of the distal radius. *Orthop Clin North Am* 1993;24:301-307.
23. DePalma A: Comminuted fractures of the distal end of the radius treated by ulnar pinning. *J Bone Joint Surg Am* 1952;34:651-662.
24. Mortier JP, Kuhlmann JN, Richet C, Baux S: Horizontal cubito-radial pinning in fractures of the distal radius including a postero-internal fragment. *Rev Chir Orthop Repar Appar Mot* 1986;72:567-572.
25. Rayhack JM, Langworthy JN, Belsole RJ: Transulnar percutaneous pinning of displaced distal radial fractures: A preliminary report. *J Orthop Trauma* 1989;3:107-114.
26. Epinette JA, Lehut JM, Cavenaile M, Bouretz JC, Decoulx J: Pouteau-Colles fracture: Double-closed "basket-like" pinning according to Kapandji. Apropos of a homogeneous series of 70 cases. *Ann Chir Main* 1982;1:71-83.
27. Chia B, Catalano LW III, Glickel SZ, Barron OA, Meier K: Percutaneous pinning of distal radius fractures: An anatomic study demonstrating the proximity of K-wires to structures at risk. *J Hand Surg Am* 2009;34:1014-1020.
28. Benoist LA, Freeland AE: Buttress pinning in the unstable distal radial fracture: A modification of the Kapandji technique. *J Hand Surg Br* 1995;20:82-96.
29. Grewal R, Perey B, Wilmink M, Stothers K: A randomized prospective study on the treatment of intra-articular distal radius fractures: Open reduction and internal fixation with dorsal plating versus mini open reduction, percutaneous fixation, and external fixation. *J Hand Surg Am* 2005;30:764-772.

30. Koval KJ, Harrast JJ, Anglen JO, Weinstein JN: Fractures of the distal part of the radius: The evolution of practice over time. Where's the evidence? *J Bone Joint Surg Am* 2008;90: 1855-1861.

31. McQueen MM: Non-spanning external fixation of the distal radius. *Hand Clin* 2005;21:375-380.

32. Winemaker MJ, Chinchalkar S, Richards RS, Johnson JA, Chess DG, King GJ: Load relaxation and forces with activity in Hoffman external fixators: A clinical study in patients with Colles' fractures. *J Hand Surg Am* 1998;23:926-932.

33. Sun JS, Chang CH, Wu CC, Hou SM, Hang YS: Extra-articular deformity in distal radial fractures treated by external fixation. *Can J Surg* 2001;44:289-294.

34. Fernandez DL, Wolfe SW: Distal radius fractures, in Green DP, Hotchkiss RN, Pederson WC, Wolfe SW, eds: *Green's Operative Hand Surgery,* ed 5. New York, NY, Churchill Livingstone, 2005, pp 645-710.

35. Jakob M, Rikli DA, Regazzoni P: Fractures of the distal radius treated by internal fixation and early function: A prospective study of 73 consecutive patients. *J Bone Joint Surg Br* 2000;82:340-344.

36. Ring D, Jupiter JB, Brennwald J, Büchler U, Hastings H II: Prospective multicenter trial of a plate for dorsal fixation of distal radius fractures. *J Hand Surg Am* 1997;22: 777-784.

37. Ladd AL, Pliam NB: Use of bone-graft substitutes in distal radius fractures. *J Am Acad Orthop Surg* 1999;7: 279-290.

38. Ladd AL, Pliam NB: The role of bone graft and alternatives in unstable distal radius fracture treatment. *Orthop Clin North Am* 2001;32:337-351.

39. Hartigan BJ, Cohen MS: Use of bone graft substitutes and bioactive materials in treatment of distal radius fractures. *Hand Clin* 2005;21:449-454.

40. Seitz WH Jr, Froimson AI, Leb R, Shapiro JD: Augmented external fixation of unstable distal radius fractures. *J Hand Surg Am* 1991;16:1010-1016.

41. Rogachefsky RA, Ouellette EA, Sun S, Applegate B: The use of tricorticocancellous bone graft in severely comminuted intra-articular fractures of the distal radius. *J Hand Surg Am* 2006;31:623-632.

42. Rajan GP, Fornaro J, Trentz O, Zellweger R: Cancellous allograft versus autologous bone grafting for repair of comminuted distal radius fractures: A prospective, randomized trial. *J Trauma* 2006;60:1322-1329.

43. Younger EM, Chapman MW: Morbidity at bone graft donor sites. *J Orthop Trauma* 1989;3:192-195.

44. Geissler WB, Freeland AE, Savoie FH, McIntyre LW, Whipple TL: Intracarpal soft-tissue lesions associated with an intra-articular fracture of the distal end of the radius. *J Bone Joint Surg Am* 1996;78:357-365.

45. Lindau T, Arner M, Hagberg L: Intraarticular lesions in distal fractures of the radius in young adults: A descriptive arthroscopic study in 50 patients. *J Hand Surg Br* 1997;22: 638-643.

46. Richards RS, Bennett JD, Roth JH, Milne K Jr: Arthroscopic diagnosis of intra-articular soft tissue injuries associated with distal radial fractures. *J Hand Surg Am* 1997;22:772-776.

47. Forward DP, Lindau TR, Melsom DS: Intercarpal ligament injuries associated with fractures of the distal part of the radius. *J Bone Joint Surg Am* 2007;89:2334-2340.

48. Rosenthal DI, Schwartz M, Phillips WC, Jupiter J: Fracture of the radius with instability of the wrist. *AJR Am J Roentgenol* 1983;141:113-116.

49. Stoffelen D, De Mulder K, Broos P: The clinical importance of carpal instabilities following distal radial fractures. *J Hand Surg Br* 1998;23: 512-516.

50. Tang JB: Carpal instability associated with fracture of the distal radius: Incidence, influencing factors and pathomechanics. *Chin Med J (Engl)* 1992; 105:758-765.

51. Akahane M, Ono H, Nakamura T, Kawamura K, Takakura Y: Static scapholunate dissociation diagnosed by scapholunate gap view in wrists with or without distal radius fractures. *Hand Surg* 2002;7:191-195.

52. Wright TW, Del Charco M, Wheeler D: Incidence of ligament lesions and associated degenerative changes in the elderly wrist. *J Hand Surg Am* 1994;19:313-318.

53. Short WH, Werner FW, Green JK, Masaoka S: Biomechanical evaluation of the ligamentous stabilizers of the scaphoid and lunate: Part II. *J Hand Surg Am* 2005;30:24-34.

54. Theumann NH, Etechami G, Duvoisin B, et al: Association between extrinsic and intrinsic carpal ligament injuries at MR arthrography and carpal instability at radiography: Initial observations. *Radiology* 2006;238: 950-957.

55. Werner FW, Short WH, Green JK, Evans PJ, Walker JA: Severity of scapholunate instability is related to joint anatomy and congruency. *J Hand Surg Am* 2007;32:55-60.

56. Cooney WP III, Dobyns JH, Linscheid RL: Complications of Colles' fractures. *J Bone Joint Surg Am* 1980; 62:613-619.

57. Doig SG, Rao SG, Carvell JE: Late carpal instability associated with dorsal distal radial fracture. *Injury* 1991; 22:486-488.

58. Dobyns JR, Linscheid RL, Chao EYS, Weber ER, Swanson GE: Traumatic instability of the wrist. *Instr Course Lect* 1975;24:182-199.

59. Brown IW: Volar intercalary carpal instability following a seemingly innocent wrist fracture. *J Hand Surg Br* 1987;12:54-56.

60. Lozano-Calderón SA, Doornberg J, Ring D: Fractures of the dorsal articular margin of the distal part of the radius with dorsal radiocarpal subluxation. *J Bone Joint Surg Am* 2006;88: 1486-1493.

61. Taleisnik J, Watson HK: Midcarpal instability caused by malunited frac-

tures of the distal radius. *J Hand Surg Am* 1984;9:350-357.

62. Park MJ, Cooney WP III, Hahn ME, Looi KP, An KN: The effects of dorsally angulated distal radius fractures on carpal kinematics. *J Hand Surg Am* 2002;27:223-232.

63. Mudgal C, Hastings H: Scapholunate diastasis in fractures of the distal radius. Pathomechanics and treatment options. *J Hand Surg Br* 1993; 18:725-729.

64. Smith DW, Henry MH: Comprehensive management of soft-tissue injuries associated with distal radius fractures. *J Am Soc Surg Hand* 2002;2: 153-164.

65. Tang JB: Carpal instability associated with fracture in distal radius. *Zhonghua Wai Ke Za Zhi* 1994;32:82-86.

66. Laulan J, Bismuth JP: Intracarpal ligamentous lesions associated with fractures of the distal radius: Outcome at one year. A prospective study of 95 cases. *Acta Orthop Belg* 1999;65: 418-423.

67. Batra S, Gupta A: The effect of fracture-related factors on the functional outcome at 1 year in distal radius fractures. *Injury* 2002;33: 499-502.

68. Weiss CB: Intercarpal ligament injuries associated with fractures of the distal part of the radius. *J Bone Joint Surg Am* 2008;90:1169-1170.

69. Owers KL, Lee J, Khan N, Healy J, Eckersley R: Ultrasound changes in the extensor pollicis longus tendon following fractures of the distal radius: A preliminary report. *J Hand Surg Eur Vol* 2007;32:467-471.

70. Turner RG, Faber KJ, Athwal GS: Complications of distal radius fractures. *Orthop Clin North Am* 2007;38: 217-228, vi.

71. Kambouroglou GK, Axelrod TS: Complications of the AO/ASIF titanium distal radius plate system (pi plate) in internal fixation of the distal radius: A brief report. *J Hand Surg Am* 1998;23:737-741.

72. Lowry KJ, Gainor BJ, Hoskins JS: Extensor tendon rupture secondary to the AO/ASIF titanium distal radius plate without associated plate failure: A case report. *Am J Orthop* 2000;29: 789-791.

73. Rozental TD, Beredjiklian PK, Bozentka DJ: Functional outcome and complications following two types of dorsal plating for unstable fractures of the distal part of the radius. *J Bone Joint Surg Am* 2003;85: 1956-1960.

74. Sánchez T, Jakubietz M, Jakubietz R, Mayer J, Beutel FK, Grünert J: Complications after pi plate osteosynthesis. *Plast Reconstr Surg* 2005;116:153-158.

75. Ruch DS, Papadonikolakis A: Volar versus dorsal plating in the management of intra-articular distal radius fractures. *J Hand Surg Am* 2006;31: 9-16.

76. Rein S, Schikore H, Schneiders W, Amlang M, Zwipp H: Results of dorsal or volar plate fixation of AO type C3 distal radius fractures: A retrospective study. *J Hand Surg Am* 2007;32:954-961.

77. Bell JS, Wollstein R, Citron ND: Rupture of flexor pollicis longus tendon: A complication of volar plating of the distal radius. *J Bone Joint Surg Br* 1998;80:225-226.

78. Nunley JA, Rowan PR: Delayed rupture of the flexor pollicis longus tendon after inappropriate placement of the pi plate on the volar surface of the distal radius. *J Hand Surg Am* 1999;24: 1279-1280.

79. Drobetz H, Kutscha-Lissberg E: Osteosynthesis of distal radial fractures with a volar locking screw plate system. *Int Orthop* 2003;27:1-6.

80. Douthit JD: Volar plating of dorsally comminuted fractures of the distal radius: A 6-year study. *Am J Orthop* 2005;34:140-147.

81. Orbay JL, Touhami A: Current concepts in volar fixed-angle fixation of unstable distal radius fractures. *Clin Orthop Relat Res* 2006;445:58-67.

82. Rozental TD, Blazar PE: Functional outcome and complications after volar plating for dorsally displaced, unstable fractures of the distal radius. *J Hand Surg Am* 2006;31:359-365.

83. Arora R, Lutz M, Hennerbichler A, Krappinger D, Espen D, Gabl M: Complications following internal fixation of unstable distal radius fracture with a palmar locking-plate. *J Orthop Trauma* 2007;21:316-322.

84. Klug RA, Press CM, Gonzalez MH: Rupture of the flexor pollicis longus tendon after volar fixed-angle plating of a distal radius fracture: A case report. *J Hand Surg Am* 2007;32: 984-988.

85. Rampoldi M, Marsico S: Complications of volar plating of distal radius fractures. *Acta Orthop Belg* 2007;73: 714-719.

86. Cross AW, Schmidt CC: Flexor tendon injuries following locked volar plating of distal radius fractures. *J Hand Surg Am* 2008;33:164-167.

87. Simic PM, Robison J, Gardner MJ, Gelberman RH, Weiland AJ, Boyer MI: Treatment of distal radius fractures with a low-profile dorsal plating system: An outcomes assessment. *J Hand Surg Am* 2006;31: 382-386.

88. Buzzell JE, Weikert DR, Watson JT, Lee DH: Precontoured fixed-angle volar distal radius plates: A comparison of anatomic fit. *J Hand Surg Am* 2008;33:1144-1152.

89. Cohen MS, Turner TM, Urban RM: Effects of implant material and plate design on tendon function and morphology. *Clin Orthop Relat Res* 2006; 445:81-90.

90. Sinicropi SM, Su BW, Raia FJ, Parisien M, Strauch RJ, Rosenwasser MP: The effects of implant composition on extensor tenosynovitis in a canine distal radius fracture model. *J Hand Surg Am* 2005;30:300-307.

91. Clement H, Pichler W, Nelson D, Hausleitner L, Tesch NP, Grechenig W: Morphometric analysis of lister's tubercle and its consequences on volar plate fixation of distal radius fractures. *J Hand Surg Am* 2008;33: 1716-1719.

92. Smith DW, Henry MH: The 45 degrees pronated oblique view for volar fixed-angle plating of distal radius fractures. *J Hand Surg Am* 2004;29: 703-706.

93. Soong M, Got C, Katarincic J, Akelman E: Fluoroscopic evaluation of intra-articular screw placement during locked volar plating of the distal radius: A cadaveric study. *J Hand Surg Am* 2008;33:1720-1723.

94. Thomas AD, Greenberg JA: Use of fluoroscopy in determining screw overshoot in the dorsal distal radius: A cadaveric study. *J Hand Surg Am* 2009;34:258-261.

95. Dyer G, Lozano-Calderon S, Gannon C, Baratz M, Ring D: Predictors of acute carpal tunnel syndrome associated with fracture of the distal radius. *J Hand Surg Am* 2008;33:1309-1313.

96. Schnetzler KA: Acute carpal tunnel syndrome. *J Am Acad Orthop Surg* 2008;16:276-282.

97. Geissler WB, Fernandez DL, Lamey DM: Distal radioulnar joint injuries associated with fractures of the distal radius. *Clin Orthop Relat Res* 1996;327:135-146.

98. MacDermid JC, Donner A, Richards RS, Roth JH: Patient versus injury factors as predictors of pain and disability six months after a distal radius fracture. *J Clin Epidemiol* 2002; 55:849-854.

99. Gliatis JD, Plessas SJ, Davis TR: Outcome of distal radial fractures in young adults. *J Hand Surg Br* 2000;25: 535-543.

100. Kreder HJ, Hanel DP, Agel J, McKee MD, Trumble TE: A randomized controlled trial of indirect reduction and percutaneous fixation versus open reduction and internal fixation for displaced intraarticular distal radius fractures. *18th Annual Meeting.* Rosemont, IL, Orthopaedic Trauma Association, 2002. http://www.hwbf.org/ota/am/ota02/otapa/OTA02067.htm. Accessed August 14, 2009.

101. Kihara H, Palmer AK, Werner FW, Short WH, Fortino MD: The effect of dorsally angulated distal radius fractures on distal radioulnar joint congruency and forearm rotation. *J Hand Surg Am* 1996;21:40-47.

102. Flinkkilä T, Raatikainen T, Kaarela O, Hämäläinen M: Corrective osteotomy for malunion of the distal radius. *Arch Orthop Trauma Surg* 2000;120:23-26.

103. Prommersberger KJ, Van Schoonhoven J, Lanz UB: Outcome after corrective osteotomy for malunited fractures of the distal end of the radius. *J Hand Surg Br* 2002;27:55-60.

104. Prommersberger KJ, Froehner SC, Schmitt RR, Lanz UB: Rotational deformity in malunited fractures of the distal radius. *J Hand Surg Am* 2004;29: 110-115.

105. Adams BD: Effects of radial deformity on distal radioulnar joint mechanics. *J Hand Surg Am* 1993;18: 492-498.

106. May MM, Lawton JN, Blazar PE: Ulnar styloid fractures associated with distal radius fractures: Incidence and implications for distal radioulnar joint instability. *J Hand Surg Am* 2002;27: 965-971.

107. Ruch DS, Yang CC, Smith BP: Results of acute arthroscopically repaired triangular fibrocartilage complex injuries associated with intra-articular distal radius fractures. *Arthroscopy* 2003;19:511-516.

108. Ruch DS, Lumsden BC, Papadonikolakis A: Distal radius fractures: A comparison of tension band wiring versus ulnar outrigger external fixation for the management of distal radioulnar instability. *J Hand Surg Am* 2005;30:969-977.

109. Gaebler C, McQueen MM: Ulnar procedures for post-traumatic disorders of the distal radioulnar joint. *Injury* 2003;34:47-59.

110. Souer JS, Ring D, Matschke S, Audige L, Marent-Huber M, Jupiter JB; AOCID Prospective ORIF Distal Radius Study Group: Effect of an unrepaired fracture of the ulnar styloid base on outcome after plate-and-screw fixation of a distal radial fracture. *J Bone Joint Surg Am* 2009;91: 830-838.

111. Young BT, Rayan GM: Outcome following nonoperative treatment of displaced distal radius fractures in low-demand patients older than 60 years. *J Hand Surg Am* 2000;25:19-28.

112. Fernandez DL: Correction of post-traumatic wrist deformity in adults by osteotomy, bone-grafting, and internal fixation. *J Bone Joint Surg Am* 1982; 64:1164-1178.

113. Fernandez DL: Radial osteotomy and Bowers arthroplasty for malunited fractures of the distal end of the radius. *J Bone Joint Surg Am* 1988;70: 1538-1551.

114. Jupiter JB, Ring D: A comparison of early and late reconstruction of malunited fractures of the distal end of the radius. *J Bone Joint Surg Am* 1996;78:739-748.

115. Lafontaine M, Hardy D, Delince P: Stability assessment of distal radius fractures. *Injury* 1989;20:208-210.

116. McQueen MM, MacLaren A, Chalmers J: The value of remanipulating Colles' fractures. *J Bone Joint Surg Br* 1986;68:232-233.

117. Jupiter JB, Ring D, Weitzel PP: Surgical treatment of redisplaced fractures of the distal radius in patients older than 60 years. *J Hand Surg Am* 2002; 27:714-723.

118. Trumble TE, Wagner W, Hanel DP, Vedder NB, Gilbert M: Intrafocal (Kapandji) pinning of distal radius fractures with and without external fixation. *J Hand Surg Am* 1998;23:381-394.

119. Agee JM: External fixation: Technical advances based upon multiplanar ligamentotaxis. *Orthop Clin North Am* 1993;24:265-274.

120. McQueen MM: Redisplaced unstable fractures of the distal radius: A randomised, prospective study of bridging versus non-bridging external fixation. *J Bone Joint Surg Br* 1998;80: 665-669.

121. Fernandez DL, Ring D, Jupiter JB: Surgical management of delayed

union and nonunion of distal radius fractures. *J Hand Surg Am* 2001;26: 201-209.

122. Finsen V, Aasheim T: Initial experience with the Forte plate for dorsally displaced distal radius fractures. *Injury* 2000;31:445-448.

123. Fernandez DL, Capo JT, Gonzalez E: Corrective osteotomy for symptomatic increased ulnar tilt of the distal end of the radius. *J Hand Surg Am* 2001;26:722-732.

124. Marx RG, Axelrod TS: Intraarticular osteotomy of distal radial malunions. *Clin Orthop Relat Res* 1996;327: 152-157.

125. Ring D, Prommersberger KJ, González del Pino J, Capomassi M, Slullitel M, Jupiter JB: Corrective osteotomy for intra-articular malunion of the distal part of the radius. *J Bone Joint Surg Am* 2005;87:1503-1509.

126. Thivaios GC, McKee MD: Sliding osteotomy for deformity correction following malunion of volarly displaced distal radial fractures. *J Orthop Trauma* 2003;17:326-333.

127. Ring D, Roberge C, Morgan T, Jupiter JB: Osteotomy for malunited fractures of the distal radius: A comparison of structural and nonstructural autogenous bone grafts. *J Hand Surg Am* 2002;27:216-222.

128. Orbay JL, Badia A, Indriago IR, et al: The extended flexor carpi radialis approach: A new perspective for the distal radius fracture. *Tech Hand Up Extrem Surg* 2001;5:204-211.

129. Orbay JL, Fernandez DL: Volar fixation for dorsally displaced fractures of the distal radius: A preliminary report. *J Hand Surg Am* 2002;27: 205-215.

130. Orbay JL, Indriago I, Badia A, Khouri RK, Gonzalez E, Fernandez DL: Corrective osteotomy of dorsally mal-united fractures of the distal radius via the extended FCR approach. *J Hand Surg Am* 2003;28(suppl 1):2.

131. Henry M: Immediate mobilisation following corrective osteotomy of distal radius malunions with cancellous graft and volar fixed angle plates. *J Hand Surg Eur Vol* 2007;32:88-92.

132. Malone KJ, Magnell TD, Freeman DC, Boyer MI, Placzek JD: Surgical correction of dorsally angulated distal radius malunions with fixed angle volar plating: A case series. *J Hand Surg Am* 2006;31:366-372.

133. Prommersberger KJ, Ring D, del Pino JG, Capomassi M, Slullitel M, Jupiter JB: Corrective osteotomy for intra-articular malunion of the distal part of the radius: Surgical technique. *J Bone Joint Surg Am* 2006;88(suppl 1 pt 2):202-211.

134. Shea K, Fernandez DL, Jupiter JB, Martin C Jr: Corrective osteotomy for malunited, volarly displaced fractures of the distal end of the radius. *J Bone Joint Surg Am* 1997;79:1816-1826.

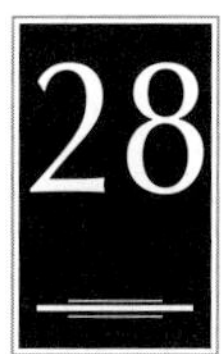

The Treatment of Complex Fractures and Fracture-Dislocations of the Hand

Jesse B. Jupiter, MD
Hill Hastings II, MD
John T. Capo, MD

Abstract

Most fractures of the phalanges or metacarpals are amenable to closed treatment, with favorable outcomes. However, two groups of complex fractures are difficult to diagnose and treat. The first group includes unicondylar and bicondylar fractures, fracture-dislocations, and fracture-related instability of the proximal interphalangeal joint. Fracture-dislocations can be treated with splinting or surgical intervention. Microscrews and condylar plates have added considerably to the ability to securely fix small articular fractures and fracture-dislocations about the proximal interphalangeal joint. Some unstable fracture-dislocations are characterized by loss of the volar aspect of the articular surface of the base of the middle phalanx; they can be treated by using a sculpted osseous articular graft from the dorsal hamate. The second group includes displaced diaphyseal fractures associated with a soft-tissue injury, instability, or multiple fracturing. Articular fractures and fracture-dislocations at the base of the metacarpal also can be difficult to diagnose and treat.

Instr Course Lect 2010;59:333-341.

Intra-articular fractures and fracture-dislocations of the proximal interphalangeal joint and metacarpal fractures and fracture-dislocations are two groups of complex fractures that can be difficult to treat. The treatment options include splinting, surgery, and plate-screw fixation.

Dr. Jupiter or an immediate family member serves as an unpaid consultant to Synthes; has received research or institutional support from Aircast-DJ Orthopaedics, Biomet, Hand Innovations, Linvatec, Mitek, SBI, Synthes, Wright Medical Technology, and Zimmer; and has received nonincome support (such as equipment or services), commercially derived honoraria, or other non–research-related funding (such as paid travel) from Saunders-Mosby-Elsevier and Wolters Kluwer Health–Lippincott Williams & Wilkins. Dr. Hastings or an immediate family member serves as a board member, owner, officer, or committee member of the Indiana Hand Center and has received royalties from Biomet. Dr. Capo or an immediate family member has received royalties from Wright Medical Technology; serves as a paid consultant to or is an employee of Wright Medical Technology; and has received research or institutional support from Synthes.

Intra-articular Fractures and Fracture-Dislocations of the Proximal Interphalangeal Joint

Unicondylar Fractures

Weiss and Hastings[1] identified four types of intra-articular unicondylar fractures of the distal aspect of the proximal phalanx[2] (Figure 1). Type I, the most common, is an oblique palmar fracture caused by a rotatory and lateral deviation force to the proximal interphalangeal (PIP) joint, which creates a short oblique fracture in both the sagittal and frontal planes. Type II is a long fracture in the sagittal plane caused by an isolated, laterally applied force to the PIP joint. The mechanism of type I and type II unicondylar fractures is shown in Figure 2. Type III, a dorsal osteochondral fracture, and type IV, a palmar osteochondral fracture, are much less common.

A nondisplaced fracture or a fracture that is displaced less than 1 mm is treated with splint immobilization and close observation. These fractures are inherently unstable and can become significantly displaced; Hastings and Carroll[3] found that five of seven

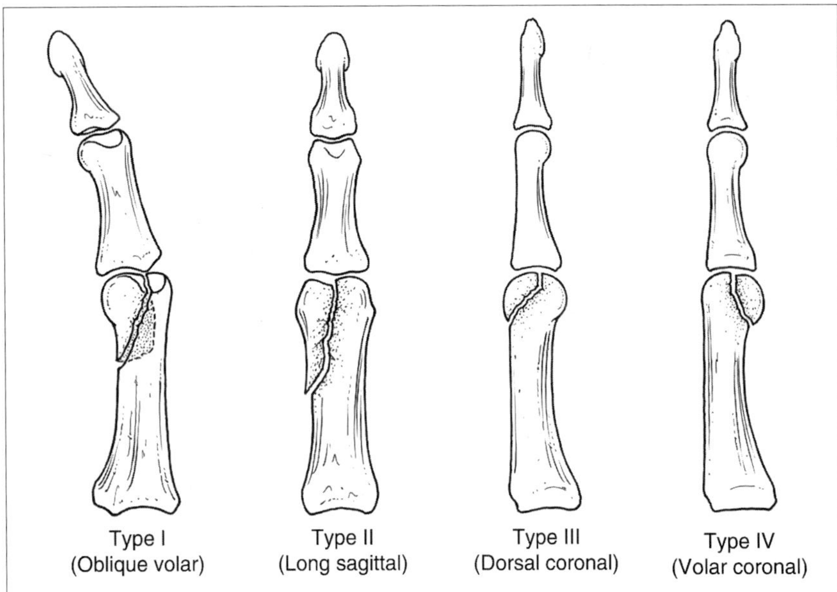

Figure 1 Schematic diagram of the Weiss and Hastings classification of unicondylar fractures of the proximal interphalangeal joint. (Copyright Gary Schnitz, Indiana Hand Center.)

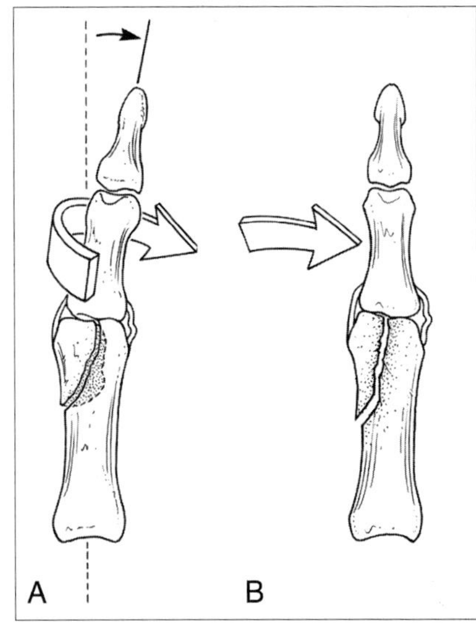

Figure 2 Schematic diagrams showing the mechanism of type I and type II unicondylar fractures. Lateral force is applied to the middle phalanx, with rotation in type I **(A)** and without rotation in type II **(B).** (Copyright Gary Schnitz, Indiana Hand Center.)

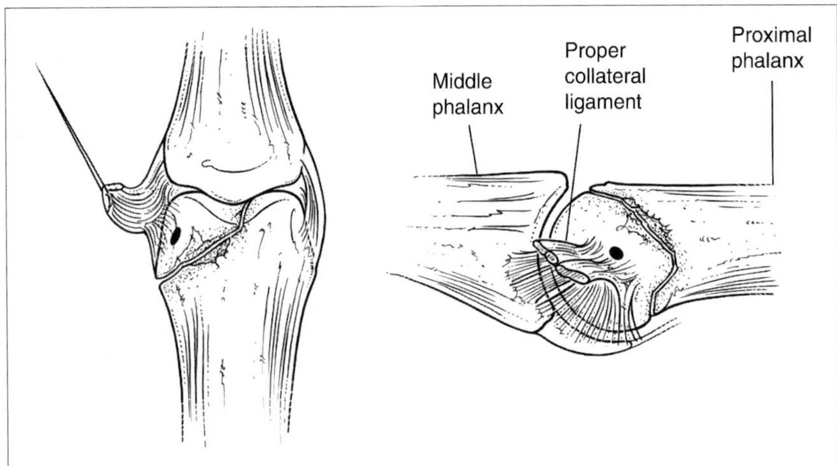

Figure 3 Schematic diagram showing PIP joint flexion, which allows drill and subsequent screw placement proximal to the proper collateral ligament and through the more palmar aspect of the fracture fragment. Black oval = entry site for screw placement. (Copyright Gary Schnitz, Indiana Hand Center.)

nondisplaced unicondylar fractures treated with immobilization became displaced and required surgical treatment. A type I fracture is particularly susceptible to displacement, and therefore percutaneous Kirschner wire fixation is recommended. The use of two small Kirschner wires is preferred to a single larger wire. Active range-of-motion exercises are initiated by 3 weeks, with passive motion by 6 weeks.

An irreducible type I fracture should be treated with open reduction and internal fixation, using 1.0-mm or 1.3-mm screws. A dorsolateral surgical exposure is used. The extensor mechanism should not be disrupted; instead, it should be retracted to facilitate a dorsal PIP capsulotomy for joint surface inspection. The optimal screw fixation is distal and deep to the appropriate collateral ligament. The screw is directed toward the opposite side of the phalanx so it will exit proximal to the opposite collateral ligament (Figure 3). Additional screws are required for fixation of a large type I or long type II unicondylar fracture (Figure 4).

A very small type III fracture fragment should be excised. A type IV fracture requires surgical fixation with a small Kirschner wire or screw. Weiss and Hastings[1] reviewed 38 unicondylar fractures treated surgically. At an average 3-year follow-up, the average joint extension was 14°, and flexion was 86°. Patients with a type IV fracture had the poorest outcome.

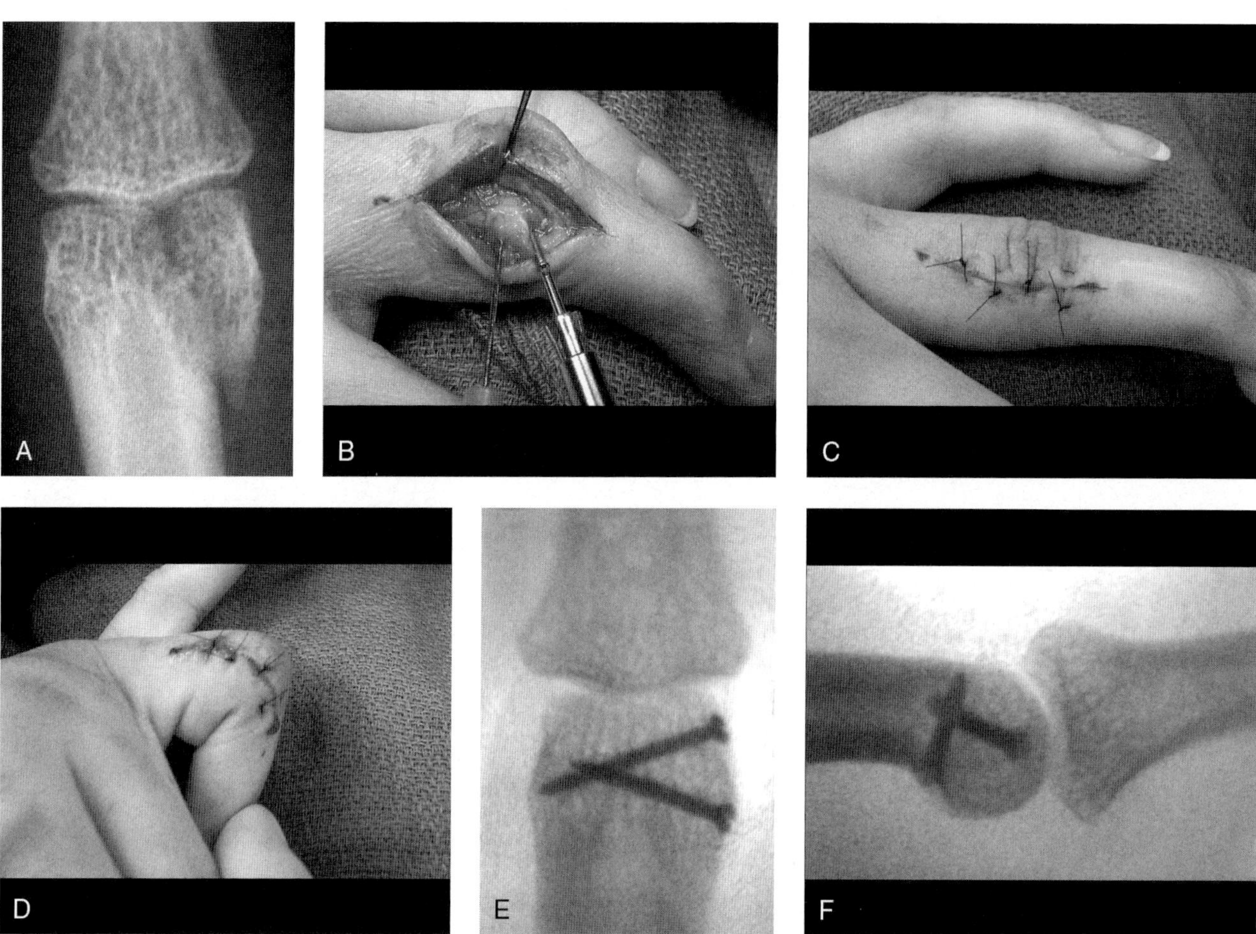

Figure 4 **A,** AP radiograph showing a large type I unicondylar fracture. **B,** Intraoperative photograph showing the placement of microscrews distal and proximal to the collateral ligament. **C,** Photograph showing the incision and joint extension after fracture fixation. **D,** Photograph showing joint flexion after internal fixation. Postoperative AP **(E)** and lateral **(F)** radiographs.

Bicondylar Fractures

Fractures involving both condyles of the head of the proximal phalanx are classified as T condylar, Y condylar, or lambda, based on their orientation. A nondisplaced fracture is treated nonsurgically. A displaced fracture requires open reduction and stable internal fixation with miniscrews, either alone or in combination with a small plate (Figure 5). The fracture is best exposed using a central tendon-splitting approach. An open fracture with a larger, more unstable fracture fragment especially can benefit from the addition of plate fixation (Figure 6). A stable fixation permits active rehabilitation.

Fracture-Dislocations

PIP fracture-dislocations were classified by Hastings[4] based on the articular involvement of the volar base of the middle phalanx (Figure 7). Injuries with less than 30% involvement generally are stable, with joint congruity through the full range of motion. If the fracture fragment involves 30% to 50% of the palmar articular base of the middle phalanx, the joint stability is less predictable and more tenuous, even if it is possible to manually reduce the joint with less than 30° of flexion. An unstable fracture-dislocation involves more than 50% of the palmar articular surface, and more than 30° of flexion is required to maintain joint congruity.

As described by McElfresh and associates,[5] the outcome of a PIP fracture-dislocation treated with closed reduction and splint or cast immobilization depends on the accuracy of the joint reduction (Figure 8). The concavity of the articular base of the middle phalanx, as seen on a lateral radiograph, must match the convexity of the head of the proximal phalanx. A relative

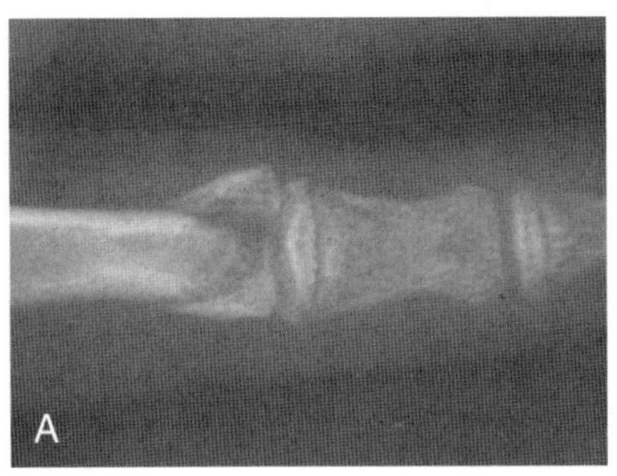

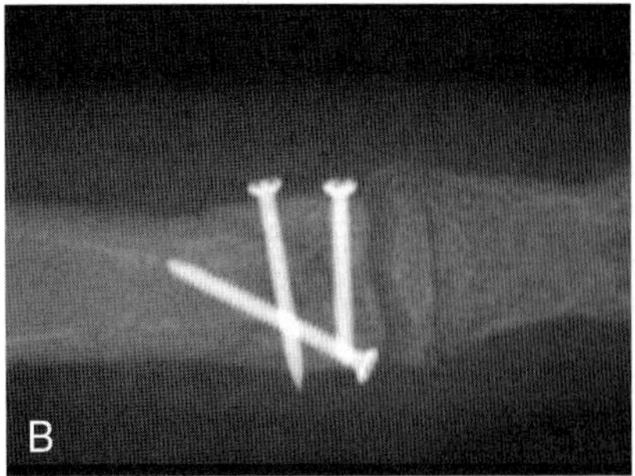

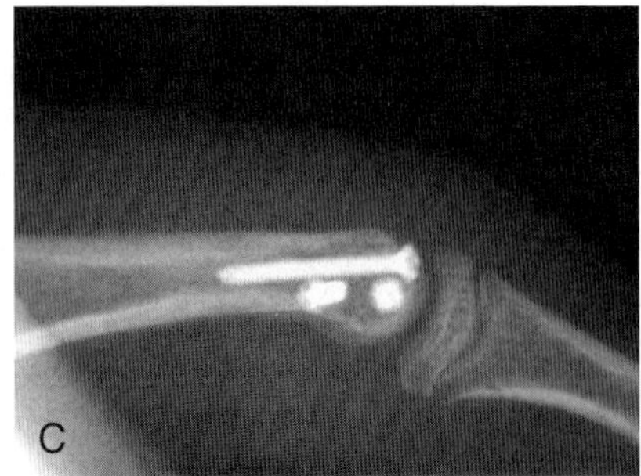

Figure 5 **A,** AP radiograph showing a T-condylar fracture. AP **(B)** and lateral **(C)** radiographs showing fixation with 1.0-mm screws.

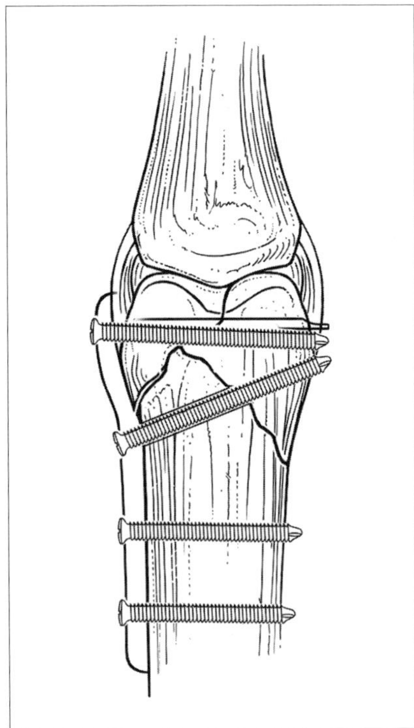

Figure 6 Schematic diagram showing condylar plate fixation of a T-condylar fracture. (Copyright Gary Schnitz, Indiana Hand Center.)

widening of the dorsal aspect of the joint (the so-called V sign) suggests residual dorsal subluxation.

An unstable PIP fracture-dislocation can be treated with closed reduction and percutaneous Kirschner wire fixation, static or dynamic traction (Figure 9), open reduction and internal fixation (Figure 10), palmar plate arthroplasty (Figure 11), or, for late treatment, osteotomy. The least invasive method should be attempted. The palmar plate arthroplasty described by Eaton and Malerich[6] has a predictable result if the fracture fragment is less than 30% of the articular surface of the base of the middle phalanx. Several investigators have reported that dynamic external fixation is a reliable, minimally invasive method of treating a very unstable PIP fracture-dislocation.[7,8] Hastings and Ernst[7] noted that the PIP joint has a relatively unifocal axis of motion, which allows a dynamic hinged fixator to provide stability while permitting motion (Figure 12). The application of a dynamic external fixator is especially useful with a pilon fracture-dislocation, which is characterized by comminution of the dorsal, palmar, and central portions of the articular base of the middle phalanx (Figure 13).

Several methods have been suggested for reconstructing the palmar aspect of the base of the middle phalanx. If the articular impaction is less than 2 mm, the thickness of the palmar plate interposed into the joint may establish stability. For an established malunion of the palmar base of the middle phalanx, osteotomy and elevation of the depressed fragment along with a supporting bone graft has been successful.[9]

A segment of the dorsal aspect of the ipsilateral hamate has been used to replace a deficient palmar articu-

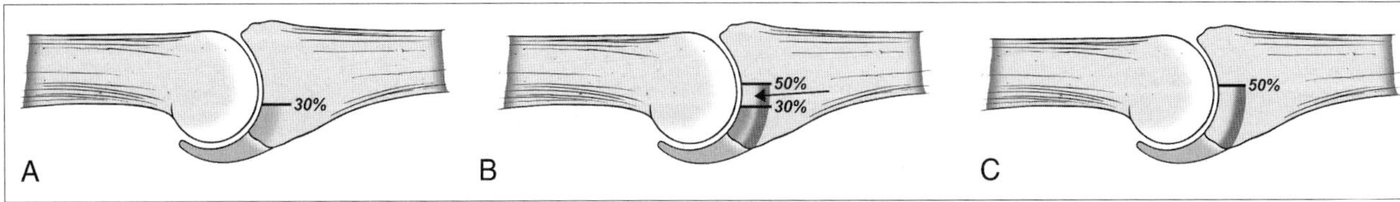

Figure 7 Schematic diagrams showing the Kiefhaber modification of the Hastings classification of PIP fracture-dislocations. **A,** A stable fracture dislocation, involving less than 30% of the joint. **B,** A tenuously stable fracture, involving 30% to 50% of the joint (*arrow*). **C,** An unstable fracture, involving more than 50% of the joint. (Copyright Gary Schnitz, Indiana Hand Center.)

lar buttress. Anatomic studies by Capo and associates[10] found that the hamate has a central ridge and a bicondylar facet with articular contours similar to those of the base of the middle phalanx (Figure 14). Removing a central portion of the hamate was found not to induce dislocation or create carpometacarpal joint instability. This hemihamate resurfacing arthroplasty has been clinically studied by several researchers.[4,10-12] Capo and associates[10] found that the hemihamate graft had united in all 10 studied fractures at an average 33-month follow-up; the average PIP extension lag was 27°, and the average flexion was 91° (Figure 15). Williams and associates[11] found an average arc of 85° of PIP motion in 13 patients.

Metacarpal Fractures and Fracture-Dislocations

Most metacarpal fractures are amenable to treatment without surgery. However, surgical intervention is required if any of the following are present: unacceptable alignment after a closed reduction (defined as angulation of more than 10° deformity of the second or third metacarpal), causing an overlap of digits or shortening of more than 5 mm; a multiple metacarpal fracture; an open fracture; complex upper extremity trauma; or neurovascular or tendon injury.[13,14]

Diaphyseal Fractures

The treatment of a metacarpal shaft fracture depends on the fracture pattern. Percutaneous Kirschner wire fixation (intramedullary or into the adjacent metacarpals), open reduction and internal fixation, or external skeletal fixation can be used if surgical treatment is necessary.[15-17] Intramedullary percutaneous wire fixation is best used for a displaced transverse fracture. The wire can be introduced antegrade through the base or head of the involved metacarpal for a stable fixation. Supplemental splinting is

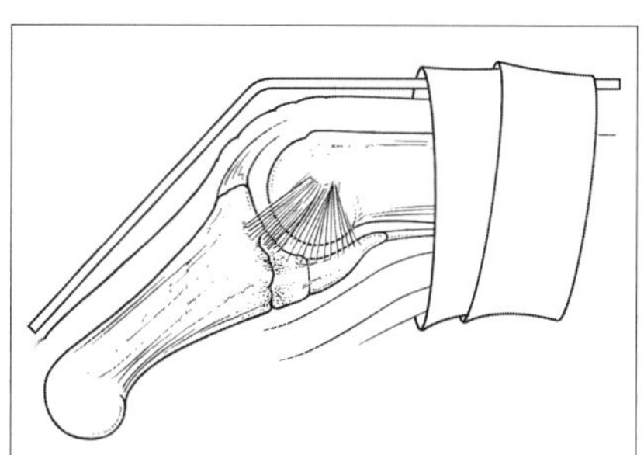

Figure 8 Schematic diagram showing dorsal block splinting of a stable or tenuously stable PIP fracture-dislocation. The splint should include the metacarpophalangeal joint in slight flexion and the wrist in slight extension. (Copyright Gary Schnitz, Indiana Hand Center.)

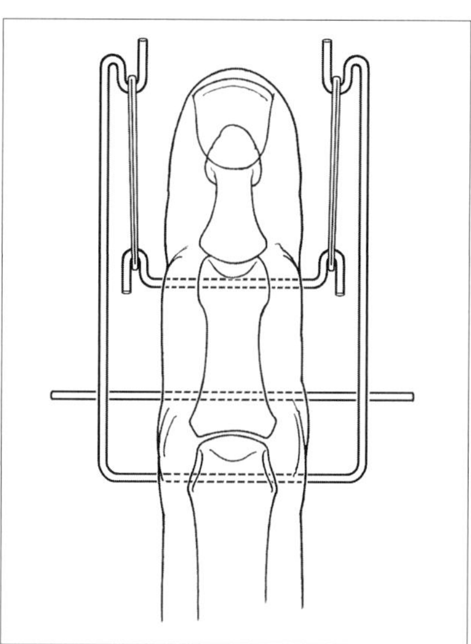

Figure 9 Schematic diagram showing dynamic traction for a fracture of the articular base of the middle phalanx using a Suzuki traction device. (Copyright Gary Schnitz, Indiana Hand Center.)

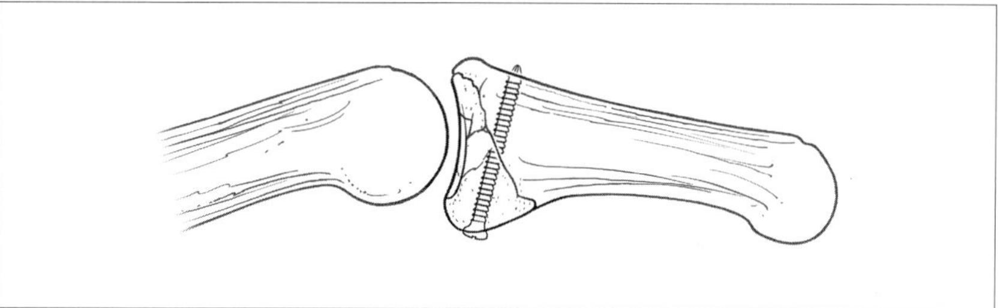

Figure 10 Schematic diagram showing screw fixation of a fracture-dislocation of the articular base of the middle phalanx. (Copyright Gary Schnitz, Indiana Hand Center.)

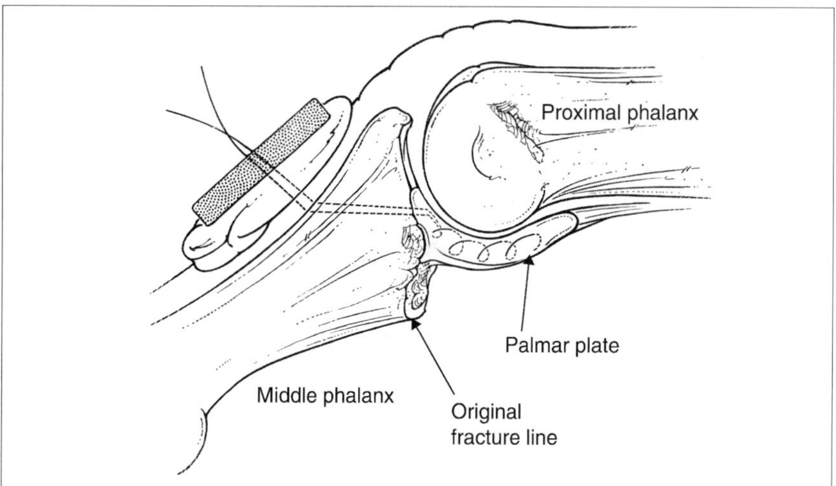

Figure 11 Schematic diagram showing a palmar plate interposition arthroplasty with button-and-suture fixation. (Copyright Gary Schnitz, Indiana Hand Center.)

required to achieve rotational control. To enhance rotational stability, the so-called bouquet technique is used, in which multiple pins are placed antegrade through the proximal flare and the pins diverge in the metacarpal head.[18] Transverse wire placement into an adjacent intact metacarpal is best used for a displaced fracture of the second or fifth metacarpal.[19]

Interfragmentary screws can be used alone for stable internal fixation of a long oblique or spiral fracture. The ideal fracture length for achieving stability with interfragmentary screws alone is at least twice the diameter of the bone; the screws must lie perpendicular to the fracture plane to minimize instability from shear forces. The surgical exposure must disrupt as little of the soft-tissue attachment as possible to preserve the vascularity of the bone (Figure 16).

Plate and screw fixation is best used for stable internal fixation of a transverse or short oblique fracture, especially if it is associated with soft-tissue trauma or multiple metacarpal fractures (Figure 17). Straight linear incisions minimize the risk of venous and lymphatic injury and provide ex-

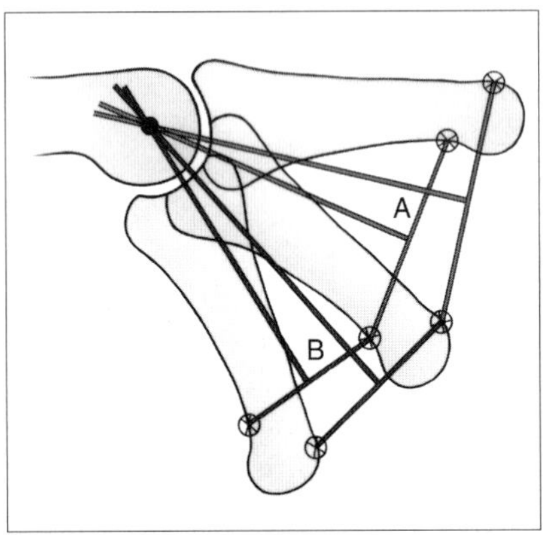

Figure 12 Schematic diagram showing an analysis of the instant center of motion of the PIP joint, which was found to have a relatively fixed axis in flexion **(A)** and extension **(B)**. (Copyright Gary Schnitz, Indiana Hand Center.)

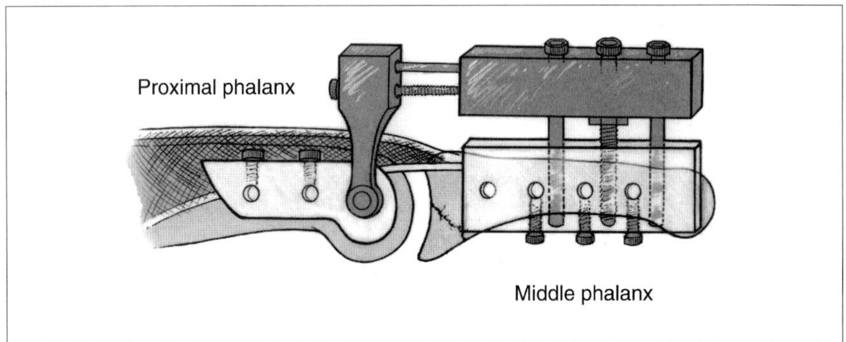

Figure 13 Schematic diagram showing dynamic external fixation of a pilon comminuted fracture-dislocation involving the entire base of the middle phalanx. (Copyright Gary Schnitz, Indiana Hand Center.)

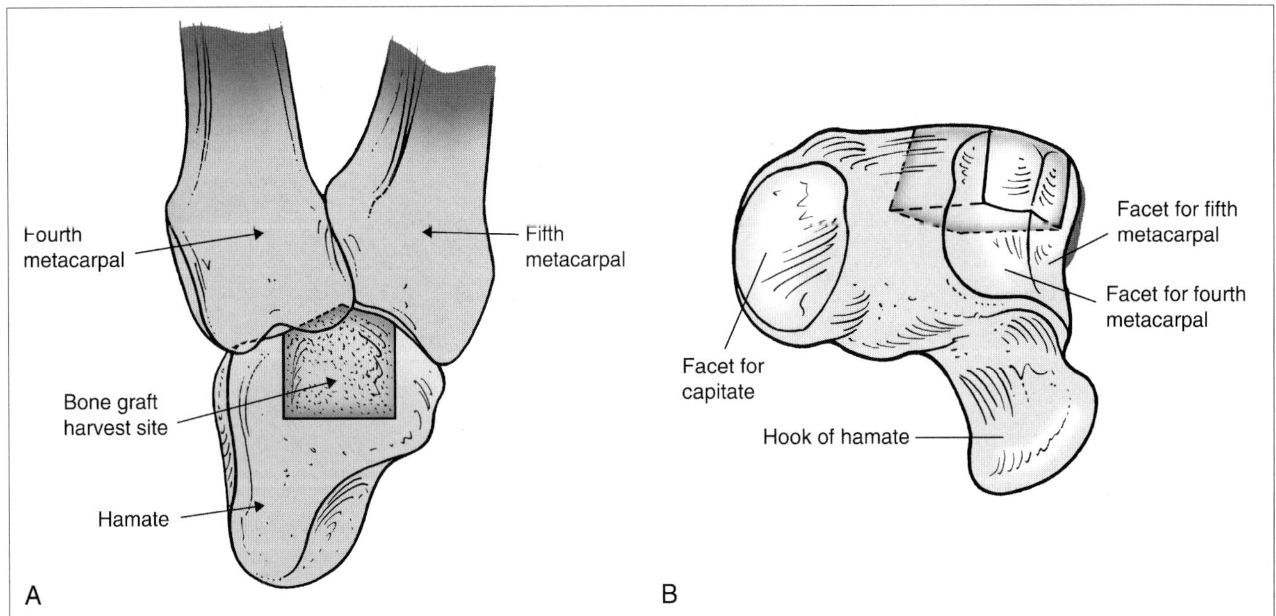

Figure 14 Schematic diagrams showing AP **(A)** and lateral **(B)** views of the harvest site for a dorsal hamate osteochondral graft. The articular surfaces of the fourth and fifth carpometacarpal joints provide a bicondylar articular base for the middle phalanx. (Copyright Gary Schnitz, Indiana Hand Center.)

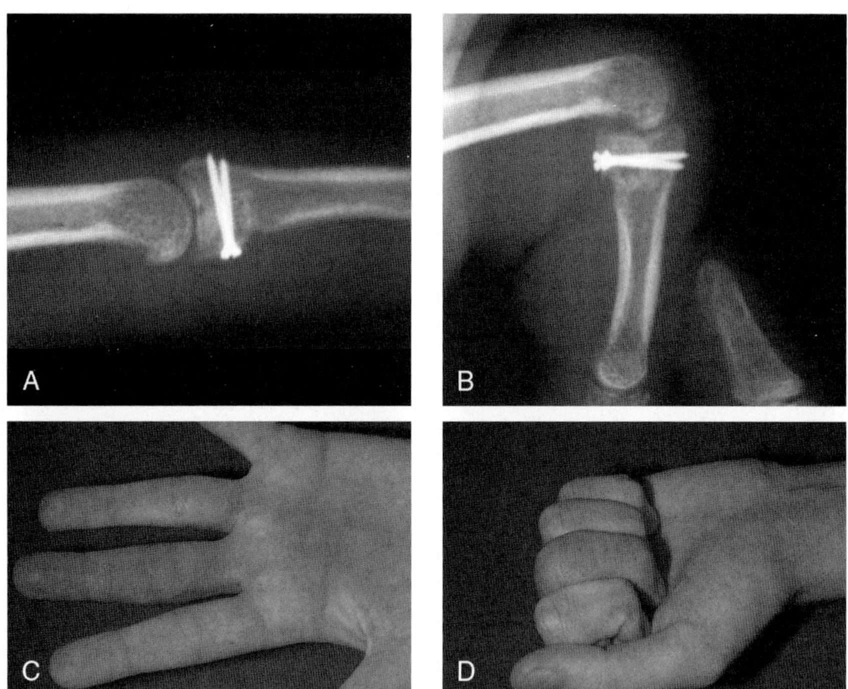

Figure 15 A hemihamate replacement 5 weeks after arthroplasty. Lateral radiographs show extension **(A)** and flexion **(B)**. Clinical photographs show joint extension **(C)** and flexion **(D)**.

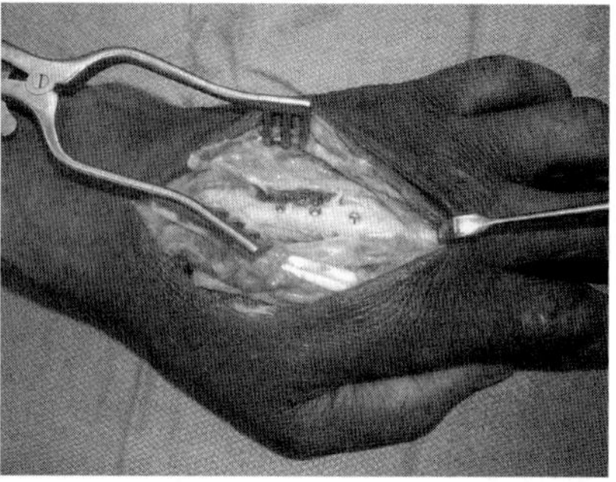

Figure 16 Clinical photograph showing a long oblique fracture of the third metacarpal. The fracture length is approximately three times the bone diameter. The fracture has been fixed with one 1.3-mm and two 1.5-mm screws.

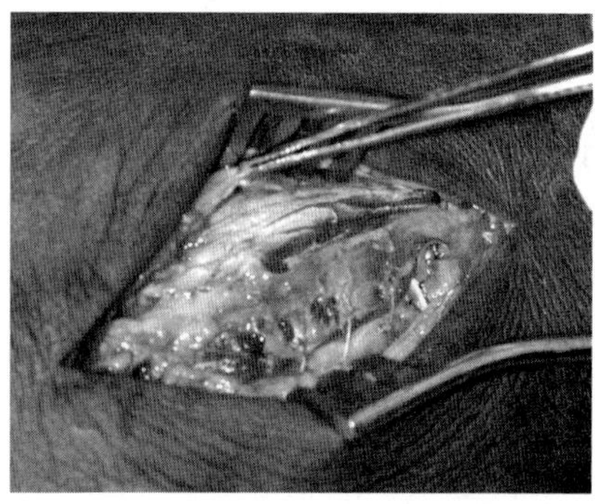

Figure 17 Clinical photograph of a displaced transverse metacarpal fracture, showing the periosteum and interosseous muscle fascia closed over a titanium blade plate. Most of the plate was covered to provide a soft-tissue layer for optimal tendon gliding.

tensile exposures. To expand the exposures, the extensor tendons are retracted or the juncturae tendineae are cut. At the completion of internal fixation, the surgeon must ensure that the digital cascade is normal and no rotatory deformity exists.

Metacarpal Base Fractures

Fractures at the base of the metacarpal can be complicated by soft-tissue injury, intra-articular fracture-dislocation, or limited cortical integrity. CT scans may be required to identify the injury. An intra-articular fracture at the base of the fifth metacarpal is especially difficult to treat; it sometimes is considered a reverse Bennett fracture. (See chapter 29 for a description of the Bennett fracture.) The fracture may be unstable because of the deforming force of the extensor carpi ulnaris, which inserts at the base of the metacarpal. A displaced, impacted, or comminuted fracture requires realignment and stabilization with percutaneous Kirschner wires or open reduction and direct realignment of the articular surface (Figure 18).

A fracture-dislocation extending beyond the fifth metacarpal base may be difficult to identify on standard AP and lateral radiographs. A pronated 30° lateral view may provide some evidence of displacement at the metacarpal base because in all views the dorsal cortex of the metacarpal base must be collinear with the distal carpal bones. CT scanning often is optimal for appreciating the displacement and any articular incongruity. The injury may be the result of a high-energy trauma with associated soft-tissue swelling, and cast immobilization after a closed reduction may not provide sufficient support. Stabilization with percutaneous Kirschner wires is preferable, in conjunction with cast immobilization.

Summary

Advances in the understanding of PIP fractures and fracture-dislocations have led to improved outcomes after treatment. The PIP joint requires a palmar buttress for overall stability. Instability is common in a fracture of the palmar base of the middle phalanx that exceeds 40% of the articular surface; a percutaneous method, traction, or open reduction is used. Late treat-

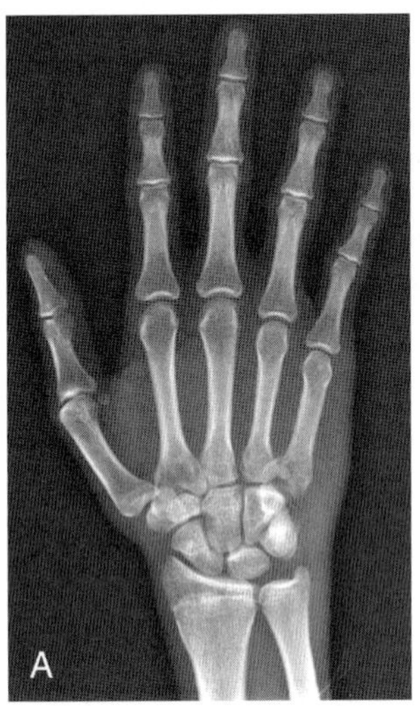

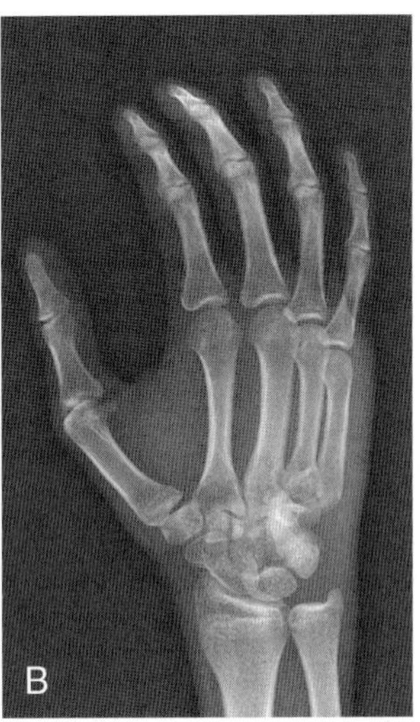

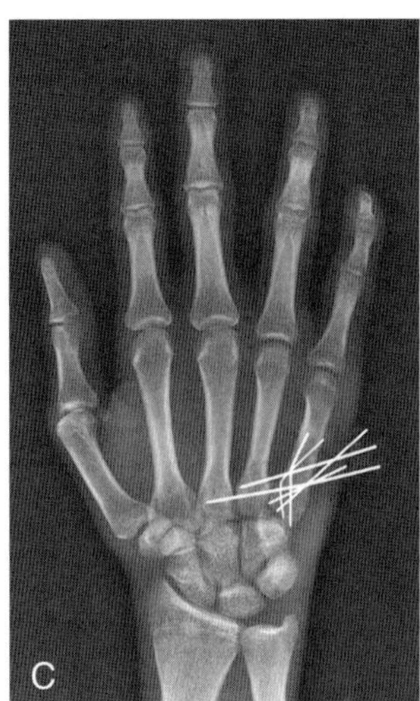

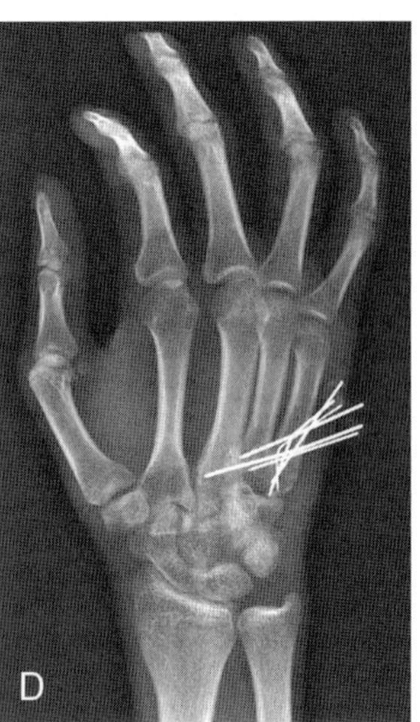

Figure 18 **A,** AP radiograph showing a comminuted intra-articular fracture of the base of the fifth metacarpal. **B,** 30° pronation view radiograph showing subluxation of the metacarpal shaft. **C,** Postsurgical AP radiograph showing an anatomic reduction of the articular fracture with Kirschner wires. **D,** Oblique radiograph showing reduction of the metacarpal shaft, with the dorsal cortex of the fifth metacarpal aligned with the dorsal cortex of the hamate.

ment may require articular reconstruction using a graft from the hamate.

A displaced metacarpal fracture or fracture-dislocation can result in a loss of digital motion, malalignment, or a complication related to surgical intervention. Whenever possible, a percutaneous method of stabilization should be used to avoid trauma to the soft tissue during open reduction or irritation of overlying extensor tendons during internal fixation.

References

1. Weiss AP, Hastings H II, Distal unicondylar fractures of the proximal phalanx. *J Hand Surg Am* 1993;18: 594-599.

2. Hastings H: Open reduction internal fixation: Unicondylar fractures of the head of the proximal phalanx, in Strickland J, Graham T, eds: *The Hand*, ed 2. Philadelphia, PA, Lippincott Williams & Wilkins, 2005, pp 47-60.

3. Hastings H II, Carroll C IV: Treatment of closed articular fractures of the metacarpophalangeal and proximal interphalangeal joints. *Hand Clin* 1988;4:503-527.

4. Hastings H: Hemi-hamate resurfacing arthroplasty for salvage of selected fracture-dislocations of the proximal interphalangeal joint, in Strickland J, Graham T, eds: *The Hand*, ed 2. Philadelphia, PA, Lippincott Williams & Wilkins, 2005, pp 61-74.

5. McElfresh EC, Dobyns JH, O'Brien ET: Management of fracture-dislocation of the proximal interphalangeal joints by extension-block splinting. *J Bone Joint Surg Am* 1972;54:1705-1711

6. Eaton RG, Malerich MM: Volar plate arthroplasty of the proximal interphalangeal joint: A review of ten years' experience. *J Hand Surg Am* 1980;5: 260-268.

7. Hastings H II, Ernst JM: Dynamic external fixation for fractures of the proximal interphalangeal joint. *Hand Clin* 1993;9:659-674.

8. Krakauer JD, Stern PJ: Hinged device for fractures involving the proximal interphalangeal joint. *Clin Orthop Relat Res* 1996;327:29-37.

9. Zemel NP, Stark HH, Ashworth CR, Boyes JH: Chronic fracture-dislocation of the proximal interphalangeal joint: Treatment by osteotomy and bone graft. *J Hand Surg Am* 1981;6:447-455.

10. Capo JT, Hastings H II, Choung E, et al: Hemicondylar hamate replacement arthroplasty for proximal interphalangeal joint fracture-dislocations: An assessment of graft suitability. *J Hand Surg Am* 2008;33:733-739.

11. Williams RM, Kiefhaber TR, Sommerkamp TG, Stern PJ: Treatment of unstable dorsal proximal interphalangeal fracture/dislocations using a hemi-hamate autograft. *J Hand Surg Am* 2003;28:857-865.

12. Williams RM, Hastings H II, Kiefhaber TR: PIP fracture/dislocation treatment technique: Use of a hemi-hamate resurfacing arthroplasty. *Tech Hand Up Extrem Surg* 2002;6:185-192.

13. Meunier MJ, Hentzen E, Ryan M, Shin AY, Lieber RL: Predicted effects of metacarpal shortening on interosseous muscle function. *J Hand Surg Am* 2004;29:689-693.

14. Strauch RJ, Rosenwasser MP, Lunt JG: Metacarpal shaft fractures: The effect of shortening on the extensor tendon mechanism. *J Hand Surg Am* 1998;23:519-523.

15. Kawamura K, Chung KC: Fixation choices for closed simple unstable oblique phalangeal and metacarpal fractures. *Hand Clin* 2006;22:287-295.

16. Sohn RC, Jahng KH, Curtiss SB, Szabo RM: Comparison of metacarpal plating methods. *J Hand Surg Am* 2008;33:316-321.

17. Orbay J: Intramedullary nailing of metacarpal shaft fractures. *Tech Hand Up Extrem Surg* 2005;9:69-73.

18. Capo JT, Hastings H II: Metacarpal and phalangeal fractures in athletes. *Clin Sports Med* 1998;17:491-511.

19. Galanakis I, Aligizakis A, Katonis P, Papadokostakis G, Stergiopoulos K, Hadjipavlou A: Treatment of closed unstable metacarpal fractures using percutaneous transverse fixation with Kirschner wires. *J Trauma* 2003;55: 509-513.

Fractures of the Base of the Thumb Metacarpal

Jerry I. Huang, MD
Diego L. Fernandez, MD

Abstract

The thumb trapeziometacarpal joint is a saddle joint that is subject to high compressive forces during prehensile hand function. Fractures to the base of the thumb metacarpal occur commonly following axial load to a partially flexed thumb. Although reduction is easily performed, severe deforming forces act to displace the fractures into a varus and shortened position. Most extra-articular fractures can be treated with closed reduction and cast immobilization. Angulation up to 30° can be tolerated because of the substantial compensatory motion at the thumb carpometacarpal joint. In Bennett fractures, good functional results are observed even with residual deformity and articular incongruity. However, the goal of treatment for intra-articular fractures should be the anatomic reduction of the joint surface with less than 1 mm of articular step-off to minimize the long-term risk of posttraumatic arthritis. Most Bennett fractures can be treated with closed reduction with percutaneous Kirschner wire fixation. Fractures with large Bennett fragments and Rolando fractures should be treated with open reduction and internal fixation to allow anatomic reduction with rigid fixation and early range of motion. Comminuted intra-articular fractures are challenging injuries that are best treated with application of an external fixator with limited open reduction and internal fixation, followed by bone grafting of metaphyseal bone defects if necessary.

Instr Course Lect 2010;59:343-356.

In 1882, Edward Bennett exhibited, in the Pathological Museum in Dublin, six cadaver specimens with united fractures involving the palmar base of the thumb metacarpal.[1] Bennett noted the most common fracture involving the base of the thumb metacarpal was a reproducible fracture pattern that involved "partial luxation of the metacarpal bone" from the palmar ulnar articular fragment at the base of the metacarpal that remained attached to the trapezium. In a clinical study in 1886, he recognized the disabling effects of this injury and recommended careful reduction and splint immobilization for a minimum of 4 weeks.[2] Despite improvements in understanding the anatomy and biomechanics of the thumb trapeziometacarpal joint and descriptions of numerous surgical techniques, controversy remains concerning the best treatment option for this common injury and its long-term consequences.

The quality of reduction and articular congruity correlate well with the development of posttraumatic arthritis; however, there has been no direct correlation between the development of arthritic changes and patient symptomatology.[3-6] Even in poorly reduced fractures, most patients have a satisfactory subjective outcome with minimal disability.[5-7] Blum[8] postulated that the articular changes from a malreduced fracture form a new joint mortise that acts as a ball-and-socket joint with structural improvement and a "more desirable end result than perfect reposition." A 1997 study using a cadaver model of a simulated Bennett fracture with 2 mm of articular incongruity showed that the contact area between the thumb metacarpal and the trapezium shifted dorsally but did not result in pathologic concentration of contact pressures at the margins of the articular step-off.[9]

Neither of the following authors nor any immediate family member has received anything of value from or owns stock in a commercial company or institution related directly or indirectly to the subject of this chapter: Dr. Huang and Dr. Fernandez.

Anatomy

The articular surfaces of the thumb metacarpal and trapezium form a reciprocating double concave-convex saddle joint. Using a three-dimensional model, Cooney and associates[10] described the true motion of the trapeziometacarpal joint occurring primarily in two planes (flexion-extension in the plane of the central ridge of the trapezium and abduction-adduction perpendicular to this plane). Based on a radiographic study of 19 normal subjects, the average arc of motion is 53° for flexion-extension and 42° for abduction-adduction perpendicular to this plane. Zancolli and associates[11] described thumb trapeziometacarpal motion as the simple angular movements of radial abduction–ulnar adduction and palmar abduction–dorsal adduction relative to the plane of the hand, as well as compound rotational movements of opposition (circumduction ulnarly and palmarly with thumb pronation) and retropulsion (radial and dorsal circumduction with thumb supination). During normal thumb function, axial rotation along the longitudinal axis of the thumb metacarpal is limited by joint geometry and capsuloligamentous soft-tissue constraints. For most prehensile hand functions, the thumb assumes a pronated, flexed, and adducted position. In thumb adduction and flexion, there is close contact between the articulating surfaces, and the trapeziometacarpal joint is tightly constrained. In contrast, with the thumb maximally abducted and extended, there is limited articular contact and increased range of motion. Further dynamic stability is conferred through compressive forces provided by extrinsic muscles. Trapeziometacarpal joint geometry precludes independent axial rotation. Thumb pronation is accompanied by flexion at the carpometacarpal (CMC) joint, whereas thumb supination is accompanied by extension at this joint.

There are five main ligaments that guide axial rotation and act as static stabilizers to the trapeziometacarpal joint.[12] The most important of these is the palmar beak or anterior oblique ligament, which is an intracapsular ligament that originates from the palmar tubercle of the trapezium and inserts onto the ulnopalmar base of the thumb metacarpal.[12,13] The palmer beak ligament is the primary stabilizer of the thumb trapeziometacarpal joint and acts to prevent dorsoradial subluxation and limit thumb pronation.[12-15] There also are two other intracapsular ligaments. The posterior oblique ligament of Haines originates from the dorsoulnar aspect of the trapezium and inserts onto the ulnar beak of the thumb metacarpal, whereas the triangular dorsoradial ligament extends from the dorsoradial tubercle of the trapezium to insert over a wide area on the dorsal rim of the thumb metacarpal.[13] The dorsal ligament complex pronates the thumb and stabilizes the thumb metacarpal during pulp pinch.[11] The first intermetacarpal ligament is an extracapsular ligament that originates from the dorsal aspect of the second metacarpal base and traverses in a radial and palmar direction to insert onto the palmar ulnar tubercle of the trapezium. The ligament is taut during abduction and opposition, and primarily resists thumb supination.[12] The ulnar collateral ligament is a thick extracapsular ligamentous band that extends from the trapezial crest to the ulnar beak of the thumb metacarpal.[12]

In normal prehensile hand functions, pinch forces are between 1 and 10 kg, whereas grasping forces average between 5 and 20 kg. The thumb metacarpal assumes a position of adduction-flexion during lateral pinch, midposition during tip pinch, and abduction-extension during grasp. Cooney and Chao[16] showed that during lateral pinch, joint compressive forces reach 12 kg at the trapeziometacarpal joint for every 1 kg of pinch force, whereas extrinsic and intrinsic tendons sustain forces as high as 30 and 50 kg, respectively. Compression forces at the trapeziometacarpal joint can reach forces as high as 120 kg during grasping activities, with extrinsic tendon forces reaching up to 50 kg.

Several deforming forces act on the thumb metacarpal. In an extra-articular fracture involving the base of the thumb metacarpal, the abductor pollicis longus extends the proximal fragment, whereas the adductor pollicis and intrinsic thenar muscles act to pull the distal fragment into a varus and flexed position, respectively. In a Bennett fracture, the ulnopalmar fragment remains attached while the remaining metacarpal is pulled dorsally, radially, and proximally by the abductor pollicis longus. Distally, the adductor pollicis again pulls the distal aspect of the thumb metacarpal into a varus position (Figure 1).

Classification

Fractures involving the base of the thumb metacarpal are generally classified as extra-articular and intra-articular and are further subdivided based on the severity of the articular involvement (Figure 2). Extra-articular fractures are usually transverse or involve a short oblique pattern.

In a Bennett fracture, the ulnopalmar articular fragment at the base of the thumb metacarpal remains

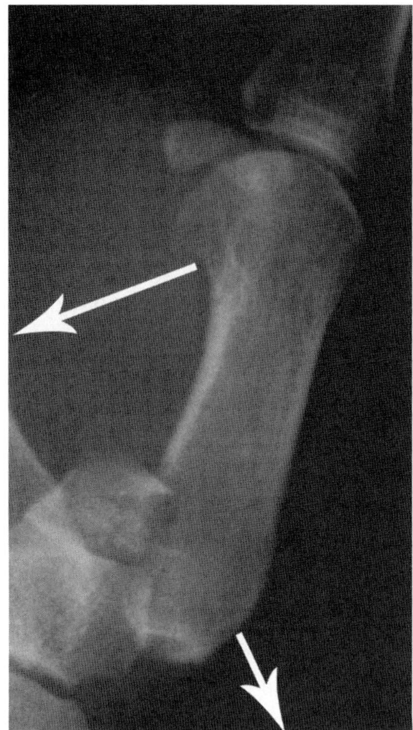

Figure 1 Radiograph of a Bennett fracture with arrows showing the severe deforming forces that act on the thumb metacarpal. The abductor pollicis longus displaces the thumb metacarpal dorsally, radially, and proximally. The direction of pull of the abductor pollicis longus is shown by the short arrow. The adductor pollicis acts to pull the distal aspect of the thumb metacarpal into varus. The direction of pull of the adductor pollicis is shown by the long arrow.

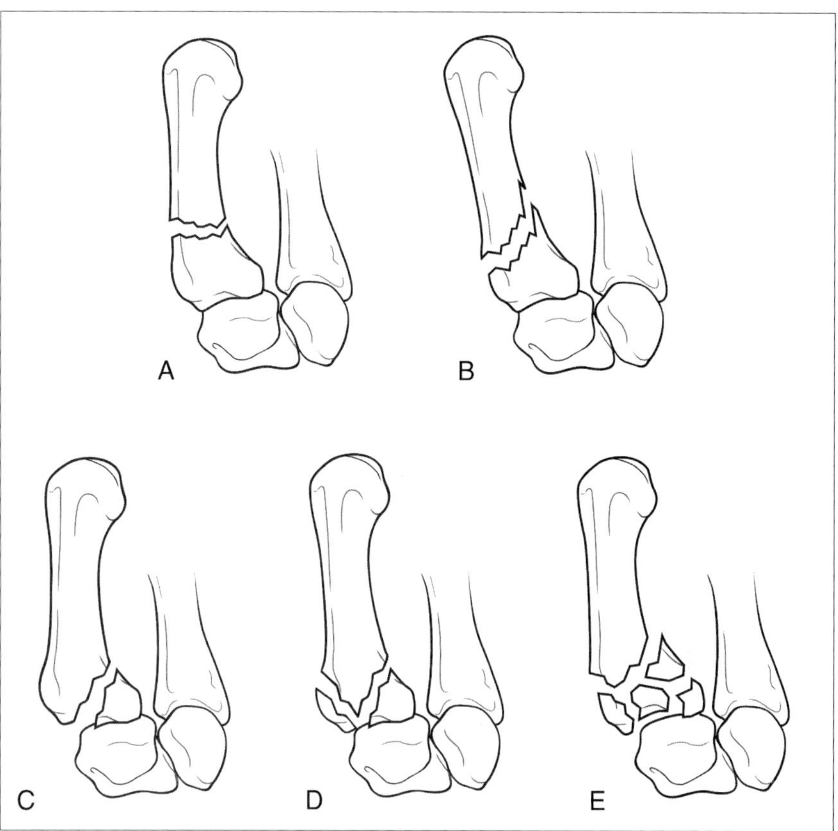

Figure 2 Illustration showing the classification of fractures of the base of the thumb metacarpal. Fractures can be classified as extra-articular or intra-articular. Extra-articular fractures are classified as transverse **(A)** or oblique **(B)**. Intra-articular fractures are classified as Bennett **(C)**, Rolando **(D)**, or comminuted **(E)** fractures.

attached to the trapezium through the palmar beak ligament while the remainder of the thumb metacarpal is subluxated dorsoradially and proximally. Gedda[17] further classified Bennett fractures into type I fractures, which involve a large articular fragment with subluxation of the metacarpal; type II fractures, with metaphyseal impaction but no metacarpal subluxation or dislocation; and type III fractures, with a small avulsion fragment and dislocation of the trapeziometacarpal joint. A Bennett fracture is a fracture-dislocation that often includes subchondral cancellous bone impaction, cartilage abrasion, and a limited area of metaphyseal (ulnar) comminution (Figure 3).

In 1910, Rolando[18] described three cases of intra-articular Y fractures, which involved a separate fracture of the dorsal articular process in addition to the palmar beak fragment seen in Bennett fractures. A Rolando fracture is now classically described as a Y- or T-shaped intra-articular fracture involving the base of the thumb metacarpal with two articular fragments. Since the original description in 1910, the term Rolando fracture often has been used to include all comminuted intra-articular fractures of the base of the thumb. The authors of this chapter believe in treating the Rolando fracture as a separate entity and view comminuted intra-articular fractures as a completely different fracture type.

Radiographic Evaluation

To accurately assess articular involvement of the thumb CMC joint, appropriate radiographs of the injured thumb are needed. Standard PA, oblique, and lateral radiographs of the injured thumb should be routinely obtained. In addition, Billing and Gedda[19] described a true lateral view of the trapeziometacarpal joint. The palmar aspect of the hand is placed flat on the cassette followed by pronation of the hand and wrist

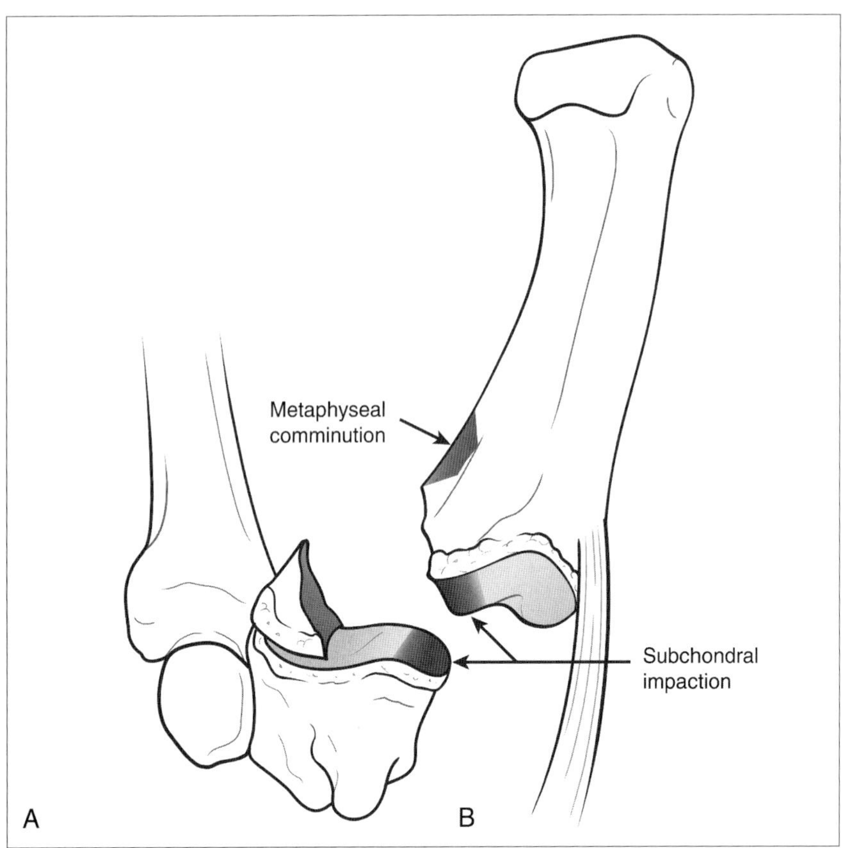

Figure 3 Bennett fractures are fracture-dislocations that include subchondral cancellous bone impaction, cartilage abrasion, and limited metaphyseal comminution ulnarly. **A,** Index metacarpal. **B,** Thumb metacarpal.

20° to 30°. The x-ray tube is then directed proximally 15° to 20° from vertical and centered over the trapeziometacarpal joint. Preoperative and intraoperative traction radiographs allow the surgeon to assess the fracture fragments in cases of articular comminution and the efficacy of ligamentotaxis on indirect reduction. CT scans of the thumb with three-dimensional reconstructions are helpful in preoperative treatment planning for severely comminuted intra-articular fractures and malunions.

Extra-articular Fractures

Most extra-articular fractures of the thumb metacarpal occur at the proximal metadiaphyseal junction and present with a transverse or short oblique pattern. The deforming forces usually result in varus and flexion angulation of the thumb metacarpal secondary to the pull of the adductor pollicis and intrinsic thenar muscles. Unlike the central metacarpals, the thumb metacarpal does not have suspensory protection from the intermetacarpal ligaments to limit shortening. With shortening and adduction of the thumb metacarpal, the thumb webspace is compromised, with resultant loss of effective grasping and pinch. However, compensatory CMC motion allows for some mild residual deformity without significant functional limitations. Angulation of 20° to 30° can generally be tolerated; however, angulation greater than 30° is often accompanied by compensatory hyperextension of the thumb metacarpophalangeal joint and should be corrected.[20]

Open reduction for an extra-articular thumb metacarpal fracture is rarely indicated. Closed reduction is generally accomplished by longitudinal traction, thumb abduction and extension, and downward pressure on the apex of the fracture. Reduction is usually stable and easily maintained in a thumb spica cast for 4 weeks. Percutaneous Kirschner wire (K-wire) fixation across the fracture site is used if the fracture is unstable and satisfactory reduction cannot be maintained. If direct K-wire fixation is not possible, intermetacarpal or transarticular fixation may be necessary. Open reduction with plate fixation should be considered in patients who want to avoid prolonged cast immobilization.

Bennett Fractures

The importance of accurate reduction of Bennett fracture-dislocations of the thumb metacarpal was advocated by Edward Bennett in his initial clinical series in 1886.[2] The reduction maneuver involves longitudinal traction with abduction, extension, and pronation of the thumb with downward pressure on the base of the thumb metacarpal. Although the reduction maneuver is well described and easy to perform, maintenance of reduction is difficult because of the deforming forces acting on the thumb metacarpal.

To help maintain length and prevent varus collapse, Robinson[21] pioneered the use of continuous skin traction in combination with splint immobilization. This innovative technique led to the subsequent development of other techniques to conservatively manage Bennett fractures by incorporating traction with cast immobilization, including the use of a Thomas splint and skeletal traction.[22-24]

Early reports of nonsurgical treatment of Bennett fractures showed that loss of reduction and malunions are extremely common, with resultant posttraumatic arthritis.[5,7,17,25,26] However, some authors have shown that high patient satisfaction and minimal disability could be expected despite some loss of motion and radiographic evidence of degenerative changes at the thumb trapeziometacarpal joint.[7,25] Based on their observations, more complex and invasive treatment methods were not justified. Blum[8] reported that the interspace between the palmar ulnar fragment and the body of the thumb metacarpal fills with callus, leading to a new joint mortise that was stable and allowed for full range of motion of the thumb with good grip strength. Based on these observations, he recommended simple physiotherapy with heat treatment and elastic bandaging, activities as tolerated for 2 weeks, then a full return to work. In a study of 31 patients, Pollen[27] demonstrated the efficacy of closed reduction and proper splint application in the maintenance of excellent reduction in 29 of 31 Bennett fractures. He suggested that poor technique and inexperience of the treating physician were important causes of inadequate reduction and the failure of nonsurgical management.

The long-term outcome of nonsurgical management of patients with Bennett fractures was evaluated by Livesley[26] in 17 patients at a mean follow-up of 26 years. All patients had loss of thumb abduction and extension and a decrease in grip strength. Twelve patients had persistent gross deformity of the hand secondary to dorsoradial subluxation of the thumb metacarpal. Seven patients were asymptomatic, and six patients had severe pain requiring activity modification and the use of the other hand in grasping activities. Radiographs showed persistent subluxation of the trapeziometacarpal joint in 13 patients, and stage II and III degenerative changes in 14 of 17 patients. Although the thumb is a non–weight-bearing joint, high joint compressive forces are experienced by the trapeziometacarpal joint during prehensile hand function.[16] In the long term, loss of articular congruity leads to progressive deterioration and symptomatic arthritis.

Gedda and Moberg[28] believed that open treatment of these injuries and anatomic restoration of the articular surface decreases the risk of posttraumatic arthritis and improves patient function.[17] However, they conceded that most patients with degenerative radiographic changes remain asymptomatic and are able to return to full function. In a retrospective study, Thurston and Dempsey[6] reviewed the clinical and radiographic outcomes of 21 Bennett fractures and reported that those with less than 1 mm of fracture displacement had superior results. Similarly, Oosterbos and de Boer[5] observed residual articular step-off in six of seven patients with posttraumatic arthrosis of the trapeziometacarpal joint.

A mixed cohort of patients with Bennett fractures treated with surgical and nonsurgical methods were analyzed by Kjaer-Petersen and associates[3] to determine the relationship between the quality of reduction and the development of symptomatic arthritis. At a mean follow-up of 7.3 years, 15 of 18 patients with excellent fracture reduction (< 1 mm step-off) were asymptomatic, whereas only 6 of 13 patients with residual displacement were asymptomatic. Radiographic evidence of arthritic changes was present in eight of nine patients with residual irregularity of the articular surface. Arthritic changes were seen in only 3 of 14 patients with excellent fracture reduction. Closed reduction and cast immobilization was effective in 2 of 10 displaced fractures. In a retrospective view of 18 patients by Timmenga and associates,[4] arthritic changes were present in all patients at a mean follow-up of 10.8 years; however, the quality of reduction correlated strongly with the severity of the degenerative changes.

Regardless of the choice of management, the goals of treatment for patients with Bennett fractures are to (1) restore the anatomic congruity of the joint surface, (2) maintain motion and normal kinesiology of the trapeziometacarpal saddle joint, (3) prevent development of posttraumatic arthritis, and (4) preserve the width of the thumb-index finger webspace.

Surgical Options

Various surgical techniques have been described for treating Bennett fractures, including closed reduction with K-wire fixation and open reduction with internal fixation. In general, the size of the articular fragment dictates the method of fixation (Figure 4). When the Bennett fragment is less than 15% to 20% percent of the articular surface, closed reduction with percutaneous pinning is indicated.

Numerous configurations and techniques have been described for percutaneous pinning of Bennett fractures (Figure 5). The Bennett

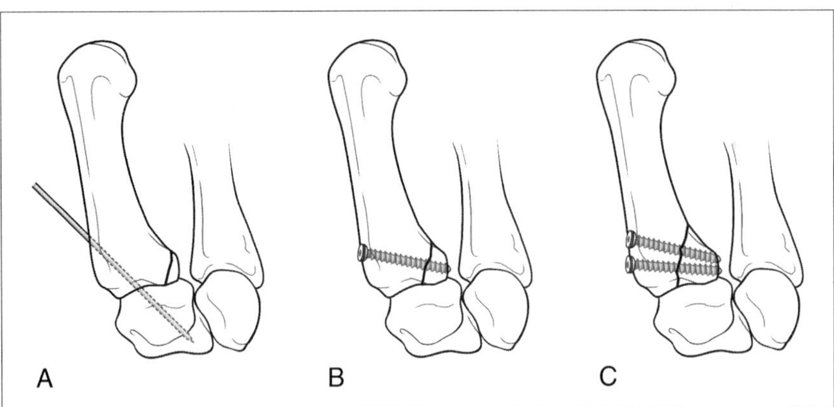

Figure 4 Illustration showing fixation of Bennett fragments. In general, the size of the Bennett fragment dictates the type of fixation chosen. **A,** If the fragment is less than 15% to 20% of the articular surface, closed reduction with percutaneous pinning is recommended. **B** and **C,** Fragments larger than 25% of the articular surface are usually amenable to open reduction and internal fixation with lag screws.

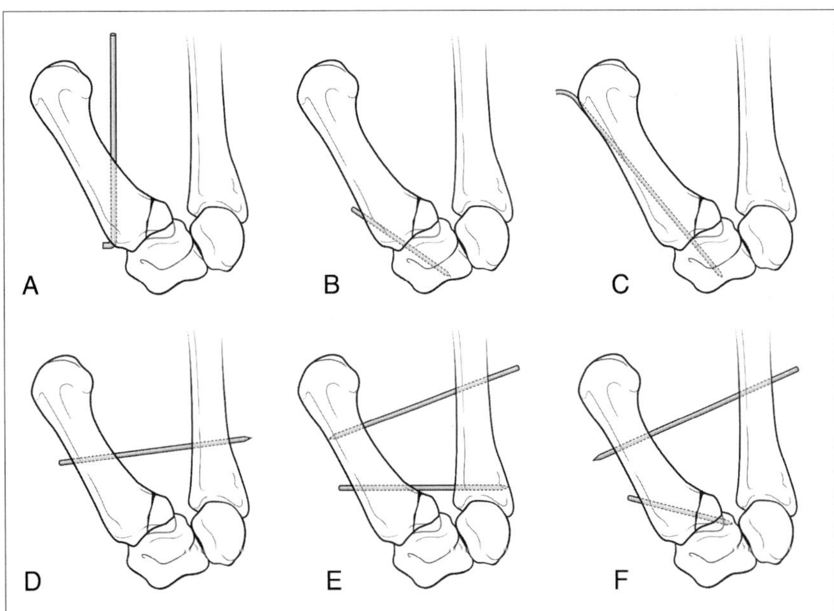

Figure 5 Illustration showing various methods for pinning Bennett fractures. **A,** Traction pinning. **B** and **C,** Transarticular pinning. **D** and **E,** Intermetacarpal pinning. **F,** Direct intermetacarpal pinning.

fragment is often very small, making direct pinning across the fracture site difficult. One technique stabilized the thumb metacarpal by intermetacarpal pinning to the second metacarpal and was later modified to include a second K-wire.[29-32] Axial fixation of the reduced metacarpal with a transarticular pin across the trapeziometacarpal joint was advocated by Wagner.[33,34] Wiggins and associates[35] described a variation on this technique with the introduction of a pin through the metacarpal head, down the shaft, and then across the CMC joint of the thumb.

Other authors described a technique of skeletal traction through an oblique K-wire placed through the thumb metacarpal that helps maintain length and prevents varus collapse.[23,24,36] This technique has largely been abandoned for treating Bennett fractures but remains useful as an option in treating comminuted intra-articular thumb metacarpal fractures.[37]

Several authors have used closed reduction and K-wire fixation to achieve anatomic or near-anatomic reduction of Bennett fractures and good functional results with no activity limitations.[32,38] In a retrospective review of 32 patients, Lutz and associates[39] compared Bennett fractures treated with closed reduction and percutaneous pinning with those treated with open reduction and internal fixation. The authors used the Wagner technique of placing a single K-wire across the trapeziometacarpal joint without supplemental intermetacarpal pinning. Although there was no difference in clinical outcomes or radiographic evidence of posttraumatic arthritis, the group with K-wire fixation had a significantly higher incidence of an adduction deformity compared with the group treated with open reduction. Using Iselin's technique of intermetacarpal pinning, Dartee and associates[32] reported good functional results (no restrictions in activities or delicate hand movement) in 32 of 33 patients.

If treated acutely, most Bennett fractures can be adequately managed with closed reduction with percutaneous pinning. The ability to achieve anatomic or near anatomic reduction is assessed intraoperatively with fluoroscopic imaging. With the thumb metacarpal reduced in an abducted, extended, and pronated position, a transarticular

K-wire is placed from the radial aspect of the base of the metacarpal and directed proximally and ulnarly across the trapeziometacarpal joint. To achieve additional stability, help maintain the thumb webspace, and prevent an adduction deformity, one or two additional intermetacarpal K-wires are placed into the base of the index finger metacarpal. A short thumb spica cast (with the interphalangeal joint free) is applied. The K-wires and the cast are removed after 4 to 6 weeks. Therapy for range of motion is initiated following removal of the pins.

If satisfactory reduction is not possible with closed methods, open reduction is mandatory. Achieving anatomic reduction should be the goal to prevent the development of posttraumatic arthritis.[4] Superior outcomes have been shown to correlate with anatomic reduction with less than 1 mm of residual displacement.[3,6]

Treating Bennett's fractures with open reduction and direct fixation was first advocated by Gedda and Moberg in 1953.[28] Based on their observations, patients with anatomic reductions through an open approach had less pain and less radiographic evidence of arthritis compared with those treated with closed methods. Heim[40] proposed the concept of rigid fixation of a Bennett fragment and the advantages of early motion. Several authors have described successful open reduction and screw fixation (with conventional and headless Herbert screws) of Bennett fractures.[40-47] When the fragment is greater than 25% to 30% of the articular surface, open reduction with rigid internal fixation allows for early cast removal and the initiation of therapy for active range of motion.

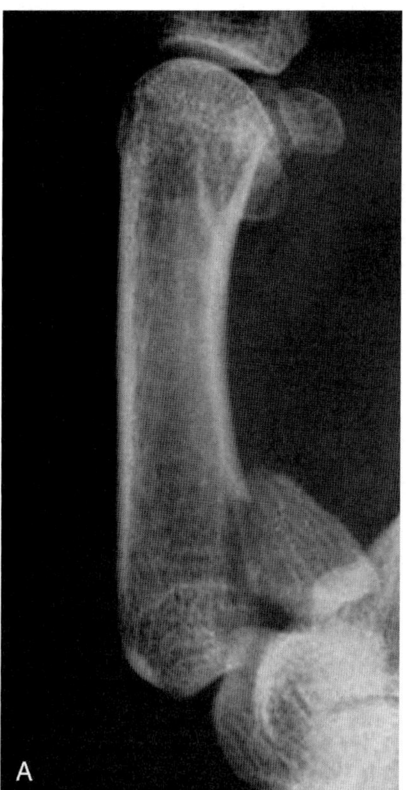

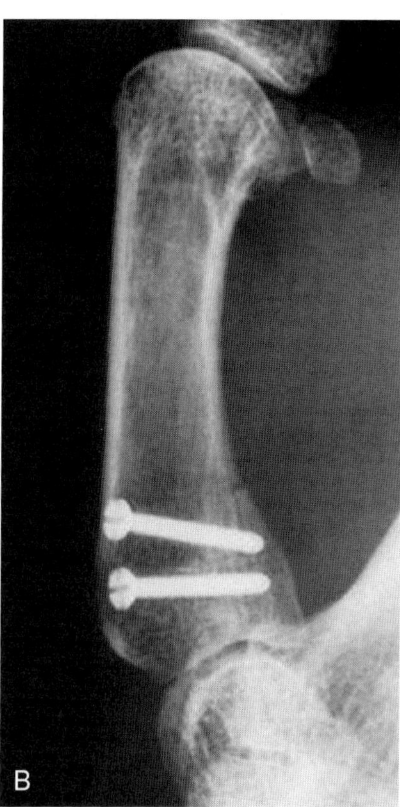

Figure 6 Radiographs showing a Bennett fracture with a large ulnopalmar fragment. **A,** Preoperative view. **B,** The fracture was treated with two lag screws placed from dorsal to volar.

The Authors' Preferred Technique

The authors of this chapter prefer surgical exposure through a longitudinal radiopalmar incision centered over the saddle joint in the interval between the abductor pollicis longus and thenar muscles or between slips of the accessory abductor pollicis longus tendons. Alternatively, a Wagner J-shaped incision can be made with curvilinear extension ulnarly to the radial aspect of the flexor carpi radialis tendon.[33] Branches of the superficial radial nerve are identified and carefully mobilized and protected. The thenar musculature is elevated subperiosteally off the volar aspect of the thumb metacarpal. The joint capsule is sharply incised to adequately visualize the fracture fragment and articular surface. Reduction is performed and maintained with a bone hook or bone reduction clamp, followed by provisional fixation with a K-wire. If the fragment is large, a 2.0-mm or 2.7-mm lag screw or a Herbert screw is placed from dorsal to volar for rigid fixation. Placement of two smaller screws is preferred to placement of a single larger screw (Figure 6). Alternatively, if the fragment is too small, secure fixation may be possible only with multiple 1.0-mm K-wires. Accurate placement of the lag screw centrally across the fracture site is accomplished with the inside-out technique (Figure 7). With the thumb maximally supinated, the fracture fragments are well visualized. The gliding hole is drilled from inside-out. Next, the thumb metacarpal is pronated to

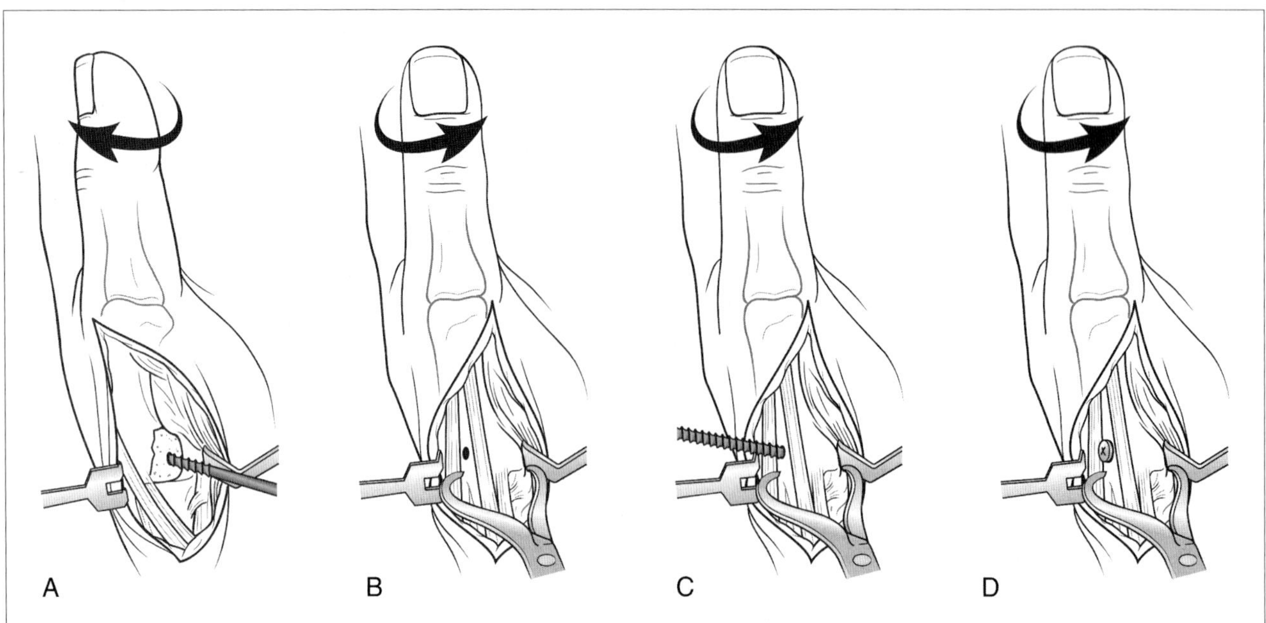

Figure 7 Accurate placement of the lag screw centrally is accomplished with the inside-out technique. The thumb metacarpal is supinated with drilling of the gliding hole **(A)**. Next, the thumb is pronated and reduced with a reduction clamp **(B)** followed by placement of the lag screw **(C** and **D)**.

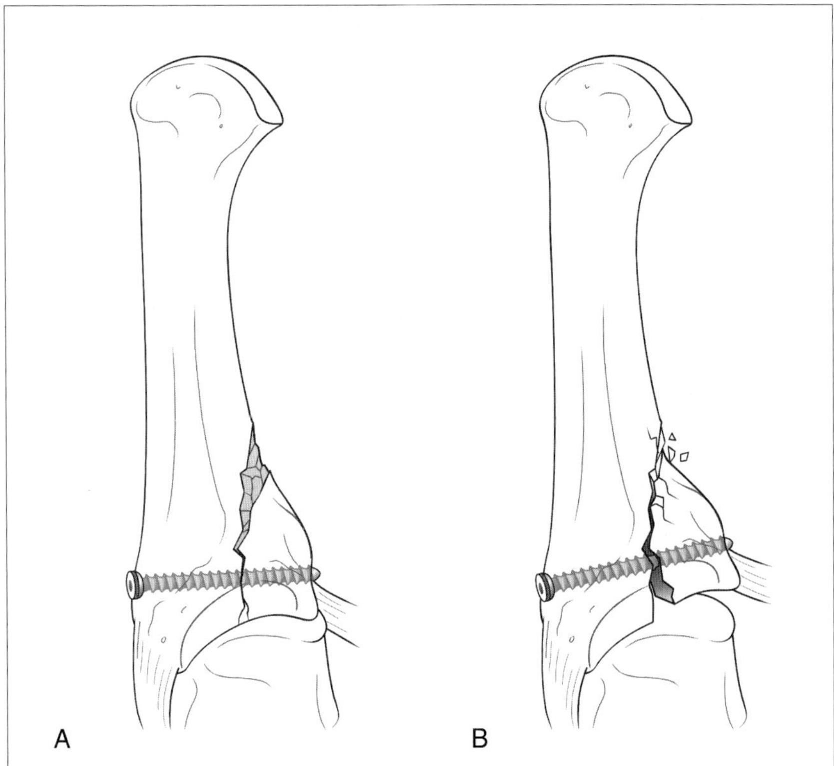

Figure 8 A common pitfall is the use of a lag screw in cases of marginal impaction. In these situations, a locking plate construct would provide more stable support. **A,** Illustration showing comminution of the metaphyseal bone. **B,** Illustration showing loss of reduction caused by metaphyseal comminution.

reduce the fragment. A lag screw is placed through the gliding hole using standard AO technique.

A common surgical pitfall is the failure to recognize the region of metaphyseal comminution just distal to the articular fragment. With lack of cortical continuity ulnarly, lag screw fixation will cause further fracture displacement with varus collapse and loss of articular congruity (Figure 8). To provide adequate stability, rigid fixation with a locking plate construct is recommended.

Postoperatively, the use of rigid fixation allows the patient to be cast free. If fixation is stable, a thumb spica splint is placed for patient comfort with the interphalangeal joint free. Active range-of-motion exercises are then initiated, with removal of the splint at 5 to 7 days.

Malunions

Patients with malunited Bennett fractures usually present with articular incongruity and characteristic shortening and varus collapse of the thumb metacarpal.[7,25,26] In addition to an increased risk of developing posttraumatic arthritis, patients usually lose thumb abduction and extension and have decreased grasping and pinching ability secondary to the loss of the thumb webspace.

Clinkscales[48] described the use of a closing wedge osteotomy at the base of the thumb metacarpal to treat CMC joint instability, correct residual varus deformity, and restore the thumb webspace. Bunnell[49] recognized the necessity for anatomic restoration of the thumb trapeziometacarpal joint and advocated an intra-articular osteotomy with rigid fixation of the fragments. Vasko[50] treated three old, unreduced Bennett fractures and was successful in restoring the normal joint mortise; he reported excellent functional results at follow-up. In 1997, Jebson and Blair[51] reported on the treatment of two young laborers with symptomatic malunited Bennett fractures with an intra-articular osteotomy. At 24- and 40-month postoperative follow-up, they reported significant pain relief and improved range of motion, grip strength, and pinch strength. The authors promoted this technique for the treatment of young patients with symptomatic malunited Bennett fractures with a large volar fragment and no radiographic evidence of degenerative changes. Older patients with malunions and those with symptomatic posttraumatic arthritis are candidates for thumb CMC fusion or trapeziectomy with interposition arthroplasty.[14,15,52-54]

Rolando Fractures

In 1910, Rolando[18] described a series of 12 thumb metacarpal fractures in which he noticed three cases of a new fracture pattern that involved a Y-shaped intra-articular split of the base of the metacarpal. The injuries occurred following an axial load to the thumb metacarpal with the thumb in an adducted position. In addition to the Bennett fragment involving the ulnopalmar aspect of the articular surface, there was a separate dorsoradial articular fragment. Classically, the fracture pattern involved a Y- or T-shaped intra-articular split either in the frontal or sagittal plane. Although the term Rolando fracture is often used to include all comminuted intra-articular fractures of the base of the thumb metacarpal, a Rolando fracture should be distinguished from comminuted intra-articular fractures, which pose a more difficult treatment challenge. Options for treating a Rolando fracture include open reduction and internal fixation, oblique skeletal traction, and external fixation.[36,37,42,55-57]

In a 1992 study, Proubasta[57] treated five Rolando fractures with closed reduction through longitudinal traction and ligamentotaxis followed by the application of a uniplanar external fixator with two pins each in the trapezium and thumb metacarpal for 6 weeks. This technique is simple and minimally invasive. At 3 months, all patients were pain free, with full thumb range of motion. However, the quality of reduction was not assessed in the study, and long-term outcomes are not available. The quality of reduction in intra-articular fractures involving the base of the thumb metacarpal has been shown to correlate with the long-term development of arthritic changes.[3,4,6]

Langhoff and associates[56] reviewed 17 Rolando fractures, which included 13 classic T- or Y-shaped Rolando fractures, 1 double-Bennett fracture, and 3 comminuted fractures. Of the 14 displaced fractures, 3 were treated with percutaneous K-wire fixation, and 11 were treated with open reduction and internal fixation. At a mean follow-up of 5.8 years, 9 of the 15 patients available for follow-up were asymptomatic, with no physical disability. Radiographs at follow-up were available for 11 patients and showed arthritic changes in 6 and irregularities in the joint surface in the other 5 patients. The quality of reduction did not correlate with the development of posttraumatic arthritis or the presence of symptoms. However, based on their experiences, good to excellent reduction was possible in almost all cases with open reduction and internal fixation, whereas an anatomic reduction was not possible in those treated with closed reduction with percutaneous pinning. Langhoff and associates[56] recommend open reduction and rigid fixation of the fragments if the fractures are not severely comminuted and the fragments are of adequate size to allow anatomic restoration of the articular surface.

The extent of fracture comminution is often discovered to be more severe on intraoperative evaluation than had been suggested by radiographic studies. In addition to the standard dorsoradial and ulnopalmar fragments, there is commonly a separate avulsion fracture of the abductor pollicis longus tendon insertion. CT scans are helpful in assessing the articular surface and in making surgical decisions; however, if the fragments are of sufficient size, open reduction and internal fixation should be attempted to achieve an anatomic reduction and rigid fixation. Surgical exposure is performed with a standard longitudinal incision as was previously decribed. In the more common sagittal

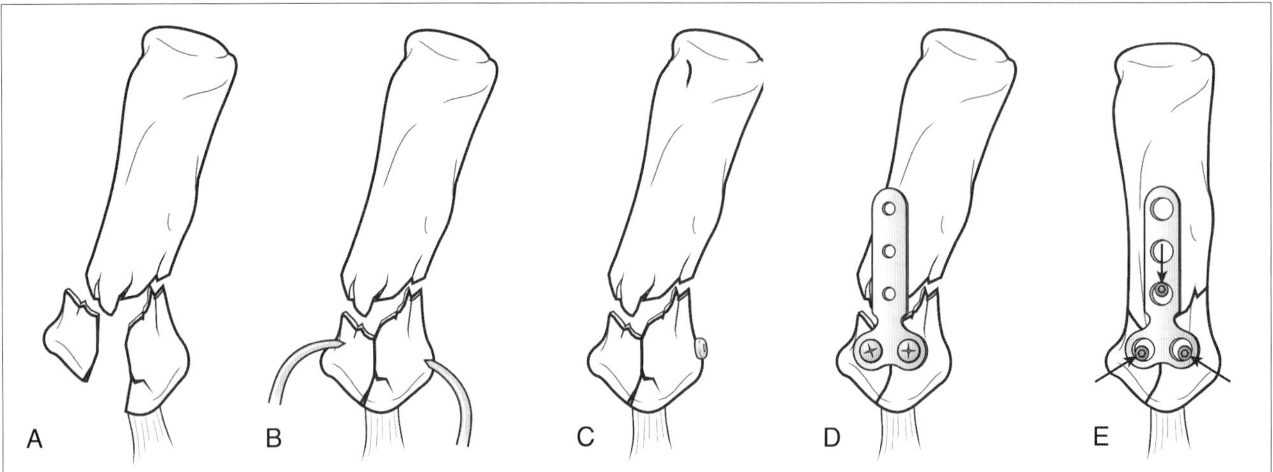

Figure 9 Illustration showing the stepwise reduction of a sagittal split in a Rolando fracture. **A** through **C,** The joint surface is reduced. **D,** A T-shaped plate is placed. **E,** Screws are placed eccentrically to allow compression of the articular fragments and metacarpal shaft.

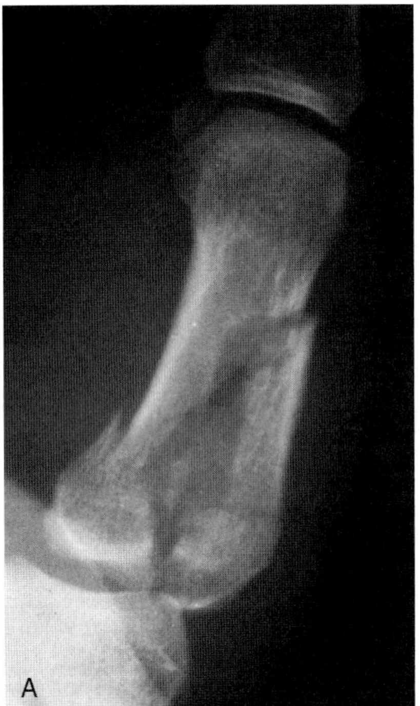

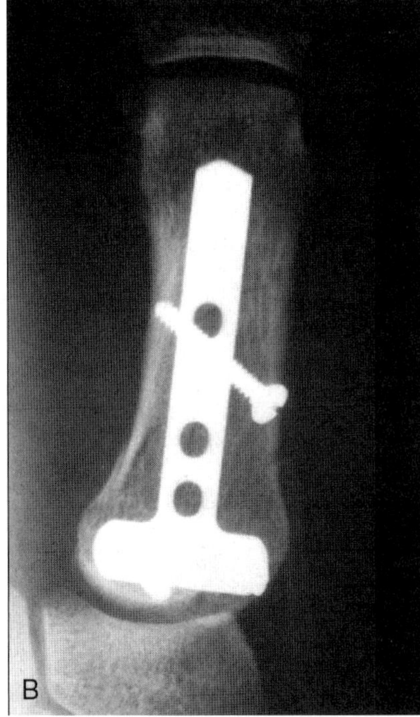

Figure 10 Preoperative **(A)** and postoperative **(B)** radiographs showing a sagittal split Rolando fracture with shaft extension treated with a T-plate.

split, reduction of the articular fragments is first performed with a bone reduction clamp, followed by provisional fixation with K-wires, and definitive fixation with a T-plate (Figures 9 and 10). The plate is precontoured to the thumb metacarpal base. Interfragmentary compression of the articular fragments is achieved by placing screws at the base of the metacarpal in an eccentric fashion. Compressing the metacarpal shaft to the base also can be achieved with eccentric screws placed distally over the proximal portion of the metacarpal shaft. In the less common frontal split, a stepwise reduction is recommended, with alignment of the metacarpal shaft with the ulnopalmar fragment that is still attached to the trapezium, followed by reduction of the dorsal articular fragment (Figure 11). The authors of this chapter prefer fixation with a minicondylar blade plate or locking plate construct for this fracture pattern.

Comminuted Intra-articular Fractures

Comminuted intra-articular fractures of the base of the thumb metacarpal usually occur from a high-energy injury and are usually accompanied by severe soft-tissue trauma. These injuries pose several technical challenges, including disimpaction of multiple articular fragments, difficulty in achieving stable fixation of multiple small fragments, and metaphyseal comminution with associated bone loss (Figures 12 and 13). Moreover, an extensile exposure risks further soft-tissue injury and devascularization of the fracture fragments. The small size of the fragments precludes the use of interfragmentary compression and complicates the aim of stabilizing the articular surface to the metacarpal shaft.

Gelberman and associates[37] described the use of Thoren's oblique traction technique in treating these complex injuries and achieving satisfactory results. The traction device allows for longitudinal pull and an ulnar directed vector on the thumb metacarpal to counteract the shortening and varus-deforming forces from the thumb abductor pollicis longus and adductor pollicis muscles. The technique is appealing in its simplicity and is minimally invasive. Early motion in the thumb interphalangeal joint is possible with the Thoren technique. Patients treated with this technique achieved pain-free range of motion and full use of the hand 8 to 10 weeks after injury.[37]

Indirect reduction with ligamentotaxis and placement of an external fixator is often the best treatment option. Techniques for external fixation include the use of a quadrilateral frame with pins in the thumb and index finger metacarpals, an uniplanar frame with pins in the thumb metacarpal and trapezium, and a triangular Hoffman frame with pins in the distal radius, the thumb metacarpal, and the index finger metacarpal.[57-60] Büchler and associates[58] advocated the application of the orthopaedic principles described by Rüedi and Allgower[61] for the treatment of tibial pilon fractures to treat severely comminuted intra-articular fractures of the base of the thumb metacarpal. These principles are (1) restoration of length, (2) anatomic reduction of the articular surface with limited internal fixation, (3) bone grafting for metaphyseal defects, and (4) neutralization of deforming forces. Ten patients with comminuted intra-articular fractures of the base of the thumb metacarpal were treated with application of a quadrilateral external fixator between the thumb and index finger metacarpals combined with limited open reduction and internal fixation of the articular surface. Eight of the 10 patients had a large metaphyseal bone defect volarly that required bone grafting. Büchler and associates[58] were able to achieve good functional results (minimal symptoms and disability) in nine patients. One patient had persistent disability

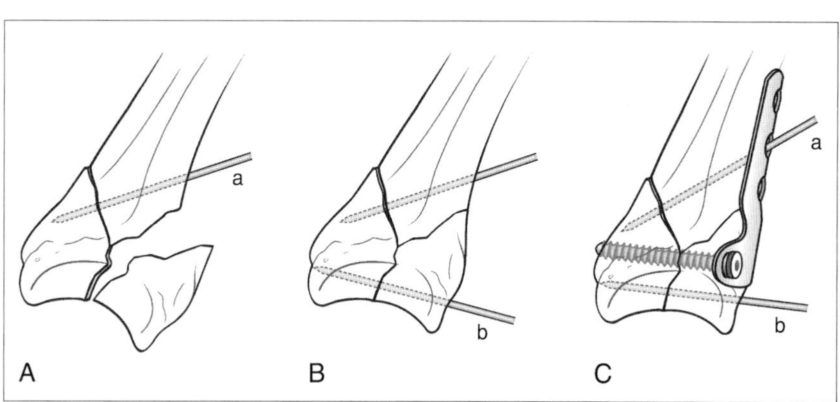

Figure 11 **A,** The stepwise reduction of a frontal split Rolando fracture involves reduction of the metacarpal shaft to the volar beak fragment with a pin (a). **B,** This is followed by reduction of the dorsoradial fragment with a pin (b). **C,** Plate fixation with a minicondylar plate or locking plate is recommended.

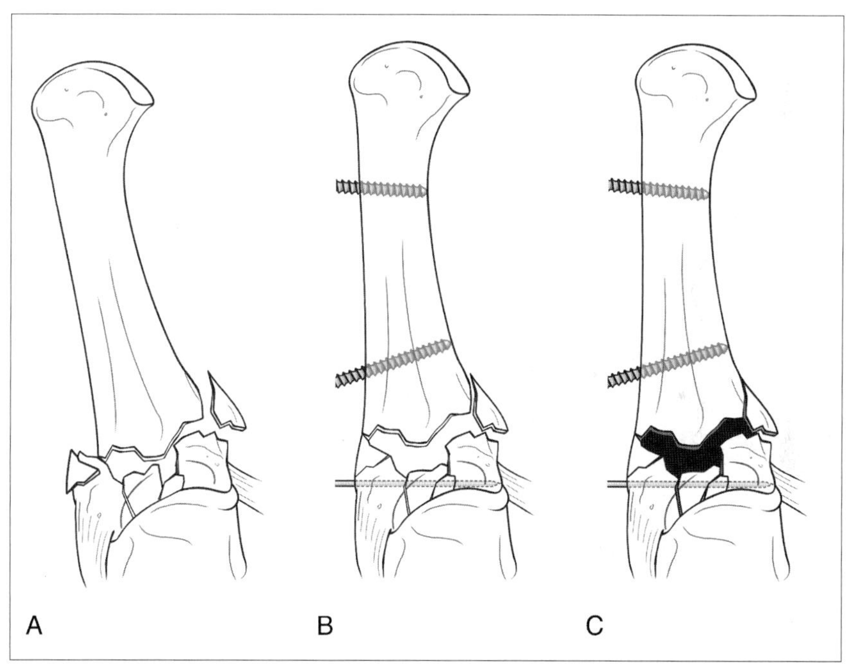

Figure 12 Comminuted intra-articular fractures **(A)** require disimpaction and limited fixation of the articular surface with placement of an external fixator **(B)** and bone grafting of metaphyseal bone defects **(C)** in a stepwise fashion.

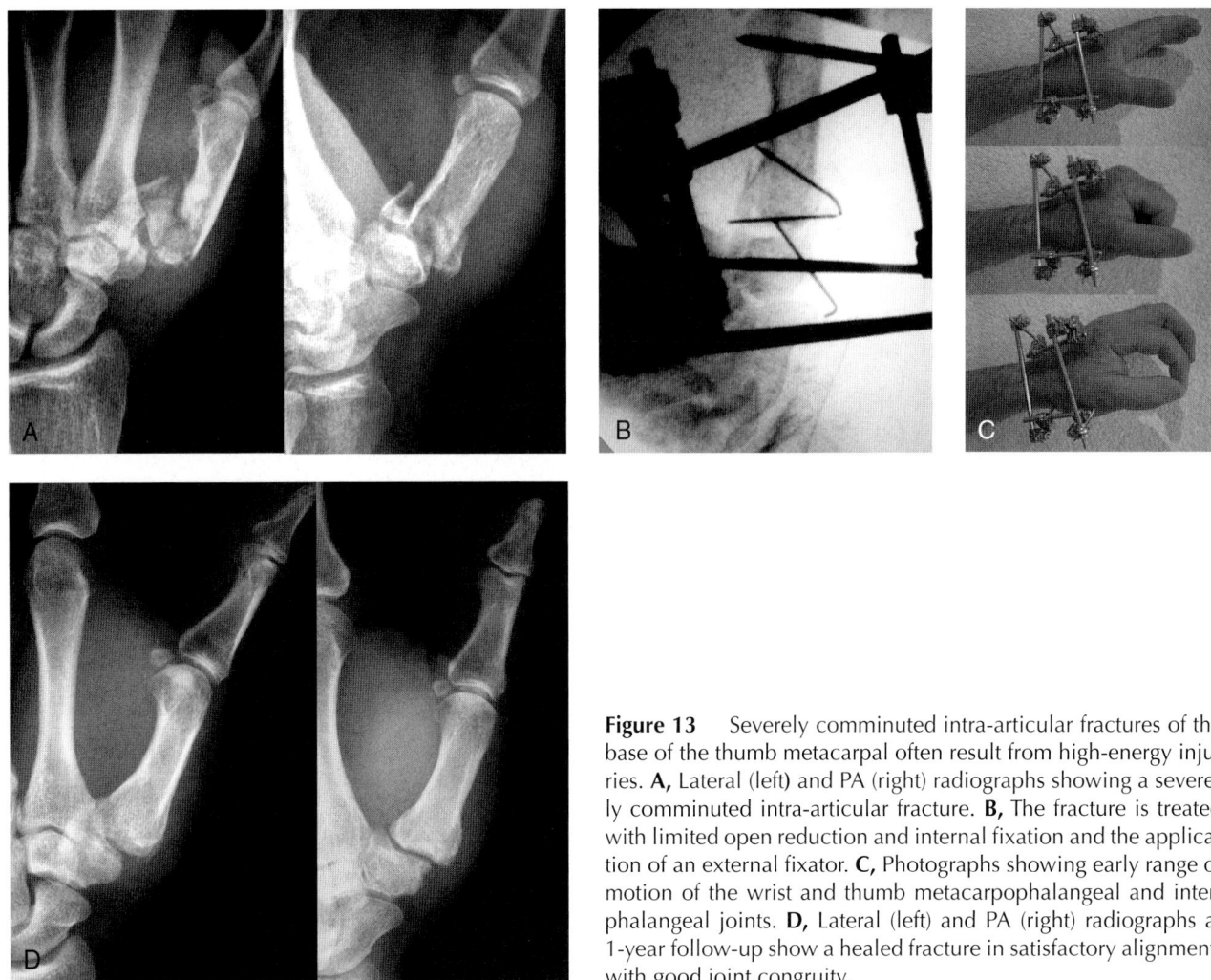

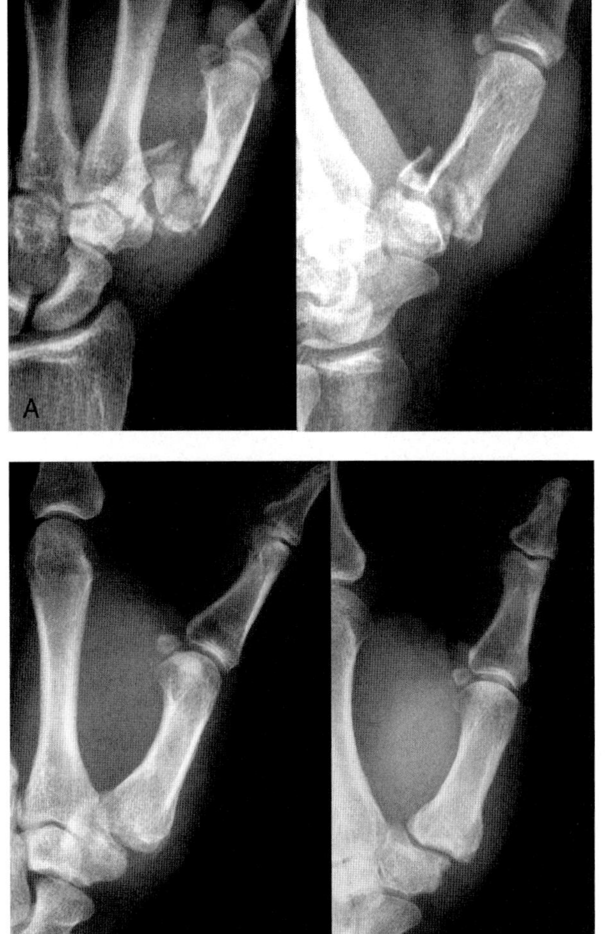
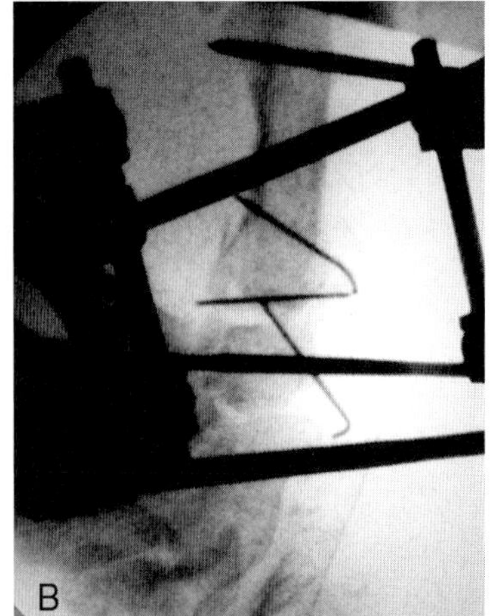
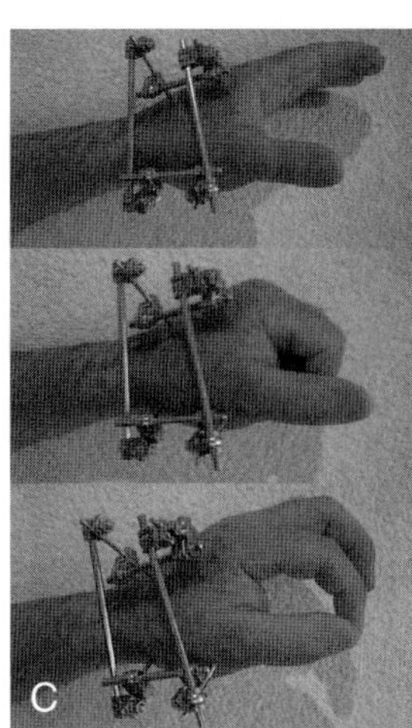

Figure 13 Severely comminuted intra-articular fractures of the base of the thumb metacarpal often result from high-energy injuries. **A,** Lateral (left) and PA (right) radiographs showing a severely comminuted intra-articular fracture. **B,** The fracture is treated with limited open reduction and internal fixation and the application of an external fixator. **C,** Photographs showing early range of motion of the wrist and thumb metacarpophalangeal and interphalangeal joints. **D,** Lateral (left) and PA (right) radiographs at 1-year follow-up show a healed fracture in satisfactory alignment, with good joint congruity.

and required a job change. One patient required revision surgery for a repeat injury; the other patients healed uneventfully without loss of reduction. Compared with the contralateral, uninjured side, radial abduction was 89%, grip strength 81%, and key pinch 88%.

Summary

Although the thumb trapeziometacarpal joint is a non–weight-bearing joint, significant compressive forces are transmitted during prehensile hand function. Good functional results correlate with early treatment and the quality of the reduction. Regardless of the preferred technique, the goals of treatment should be the anatomic restoration of the articular surface to decrease the long-term risk of posttraumatic arthritis. In Bennett fractures, successful treatment can be achieved in most patients with closed reduction with percutaneous pinning. With larger fragments and Rolando fractures, open reduction and internal fixation allows for anatomic reduction and rigid fixation. The ability to initiate early therapy with active range of motion should be considered in the treatment algorithm.

References

1. Bennett EH: Fractures of the metacarpal bones. *Dublin J Med Sci* 1882; 73:72-75.
2. Bennett EH: On fracture of the metacarpal bone of the thumb. *BMJ* 1886; 2:12-13.
3. Kjaer-Petersen K, Langhoff O, Andersen K: Bennett's fracture. *J Hand Surg Br* 1990;15:58-61.
4. Timmenga EJ, Blokhuis TJ, Maas M, Raaijmakers EL: Long-term evaluation of Bennett's fracture: A comparison between open and closed reduction. *J Hand Surg Br* 1994;19:373-377.
5. Oosterbos CJ, de Boer HH: Nonoperative treatment of Bennett's frac-

ture: A 13-year follow-up. *J Orthop Trauma* 1995;9:23-27.

6. Thurston AJ, Dempsey SM: Bennett's fracture: A medium to long-term review. *Aust N Z J Surg* 1993;63: 120-123.
7. Cannon SR, Dowd GS, Williams DH, Scott JM: A long-term study following Bennett's fracture. *J Hand Surg Br* 1986;11:426-431.
8. Blum L: The treatment of Bennett's fracture-dislocation of the first metacarpal bone. *J Bone Joint Surg Am* 1941;23:578-580.
9. Cullen JP, Parentis MA, Chinchilli VM, Pellegrini VD Jr: Simulated Bennett fracture treated with closed reduction and percutaneous pinning: A biomechanical analysis of residual incongruity of the joint. *J Bone Joint Surg Am* 1997;79:413-420.
10. Cooney WP III, Lucca MJ, Chao EY, Linscheid RL: The kinesiology of the thumb trapeziometacarpal joint. *J Bone Joint Surg Am* 1981;63:1371-1381.
11. Zancolli EA, Zaidenberg C, Zancolli E Jr: Biomechanics of the trapeziometacarpal joint. *Clin Orthop Relat Res* 1987;220:14-26.
12. Imaeda T, An KN, Cooney WP III, Linscheid R: Anatomy of trapeziometacarpal ligaments. *J Hand Surg Am* 1993;18:226-231.
13. Haines RW: The mechanism of rotation at the first carpo-metacarpal joint. *J Anat* 1944;78:44-46.
14. Eaton RG, Lane LB, Littler JW, Keyser JJ: Ligament reconstruction for the painful thumb carpometacarpal joint: A long-term assessment. *J Hand Surg Am* 1984;9:692-699.
15. Eaton RG, Littler JW: A study of the basal joint of the thumb: Treatment of its disabilities by fusion. *J Bone Joint Surg Am* 1969;51:661-668.
16. Cooney WP III, Chao EY: Biomechanical analysis of static forces in the thumb during hand function. *J Bone Joint Surg Am* 1977;59:27-36.
17. Gedda KO: Studies on Bennett's fracture: Anatomy, roentgenology, and therapy. *Acta Chir Scand Suppl* 1954; 193:1-114.
18. Rolando S: Fracture de la base du premier metacarpien, et principalement sur une variete non encore decreite. *Presse Med* 1910;33:303.
19. Billing L, Gedda KO: Roentgen examination of Bennett's fracture. *Acta Radiol* 1952;38:471-476.
20. Stern PJ: Fractures of the metacarpals and phalanges, in Green DP, Hotchkiss RN, eds: *Operative Hand Surgery*, ed 3. New York, NY, Churchill-Livingston, 1993, pp 695-758.
21. Robinson S: The Bennett fracture of the first metacarpal bone: Diagnosis and treatment. *Boston Med and Surg J* 1908;158:275.
22. Roberts N: Fractures of the phalanges of the hand and metacarpals. *Proc R Soc Med* 1938;31:793-798.
23. Spangberg O, Thoren L: Bennett's Fracture: A method of treatment with oblique traction. *J Bone Joint Surg Br* 1963;45:732-736.
24. Thoren L: A new method of extension treatment in Bennett's fracture. *Acta Chir Scand* 1956;110:485-493.
25. Griffiths JC: Fractures at the base of the first metacarpal bone. *J Bone Joint Surg Br* 1964;46:712-719.
26. Livesley PJ: The conservative management of Bennett's fracture-dislocation: A 26-year follow-up. *J Hand Surg Br* 1990;15:291-294.
27. Pollen AG: The conservative treatment of Bennett's fracture-subluxation of the thumb metacarpal. *J Bone Joint Surg Br* 1968;50:91-101.
28. Gedda KO, Moberg E: Open reduction and osteosynthesis of the so-called Bennett's fracture in the carpometacarpal joint of the thumb. *Acta Orthop Scand* 1953;22:249-257.
29. Iselin M, Blanguenon S, Benoist D: Fractures des la base du premier metacarpien. *Meem Acad Chir* 1956; 82:771-774.
30. Johnson EC: Fractures of the base of the thumb: A new method of fixation. *JAMA* 1944;126:27-28.
31. Sedel L: Treatment of fractures of the base of the first metacarpal using double intermetacarpal pinning. *Acta Orthop Belg* 1973;39:1087-1099.
32. Dartee DA, Brink PR, van Houtte HP: Iselin's operative technique for thumb proximal metacarpal fractures. *Injury* 1992;23:370-372.
33. Wagner CJ: Method of treatment of Bennett's fracture dislocation. *Am J Surg* 1950;80:230-231.
34. Wagner CJ: Transarticular fixation of fracture-dislocations of the first metacarpal-carpal joint. *West J Surg Obstet Gynecol* 1951;59:362-365.
35. Wiggins HE, Bundens WD Jr, Park BJ: A method of treatment of fracture-dislocations of the first metacarpal bone. *J Bone Joint Surg Am* 1954;36: 810-819.
36. Thoren L: Basal fractures of the first metacarpal bone: A method of treatment by extension. *Acta Orthop Scand* 1957;27:40-48.
37. Gelberman RH, Vance RM, Zakaib GS: Fractures at the base of the thumb: Treatment with oblique traction. *J Bone Joint Surg Am* 1979;61: 260-262.
38. van Niekerk JL, Ouwens R: Fractures of the base of the first metacarpal bone: Results of surgical treatment. *Injury* 1989;20:359-362.
39. Lutz M, Sailer R, Zimmermann R, Gabl M, Ulmer H, Pechlaner S: Closed reduction transarticular Kirschner wire fixation versus open reduction internal fixation in the treatment of Bennett's fracture dislocation. *J Hand Surg Br* 2003;28:142-147.
40. Heim U: Rigid osteosynthesis in the treatment of fractures of the first metacarpal. *Acta Orthop Belg* 1973;39: 1078-1086.
41. Crawford GP: Screw fixation for certain fractures of the phalanges and metacarpals. *J Bone Joint Surg Am* 1976;58:487-492.
42. Foster RJ, Hastings H II: Treatment of Bennett, Rolando, and vertical intraarticular trapezial fractures. *Clin Orthop Relat Res* 1987;214:121-129.

43. Freeland AE, Geissler WB, Weiss AP: Surgical treatment of common displaced and unstable fractures of the hand. *Instr Course Lect* 2002;51: 185-201.

44. Hughes AW: Bennett's fractures fixed using the Herbert scaphoid screw. *J R Coll Surg Edinb* 1985;30:231-233.

45. Stromberg L: Compression fixation of Bennett's fracture. *Acta Orthop Scand* 1977;48:586-591.

46. Howard FM: Fractures of the basal joint of the thumb. *Clin Orthop Relat Res* 1987;220:46-51.

47. Massart P, Bezes H: Screw or miniplate fixation in fractures of the first metacarpal: Experience with thirty-nine cases. *Ann Chir Main* 1982;1: 293-300.

48. Clinkscales GS Jr: Complications in the management of fractures in hand injuries. *South Med J* 1970;63: 704-707.

49. Bunnell S: *Surgery of the Hand*, ed 2. Philadelphia, PA, JB Lippincott, 1948, pp 712-715.

50. Vasko JR: An operation for old unreduced Bennett's fracture. *J Bone Joint Surg Am* 1947;29:753-756.

51. Jebson PJ, Blair WF: Correction of malunited Bennett's fracture by intra-articular osteotomy: A report of two cases. *J Hand Surg Am* 1997;22: 441-444.

52. Carroll RE: Arthrodesis of the carpometacarpal joint of the thumb: A review of patients with a long postoperative period. *Clin Orthop Relat Res* 1987;220:106-110.

53. Eaton RG, Littler JW: Ligament reconstruction for the painful thumb carpometacarpal joint. *J Bone Joint Surg Am* 1973;55:1655-1666.

54. Hartigan BJ, Stern PJ, Kiefhaber TR: Thumb carpometacarpal osteoarthritis: Arthrodesis compared with ligament reconstruction and tendon interposition. *J Bone Joint Surg Am* 2001; 83:1470-1478.

55. Bruske J, Bednarski M, Niedzwiedz Z, Zyluk A, Grzeszewski S: The results of operative treatment of fractures of the thumb metacarpal base. *Acta Orthop Belg* 2001;67:368-373.

56. Langhoff O, Andersen K, Kjaer-Petersen K: Rolando's fracture. *J Hand Surg Br* 1991;16:454-459.

57. Proubasta IR: Rolando's fracture of the first metacarpal: Treatment by external fixation. *J Bone Joint Surg Br* 1992;74:416-417.

58. Büchler U, McCollam SM, Oppikofer C: Comminuted fractures of the basilar joint of the thumb: Combined treatment by external fixation, limited internal fixation, and bone grafting. *J Hand Surg Am* 1991;16: 556-560.

59. Nonnenmacher J: Osteosynthesis of fractures of the base of the first metacarpal by an external fixator. *Ann Chir Main* 1983;2:250-257.

60. Schuind F, Noorbergen M, Andrianne Y, Burny F: Comminuted fractures of the base of the first metacarpal treated by distraction-external fixation. *J Orthop Trauma* 1988;2: 314-321.

61. Rüedi TP, Allgöwer M: The operative treatment of intra-articular fractures of the lower end of the tibia. *Clin Orthop Relat Res* 1979;138: 105-110.

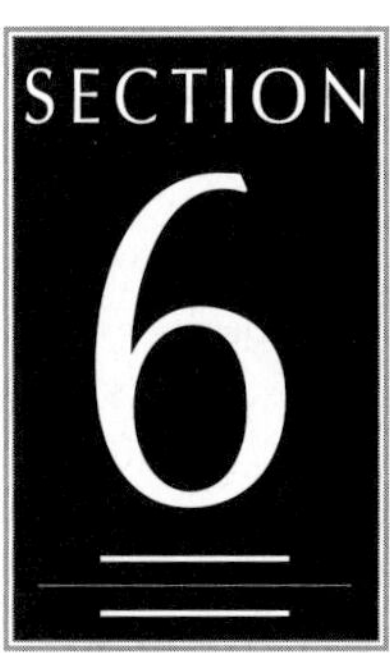

Section 6

Foot and Ankle

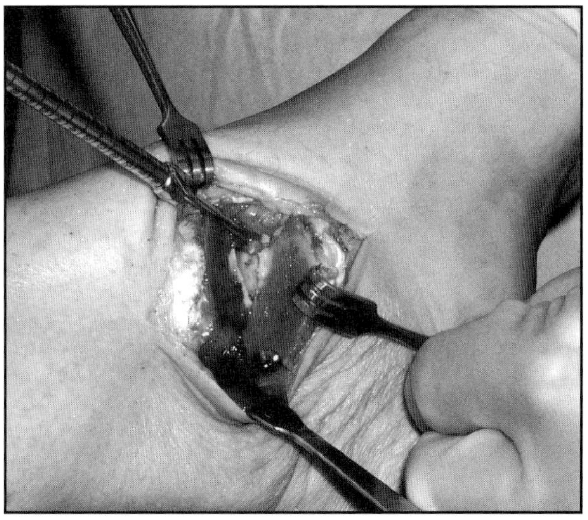

End-Stage Ankle Arthritis: Magnitude of the Problem and Solutions

Mark Glazebrook, PhD, MD, FRCSC

Abstract

Patients with end-stage ankle arthritis have a significantly compromised health-related quality of life. Nonsurgical treatments for end-stage ankle arthritis should be considered prior to surgery. Currently, the most accepted surgical treatment is ankle arthrodesis. The shortcomings of ankle arthrodesis, such as increased rates of ipsilateral periarticular arthritis and the possible long-term need for amputation, have cast doubt on the success of this treatment for end-stage ankle arthritis. Newer second and third generation total ankle arthroplasty prostheses have shown positive short- and medium-term results. An examination of the available literature provides good evidence to support ankle arthrodesis and total ankle arthroplasty for treating patients with end-stage ankle arthritis. Other treatment options, including ankle osteotomies, ankle osteochondral allograft transplantation, and distraction arthroplasty, require further study by surgeons with advanced training in these procedures.

Instr Course Lect 2010;59:359-365.

Arthritis is a debilitating chronic disease associated with pain and dysfunction; in patients with advanced disease, muscle atrophy, joint contractures, and limb deformity may occur.[1] More than 22 million people in North America are currently living with osteoarthritis.[1-3] The World Health Organization estimates that 80% of people with osteoarthritis experience restricted movement and 25% cannot perform some activities of daily living.[2] In 1995, an estimated 44 million North Americans had some form of arthritis, and this number is expected to increase to 66 million by 2020.[2] Approximately 6% to 13% of all osteoarthritis occurs in the ankle joint; however, there is limited data documenting common characteristics, general health, severity of pain, and loss of function in these patients.[1,4,5] A recent report has suggested that severe debilitation and reduction in the quality of life is caused by end-stage ankle arthritis.[5]

A recent study compared the health-related quality of life of patients with end-stage ankle arthritis to a similar cohort of patients with end-stage hip arthrosis,[6] a condition with well-established severe effects on the health-related quality of life.[7-11] This level I prognostic study used the Medical Outcomes Study 36-Item Short Form (SF-36) generic clinical outcome scale to assess health-related quality of life.[6] The patients in both cohorts scored approximately 2 standard deviations below normal population scores for all symptoms and functional SF-36 subscale scores. All differences between ankle and hip SF-36 subscale scores were less than four points. Patients with ankle disease had worse mental and general health scores, and poorer scores based on assessments of physical limitations with work and daily activities. The authors concluded that the mental and physical disabilities caused by end-stage ankle arthrosis were at least as severe as those observed in patients with end-stage hip arthrosis. The sufficient evidence support-

Dr. Glazebrook or an immediate family member serves as a paid consultant to or is an employee of DePuy and ConMed Linvatec; has received research or institutional support from Arthrex, Biomimetic, and DePuy; and owns stock or stock options in Smith & Nephew, Stryker, and Wright Medical Technology.

Table 1
Treatment Options for Ankle Arthritis

Nonsurgical
Activity modification
Bracing
Injectables (corticosteroids and viscosupplementation)
Medications (analgesics and anti-inflammatory drugs)
Nutritional supplements (chondroitin and glucosamine)
Patient education
Physical therapy
Shoe wear modifications (for example, rocker-bottom shoe wear)
Shoe orthotics
Weight reduction

Surgical
Arthrodesis
Arthroplasty
Arthroscopy
Distraction arthroplasty
Osteochondral allograft transplantation
Osteotomy

ing the dramatic effect that end-stage ankle arthritis has on health-related quality of life has resulted in an increasing focus on effective treatment options.

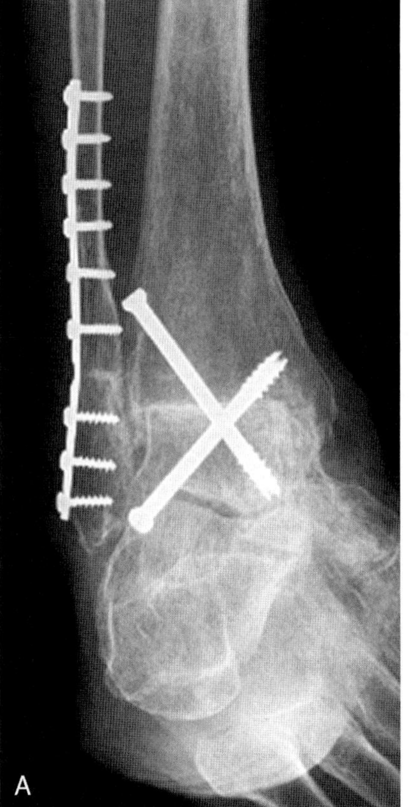

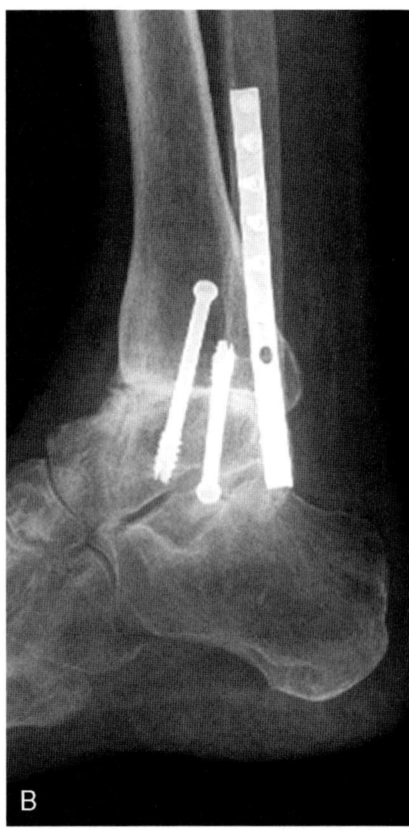

Figure 1 Postoperative AP **(A)** and lateral **(B)** radiographs of an anatomic ankle arthrodesis.

Nonsurgical Treatment Options

Most nonsurgical treatment modalities for ankle arthritis are focused on reducing pain and improving motion and function. Current nonsurgical treatments for ankle arthritis are listed in Table 1. Nonsurgical treatment options have a limited role in the treatment of end-stage ankle arthritis because of the advanced nature of the disease and are not a primary focus of this chapter. However, nonsurgical treatments for patients with end-stage ankle arthritis should be considered prior to surgical treatment. The current literature that supports most nonsurgical treatments for ankle arthritis primarily use lesser quality, level IV studies. A systematic review of the current literature is needed to determine the level of evidence available to determine the grade of recommendation of nonsurgical options for treating ankle arthritis.

Surgical Treatment Options

Ankle Arthrodesis

Currently, the most accepted surgical treatment for end-stage ankle arthritis is ankle arthrodesis (Figure 1). Evidence in the literature ranging from level I to IV studies support a grade A recommendation (good evidence with consistent findings from level I studies) or at least a grade B recommendation (fair evidence with consistent findings in level II or III studies) for the use of ankle arthrodesis in treating end-stage ankle arthritis.

In a recent systematic review of the literature, Haddad and associates[12] examined the intermediate and long-term outcomes of ankle arthrodesis and total ankle arthroplasty. This review included 39 papers (1,262 patients) on ankle arthrodesis for the treatment of end-stage ankle arthritis. Evidence levels ranged from I to IV. The results included a mean American Orthopaedic Foot and Ankle Society joint-specific clinical outcome score of 75.6 (range, 71.6 to 79.6; confidence interval, 95%). The complications rate was acceptable, with revision rates less than 10% and an infection rate of less than 5%. However, the 5% reported amputation rate is reason for concern.

Recently, ankle arthrodesis has been associated with arthritic changes in the ipsilateral tarsometatarsal and subtalar joints. Several level III long-term studies reported a high incidence of ipsilateral hindfoot arthritis following ankle arthrodesis, particularly of the subtalar joint.[13-18] It can be concluded that long-term follow-up of patients with ankle arthritis and/or ankle arthrodesis show a high incidence of ipsilateral hindfoot arthritis, with the subtalar joint most commonly affected. Level III evidence shows that the presence of ipsilateral hindfoot arthritis compromises the functional outcome of the patient following ankle arthrodesis.[16,19] None of the long-term studies demonstrated an increased incidence of knee or metatarsophalangeal arthritis on either the ipsilateral or contralateral extremities.[15,20]

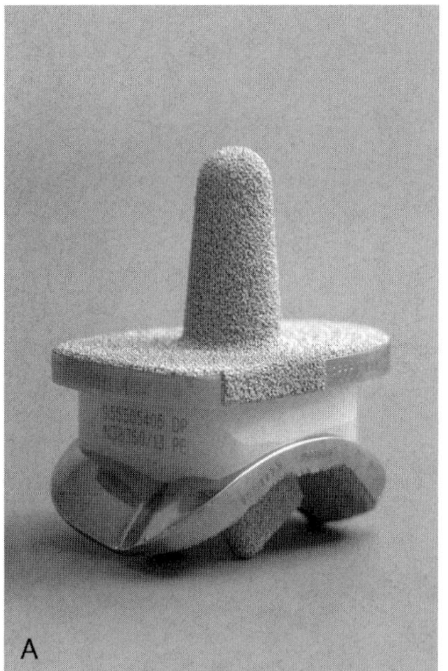

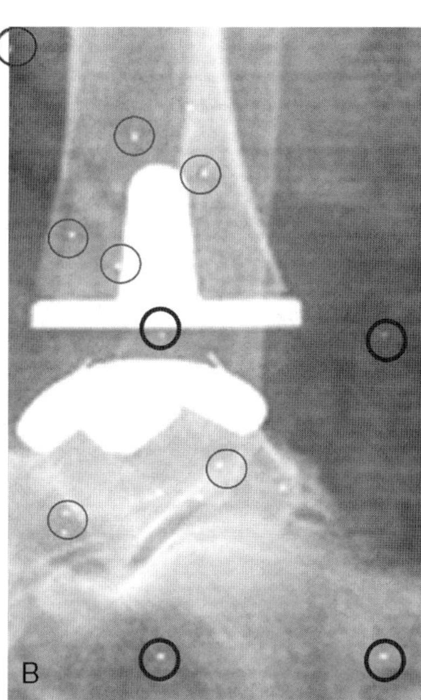

Figure 2 **A,** A third generation Mobility total ankle prosthesis. **B,** Postoperative radiograph of the Mobility ankle prosthesis with radiostereometric analysis beads circled (unbolded in patient and bolded in calibration box between the patient and x-ray detector).

Ankle Arthroplasty

Shortcomings of ankle arthrodesis, such as increased rates of ipsilateral periarticular arthritis and possible long-term amputation, have cast doubt on the success of this procedure for treating patients with end-stage ankle arthritis. Newer second and third generation total ankle arthroplasty prostheses (Figure 2) have shown positive short- and medium-term results in North America and Europe.[21-24] These new second and third generation implants (for example, the Agility Ankle and the Mobility Ankle [DePuy, Warsaw, IN]; the Buechel-Pappas Ankle and the Low Contact Stress Ankle [Endotec, South Orange, NJ]; the Hintegra Ankle [New Deal SA, Lyon, France]; and the Scandinavian Total Ankle Replacement—STAR [W. Link GmbH and Co, Hamburg, Germany]) have improved design features, including three components, mobile bearings, and nonconstrained and noncemented components.

The intermediate outcomes for the treatment of end-stage ankle arthritis with total ankle arthroplasty are superior to those of ankle arthrodesis. This is due in part to the fact that outcome studies on ankle arthroplasty are more recent and still include only intermediate-term results. Comparative prospective studies and long-term outcomes are lacking.

In a review by Haddad and associates[12] of the intermediate-term outcomes for total ankle arthroplasty for treating end-stage ankle arthritis, 10 papers (852 patients) were identified that provided mainly level II to level IV evidence. The results included a mean American Orthopaedic Foot and Ankle Society joint-specific clinical outcome score of 78.2 (range, 71.9 to 84.5; confidence interval, 95%). The complications rate was acceptable, with a revision rate of 7% and a 1% amputation rate.

Another review focused on survival and complication rates of total ankle arthroplasties by examining 20 studies on the short- and intermediate-term outcomes from a 10-year time period (1997 to 2007); each study had a sample size of at least 25 patients who were treated with total ankle arthroplasty for end-stage ankle arthritis.[25] Failed total ankle arthroplasties in this review ranged from 1.3% to 32.3%, with an overall mean of 12.4% failure at 64 months. Complications of total ankle arthroplasty were identified and included deep infection, aseptic loosening, and implant failure, which are considered high-grade complications because they result in an implant failure rate of more than 50%. Technical errors, subsidence, and postoperative bone fracture were considered medium-grade complications, whereas intraoperative bone fractures and wound healing problems

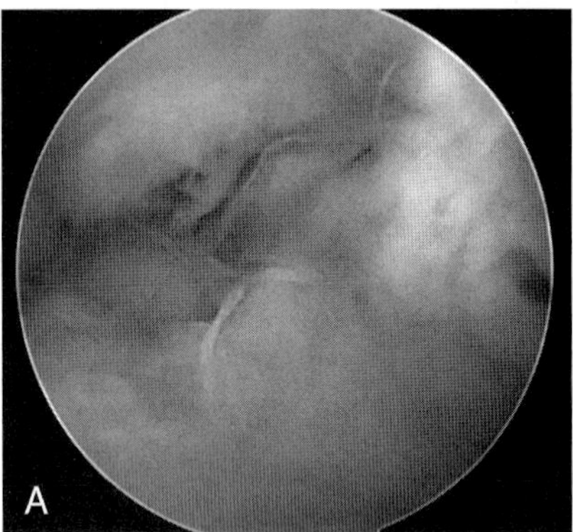

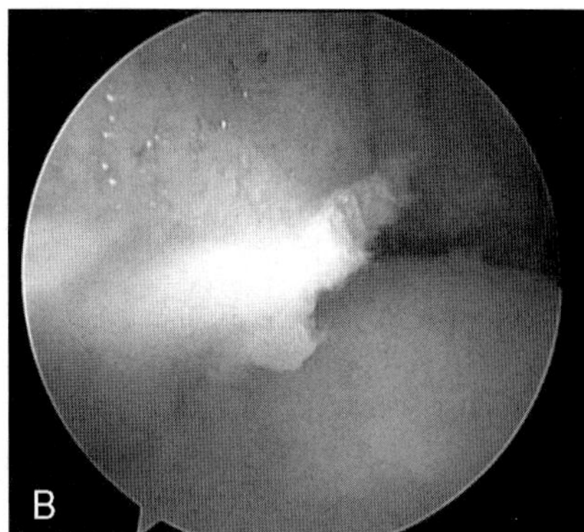

Figure 3 Intraoperative photographs of an ankle arthroscopy before **(A)** and after **(B)** anterior débridement of soft tissue and bone impingement.

were considered low-grade complications.

The literature supports total ankle arthroplasty for the treatment of end-stage ankle arthritis with respect to efficacy and safety based on intermediate-term follow-up with level II to IV evidence in favor of a grade B recommendation.

Ankle Arthroscopy

Ankle arthroscopy often has been used to treat patients with anterior soft-tissue and/or bony impingement from ankle arthritis (Figure 3). Patients should be carefully selected for ankle arthroscopy because those with ankle arthritis and no evidence of impingement are unlikely to benefit from the procedure. For example, Ogilvie-Harris and Sekyi-Otu[26] reviewed 32 patients treated with arthroscopic débridement for ankle osteoarthrosis; 17 improved, and only 2 were restored to normal function. In a study by Amendola and associates,[27] patients treated with arthroscopic débridement for ankle osteoarthritis or generalized chondromalacia showed poor results, with only 2 of 11 patients benefiting from the procedure. Cerulli and associates[28] and Martin and associates[29] also reported poor results in their studies on ankle arthroscopy. Based on the above studies, arthroscopic débridement for advanced ankle osteoarthritis without evidence of anterior impingement is not indicated. This represents a grade C recommendation against arthroscopic treatment based on the lack of available evidence-based literature.

There is evidence for the efficacy of ankle arthroscopy in patients with bony and/or soft-tissue impingement, with many level IV studies and at least six level III or better studies showing consistent support for ankle arthroscopy in those with impingement.[30-35] Most of these studies did not report the coexistence of advanced arthritis. Although arthroscopic débridement for soft-tissue or bony impingement is supported by evidence in the literature, it is important ensure that impingement rather than arthritis is the cause of the symptoms.

Ankle Osteotomy

Limited data support the use of osteotomies about the ankle for treating ankle arthritis with deformity. Six level IV studies suggest that supramalleolar osteotomies are beneficial in treating ankle arthritis with deformity and have acceptable complication rates.[36-41] Because of the limited number of evidence-based studies, the grade of recommendation is currently incomplete, with insufficient evidence for or against ankle osteotomies for the treatment of arthritis with deformity. This technique is promising and deserves further investigation with prospective comparative studies.

Ankle Osteochondral Allograft Transplantation

The outcomes of fresh osteochondral allograft transplantation for end-stage ankle arthritis have been reported in at least four level IV studies.[42-45] In a study by Gross and associates,[42] six of nine talar allograft transplants had survived at 11-year follow-up. In two other studies from the same institution, successful outcomes were reported in 6 of 11 patients[44] and 10 of 12 patients.[45] However, in the largest and most recent study, Jeng and associates[43] reported on 29 patients (mean age, 41 years; mean follow-up, 2 years) treated with an osteochondral total ankle transplant. At follow-up, 14 of the 29 transplants had been revised with another ankle transplant, prosthetic total ankle arthroplasty, or bone block arthrodesis. Six of the remaining 15 transplants were deemed to be radiographic failures because of allograft fracture, allograft collapse, or progressive loss of joint space. The remaining nine allograft transplantations (31%) were considered successful. Based on the limited and conflicting level IV evidence available, there is no support for or against the use of osteochondral allografts for treating end-stage ankle arthritis.

Ankle Distraction Arthroplasty

Articular distraction of the ankle

joint with an external fixation device recently has been advocated for end-stage ankle arthritis in patients who are candidates for arthrodesis. The procedure involves application of a ringed external fixator to the distal tibia and foot after open or arthroscopic débridement. A review of the literature showed 11 articles, 7 of which were based on expert opinion.[15,46-51] Three of the four remaining studies were level IV studies.[52-54]

The only level II study by Marijnissen and associates[55] reported significant clinical benefits in 43 of the 57 patients (75%) studied. Interestingly, a randomized trial in a subset of 17 patients showed joint distraction achieved significantly better results than débridement.

Although ankle distraction arthroplasty holds promise, especially in younger patients, data supporting a successful outcome are limited. There is a need for evidence-based literature by surgeons with advanced training in external fixation procedures.

Future Directions

A review of treatment options for end-stage ankle arthritis shows no clear consensus for treatment. Even when considering the well-supported surgical treatments of ankle arthrodesis and total ankle arthroplasty, there are no clear indicators on which procedure is best for an individual patient. It is likely that many of these procedures may prove to be the preferred treatment for an individual patient based on the unique characteristics of that patient. For example, many surgeons would agree that a patient with end-stage ankle arthritis and concurrent subtalar arthritis may be best treated with a motion-sparing surgical treatment such as total ankle arthroplasty. However, in a younger patient, it could be argued that total ankle arthroplasty is relatively contraindicated because of its limited longevity and a lack of well-established revision techniques. In a young patient, some surgeons would consider distraction arthroplasty, which would be more suitable as a temporizing procedure. Other surgeons may believe that total ankle arthroplasty is a viable option for a young patient because it should theoretically spare the periarticular joints and leave ankle arthrodesis as a viable salvage procedure. After failed arthroplasty, arthrodesis can be successful in achieving pain relief with acceptable complication rates.[56]

With promising options but limited evidence-based support from the literature, it is clear that more clinical research is necessary to advance the surgical care of patients with end-stage ankle arthritis. Well-designed randomized controlled trials are the preferred method for this research. However, reporting of results in lower quality level II to IV studies should not be dismissed because large numbers of lesser quality studies will often provide necessary preliminary data required to guide the more definitive level I studies. All clinical outcome studies should be competently performed and should include a record or classification of individual patient characteristics that will be important in correlating clinical outcomes. This will allow the potential identification of a more tailored approach to the surgical treatment of end-stage ankle arthritis that is based on preoperative patient characteristics.

Newer research techniques such as radiostereometric analysis (Figure 2), a technique that uses small tantalum bead placement to serve as reference points to monitor micromotion of various prosthesis segments, should be embraced[57] (DM Veljkovic, MD, Toronto, Canada, unpublished data presented at the American Orthopaedic Foot and Ankle Society annual summer meeting, 2007). This research technique will accelerate the evaluation of new prosthesis designs because it allows early detection of prosthetic components that are at risk for aseptic loosening and premature failure.[58] This improved sensitivity will shorten study times from approximately 10 years to 2 years and will dramatically reduce the study subject sample size required to assess fixation of new implant technology from thousands of subjects to fewer than 100. The benefits of such research are accelerated product development and minimization of patient risk.

Summary

End-stage ankle arthritis is a growing problem that has dramatic negative effects on a patient's health-related quality of life. Treatment options include nonsurgical modalities that should be attempted prior to surgery. If nonsurgical treatment options fail, surgical techniques that have evidence-based support, such as ankle arthrodesis and total ankle arthroplasty, should be considered. Other surgical techniques, such as distraction arthroplasty and allograft ankle transplantation, should be evaluated in well-designed studies performed by orthopaedic surgeons with advanced training in the techniques. Future investigations should include well-designed clinical and biomechanical studies that identify the most important patient characteristics that correlate with optimal outcomes for specific surgical treatments for end-stage ankle arthritis.

References

1. Buckwalter JA, Saltzman C, Brown T: The impact of osteoarthritis: Implications for research. *Clin Orthop Relat Res* 2004;427(suppl): S6-S15.
2. Lawrence RC, Helmick CG, Arnett FC, et al : Estimates of the prevalence of arthritis and selected musculoskeletal disorders in the United States. *Arthritis Rheum* 1998;41:778-799.
3. Badley EM: Arthritis in Canada: What do we know and what should we know? *J Rheumatol Suppl* 2005;72: 39-41.
4. Thomas RH, Daniels TR: Ankle arthritis. *J Bone Joint Surg Am* 2003;85: 923-936.
5. Agel J, Coetzee JC, Sangeorzan BJ, Roberts MM, Hansen ST Jr: Functional limitations of patients with end-stage ankle arthrosis. *Foot Ankle Int* 2005;26:537-539.
6. Glazebrook M, Daniels T, Younger A, et al: Comparison of health-related quality of life between patients with end-stage ankle and hip arthrosis. *J Bone Joint Surg Am* 2008;90:499-505.
7. Croft P, Lewis M, Wynn Jones C, Coggon D, Cooper C: Health status in patients awaiting hip replacement for osteoarthritis. *Rheumatology (Oxford)* 2002;41:1001-1007.
8. Bachmeier CJ, March LM, Cross MJ, et al: A comparison of outcomes in osteoarthritis patients undergoing total hip and knee replacement surgery. *Osteoarthritis Cartilage* 2001;9:137-146.
9. Boardman DL, Dorey F, Thomas BJ, Lieberman JR: The accuracy of assessing total hip arthroplasty outcomes: A prospective correlation study of walking ability and 2 validated measurement devices. *J Arthroplasty* 2000;15:200-204.
10. Salaffi F, Carotti M, Grassi W: Health-related quality of life in patients with hip or knee osteoarthritis: Comparison of generic and disease-specific instruments. *Clin Rheumatol* 2005;24:29-37.
11. Arokoski MH, Haara M, Helminen HJ, Arokoski JP: Physical function in men with and without hip osteoarthritis. *Arch Phys Med Rehabil* 2004;85:574-581.
12. Haddad SL, Coetzee JC, Estok R, Fahrbach K, Banel D, Nalysnyk L: Intermediate and long-term outcomes of total ankle arthroplasty and ankle arthrodesis: A systematic review of the literature. *J Bone Joint Surg Am* 2007;89:1899-1905.
13. Ahlberg A, Henricson AS: Late results of ankle fusion. *Acta Orthop Scand* 1981;52:103-105.
14. Boobbyer GN: The long-term results of ankle arthrodesis. *Acta Orthop Scand* 1981;52:107-110.
15. Coester LM, Saltzman CL, Leupold J, Pontarelli W: Long-term results following ankle arthrodesis for post-traumatic arthritis. *J Bone Joint Surg Am* 2001;83:219-228.
16. Fuchs S, Sandmann C, Skwara A, Chylarecki C: Quality of life 20 years after arthrodesis of the ankle: A study of adjacent joints. *J Bone Joint Surg Br* 2003;85:994-998.
17. Mazur JM, Schwartz E, Simon SR: Ankle arthrodesis: Long-term follow-up with gait analysis. *J Bone Joint Surg Am* 1979;61:964-975.
18. Morrey BF, Wiedeman GP Jr: Complications and long-term results of ankle arthrodeses following trauma. *J Bone Joint Surg Am* 1980;62:777-784.
19. Buchner M, Sabo D: Ankle fusion attributable to posttraumatic arthrosis: A long-term followup of 48 patients. *Clin Orthop Relat Res* 2003;406: 155-164.
20. Sheridan BD, Robinson DE, Hubble MJ, Winson IG: Ankle arthrodesis and its relationship to ipsilateral arthritis of the hind- and mid-foot. *J Bone Joint Surg Br* 2006;88:206-207.
21. Buechel FF Sr, Buechel FF Jr, Pappas MJ: Twenty-year evaluation of cementless mobile-bearing total ankle replacements. *Clin Orthop Relat Res* 2004;424:19-26.
22. Hintermann B, Valderrabano V, Knupp M, Horisberger M: The Hintegra ankle: Short- and mid-term results. *Orthopade* 2006;35:533-545.
23. Knecht SI, Estin M, Callaghan JJ, et al: The Agility total ankle arthroplasty: Seven to sixteen-year follow-up. *J Bone Joint Surg Am* 2004;86: 1161-1171.
24. Kofoed H: Scandinavian Total Ankle Replacement (STAR). *Clin Orthop Relat Res* 2004;424:73-79.
25. Glazebrook M, Arsenault K, Dunbar M: An evidence based classification of complications in total ankle arthroplasty, in Wright JG, ed: *Evidence-Based Orthopaedics*. Philadelphia, PA, Elsevier, 2008.
26. Ogilvie-Harris DJ, Sekyi-Otu A: Arthroscopic debridement for the osteoarthritic ankle. *Arthroscopy* 1995;11: 433-436.
27. Amendola A, Petrik J, Webster-Bogaert S: Ankle arthroscopy: Outcome in 79 consecutive patients. *Arthroscopy* 1996;12:565-573.
28. Cerulli G, Caraffa A, Buompadre V, Bensi G: Operative arthroscopy of the ankle. *Arthroscopy* 1992;8:537-540.
29. Martin DF, Baker CL, Curl WW, Andrews JR, Robie DB, Haas AF: Operative ankle arthroscopy: Long-term followup. *Am J Sports Med* 1989;17: 16-23.
30. Baums MH, Kahl E, Schultz W, Klinger HM: Clinical outcome of the arthroscopic management of sports-related "anterior ankle pain": A prospective study. *Knee Surg Sports Traumatol Arthrosc* 2006;14:482-486.
31. Han SH, Lee JW, Kim S, Suh JS, Choi YR: Chronic tibiofibular syndesmosis injury: The diagnostic efficiency of magnetic resonance imaging and comparative analysis of operative treatment. *Foot Ankle Int* 2007;28: 336-342.
32. Kim SH, Ha KI: Arthroscopic treatment for impingement of the anterolateral soft tissues of the ankle. *J Bone Joint Surg Br* 2000;82:1019-1021.

33. Scranton PE Jr, McDermott JE: Anterior tibiotalar spurs: A comparison of open versus arthroscopic debridement. *Foot Ankle* 1992;13:125-129.

34. Takao M, Uchio Y, Naito K, Kono T, Oae K, Ochi M: Arthroscopic treatment for anterior impingement exostosis of the ankle: Application of three-dimensional computed tomography. *Foot Ankle Int* 2004;25:59-62.

35. van Dijk CN, Verhagen RA, Tol JL: Arthroscopy for problems after ankle fracture. *J Bone Joint Surg Br* 1997;79:280-284.

36. Benthien RA, Myerson MS: Supramalleolar osteotomy for ankle deformity and arthritis. *Foot Ankle Clin* 2004;9:475-487.

37. Cheng YM, Huang PJ, Hong SH, et al: Low tibial osteotomy for moderate ankle arthritis. *Arch Orthop Trauma Surg* 2001;121:355-358.

38. Neumann HW, Lieske S, Schenk K: Supramalleolar, subtractive valgus osteotomy of the tibia in the management of ankle joint degeneration with varus deformity. *Oper Orthop Traumatol* 2007;19:511-526.

39. Takakura Y, Takaoka T, Tanaka Y, Yajima H, Tamai S: Results of opening-wedge osteotomy for the treatment of a post-traumatic varus deformity of the ankle. *J Bone Joint Surg Am* 1998;80:213-218.

40. Takakura Y, Tanaka Y, Kumai T, Tamai S: Low tibial osteotomy for osteoarthritis of the ankle: Results of a new operation in 18 patients. *J Bone Joint Surg Br* 1995;77:50-54.

41. Tanaka Y, Takakura Y, Hayashi K, Taniguchi A, Kumai T, Sugimoto K: Low tibial osteotomy for varus-type osteoarthritis of the ankle. *J Bone Joint Surg Br* 2006;88:909-913.

42. Gross AE, Agnidis Z, Hutchison CR: Osteochondral defects of the talus treated with fresh osteochondral allograft transplantation. *Foot Ankle Int* 2001;22:385-391.

43. Jeng CL, Kadakia A, White KL, Myerson MS: Fresh osteochondral total ankle allograft transplantation for the treatment of ankle arthritis. *Foot Ankle Int* 2008;29:554-560.

44. Meehan R, McFarlin S, Bugbee W, Brage M: Fresh ankle osteochondral allograft transplantation for tibiotalar joint arthritis. *Foot Ankle Int* 2005;26:793-802.

45. Tontz WL Jr, Bugbee WD, Brage ME: Use of allografts in the management of ankle arthritis. *Foot Ankle Clin* 2003;8:361-373.

46. Buckwalter JA: Joint distraction for osteoarthritis. *Lancet* 1996;347:279-280.

47. Martin RL, Stewart GW, Conti SF: Posttraumatic ankle arthritis: An update on conservative and surgical management. *J Orthop Sports Phys Ther* 2007;37:253-259.

48. Paley D, Lamm BM: Ankle joint distraction. *Foot Ankle Clin* 2005;10:685-698.

49. van Roermund PM, Lafeber FP: Joint distraction as treatment for ankle osteoarthritis. *Instr Course Lect* 1999;48:249-254.

50. van Roermund PM, Marijnissen AC, Lafeber FP: Joint distraction as an alternative for the treatment of osteoarthritis. *Foot Ankle Clin* 2002;7:515-527.

51. van Valburg AA, van Roermund PM, Lammens J, et al: Can Ilizarov joint distraction delay the need for an arthrodesis of the ankle? A preliminary report. *J Bone Joint Surg Br* 1995;77:720-725.

52. Ploegmakers JJ, van Roermund PM, van Melkebeek J, et al: Prolonged clinical benefit from joint distraction in the treatment of ankle osteoarthritis. *Osteoarthritis Cartilage* 2005;13:582-588.

53. van Valburg AA, van Roermund PM, Marijnissen AC, et al: Joint distraction in treatment of osteoarthritis: A two-year follow-up of the ankle. *Osteoarthritis Cartilage* 1999;7:474-479.

54. van Valburg AA, van Roermund PM, Marijnissen AC, et al: Joint distraction in treatment of osteoarthritis (II): Effects on cartilage in a canine model. *Osteoarthritis Cartilage* 2000;8:1-8.

55. Marijnissen AC, Van Roermund PM, Van Melkebeek J, et al: Clinical benefit of joint distraction in the treatment of severe osteoarthritis of the ankle: Proof of concept in an open prospective study and in a randomized controlled study. *Arthritis Rheum* 2002;46:2893-2902.

56. Kitaoka HB, Romness DW: Arthrodesis for failed ankle arthroplasty. *J Arthroplasty* 1992;7:277-284.

57. Carlsson A, Markusson P, Sundberg M: Radiostereometric analysis of the double-coated STAR total ankle prosthesis: A 3-5 year follow-up of 5 cases with rheumatoid arthritis and 5 cases with osteoarthrosis. *Acta Orthop* Scand 2005;76:573-579.

58. Kiss J, Murray DW, Turner-Smith AR, Bulstrode CJ: Roentgen stereophotogrammetric analysis for assessing migration of total hip replacement femoral components. *Proc Inst Mech Eng [H]* 1995;209:169-175.

Total Ankle Replacement Systems Available in the United States

J. Chris Coetzee, MD, FRCSC
James K. DeOrio, MD

Abstract

Ankle replacement continues to be a viable option for treating patients with ankle arthritis. Over the past 10 years, there has been a significant increase in the number of ankle replacement systems available for use. Current controversy centers on whether fixed- or mobile-bearing devices are most advantageous. Most total ankle systems used outside the United States are mobile-bearing devices, whereas ankle replacement systems used in the United States are all essentially fixed-bearing devices.

Not all ankles with degenerative changes are amenable to replacement surgery, and several exclusion criteria are well documented. Ankle replacement is especially complicated because of the ankle's proximity to the foot and the important role that the balance and alignment of the foot play in the success of the ankle replacement. Foot deformities should be treated before or at the time of ankle replacement surgery. Ignoring foot deformities can lead to failure of the ankle replacement.

It is also of paramount importance to consider the stability of the ankle ligaments. An unstable ankle with a varus or valgus deformity of more than 20° is probably not amenable to ankle replacement. There are currently no reliable options to predictably reconstruct the lateral or medial ligaments in these severe deformities.

It is important to be aware of the ankle replacement systems currently available in the United States and understand the key features of each design. Devices approved by the US Food and Drug Administration, a device that is awaiting approval, and a device that is being evaluated by the Food and Drug Administration in a prospective randomized clinical trial are discussed, along with an objective comparison of fixed- and mobile-bearing devices.

Instr Course Lect 2010;59:367-374.

Dr. Coetzee or an immediate family member has received royalties from Arthrex and DePuy; is a member of a speakers' bureau or has made paid presentations on behalf of Arthrex and DePuy; serves as a paid consultant to or is an employee of DePuy and Arthrex; and has received research or institutional support from DePuy. Dr. DeOrio or an immediate family member has received royalties from Merete; is a member of a speakers' bureau or has made paid presentations on behalf of Tornier, INBONE, Merete, SBI, Integra, and Wright Medical Technologies; serves as a paid consultant to or is an employee of INBONE, Integra, Merete, SBI, and Wright Medical Technologies; has received research or institutional support from Tornier, INBONE, Merete, SBI, Integra, and Synthes; and has stock or stock options held in INBONE.

Ankle replacements are becoming a mainstream treatment option for patients with ankle arthritis. Currently, there are 23 different ankle replacement systems in existence worldwide; the proliferation of ankle replacement designs may result in even wider use in the future.

Conflicting reports exist regarding improved midterm and longer term outcomes of second-generation ankle implants compared with the first-generation ankle implants used in the 1970s. Recent studies also describe potential complications with total ankle replacement surgery. Orthopaedic surgeons should be knowledgeable about the various systems available, should be aware of the pitfalls of ankle replacement surgery, and should know how to treat challenging ankle disorders, especially those involving varus and valgus deformities. The greater the varus or valgus deformity, the more difficult is the ankle replacement procedure, and the less predictable is the outcome.

Range of Motion

Several important factors should be considered when discussing potential ankle replacement surgery with a patient. Generally, the eventual postoperative range of motion (ROM) is largely determined by the preoperative ROM. On average, there is only a 5° improvement in the preoperative ROM.[1] This relatively small improvement is believed to result from the significant role that the soft-tissue envelope around the ankle has in ROM. For example, a patient with a severe pilon fracture treated with multiple surgeries will usually have a very stiff, rigid soft-tissue envelope compared with a patient with idiopathic degenerative joint disease and no prior surgeries.

Foot Alignment

A stable plantigrade foot is essential to successful ankle replacement. A cavovarus foot is common in patients with varus ankle deformities, and a planovalgus foot is common in those with valgus deformities. Chronic posterior tibial tendon dysfunction is common in patients with secondary foot deformities associated with a valgus ankle. In patients with varus ankles, the peroneal tendons may be compromised. Failure to treat these disorders will compromise the long-term outcome of the ankle replacement. Preoperative radiographs to diagnose cavovarus and planovalgus feet should include weight-bearing images. The lateral ankle view, in particular, should include the entire foot.

Varus and Valgus Deformities

As surgeons gain experience in total ankle arthroplasty, there is a tendency to attempt treatment of more complex deformities, including varus and valgus ankles. The difficulty in treating these deformities should never be underestimated. Occasionally, a varus or valgus deformity will result from pure bony erosion, but in many instances there will be an element of ligamentous imbalance and, often, elements of both erosion and imbalance. If the imbalance is not corrected at the time of surgery, the life span of the implant will be compromised.[2]

Varus Ankles

As previously mentioned, both foot and ankle alignment should be treated before ankle replacement surgery. A supramalleolar deformity may be present; however, in some patients, hindfoot varus requires correction. After all the extra-articular deformities are treated, the surgeon can concentrate on the ankle. Not all varus ankles result from the same etiology. A varus deformity can result from bone erosion alone or a combination of bone erosion and lateral instability, or it may be caused primarily by ligamentous instability.

Alvine developed a useful classification system to quantify varus deformities, with stages ranging for those with minimal deformity (stage 1) to severe instability and secondary deformities (stage 3).[3] A simple Broström ligament repair is never sufficient to correct instability as part of an ankle replacement procedure.[3] Other treatment options include the use of a split or complete peroneus brevis tendon in an anatomic reconstruction, anatomic allograft reconstruction, or nonanatomic repair using allograft or peroneus brevis tendon.[3] Stage 1 varus deformity can usually be corrected with a lateral ligament repair alone. Stage 3 deformities usually require subtalar fusion and other procedures prior to ankle replacement. Patients with stage 3 deformities are not candidates for routine ankle replacements.[4]

In ankles with stage 2 varus deformity, the medial malleolus is often eroded, and there is shortening and contracture of the deltoid ligament, medial capsule, and tibialis posterior tendon sheath. There is often a large buildup of osteophytes in the lateral gutter, specifically the lateral side of the talus. Bone overgrowth in the gutters should be removed to allow rotation of the talus back into the mortise. The osteophytes are removed from the lateral talus and medial fibula. If it is still not possible to rotate the talus back into place, it can be assumed that the medial structures are tight. The deep deltoid is released from the talus by sliding an osteotome or knife down the medial border of the talus until the entire deep portion is released. It is advisable not to release the entire deltoid because it may leave the medial complex completely unstable.

An alternative to a deltoid release is a medial malleolar distal sliding osteotomy.[5] Distal displacement of the medial malleolus creates functional lengthening of the deltoid without destabilizing the deltoid. Alternatively, the periosteum above the deltoid can be lifted off the tibia and the entire deltoid peeled off the medial malleolus, thus leaving it intact as a continuous sleeve (similar to the technique used on the medial collateral ligament in a varus knee replacement).[6]

After the ankle joint is mobile and passively correctable to neutral in the ankle mortise, hindfoot alignment is evaluated. If there is a tendency to a varus deformity below the ankle, a lateralizing or lateral closing wedge calcaneal osteotomy should be done to improve the mechanical axis of the ankle and subsequent lateral ligament repair. If there is a true calcaneus varus, a lateral closing wedge osteotomy is done and immobilized with a staple or screw. If the plan is to move the mechanical axis more laterally to protect the lateral ligament repair, a lateralizing calcaneal osteotomy is done.

Valgus Instability

Ankles with valgus instability can be even more difficult to balance than varus ankles. In mild to moderate deformities, treatment can include a medializing calcaneal osteotomy, posterior tibial tendon repair and augmentation with flexor digitorum longus, and gastrocnemius slide and medial ray stabilization if indicated.[7,8] Because there is no reliable local tissue to repair or reconstruct the deltoid ligament, reconstruction with nonnative tissue is needed. A double strand allograft deltoid reconstruction has been proposed as the best option.[9]

Table 1
Ankle Prostheses Currently FDA Approved or Seeking FDA Approval for Implantation in the United States

Prosthesis	Manufacturer
*Agility Total Ankle System	DePuy Orthopaedics (Warsaw, IN)
*INBONE (formerly Berkeley, formerly Topez) Total Ankle Replacement System	Wright Medical Technologies (Arlington, TN)
*Salto-Talaris Anatomic Ankle Prosthesis	Tornier (Stafford, TX)
†STAR	Small Bone Innovations (Morrisville, PA)
†Mobility	DePuy Orthopaedics

*Cemented prostheses are FDA approved (used off-label without cement).
†The STAR prosthesis (waiting for final FDA approval) and the Mobility prosthesis (being used in an FDA study) are intended to be used without cement.

Inclusion and Exclusion Criteria for Total Ankle Replacement

There are no uniform inclusion and exclusion criteria to determine if total ankle replacement is the most appropriate treatment. The choice is based on the patient's preference after receiving consultation and recommendations from the treating surgeon. Some guidelines can help the surgeon in making the appropriate treatment recommendations. Total ankle replacement is indicated in patients who are older than 50 years, have a body mass index less than 35, have advanced degenerative joint disease, or have advanced rheumatoid arthritis. Total ankle replacement is not recommended for patients with diabetes, especially insulin-dependent diabetes with no pulses; those with talar osteonecrosis that is not resectable at the time of arthroplasty; and patients with neurologic deficits resulting in motor loss of ankle muscles or sensory impairment of the foot and ankle. It also is contraindicated in patients with significant vascular insufficiency, inadequate skin or soft-tissue quality that would prevent reliable wound closure and healing, and those with ligamentous instability with more than 20° varus or valgus that could be difficult to correct.

Background on Implant Designs

For approximately 10 years, the two-piece, fixed-bearing, Agility Total Ankle (DePuy Orthopaedics, Warsaw, IN) was the only ankle approved by the Food and Drug Administration (FDA) for use in the United States. Outside this country, essentially all the ankle replacement systems are three-piece designs with a mobile polyethylene bearing. The reason for the lack of mobile-bearing devices in the United States is that fixed-bearing devices can "piggyback" the FDA approval already granted to historic (pre-1986) total ankle arthroplasty devices, whereas a mobile-bearing ankle would require an expensive and time-consuming FDA investigational device evaluation. Currently, debate continues on the virtues of fixed- versus mobile-bearing ankles, with no objective data to support the superiority of either type of device.

In addition to the Agility ankle prosthesis, there are other fixed-bearing devices that have FDA approval or that are seeking FDA approval for implantation in the United States (Table 1). The Scandinavian Total Ankle Replacement (STAR; Small Bone Innovations, Morrisville, PA) is a mobile-bearing ankle that is awaiting final approval from the FDA. The Mobility ankle (DePuy) is currently being used in an FDA prospective randomized clinical trial in an attempt to gain approval.

Two-Component Designs

Agility Total Ankle System

Two-component ankle prosthesis designs differ dramatically from each other (Figure 1). The Agility Total Ankle was designed by Alvine and has been in use longer (since 1984) than any other total ankle replacement system in the United States. The basic design includes six sizes of matching tibial and talar components. The titanium alloy tibial component has an ingrowth surface that simultaneously rests on the tibia and inner sides of the medial malleolus and fibula. Proper positioning requires resection of the

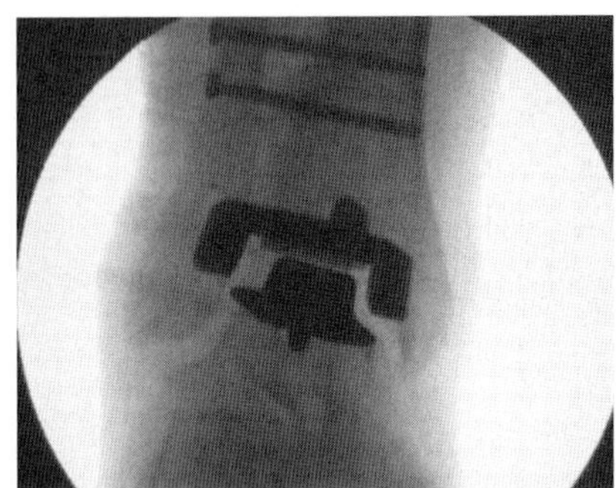

Figure 1 Fluoroscopic image of the Agility LP Total Ankle, a two-component, fixed-bearing design. It should be noted that the asymmetry of the component is a result of the angle of the x-ray projection and is of no consequence.

articular surfaces of both malleoli to place the metal against cancellous bone. This procedure necessitates fusion of the syndesmosis, which has proven to be both an asset and a pitfall. The fusion allows a larger area of bone for ingrowth but also results in a possible complication (nonunion of the syndesmosis) that is unique to the Agility Ankle and can lead to a higher failure rate for the prosthesis.[10] The largest study of the Agility Total Ankle included more than 300 ankles and showed a revision rate of 28% (for all reasons) and an overall 5-year implant survival rate of 80%.[11]

The dome of the talus is removed and replaced with a cobalt-chromium dome component. The redesigned (Agility LP) talar component provides a wider base that covers the entire cut surface of the talus to prevent subsidence of the talar component. The Agility LP has a front-loading insert instead of the previous bottom-loading system, which greatly simplifies exchange of the insert and also provides a better locking mechanism. Standard revision components are available for the talar and polyethylene components. The revision talus has a larger true rectangular base and a 2-mm greater vertical thickness. The new Agility LP talar component has largely replaced the older Agility revision talar component and is the preferred revision component for Agility Ankles. The Agility LP talar component can be used in only a limited number of ankle prostheses revision procedures because some prostheses require custom talar components.

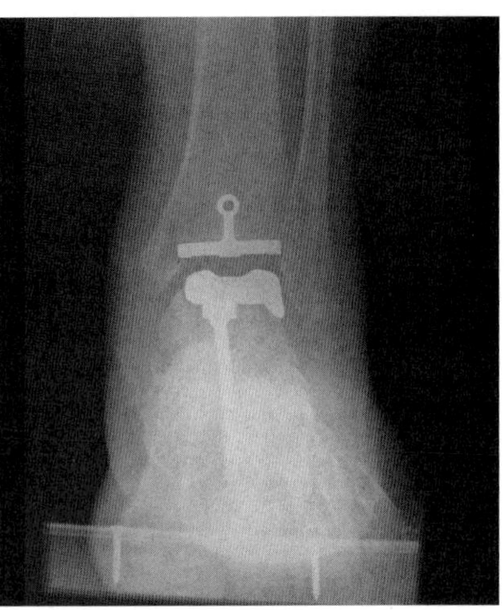

Figure 2 AP radiograph showing the Salto-Talaris ankle, a two-component, fixed-bearing design. The talar component has a 10-mm barrel into the talus and a lateral flare for stability. In this case, subtalar fusion was added, and a screw was placed anterior to the talar component into the calcaneus.

The polyethylene component has half columns on the side; this allows replacement of the polyethylene without removing the tibial component. A thicker polyethylene revision component (2 mm) also is available. These components may be used to increase the total height of the revision prosthesis by 4 mm. More extensive revision components are available on a custom basis and include stemmed talar and tibial components. Motion is constrained by the implant's articulating surfaces and the periankle ligaments.

Video 31.1: Agility Total Ankle Arthroplasty. Charles L. Saltzman, MD; Frank G. Alvine, MD; Steven L. Haddad, MD (53 min)

Salto-Talaris Anatomic Ankle Prosthesis and Salto Total Ankle Prosthesis

The Salto-Talaris Anatomic Ankle (Tornier, Stafford, TX) design is based on the Salto (Tornier) ankle system (Figure 2). The Salto-Talaris Anatomic Ankle received FDA approval in November 2006. The Salto ankle system is used internationally as a mobile-bearing ankle, but the design was changed to a fixed-bearing prosthesis for the US market. Both the Salto and the Salto-Talaris Anatomic Ankle systems involve resurfacing of the lateral talar side and do not alter the medial ankle articulation. The talar component has an anatomic design with a smaller medial than lateral radius, is made of cobalt chromium, and has a titanium spray coating. Only the Salto ankle prosthesis has a hydroxyapatite coating and an optional unique, high-density polyethylene button that may be implanted on the medial surface of the fibula. The button may be used when there is severe wear in the lateral gutter of the ankle; however, this option is used infrequently.

The Salto and Salto-Talaris prostheses have a pedestal-like stem that is inserted into the distal tibial. The polyethylene component in the Salto-Talaris (mobile in the Salto ankle) slides and locks into the tibial-side component. Final seating of the tibial component is determined with the talar trial component in place. The tibial component is allowed to rotate and find its ideal location, where it produces the greatest conformity with the talar component and the least rotation between the components. The hole for the pedestal is then created. In practice, however, there is usually very little and sometimes no motion of the tibial component, which is wedged between the malleoli.

As previously mentioned, the reason for the change from a mobile-bearing to a fixed-bearing design was to permit an easier and more cost-effective introduction of the prosthesis into the US market. At present, there is no independent study that compares fixed- versus mobile-bearing ankle designs. A study by the manufacturer supported the two-component design over the three-component design after radiographic analysis showed that the free-floating polyethylene component moved only 1 mm in 3 of 20 ankle specimens.[12] In the 17 other specimens, the polyethylene spacer was locked in place by heterotopic bone. The study did not provide information on how long it took for the polyethylene component to lock in place or if the initial motion of the polyethylene component was important in determining its final position. A more recent study comparing the translational and rotational motion between components of the Salto implant showed that the rotational motion played a more dominant role in the kinematics of the prosthesis.[12]

It is possible that the mobile bearing is only mobile for a limited period of time until scarring occurs around the bearing. It is not clear how important this initial mobility is in obtaining the most suitable relationship of the tibial and talar components.

INBONE Total Ankle System

The INBONE total ankle system (Wright Medical Technologies, Arlington, TN) differs from the previously described ankle replacement systems (Figure 3). For implantation, the system requires immobilization of the leg in a holder with pin fixation. After correct positioning is assured with multiple fluoroscopic reviews, a hole (approximately 6 mm) is drilled in the plantar surface of the calcaneus, through the talus, and into the tibia. The tibia is reamed by a special reamer that is placed onto the rod inside the ankle and driven upward into the tibia. The talar stem hole is then drilled. The cylindrical tibial components (usually four components are used but more are needed if a longer stem is desired) are inserted one by one and screwed into each other, followed by the tibial tray, the stemmed talar component, and the polyethylene component.

The INBONE total ankle system does not resurface either side of the talus. A long calcaneal talar stem is available on a custom basis. At early follow-up, one of the authors and his coworkers at Duke University with extensive experience with the INBONE ankle reported a 5% rate of significant complications in more than 150 total ankle replacements. Significant complications included medial malleolar fractures (2%), serious wound problems requiring flaps in two ankles, and deep infection in three ankles (which required amputation in two patients). Minor wound problems also occurred in eight patients. (J DeOrio, MD, unpublished data).

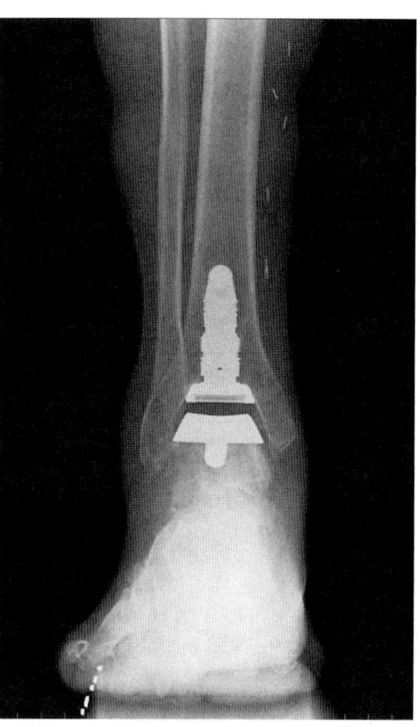

Figure 3 AP weight-bearing radiograph showing the INBONE total ankle system, a fixed-bearing, two-component design. It is the only system that uses an intramedullary guide system for bone cuts.

Three-Component Mobile-Bearing Designs

The three-component ankle replacement systems with a mobile polyethylene component along with the names of their manufacturers are shown in Table 2. The ankle replacement systems share both similarities and differences. All incisions for ankle replacement surgery are made into the anterior aspect of the ankle, except for the ESKA Ankle, which is inserted from the lateral side and requires a fibular osteotomy, and the Eclipse, which can be inserted through either a medial or lateral approach. The choice of ankle replacement often depends on the surgeon's preference and experience.

Mobility Total Ankle System

The Mobility Total Ankle System was developed by a design team of surgeons in collaboration with the manufacturer (Figure 4). Although the Mobility Total Ankle was first implanted in September 2003 in Wrightington, England, it became commercially available in October

Table 2
Three-Component Ankle Replacement Systems With a Mobile Polyethylene Component

Implant	Manufacturer (Name and Location)
Scandinavian Total Ankle Replacement (STAR)	Small Bone Innovations (Morrisville, PA)
Buechel-Pappas Total Ankle System	Endotec (South Orange, NJ)
ESKA Ankle	ESKA Implants (Lübeck, Germany)
HINTEGRA Total Ankle Prosthesis	Newdeal France and International (Lyon, France)
Salto Total Ankle Prosthesis	Tornier (Stafford, TX)
BOX Total Ankle Replacement	Finsbury Orthopaedics (Leatherhead, England)
Mobility	DePuy Orthopaedics (Warsaw, IN)
Corin Ankle Replacement	Corin Group PLC (Cirencester, England)
Albatros	Groupe Lepine (Lyon, France)
Ramses	Maîtrise Orthopédique (Paris, France)
Ankle Evolution System	Biomet (Dordrecht, The Netherlands)
CCI Evolution	Van Straten Medical (Amsterdam, The Netherlands)
TARIC Ankle Joint Prosthesis	Implantcast (Buxtehude, Germany)
Alphamed Orthner	Alphamed Medizintechnik Fischer (Lassnitzhöhe, Austria)
German Ankle System	Arge Medizintechnik (Hannovera, Germany)

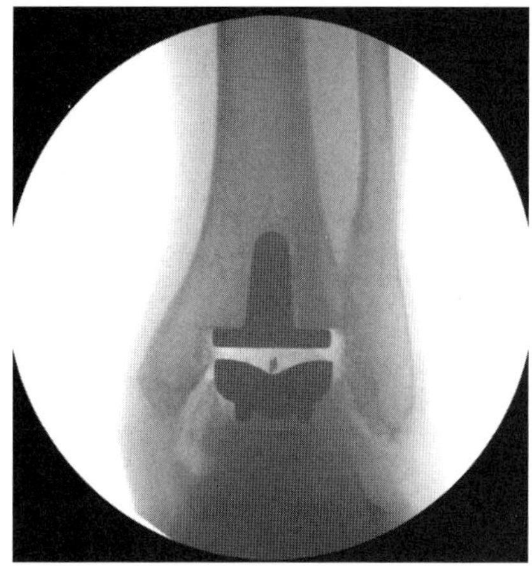

Figure 4 Fluoroscopic image of the Mobility ankle, a three-component, mobile-bearing, noncemented ankle replacement.

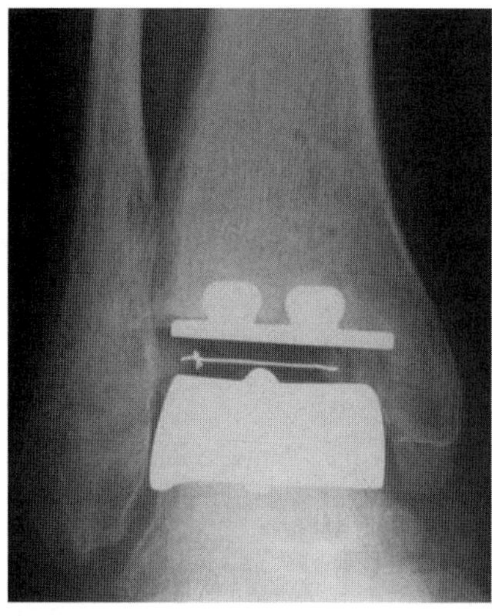

Figure 5 AP radiograph of the STAR prosthesis, a mobile-bearing, three-component design.

2004. Five hundred forty Mobility Total Ankle Systems were implanted in 2005, and 970 and 1,200 were implanted in 2006 and 2007, respectively. The device has been approved for general use in most of the world, including Europe, Australia, New Zealand, South Africa, and Canada. An FDA study for approval in the United States began in 2006. The Mobility is a three-component, cementless, unconstrained, mobile-bearing prosthesis. It features a short conical stem on the tibial component. It has a long plate that provides primary fixation to the tibia and allows rotational adjustment of the tibial component. The polyethylene insert has fully conforming congruent surfaces, and the talar component has a resurfacing three-plane contact area with the talus, a deep talar sulcus, and short and deep anterior talar fins. The metal that lies adjacent to the bone has a spray coating of titanium.

Data from 200 cases with 1-year follow-up showed that pain, measured with a visual analog scale, ranged from a preoperative mean score of 8.1 to a postoperative mean score of 1.4 (PL Wood, P Rippstein, unpublished data presented at the EFORT meeting, Nice, France, 2008). Postoperative complications included two patients with delayed wound healing, one with deep infection (the patient underwent an arthroscopic débridement and had antibiotic therapy for 6 months with the prosthesis in place), two patients with stress fractures in the medial malleolus, and two with aseptic loosening of the tibial component at 6 months from an unknown cause.

Scandinavian Total Ankle Replacement

The STAR is the prototypic, three-component, ankle replacement design (Figure 5). It was created by Kofoed in 1981 as a smooth, two-component, cemented design.[13] The design was changed over time and has evolved into a three-component, meniscal-bearing (mobile-bearing) ingrowth design. The tibial component is a trapezoidal tray (wider in the front) and has two cylinders with ridges to secure it to the bone. The talar component is a symmetric convex partial cylinder that is the average width of the medial and lateral radii. The talar dome curves and has two sides that articulate with the malleoli. The talar component has a fin that inserts into the talus and a protruding central dorsal extension that fits into a high-density polyethylene congruent spacer. The spacer is concave on the bottom and articulates with the domed talar component. It is flat on the top and glides on the flat tibial component. The cobalt-chromium metal surfaces have a titanium spray coating for bony ingrowth. A hydroxyapatite coating also can be applied. The talus is available in five sizes, and the tibial component is available in 30- to 45-mm lengths (5-mm increments) with little change in the width. The polyethylene component is 6 to 10 mm thick (sized in 1-mm increments).

A stemmed revision component for the tibia is available, and thicker polyethylene revision components are available (11- to 15-mm thickness, 1-mm increments). Implantation of this system in 200 ankles with a mean follow-up of 46 months (range, 24 to 101 months) showed a 5-year implant survival rate of 93%. A second surgery (for any reason) was performed in 20 ankles.[14]

Summary

Direct comparison of the outcomes of ankle replacement systems is difficult, not only because of the relatively small number of cases but also because of the difficulty of doing prospective randomized studies with different ankle systems. A current ongoing FDA randomized clinical trial using the Agility Total Ankle and the Mobility Total Ankle system will provide an opportunity to compare mobile- and fixed-bearing designs.

Because of the long, steep learning curve required for all ankle replacement procedures, it is believed that few surgeons are willing or treat enough patients needing ankle replacement to warrant the use of multiple systems. There are unanswered questions regarding the need for resurfacing the sides of the talus, the use of fixed- versus mobile-bearing devices, the best surgical approach, the need for coating components to improve bone ingrowth, and the best revision options if the primary replacement fails.

Edge loading of the polyethylene is also a concern because it may cause wear, leading to osteolysis. Newer designs such as the Mobility Total Ankle system have an upward sloping polyethylene component to decrease the chance of polyethylene contact with the edge of the tibial component. A conforming two-component design has greater inherent stability; however, it is unknown if polyethylene wear or the mobile-bearing design more frequently leads to osteolysis.

The initial fixation of components is important because it allows ingrowth of bone into metal. Thus, components with increased metal-bone interface (for example, those with stemmed components) may be more stable and allow more rapid bony ingrowth than systems that have a lower metal-bone interface.

Ankle replacement procedures will never become as prevalent as hip and knee replacement procedures. Even though ankle replacement is a more complex procedure and fewer ankles require replacement, it is still important for orthopaedic surgeons to be aware of available total ankle replacement systems.

References

1. Coetzee JC, Castro MD: Accurate measurement of ankle range of motion after total ankle arthroplasty. *Clin Orthop Relat Res* 2004;424:27-31.
2. Tarr RR, Resnick CT, Wagner KS, Sarmiento A: Changes in tibiotalar joint contact areas following experimentally induced tibial angular deformities. *Clin Orthop Relat Res* 1985;199: 72-80.
3. Coetzee JC: Management of varus or valgus ankle deformity with ankle replacement. *Foot Ankle Clin* 2008;13: 509-520.
4. Smith R, Wood PL: Arthrodesis of the ankle in the presence of a large deformity in the coronal plane. *J Bone Joint Surg Br* 2007;89:615-619.
5. Cornelis Doets H, van der Plaat LW, Klein JP: Medial malleolar osteotomy for the correction of varus deformity during total ankle arthroplasty: Results in 15 ankles. *Foot Ankle Int* 2008; 29:171-177.
6. Verdonk PC, Pernin J, Pinaroli A, Ait Si Selmi T, Neyret P: Soft tissue balancing in varus total knee arthroplasty: An algorithmic approach. *Knee Surg Sports Traumatol Arthrosc* 2009; 17(6):660-666.
7. Myerson MS, Corrigan J, Thompson F, Schon LC: Tendon transfer combined with calcaneal osteotomy for treatment of posterior tibial tendon insufficiency: A radiological investigation. *Foot Ankle Int* 1995;16: 712-718.
8. Sizensky JA, Marks RM: Medial-sided bony procedures: Why, what, and how? *Foot Ankle Clin* 2003;8: 539-562.
9. Dedhia S, Zhang L, Yupeng R, Rotstein J, Haddad SL: Abstract: Deltoid ligament reconstruction: A biomechanical analysis. *75th Annual Meeting Proceedings*. Rosemont, IL, American Academy of Orthopaedic Surgeons, 2008, pp 512-513.
10. Knecht SI, Estin M, Callaghan JJ, et al: The Agility total ankle arthroplasty: Seven to sixteen-year follow-

up. *J Bone Joint Surg Am* 2004;86: 1161-1171.

11. Spirt AA, Assal M, Hansen ST Jr: Complications and failure after total ankle arthroplasty. *J Bone Joint Surg Am* 2004;86:1172-1178.
12. Leszko F, Komistek RD, Mahfouz MR, et al: In vivo kinematics of the Salto total ankle prosthesis. *Foot Ankle Int* 2008;29:1117-1125.
13. Kofoed H: Scandinavian Total Ankle Replacement (STAR). *Clin Orthop Relat Res* 2004;424:73-79.
14. Wood PL, Deakin S: Total ankle replacement: The results in 200 ankles. *J Bone Joint Surg Br* 2003;85:334-341.

Video Reference

31.1: Saltzman CL, Alvine FG, Haddad SL: Video. Agility total ankle arthroplasty, in Alvine FG, Haddad SL, eds: *JBJS-A, DVD*. Rosemont, IL, American Academy of Orthopaedic Surgeons, 2004.

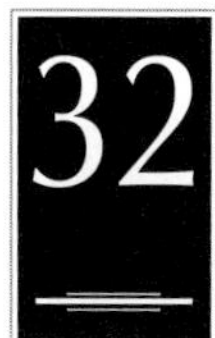

The Natural History of Osteochondral Lesions in the Ankle

C. Niek van Dijk, MD, PhD
Mikel L. Reilingh, MD
Maartje Zengerink, MD
Christiaan J.A. van Bergen, MD

Abstract

Most osteochondral lesions (defects) of the talar dome are caused by trauma, which may be a single event or repeated, less intense events (microtrauma). A lesion may heal, remain asymptomatic, or progress to deep ankle pain on weight bearing, prolonged joint swelling, and the formation of subchondral bone cysts. During loading, compression of the cartilage forces water into the microfractured subchondral bone. The increased flow and pressure of fluid in the subchondral bone can cause osteolysis and the slow development of a subchondral cyst. The pain does not arise from the cartilage lesion but most likely is caused by repetitive high fluid pressure during walking and a concomitant decrease in pH produced by osteoclasts, which sensitize the highly innervated subchondral bone. Prevention of further degeneration depends on several factors, including the repair of the subchondral bone plate and the correct alignment of the ankle joint.

Instr Course Lect 2010;59:375-386.

An osteochondral lesion (defect) of the talus involves the talar articular cartilage and its subchondral bone. Trauma is known to be an important etiologic factor, but idiopathic osteochondral ankle lesions also occur.[1] The trauma causing the lesion can be a single event or a series of less intense microtraumas.[2-4] The lesion initially may consist only of cartilage damage caused by shearing stresses, with the subchondral bone left intact. Bone contusion following high-impact force also can cause a lesion, and ischemia is a possible etiologic factor.[2,5-7]

The most common location of an osteochondral lesion in a patient with ankle trauma is the anterolateral or posteromedial side of the talar dome. Lateral lesions usually are shallow and oval and caused by a shear mechanism. In contrast, medial lesions usually are deep and cup shaped and caused by torsional impaction and axial loading.[8-13]

The etiology and pathogenesis of osteochondral lesions of the talus are not fully understood. Invasive and costly surgical treatments increasingly are the focus of research, while research into the pathogenesis of the lesions has been somewhat neglected. To more effectively treat osteochondral lesions of the talus, more should be known about its natural history.

An osteochondral lesion may have a sudden onset, but a subchondral cyst most often develops slowly. Some lesions remain asymptomatic and inert, but others eventually cause pain on weight bearing, are characterized by persistent bone edema visible on MRI, and result in the formation of a subchondral cyst. Understanding this process could lead to the development of strategies for preventing progressive joint damage.

Etiology

It is widely accepted that traumatic insult is the most important

Neither Dr. van Dijk, Dr. Reilingh, Dr. Zengerink, Dr. van Bergen nor any immediate family members have received anything of value from or own stock in a commercial company or institution related directly or indirectly to the subject of this chapter.

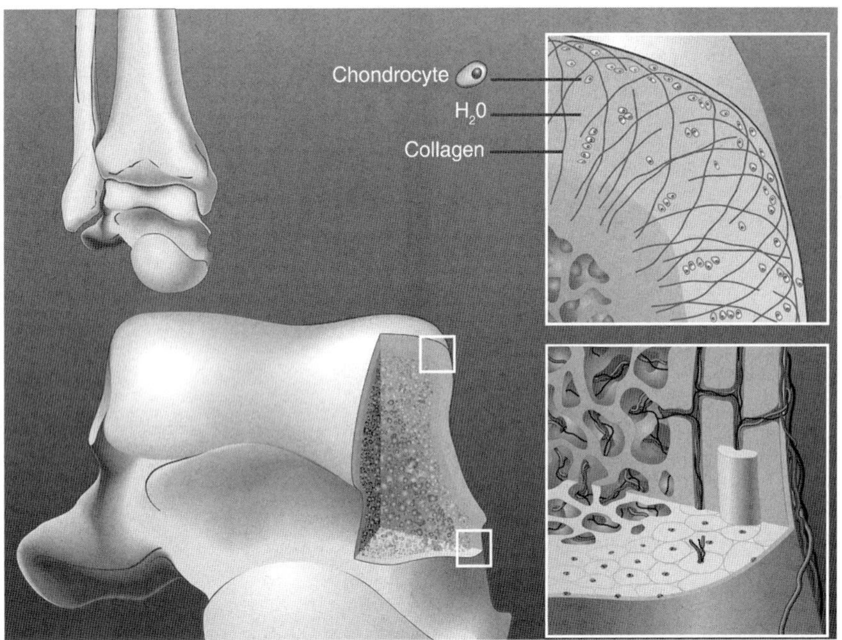

Figure 1 Illustrations showing the normal anatomy of the ankle cartilage, the subchondral plate, and the subchondral bone area. The cartilage consists of chondrocytes that lie groupwise in lacunae of the extracellular matrix, which contains collagen fibers in an arcwise configuration, hyaluronic acid, proteoglycans, and 75% water (upper right). Magnified illustration of the vascularization and innervation of the talus (lower right). Within each osteon, a hollow tube known as a haversian canal runs longitudinally down the center of the osteon. It contains an arteriole, a venule, and a lymphatic duct to provide the vascular and lymphatic drainage of compact bone.

etiologic factor in an osteochondral talar lesion. Trauma was reported in 93% to 98% of lateral talar lesions and 61% to 70% of medial lesions.[11,13] However, not all patients report a history of ankle injury.[14] The etiology of a nontraumatic, idiopathic lesion may involve ischemia, necrosis, or genetics.[2] Osteochondral lesions of the talus have been described in identical twins and siblings.[15-17] The defect is bilateral in 4% to 7% of patients.[8,9]

The three categories of traumatic cartilage injuries are microdamage or blunt trauma damage, chondral fracture, and osteochondral fracture.[18] Ankle sprains have a prominent role in traumatic osteochondral lesions. Rotation of the talus inside the ankle mortise during an ankle sprain can damage the cartilage lining, leading to bruising and subsequent softening of the cartilage or cracking of the cartilage with subsequent delamination.

Separation in the upper layer of the cartilage occurs as a result of shearing forces. Alternatively, separation may occur in the subchondral bone, giving rise to a subchondral bone lesion. Fragments may break off and float loose in the ankle joint, or they may remain partially attached and stay in position. The lesions can either heal and remain asymptomatic or progress to subchondral bone cyst formation, causing pain on weight bearing.

Berndt and Harty[8] reproduced lateral defects in cadaver ankles by strongly inverting a dorsiflexed ankle. As the foot was inverted on the leg, the lateral border of the talar dome was compressed against the face of the fibula. When the lateral ligament ruptured, avulsion of the chip began. With the use of excessive inverting force, the talus within the mortise was rotated laterally in the frontal plane, impacting and compressing the lateral talar margin against the articular surface of the fibula. A portion of the talar margin was sheared off from the main body of the talus, causing the lateral lesion. A medial lesion was reproduced by plantar flexing the ankle in combination with slight anterior displacement of the talus on the tibia, inversion, and internal rotation of the talus on the tibia.

Cartilage and Bone Anatomy

Cartilage consists of chondrocytes that lie groupwise in the lacunae of the extracellular matrix. The cartilaginous matrix consists of collagen, hyaluronic acid, proteoglycans, and a small quantity of glycoproteins (Figure 1). Its elasticity is based on the electrostatic connections between collagen fibers and the glycosaminoglycan (GAG) side chains of the proteoglycans, the water contained by the negatively loaded GAGs of the central protein of the proteoglycans, and the flexibility and sliding qualities of the collagen fibers. Cartilage is avascular and is nourished by the intra-articular fluid; the tissue fluid of the cartilage matrix, which accounts for approximately 75% of the total weight of the cartilage, functions as a transport medium. Cartilage does not contain lymph vessels or nerves and has a slow metabolism.[19] In healthy cartilage, the GAG side chains of the proteoglycans have an important role in elasticity and maintenance of the 75% water content.

Compact bone acts as the main weight-bearing pillar of the skeleton. It is not a solid tissue but rather an aggregation of osteons. Each osteon is a multicellular unit composed of groups of concentric calcified cylinders, each of which is composed of bone matrix proteins that form long cylinder-shaped structures oriented parallel to the long axis of the bone.[20]

Clinical Presentation

It is important to differentiate the symptoms of acute and chronic osteochondral lesions of the talus.[21] The symptoms of a nondisplaced acute lesion often are not recognized because of swelling and pain from the lateral ligament lesion. The initial radiographic findings often are negative; only large lesions may be visible. Swelling, limited range of motion, and pain on weight bearing may persist after the symptoms of the ligament injury have resolved. If the symptoms continue more than 4 to 6 weeks, an osteochondral defect should be suspected. Locking and catching are symptoms of a displaced fragment.

The typical symptom of a chronic lesion is persistent or intermittent deep ankle pain during or after activity.[22] Reactive swelling or stiffness may be present. Most patients have normal range of motion without swelling or tenderness on palpation. They have no signs of synovitis, and the joint temperature is normal. However, the absence of swelling, locking, or catching does not rule out the presence of an osteochondral defect.

The natural history of an osteochondral lesion of the talus is usually benign, regardless of whether it is treated. Only 1 of 38 patients was found to have radiographic progression at 10-year follow-up.[23] Ankle arthrodesis is rare after osteochondral lesions of the talus.[22,23]

Histopathology

Koch and associates[24] studied cartilage and bone morphology in osteochondral defects of the knee. Cylinders were harvested from osteochondral areas in 30 patients during cartilage-bone transplantation. In the cartilage of these diseased samples, a loss of acidic GAG from the extracellular matrix and a decrease in the number of chondrocytes were found. Hyaline cartilage often was replaced by fibrocartilage. All samples had fractured areas in the subchondral and underlying cancellous bone. Subchondral bone remodeling and areas of enhanced bone resorption were common. Osteoclasts typically were located in lacunae at the cancellous bone trabeculae, where they digested the subchondral bone plate and adjacent trabeculae. Areas of newly formed osteoid attempted to compensate for the loss of bone stock. Although collagen fiber bundles normally do not cross the subchondral bone plate, as was stated by Koch and associates,[24] they found that fibrous tissue connected the osteochondrotic cartilage to subchondral bone as a secondary change. The cancellous bone underneath the subchondral plate showed sclerosis to a varying extent.

According to Koch and associates,[24] all of the morphologic features suggest that the main area of action is around the subchondral bone plate. Large numbers of osteoclasts that apparently are digesting parts of the bone plate lie close to osteoblasts that apparently are compensating for bony instabilities by remodeling the bone stock. Paralleling a general loss of proteoglycans from the superficial layers of the extracellular cartilage matrix, there is an increase in the quantity of chondroitin sulfates and keratan sulfate in deep cartilage layers and the subchondral bone. The amount of GAG (the cartilage substance that is coresponsible for the containment of water) is decreased in damaged cartilage.

Joint Congruence and Cartilage Thickness

The cartilage of the talar dome is thin in comparison with the cartilage of other articulating surfaces. The average cartilage thickness of the talar dome is 1.11 mm (± 0.28 mm) in women and 1.35 mm (± 0.22 mm) in men.[25,26] In 1891, Braune and Fischer[27] proposed that articular cartilage is thicker in regions of low congruence. Simon and associates[28] related joint congruence to cartilage thickness. They calculated congruence ratios for canine joints by dividing the average length of the congruent surface by the average length of the total articular surface. The ankle (with the thinnest articular cartilage) had the highest ratio, and the knee (with the thickest cartilage) had the lowest ratio. Shepherd and Seedhom[26] conducted a similar study with human cadaver specimens. The average thickness of the cartilage in the ankle, hip, and knee joints was 1.2 mm (range, 1.0 to 1.6 mm), 1.6 mm (1.4 to 2.0 mm), and 2.2 mm (1.7 to 2.6 mm), respectively. The thickness of the cartilage appeared to be related to the congruence of a joint. Shepherd and Seedhom[26] hypothesized that congruent joint surfaces, such as those in the ankle and elbow, are covered only by thin articular cartilage because the compressive loads are spread over a wide area, decreasing local joint stresses and eliminating the necessity for large cartilaginous deformations. Incongruent joints

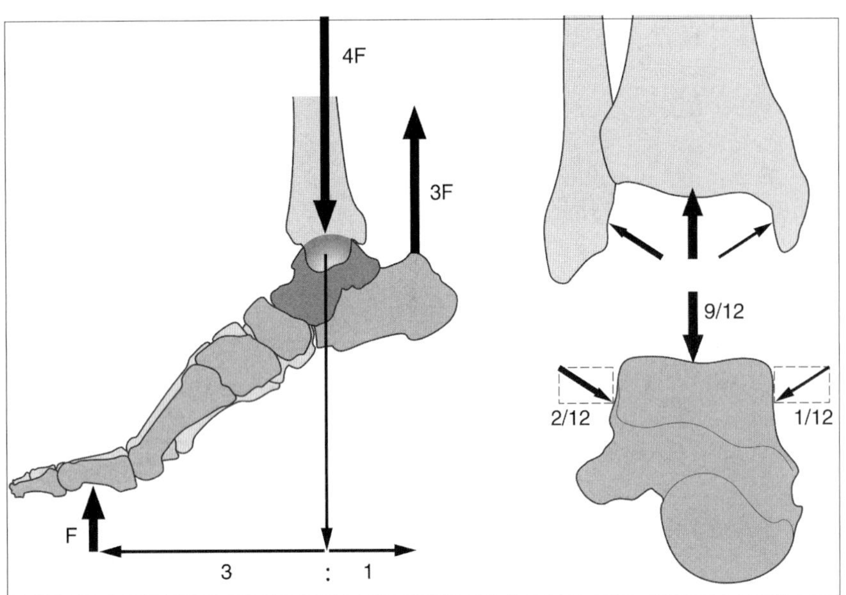

Figure 2 Schematic diagrams showing the calculation of load transmission through the ankle joint during walking. Approximately one sixth of the load across the ankle is transmitted through the talofibular facet, and the remaining load is transmitted through the tibiotalar articulation. F = force. Arrows show the distribution of forces.

are covered by thicker cartilage, which more easily deforms, thereby increasing the load-bearing area and decreasing the stress per unit area.

Cartilage and Loading

The load-bearing area of the ankle joint is relatively small compared to the forces it conducts. Procter and Paul[29] calculated the load on the ankle joint as 3.9 times body weight at heel rise during the stance phase of walking (Figure 2);[30] Mow and associates[31] measured a load of 5.0 times body weight at heel rise. For example, according to the data of Proctor and Paul,[29] the force on the talus with every step taken by a person weighing 75 kg is 2,865 N (3.9 × 75 kg × 9.8 m/s^2 [acceleration on Earth] = 2,865 N). The average tibiotalar contact area[32] is estimated to be 4.4 cm^2. Therefore, the average load on the articular cartilage during the stance phase can be calculated as 650 N/cm^2. During running, this load increases multiple times.

When the contact surface areas decrease in size, the load on the remaining cartilage increases, as occurs after an ankle fracture malunion. Ramsey and Hamilton[32] found that a 1-mm lateral talar shift reduces the contact area by 42%, and a 2-mm lateral shift reduces the contact area by 58%. For a person weighing 75 kg, the average load per square centimeter after a 2-mm lateral shift is increased from 650 to 1,590 N (Figure 3). A 2-mm shift therefore should be surgically corrected because of the high risk of degenerative changes.[33] A 1-mm shift generally is considered acceptable; the implication is that if the ankle is normally aligned, the talar cartilage can adapt to an increase in load as great as 40%.

An average osteochondral talar defect measures 0.85 cm^2 on MRI;[34] however, the size of the defect may be overestimated on MRI because of bone edema. CT was used to measure the size of 52 consecutive lesions; an average defect size of 0.65 cm^2 (range, 0.5 to 0.8 cm^2) was found (M Zengerink, MD, and CN van Dijk, MD, PhD, unpublished data, 2006.) Débridement of an osteochondral talar defect with a diameter of 0.65 cm^2 increases the load on the remaining talar cartilage by 15% (Figure 3). Such an increase in load probably is not large enough to cause damage to the remaining cartilage in a normally aligned ankle. However, any varus or valgus malalignment increases the likelihood of cartilage damage.[35]

Radin and Rose[36] argued that articular cartilage, by virtue of its thinness, is not a good shock absorber in terms of reducing the peak impact force. Although the underlying bone is much stiffer than the articular cartilage, it also is much longer, and therefore its total compliance exceeds that of the cartilage. Nonetheless, the peak stresses at the joint surface are greatly reduced through the redistribution and deformation of cartilage. The talus is a compact bone, in comparison to a long bone such as the tibia, and the peak impact force can be distributed only over a small volume of bone. The small volume of the talus, combined with its thin cartilage, may explain why osteochondral defects are more common on the talar dome than in the tibial plafond.

Thin cartilage is less elastic than thick cartilage. Shepherd and Seedhom[26] suggested an inverse relationship between mean cartilage thickness and mean compressive modulus; that is, thin cartilage has a high compressive modulus. Measurement of cartilage from human cadaver specimens and specimens from several other species led to the conclusion that the two factors contributing to cartilage deformability are its thickness and intrinsic elasticity. There is a curvilinear relationship between the magnitude of the deformation and the thickness of the articular cartilage under each level of loading. Li and associates[37] measured a deformation in congruent ankle joints of 24% to 38% after 20 seconds of continuous static loading between 700 and 820 N (Figure 4).

Because the talar cartilage is thin and therefore relatively inelastic, it is susceptible to cartilage lesions and microfractures in the underlying bone when it is exposed to high-impact forces. However, osteochondral defects also occur in joints with thicker cartilage, where the development of a defect probably is related to factors including impact force and shearing stress.

Cartilage is able to withstand compressive stress because of the interaction of its liquid and solid components. The liquid is a dialysate of synovial fluid that is incompressible but able to flow. However, this fluid must be contained if it is to withstand the compressive loads that joints sustain. The cartilage matrix resembles a sponge with directional pores; the small diameter of these functional pores and their arrangement in circuitous tunnels (created by the hydrophilic collagen proteoglycan matrix components) prevents large molecules from entering the cartilage and offers considerable resistance to interstitial fluid flow. These characteristics provide adequate containment for the fluid to support the load. Only a part of the joint is compressed or bearing a load at a specific time. When one part of the joint is in compression, the adjacent area is being stretched and pulled apart. Liquid flows from the loaded area to the unloaded area. In a healthy joint, the liquid is not able to enter the subchondral plate and flows only to adjacent cartilage. Fluid in cartilage, whether extrafibrillar or intrafibrillar, is freely exchangeable.[38] Herberhold and associates[39] studied patellar and femoral compression during a 4-hour continuous static loading of 150% of body weight. In patellar cartilage, the maximal thickness reduction was 57% (±15%), with a volume change of more than 30%. These findings suggest that more than 50% of the interstitial fluid was displaced from the matrix.

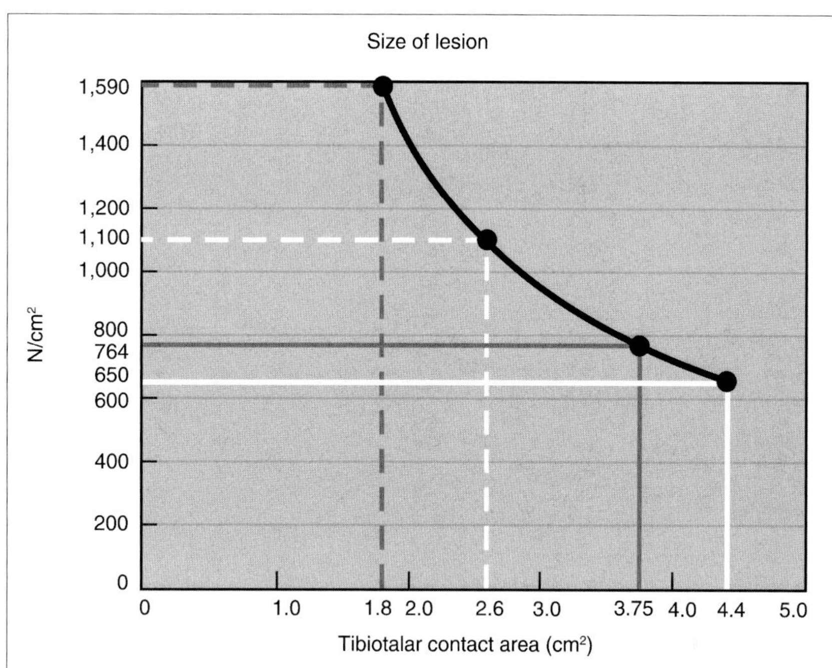

Figure 3 Graph showing load in relation to tibiotalar contact (black line). The white line represents the average tibiotalar contact area of 4.4 cm^2 for a 75-kg person during the normal stance phase of walking. The dashed white represents the same person with a tibiotalar contact area diminished by 42% to 2.6 cm^2, as would occur after an ankle fracture with 1 mm of lateral displacement of the talus and fibula. The gray dashed line represents the same person with a tibiotalar contact area diminished by 58% to 1.8 cm^2, as would occur after an ankle fracture with 2 mm of lateral displacement of the talus and fibula. The gray line represents a person weighing 75 kg with an osteochondral defect measuring 0.65 cm^2; the average load on the remaining cartilage is increased from 650 to 764 N/cm^2.

Traumatic microfractures of the subchondral bone plate allow the liquid not only to flow within the cartilage but also to enter the subchondral bone through the microfractured area. Damaged subchondral bone is less able to support the overlying cartilage,[40] and cartilage that is not supported by the underlying bone plate loses proteoglycans and glycoprotein.[19,36] The loss of negatively loaded GAG side chains and hydrophilic proteoglycans causes a decrease in water containment, and the liquid more easily flows to other places. Every step or other load-bearing activity causes liquid to be pressed out of the cartilage and into the microfractured areas of the subchondral bone (Figure 5). Continuously high fluid

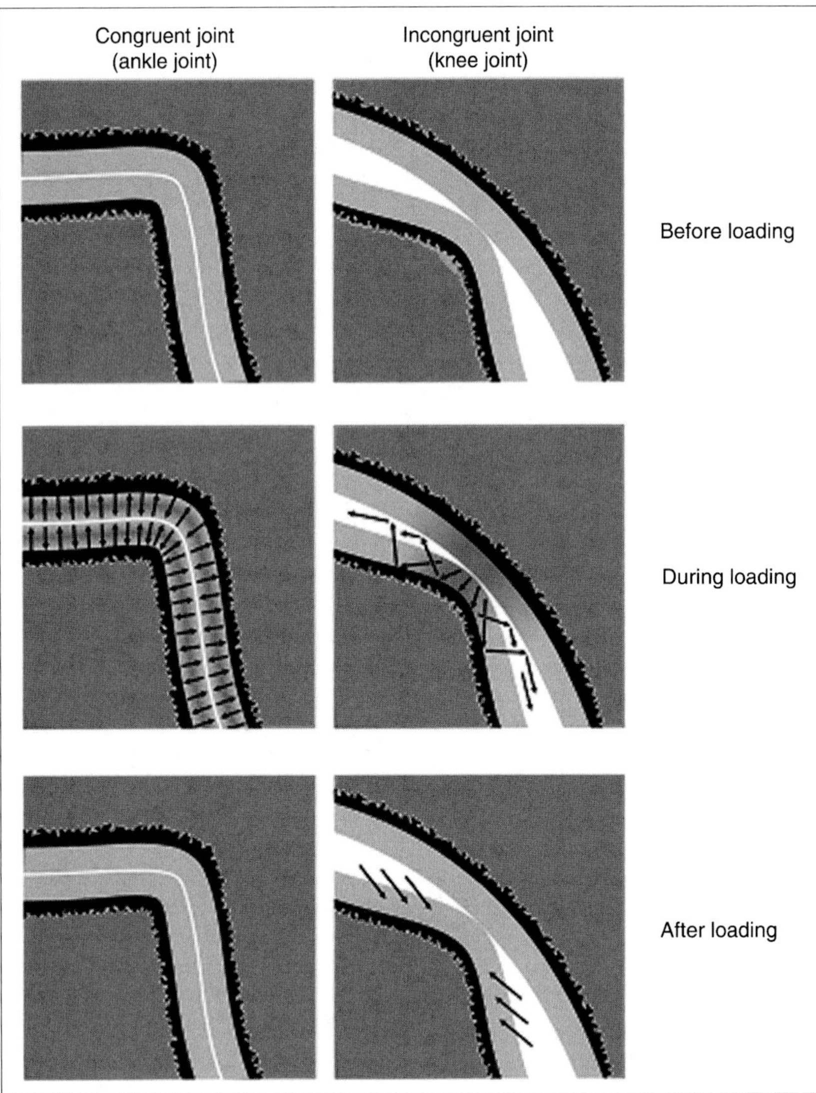

Figure 4 Schematic comparison of the deformation of cartilage in a congruent (ankle) and incongruent (knee) joint before, during, and after loading. Arrows = direction of fluid flow under pressure of weight bearing. White areas = joint space filled with synovial fluid. Dark gray areas = bone marrow. Light gray areas = cartilage. Black areas = subchondral bone plate.

pressure has been proved to cause osteolysis. Intermittently or continuously high local pressure can interfere with normal bone perfusion and lead to osteonecrosis, bone resorption, and formation of lytic areas[41-45] (Figure 6).

Irie and associates[46] studied calcitonin gene-related peptide (CGRP) in bone tissue nerve fibers and its involvement in bone remodeling. The effect of CGRP on bone remodeling may in part result from its action in regulating local blood flow. High fluid pressures may excite CGRP-containing nerve fibers, thereby diminishing blood flow through bone and causing osteolysis. Subchondral bone may be exposed because the overlying cartilage was sheared off or the cartilage-bone interface was damaged at a microscopic level, and it is subject to continuously high fluid pressures that cause osteolysis and subsequent large osteochondral talar lesions.[45,47,48] A vicious circle begins, in which damage to the overlying cartilage leads to subchondral bone damage, and the cartilage is further damaged because the underlying bone is unable to provide support.

The Causes of Pain

Several factors can cause pain from an osteochondral lesion of the talus. Increased intraosseous pressure has been reported as a cause of pain and has been associated with joint degeneration;[41,42,44] medullary decompression can be used to decrease the intraosseous pressure.[49,50]

Intra-articular pressure is a cause of pain in degenerative joint disease. Goddard and Gosling[51] found a linear correlation between pain in osteoarthritis and resting intra-articular pressure of the synovial fluid. Bünger and associates[52] found a connection between synovial hypertrophy and high intra-articular pressure in arthritis. However, patients with a localized osteochondral talar defect typically do not have relevant joint effusion, and therefore it is unlikely that increased intra-articular pressure contributes to their pain.

Nerve endings can be found in the synovium and the joint capsule; the joint capsule and soft tissue around the joint are important in triggering nociception. The upregulation of substance P and CGRP-positive neurons in response to arthritic changes suggests a mechanism involving neuropeptides in the maintenance of painful degenerative joint disease.[53] The synovium of the anterior ankle joint lies directly under the skin and can easily be palpated. Patients with an osteochondral

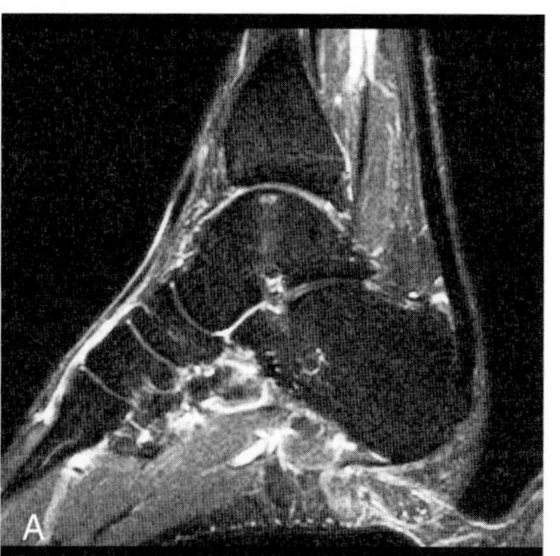

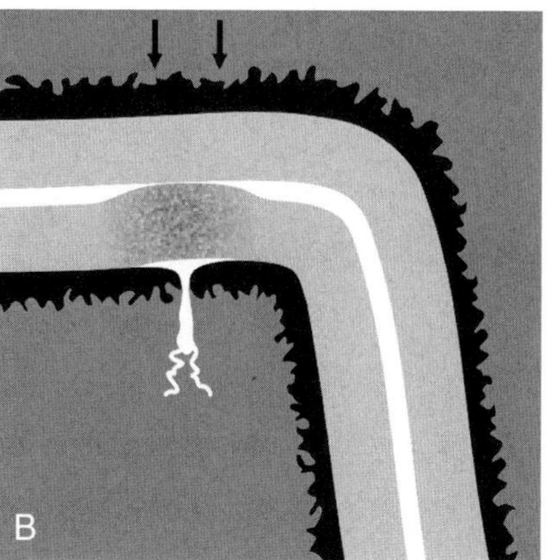

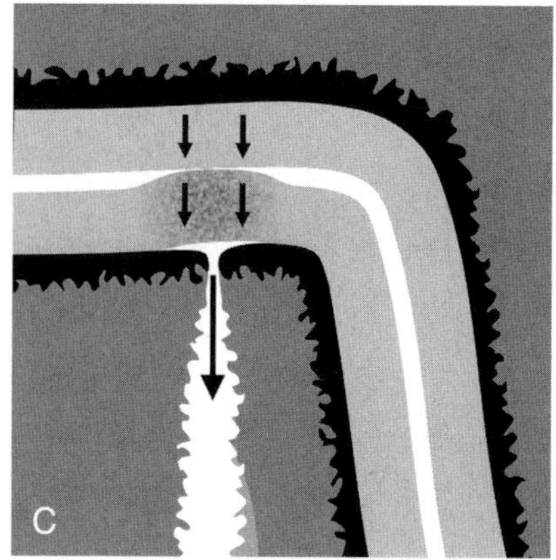

Figure 5 **A,** Sagittal T2-weighted MRI of an ankle with an osteochondral defect. The vertical configuration of the water column (seen in the center of the talus) suggests that the water is pumped directly caudal under high pressure, perpendicular to the talar joint surface. Schematic diagrams of fissures in the cartilage and the subchondral bone plate of an unloaded ankle **(B)** and a loaded ankle **(C)** are shown. The small black arrows show the direction of the force. When the ankle is loaded, water is squeezed out of the cartilage into the subchondral bone. The large black arrow shows the movement of water. The diameter of the opening of the subchondral bone plate determines the pressure of the fluid flow (the smaller the diameter, the higher the pressure). White areas = joint space filled with synovial fluid. Dark gray areas = bone marrow. Light gray areas = cartilage. Black areas = subchondral bone plate.

talar lesion generally do not have much synovitis, and usually they can differentiate secondary synovial pain from the disabling deep ankle pain caused by the osteochondral defect. Their deep ankle pain occurs during weight bearing and cannot be reproduced during physical examination. The nerve endings in the subchondral bone are the most probable cause of this pain.[20]

The hollow haversian canal that runs longitudinally down the center of each osteon in compact bone contains an arteriole, a venule, and a lymphatic duct for vascular and lymphatic drainage. The Volkmann canals run perpendicular to and connect the haversian canals (Figure 1). Mach and associates[20] found that not all osteons are innervated in mouse femora. The likelihood of an osteon being innervated is greatest in the proximal head, followed by the distal head and the diaphysis of the femur. The presence of CGRP-immunoreactive nerve fibers and RT-97 (clone name of neurofilament)–immunoreactive nerve fibers suggests that the mineralized bone, bone marrow, and the periosteum are innervated by both unmyelinized and myelinized fibers. These fibers contain A-β, A-δ, and C fibers that can conduct sensory input from the periphery to the spinal cord. In general, Mach and associates[20] found the highest density of sensory and sympathetic fibers in the areas of mineralized bone that underwent the greatest mechanical stress and loading, had the highest metabolic rate, and were the most vascularized. The abundant innervation of bone marrow may explain the pain experienced by patients with bone disease before bone destruction or periosteal involvement appears on radiographs. Many of the primary efferent nerves that innervate mineralized bone have acid registration ion channels, and it is likely that a decrease in pH (caused by osteoclasts) at the mineralized bone interface can activate these channels. Pain probably develops as a rise in fluid pressure, and a decrease in pH excites the nerve fibers present in bone.

The Natural History of Types of Osteochondral Ankle Lesions

Several factors may play a role in the natural history of osteochondral lesions. A decrease in the high joint congruence of the ankle joint increases the contact pressure per area. Greater displacement also corresponds to increasing contact pressure.[32] Thordarson and associates[54] confirmed that substantial displacement of the fibula (as much as 2 mm of shortening or lateral shift, or as much as 5° of external rotation) increases the contact pressures in the ankle joint. Long-term follow-up studies showed that patients with a persistent displaced ankle fracture had a poorer long-term result than those without persistent displace-

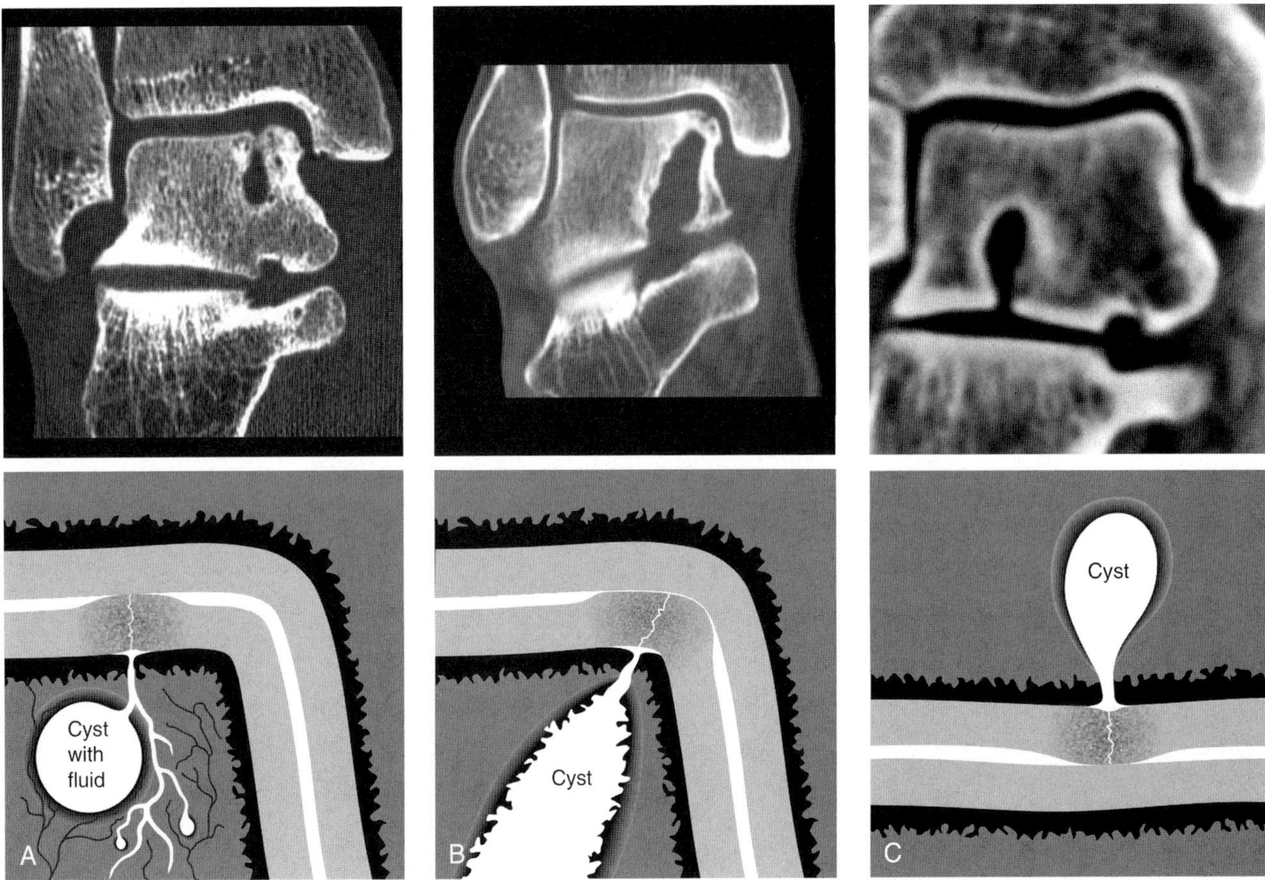

Figure 6 A through **C,** Coronal CT scans (upper row) with corresponding schematic diagrams (lower row), showing the ankles of three patients (age 26 to 37 years) who had deep ankle pain of 5 to 12 years' duration. An opening in the subchondral bone plate can be seen in all three CT scans, with subchondral osteolysis that has developed into a subchondral cyst. **A,** The coronal CT scan shows a cystic lesion in the talar body, with the corresponding diagram indicating the supposed mechanism of cyst formation. **B,** In this patient, the cyst has extended into the subtalar joint. **C,** In this patient, sclerosis is visible around the subtalar cyst. Lower rows (**A** through **C**): white areas = joint space filled with synovial fluid; dark gray areas = bone marrow; light gray areas = cartilage; and black areas = subchondral bone plate.

ment.[33] Therefore, displacement or malalignment of the fibula should not be accepted after an injury.

Varus or valgus malalignment also may play an important role by increasing the contact pressure in some areas of the ankle. Biomechanical experiments showed that in varus and supination, the maximal pressure is on the medial border of the talus; in valgus and pronation, the maximal pressure is on the lateral border of the talus.[55] Because increased pressure on an existing osteochondral defect may negatively influence the natural history of the lesion,[40] it is important to detect malalignment in patients with an osteochondral talar defect.

Understanding the different types of osteochondral talar defects provides clues to the development of these lesions. A superficial lesion consists of sheared-off flakes with an intact subchondral bone plate (Figure 7). In a more severe lesion, the subchondral bone is damaged, as with microfractures and bone bruises. Bone bruises are seen as a decreased signal intensity on T1-weighted MRI studies and as an elevated intensity on T2-weighted MRI studies of the bone marrow. The reticular type of bone bruise is not continuous with the adjacent articular surface[6,56,57] (Figure 8). In general, this type of bone bruise heals normally; healing occurs from the periphery to the center.[58] The geographic type of bone bruise, which is continuous with the adjacent articular surface, is associated with osteochondral talar lesions (Figure 9). Spontaneous healing is impaired or absent, possibly because

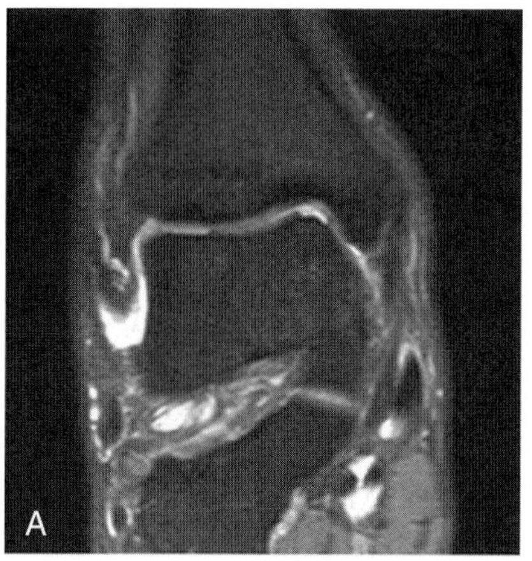

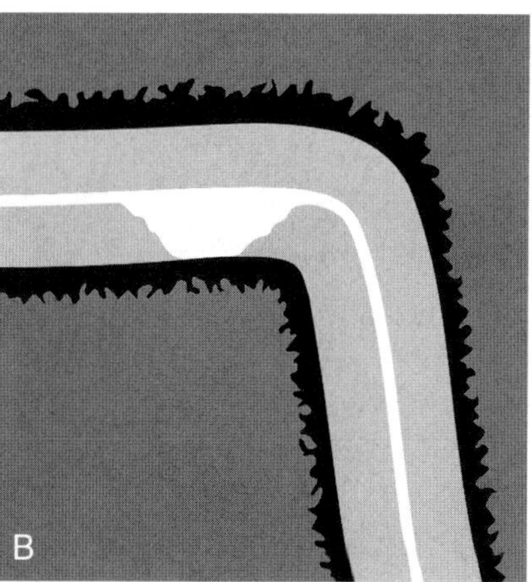

Figure 7 **A,** MRI scan showing a cartilage lesion of the medial talar dome. The subchondral bone plate has remained intact, and there is no sign of bone bruising. **B,** Schematic diagram showing a fragment that probably was sheared from the underlying bone. White areas = joint space filled with synovial fluid. Dark gray areas = bone marrow. Light gray areas = cartilage. Black areas = subchondral bone plate.

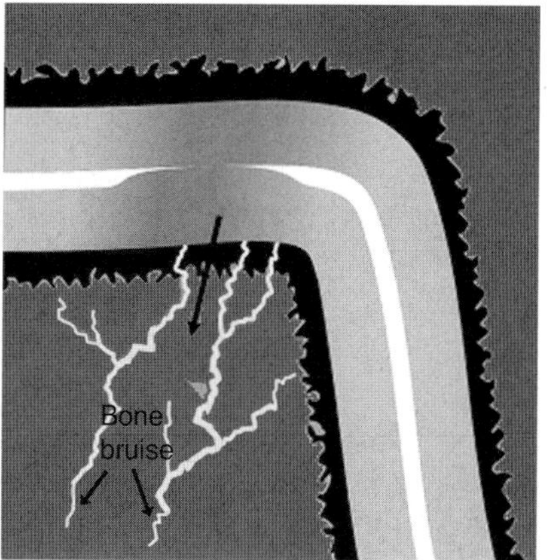

Figure 9 Schematic diagram showing the geographic type of bone bruise, which is continuous with the adjacent articular surface. Healing depends on the healing of the subchondral bone plate. Long black arrow shows fluid flow under pressure from weight bearing. Water can enter the subchondral bone only when there is a defect in the subchondral bone plate. White areas = joint space filled with synovial fluid. Dark gray areas = bone marrow. Light gray areas = cartilage. Black areas = subchondral bone plate.

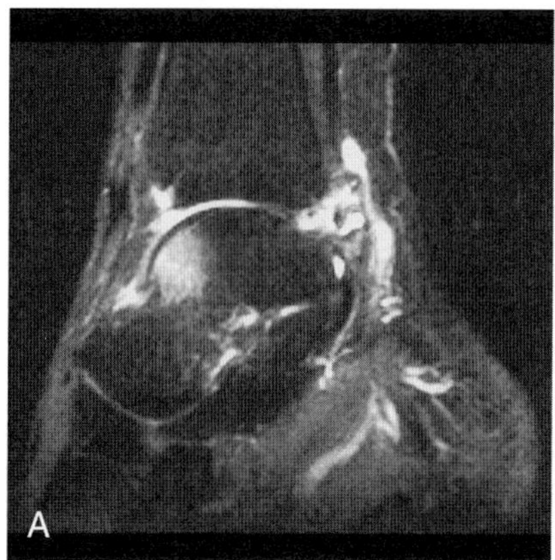

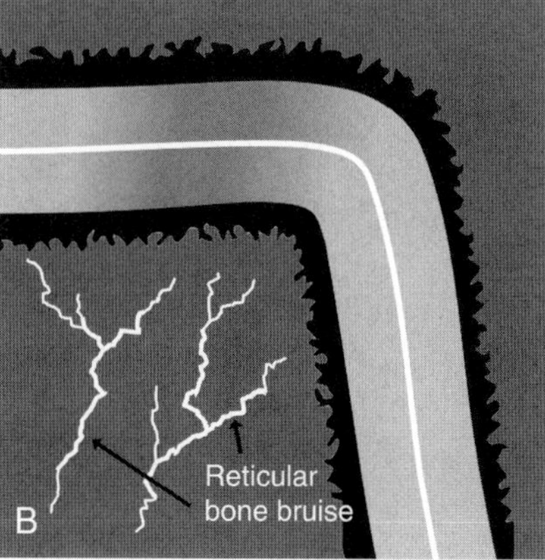

Figure 8 **A,** Sagittal T2-weighted MRI of an ankle with a reticular bone bruise. The white area in the anterior talus represents bone edema. **B,** Schematic diagram of a reticular bone bruise with an intact subchondral bone plate. This type of bone bruise heals from the periphery to the center without complications. White areas = joint space filled with synovial fluid. Dark gray areas = bone marrow. Light gray areas = cartilage. Black areas = subchondral bone plate.

the cartilaginous water content is forced into the persistent fissure in the bone plate underneath.[6,57,59] Healing of an osteochondral fragment may be precluded by intermittent fluid flow around the fragment (Figure 10).

Next to the described intraosseous pressure by direct cartilaginous fluid pressure, subchondral cyst formation has been hypothesized to be caused by the damaged cartilage functioning as a valve.[60] The valve mechanism may allow intrusion of fluid from the joint space into the subchondral bone but not in the opposite direction. During the weight-bearing phase of the gait, there is full contact between major parts of the talar and tibial cartilage, with most contact over the talar shoulders;[61] the theoretically identical pressures in the opposing talar and tibial cartilage may force fluid in the direction of the least resistance, which is to the damaged subchondral bone. Backflow is prevented by the direct contact of opposing cartilage. During joint unloading, the joint space fluid may reenter the articular cartilage. During the next weight-bearing cycle, the fluid again intrudes into the subchondral bone. This repetitive mechanism can lead to a vicious circle in which the shift of synovial fluid into the damaged subchondral talar bone slowly results in the formation of a subchondral cyst.

Summary

Most osteochondral talar lesions are caused by trauma. They may heal and remain asymptomatic or may progress to subchondral cysts with

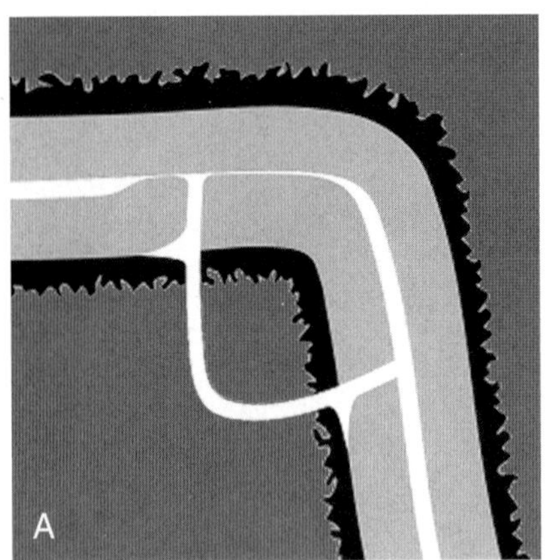

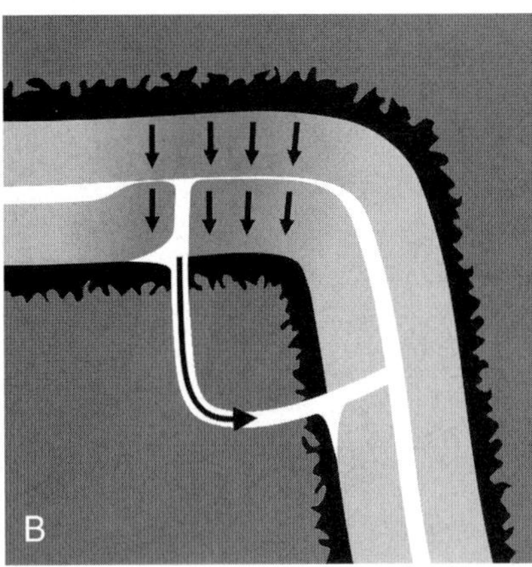

Figure 10 Schematic diagrams showing a loose osteochondral fragment when the ankle is unloaded **(A)** and loaded **(B)**. Healing under loading may be precluded by intermittent fluid flow around the fragment. Small arrows show the direction of force during loading. The large arrow represents the movement of synovial fluid during loading. White areas = joint space filled with synovial fluid. Dark gray areas = bone marrow. Light gray areas = cartilage. Black areas = subchondral bone plate.

deep ankle pain on weight bearing. The pain in osteochondral lesions is most probably caused by a local rise in fluid pressure with every step, which sensitizes the highly innervated subchondral bone. The development of symptoms and subchondral cysts depends on the type of defect (in particular, involvement of the subchondral bone), joint congruence, alignment, impact force, and shearing stress.

Cartilage has a liquid and a solid component that enables it to withstand compressive stress. A congruent joint surface, such as the ankle, is covered by thin articular cartilage. Incongruent joints, such as the knee, are covered by thicker cartilage. There is a curvilinear relationship between the cartilage thickness and deformation. Thick cartilage easily deforms, thereby increasing the load-bearing area and decreasing the stress area.

Fluid from the damaged cartilage can be forced into the microfractured subchondral bone plate during loading. This intermittent local rise in fluid pressure will cause osteolysis and the eventual formation of a subchondral cyst. Malalignment of the ankle joint may aggravate this process by increasing local pressure in specific locations of the ankle.

Acknowledgments

L. Blankevoort, PhD, is gratefully acknowledged for his advice during the preparation of this chapter. I.E.M. Kos is gratefully acknowledged for the preparation of the figures.

References

1. van Bergen CJ, de Leeuw PA, van Dijk CN: Potential pitfall in the microfracturing technique during the arthroscopic treatment of an osteochondral lesion. *Knee Surg Sports Traumatol Arthrosc* 2009;17:184-187.
2. Schachter AK, Chen AL, Reddy PD, Tejwani NC: Osteochondral lesions of the talus. *J Am Acad Orthop Surg* 2005;13:152-158.
3. Bruns J: Osteochondrosis dissecans. *Orthopade* 1997;26:573-584.
4. Ray R, Coughlin E. Osteochondritis dissecans of the talus. *J Bone Joint Surg* 1947;29:697-706.
5. Quinn TM, Allen RG, Schalet BJ, Perumbuli P, Hunziker EB: Matrix and cell injury due to sub-impact loading of adult bovine articular cartilage explants: Effects of strain rate and peak stress. *J Orthop Res* 2001;19:242-249.
6. Vellet AD, Marks PH, Fowler PJ, Munro TG: Occult posttraumatic osteochondral lesions of the knee: Prevalence, classification, and short-term sequelae evaluated with MR imaging. *Radiology* 1991;178:271-276.
7. Torzilli PA, Grigiene R, Borrelli J Jr, Helfet DL: Effect of impact load on articular cartilage: Cell metabolism and viability, and matrix water content. *J Biomech Eng* 1999;121:433-441.
8. Berndt AL, Harty M: Transchondral fractures (osteochondritis dissecans) of the talus. *J Bone Joint Surg Am* 1959; 41:988-1020.
9. Canale ST, Belding RH: Osteochondral lesions of the talus. *J Bone Joint Surg Am* 1980;62:97-102.
10. Chen DS, Wertheimer SJ: Centrally located osteochondral fracture of the talus. *J Foot Surg* 1992;31:134-140.
11. Flick AB, Gould N: Osteochondritis dissecans of the talus (transchondral fractures of the talus): Review of the literature and new surgical approach for medial dome lesions. *Foot Ankle* 1985;5:165-185.
12. Stone JW: Osteochondral lesions of the talar dome. *J Am Acad Orthop Surg* 1996;4:63-73.
13. Verhagen RA, Struijs PA, Bossuyt PM, van Dijk CN: Systematic review of treatment strategies for osteochondral defects of the talar dome. *Foot Ankle Clin* 2003;8:233-242.
14. Ferkel RD, Scranton PE Jr: Arthroscopy of the ankle and foot. *J Bone Joint Surg Am* 1993;75:1233-1242.
15. Anderson DV, Lyne ED: Osteochondritis dissecans of the talus: Case report on two family members. *J Pediatr Orthop* 1984;4:356-357.
16. Erban WK, Kolberg K: Simultaneous mirror image osteochondrosis dissecans in identical twins. *Rofo* 1981; 135:357.

17. Woods K, Harris I: Osteochondritis dissecans of the talus in identical twins. *J Bone Joint Surg Br* 1995;77:331.

18. Frenkel SR, Di Cesare PE: Degradation and repair of articular cartilage. *Front Biosci* 1999;4:D671-D685.

19. Junqueira L, Carneiro J, Kelly R: *Functionele Histologie*, ed 11. Maarssen, Netherlands, Elsevier, 2007, pp 140-147.

20. Mach DB, Rogers SD, Sabino MC, et al: Origins of skeletal pain: Sensory and sympathetic innervation of the mouse femur. *Neuroscience* 2002;113: 155-166.

21. Zengerink M, Szerb I, Hangody L, Dopirak RM, Ferkel RD, van Dijk CN: Current concepts: Treatment of osteochondral ankle defects. *Foot Ankle Clin* 2006;11:331-359.

22. Ferkel RD, Zanotti RM, Komenda GA, et al: Arthroscopic treatment of chronic osteochondral lesions of the talus: Long-term results. *Am J Sports Med* 2008;36:1750-1762.

23. Schuman L, Struijs PA, van Dijk CN: Arthroscopic treatment for osteochondral defects of the talus: Results at follow-up at 2 to 11 years. *J Bone Joint Surg Br* 2002;84:364-368.

24. Koch S, Kampen WU, Laprell H: Cartilage and bone morphology in osteochondritis dissecans. *Knee Surg Sports Traumatol Arthrosc* 1997;5:42-45.

25. Sugimoto K, Takakura Y, Tohno Y, Kumai T, Kawate K, Kadono K: Cartilage thickness of the talar dome. *Arthroscopy* 2005;21:401-404.

26. Shepherd DE, Seedhom BB: Thickness of human articular cartilage in joints of the lower limb. *Ann Rheum Dis* 1999;58:27-34.

27. Braune W, Fischer O: *Die Bewegungen des Kniegelenks nach einer neuen Methode am lebenden Menschen gemessen*. Leipzig, Germany, S. Hirzel, 1891, pp 75-150.

28. Simon WH, Friedenberg S, Richardson S: Joint congruence: A correlation of joint congruence and thickness of articular cartilage in dogs. *J Bone Joint Surg Am* 1973;55:1614-1620.

29. Procter P, Paul JP: Ankle joint biomechanics. *J Biomech* 1982;15:627-634.

30. Lambert KL: The weight-bearing function of the fibula: A strain gauge study. *J Bone Joint Surg Am* 1971;53: 507-513.

31. Mow VC, Flatow EL, Ateshian GA: Biomechanics, in Buckwalter JA, Einhorn TA, Simon SB, eds: *Orthopaedic Basic Science*, ed 2. Rosemont, IL, American Academy of Orthopaedic Surgeons, 2000, pp 133-180.

32. Ramsey PL, Hamilton W: Changes in tibiotalar area of contact caused by lateral talar shift. *J Bone Joint Surg Am* 1976;58:356-357.

33. Joy G, Patzakis MJ, Harvey JP Jr: Precise evaluation of the reduction of severe ankle fractures. *J Bone Joint Surg Am* 1974;56:979-993.

34. Elias I, Zoga AC, Morrison WB, Besser MP, Schweitzer ME, Raikin SM: Osteochondral lesions of the talus: Localization and morphologic data from 424 patients using a novel anatomical grid scheme. *Foot Ankle Int* 2007;28:154-161.

35. Tarr RR, Resnick CT, Wagner KS, Sarmiento A: Changes in tibiotalar joint contact areas following experimentally induced tibial angular deformities. *Clin Orthop Relat Res* 1985; 199:72-80.

36. Radin EL, Rose RM: Role of subchondral bone in the initiation and progression of cartilage damage. *Clin Orthop Relat Res* 1986;213:34-40.

37. Li G, Wan L, Kozanek M: Determination of real-time in-vivo cartilage contact deformation in the ankle joint. *J Biomech* 2008;41:128-136.

38. Maroudas A, Schneiderman R: "Free" and "exchangeable" or "trapped" and "non-exchangeable" water in cartilage. *J Orthop Res* 1987;5:133-138.

39. Herberhold C, Faber S, Stammberger T, et al: In situ measurement of articular cartilage deformation in intact femoropatellar joints under static loading. *J Biomech* 1999;32:1287-1295.

40. Buckwalter JA, Mankin HJ: Articular cartilage: Degeneration and osteoarthritis, repair, regeneration, and transplantation. *Instr Course Lect* 1998;47: 487-504.

41. Aspenberg P, Van der Vis H: Migration, particles, and fluid pressure: A discussion of causes of prosthetic loosening. *Clin Orthop Relat Res* 1998; 352 :75-80.

42. Astrand J, Skripitz R, Skoglund B, Aspenberg P: A rat model for testing pharmacologic treatments of pressure-related bone loss. *Clin Orthop Relat Res* 2003;409:296-305.

43. Schmalzried TP, Akizuki KH, Fedenko AN, Mirra J: The role of access of joint fluid to bone in periarticular osteolysis: A report of four cases. *J Bone Joint Surg Am* 1997;79: 447-452.

44. van der Vis HM, Aspenberg P, Marti RK, Tigchelaar W, Van Noorden CJ: Fluid pressure causes bone resorption in a rabbit model of prosthetic loosening. *Clin Orthop Relat Res* 1998;350:201-208.

45. Dürr HD, Martin H, Pellengahr C, Schlemmer M, Maier M, Jansson V: The cause of subchondral bone cysts in osteoarthrosis: A finite element analysis. *Acta Orthop Scand* 2004;75: 554-558.

46. Irie K, Hara-Irie F, Ozawa H, Yajima T: Calcitonin gene-related peptide (CGRP)-containing nerve fibers in bone tissue and their involvement in bone remodeling. *Microsc Res Tech* 2002;58:85-90.

47. Rangger C, Kathrein A, Freund MC, Klestil T, Kreczy A: Bone bruise of the knee: Histology and cryosections in 5 cases. *Acta Orthop Scand* 1998;69: 291-294.

48. Yamamoto T, Bullough PG: Spontaneous osteonecrosis of the knee: The result of subchondral insufficiency fracture. *J Bone Joint Surg Am* 2000;82: 858-866.

49. Kiaer T, Pedersen NW, Kristensen KD, Starklint H: Intra-osseous pressure and oxygen tension in avascular necrosis and osteoarthritis of the hip. *J Bone Joint Surg Br* 1990;72:1023-1030.

50. Specchiulli F, Capocasale N, Laforgia R, Solarino GB: The surgical treatment of idiopathic osteonecrosis of the femoral head. *Ital J Orthop Traumatol* 1987;13:345-351.

51. Goddard NJ, Gosling PT: Intra-articular fluid pressure and pain in osteoarthritis of the hip. *J Bone Joint Surg Br* 1988;70:52-55.

52. Bünger C, Harving S, Hjermind J, Bünger EH: Relationship between intraosseous pressures and intra-articular pressure in arthritis of the knee: An experimental study in immature dogs. *Acta Orthop Scand* 1983; 54:188-193.

53. Saxler G, Löer F, Skumavc M, Pförtner J, Hanesch U: Localization of SP- and CGRP-immunopositive nerve fibers in the hip joint of patients with painful osteoarthritis and of patients with painless failed total hip arthroplasties. *Eur J Pain* 2007;11:67-74.

54. Thordarson DB, Motamed S, Hedman T, Ebramzadeh E, Bakshian S: The effect of fibular malreduction on contact pressures in an ankle fracture malunion model. *J Bone Joint Surg Am* 1997;79:1809-1815.

55. Bruns J, Rosenbach B: Pressure distribution at the ankle joint. *Clin Biomech (Bristol, Avon)* 1990;5:153-161.

56. Bretlau T, Tuxoe J, Larsen L, Jorgensen U, Thomsen HS, Lausten GS: Bone bruise in the acutely injured knee. *Knee Surg Sports Traumatol Arthrosc* 2002;10:96-101.

57. Nakamae A, Engebretsen L, Bahr R, Krosshaug T, Ochi M: Natural history of bone bruises after acute knee injury: Clinical outcome and histopathological findings. *Knee Surg Sports Traumatol Arthrosc* 2006;14:1252-1258.

58. Davies NH, Niall D, King LJ, Lavelle J, Healy JC: Magnetic resonance imaging of bone bruising in the acutely injured knee: Short-term outcome. *Clin Radiol* 2004;59:439-445.

59. Roemer FW, Bohndorf K: Long-term osseous sequelae after acute trauma of the knee joint evaluated by MRI. *Skeletal Radiol* 2002;31:615-623.

60. Scranton PE Jr, McDermott JE: Treatment of type V osteochondral lesions of the talus with ipsilateral knee osteochondral autografts. *Foot Ankle Int* 2001;22:380-384.

61. Millington S, Grabner M, Wozelka R, Hurwitz S, Crandall J: A stereophotographic study of ankle joint contact area. *J Orthop Res* 2007;25:1465-1473.

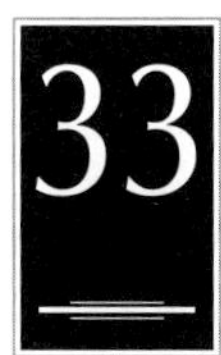

Surgical Treatment of Osteochondral Lesions of the Talus

Richard D. Ferkel, MD
Pierce E. Scranton Jr, MD
James W. Stone, MD
Brian S. Kern, MD

Abstract

When conservative treatment is unsuccessful, there are many surgical options to treat patients with symptomatic chronic osteochondral lesions of the talus. The chosen treatment depends on the patient's symptoms, clinical examination findings, preoperative imaging results, and whether prior surgery was unsuccessful. It is important to be aware of treatment alternatives such as marrow stimulation, osteochondral autograft or allograft plugs, autologous chondrocyte implantation, and newer techniques currently being investigated outside the United States.

Instr Course Lect 2010;59:387-404.

An osteochondral lesion of the talus may occur in any location over the talar articular surface; however, these lesions usually occur on the posteromedial or anterolateral talar dome. The anterolateral lesions are most commonly associated with acute trauma, such as a severe sprain, usually with only a small flake of bone attached to the articular cartilage fragment. In contrast, the posteromedial lesions tend to be more chronic in nature with a larger piece of associated necrotic bone and may have associated cystic degeneration of the subchondral bone. Although some lesions may be treated nonsurgically, especially nonseparated lesions in skeletally immature patients, studies dating to the mid 1900s suggest that surgical treatment is appropriate for most lesions.[1,2] Berndt and Harty[2] suggested a classification scheme that defined an increasing degree of fragment separation from stage I to stage IV based on clinical and radiographic analysis and recommended surgical treatment of most patients with stage III or IV separated lesions. Newer classification schemes using CT or MRI evaluation allow more precise assessment of talar osteochondral lesions for both clinical treatment and research comparisons.[3-5] An arthroscopic classification of osteochondral lesions also has been developed.[6] Open surgery for débridement of these lesions has largely been replaced by arthroscopic techniques that allow a minimally invasive approach with less morbidity and faster rehabilitation.

Indications for Surgery

Indications for surgery are determined by the patient's symptoms, the stage of the lesion, and the absence of improvement with conservative treatment (Table 1). The traditional treatment of a symptomatic osteochondral lesion of the talus involves excision of the bony fragment and some type of treatment of the bony base. Options for treatment of

Dr. Ferkel or an immediate family member has received royalties from Smith & Nephew; serves as a paid consultant or is an employee of Smith & Nephew; and has received research or institutional support from Mitek and Smith & Nephew. Dr. Scranton or an immediate family member has received royalties from Arthrex and has received research or institutional support from Arthrex. Dr. Stone or an immediate family member serves as a paid consultant to or is an employee of Smith & Nephew and has stock or stock options held in Johnson & Johnson, Procter & Gamble, GE Healthcare, Medtronic, and Pfizer. Neither Dr. Kern nor any immediate family members have received anything of value from or own stock in a commercial company or institution related directly or indirectly to the subject of this chapter.

Table 1
Surgical Indications for Osteochondral Lesions of the Talus

All CT or MRI stage I or II lesions that fail nonsurgical treatment
All CT or MRI stage III lesions in children younger than age 18 years that fail nonsurgical treatment
All CT or MRI stage III symptomatic lesions in adults
All CT or MRI stage IV lesions in adults and children

the base include abrasion, drilling, and microfracture. The goals of this treatment method are to remove the loose osteoarticular fragment, which may contribute to pain and mechanical symptoms; stabilize the bone and articular cartilage at the margins of the lesion; and create an environment that maximizes the likelihood of developing fibrocartilaginous repair tissue over the bony base.

Arthroscopic Techniques

Most osteochondral lesions of the talar dome, including posteromedial lesions, can be approached arthroscopically. Although 4-mm-diameter arthroscopes that are used for large joint arthroscopy can be used to visualize the anterior compartment of the ankle joint, complete joint access is facilitated using a 2.7-mm-diameter arthroscope, which decreases the risk of iatrogenic articular cartilage injury. The patient is supine on the operating table under general, spinal, or epidural anesthesia, with the ipsilateral hip and knee flexed and supported by a well-padded leg holder. The noninvasive ankle distractor is applied and the joint approached using routine anteromedial, anterolateral, and posterolateral portals. Inflow is initially placed through the posterolateral portal, but this portal also may be used to visualize lesions located on the far posterior talar dome and for introducing instruments and motorized débriders and abraders. A complete 21-point examination of the ankle is initially performed to assess the entire ankle joint.[7]

Drilling of an Intact Osteochondral Lesion of the Talar Dome

The lesion, whether medial or lateral, is first identified and its extent is confirmed under direct visualization. The arthroscopic probe is used to examine the junction of the normal articular cartilage and the abnormal articular cartilage. In the rare instance when the articular cartilage appears normal on arthroscopic viewing and when there is no definite loose bony fragment, in situ drilling may be the preferred procedure. Drilling may be performed using one of three techniques.

If there is an anterolateral lesion or if a medial lesion has a relatively anterior location, drilling may be performed using one of the standard anterior portals or using an accessory portal located adjacent to the tibia whose position is guided using a hypodermic needle to obtain the optimal approach angle to the lesion. A 0.062-inch Kirschner wire is advanced through a small cannula, and multiple drill holes are placed at approximately 5-mm intervals. It is always important to irrigate the pin while drilling to prevent thermal necrosis.

For posteromedial lesions inaccessible through the anterior portal, two options exist. A transmedial malleolar portal may be used; the wire is drilled through the medial malleolus using a drill guide and multiple penetrations are made into the lesion. Although this approach is relatively easy to perform, the required penetration of the normal articular cartilage of the tibial plafond/medial malleolus makes this approach less desirable. Damage to normal articular cartilage of the plafond can be obviated by using the distal to proximal transtalar drilling technique (Figure 1). The Kirschner wire is introduced through the sinus tarsi using a drill guide and advanced retrograde into the lesion until just beneath the articular cartilage of the talar dome. Multiple drillings can be performed using a guide.

Débridement and Microfracture of an Unstable Osteochondral Lesion of the Talar Dome

Most posteromedial talar dome lesions can be approached with the arthroscope in the anterolateral portal, the inflow in the posterolateral portal, and the instruments placed in the anteromedial portal. The 70° arthroscope may be useful for visualizing far posterior lesions or for visualizing the extent of the lesion in the medial gutter. The extent of the lesion is determined by visualization and palpation with a probe; the unstable nature of the lesion is confirmed by ballottement with the probe. The lesion is elevated with the probe, a freer elevator, a curet, or a similar instrument. A portion of the articular cartilage is generally attached to a piece of unstable subchondral bone, and the major fragment or fragments can be removed with a small loose-body forceps. A significant amount of necrotic bone is usually found beneath the major bony fragment; this material is easily removed from the normal subchondral bone using an angled curet. It is important to define and remove all the unstable necrotic bone, not only on the horizontal surface of the talar dome but also along the vertical surface in the medial gutter. Failure to remove all unstable bone will result in persistent symptoms, and the sur-

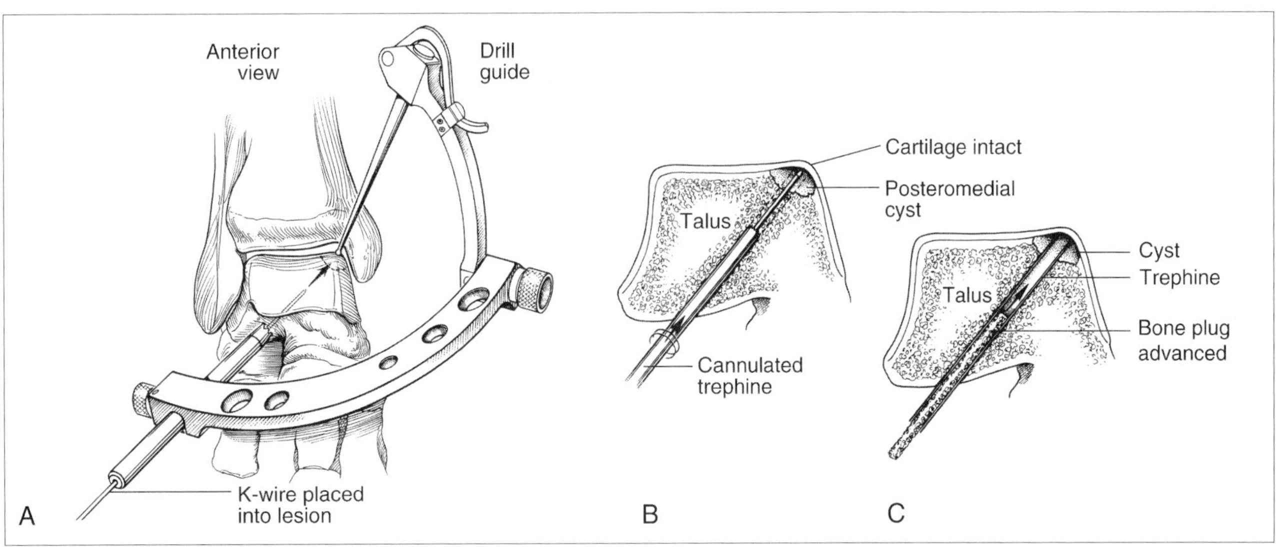

Figure 1 Illustration of the transtalar drilling of an osteochondral lesion of the medial dome of the talus. **A,** A Kirschner wire is inserted using a drill guide by drilling from the sinus tarsi posteromedially. **B,** A cannulated trephine is used to core out the bone from the lateral aspect of the talus into the area of the osteochondral defect. **C,** Using a plunger, the bone plug is advanced into the area of the osteochondral lesion.

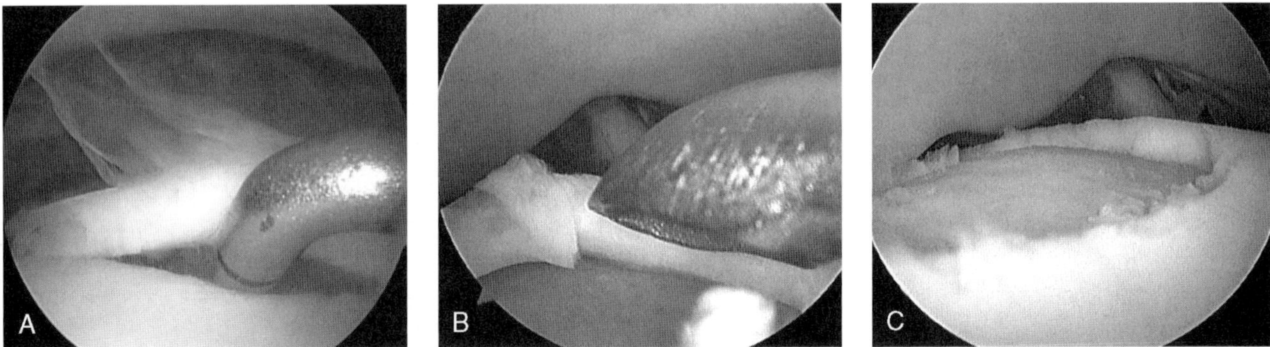

Figure 2 Arthroscopic views of a medial lesion with chondral delamination and minimal subchondral bone involvement. **A,** Elevation of chondral fragment with probe. **B,** Débridement of an osteochondral talar lesion using a curet. **C,** The lesion after débridement.

gical procedure will not relieve pain. The articular cartilage margins must be débrided until healthy, well-attached articular cartilage margins are established (Figure 2).

After débriding all necrotic bone and stabilizing the peripheral articular cartilage, the viability of the subchondral bone should be assessed by decreasing the inflow pressure (and deflating the tourniquet if it has been inflated for the débridement) and observing bleeding from the entire bony bed. If adequate bleeding is not present, then the base of the lesion may be further débrided using a motorized abrader or by microfracture of the base using specially designed awls that are available in several angulations (Figure 3).

The term microfracture describes a technique initially applied to chondral defects of the femoral condyle in which the defect is débrided to the level of the calcified cartilage, not into the cancellous bone, and then the subchondral plate is penetrated with awls rather than drilled.[8] As applied to lesions of the talar dome, the technique is not usually a true microfracture because treatment of most lesions involves removal of necrotic subchondral bone to the level of cancellous bone, with removal of the subchondral bone plate.

Access to a posteromedial osteochondral lesion of the talus can be problematic, particularly when the patient's ankle is tight and access is difficult or if the lesion is located very posteromedially. In these

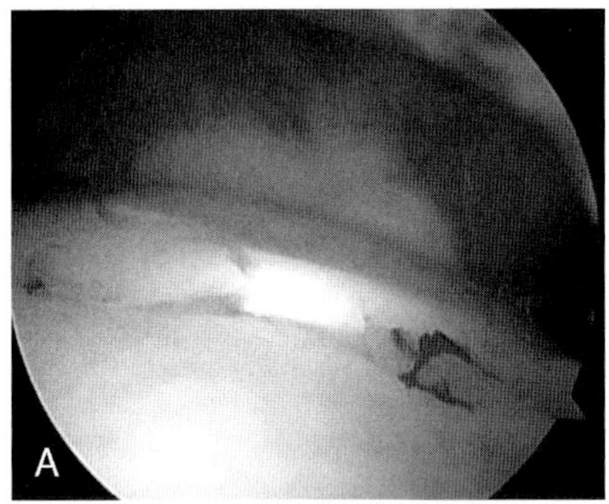

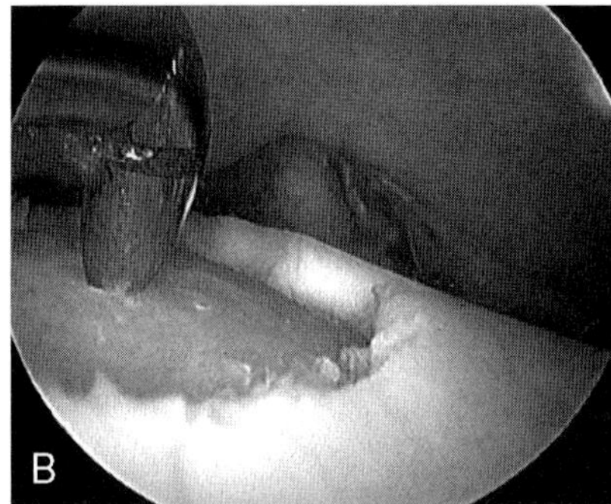

Figure 3 **A,** Arthroscopic view of a separated osteochondral lesion of the lateral talar dome in a right ankle. **B,** Arthroscopic view of microfracture of a posterior lesion with a 90° awl. Many angled awls are available.

instances, the arthroscope should be inserted through the posterolateral portal to visualize the posteromedial osteochondral lesion of the talus. The lesion is excised through the anteromedial portal using the extra space provided by the notch of Harty by using ring and curved curets and graspers as well as a shaver. Using both the 30° and 70° arthroscopes through the posterolateral portal, the lesion can be clearly seen and microfracture and/or transmalleolar or transtalar drilling can be used.

After débridement with abrasion, drilling, or microfracture, the ankle is immobilized in a short leg posterior splint for approximately 1 week and then the sutures are removed. For patients with smaller lesions (approximately < 1 cm in diameter), weight bearing can be increased as tolerated and range-of-motion exercises can begin. For larger lesions (approximately > 1 cm in diameter), patients are instructed not to bear weight for 4 to 6 weeks; weight bearing is then advanced as tolerated. Range-of-motion exercises can be enhanced using a continuous passive motion machine during the non–weight-bearing period. Physical therapy may be used to increase range of motion and strengthening as tolerated.

Treatment Results for Talar Dome Lesions

Many studies have documented the results of treating talar dome lesions with débridement combined with abrasion, drilling, or microfracture.[6,8-13] Most were level III or IV studies (case control studies, retrospective comparative studies, systematic reviews of level III studies, or case series). There are no level I high quality, prospective randomized controlled trials of these treatment methods.

In addition to the fact that most studies of talar dome lesions are retrospective and nonrandomized and are therefore less definitive, several other factors contribute to the difficulty in assessing the clinical significance of studies of osteochondral lesions of the talar dome. Most studies include both medial and lateral lesions, which have different etiologies and different clinical outcomes based solely on their locations. Lateral lesions have better results with traditional treatments, which include either internal fixation or simple excision. In contrast, treatment results of posteromedial lesions are not as predictable. Inclusion of medial and lateral lesions in the same study may skew the study toward better results than if medial lesions alone were analyzed.

Most studies do not control for lesion size and may include relatively small lesions with a high likelihood of successful outcomes or larger lesions with a propensity for poorer outcomes. The size of the bony lesion is often overestimated on MRI scans because edema is accentuated, whereas CT scans more accurately assess the precise size of the bony fragment or associated cyst. The use of multiple measures of clinical outcome, including multiple grading scales ranging from the simplistic (excellent/good/poor) to comprehensive (the American Orthopaedic Foot and Ankle Society [AOFAS] hindfoot scoring system) also makes comparisons among studies difficult.

Studies have been performed assessing the results of traditional treatment of osteochondral lesions of the talar dome with excision combined with some form of treatment of the base of the lesion.[6,9-14] Flick and Gould[9] reported on 19 patients treated with open excision of the bony fragment with curettage and drilling of the bony bed and reported 79% good or excellent results. In 1989, Angermann and Jensen[10] reported on 20 patients followed for 9 to 15 years after excision and drilling of osteochondral lesions of the talar dome. Eighty-five percent of patients showed improvement at short-term follow-up, although the results deteriorated over time. Kelbérine and Frank[11] reported on 48 patients with either anterolateral loose fragments or posteromedial lesions. They reported good results in 16 of 18 patients with lateral lesions and good or excellent results in 20 of 30 patients with chronic lesions. Ogilvie-Harris and Sarrosa[12] reported on 33 patients treated with fragment excision and abrasion of the base (average follow-up, 7.4 years) and found good or excellent results in all categories of the postoperative evaluation for pain, swelling, stiffness, and limp.

More recently, Takao and associates[13] performed a prospective study of 39 patients treated with in situ drilling of intact talar dome lesions and 30 patients treated with débridement and drilling of talar dome lesions. Arthroscopic reevaluation was performed at 1 year after the index procedure to evaluate the quality of the articular surface. In the in situ drilling group, improvement of articular cartilage quality was reported in 28% of patients and cartilage deterioration occurred in 41%. In those treated with débridement and drilling of talar dome lesions, 93% showed improvement in articular cartilage quality.

Ferkel and associates[6] reported on 50 patients with chronic talar dome lesions with an average 6-year follow-up. Four patients were treated with drilling of lesions in situ, 6 patients had excision with abrasion, and 40 patients were treated with excision and drilling. Based on the Alexander scale, 72% of patients had excellent or good results, 20% fair results, and 8% poor results. Results deteriorated in 6 of 17 patients (35%) who were followed for more than 5 years.

Gobbi and associates[14] compared three groups of patients with osteochondral lesions of the talar dome—11 patients were treated with chondroplasty, 10 with microfracture, and 12 with osteoarticular autografting. They reported no clinical difference among the groups at final follow-up; however, the study illustrates the difficulties in evaluating study methodology. When published, the study was labeled level I evidence. Careful reading of the materials and methods, however, suggested that it may have been a retrospective study and therefore a level III or IV study. The authors later suggested that it presented level II evidence. The validity of the study was further weakened by the randomization method in which patients were pseudorandomized because the specific treatment they received depended on which physician provided treatment; this was not a true blinded randomization method. In addition, those patients treated with osteoarticular autografting did not have medial malleolar osteotomies, suggesting that the lesions were quite anterior in location and atypical of the posterior lesions that are more problematic to treat.

There are no studies in the ankle literature in which the pathology of the repaired tissue after débridement and drilling or microfracture is compared with another treatment modality, such as osteoarticular autografting or autologous chondrocyte implantation (ACI), which attempts to replace the diseased articular cartilage with new articular cartilage. In literature on the knee, Knutsen and associates[15] performed a prospective, randomized study comparing the treatment of symptomatic osteochondral lesions of the medial femoral condyle with either microfracture or ACI. They reported no clinical or radiographic differences in the two groups at 2- and 5-year follow-up, as well as no differences in the pathology of the healing tissue in the two groups.

Verhagen and associates[8] reviewed electronic databases from 1966 to 2000, including 39 studies (no randomized studies) that reported on the treatment of talar dome lesions. Patients could be classified into four treatment groups: nonsurgical treatment, excision alone, excision with curettage, and excision combined with curettage and drilling. Nonsurgical treatment yielded a success rate of 45%, whereas excision of the fragment alone resulted in a success rate of 38%. Excision with curettage achieved a success rate of 78%; excision, curettage and drilling showed a success rate of 86%. This retrospective analysis of 39 studies suggests that, at medium-term follow-up, traditional treatment with excision combined with either curettage or drilling of the base will yield approximately 80% good to excellent results in treating talar dome lesions.

Most osteochondral defects of the talar dome that are not responsive to nonsurgical treatment or that initially display clinical or radiographic signs of fragment separation are appropriately treated with some form of fragment débridement with abrasion, drilling, or microfracture. The available literature suggests approximately 80% of patients have medium-term good or excellent results.[16,17]

Autograft or Allograft Treatment

Classification

From the standpoint of treatment, the principles of the original Berndt and Harty[2] stage I to IV classification of talar lesions are still valid.[18] With the discovery of large cystic subchondral talar defects seen with new imaging techniques, it was determined that these cavities would require some form of bone grafting to fill the structural defect. In keeping with the treatment classification of Berndt and Harty,[2] these cystic le-

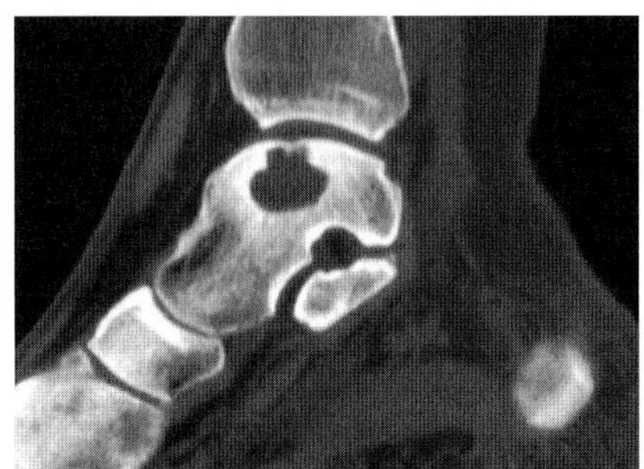

Figure 4 Sagittal CT scan showing a type Va osteochondral lesion of the talus.

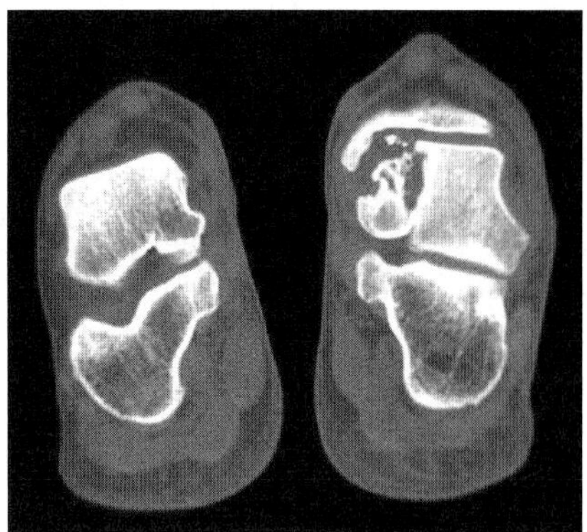

Figure 5 Coronal CT scan of a type Vb osteochondral lesion of the talus.

sions have been designated as stage V lesions.[19,20] Stage V lesions are divided into stage Va and stage Vb, based on the presence or absence of talar structural integrity. Stage Va lesions represent cystic defects within a structurally stable talus (Figure 4), whereas stage Vb lesions represent larger defects with structural collapse[21] (Figure 5).

Considerations and Imaging

Generally, treatment is delayed because of the time lag between the original traumatic ankle injury and the eventual recognition that a symptomatic osteochondral lesion of the talus is present. It may take many months from the time of injury for talar symptoms to develop. Symptoms may be multifactorial and can include pain associated with the pressure of synovial fluid intrusion into the subchondral bone, pain and synovitis from mechanical catching of loose articular flaps, or actual mechanical collapse of a portion of the talus. One report showed that 80% of the patients presenting for surgical treatment had symptoms for more than 1 year before the diagnosis of a talar lesion.[22] Appropriate imaging studies are imperative for diagnosis and treatment planning.

Plain radiographs may be nondiagnostic. A technetium Tc 99m scan with pinhole collimation can localize an osteochondral lesion of the talus in patients with normal radiographs but nonspecific ankle pain that persists for many months after injury. Additional imaging is then necessary. Before choosing an imaging study, the physician should be aware of the advantages and disadvantages of CT or MRI. A CT scan can reveal osseous defects but may not detect articular surface pathology. An MRI scan can show articular surface defects, subchondral edema, or cystic defects but may be interpreted as showing more pathologic involvement (edema) of the talus than is clinically significant.

In patients in whom an osteochondral lesion of the talus is diagnosed and who do not respond to conservative treatment with no weight bearing and ankle immobilization, MRI is recommended as an initial imaging test. If MRI suggests a large cystic talar defect, a CT scan should be obtained as a planning tool for determining the size of the needed osteochondral graft.

Autograft Treatment for Stage Va Cystic Lesions (Diameter 9 to 15 mm)

Larger symptomatic cystic lesions of the talus have poorer results with conventional microfracture, débridement, or cancellous grafting.[23,24] As a consequence, it is reasonable to consider treating these larger lesions with a one-step cored osteochondral graft or osteochondral autograft transplant system (OATS). In effect, the structural defect is drilled out and neovascularization may be stimulated from the base of the newly drilled defect. The drilled defect is replaced with a matched osteochondral graft harvested either arthroscopically or by arthrotomy from the ipsilateral knee joint. In a study of 50 consecutive patients (mean follow-up, 36 months), 90% had good to excellent results with mean Karlsson-Peterson ankle scores improving from 24 to 83 points.[22] No nonunions or malunions occurred in the 26 patients who required a medial malleolar osteotomy for exposure. At final follow-up, none of the patients had symptoms from the autograft that was arthroscopically harvested from the trochlear region of the knee.

The trochlea and sulcus terminalis regions of the knee joint are ideal for an OATS donor graft. The corner of the trochlear notch can closely match shoulder lesions in the talus. The flatter sulcus terminalis region can be used for dome surface grafting. If the surgeon chooses to perform a knee arthrotomy to obtain graft material, using the superolateral trochlear region has been associated with later symptoms of a painful chondromalacia patella. If an arthrotomy is used, it is recommended that the knee be flexed to harvest graft material from the trochlear region as described. If the graft is harvested from the superior trochlear region, the surgeon should perform a lateral retinacular release to decompress the patellofemoral joint at the location of the graft harvest.

The surgical technique for treating osteochondral lesions of the talus with or without a malleolar osteotomy has been extensively described in the literature.[22] Some useful technical tips include the need for proper visualization of the entire medial malleolus, tendons, and joint if a medial malleolar osteotomy is necessary. Small Hohmann-type retractors provide adequate exposure and protection of the tendons and deeper neurovascular structures. The osteotomy must come in at approximately a 45° angle, ending exactly at the junction of the weight-bearing surface of the tibial plafond and the corner of the medial malleolar border of the colliculus. If the angle is too flat or too acute, the residual tibial border will restrict access to the talus. Manual valgus levering of the heel by the assisting surgeon will help to adequately expose the talar surface. The articular disruption is usually easily visualized. One of the authors (PES) prefers to drill into the defect using an acorn drill, drilling over a Beath pin driven into the center of the lesion (Figure 6).

Another important consideration is orienting and matching the length of the donor graft. It is vital to know the exact depth of the recipient hole in the talus. Also, to facilitate graft introduction into the recipient hole, the graft should be carefully tapered with a rongeur. The depth of the hole and the length of graft must match precisely. A graft that is even 1 mm proud will shear off at the articular surface or gouge the tibial plafond. By tapering the tip of the graft, on introduction it can be oriented to create the optimal match with the curved contour of the talus. A graft with a tapered tip will facilitate graft rotation before impaction into the recipient hole for optimal alignment. If the graft is slightly proud, a tapered graft with a fine-pointed tip will allow gentle impaction to accomplish a finished fit. Applying too much force to impact the graft can cause chondrocyte damage or actual shearing at the tidemark.[25] Precise measuring and tapering of the graft are crucial to a satisfactory fit.

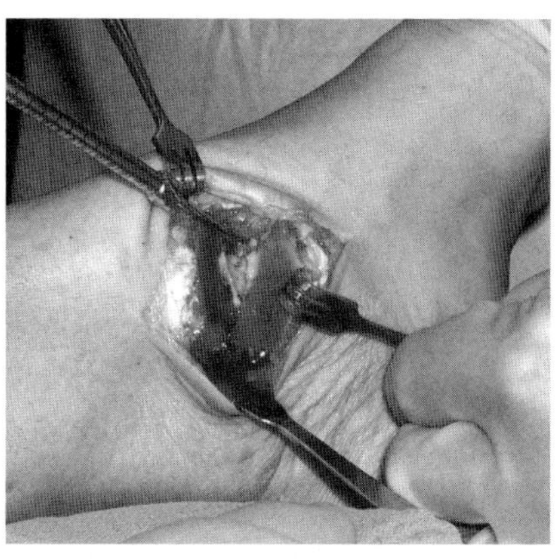

Figure 6 Intraoperative view of the osteochondral lesion of the left ankle shown in Figure 3 with the medial malleolus reflected inferiorly to expose the talar lesion. A Beath pin has been driven into the center of the lesion, and a cannulated acorn drill bit is ready to drill into the defect.

Single autografts or multiple nested grafts may be used. In one patient, one of the authors (PES) used three autografts harvested from the 9 o'clock, 12 o'clock, and 3 o'clock positions on the trochlea; however, usually only one autograft is necessary. For example, in an irregular 12-mm osteochondral lesion of the talus, drilling into the lesion's center with a 10-mm acorn drill over a Beath pin will create cancellous slurry that will fill the talar defect. A single 10-mm OATS donor graft will be sufficient. Irregular lesions that are not wider than 12 mm and not longer than 16 mm can be treated with two nested grafts (Figure 7).

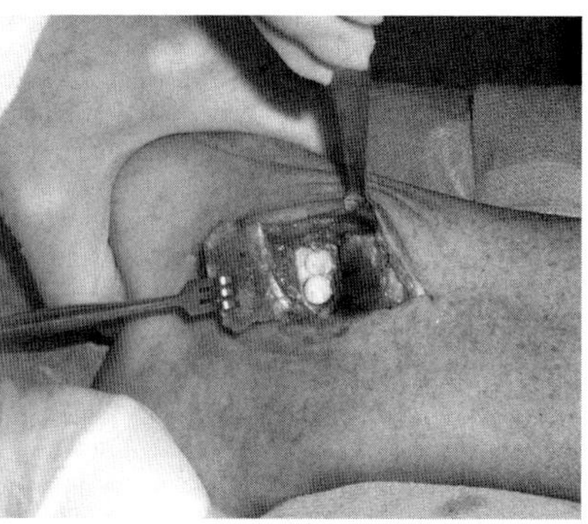

Figure 7 Photograph of a right ankle with reflected medial malleolus and two nested autografts.

Allograft Treatment for Stage Va and Vb Cystic Lesions (Diameter > 15 mm)

Cystic lesions measuring greater than 12 mm × 16 mm will require at least two nested grafts. Most patients cannot tolerate the morbidity of harvesting two 10-mm grafts from the same knee joint. In stage Vb defects, the talar lesion is so large that there is structural collapse of the talus and an en bloc allograft is more appropriate. The literature on allograft treatment of bone defects is fairly recent and most involves reports on allograft success in treating tibial or femoral defects associated with tumors or bone loss.[24] Two studies report an approximate 66% success rate with an average length of follow-up of 7 years in one study and 11 years in the other.[26,27] In selecting allografts, it is important that the donor tissue be used within 21 days of harvest and that it closely match the size and contour requirements for the recipient bone. Allografts used more than 21 days after harvest are unlikely to have viable chondrocytes and will probably result in a failed procedure.[28]

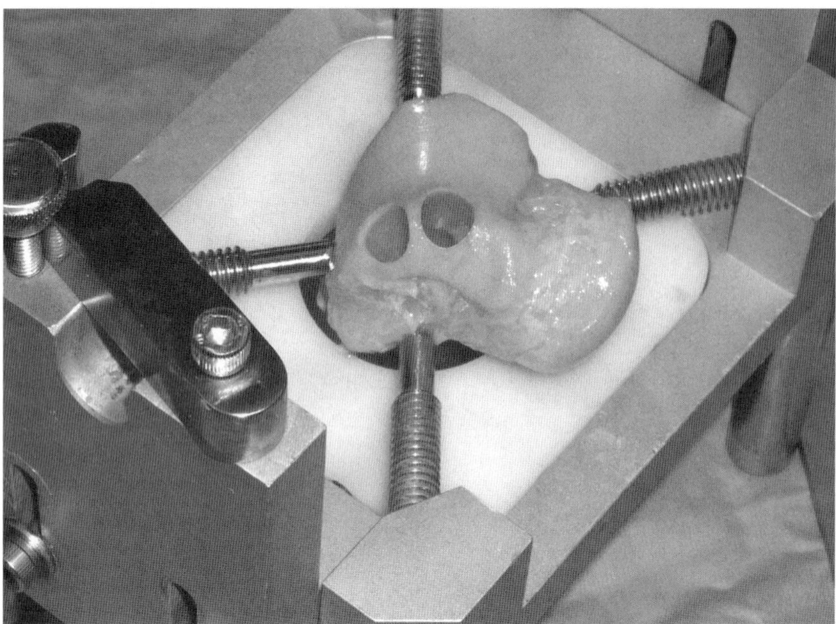

Figure 8 Photograph of a fresh allograft talus illustrating the options for multiple donor grafts.

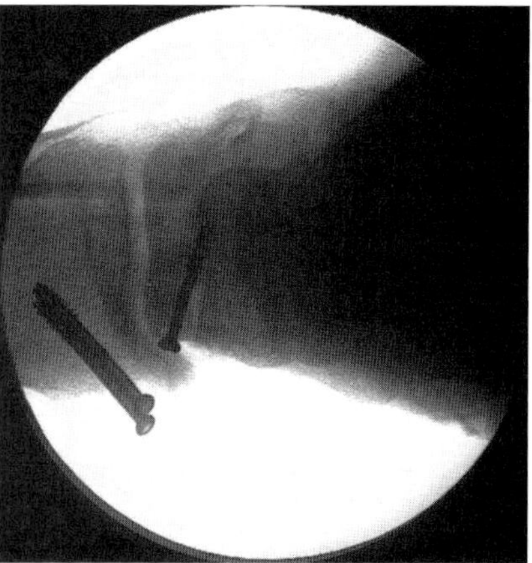

Figure 9 Postoperative AP radiograph of an en bloc talar allograft.

Another advantage of using allografts is that either a femoral condyle or a whole talus may be used. Using an allograft condyle allows the surgeon to exactly match the contour of the talar defect. The tidemark may not match, but this is not clinically important.[29] Either a condyle or a fresh talus will allow for multiple harvested donor cores to fill larger lesions (Figure 8).

In talar defects in which the structural integrity of the talus is lost, it is necessary to consider an en bloc graft. Invariably, the medial malleolus will require an osteotomy for adequate exposure. The fresh talar allograft must match the size of the recipient talus, or the curved donor talar dome will mismatch the host and joint incongruity will result. Measurements should be exact; however, initially erring on the side of too large a donor graft is preferable so that it can be trimmed as necessary for articular congruity. A graft that is initially too small is unsalvageable. Fixation is secured with countersunk small fragment or 4.0-mm screws, with cannulated 4.0-mm medial screws used for the medial malleolus (Figure 9).

Allografts are rarely needed to treat osteochondral lesions of the talus. In the experience of one of the authors (PES) who has performed more than 150 OATS procedures since 2000, only nine patients have required an allograft for a talar defect. Two patients required en bloc replacement grafts and the other seven had two or three nested, cored, donor grafts. No patient required an arthrodesis, although two required revision surgery. One of the two patients treated with an en bloc graft required arthroscopic débridement and an arthrotomy with screw removal, and the other patient was treated with arthroscopic lysis for anterior adhesions in the ankle. All patients were able to participate in mild recreational activities, although one of the patients treated with the en bloc graft had to quit participation in AAA professional baseball. Considering that each of these patients had been advised that they would probably require ankle arthrodesis, the results at an average follow-up of 3.5 years are considered good.

Conclusion

The treatment of stage Va or Vb lesions is demanding. Adequate imaging and surgical planning are imperative. Because these are large lesions, most of the patients treated already have been advised of the probable need for ankle arthrodesis. Autograft reconstruction of the defect from the ipsilateral knee has been successful in salvage surgery, with 90% good to excellent results in the first 50 patients treated by one of the authors (PES). In large defects, results using allografts have been very good. If autograft or allograft reconstruction is not successful, salvage ankle arthrodesis remains a treatment option.

Autologous Chondrocyte Implantation

Definition

ACI techniques have been evolving since 1965 when Smith[30] first isolated and grew chondrocytes in culture. First generation ACI is defined as implantation of in vitro cultured autologous chondrocytes using a periosteal tissue cover after expansion of isolated chondrocytes. Brittberg and associates[31] originally described the early results of ACI treatment of osteochondral lesions in the knee. At 2-year follow-up, good or excellent outcomes were reported in 14 of 16 patients. Since then, ACI has been used to treat more than 25,000 patients. Ninety-five percent of ACI treatments have been in the knee, 3% in the ankle, and 2% in other joints. Based on promising early results with ACI in the knee, surgeons have begun to evaluate outcomes after ACI for an osteochondral lesion of the talus.

Newer methods have been developed for using ACI. In second generation ACI treatments, the cartilage cells are inserted under a tissue patch or onto a carrier scaffold, whereas in third generation treatments, carrier-free immature cartilage tissue is placed over the defect.

Preoperative Considerations

The evaluation of patients who have chronic osteochondral lesions of the talus begins with a thorough history and physical examination in addition to plain radiographs, including AP, mortise, and lateral views. Weight-bearing and stress radiographs are obtained as needed. CT scans in the coronal and axial planes with sagittal reconstructions to measure the exact size of the lesion and assess the cortical outlines are used. MRI is helpful in assessing the quality of the overlying articular cartilage and in detecting subchondral cysts; however, the size of lesion may be overestimated. Osteochondral lesions of the talus are then classified based on a recognized CT classification system.[32]

For patients with osteochondral lesions of the talus who remain symptomatic after ankle arthroscopy with excision, curettage, and drilling or microfracture, ACI is considered a viable treatment option. Indications for ACI in the ankle are shown in Table 2. Age 55 years was chosen as an upper age limit for ACI because articular chondrocytes may become senescent with advancing age.[33]

Relative contraindications to ACI are bipolar lesions or diffuse degenerative joint changes. ACI is not typically offered as an initial treatment to patients who have an osteochondral lesion of the talus; however, patients who have a large lesion and significant subchondral cystic changes may be candidates for ACI using the "sandwich technique" as the initial surgical treatment because these lesions respond poorly with marrow stimulation techniques alone.[29] Advanced osteoarthritis is an absolute contraindication to ACI. Skeletal malalignment and ligamentous instability also are absolute contraindications unless they are concomitantly corrected at the time of surgery.

Table 2
Indications for ACI in the Ankle

Patient age of 15 to 55 years
Focal defect > 1 cm^2
Unipolar lesion (only talus)
Contained lesion
Failure of previous surgery
Large lesions with subchondral cystic changes in primary cases

Surgical Technique

The surgical technique described is for first generation ACI in the United States and is similar to the technique of Baums and associates.[34] ACI is a staged procedure. The initial surgery consists of ipsilateral knee arthroscopy for cartilage harvesting. Articular cartilage is harvested from non–weight-bearing surfaces such as the intercondylar notch. Approximately 200 to 300 mg of cartilage are harvested with the use of curets. The specimen is sent to Genzyme Tissue Repair Laboratories (Cambridge, MA; the only laboratory providing this service) for chondrocyte isolation and proliferation. Recently, Giannini and associates[35] reported good results using the detached osteochondral fragment as the source of cells. Taking a biopsy sample from a non–weight-bearing area of the normal portion of the talus also has been advocated.[36]

Ankle arthroscopy is performed at the time of the chondrocyte harvest to assess the size of the osteochondral talar lesion and the status of the surrounding articular cartilage and treat other pathology not amenable to treatment through the planned malleolar osteotomy. A 21-point diagnostic examination is performed to assess the talar lesion and evaluate the remainder of the joint for concomitant pathology.[7] The cells are sent to a laboratory using a proprietary method to cultivate a tenfold increase in chondrocytes (10 to 12 million cells) and are then ready for implantation.

After cell preparation, the patient returns to the operating room at least 4 weeks after the harvesting procedure for the second stage of the procedure. A medial or lateral malleolar osteotomy is necessary to provide access for the ACI procedure. The level of the osteotomy is determined intraoperatively with the assistance of fluoroscopy and preoperative scans. It is essential that the osteotomy be carried far enough medially or laterally to provide adequate access to the osteochondral talar lesion[37] (Figure 10). Drill holes for malleolar fixation are created

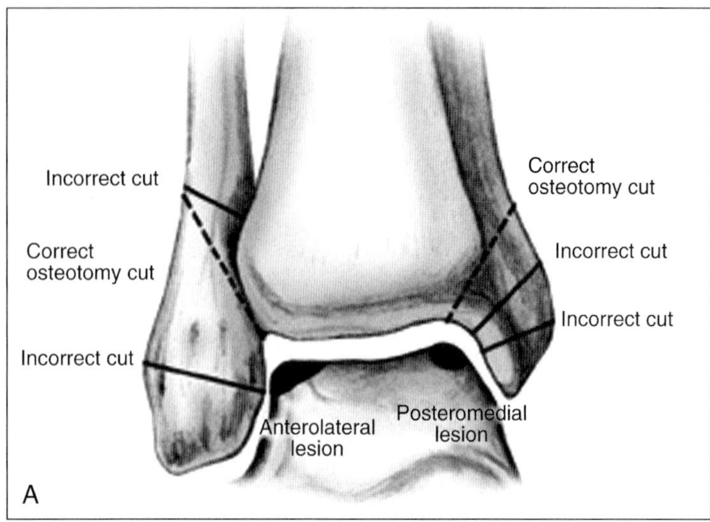

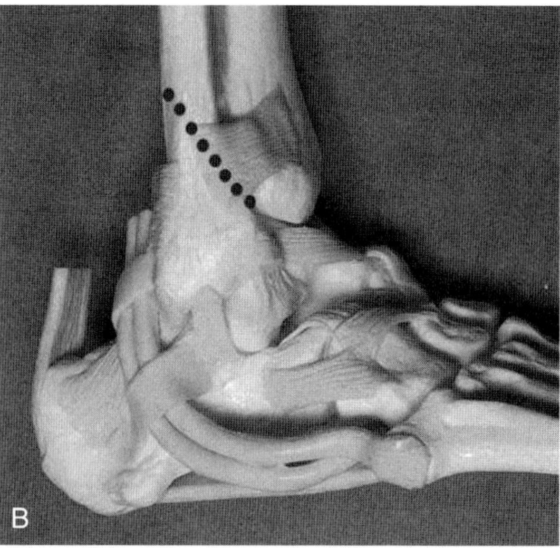

Figure 10 Illustrations showing the correct (dashed lines) and incorrect (solid lines) techniques for a malleolar osteotomy. **A,** It is critical that the osteotomy of the medial or lateral malleolus is performed at the correct level to allow exposure of the entire osteochondral lesion and permit periosteal suturing. **B,** Side view of the correct plane of the lateral malleolar osteotomy to permit access to the lateral talar dome osteochondral lesion. (Reproduced with permission from Richard D. Ferkel, MD, Van Nuys, CA.)

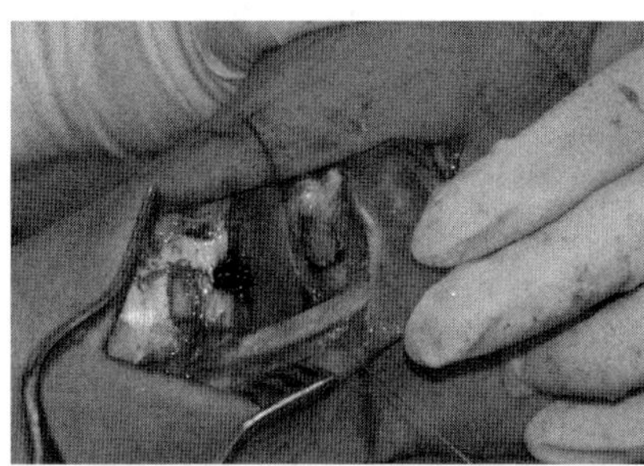

Figure 11 Intraoperative view of a left ankle after the periosteum has been secured with suture.

before the osteotomy. The osteotomy is initiated with a saw and completed with an osteotome under direct visualization. The medial malleolus is hinged inferiorly on the deltoid ligament, and the fibula is hinged posteriorly after release of the anterior inferior tibiofibular ligament and the anterior talofibular ligament.

The malleolus is retracted to provide direct visualization of the osteochondral lesion. All pathologic fibrous and cartilaginous tissue is débrided. A No. 15 blade is used to make a vertical incision at the periphery of the defect. The subchondral bone should not be penetrated during this step because this would enable marrow elements to contaminate the cultured chondrocyte population.

The periosteal graft is then obtained from the ipsilateral proximal or distal tibia. A template of the osteochondral talar lesion is created to guide the shape and size of the periosteal resection. The periosteal graft is typically oversized by 1 to 2 mm. The noncambium layer is marked and the graft is stored in a moist sponge to prevent shrinkage. The tourniquet is released and hemostasis is obtained.

With the cambium side facing toward bone, the periosteal graft is placed over the defect and secured with multiple 5.0 or 6.0 polyglycolic acid sutures. The sutures are spaced 3 mm apart and the knots are tied over the graft (Figure 11). Fibrin glue is placed at the interface to help seal the graft. A small opening at the interface is left patent so that an angiocatheter can be placed into the osteochondral lesion to inject the chondrocytes. Saline is injected to confirm that a watertight compartment has been created; the saline is subsequently aspirated from the defect. It is critical to ensure that the periosteal graft does not adhere to the surface of the defect during saline removal. The cultured chondrocytes are then placed into the defect, and the insertion site is closed with the last polyglycolic acid suture and fibrin glue.

When there is a cystic defect in the subchondral bone, a "sandwich procedure" may be necessary. The cartilage of the defect is prepared as previously described. The cystic lesion is débrided with curets and a burr. Autogenous bone graft is obtained from the iliac crest, the proximal tibia, or the calcaneus. After the base of the osteochondral talar lesion is drilled, the bone graft is impacted into the defect to the level of subchondral bone. In the sandwich procedure, two peri-

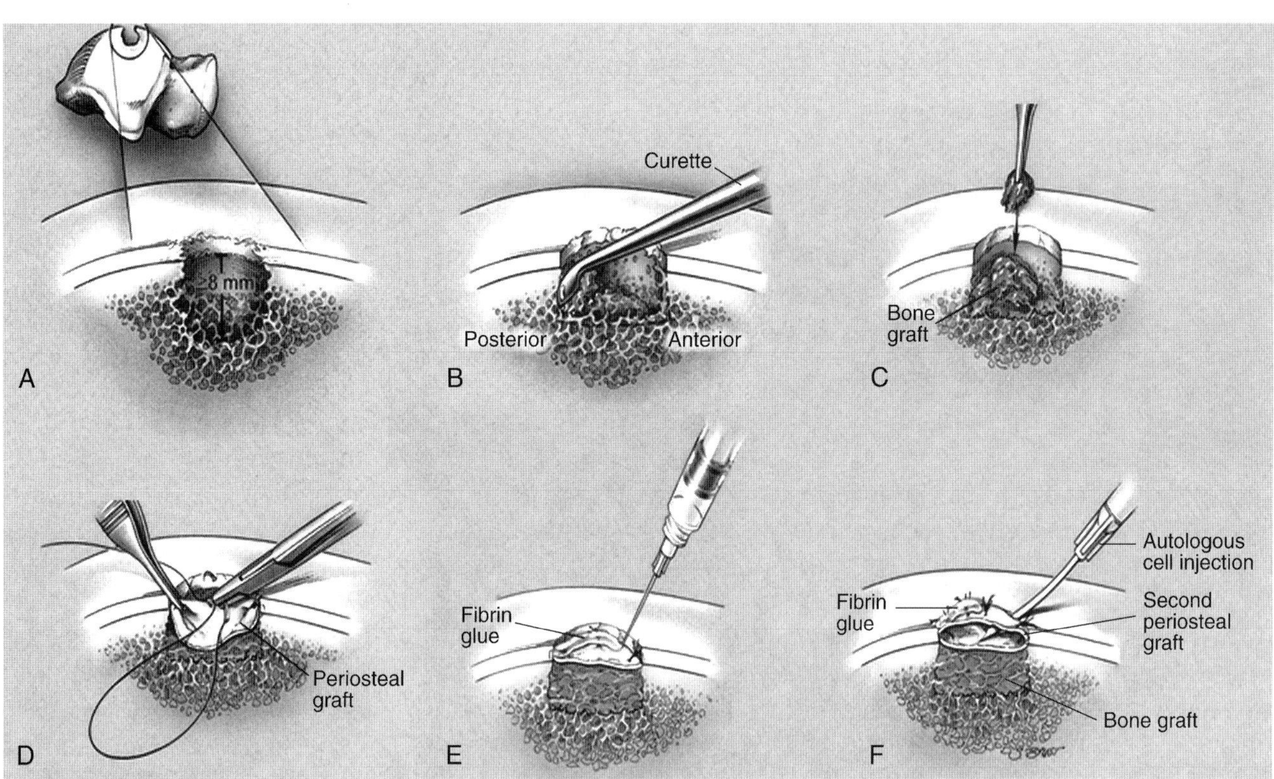

Figure 12 The sandwich procedure. The cystic lesion is removed, and bone is grafted. Two periosteal grafts are inserted over the bone graft and the cells are inserted in between. **A,** The 8-mm deep cystic osteochondral lesion of the talus is shown. **B,** Curettage of the cystic lesion is carried out. **C,** The bone graft is inserted into the cystic hole. **D,** The periosteum is sewn with the cambium side up over the bone graft. **E,** The top layer of the periosteum is inserted with the cambium side down and is then sealed with fibrin glue. **F,** The autologous cells are inserted between the two periosteal layers. (Reproduced with permission from Richard D. Ferkel, MD, Van Nuys, CA.)

osteal grafts are necessary. The first graft is placed over the bone graft with the cambium side facing toward the articular surface. The second periosteal patch is sewn over the cartilage defect with the cambium side down; the remainder of the procedure is completed as previously described (Figure 12).

After completion of ACI, the osteotomy site is reduced, and internal fixation is performed using the predrilled screw holes. The authors use three 4.0 AO cannulated screws for medial malleolar fixation and a one third tubular plate and two lag screws for fixation of the lateral malleolar osteotomy. Titanium implants are preferred to allow future MRI compatibility. The medial and lateral capsule and ligaments are repaired as needed, and routine wound closure is performed. The leg is placed in a well-padded short leg cast.

Rehabilitation

The patient remains in a well-padded short leg cast during the immediate postoperative period and does not bear weight. At 2 weeks postoperatively, the sutures are removed and the patient is placed in a controlled action motion walker boot. Partial weight bearing, limited to 30 lb, is permitted at this time. Gentle ankle range-of-motion exercises also begin at this time and are performed four to five times per day. Weight bearing is advanced based on radiographic evidence of osteotomy healing. At 6 weeks, the patient discontinues the use of the controlled action walker boot and transitions to a lace-up, figure-of-8 brace that may be worn with a comfortable shoe. Formal physical therapy in a pool and on land begins at 6 weeks and consists of four phases: the proliferation phase (< 6 weeks), the transition phase (6 to 12 weeks), the remodeling phase (12 to 32 weeks), and the maturation phase (32 to 52 weeks). Low-impact athletic activities such as cycling and skating may be started at 4 to 6 months. Repetitive impact activities such as jogging and aerobics can be resumed at 6 to 8 months. Return to high-level sports, such as basketball and football, is permitted at 12 months after surgery.[38]

Results

Giannini and associates[39] described eight patients treated with ACI, none had previous surgery. After 2 years of follow-up, the overall AOFAS ankle scores averaged 91 points. Three of the patients were able to resume full participation in sports activities. Immunohistochemistry studies after second-look arthroscopy showed evidence of hyaline-like tissue and type II collagen in each patient.

Petersen and associates[40] reported on 25 patients treated with ankle ACI who were followed for a mean of 45 months. Eleven patients had good or excellent results, and 12 patients considered their conditions to be improved. No scoring system was used to assess the outcomes.

Whittaker and associates[41] studied 10 patients with stable ankles with isolated osteochondral full-thickness defects of the talus who were treated with ACI using cartilage taken from the knee and were prospectively reviewed at a mean follow-up of 23 months (range, 12 to 54 months). The mean age of the patients was 42 years (range, 18 to 62 years) and the mean area of the lesions was 1.95 cm^2 (range, 1 to 4 cm^2) based on intraoperative measurements. All 10 patients received ACI for disabling pain and swelling for a median of 2 years; 6 had previous surgery. Nine of the 10 patients (90%) were pleased or extremely pleased with the surgery, a result that was maintained at 4-year follow-up. The mean Mazur ankle score increased 23 points (from 51 of 90 points preoperatively to 74 of 90 points at a mean follow-up of 23 months). The Lysholm knee score returned to the preoperative level at 1 year in three patients, with the remaining seven showing a score reduction of 15% at 1 year, suggesting donor-site morbidity. In nine patients, a second-look arthroscopic examination at 1 year showed filled defects and stable cartilage. Full-thickness biopsies obtained in five patients showed hyaline cartilage was present in some regions of two biopsies, with the three remaining samples being fibrocartilage. Fibrous tissue was not present in any of the samples. Seventy percent of the patients had donor site symptoms in the knee.

Baums and associates[42] reported on a prospective study using ACI in the talus of 12 patients (7 female and 5 male patients; mean age, 29.7 years). The mean size of the lesion was 2.3 cm^2. Follow-up at a mean of 63 months was performed using the Hannover ankle score, the AOFAS ankle-hindfoot score, a visual analog scale for pain, and MRI evaluation. There was a significant improvement in the Hannover score (40 preoperatively to 86 at follow-up) with seven excellent results, four good results, and one satisfactory result. The AOFAS mean score was 88.4 compared with 43.5 preoperatively. MRI evaluation showed a nearly congruent joint surface in seven patients, discrete irregularities in four, and an incongruent surface in one. The patients who had been involved in competitive sports were able to return to their full activity level. None of the patients required second-look arthroscopy because of their good clinical results.

One of the authors (RDF) has performed ACI on 32 patients (16 males and 16 females; mean age, 35 years; range, 18 to 54 years) who had at least one prior surgery for osteochondral lesions of the talus. Twenty-five patients had medial lesions, and 7 had lateral lesions. Eight patients had a sandwich procedure. Twenty-five of the 32 patients (78%) had an arthroscopic second-look procedure without biopsy.

The initial 11 patients were formally evaluated. Four of these patients had lesions in the right ankle and seven in the left ankle.[38] The talar lesion was medial in nine patients and lateral in two. The average size of the lesion was 21 × 13 mm (2.73 cm^2) (range, length = 10 to 20 mm; width = 8 to 15 mm). Six of the 11 patients with medial osteochondral talar lesions required a sandwich procedure. Nine of 11 patients had good or excellent results, and 2 had fair results. No patient had a poor outcome. The preoperative Tegner activity level score was 1.3 ± 1.0. Postoperatively, this value improved to 4.0 ± 1.6. The AOFAS score improved from 47.4 preoperatively to 84.3 postoperatively.[38]

Second-look arthroscopy showed complete coverage of the defect in all patients. The cartilage at the repair site was observed to be softer than the surrounding native articular cartilage and was graded I, II, or III. A correlation was observed between firmness of the graft and the total length of time from tissue implantation to second-look arthroscopy. The grafts seemed to become stiffer as a function of time, and the more mature grafts felt similar to the surrounding native articular cartilage on palpation (Figure 13). Periosteal overgrowth was reported in 2 of the 11 patients. To date, no donor site morbidity or other complications have been reported in this group of patients.

Complications of First Generation ACI

Complications associated with first generation ACI include periosteal hypertrophy, delamination, and graft

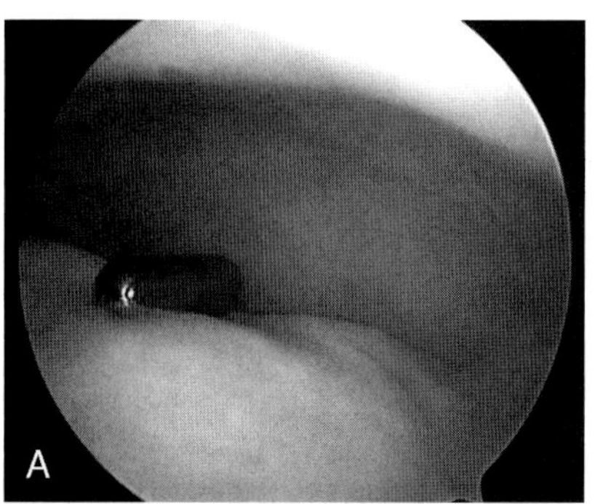

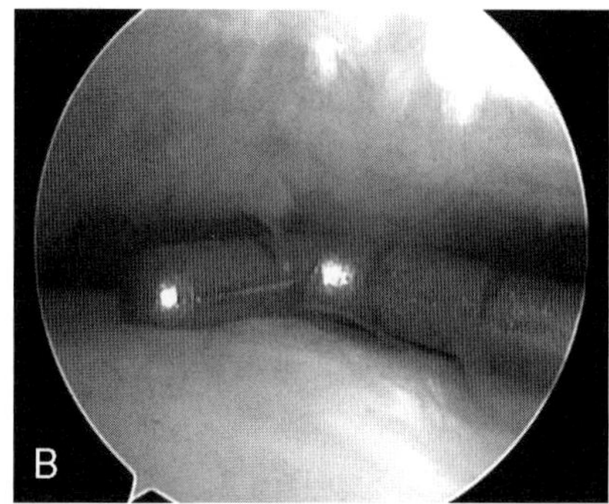

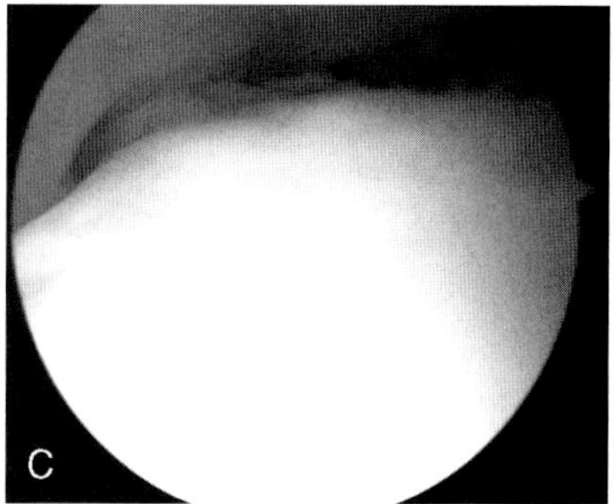

Figure 13 Second-look arthroscopy after an ACI procedure. **A,** At 9-month follow-up the articular cartilage is soft and ballotable. **B,** At 17-month follow-up the cartilage was medium firm. **C,** At 48-month follow-up the cartilage was firm.

failure. Wood and associates[43] estimated a 3.8% complication rate (285 of 7,500 procedures) in the knee, including 52 of 294 patients with graft hypertrophy. Kreuz and associates[44] developed a classification for graft hypertrophy in the knee. No studies are currently available for the ankle.

Second Generation ACI

Newer technologies for ACI have been developed to lower costs, avoid a second surgery, diminish donor site morbidity, and alleviate periosteal hypertrophy. These procedures are being performed outside the United States and are not currently approved by the US Food and Drug Administration (FDA). The second generation ACI procedures include the use of a membrane patch or cells seeded onto a scaffold membrane.[45] These techniques potentially alleviate periosteum complications, prevent potential cell leakage and uneven distribution of cells, are easier to handle, and allow for efficient and complete integration with surrounding cartilage.[45]

Ideally, a scaffold membrane should be biocompatible, noncytotoxic, biodegradable, permeable, mechanically stable, reproducible, readily available, capable of supporting and holding cells, and versatile for use in full- and partial-thickness lesions.[45] Scaffold materials for the repair of chondral and osteochondral defects are shown in Table 3.

Table 3
Scaffold Materials for the Repair of Chondral and Osteochondral Defects

Biologic polymers	Collagen
	Fibrin
	Alginates
	Agarose
	Hyaluronan
	Chitosan
	Collagen/glycosaminoglycan
Synthetic polymers	Polylactic acid
	Polyglycolic acid
	Polycaprolactone
	Carbon fiber
	Teflon
	Dacron
Other	Calcium phosphates
	Hydroxyapatite
	Demineralized bone matrix
	Devitalized cartilage
	Periosteum
	Bioactive glass

Collagen-covered ACI (CACI or ACI-C) has been popularized in Europe. It involves the use of a porcine type I/III bilayer collagen membrane or matrix. Chondro-Gide (Geistlich, Wolhusen, Germany) is a bilayer membrane with one compact and one porous surface and takes the place of periosteum. Cells are injected under the membrane or the membrane can be sewn over a cartilage defect after microfracture of the defect (termed autologous matrix induced chondrogenesis). Gooding and associates[46] compared ACI with a periosteal cover with ACI-C and found no difference in outcome, but the periosteum group required 36% graft shaving, whereas the collagen

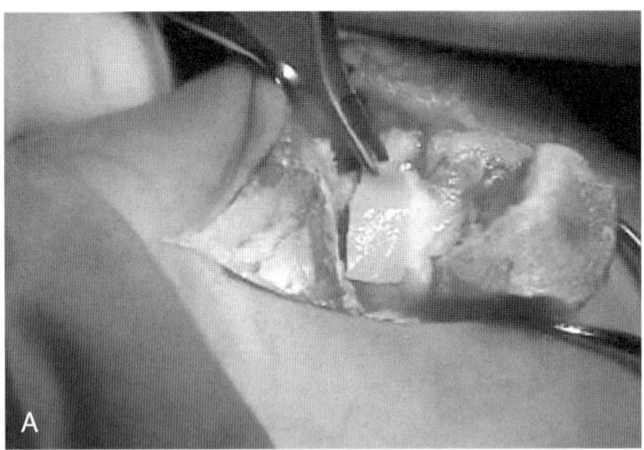

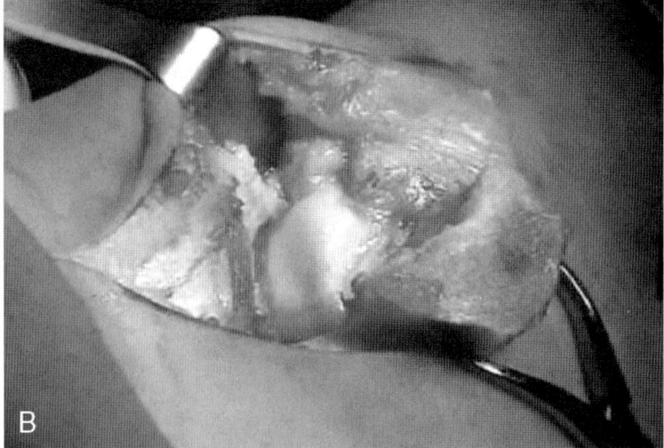

Figure 14 MACI procedure in a left ankle after a medial malleolar osteotomy. **A,** The MACI graft is sized and then cut to fit the osteochondral lesion defect. **B,** The MACI graft is applied over the osteochondral lesion site and secured with fibrin glue. (Courtesy of Pedro Guillen, MD, and Steve Abelow, MD, Lake Tahoe, CA.)

membrane group required no shaving. Other authors have shown good results in knees with this technology.[47-49] More recently, investigators have seeded the chondrocytes onto the Chondro-Gide directly.

Matrix-Induced Autologous Chondrocyte Implantation

Matrix-induced autologous chondrocyte implantation (MACI; Genzyme, Cambridge, MA) is a membrane that is widely used outside the United States. Chondrocytes from the patient are expanded in vitro and then seeded onto a bioabsorbable type I/III collagen membrane in the operating room before implantation.[50,51] Chondro-Gide and other materials are currently being used in this technique. The MACI construct is absorbable, tear resistant, and implanted via a malleolar osteotomy, a miniopen incision, or arthroscopically (Figure 14). The membrane is maintained with fibrin glue and, in some cases, with pins, absorbable anchors, or sutures. Short-term results of outcomes after MACI for osteochondral lesions of the talus are encouraging[52,53] (P Guillen, MD, Palm Desert, CA, unpublished data presented at the American Association of Nurse Anesthetists fall course, 2004).

Hyaluronic Acid-Based Scaffold

Hyalograft C (Fidia Advanced Biopolymers, Abano Terme, Italy) is a graft that uses a hyaluronic acid-based scaffold. The scaffold is biocompatible and fully resorbs in 3 months with controllable degradation rates; the main by-product is hyaluronan, a sugar.[45] Cells are isolated and expanded as in regular ACI and then absorbed onto the scaffold at a density of 1 million cells/cm^2, resulting in a total of 4 million seeded cells/cm^2 per graft.[45] Basic science studies have shown that this scaffold promotes maintenance of a chondrocyte phenotype with a decrease in type I collagen and *Sox9* production as well as an increase in type II collagen and aggrecans.[54] Adhesive properties of the graft hold it in place.

Giannini and associates[55] have extensive experience using the Hyalograft C scaffold. In a recent study, 46 patients with a mean age of 31 years (range, 20 to 47 years) were surgically treated for posttraumatic talar dome lesions. Ankle arthroscopy was performed first with cartilage harvested from the detached osteochondral fragment or margins of the lesion. Chondrocytes were then cultured and implanted on a Hyalograft C scaffold. In the second step of surgery, the Hyalograft C membrane was arthroscopically implanted into the lesion. Lesions larger than 5 mm deep were first filled with autologous cancellous bone. The results showed a preoperative AOFAS score of 57; at 12-month follow-up, the mean AOFAS score was 87, and at 36 months, the mean score was 90. Histologic examinations revealed hyaline-like cartilage regeneration.

Polymer Fleeces

Polylactic acid and polyglycolic acid polymer fleeces are available in two sizes, 2 × 1 cm and 3 × 2 cm. These scaffolds are implanted arthroscopically.[45] Erggelet and associates[56] used polylactic acid and polyglycolic acid scaffolds in the knees of 102 patients and reported an improvement in Lysholm scores (from 48 to 78), the Knee Injury and Osteoarthritis

Outcome Score quality of life rating (from 29 to 51), and Cincinnati Knee Rating Scale scores (from 3.7 to 6.4). However, published results are still pending; to date there are no known studies regarding the use of these scaffolds to treat lesions of the talus.

Table 4
Guideline for Treating Osteochondral Talar Lesions

Lesion	Treatment
Type 1: asymptomatic lesion, low-symptomatic lesion	Conservative
Type 2: symptomatic lesion ≤ 10 mm	Débridement and drilling/microfracture
Type 3: symptomatic lesion 11 to 14 mm	Consider débridement and drilling/microfracture, fixation, an osteochondral graft, or ACI
Type 4: symptomatic lesion ≥ 15 mm*	Consider fixation, graft, or ACI
Type 5: large talar cystic lesion*	Consider retrograde drilling ± bone graft or ACI with a sandwich procedure or osteochondral transplant
Type 6: secondary lesion*	Consider osteochondral transplant

*For types 4 through 6, débridement and bone marrow stimulation can be considered a treatment option.

Other Technologies

Cartipatch (TBF Tissue Engineering, Bron, France) is a monolayer expanded cartilage cell product that is combined with a novel alginate-agarose hydrogel to improve cell phenotypic stability and promote the ease of surgical handling.[57] Implantation into the knee has achieved significant clinical improvement at 2-year follow-up with predominantly hyaline cartilage-like repair tissue.[57]

NeoCart (developed at the Brigham and Woman's Hospital in conjunction with Histogenics, Waltham, MA) is a novel technology in which a patient's chondrocytes are grown in a two-dimensional culture in vitro. These autologous chondrocytes are then placed in a bovine collagen gel/sponge construct and treated in vitro with hydrostatic pressure, followed by static culture before implantation. This three-dimensional culture occurs under dynamic as well as static conditions. The result is that the chondrocytes redifferentiate and produce extracellular matrix, mostly type II collagen, in addition to significantly increasing the glycosaminoglycans and DNA content compared with a static culture. The construct is fixed with proprietary collagen/polyethylene glycol-based glue only. A phase I FDA study of 10 patients treated with NeoCart has been completed at the University of California, San Francisco, and Oregon Health and Sciences University. The authors reported promising results.[45] A phase II multicenter trial comparing the safety and preliminary efficacy of NeoCart with those of conventional microfracture therapy is beginning in the United States.[58]

Cartilage regeneration systems (CaReS; Ars Arthro AG, Esslingen, Germany) uses an acellular three-dimensional collagen matrix seeded with cartilage secured on the cartilage defect with fibrin glue. No studies have been published to date, but early investigations are being conducted at the Cleveland Clinic.[59]

Another new technology called Chondrosphere (Co.don AG, Teltow, Germany) uses autologous in vitro, de novo synthesized cartilage aggregated together with cultured, load-differentiated, highly concentrated viable chondrocytes. Chondrosphere adheres and remodels at the cartilage defect, followed by active migration of cartilage cells.[59]

Future Scaffolds

Bioactive and spatially oriented scaffolds are two new approaches being investigated that could dramatically improve clinical results.[45] Bioactive scaffolds provide signals (such as growth factors) to chondrocytes that promote proliferation and production of extracellular matrix components.[60,61] Spatially oriented scaffolds direct cells to create cartilage tissue with a spatial structure similar to that of normal articular cartilage.[62,63]

Third Generation ACI

Third generation ACI is autologous de novo cartilage transplantation in which no scaffold is present. As the optimal scaffold for cartilage repair has yet to be developed, scaffold-free cartilage implants may prevent the complications caused by suboptimal scaffolds.[64] Results of a recent study on cartilage defects in the femoral condyle of sheep showed that third generation ACI is a promising development in the field of biologic cartilage regeneration.[64]

Summary

The search for the ideal technique to treat osteochondral lesions of the talus is ongoing. No technique replicates the structure and function of hyaline cartilage. The authors recommend that the size and nature of the lesion be used as the main indication for treatment[65] (Table 4). Future research will determine if newer techniques will solve this challenging therapeutic dilemma.

References

1. Ray RB, Coughlin EJ: Osteochondritis dissecans of the talus. *J Bone Joint Surg* 1947;29:697-710.
2. Berndt AL, Harty M: Transchondral fractures (osteochondritis dissecans) of the talus. *J Bone Joint Surg Am* 1959; 41:988-1020.
3. Ferkel RD, Sgaglione NA: Arthroscopic treatment of osteochondral lesions of the talus: Long term results. *Orthop Trans* 1993-1994;17:1011.
4. Anderson IF, Crichton KJ, Grattan-Smith T, Cooper RA, Brazier D: Osteochondral fractures of the dome of the talus. *J Bone Joint Surg Am* 1989; 71:1143-1152.
5. Dipola JD, Nelson DW, Colville MR: Characterizing osteochondral lesions by magnetic resonance imaging. *Arthroscopy* 1991;7:101-104.
6. Ferkel RD, Zanotti RM, Komenda GA, et al: Arthroscopic treatment of chronic osteochondral lesions of the talus. *Am J Sports Med* 2008;36:1750-1762.
7. Ferkel RD: *Arthroscopic Surgery: The Foot and Ankle*. Philadelphia, PA, Lippincott, 1996.
8. Verhagen RA, Struijs PA, Bossuyt PM, van Dijk CN: Systematic review of treatment strategies for osteochondral defects of the talar dome. *Foot Ankle Clin* 2003;8:233-242.
9. Flick AB, Gould N: Osteochondritis dissecans of the talus (transchondral fractures of the talus): Review of the literature and new surgical approach for medial dome lesions. *Foot Ankle* 1985;5:165-185.
10. Angermann P, Jensen P: Osteochondritis dissecans of the talus: Long-term results of surgical treatment. *Foot Ankle* 1989;10:161-163.
11. Kelbérine F, Frank A: Arthroscopic treatment of osteochondral lesions of the talar dome: A retrospective study of 48 cases. *Arthroscopy* 1999;15:77-84.
12. Ogilvie-Harris DJ, Sarrosa EA: Arthroscopic treatment of osteochondritis dissecans of the talus. *Arthroscopy* 1999;15:805-808.
13. Takao M, Uchio Y, Kakimaru H, Kumahashi N, Ochi M: Arthroscopic drilling with debridement of remaining cartilage for osteochondral lesions of the talar dome in unstable ankles. *Am J Sports Med* 2004;32:332-336.
14. Gobbi A, Francisco RA, Lubowitz JH, Allegra F, Canata G: Osteochondral lesions of the talus: Randomized controlled trial comparing chondroplasty, microfracture, and osteochondral autograft transplantation. *Arthroscopy* 2006;22:1085-1092.
15. Knutsen G, Drogset JO, Engebretsen L, et al: A randomized trial comparing autologous chondrocyte implantation with microfracture: Findings at five years. *J Bone Joint Surg Am* 2007;89:2105-2112.
16. Giannini S, Vannini F: Operative treatment of osteochondral lesions of the talar dome: Current concepts review. *Foot Ankle Int* 2004;25:168-175.
17. Stone JW: Osteochondral lesions of the talar dome. *J Am Acad Orthop Surg* 1996;4:63-73.
18. Konig F: Uber freie koper in den gelenken. *Dtsch Z Chir* 1888;27:90-109.
19. Scranton PE Jr, McDermott JE: Treatment of type V osteochondral lesions of the talus with ipsilateral knee osteochondral grafts. *Foot Ankle Int* 2001;22:380-384.
20. Hepple S, Winson IG, Glew D: Osteochondral lesions of the talus: A revised classification. *Foot Ankle Int* 1999;20:789-793.
21. Ferkel RD: Arthroscopic treatment of osteochondral lesions, soft-tissue impingement and loose bodies, in Pfeffer GB, ed: *Chronic Ankle Pain in the Athlete*. Rosemont, IL, American Academy of Orthopaedic Surgeons, 2000, pp 43-70.
22. Scranton PE Jr, Frey CC, Feder KS: Outcome of osteochondral autograft transplantation for type-V cystic osteochondral lesions of the talus. *J Bone Joint Surg Br* 2006;88:614-619.
23. Robinson DE, Winson IG, Harries WJ, Kelly AJ: Arthroscopic treatment of osteochondral lesions of the talus. *J Bone Joint Surg Br* 2003;85:989-993.
24. Kolker D, Murray M, Wilson M: Osteochondral defects of the talus treated with autologous bone grafting. *J Bone Joint Surg Br* 2004;86: 521-526.
25. Borazjani BH, Chen AC, Bae WC, et al: Effect of impact on chondrocyte viability during insertion of human osteochondral grafts. *J Bone Joint Surg Am* 2006;88:1934-1943.
26. Fitzpatrick PL, Morgan DA: Fresh osteochondral allografts: A 6-10-year review. *Aust N Z J Surg* 1998;68:573-579.
27. Beaver RJ, Mahomed M, Backstein D, Davis A, Zukor DJ, Gross AE: Fresh osteochondral allografts for post-traumatic defects in the knee: A survivorship analysis. *J Bone Joint Surg Br* 1992;74:105-110.
28. Malinin T, Temple HT, Buck BE: Transplantation of osteochondral allografts after cold storage. *J Bone Joint Surg Am* 2006;88:762-770.
29. Kumai T, Takahura Y, Higashiyama I, Tamai S: Arthroscopic drilling for the treatment of osteochondral lesions of the talus. *J Bone Joint Surg Am* 1999; 81:1229-1235.
30. Smith AV: Survival of frozen chondrocytes isolated from cartilage of adult mammals. *Nature* 1965;205: 782-784.
31. Brittberg M, Lindahl A, Nilsson A, Ohlsson C, Isaksson O, Peterson L: Treatment of deep cartilage defects in the knee with autologous chondrocyte transplantation. *N Engl J Med* 1994;331:889-895.
32. Ferkel RD, Sgaglione NA, Del Pizzo W: Arthroscopic treatment of osteochondral lesions of the talus: Techniques and results. *Orthop Trans* 1990;14:172.
33. Buckwalter JA: Articular cartilage injuries. *Clin Orthop Relat Res* 2002; 402 :21-37.

34. Baums MH, Heidrich G, Schultz W, Steckel H, Kahl E, Klingler HM: The surgical technique of autologous chondrocyte transplantation of the talus with use of a periosteal graft: Surgical technique. *J Bone Joint Surg Am* 2007;89:170-182.

35. Giannini S, Buda R, Grigolo B, Vannini F, De Franceschi L, Facchini A: The detached osteochondral fragment as a source of cells for autologous chondrocyte implantation (ACI) in the ankle joint. *Osteoarthritis Cartilage* 2005;13:601-607.

36. Sammarco GJ, Makwana NK: Treatment of talar osteochondral lesions using local osteochondral graft. *Foot Ankle Int* 2002;23:693-698.

37. Bazaz R, Ferkel RD: Treatment of osteochondral lesions of the talus with autologous chondrocyte implantation. *Tech Foot Ankle Surg* 2004;3: 45-52.

38. Nam EK, Ferkel RD, Applegate GR: Autologous chondrocyte implantation of the ankle: A 2- to 5-year follow-up. *Am J Sports Med* 2009;37: 274-284.

39. Giannini S, Vannini F, Buda R: Osteoarticular grafts in the treatment of OCD of the talus: Mosaicplasty versus autologous chondrocyte transplantation. *Foot Ankle Clin* 2002;7: 621-633.

40. Petersen L, Brittberg M, Lindahl A: Autologous chondrocyte transplantation of the ankle. *Foot Ankle Clin* 2003;8:291-303.

41. Whittaker JP, Smith G, Makwana N, et al: Early results of autologous chondrocyte implantation in the talus. *J Bone Joint Surg Br* 2005;87: 179-183.

42. Baums MH, Heidrich G, Schultz W, Steckel H, Kahl E, Klingler HM: Autologous chondrocyte transplantation for treating cartilage defects of the talus. *J Bone Joint Surg Am* 2006;88:303-308.

43. Wood JJ, Malek MA, Frassica FJ, et al: Autologous cultured chondrocytes: Adverse events reported to United States Food and Drug Administration. *J Bone Joint Surg Am* 2006;88: 503-507.

44. Kreuz PC, Steinwachs M, Erggelet C, et al: Classification of graft hypertrophy after autologous chondrocyte implantation of full-thickness chondral defects in the knee. *Osteoarthritis Cartilage* 2007;15:1339-1347.

45. Safran MR, Kim H, Zaffagnini S: The use of scaffolds in the management of articular cartilage injury. *J Am Acad Orthop Surg* 2008;16:306-311.

46. Gooding CR, Bartlett W, Bentley G, Skinner JA, Carrington R, Flanagan A: A prospective, randomised study comparing two techniques of autologous chondrocyte implantation for osteochondral defects in the knee: Periosteum covered versus type I/III collagen covered. *Knee* 2006;13: 203-210.

47. Robertson WB, Fick D, Wood DJ, Linklater JM, Zheng MH, Ackland TR: MRI and clinical evaluation of collagen-covered autologous chondrocyte implantation (CACI) at two years. *Knee* 2007;14:117-127.

48. Steinwachs M, Kreuz PC: Autologous chondrocyte implantation in chondral defects of the knee with a type I/III collagen membrane: A prospective study with a 3-year follow-up. *Arthroscopy* 2007;23:381-387.

49. Krishnan SP, Skinner JA, Carrington RW, Flanagan AM, Briggs TW, Bentley G: Collagen-covered autologous chondrocyte implantation for osteochondritis dissecans of the knee: Two- to seven-year results. *J Bone Joint Surg Br* 2006;88:203-205.

50. Masuda K, Sah R, Hejna M, Thonar E: A novel two-step method for the formation of tissue-engineered cartilage by mature bovine chondrocytes: The alginate-recovered-chondrocyte (ARC) method. *J Orthop Res* 2003;21:139-148.

51. Guillen P, Abelow SP, Fernandez Jaen T: Abstract: Matrix/ membranous autologous chondrocyte implantation for the treatment of large chondral defects in the knee and ankle, in *Final Program*. Rosemont, IL, American Orthopaedic Society for Sports Medicine, 2005, p 145.

52. Ronga M, Grassi FA, Montoli C, et al: Treatment of chondral defects by matrix-guided autologous chondrocyte implantation (MACI). *Foot Ankle Surg* 2005;11:29-31.

53. Basad E, Sturz H, Steinmeyer J: Treatment of chondral defects by matrix-guided autologous chondrocyte implantation (MACI), in Hendrich C, Noth U, Eulert J, eds: *Cartilage Surgery and Future Perspectives*. Berlin, Germany, Springer-Verlag, 2003, pp 49-56.

54. Grigolo B, Lisignoli G, Piacentini A, et al: Evidence for redifferentiation of human chondrocytes grown on a hyaluronan-based biomaterial (HYAff11): Molecular, immunohistochemical and ultrastructural analysis. *Biomaterials* 2002;23:1187-1195.

55. Giannini S, Buda R, Vannini F, Di Caprio F, Grigolo B: Arthroscopic autologous chondrocyte implantation in osteochondral lesions of the talus: Surgical technique and results. *Am J Sports Med* 2008;36:873-880.

56. Erggelet C, Sittinger M, Lahm A: The arthroscopic implantation of autologous chondrocytes for the treatment of full-thickness cartilage defects of the knee joint. *Arthroscopy* 2003;19: 108-110.

57. Selmi TAS, Verdonk P, Chambat P, et al: Autologous chondrocyte implantation in a novel alginate-agarose hydrogel: Outcome at two years. *J Bone Joint Surg Br* 2008;90:597-604.

58. Kim HT, Zaffagnini S, Mizuno S, Abelow S, Safran MR: A peek into the possible future of management of articular cartilage injuries: Gene therapy and scaffolds for cartilage repair. *J Orthop Sports Phys Ther* 2006;36:765-773.

59. Zanasi S, Brittberg M, Marcacci M: *Basic Science, Clinical Repair and Reconstruction of Articular Cartilage Defects: Current Status and Prospects*. Bologna, Italy, Timeo, 2006.

60. Strauss EJ, Goodrich LR, Chen CT, Hidaka C, Nixon AJ: Biochemical and biomechanical properties of le-

sion and adjacent articular cartilage after chondral defect repair in an equine model. *Am J Sports Med* 2005; 33:1647-1653.

61. Chou CH, Cheng WT, Lin CC, Chang CH, Tsai CC, Lin FH: TGF-beta1 immobilized tri-co-polymer for articular cartilage tissue engineering. *J Biomed Mater Res B Appl Biomater* 2006;77:338-348.

62. Zehbe R, Libera J, Gross U, Schubert H: Short-term human chondrocyte culturing on oriented collagen coated gelatine scaffolds for cartilage replacement. *Biomed Mater Eng* 2005; 15:445-454.

63. Woodfield TB, Van Blitterswijk CA, De Wijn J, Sims TJ, Hollander AP, Riesle J: Polymer scaffolds fabricated with pore-size gradients as a model for studying the zonal organization within tissue-engineered cartilage constructs. *Tissue Eng* 2005;11: 1297-1311.

64. Jubel A, Andermahr J, Schiffer G, et al: Transplantation of de novo scaffold-free cartilage implants into sheep knee chondral defects. *Am J Sports Med* 2008;36:1555-1564.

65. Zengerink M, Szerb I, Hangody L, Dopirak RM, Ferkel RD, van Dijk CN: Current concepts: Treatment of osteochondral ankle defects. *Foot Ankle Clin* 2006;11:331-359.

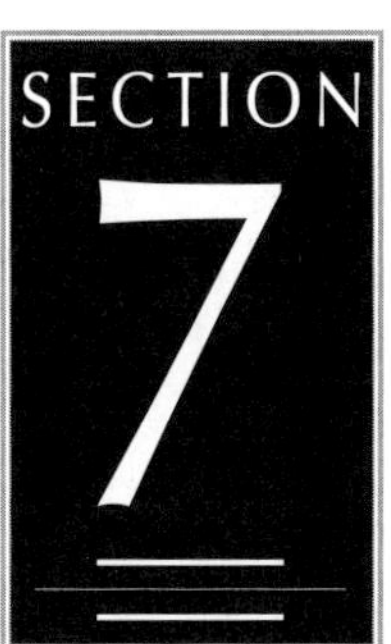

Spine

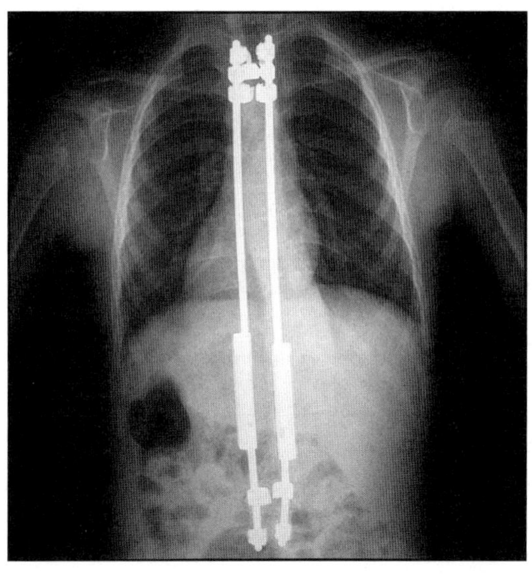

Approaches for the Very Young Child With Spinal Deformity: What's New and What Works

Behrooz A. Akbarnia, MD
Laurel C. Blakemore, MD
Robert M. Campbell Jr, MD
John P. Dormans, MD, FACS

Abstract

Treating very young children with spinal deformities is challenging and complex, and it entails risks. The consequences of surgical treatment can be profound, with lifelong implications. The recent focus on "fusionless" surgery and spinal column lengthening strategies, such as growing rod instrumentation and the use of a Vertical Expandable Prosthetic Titanium Rib, illustrate the current understanding of the importance of spinal growth and lung development in infants and young children.

Instr Course Lect 2010;59:407-424.

Treating children who have a spinal deformity is complex and entails challenges and risks. The surgical outcome can have profound, lifelong implications for the patient. The recent focus on "fusionless" surgery and strategies for spinal column lengthening, such as the use of growing rod instrumentation or the Vertical Expandable Prosthetic Titanium Rib (VEPTR; Synthes Spine, West Chester, PA), emphasizes the recognition of the importance of spinal growth and lung development in children 16 years or younger. This chapter reviews the current knowledge and treatment options for young patients with spinal deformity.

Indications, Applications, and Clinical Experience With Growing Rods

The surgical treatment of progressive, early onset scoliosis is challenging and requires expertise, not only in the management of the spinal deformity but also for associated conditions such as pulmonary disorders, which commonly occur in these children. Surgery should be considered when nonsurgical management, including casting and bracing, is not indicated or fails to arrest the progression of the deformity. Fusion options include spinal fusion (posterior, anterior, or combined) and hemiepiphysiodesis. Nonfusion methods continue to evolve and are primarily aimed at curve correction while simultaneously preserving, directing, and/or stimulating spine and chest wall growth.[1-3]

Dr. Akbarnia or an immediate family member serves as a board member, owner, officer, or committee member of the Scoliosis Research Society, the Orthopaedic Research and Education Foundation, the Growing Spine Study Group, the San Diego Center for Spinal Disorders, and the San Diego Spine Foundation; has received royalties from DePuy and K2M; is a member of a speakers' bureau or has made paid presentations on behalf of Nuvasive, Stryker, K2M, and DePuy; serves as a paid consultant to or is an employee of DePuy, Nuvasive, K2M, and Ellipse Technologies; has received research or institutional support from DePuy, Medtronic Sofamor Danek, and Nuvasive; and has stock or stock options held in Nuvasive and Allez Spine. Dr. Blakemore or an immediate family member serves as a paid consultant to or is an employee of Globus Medical, OrthoPediatrics, and K2M. Dr. Campbell has received royalties from Synthes and is a member of a speakers' bureau or has made paid presentations on behalf Synthes. Dr. Dormans or an immediate family member serves as a board member, owner, officer, or committee member of the Pediatric Orthopaedic Society of North America, Orthopaedic Overseas, the American Academy of Orthopaedic Surgeons, the National Children's Cancer Study Group, and SICOT USA; serves as an unpaid consultant to Medtronic and Globus Medical; has received research or institutional support from Brookes Publishing, Elsevier, Mosby, and Synthes; and has received nonincome support (such as equipment or services), commercially derived honoraria, or other non–research-related funding (such as paid travel) from Brookes Publishing, Mosby, and Elsevier.

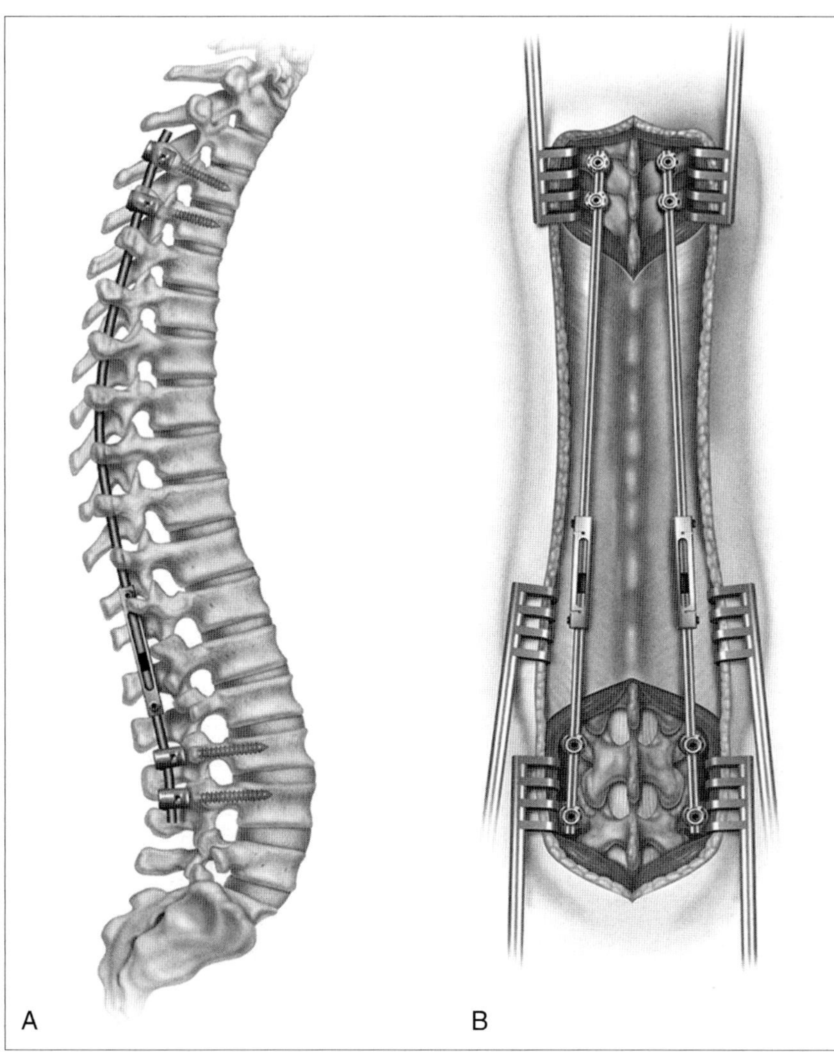

Figure 1 Lateral **(A)** and AP **(B)** illustrations of the dual growing rod technique for treating early onset scoliosis. Both hooks and screws can be used in upper and/or lower foundations. A transverse connector is recommended between the two rods when an all-hook foundation is used.

These procedures are divided in three groups: (1) distraction-based procedures using single or dual growing rods and VEPTR where the correction is achieved mainly by distraction; (2) growth-guided procedures such as Luque trolley or Shilla procedures in which the growth is directed but the spine but is not distracted; and (3) compression-based anterior procedures such as stapling or tethering, which have been used in older children.

Dual Rod Technique

In the dual rod technique, subperiosteal dissection, through one or two midline skin incisions, is performed only at the upper and lower anchor sites of the construct. At the upper end, hooks and/or screws are placed in a claw pattern spanning two or three vertebral levels (depending on the anatomic site and bone quality) to allow for maximal stability. Similar pedicle screw or hook anchors are used at the caudal end. These sites are called the foundations of the construct. Rods in each side are then measured and cut into upper and lower segments, contoured, placed on each side of the spine, and connected to the foundations (Figure 1). A transverse connector is added at the level of each foundation, especially when hooks alone are used. Mahar and associates[4] reported that transverse connectors add significant stability to the construct in the absence of pedicle screws. Limited fusions are performed at the site of the foundations with the use of local bone or synthetic graft. The upper and lower rods are linked by two tandem connectors placed at the thoracolumbar junction or by two or more side-to-side connectors. Rods can be placed submuscularly or subcutaneously; however, recent studies report more wound-related complications with no significant benefits when rods are placed subcutaneously (BA Akbarnia, MD, and associates, San Diego, CA, unpublished data, 2008). Bracing is typically used for 6 months until solid fusion is achieved, after which it is discontinued unless there is a specific concern about bone quality or the stability of the construct (Figure 2).

After initial placing of the construct, lengthening procedures are performed at 6-month intervals. Patients treated with more frequent lengthening procedures (≤ 6 months) have shown better correction of scoliosis and greater spinal growth compared with those treated with less frequent lengthening procedures (> 6 months)[5] (Figure 3). In a study by the Growing Spine Study Group, continuous T1 through S1 growth was confirmed with repeated lengthening procedures; however, this gain tends to decrease with each subsequent lengthening procedure over time (DL Skaggs, MD, and associates, Los Angeles, CA, unpublished data, 2009). Spinal cord monitoring is used for patients treated with growing rod surgery. Sankar and associates[6] reported a 0.8%, 0.6%, and 0.3% incidence of transient neurologic complications for the initial placement of the construct, implant exchange, and the lengthening procedure, respectively. No permanent neurologic changes were reported in 782 growing rod surgeries.

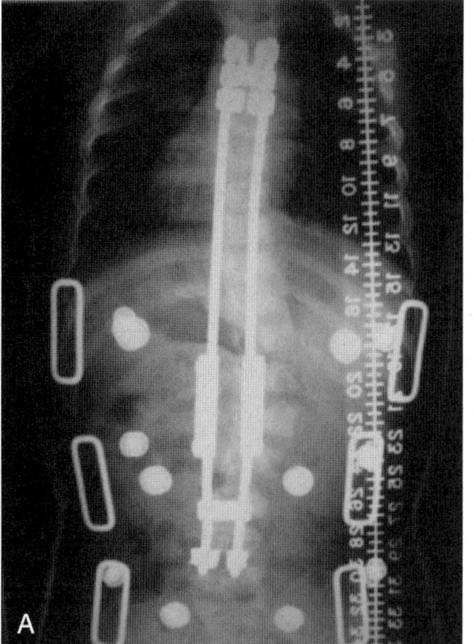

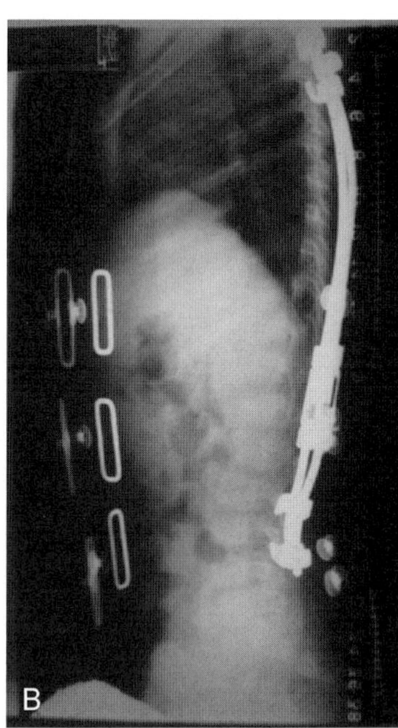

Figure 2 Postoperative AP **(A)** and lateral **(B)** radiographs of the spine of a child with scoliosis taken after initial surgical treatment with the dual rod technique. The radiographs were taken with the patient in a brace, which will be worn for 6 months.

Results

A 2005 study reported initial minimum 2-year follow-up data from the Growing Spine Study Group on patients with early onset scoliosis treated with the dual growing rod technique.[3] The mean age of patients at the time of the initial surgery was 5.4 years; patients had a mean of 6.6 lengthening procedures during the treatment period. The mean Cobb angle was 82° preoperatively, 38° at the initial postoperative visit, and 36° at the most recent follow-up or after final fusion. Growth of the spine approached normal levels with an average of 1.21 cm per year. Seven patients who were followed to final fusion had a mean of 11.8 cm of total spinal growth during treatment.

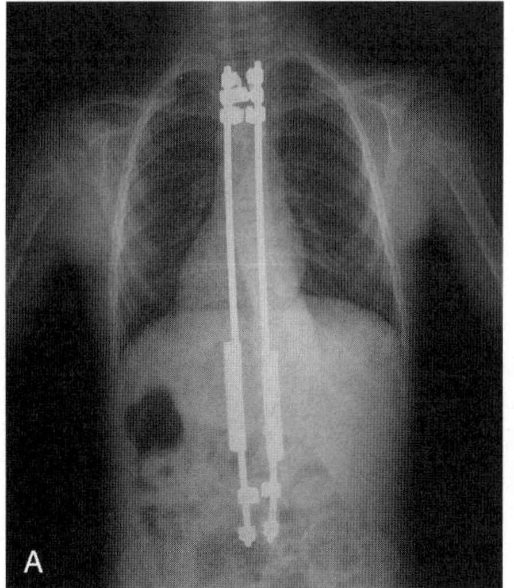

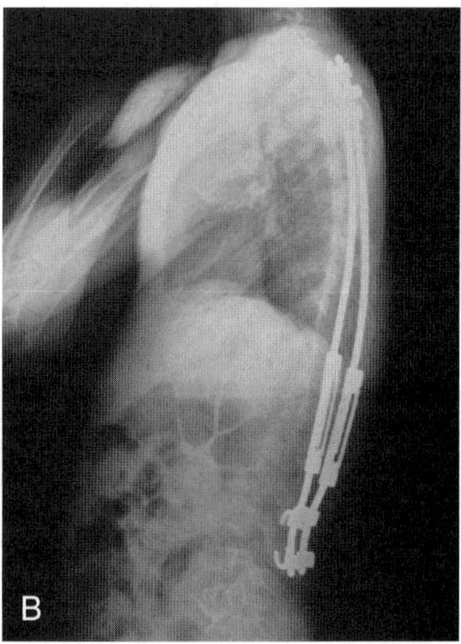

Figure 3 AP **(A)** and lateral **(B)** radiographs of the patient shown in Figure 2 after 52 months of treatment and eight lengthening procedures.

A study by Thompson and associates[7] also supports the use of dual rod instrumentation. Twenty-eight patients in the study were divided into three groups based on treatment with (1) a single rod with anterior and posterior apical fusion (5 patients), (2) a single rod without apical fusion (16 patients), and (3) a dual rod without apical fusion (7 patients). All patients were followed until final fusion was achieved. Although the authors determined that the single and dual rod techniques were effective at correcting the curve and allowing spinal growth, the dual rod system not only improved the curve but also better maintained the initial correction and facilitated increased spinal growth. Because short apical fusion was associated with curve stiffening, the crankshaft phenomenon, and a higher incidence of complications, the authors questioned the effect of combining apical fusion with either of the growing rod techniques in treating patients with early onset scoliosis.

Complications

In a recent study of 143 patients treated with 910 growing rod surgeries, Bess and associates[8] reported 177 complications in 83 patients. The complication rate per surgery was less than 20%. Fewer patients treated with dual rod instrumentation had implant-related unplanned surgeries than patients treated with a single rod. There also were fewer total implant-related unplanned surgeries in those treated with dual rods versus single rods. Subcutaneous placement of the rod resulted in more complications per patient and more wound problems than submuscular placement. In the dual rod group, subcutaneous placement of the rods resulted in more complications per patient, including wound complications, prominent implants, and more instances of implant-related unplanned surgery than in those with submuscular rod placement. It was concluded that the complication rate per growing rod procedure was comparable to the rate in other surgical treatments of scoliosis. Complications are likely caused by the multiple procedures that are necessary with current growing rod techniques.[8]

Contraindications for Treatment With Growing Rod Techniques

The goals of growing rod treatment are to allow spine and thoracic growth while correcting and/or maintaining the deformity. These techniques should be avoided if these goals cannot be achieved. Based on the initial experience of the chapter's authors and short-term follow-up results, growing rod techniques are contraindicated in children with very stiff congenital curves with rib fusions and thoracic insufficiency, older children with minimal remaining growth, and children who are too young for instrumentation or have very soft bone. Curve flexibility can be increased by applying preoperative traction or using various methods of surgical release. This treatment method is complex and requires an experienced surgeon and a patient with an informed and cooperative family. Patients with severe congenital curves with fused ribs and thoracic insufficiency syndrome may be candidates for other treatment methods, such as VEPTR. The final treatment decision should be based on an assessment of the risks and benefits and discussions with the patient's family.

Some patients with deformities, such as congenital anomalies of the spine, may not have significant remaining growth potential; however, in select patients, the growing rod technique may prevent the deformity from worsening and provide ongoing internal support. The first report of the use of growing rods in congenital scoliosis from the Growing Spine Study Group showed that growing rods are safe and effective in treating congenital spinal deformities.[9] Mean curves improved from 65° to 45° after the initial treatment and to 47° at the last follow-up or after final fusion was achieved; average spinal growth was 12 mm per year. During the treatment period, complications occurred in 8 of the 19 patients (42%). Although there was less correction obtained at the initial surgery compared with reports of the use of this technique in other etiologies, there was minimal loss of correction, near normal growth of the spine, and improvement in the space available for the lungs during the treatment period. There were no neurologic complications in this group of patients with various types of congenital deformities. Growing rod systems also have been successfully used for treating scoliosis in patients with myelomeningocele and Marfan syndrome[10] (R McCarthy, MD, and associates, Little Rock, AR, unpublished data, 2008).

The success of growing rod system procedures can be improved if the patient's family is willing to cooperate with the treatment regimen, is aware of the length of the treatment period, and understands possible complications.

Early onset scoliosis remains one of the most challenging pediatric spinal disorders. Historical data have shown that untreated curves have the potential for serious cardiopulmonary and skeletal complications and even death.[11,12] Observation, casting, orthotic use, traction, and surgical treatment are options for managing early onset scoliosis. Surgical treatment should be considered for patients who do not meet the criteria for observation or orthotic management or those who have been unsuccessfully treated with orthotics.

Although current growing rod techniques attempt to allow spinal growth and prevent curve progression, the patient needs many surgical procedures before definitive spinal fusion. Reducing the frequency of these surgeries or eliminating the need for repeat surgeries without sacrificing growth or correction should be the primary goals of new treatment methods. New techniques are emerging that avoid multiple surgical procedures. The Shilla procedure, developed by McCarthy and associates,[13] attempts to eliminate the need for multiple surgeries while allowing continued spinal growth and correction of the three-dimensional deformity. The apex of the curve is fused; at the upper and lower ends of the rod, the screws are attached but not fixed to the rod to allow the rod to slide with growth of the spine. The goal is to remove the implants after the patient has reached skeletal maturity. This is a growth-directed procedure and does not provide any growth stimulation such as that provided by distraction-based methods; however, the Shilla procedure reduces the number of surgeries required by other techniques. The Shilla procedure is new, and, at this time, no patients have completed treatment. Because there is minimal experience available with anterior fusionless techniques or VEPTR in patients with idiopathic infantile scoliosis or early onset scoliosis without congenital anomalies, the growing rod technique remains the principal surgical option for this patient population. The VEPTR procedure remains an effective treatment method for patients with congenital anomalies, fused ribs, and thoracic insufficiency syndrome.

There is a need for treatments that are less invasive, require fewer surgical procedures, and allow normal spinal growth and correction of the deformity. Self-lengthening rods as well as remotely controlled lengthening techniques are being developed to avoid multiple surgeries. The dual growing rod technique allows minimal restrictions to normal spinal growth and maintains spine and chest wall deformity correction in patients with progressive early onset scoliosis. Future research, with multicenter studies and longer follow-up periods, will attempt to find new solutions in the management of early onset scoliosis.

Definitive Fusion After Treatment With Growing Rods

Submuscular rod instrumentation is a powerful technique for controlling a progressive curve in a child with significant remaining growth. Ideal growth-sparing instrumentation would control alignment of progressive curves; allow the best growth of the spine and thorax, including the heart and lungs; be self-lengthening; and permit the spine to remain flexible at the conclusion of growth. Growing rod instrumentation addresses some of these concerns; however, the ideal timing for growing rod instrumentation is not yet known. The goal is to achieve maximal spinal and pulmonary growth to complete skeletal maturity or to control spinal alignment until spinal fusion would not be detrimental to thoracic growth and pulmonary function.

Estimating Spinal and Pulmonary Growth

When considering converting a growing rod instrumentation system to definitive posterior spinal fusion, the amount of remaining skeletal and thoracic growth should be considered. Traditional estimates of skeletal maturity have included the Risser sign and closure of the triradiate cartilages. More recently, epiphyseal capping has been reported to be an accurate indicator of peak height velocity in adolescent growth in males and females.[14] The thoracic spine grows an average of 1.5 cm a year from birth to age 5 years, 0.6 cm per year from age 5 to up to 10 years, and 1.2 cm per year from age 10 to 16 years.[15] Overall spinal growth in girls from the time of peak height velocity to skeletal maturity is approximately 5.7 cm; in boys, 6.2 cm. Peak height velocity typically occurs between the ages of 11 and 13 years in girls and 13 and 15 years in boys, with a 7.5-cm and an 8.5-cm per year increase in sitting height, respectively.[16] Based on this knowledge of spinal growth, the surgeon must estimate how much spinal shortening would occur with spinal fusion. Winter's formula is commonly used in this assessment.[17] To calculate the shortening effect of spinal fusion, this formula uses a factor of 0.07 multiplied by the number of spinal levels fused multiplied by the usual remaining growth expressed in centimeters. Although this formula can be used to estimate how much spinal height will be lost, it does not aid in determining the overall growth of the thorax.

Another concern of early spinal fusion in terms of trunk alignment is the crankshaft phenomenon, which is described as solid posterior fusion with an increase in the Cobb angle and rib rotation believed to be caused by continued anterior spinal growth. Two studies reported that the crankshaft phenomenon should not occur if the patient is older than 10 years and the triradiate cartilages are closed at the time of spinal fusion.[18,19] Pedicle screw instrumentation may decrease the risk of the crankshaft phenomenon in children who still have significant remaining skeletal growth. In 1996, Kioschos and associates[18] reported that a pedicle screw construct was able to overpower the crankshaft phenomenon in an immature canine model. Suk and associates[20] also described posterior spinal fusion to treat open triradiate cartilages in adolescent children using an all-pedicle screw construct and reported no instances of the crankshaft phenomenon. It is

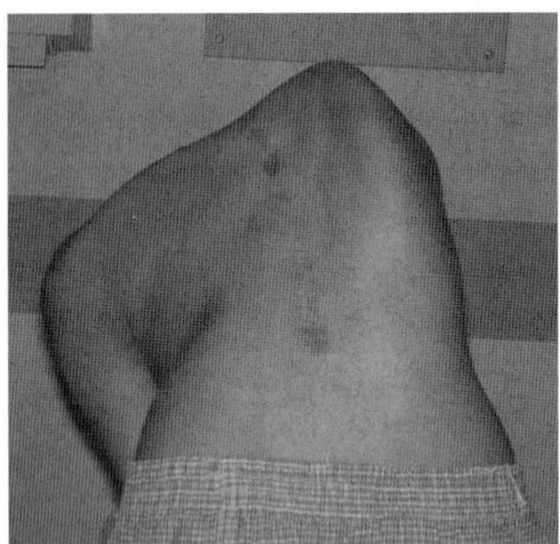

Figure 4 Photograph showing a patient with the crankshaft phenomenon after growing rod placement. The child was lost to follow-up for 2 years after submuscular rod placement in another region. Note the severe "razorback" deformity of the right thoracic cage.

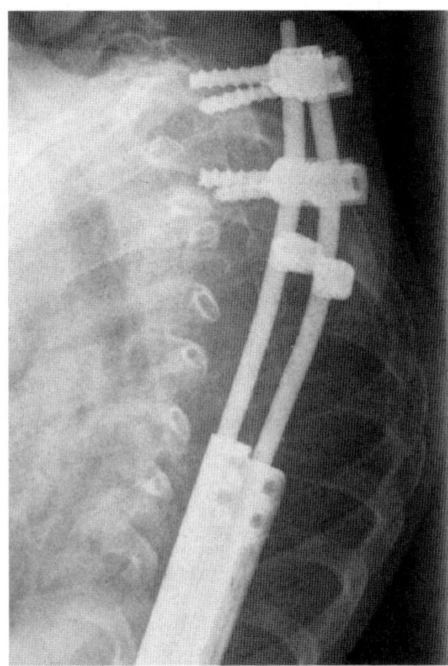

Figure 5 Lateral radiograph of the spine of a patient showing loss of proximal anchor fixation 2 years after initial submuscular rod placement. Note the development of proximal junctional kyphosis in addition to the loss of pedicle screw purchase. The patient's family had noticed increased prominence, but the patient was otherwise asymptomatic.

possible that the use of pedicle screws may not only change the indications for anterior diskectomy and fusion but may lower the age at which this definitive fusion could be safely performed without significant risk of the crankshaft phenomenon (Figure 4).

The amount of spinal growth that will allow normal growth of the thorax and lungs also must be determined. The number of alveoli reach the adult level by 8 years of age. However, by 10 years of age, rib growth is only 30% of its full circumference, and thoracic volume is only 50% of its adult level.[21] The thoracic volume doubles between the ages of 10 and 15 years. The relationship of trunk and spinal height to thoracic growth is unclear. A study by Whittaker and associates[22] suggested that the variation in chest dimensions between ethnic groups had only a trivial effect on lung function. One method, described by Emans and associates,[23] for predicting final chest size in growing children is based on the direct correlation between pelvic width and chest size. This method may be helpful in assessing the child's anticipated final chest size. However, the ultimate goal of treating spinal deformity is to allow normal or near-normal thoracic function. Further studies are needed to determine at what point in a child's growth period a posterior spinal fusion can be performed without a deleterious effect on thoracic functions.

Complications in Growth-Sparing Systems Leading to Spinal Fusion

Submuscular rod instrumentation is associated with several complications, which (when severe or recurrent) can cause the surgeon to abandon the growth-sparing technique in favor of a spinal fusion. These complications are associated with the type of implant and implant profile, loss of fixation (proximally and distally), and the generation of junctional kyphosis. Implant wound complications occur in 10% to 25% of children treated with growing rod instrumentation.[24]

Several contributing factors include the small size of these young children, which requires the relatively superficial positioning of the instrumentation and the resulting poor soft-tissue coverage, and the need for instrumentation in children with altered protective functions, such as those with cerebral palsy, paraplegia, or myelodysplasia. Because submuscular positioning of the rods is associated with fewer implant complications and infections than subcutaneous positioning, submuscular positioning is used by most surgeons. Meticulous attention to protecting soft tissues and using the lowest possible implant profile will help avoid these complications.

Loss of fixation is a relatively common complication in children treated with submuscular rod systems and is associated with poor bone quality; small, short pedicles; thin lamina; and the progressive distraction force in the posterior spine (Figure 5). Because the instrumentation spans an area of unfused spine, active children may displace the instrumentation through repeated micromotion. The repeated distractions may cause the implants to lose position proximally. In some instances, the pedicles or lamina appears to "grow away" from the spinal rods; it is unclear whether this results from a gradual reforming of bone caused by kyphosing stress. There is concern that gradual or sudden pullback of converging screws in the upper thoracic spine

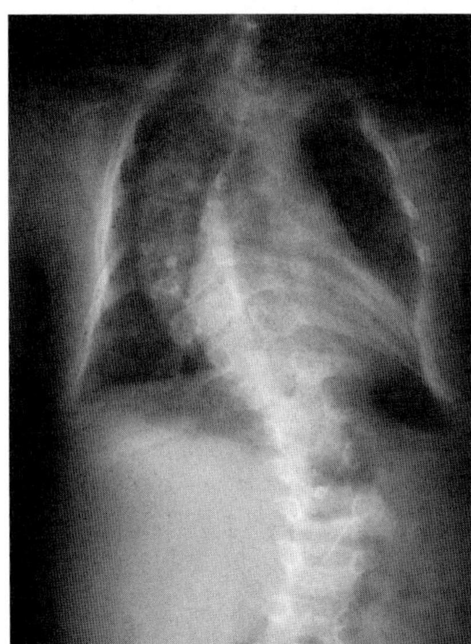

Figure 6 AP radiograph of a patient with congenital scoliosis and fused ribs. The concave hemithorax is reduced in height compared with the convex hemithorax.

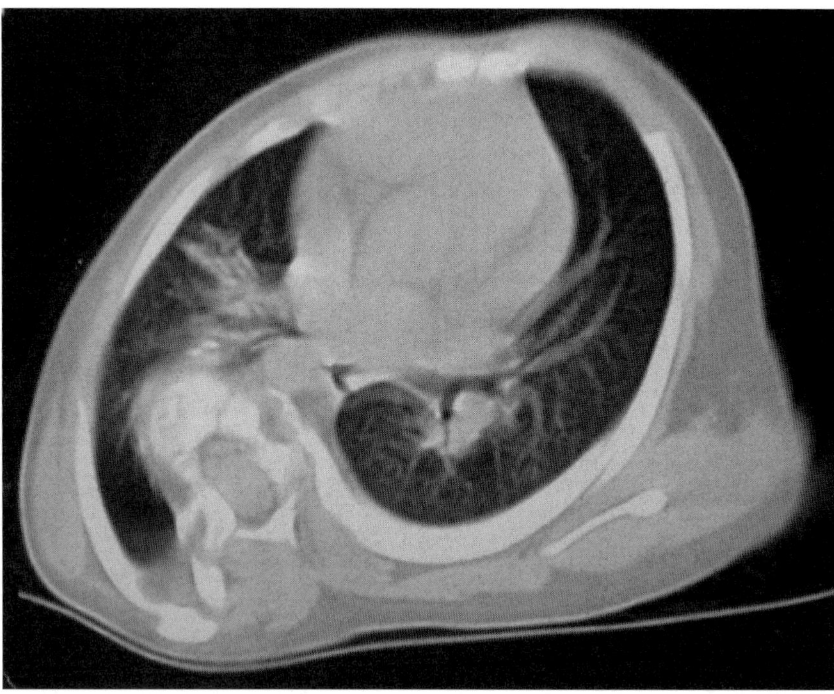

Figure 7 Transverse plane CT scan showing a windswept deformity of the chest. In this patient with scoliosis, the spine has rotated into the convex hemithorax with severe loss of lung volume, contributing to restrictive lung disease. The rib hump also is stiff, limiting the rib cage contribution to respiration. AP radiographs poorly show these important pathologic changes in the chest in patients with scoliosis.

can cause neurologic injury. Thoracic hooks also present some neurologic risk. Hooks can pull completely through the lamina but appear to have some bone underneath, suggesting that there is a gradual remodeling of the upper thoracic fusion mass as proximal kyphosis develops.

Distal loss of fixation is more common in insensate children with poor bone quality and limited anchor points, and it may be particularly problematic in a patient with myelodysplasia because the pedicles are short and splayed. Sacral hooks provide good fixation of the alar wings; however, the hooks can pull through the sacrum and cause skin problems as well as loss of fixation.

There are no definitive guidelines regarding the timing of fusion after growing rod instrumentation. In general, it is preferable to wait until peak height velocity has been achieved and the triradiate cartilages are closed. Other relative indications for proceeding with definitive fusion include gradual curve progression despite regular lengthenings at 6-month intervals, no further lengthening achieved by the time of the current lengthening procedure, and the failure of the technique because of infection or the inability to maintain adequate fixation. Akbarnia and associates[5] reported a mean age of 10 years and 3 months for patients treated with definitive fusion after submuscular dual rod instrumentation. A total of 1.66 cm per year of spinal growth was gained during treatment and the space available for the lung was close to normal on the concave side of the curvature. It appears, therefore, that definitive fusion can be achieved at age 50 years with a low likelihood of significant cardiopulmonary compromise, although outcome studies are needed for confirmation.

Technical Considerations

At the conclusion of treatment with growing rod instrumentation, surgical options include removing the growing rod and inserting new instrumentation to complete a segmental spinal instrumentation and fusion, fusion in situ without reinstrumentation, and removing the rods without performing fusion. The last option is the most appealing because, in theory, this would allow the spine to have more long-term flexibility. However, there are no real data regarding the long-term outcomes of removing rods without fusion. At the time of surgery, most surgeons will plan fusion exploration, revision of the instrumentation, and fusion of all instrumented levels. Occasionally, the

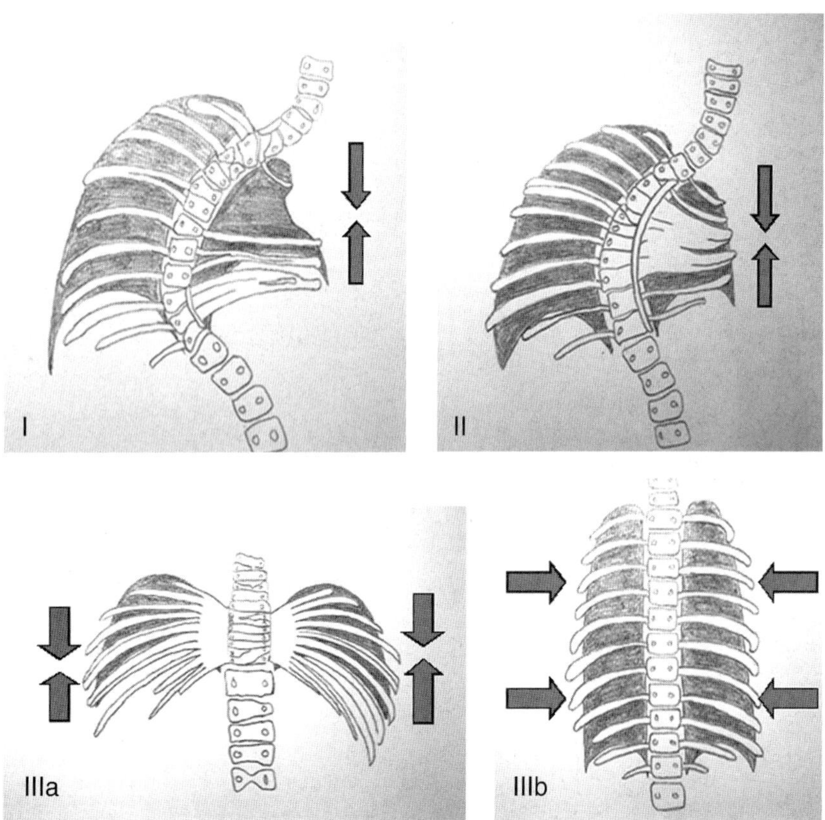

Figure 8 Campbell and associates[25] classification system for volume depletion deformities of the thorax. A type I deformity is unilateral thoracic hypoplasia caused by absent ribs and scoliosis. Type II is unilateral thoracic hypoplasia caused by fused ribs and scoliosis. A type III deformity is the more lethal global thoracic hypoplasia caused by congenital loss of height of the thorax (type IIIa) or loss of width (type IIIb), either from a congenital narrow thorax or from windswept deformity in scoliosis.

presence of significant areas of autofusion and fibrous growth leave the spine quite stiff. In these instances, the growing rod instrumentation can remain in place, and fusion can be completed using decortication and bone grafting without changing the instrumentation or attempting further correction.

To determine the ideal timing for definitive fusion, outcome assessment studies are needed. Spinal growth, thoracic growth and development, and final pulmonary function should be assessed. No studies have been performed to assess the quality of life of children treated with growth-sparing instrumentation followed by definitive fusion. When acceptable chest wall growth and the relationship of chest wall dimensions to pulmonary function are better understood, guidelines can be developed to establish the optimal time frames for discontinuing growing rod instrumentation in the patient's treatment plan.

VEPTR for Treating Thoracic Insufficiency Syndrome

There has been a resurgence of interest in growth-sparing approaches to spinal deformity in young children; these techniques include the use of growing rods and casting and are intended to control scoliosis without spinal fusion until the child is older and better suited for a definitive spinal fusion. The specific goal of these approaches, beyond increasing the length of the spine, is unclear. VEPTR expansion thoracoplasty controls spinal deformity, results in increased spinal length, and treats thoracic insufficiency syndrome (the inability of the thorax to support normal respiration or lung growth).

Historically, scoliosis in the growing child was considered a lateral curvature deformity with no adverse effect on pulmonary function, except in patients with extremely severe curves. Pulmonary function is directly dependent on the thoracic function of the diaphragm and the respiratory expansion of the rib cage. The effect of congenital anomalies (such as rib fusion in patients with congenital scoliosis) on thoracic function and lung growth are almost completely unknown. Although untreated idiopathic adolescent scoliosis with an onset relatively late in the growth phase of the thorax and the lung has little impact on long-term pulmonary function, untreated infantile scoliosis has a profound effect; mortality rates from respiratory insufficiency by age 60 years are 300% greater than normal.[11] Although patients with idiopathic adolescent scoliosis and those with infantile scoliosis have lateral curvature of the spine, there is a profound unrecognized disease component in infantile scoliosis that is responsible for the large increase in pulmonary morbidity and mortality. Campbell and associates[25] reported that, in very young patients, the disease process involves a spinal deformity and a serious three-dimensional thoracic malformation that affects the volume, symmetry, and function of the thorax and indirectly affects lung growth. The concept of thoracic insufficiency syndrome, the inability of the thorax to support normal respiration or lung growth, was introduced to explain how a spinal and chest wall deformity can degrade respiratory function or lung growth, with both affected in most patients. Thoracic insufficiency syndrome is a rare diagnosis, which is applicable only to early onset congenital and idiopathic scoliosis in which there is a concave side, volume-decreasing, chest wall deformity caused by rib fusion (Figure 6), or a transverse plane deformity resulting from the rotation of the spine into the convex hemithorax, with a reduction in lung volume (termed the windswept deformity of the rib cage) (Figure 7). In 2003, Campbell and associates[25] introduced a classification system for thoracic deformity, termed volume depletion deformities of the thorax. This system classified complex spine and chest wall abnormalities into three main categories based on the thoracic deficit and the mechanism causing the loss of lung volume (Figure 8). This biomechanical classification system is useful in analyzing the volume depletion aspect of thoracic insufficiency syndrome in patients and indicates practical treatment options.

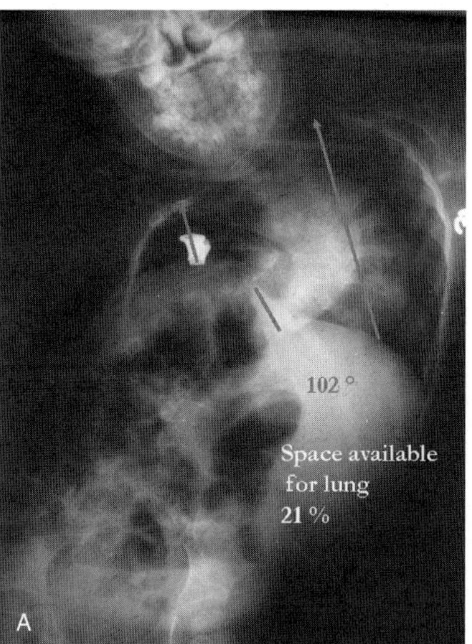

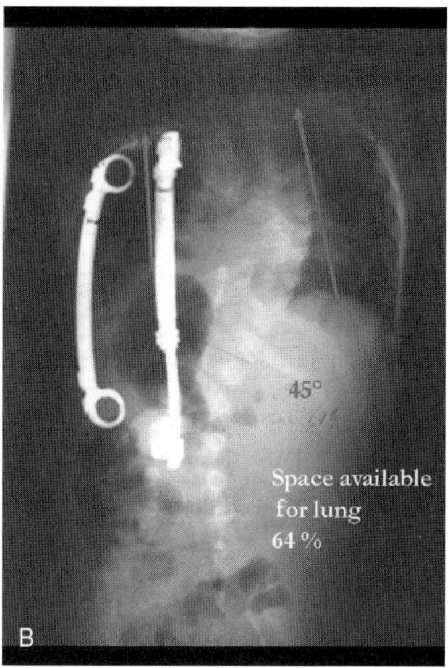

Figure 9 Preoperative **(A)** and postoperative **(B)** radiographs of a patient with fused ribs and scoliosis who was treated with a VEPTR opening wedge thoracostomy. In addition to substantial Cobb angle correction, there is a twofold increase in the space available for the lung, which gives the concave lung more room for potential growth.

VEPTR expansion thoracoplasty is most commonly used to treat congenital scoliosis and fused ribs. The concave hemithorax that is constricted by rib fusion is lengthened through transverse rib osteotomies, which indirectly corrects the scoliosis. The thoracic reconstruction is stabilized by the addition of VEPTRs. To accommodate the patient's growth, outpatient surgery is performed two times per year to expand the devices. The rationale for treatment is that in a growing child, the surgically enlarged hemithorax will likely trigger a lung "stretch reflex," causing the lung to grow to fill the new space with the underlying hemidiaphragm "powering" the larger lung.[26] In a 2004 clinical study, Campbell and associates[27] reported an increased concave lung size on radiographs after expansion thoracoplasty, with an average curve correction of 25° (Figure 9). The space available for the lung, the ratio in height of the concave lung divided by the height of the convex lung (as measured on radiographs), improved on average from 63% to 80%. Of the 22 patients, 7 had gradual asymptomatic superior migration of the VEPTR through the proximal ribs, which was treated by reseating the device into the reformed ribs. The infection rate was 1.9% per procedure. Four patients had skin slough, and two patients had transient brachial plexopathy. Monoplegia, from surgical violation of the canal, developed in one patient but almost completely resolved with time. In another study of the use of VEPTR for congenital scoliosis, Emans and associates[28] reported that the volume of the concave hemithorax improved based on the ratio of lung volumes measured on CT scans.

Because spine fusion was avoided in these patients, additional long-term global thoracic volume gains were probably achieved by the growth in height of the thoracic spine. A three-dimensional CT software program showed a highly significant average increase (7% per year) in the length of the concave side unilateral unsegmented bars.[29] Other clinical expansion thoracoplasty techniques have been developed to treat many other volume

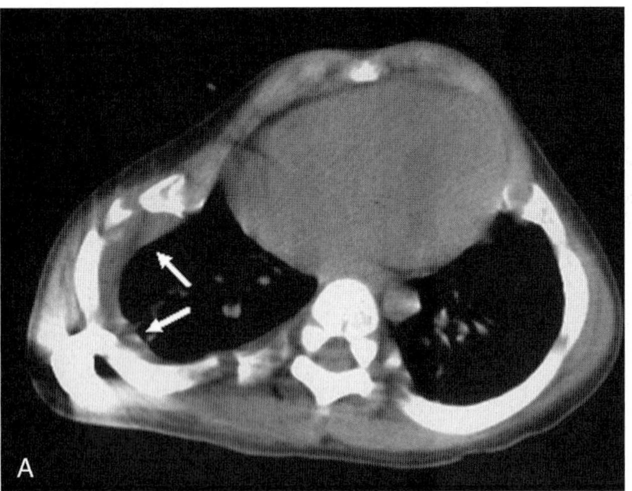

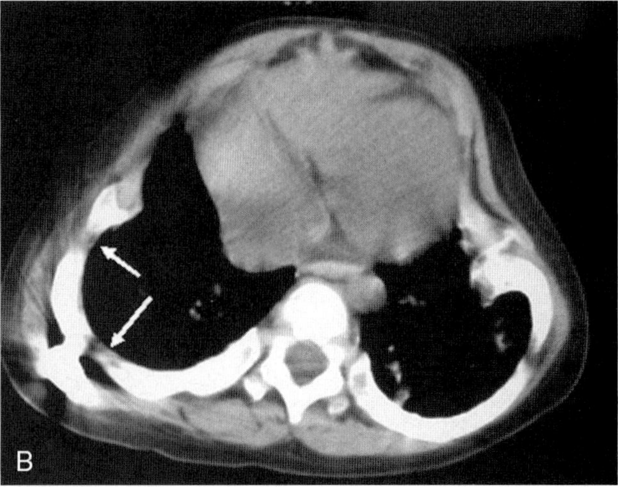

Figure 10 In a patient with Jeune syndrome, severe, often lethal restrictive lung disease occurs secondary to extreme congenital narrowing of the chest. VEPTR expansion thoracoplasty widens the chest by creating an iatrogenic central flail chest from anterior-posterior rib osteotomies of ribs 3 to 8, with a segment of the chest pulled up to a tightly curved VEPTR that functions as an arch of support. **A,** After thoracoplasty, the immediate postoperative CT scan shows the lungs are still the preoperative size, with the new thoracic volume filled with pleural effusion. **B,** At 5-month follow-up, the CT scan shows that the radiolucent lung tissue has expanded to the widened borders of the expanded chest, likely through lung growth.

depletion deformities of the thorax with similar improvements in the radiographic size of the constricted lung.[30] The increase in lung size does not appear to be based on simple postoperative mechanical stretching of the lung. After lateral expansion thoracoplasty of the often lethally narrow thorax in patients with Jeune syndrome, the acute postoperative CT scan showed that the lung did not change from the preoperative size, with the extra thoracic volume filled with pleural effusion; however, within months the lung expanded to fill the new borders of the enlarged thorax[30] (Figure 10).

Patients treated with expansion thoracoplasty appear to clinically improve, with an increase in absolute vital capacity at follow-up, especially if surgery was performed when the patient was younger than 2 years when lung growth is maximal.[26] The defining biologic nature of the radiographic increase in lung size is an enigma. It is unknown if it is an additive phenomenon, with compensatory lung growth from the addition of new alveolar cells; the result of alveolar cell hypertrophy, the mechanism for normal lung growth after the early phase of alveolar cell hyperplasia; or the result of a totally new mechanism for compensatory lung growth. Clinically, any of these mechanisms could contribute to a long-term pulmonary benefit. The absence of an understanding of events at the cellular level has been a handicap to further development of expansion thoracoplasty procedures.

The growth of the spine, the rib cage, and the lungs are interdependent. As was stated previously, the thoracic spine increases in height 1.5 cm/year from birth to 5 years of age, 0.6 cm/year from 5 to 10 years of age, and 1.2 cm/year until skeletal maturity.[15] Total thoracic volume is 6.7% of adult volume at birth, increases to 30% of adult volume at age 5 years, 50% by age 10 years, and then doubles in volume by skeletal maturity.[15] There is also a likely physiologic relationship between growth of the thoracic spine and the rib cage. In a rabbit model, Canavese and associates[31] reported a reduction in anteroposterior diameter of the thorax and a reduction in length of the sternum after a posterior thoracic spinal fusion. Early in life, the lungs increase in size largely by alveolar cell multiplication; although the end point is controversial, the increase probably continues up to age 2 years; then alveolar cell hypertrophy assumes a greater role[26] (Figure 11).[32-37] The complex growth interrelationships between the spine, the rib cage, and the lungs are extremely important but are largely unknown at the present time and require the development of a standard animal study model.

The lungs cannot grow beyond the confines of the physical dimensions of the thorax, which includes

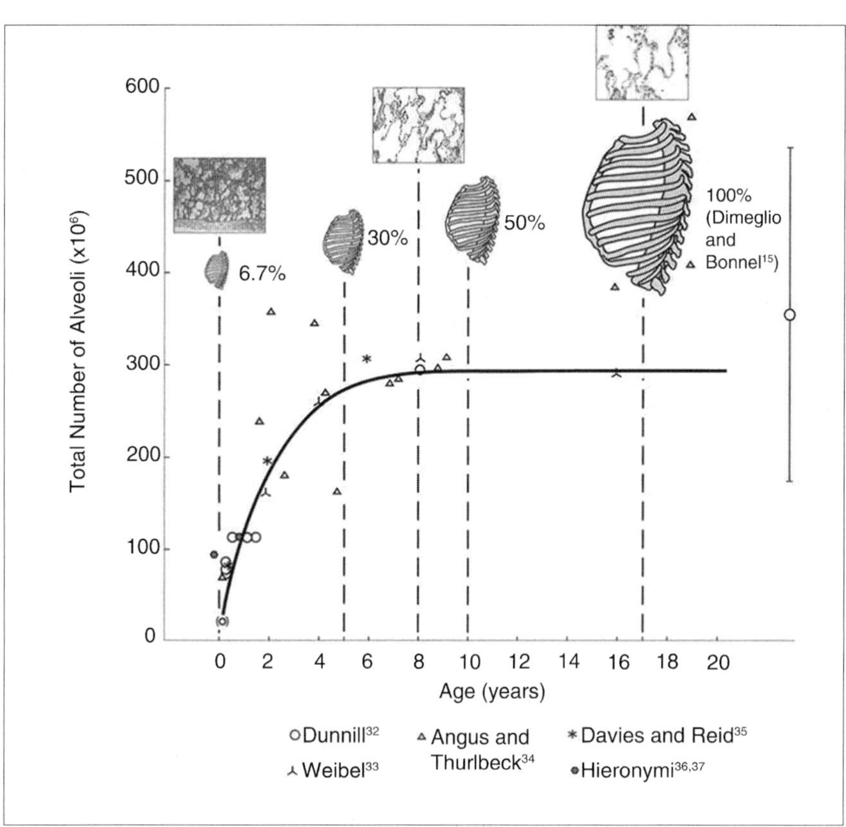

Figure 11 This graph showing lung growth by alveolar cell multiplication as a function of time is based on summaries of small autopsy studies,[32-37] with thoracic volume increases based on the reports of Dimeglio and Bonnel.[15] (Adapted from Campbell RM Jr, Smith MD: Thoracic insufficiency syndrome and exotic scoliosis. *J Bone Joint Surg Am* 2007;89:108-122.)

the spine, the rib cage, the sternum, and the diaphragm; therefore, any disease process or congenital abnormality that adversely affects the increase in volume of the thorax by limiting growth would adversely affect the growth of the lungs. The synergistic relationship between the thorax and the lungs is confirmed by natural history examples. A greater than 50% mortality rate from severe restrictive lung disease occurs in patients with Jeune syndrome, resulting from extrinsic lung hypoplasia from thoracic constriction caused by congenitally shortened ribs. A similar mortality rate has been reported in patients with spondylothoracic dysplasia, in which there is severe shortening of the rib cage, with the thoracic spine only 24% of normal height.[38] Windswept deformity of the thorax in scoliosis can cause a volume depletion deformity similar to Jeune syndrome, with extrinsic restrictive lung disease. Early fusion of the spine for scoliosis may stabilize and straighten the spine, but the loss of thoracic spinal growth from the fusion may shorten the thorax enough to produce a type of spondylothoracic dysplasia extrinsic restrictive lung disease. A study by Karol and associates[39] emphasized the need to consider thoracic insufficiency syndrome when treating patients with early onset scoliosis. The authors reported that low vital capacity, defined as less than 50% normal, was seen at follow-up in 43% of patients who received fusion early in life and was more prevalent in patients treated with proximal spine fusions, although the reason was unknown. The height of the fused thoracic spine and its contribution to thoracic volume seemed to be linked to vital capacity at follow-up. In patients with a thoracic spinal height of less than 18 cm, which is approximately normal height for a 5-year-old child, 63% of skeletally mature patients had low vital capacity. Among patients with a thoracic spinal height of 18 to 22 cm, 25% had low vital capacity. No patients with a thoracic spinal height from 22 cm to a normal measurement of 28 cm had low vital capacity. The authors suggested that growth-sparing surgical techniques should be strongly considered for young children with scoliosis, rather than traditional approaches using spinal fusion.

Other novel research on patients with thoracic insufficiency syndrome involves lung scan studies of perfusion abnormalities and quality of life instrument analysis, which has shown extremely poor results in preoperative patients with thoracic insufficiency syndrome.[40,41] Pulmonary function studies are somewhat useful but are flawed because the results summate performance of both sides of the thorax. Campbell and associates[42] recently presented dynamic lung MRI hemithorax analysis of the contribution of rib cage expansion and diaphragmatic expansion of the lungs in children with thoracic insufficiency syndrome. The authors reported differences during tidal volume respiration in rib cage expansion between convex and concave sides in early onset scoliosis and in congenital scoliosis, with the convex "rib hump" side having less motion and

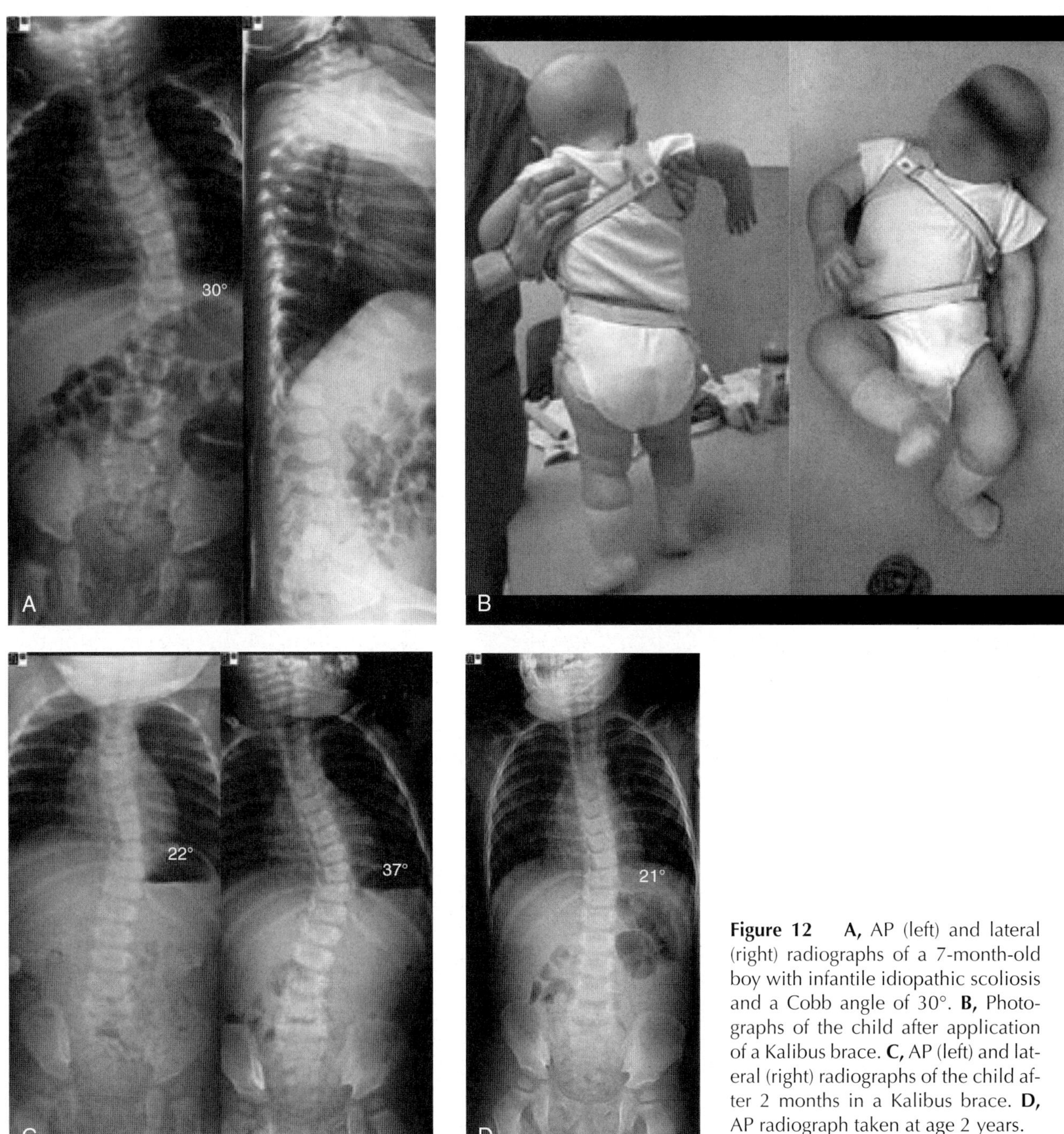

Figure 12 **A,** AP (left) and lateral (right) radiographs of a 7-month-old boy with infantile idiopathic scoliosis and a Cobb angle of 30°. **B,** Photographs of the child after application of a Kalibus brace. **C,** AP (left) and lateral (right) radiographs of the child after 2 months in a Kalibus brace. **D,** AP radiograph taken at age 2 years.

with almost absent rib cage motion bilaterally in those with kyphoscoliosis. In the future, dynamic lung MRI hemithorax analysis may aid in the preoperative evaluation of patients with thoracic insufficiency syndrome to effectively treat the most severe biomechanical disorders, assess results, and reveal new surgical strategies.

VEPTR expansion thoracoplasty is the first step in the evolution of a surgical technique to treat spinal deformity, with a growth-sparing approach, and to treat thoracic insufficiency syndrome. The VEPTR technique cannot restore motion to a fused chest wall with congenital absence of intercostal muscles, but the approach can enlarge a constricted hemithorax, probably with compensatory growth of the underlying lung in a young patient, with the enlarged lung "powered" by the action of the diaphragm. It is unclear whether the other growth-sparing approaches will treat thoracic insufficiency syndrome because patient pulmonary function tests or analyses of CT-determined lung volumes have been reported by the proponents of these methods. In time, VEPTR devices may be available with self-expanding capabilities, which will reduce the inherent morbidities of repetitive surgeries. Future devices may be capable of providing active rib cage expansion respiratory capability, in addition to simple volume increase. Regardless of the technique, the goals of any casting approach, growing rod technique, Shilla procedure, spine fusion, or VEPTR expansion thoracoplasty are not only to correct the Cobb angle of scoliosis but also to obtain the largest, most symmetric and functional thorax possible by the time the patient reaches skeletal maturity; achieving these goals will safeguard lifelong pulmonary function. The challenge is huge, but the potential benefit to pediatric patients justifies new research.

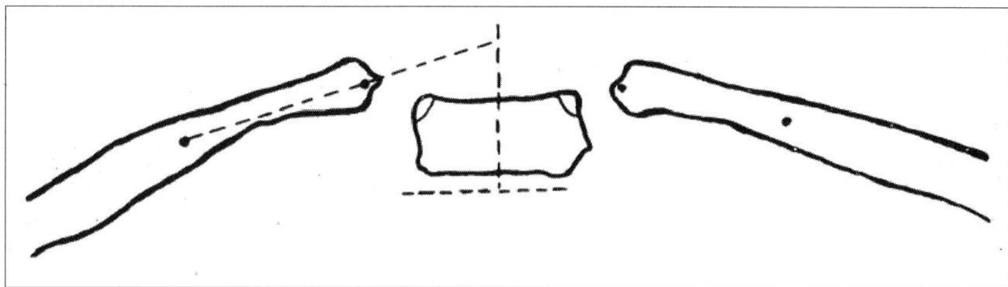

Figure 13 The rib-vertebral angle difference.

Other Treatments

Traditional scoliosis treatment options include bracing, casting, traction, true fusionless surgery (wedge osteotomies preserving growth cartilage), relative fusionless surgery (vertebral body stapling, other tethers, VEPTR, growing rods, Shilla, and true fusion surgery). Biologic manipulation also is being investigated as a treatment option.

Bracing

The Kalibus brace is used for infants with scoliosis. It is generally believed to be most effective when the child is prone or supine. When the child is sitting and standing, the brace is believed to be less functional because the straps can no longer maintain tension and the VEPTRs are no longer aligned properly. Figure 12 shows a 7-month-old male infant with infantile idiopathic scoliosis and a Cobb angle of 30° who was placed in a Kalibus brace. His rib vertebral angle difference (RVAD) was greater than 20° (Figure 13). After 2 months in a Kalibus brace, the scoliosis had improved. The child subsequently outgrew the Kalibus brace, and the curve progressed to 37°. He was placed in a second bending thoracolumbosacral Kalibus-type brace at his most recent follow-up at 2 years of age.

The RVAD is helpful in predicting curve progression and defining the natural history for children with infantile scoliosis. In patients with a RVAD of greater than 20° or more, 80% of curves are likely to progress.[43] An appropriate workup, with MRI to rule out intraspinal anomalies or other pathologies, is needed to confirm the diagnosis of idiopathic infantile scoliosis.

Casting

Casting is another option for the very young child with scoliosis. Traditional Risser casting has a high incidence of rib and mandibular deformity complications and cast sores. Recently, casting is being reconsidered as an effective treatment modality for young children with scoliosis. Traditionally, casting has included the Risser techniques (turnbuckle and localizer casting technique) and the Cotrel and Morel technique. The Mehta technique recently has been developed and is similar to the Cotrel and Morel technique, which primarily treats curves by correcting rotation. The Mehta technique is described as a "twist and shift" rather than a "push and bend" technique[43] (Figure 14). In a study of 136 patients with infantile scoliosis treated with the Mehta casting technique, 94 patients had "full correction," and 42 patients had "partial correction."[43] There are no studies comparing different types of casting, and it is unknown if the Mehta technique will result in long-term improvement.

Some curves are too large to cast. Chest wall deformity does not seem to be an issue with proper casting. Spines remain flexible, and patients appear to tolerate casting reasonably well. Curve improvement tends to occur faster in younger patients than in older patients.

Traction

Traction (halo femoral, halo pelvic, and halo gravity) is an alternative option for treating infantile scoliosis. It is one of the oldest treatment methods and is best used to obtain some correction before surgical cor-

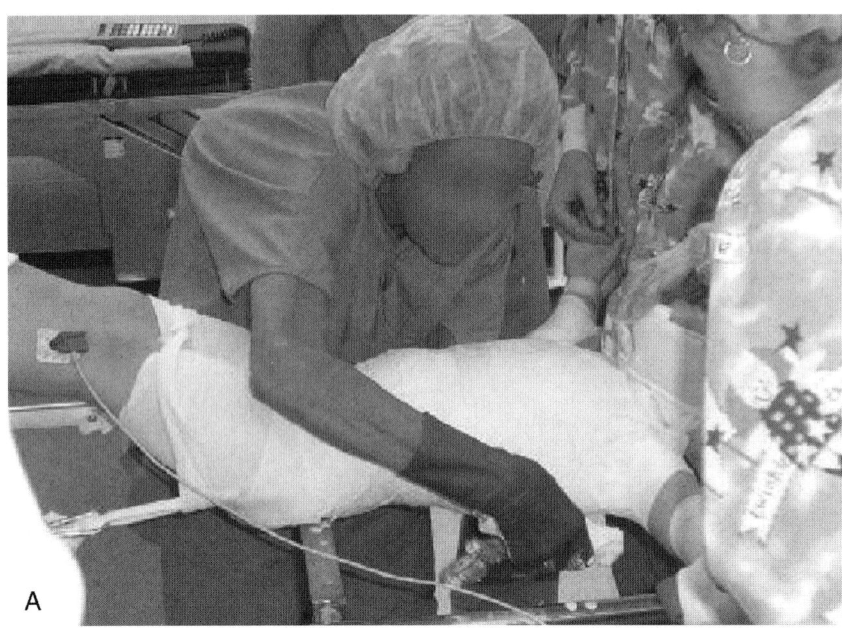

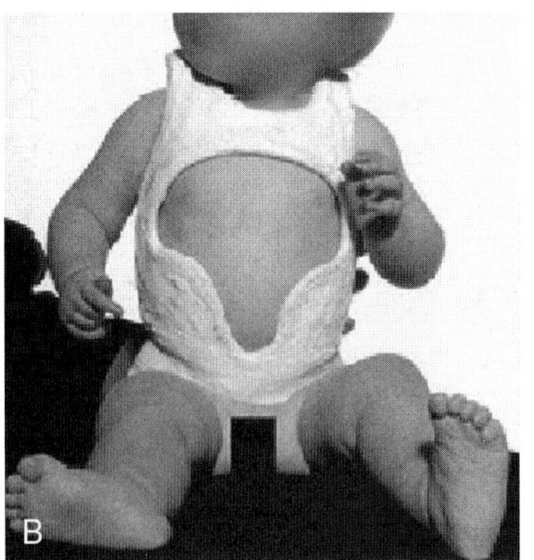

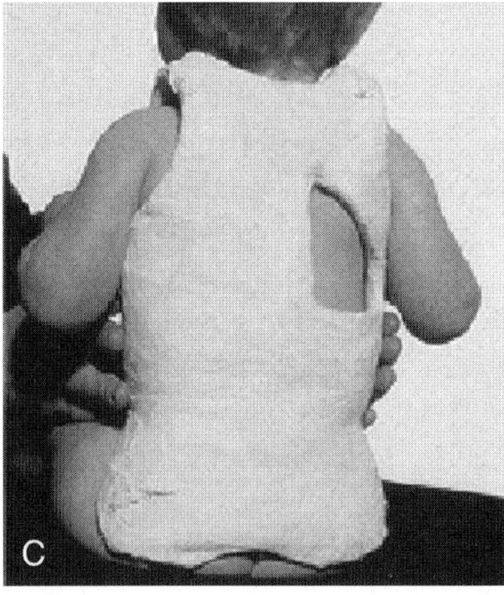

Figure 14 The Mehta technique. **A,** A casting procedure for curve correction, using a twist-and-shift rotation method. **B** and **C,** A cast used for an infant.

rection, especially for patients with severe scoliosis (> 80°) and scoliosis associated with kyphosis of the spinal column.[44]

Wedge Osteotomies

Wedge osteotomies of the spine for deformity correction are an attractive treatment option. Wedge osteotomy with removal of a wedge-shaped section of vertebra on the concave side of the spine can be combined with bridging instrumentation. This technique was evaluated using a calf model to compare wedging alone with a wedge-rod construct.[45] The wedge-rod system was much stiffer compared with the wedging procedure alone. The authors concluded that osteotomies with a wedge-rod construct for 8 to 12 weeks followed by removal of the rod could provide adequate fixation and correction of deformities. Human clinical studies also have been performed. Fourteen patients with scoliosis secondary to spinal cord injury were treated with a fusionless vertebral-body wedge osteotomy.[46] At a mean follow-up of 15 months, the average correction was 86%. There were no major complications or nonunion at the osteotomy site, and spinal mobility was maintained. Two patients had overcorrection, and the Cobb magnitude worsened in one patient. The long-term efficacy of the procedure is unknown.

Vertebral Body Stapling and Other Tethers

Vertebral body stapling is also an attractive treatment option. The staple is placed on the convex side of the anterior spine to stop development of the curve. Stapling attempts to stabilize curve progression. The idea of controlling bone growth by epiphyseal stapling was first clinically tested in the 1950s.[47] The authors concluded that stapling straightens the curve; however, the staples should eventually be removed to prevent overcorrection. Stapling also was evaluated in a study by Smith and associates.[48] Of the three patients in the study, there was no increase in the curve in the area in which the staples were placed; however, there was no decrease in the original deformity. On the unstapled vertebrae, secondary curves developed in the opposite direction of the primary curve; two of the three patients required fusion surgery after stapling.

More recently, vertebral body stapling has been performed with a nitinol (nickel titanium) staple. When cold, this metal alloy remains in a "straight" position. With warming to body temperature, the prongs clamp down into the bone in a C-shape. In a human clinical study, 10 patients with curves of less than 50° and a Risser sign of less than 2 were treated with spinal stapling.[49] Re-

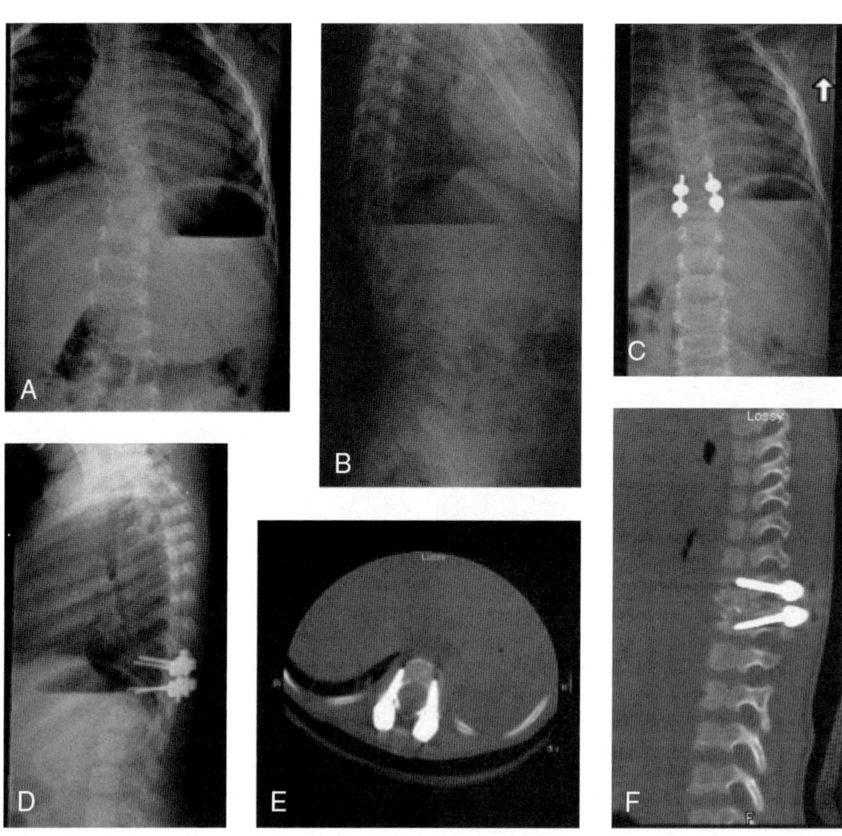

Figure 15 Hemivertebrectomy was used to treat a 2-year-old boy with congenital kyphoscoliosis and congenital scoliosis. Preoperative AP **(A)** and lateral **(B)** radiographs of the isolated segmented hemivertebra. Postoperative AP **(C)** and lateral **(D)** radiographs of the hemivertebrectomy, with limited instrumentation and fusion. **E,** CT showing pedicle screw placement in a transverse plane. **F,** Sagittal radiograph showing the position of the vertebrae after the hemivertebrectomy.

sults showed that the curve remained stable in 60% of patients and progressed in 40%. One of the 10 patients required spinal fusion. In another study, 39 patients were treated with vertebral body stapling.[50] The authors reported that patients age 8 years or older with less than 50° of preoperative curve magnitude achieved coronal curve stability at a rate of 87% at a minimum follow-up of 1 year.

Other tether materials and techniques have been used. Flexible posterior asymmetric tethers attached to bone anchors show greater efficacy in correcting curves compared with staples.[51]

Spinal Fusion

Spinal fusion is another treatment option for the very young child with spinal deformity. With posterior spinal fusion alone, there is the risk of deformity progression and "crankshafting." This risk can be lessened or prevented with combined anterior and posterior spinal fusion. This more aggressive technique, however, is associated with a loss of spine height and potential pulmonary implications for those with thoracic curvature. Definitive fusion may be used as definitive treatment in the older child (generally older than 8 to 10 years). For young patients with an open triradiate cartilage who are treated with spinal fusion, there is a risk for the development of the crankshaft phenomenon, especially with a posterior-only procedure. For these younger patients, anterior release and fusion may be needed to prevent the crankshaft phenomenon. A form of fusion is a convex hemiepiphysiodesis and fusion with or without instrumentation. This surgery has been likened to a "spot weld" and helps prevent progressive spinal imbalance and deformity in patients with less severe curves.

Hemivertebrectomy

Hemivertebrectomy for congenital scoliosis remains an effective treatment option. More commonly done as a combined anterior and posterior procedure, hemivertebrectomy can be safely done as a posterior-only procedure when performed by an experienced surgeon (Figure 15).

Shilla Procedure

The Shilla procedure, which was previously described in this chapter, is another treatment option for the very young child with a spinal deformity (Figure 16). Three "anchors" are used. The central set of anchors generally is at the apex of the curvature, and pedicle screws can be used here to derotate the spine apex. With growth, the peripheral anchors migrate on the rods away from the apex to allow for growth. The long-term efficacy of this procedure has not been determined.

Summary

The goals of treating a patient with a growing spine are correction and/or prevention of deformity progression with maintenance of correction while allowing for growth of the spine and thoracic cage to achieve optimal pulmonary growth and

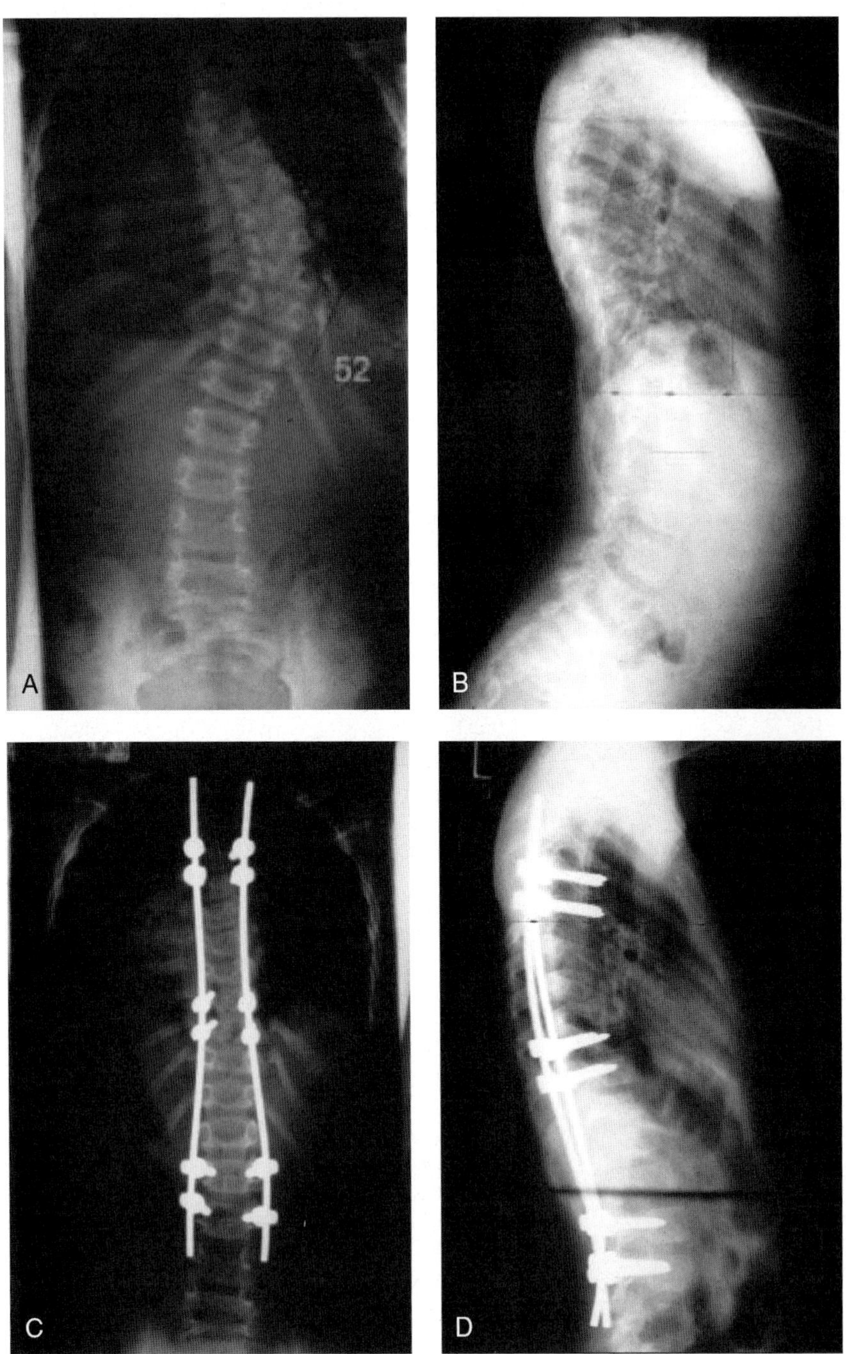

Figure 16 The Shilla procedure. Preoperative AP **(A)** and lateral **(B)** radiographs of the thoracic curve showing the curvature in the spine. Postoperative AP **(C)** and lateral **(D)** radiographs of the thoracic curve showing rod and screw placement in three segments.

function. Management principles are based on the correct diagnosis and understanding of the natural history of the spinal deformity.

The old adage that "a short straight spine is better than a short crooked spine" is no longer true. Pulmonary growth and development is as an important factor to consider when treating the very young child with a spinal deformity.

References

1. Akbarnia B, McCarthy R: Pediatric Isola instrumentation without fusion for the treatment of progressive early onset scoliosis, in McCarthy R, ed: *Spinal Instrumentation Techniques*. Chicago, IL, Scoliosis Research Society, 1998.
2. Akbarnia BA, Marks DS: Instrumentation with limited arthrodesis for the treatment of progressive early-onset scoliosis. *Spine* 2000;14:181-189.
3. Akbarnia BA, Marks DS, Boachie-Adjei O, Thompson AG, Asher MA: Dual growing rod technique for the treatment of progressive early-onset scoliosis: A multicenter study. *Spine* 2005;30:S46-S57.
4. Mahar AT, Bagheri R, Oka R, Kostial P, Akbarnia BA: Biomechanical comparison of different anchors (foundations) for the pediatric dual growing rod technique. *Spine* 2008;8: 933-939.
5. Akbarnia BA, Breakwell LM, Marks DS, et al: Dual growing rod technique followed for three to eleven years until final fusion: The effect of frequency of lengthening. *Spine* 2008;33:984-990.
6. Sankar W, Wudbhav N, Skaggs DL, et al: Neurologic risk in growing rod spine surgery in early onset scoliosis: Is neuromonitoring necessary for all cases? *Spine* 2009;34:1952-1955.
7. Thompson GH, Akbarnia BA, Kostial P, et al: Comparison of single and dual growing rod techniques followed through definitive surgery: A preliminary study. *Spine* 2005;30: 2039-2044.
8. Bess RS, Akbarnia BA, Thompson G, et al: Complications in 910 growing rod surgeries: Use of dual rods and submuscular placement of rods decreases complications. *Spine J* 2008;8: 13S-14S.

9. Elsebaie H, Yazici M, Thompson GH, et al: Abstract: Safety and efficacy of growing rods for pediatric congenital spinal deformities. Growing Spine Study Group. Second International Congress on Early Onset Scoliosis and Growing Spine. *J Child Orthop* 2009;3:145-168.

10. Sponseller P, Thompson GH, Akbarnia BA, et al: Growing rods for infantile scoliosis in Marfan syndrome. *Spine* 2009;34:1711-1715.

11. Pehrsson K, Larsson S, Oden A, Nachemson A: Long-term follow-up of patients with untreated scoliosis: A study of mortality, causes of death, and symptoms. *Spine* 1992;17:1091-1096.

12. Muirhead A, Conner AN: The assessment of lung function in children with scoliosis. *J Bone Joint Surg Br* 1985;67:699-702.

13. McCarthy R, Luhmann S, Lenke L: Abstract: Greater than two year follow-up Shilla Growth Enhancing System for the treatment of scoliosis in children. Paper presented at International Congress on Early Onset Scoliosis and Growing Spine, 2008, Montreal, QC. http://www.growingspine.org/files/abstracts-for-journal.doc. Accessed November 18, 2009.

14. Sanders JO, Khoury JG, Kishan S, et al: Predicting scoliosis progression from skeletal maturity: A simplified classification during adolescence. *J Bone Joint Surg Am* 2009;90:540-553.

15. Dimeglio A, Bonnel F: *Le Rachis en Croissance*. Paris, France, Springer, 1990.

16. Dimeglio A: Growth in pediatric orthopaedics. *J Pediatr Orthop* 2001;21: 549-555.

17. Winter RB: Scoliosis and spinal growth. *Orthop Rev* 1977;6:17-20.

18. Kioschos HC, Asher MA, Lark RG, Harner EJ: Overpowering the crankshaft mechanism: The effect of posterior spinal fusion with and without stiff transpedicular fixation on anterior spinal column growth in immature canines. *Spine* 1996;21:1168-1173.

19. Sanders JO, Little DG, Richards BS: Prediction of the crankshaft phenomenon by peak height velocity. *Spine* 1997;22:1352-1357.

20. Suk SI, Lee SM, Chung ER, Kim JH, Kim SS: Selective thoracic fusion with segmental pedicle screw fixation in the treatment of thoracic idiopathic scoliosis: More than 5-year follow-up. *Spine* 2005;30:1602-1609.

21. Charles YP, Demeglio A, Marcoul M, Bourgin JF, Marcoul A, Bozonnat MC: Influence of idiopathic scoliosis on three-dimensional thoracic growth. *Spine* 2008;33:1209-1218.

22. Whittaker AL, Sutton AJ, Beardsmore CS: Are ethnic differences in lung function explained by chest size? *Arch Dis Child Fetal Neonatal Ed* 2005; 90:F423-F428.

23. Emans JB, Ciarlo M, Callahan M, Zurakowski D: Prediction of thoracic dimensions and spine length based on individual pelvic dimensions in children and adolescents: An age-independent, individualized standard for evaluation of outcome in early onset spinal deformity. *Spine* 2005;30: 2824-2829.

24. Akbarnia BA: Management themes in early onset scoliosis. *J Bone Joint Surg Am* 2007;89:42-54.

25. Campbell RM Jr, Smith MD, Mayes TC, et al: The characteristics of thoracic insufficiency syndrome associated with fused ribs and congenital scoliosis. *J Bone Joint Surg Am* 2003;85:399-408.

26. American Thoracic Society Ad Hoc Statement Committee: Mechanisms and limits of induced postnatal lung growth. *Am J Respir Crit Care Med* 2004;170:319-343.

27. Campbell RM Jr, Smith MD, Mayes TC, et al: The effect of opening wedge thoracostomy on thoracic insufficiency syndrome associated with fused ribs and congenital scoliosis. *J Bone Joint Surg Am* 2004;86:1659-1674.

28. Emans JB, Caubet JF, Ordonez CL, Lee EY, Ciarlo M: The treatment of spine and chest wall deformities with fused ribs by expansion thoracostomy and insertion of vertical expandable prosthetic titanium rib: Growth of thoracic spine and improvement of lung volumes. *Spine* 2005;30:S58-S68.

29. Campbell RM Jr, Hell-Vocke AK: Growth of the thoracic spine in congenital scoliosis after expansion thoracoplasty. *J Bone Joint Surg Am* 2003;85: 409-420.

30. Campbell RM Jr, Smith MD: Thoracic insufficiency syndrome and exotic scoliosis. *J Bone Joint Surg Am* 2007;89:108-122.

31. Canavese F, Dimeglio A, Volpatti D, et al: Dorsal arthrodesis of thoracic spine and effects on thorax growth in prepubertal New Zealand white rabbits. *Spine* 2007;32:E443-E450.

32. Dunnill M: Postnatal growth of the lung. *Thorax* 1962;17:328-333.

33. Weibel E: *Morphometry of the Human Lung*. Berlin, Germany, Springer, 1963, p 111.

34. Angus G, Thurlbeck W: Number of alveoli in the human lung. *J Appl Physiol* 1972;32:483-485.

35. Davies G, Reid L: Growth of the alveoli and pulmonary arteries in childhood. *Thorax* 1970;25:669-681.

36. Hieronymi G: On the change in the morphology of the human lung due to aging. *Ergeb Allg Pathol Pathol Anat* 1961;41:1-62.

37. Hieronymi G: Changes in the lung structure at different ages. *Verh Dtsch Ges Pathol* 1960;44:129-130.

38. Ramírez N, Conier AS, Campbell RM Jr, Carlo S, Arroyo S, Romeu J: Natural history of thoracic insufficiency syndrome: A spondylothoracic dysplasia perspective. *J Bone Joint Surg Am* 2007;89:2663-2675.

39. Karol K, Johnston C, Mladenov K, Schochet P, Walter P, Browne R: Pulmonary function following early thoracic spine fusion in non-neuromuscular scoliosis. *J Bone Joint Surg Am* 2008;90:272-281.

40. Redding G, Song K, Inscore S, Effmann E, Campbell R: Lung function asymmetry in children with congenital and infantile scoliosis. *Spine J* 2008;8:639-644.

41. Vitale MG, Matsumoto H, Roye DP Jr, et al: Health-related quality of life in children with thoracic insufficiency syndrome. *J Pediatr Orthop* 2008;28:239-243.

42. Campbell R, Simmons J III, Joshi A, Inscore S, Doski J: Abstract: The characterization of the thoracic biomechanics of respiration in thoracic insufficiency syndrome by dynamic lung MRI: A preliminary report. Paper presented at International Congress on Early Onset Scoliosis and Growing Spine, 2008, Montreal, QC. http://www.growingspine.org/files/abstracts-for-journal.doc. Accessed November 18, 2009.

43. Mehta MH: Growth as a corrective force in the early treatment of progressive infantile scoliosis. *J Bone Joint Surg Br* 2005;87:1237-1247.

44. D'Astous J, Sanders J: Casting and traction treatment methods for scoliosis. *Orthop Clin North Am* 2007;38:477-484.

45. Betz RR, Cunningham B, Selgrath C, Drewry T, Sherman MC: Preclinical testing of a wedge-rod system for fusionless correction of scoliosis. *Spine* 2003;28:S275-S278.

46. Guille JT, Betz RR, Balsara RK, Mulcahey MJ, D'Andrea LP, Clements DH: The feasibility, safety, and utility of vertebral wedge osteotomies for the fusionless treatment of paralytic scoliosis. *Spine* 2003;28:S266-S274.

47. Nachlas IW, Borden JN: The cure of experimental scoliosis by directed growth control. *J Bone Joint Surg Am* 1951;33:24-32.

48. Smith AD, Von Lackum WH, Wylie R: An operation for stapling vertebral bodies in congenital scoliosis. *J Bone Joint Surg Am* 1954;36:342-348.

49. Betz RR, Kim J, D'Andrea LP, Mulcahey MJ, Balsara RK, Clements DH: An innovative technique of vertebral body stapling for the treatment of patients with adolescent idiopathic scoliosis: A feasibility, safety, and utility study. *Spine* 2003;28:S255-S265.

50. Betz RR, D'Andrea LP, Mulcahey MJ, Chafetz RS: Vertebral body stapling procedure for the treatment of scoliosis in the growing child. *Clin Orthop Relat Res* 2005;434:55-60.

51. Braun JT, Akyuz E, Ogilvie JW, Bachus KN: The efficacy and integrity of shape memory alloy staples and bone anchors with ligament tethers in the fusionless treatment of experimental scoliosis. *J Bone Joint Surg* 2005;87:2038-2051.

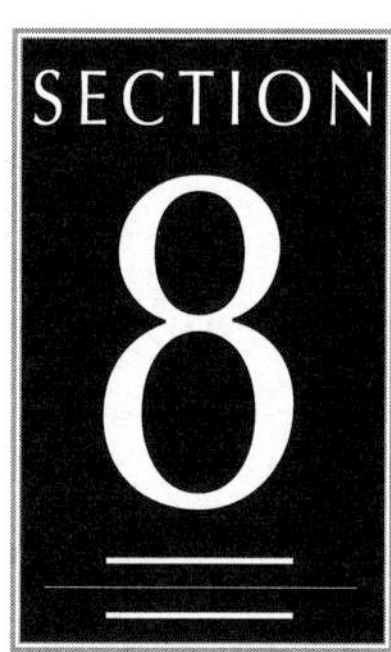

Trauma

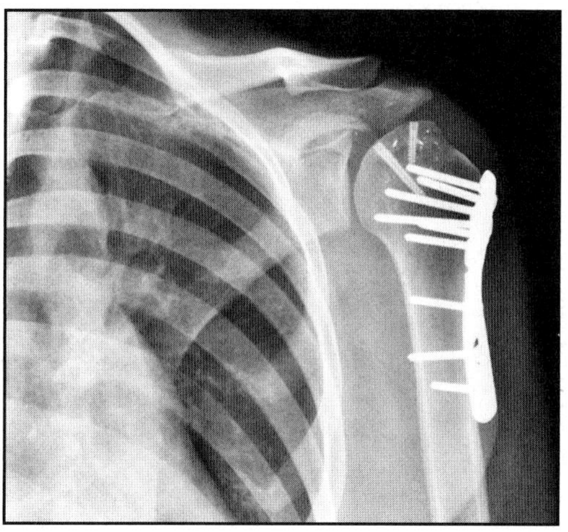

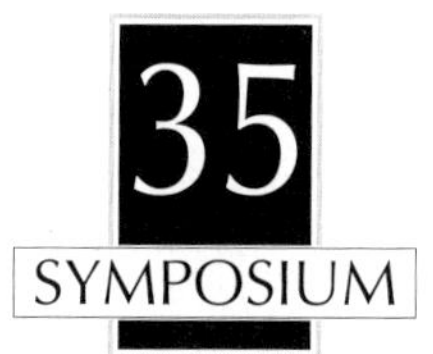

Advances in the Care of Battlefield Orthopaedic Injuries

CAPT Dana C. Covey, MD, MC, USN
Col Mark W. Richardson, MD, MC, USAF
Col Elisha T. Powell IV, MD, MC, USAF (Ret)
CDR Michael T. Mazurek, MD, MC, USN
Steven J. Morgan, MD

Abstract

Musculoskeletal wounds are the most common type of injury among survivors of combat trauma. The treatment of these wounds entails many challenges. Although methods of care are evolving, significant gaps remain as knowledge of civilian trauma is extrapolated to combat injuries. It is important to discuss issues related to the use of portable vacuum-assisted wound closure devices during transport, as well as the prevention of heterotopic ossification and the participation of civilian orthopaedic trauma experts in caring for injured service members through the Distinguished Visiting Scholar Program.

Instr Course Lect 2010;59:427-435.

More than 34,000 members of the US Armed Forces have been wounded during the ongoing wars in Iraq and Afghanistan. Most of the injuries are musculoskeletal[1,2] and result from an explosion of munitions such as mortars, rockets, rocket-propelled grenades, and improvised explosive devices (IEDs). In Iraq, IEDs have caused more than 60% of the casualties[3] (Figure 1). Currently, almost 90% of personnel wounded in Iraq survive their injuries; 10.1% die from their battlefield injuries.[4] Improvements in the survival rate correspond to improvements in the initial and later treatment of complex musculoskeletal war injuries. Treatment strategies are developing to reflect an increasing research focus on the optimal treatment of these injuries.

This chapter addresses several topics germane to the treatment of musculoskeletal injuries sustained on the battlefield, including the use of portable vacuum-assisted wound closure devices during transport, the prevention of heterotopic ossification (HO), and the participation of civilian orthopaedic trauma experts in caring for injured service members through the Distinguished Visiting Scholar Program.

The Use of Portable Vacuum-Assisted Wound Closure Devices During Medical Evacuation

Until quite recently, the in-flight use of negative pressure wound

Dr. Covey or an immediate family member has received research or institutional support from Arthrex, DJ Orthopaedics, Medtronic Sofamor Danek, Sanofi-Aventis, Stryker, Synthes, and Karl Storz. Dr. Mazurek is deceased. At the time this chapter was written, Dr. Mazurek or an immediate family member had received research or institutional support from the federally funded Orthopaedic Trauma Extremity Research Program. Dr. Morgan or an immediate family member is a member of a speakers' bureau or has made paid presentations on behalf of Smith & Nephew, Easi, and Stryker; serves as a paid consultant to or is an employee of Vision Med; has received research or institutional support from AO, Smith & Nephew, Synthes, Wyeth, and Twin Star Medical; has stock or stock options held in Johnson & Johnson and Cerapedics; and has received nonincome support (such as equipment or services), commercially derived honoraria, or other non–research-related funding (such as paid travel) from SLACK. Neither of the following authors or a member of their immediate families has receive anything of value from or owns stock in a commercial company or institution related directly or indirectly to the subject of this chapter: Dr. Richardson and Dr. Powell.

The opinions or assertions contained herein are the private views of the authors and are not to be construed as official or reflecting the views of the Department of Defense of the US government.

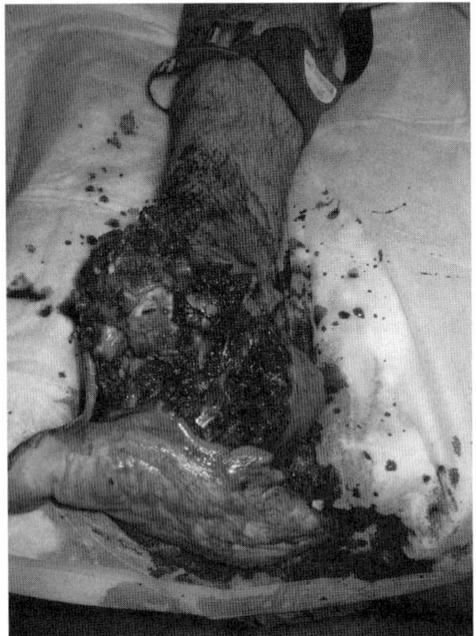

Figure 1 Clinical photograph of Gustilo and Anderson type IIIC fractures of the right leg and foot in a 25-year-old man with multiple fractures and fragment injuries caused by an IED detonation.

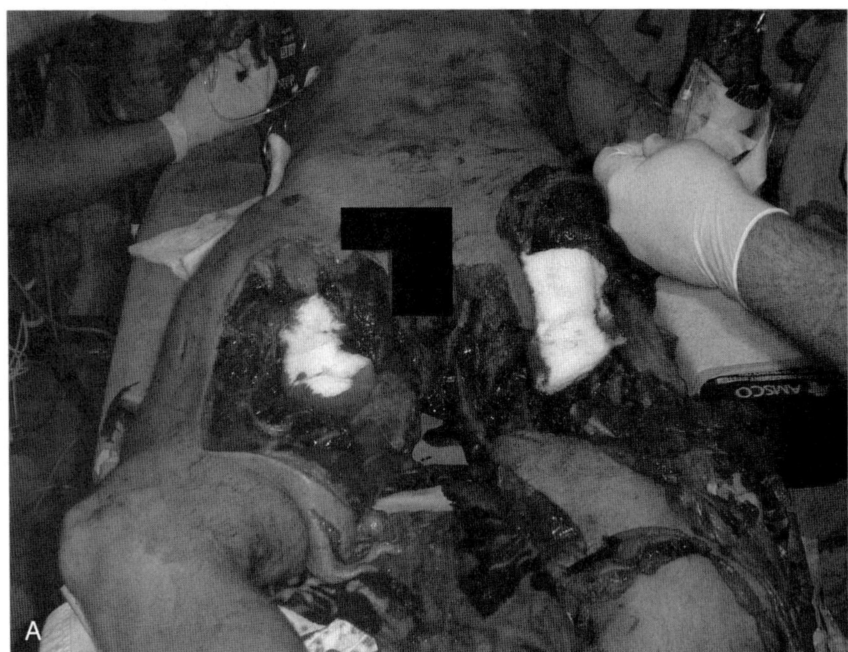

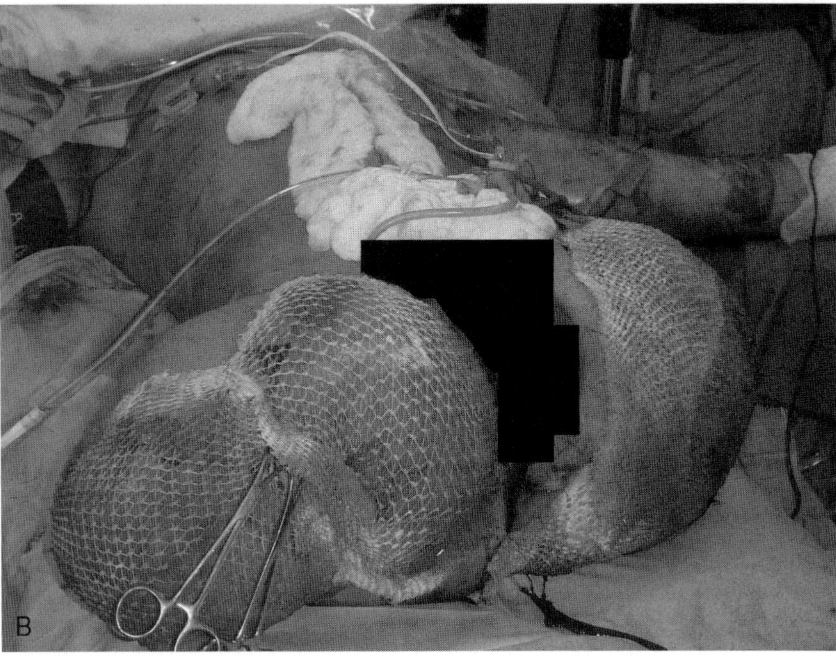

Figure 2 Clinical photographs of a 28-year-old man with severe bilateral lower extremity trauma caused by a rocket detonation at close range. **A,** The injuries before bilateral above-knee high amputations. **B,** The standard dressing illustrates the potential for leakage and wound contamination.

therapy (NPWT) was a controversial topic. The V.A.C. system (KCI, San Antonio, TX) has been successfully used in the treatment of severe ballistic wounds in military trauma hospitals in Iraq, Germany, and the United States (at care levels III, IV, and V, respectively).[5] Despite increasing acceptance in both military and civilian trauma practices,[6-18] data were not available to determine whether a vacuum-assisted wound closure device was safe to use during air transport. Recent reports of successful transport while these devices were being used have helped to resolve the controversy.[19]

NPWT has several potential advantages. Because the device maintains a closed environment that keeps the wound contained and inaccessible for dressing changes, it decreases the risk of secondary contamination. This characteristic often is considered the primary advantage of using NPWT during transport (Figures 2 and 3). NPWT has been shown to facilitate the formation of a granulation bed, with wound drainage to remove harmful exudates.[8,15] NPWT appears to resuscitate borderline tissue in the zone of stasis, and it may help wounds heal.[6,16]

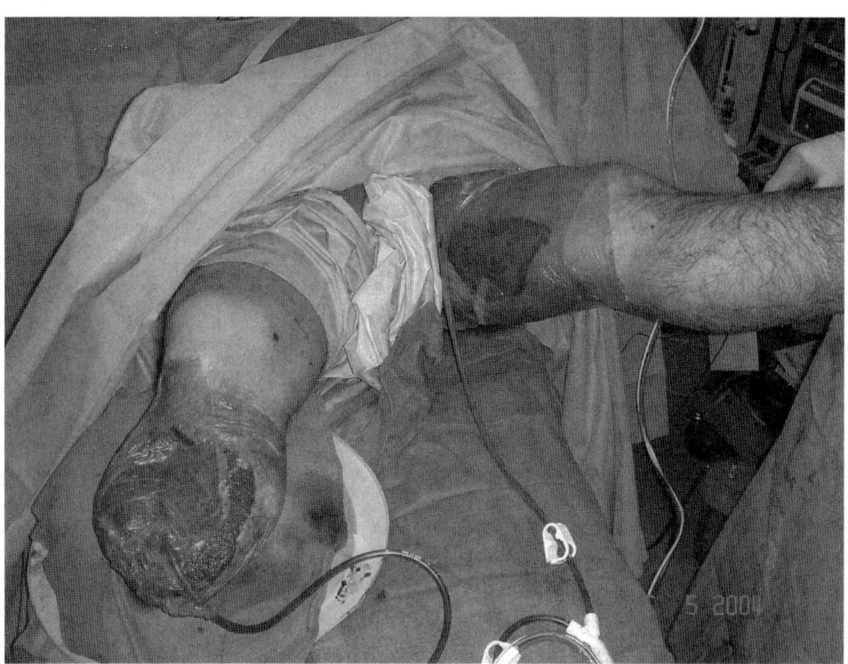

Figure 3 Clinical photograph showing the use of NPWT to separate a wound from the environment. An unreconstructible limb was treated with tissue-sparing amputation in a 15-year-old boy with a mortar-explosion blast wound.

Leininger and associates[20] reported on the use of NPWT to treat war wounds in 77 Iraqi patients at Balad Air Base, Iraq. The environment of the tent hospital was difficult, and high-energy, extremely contaminated ballistic wounds were common. Nonetheless, the infection rate was dramatically lower than previously reported anecdotal rates. NPWT was included in a 2004 protocol developed by orthopaedic trauma surgeons, which eliminated bedside dressing changes in favor of serial surgical débridements, with NPWT dressings applied in the operating room; primary wound closure with local flaps was delayed, as indicated.[7]

Opposition to the use of NPWT during air transport primarily came from surgeons at level V military medical centers in the United States because some patients had arrived at these centers with a nonfunctioning NPWT device and a septic wound. However, recently it was reported that these catastrophic failures involved the use of occlusive dressings with an improvised portable suction device not designed for NPWT.[7] Pollak and associates[19] described three potential disadvantages of the in-flight use of NPWT: the closed environment could promote an anaerobic infection if the drainage system failed; NPWT is more expensive to use than standard dressings; and using NPWT is more complex for the aeromedical evacuation crew.

Despite firmly held, contrary opinions among surgeons, there is consensus on some points related to NPWT. Because wounded coalition troops were being rapidly transported out of the conflict zone, they were not receiving NPWT and therefore possibly not being treated as well as wounded patients from the host country. For open fractures, particularly in massive blast-injury wounds, standard dressings can be difficult to change outside the operating room. However, surgeons agreed that NPWT, which does not require frequent dressing changes, can be used only if suction is applied. Most surgeons were willing to recommend the use of NPWT in transport if it could be shown almost invariably to function properly.

Concern over disparity in the care of war wounds sustained by local nationals and coalition troops was addressed in a 2006 videoconference on the use of NPWT in transport.[7] Experienced trauma surgeons from the US Army, Air Force, and Navy reached a consensus that a clinical study was needed to assess the continuous use of NPWT beginning after débridement at a level III trauma center in Iraq or Afghanistan and continuing through transport. In addition, the surgeons agreed that a study of the safety of prolonged transport from the level IV center in Germany to a level V center in the United States should be completed before the clinical efficacy of NPWT was examined. The safety study began when the portable V.A.C. Freedom system was approved for in-flight use aboard military aircraft after a 2006 airworthiness test.[7]

Pollak and associates[19] first reviewed the use of the Freedom system in transport from the combat theater to Landstuhl Regional Medical Center (LRMC) in Germany. A chart review identified 281 patients transported between October 2006 and September 2007, and 203 met the criteria for inclusion. These patients had 277 NPWT dressings at an average of 1.36 wound sites. Thirty-seven complications appeared in 36 patients, but only 1 was

Table 1
The Brooker Classification of HO in the Hip

Type	Radiographic Description
I	Islands of bone within the abductors
II	Bone spurs extending from the acetabulum and/or proximal femur, with a gap of 1 cm or more between the opposing surfaces
III	Bone spurs extending from the acetabulum and/or proximal femur with a gap of less than 1 cm between the opposing surfaces
IV	Ankylosis of the hip joint

considered major. This complication arose from an in-flight failure of NPWT; the resultant wound sepsis improved after repeat débridement at LRMC. Difficulty in using NPWT during transport was reported on seven occasions, including four occasions in which clamping of the suction was required for a prolonged period. The complication rate in these seven patients was 14%, which was slightly lower than the 18% overall complication rate. These encouraging results suggested that the use of NPWT during aeromedical evacuation is both feasible and safe. Nonetheless, skepticism remained as to the feasibility of using NPWT during transoceanic flights to the United States.

A prospective, observational, Institutional Review Board–approved pilot study recently explored the feasibility of using NPWT during aeromedical evacuation from LRMC to the United States. In-flight dressing maintenance was evaluated in 30 patients to determine whether the NPWT dressing was intact at the conclusion of the flight or had been converted to a standard dressing. The comments from the patients and aeromedical evacuation crews in the pilot project have been highly favorable, and there have been no reported adverse outcomes.[19]

Despite the encouraging results of the initial safety studies, there is reason for concern about wound sepsis resulting from device failure during prolonged transcontinental air evacuation. Treatment failed in 12 of 123 patients (10%) after an unrecognized interruption in the operation of the NPWT device (C Collinge, MD, and R Reddix, MD, Ft. Worth, TX, unpublished data, 2009). Despite appropriate and aggressive wound management, 7 of the 12 patients had significant, continuing wound complications. The noise, vibration, pressure changes, and limited space of the aeromedical evacuation environment impede the ability to recognize a device failure, and the possibility of an unrecognized interruption of therapy is a continuing issue. Before prolonged transport, antibiotic beads can be placed in the bone voids of an open fracture, under the reticulated foam of a NPWT dressing, to reduce the likelihood of wound sepsis if device failure occurs.[21] This recommendation is based on anecdotal evidence and personal opinion. However, the use of antibiotic beads may help resolve the remaining debate over the efficacy of NPWT. More importantly, it has the potential to prevent prolonged infectious complications or sepsis in military service members.

Heterotopic Ossification in Battle-Wounded Extremities

HO is defined as the formation of mature lamellar bone within tissues that normally do not have ossification, such as muscle, tendon, ligaments, and joint capsules.[22] HO is not to be confused with callus, which is bone that forms in response to a fracture and is a normal healing response. Although the earliest widely recognized descriptions of HO were associated with hip replacement, HO was first described during World War I as occurring after head trauma.[23,24] In addition to joint arthroplasty (usually total hip arthroplasty) and head injuries, HO has been associated with burns; arthropathies including ankylosing spondylitis, psoriatic arthritis, and diffuse idiopathic skeletal hyperostosis; periarticular injury to the elbow, hip, or knee; certain genetic disorders; and other trauma. HO can cause pain, decreased range of motion (either by bridging a joint or binding muscle units), and difficulty in fitting a prosthetic limb.[25] The increasing survival rates after battlefield injury have been accompanied by an increasing incidence of HO.[26]

The first system for quantifying HO was described by Brooker and associates,[27] and it is still widely used (Table 1). The Brooker classification describes the radiographic appearance of HO across the hip joint but does not assess function. The data were derived from a retrospective review of 100 consecutive total hip arthroplasties; the 21% incidence of HO was much higher than is currently found. This classification system has often been extrapolated to other joints. Letournel and associates[28] found that the overall incidence of HO was 24% after 669 acetabular fracture fixations. Increasing incidences were found with more extensile surgical exposures; patients requiring an extended iliofemoral approach had the highest incidence (57%). This finding suggests that the likelihood of developing HO is associated with progressively greater surgical trauma. Hastings and Graham[29] developed a system for classifying HO about the elbow that combined radiographic evidence with clinical range of motion (Table 2, Figure 4). Mills and Tejwani[30] developed a system to describe HO after knee dislocation (Table 3). They found that the severity of HO was associated with the overall severity of the trauma, as quantified by the Injury Severity Score. Regardless of the presence of a closed head injury, patients with a higher Injury Severity Score were more likely to have HO about the knee, and the HO was more likely be severe. In a retrospective study, Pape and associates[31] attempted to establish a correlation between HO formation and closed head injury. One group of patients had a Glasgow Coma Scale score lower than 9 and a positive head CT finding; patients in the second group had a Glasgow Coma Scale score of 9 or higher and a normal head CT finding. The Injury Severity Scores of the two patient groups were comparable (31 and 33, respectively). The rate of periarticular HO formation was 47% in the first group and 43% in the second group. These studies suggest that the formation of HO is influenced by both local and systemic factors, but the exact mechanism that triggers the cascade of events leading to HO remains poorly understood.

In 213 patients who underwent amputation after a battlefield injury, Potter and associates[25] found that the incidence of HO was 63% (134 residual limbs). The risk factors associated with the formation of HO were amputation within the zone of injury and injury from a blast mechanism; of the 147 patients with a blast injury, 117 (almost 80%) developed HO. Throughout the conflicts in Iraq and Afghanistan, most battlefield extremity injuries have been caused by explosive devices; this mechanism of injury, coupled with military surgeons' effort to preserve as much residual limb length as possible by amputating the lower extremity below the knee, can account for the high incidence of HO. Recent data suggest that high rates of

Table 2
The Hastings and Graham Classification of HO in the Elbow

Type	Functional Description*
I	No limitation of motion
IIA	Flexion-extension limitation
IIB	Pronation-supination limitation
IIC	Flexion-extension and pronation-supination limitation
III	Flexion-extension or pronation-supination ankylosis

*Radiographic HO is present in all types.

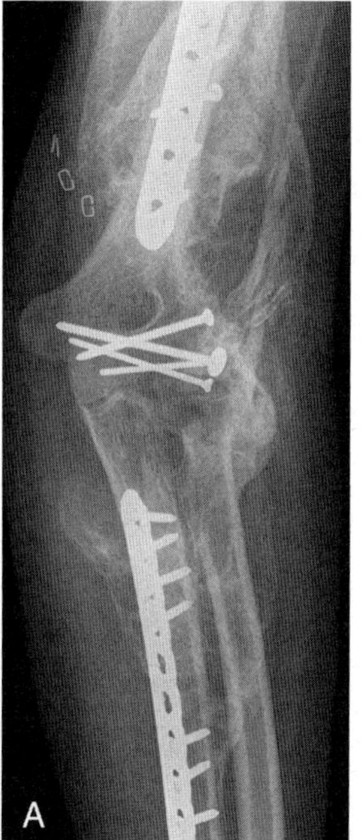

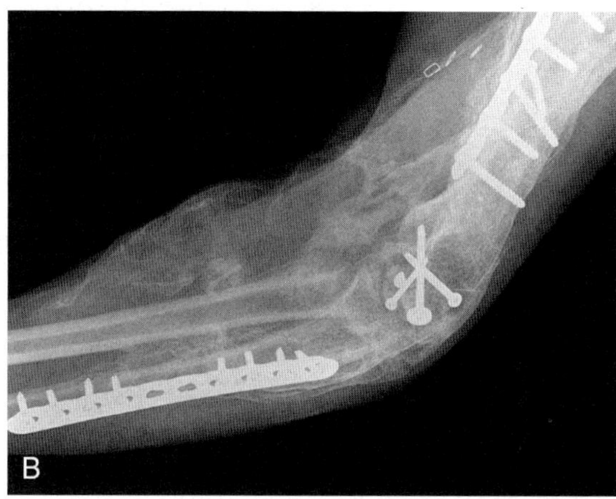

Figure 4 A 22-year-old man had multiple injuries caused by an explosive detonation. AP **(A)** and lateral **(B)** radiographs of the left elbow show Hastings and Graham type III HO after treatment of humeral and ulnar fractures using plate-and-screw constructs.

Table 3
The Mills and Tejwani Classification of HO After Knee Dislocation

Type	Radiographic Description
0	No HO
I	Medial and/or lateral collateral or capsular HO
II	Medial and/or lateral collateral or capsular HO and posterior femoral HO
III	Medial and/or lateral collateral or capsular HO and posterior tibial HO
IV	Knee-spanning (ankylosing) medial, lateral, or posterior HO

HO also are found in patients who have not undergone amputation. Forsberg and associates[32] found HO in almost 65% of 243 war-wounded patients who had undergone at least one orthopaedic procedure. Amputation was an independent risk factor, but head injury, an Injury Severity Score higher than 16, and multiple extremity involvement also were predictive of the development of HO. This finding suggests the presence of a systemic pathway that is activated more frequently and is more severe after war wounds than typical civilian traumas (Figure 4).

Nonsteroidal anti-inflammatory drugs (NSAIDs) and radiation currently are used as HO prophylaxis, but the topic is controversial. The highest level of evidence for the use of these modalities is found in research on acetabular fractures. In a prospective randomized study of the use of indomethacin and radiation therapy,[33] 11 of 150 patients (7%) developed HO after undergoing open reduction and internal fixation of an acetabular fracture through a posterior, combined, or extensile approach. In comparison, 100% of 16 patients who received no prophylaxis developed HO, including 6 (38%) who developed Brooker grade III or IV HO. Of the 150 patients, those who received NSAIDs were three times more likely to develop Brooker grade III or IV HO than those treated with radiation therapy. Karunakar and associates,[34] in a prospective randomized double-blind study, compared the use of indomethacin and a placebo in 121 consecutive patients undergoing surgical fixation of an acetabular fracture. The overall incidence of clinically significant HO was 17%; the rate was 15% among patients in the treatment group and 19% among patients in the placebo group. The difference between the two groups was not statistically significant, however, and the findings of this study bring into question the role of NSAIDs in preventing HO.

A high percentage of battlefield blast–injured patients develop HO. The current data suggest that a systemic process triggers a cascade of events leading to the development of HO masses that are painful and detrimental to function. It is questionable whether NSAIDs are effective in preventing HO. Prophylaxis with radiation therapy is impractical for most war-wounded patients because of their multiple extremity involvement. Despite the absence of any documented incidences of sarcoma after a single dose of radiation therapy, there is a theoretic risk of future malignant transformation, which must be considered before the widespread use of radiation prophylaxis.

Prevention of HO is a priority of the Orthopaedic Trauma Research Program, a federally funded grant project.[35] Preliminary research data from studies directly funded by this program were presented at the January 2009 Extremity War Injury Symposium in Washington, DC. These studies provide hope that HO formation can be halted by directly inhibiting specific receptors on the mesenchymal stem cells implicated in the process. Continued research is necessary because the number of patients with disabling HO is likely to increase as more patients survive high-energy trauma on and off the battlefield.

The Distinguished Visiting Scholar Program

The Distinguished Visiting Scholar Program (DVSP) is a collaborative effort of the Orthopaedic Trauma Association, the American Academy of Orthopaedic Surgeons, and the US Army. The program is modeled after the American College of Surgeons Visiting Trauma Surgeon Program. The DVSP regularly assigns experienced orthopaedic trauma surgeons to a military hospital for short periods of time. The program has several purposes. Military orthopaedic surgeons serving overseas are able to receive on-site training, guidance, and continuing medical education credit from experts in the treatment of extremity trauma. Visiting surgeons gain experience in the initial management of extremity war wounds. The military establishment receives a critique of extremity trauma care and patient care from a civilian perspective. In addition, the program is intended to lead to the development of US national and regional networks of orthopaedic surgeons with experience in the care of explosive or high-velocity missile injuries to the extremities, in preparation for any event requiring a high-level coordinated response.[36]

The DVSP is managed by the military subcommittee of the Orthopaedic Trauma Association, which includes civilian, active military, and retired military members. The committee is responsible for selecting the visiting scholars and administering the program. To be considered for service as a visiting scholar, a surgeon must have fellowship training in orthopaedic trauma, a minimum of 10 years of practice in orthopaedic surgery, a practice focused on orthopaedic trauma, and the ability to spend at least 2 weeks overseas.

The overseas location of the DVSP is LRMC, which has the only American College of Surgeons–accredited level II trauma center outside the continental United States. LRMC is a US Army base adjacent to Ramstein Air Force Base, the major transfer point for injured personnel in transit from Afghanistan or Iraq (Figure 5). LRMC is a full-service hospital for military personnel, their dependents, and military retirees in Europe, and it is an intermediate care facility for all patients evacuated from Iraq or Afghanistan with trauma-related or other medical conditions. All patients with traumatic extremity injuries pass through LRMC; therefore, it is the ideal location to place the visiting scholars. LRMC has orthopaedic surgeons from the Army, Navy, and Air Force who care for patients being evacuated to definitive care centers in the United States. The visiting scholars have full hospital privileges at LRMC. Because the visiting scholars are officially considered Red Cross volunteers, they are limited to providing care to US military personnel.

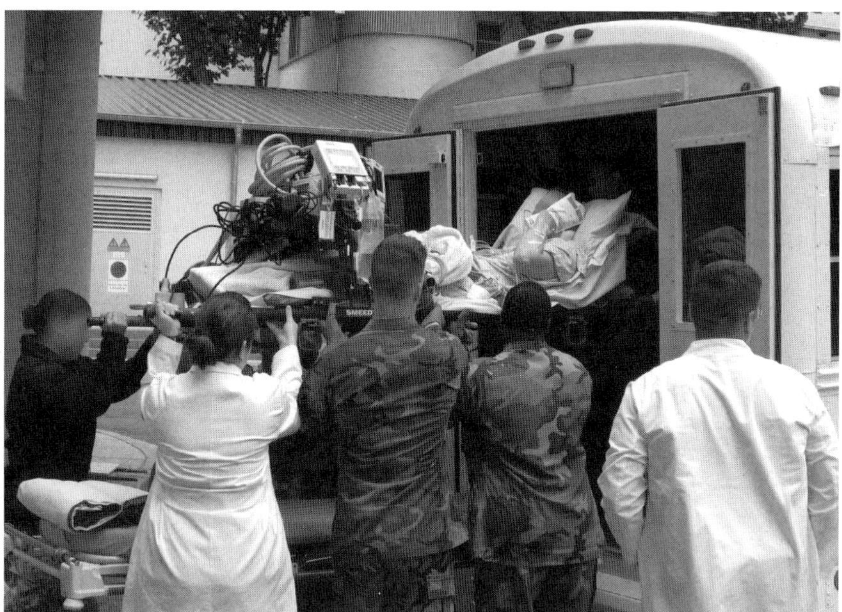

Figure 5 An injured service member is transferred from the flight line to LRMC via an ambulance bus.

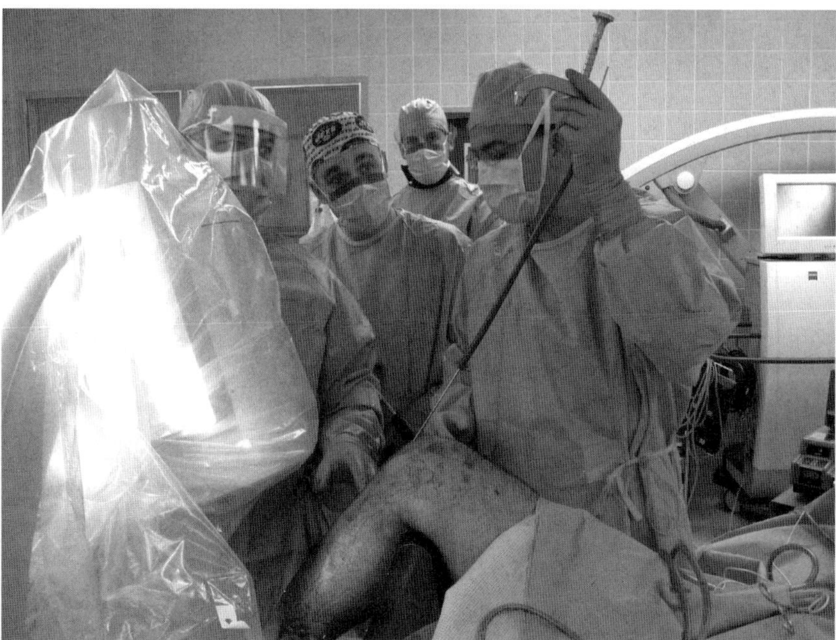

Figure 6 A visiting scholar (right) does a tibial nailing procedure with military orthopaedic surgeons.

On a daily basis, a visiting scholar first participates in the morning injury report, which is a discussion of incoming injured patients, development of surgical plans, and discharge planning for patients being transported to the United States. The scholar then participates in the surgical care of patients, thus extending the capacity and the abilities of the staff (Figure 6). The daily volume of surgical procedures ranges from none to seven, depending on the operational tempo of combat units in the conflict zones. Although most injuries are from an IED explosion, they also may result from a high-velocity gunshot, an indirect fire blast, or a motor vehicle crash. Most of the surgical care focuses on treatment of the soft-tissue injury, which often is in evolution because of the patient's rapid evacuation from the conflict zone. Definitive management of osseous injuries often is deferred until the patient returns to the United States. Most fractures have been stabilized with a temporary external fixator applied at a facility in the combat zone. The definitive osseous reconstructions done at LRMC primarily involve closed or long bone fractures. After the day's surgical procedures, the visiting scholar assists in evaluating newly admitted patients.

On a weekly basis, the visiting scholar lectures in a CME-approved format on an aspect of orthopaedic trauma care. In addition, the visiting scholar participates in a videoconference or a trauma review of selected patients with treating surgeons in forward-deployed medical units in Iraq and Afghanistan, as well as surgeons at US definitive care centers. The conference focuses on patient outcomes and quality assessment. At the completion of the rotation, the visiting scholar submits a written report of the experience, including observations on patient orthopaedic care, and receives a debriefing from the orthopaedic department director at LRMC and, on occasion, the hospital commander.

Since the inception of the DVSP in July 2007, more than 20 orthopaedic trauma surgeons have participated, and more than 20 hours of CME credit have been provided. The program has had mutually beneficial direct and indirect effects. The resources for orthopaedic trauma care at LRMC have increased, collaborative research efforts have been completed or initiated, and joint civilian and military efforts have led to increased funding for research on war-related extremity injuries.

Summary

Numerous challenges are inherent in treating patients with battlefield orthopaedic injuries, and the care of these injuries continues to evolve. Newer techniques in the management of massive soft-tissue wounds and new therapies to prevent HO can help to restore the best possible function. The current wars in Iraq and Afghanistan continue to provide a stimulus for advances in the treatment of high-energy, complex musculoskeletal traumatic injuries, and these advances are also likely to be applied in the care of civilian injuries.

References

1. US Department of Defense: DefenseLINK U.S. casualty status. http://www.defenselink.mil/news/casualty.pdf. Accessed May 18, 2009.
2. Covey DC: From the frontlines to the home front: The crucial role of military orthopaedic surgeons. *J Bone Joint Surg Am* 2009;91:998-1006.
3. US Department of Defense: Casualty summary by reason code. http://siadapp.dmdc.osd.mil/personnel/CASUALTY/gwot_reason.pdf. Accessed May 19, 2009.
4. Holcomb JB, Stansbury LG, Champion HR, Wade C, Bellamy RF: Understanding combat casualty care statistics. *J Trauma* 2006;60:397-401.
5. Bagg MR, Covey DC, Powell ET IV: Levels of medical care in the global war on terrorism. *J Am Acad Orthop Surg* 2006;14:S7-S9.
6. Webb LX, Pape HC: Current thought regarding the mechanism of action of negative pressure wound therapy with reticulated open cell foam. *J Orthop Trauma* 2008;22:S135-S137.
7. Powell ET IV: The role of negative pressure wound therapy with reticulated open cell foam in the treatment of war wounds. *J Orthop Trauma* 2008; 22:S138-S141.
8. Pollak AN: The use of negative pressure wound therapy with reticulated open cell foam for lower extremity trauma. *J Orthop Trauma* 2008;22: S142-S145.
9. Rinker B, Amspacher JC, Wilson PC, Vasconez HC: Subatmospheric pressure dressing as a bridge to free tissue transfer in the treatment of open tibia fractures. *Plast Reconstr Surg* 2008;121: 1664-1673.
10. Bhattacharyya T, Mehta P, Smith R, Pomahac B: Routine use of wound vacuum-assisted closure does not allow coverage delay for open tibia fractures. *Plast Reconstr Surg* 2008;121: 1263-1266.
11. Dedmond BT, Kortesis B, Punger K, et al: The use of negative-pressure wound therapy (NPWT) in the temporary treatment of soft-tissue injuries associated with high-energy open tibial fractures. *J Orthop Trauma* 2007; 21:11-17.
12. Gomoll AH, Lin A, Harris MB: Incisional vacuum-assisted closure therapy. *J Orthop Trauma* 2006;20: 705-709.
13. Stannard JP, Robinson JT, Anderson ER, McGwin G Jr, Volgas DA, Alonso JE: Negative pressure wound therapy to treat hematomas and surgical incisions following high-energy trauma. *J Trauma* 2006;60:1301-1306.
14. Archdeacon MT, Messerschmitt P: Modern Papineau technique with vacuum-assisted closure. *J Orthop Trauma* 2006;20:134-137.
15. Herscovici D Jr, Sanders RW, Scaduto JM, Infante A, DiPasquale T: Vacuum-assisted wound closure (VAC therapy) for the management of patients with high-energy soft tissue injuries. *J Orthop Trauma* 2003;17: 683-688.
16. Webb LX: New techniques in wound management: Vacuum-assisted wound closure. *J Am Acad Orthop Surg* 2002;10:303-311.
17. DeFranzo AJ, Argenta LC, Marks MW, et al: The use of vacuum-assisted closure therapy for the treatment of lower-extremity wounds with exposed bone. *Plast Reconstr Surg* 2001;108: 1184-1191.
18. Argenta LC, Morykwas MJ: Vacuum-assisted closure: A new method for wound control and treatment. Clinical experience. *Ann Plast Surg* 1997; 38:563-577.
19. Pollak AN, Flaherty SF, Cooper EO, Fang R, Powell ET, Ficke JR: Abstract: Use of negative pressure wound therapy during aeromedical evacuation of wounded warriors. *2009 Annual Meeting Proceedings*. Rosemont, IL, American Academy of Orthopaedic Surgeons, 2009, p 807.
20. Leininger BE, Rasmussen TE, Smith DL, Jenkins DH, Coppola C:

Experience with wound VAC and delayed primary closure of contaminated soft tissue injuries in Iraq. *J Trauma* 2006;61:1207-1211.

21. Ostermann PA, Seligson D, Henry SL: Local antibiotic therapy for severe open fractures: A review of 1085 consecutive cases. *J Bone Joint Surg Br* 1995;77:93-97.
22. Kaplan FS, Glaser DL, Hebela N, Shore EM: Heterotopic ossification. *J Am Acad Orthop Surg* 2004;12: 116-125.
23. Dejerne A, Ceiller A: Para-osteoarthropathies des paraplegiques par lesion medullaire: Etude clinique et radiographique. *Ann Med* 1918;5:497.
24. Pape HC, Marsh S, Morley JR, Krettek C, Giannoudis PV: Current concepts in the development of heterotopic ossification. *J Bone Joint Surg Br* 2004;86:783-787.
25. Potter BK, Burns TC, Lacap AP, Granville RR, Gajewski DA: Heterotopic ossification following traumatic and combat-related amputations: Prevalence, risk factors, and preliminary results of excision. *J Bone Joint Surg Am* 2007;89:476-486.
26. Covey DC, Aaron RK, Born CT, et al: Orthopaedic war injuries: From combat casualty care to definitive treatment. A current review of clinical advances, basic science, and research opportunities. *Instr Course Lect* 2008; 57:65-86.
27. Brooker AF, Bowerman JW, Robinson RA, Riley LH Jr: Ectopic ossification following total hip replacement: Incidence and a method of classification. *J Bone Joint Surg Am* 1973;55: 1629-1632.
28. Letournel E, Judet R, Elson RA: *Fractures of the Acetabulum*, ed 2. New York, NY, Springer, 1993.
29. Hastings H II, Graham TJ: The classification and treatment of heterotopic ossification about the elbow and forearm. *Hand Clin* 1994;10: 417-437.
30. Mills WJ, Tejwani N: Heterotopic ossification after knee dislocation: The predictive value of the injury severity score. *J Orthop Trauma* 2003;17: 338-345.
31. Pape HC, Lehmann U, van Griensven M, Gänsslen A, von Glinski S, Krettek C: Heterotopic ossifications in patients after severe blunt trauma with and without head trauma: Incidence and patterns of distribution. *J Orthop Trauma* 2001;15:229-237.
32. Forsberg JA, Pepek JM, Wagner S, et al: Heterotopic ossification in high-energy wartime extremity injuries: Prevalence and risk factors. *J Bone Joint Surg Am* 2009;91: 1084-1091.
33. Burd TA, Lowry KJ, Anglen JO: Indomethacin compared with localized irradiation for the prevention of heterotopic ossification following surgical treatment of acetabular fractures. *J Bone Joint Surg Am* 2001;83:1783-1788.
34. Karunakar MA, Sen A, Bosse MJ, Sims SH, Goulet JA, Kellam JF: Indometacin as prophylaxis for heterotopic ossification after the operative treatment of fractures of the acetabulum. *J Bone Joint Surg Br* 2006;88: 1613-1617.
35. United States Army Institute of Surgical Research: Orthopaedic Trauma Research Program (OTRP). http://www.usaisr.amedd.army.mil/otrp.html. Revised May 21, 2009. Accessed June 2, 2009.
36. American Academy of Orthopaedic Surgeons: Extremity War Injuries Disaster Preparedness. http://www.aaos.org/research/committee/ewi/ewi.asp. Accessed June 9, 2009.

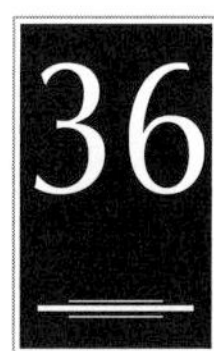

Adult Trauma: Getting Through the Night

Andrew H. Schmidt, MD
Jeffrey O. Anglen, MD, FACS
Arvind D. Nana, MD
Thomas F. Varecka, MD

Abstract

It is now recognized that the treatment of many orthopaedic injuries can be, and in many cases should be, deferred until a later date. For example, surgical repair of most fractures of the proximal and distal tibia is now delayed until soft-tissue healing has occurred. Acute treatment involves only provisionally reducing and stabilizing such fractures using a joint-spanning external fixator. However, situations occur in the emergency department in which emergency treatment, even if it is just temporizing in nature, must be done immediately. Often, such treatment is outside the comfort zone of the responsible orthopaedic surgeon, even physicians with training and experience in orthopaedic trauma. Orthopaedic surgeons will benefit from updated information on current methods for the emergency management of limb- and/or life-threatening injuries in adults. Such treatment is often provisional in nature, treating only the urgent component of the injury (such as a compartment syndrome associated with a complex tibial plateau fracture). It is important for orthopaedic surgeons to understand how to get "through the night" so that later appropriate definitive care is facilitated to optimize patient outcomes.

Instr Course Lect 2010;59:437-453.

Dr. Schmidt or an immediate family member is a board member, owner, officer, or committee member of the Orthopaedic Trauma Association; has received royalties from Smith & Nephew; is a member of a speakers' bureau or has made paid presentations on behalf of Synthes; serves as a paid consultant to or is an employee of Smith & Nephew, Twin Star Medical, Medtronic, DigiMed, and AGA; serves as an unpaid consultant to Conventus Orthopedics and Anthem Orthopedics; has received research or institutional support from Synthes, Smith & Nephew, Twin Star Medical, and Medtronic; owns stock or stock options in Twin Star Medical, Conventus Orthopedics, and the International Spine and Orthopedic Institute; and has received nonincome support (such as equipment or services), commercially derived honoraria, or other non–research-related funding (such as paid travel) from Thieme. Dr. Anglen or an immediate family member is a board member, owner, officer, or committee member of the American Board of Orthopaedic Surgery, the American College of Surgeons, and the Orthopaedic Trauma Association; has received royalties from Biomet; serves as a paid consultant to or is an employee of Stryker; has received research or institutional support from Stryker and Wyeth; and has received nonincome support (such as equipment or services), commercially derived honoraria, or other non–research-related funding (such as paid travel) from the Journal of the American Academy of Orthopaedic Surgeons. *Dr. Nana or an immediate family member is a member of a speakers' bureau or has made paid presentations on behalf of Orthofix and serves as an unpaid consultant to Advanced Orthopaedic Solutions. Dr. Varecka or an immediate family member is a member of a speakers' bureau or has made paid presentations on behalf of Synthes, Stryker, and Zimmer.*

There has been a dramatic change in the approach to the treatment of acute musculoskeletal injuries over the past decade. The previous emphasis on so-called early total care, which advocated immediate definitive repair of all injuries, has shifted to an approach emphasizing "damage control orthopaedics" for a multiply injured patient. In this new paradigm, definitive repair of fractures is delayed until the patient is stabilized physiologically, associated soft-tissue injuries (if present) have healed, and optimum resources are available. However, there remain situations in which immediate treatment may be needed, such as in a patient with a pelvic ring injury and hemodynamic instability, a compartment syndrome, or an irreducible joint dislocation with associated neurovascular compromise. In these circumstances, there may not be time to safely transfer the patient to a specialized center, and emergent treatment directed at the specific problem must be provided. Emergent treatment of open fractures, compartment syndrome, and hemodynamic instability in a patient with a pelvic fracture as well as damage control in multiply injured patients should be understood by all physicians who treat musculoskeletal injuries. Finally, a less often discussed but no less important aspect of surgical care that may affect initial treatment decisions and outcome is sleep deprivation and fatigue of the members of the surgical team.

Open Fractures

Traditionally, the initial management of open fracture wounds was débridement within 6 hours after the injury to prevent infection. That guideline was based on animal experiments performed in the 1890s and is not supported by modern human clinical studies. The Lower Extremity Assessment Project (LEAP) study, a prospective multicenter investigation of severe open lower extremity fractures, showed no relationship between the time from the injury to the surgery and subsequent infection.[1] Multiple retrospective series of open fractures have also failed to support the "6-hour rule," and recent literature reviews have revealed scant support for emergency surgical débridement of open fractures.[2-6] The current consensus favors prudent early surgery within the first 24 hours.

The initial surgical procedure for an open fracture is débridement and irrigation of the open wound. The purpose of débridement is to remove foreign material, contaminating pathogens, and devitalized host tissue. The principles of the surgical procedure include (1) extension of the traumatic wound longitudinally, with the surgeon being careful to consider options for future closure and proceeding systematically through each tissue layer from superficial to deep; (2) careful inspection of surfaces, with preservation of critical tissue such as skin and articular surfaces when possible; and (3) thorough removal of foreign material and dead tissue. Doing this well requires attention, patience, and surgical judgment. Tissue viability is dynamic, and initially it is not possible to determine precisely which tissue will survive. Usually, repeat examination is necessary to ensure adequate removal of dead tissue. Open wounds do not necessarily adequately decompress tissue compartments, and compartment syndrome is a risk with many high-energy fractures. Irrigation of open fracture wounds cleans the wound by removing additional debris and lowering the bacterial load. The irrigation volume, pressure, mode of delivery, and additives are all of potential importance, but little information is available about these parameters. Animal studies suggest that increasing the volume of fluid improves removal of particulate debris and bacteria up to a point,[7] but there are no clear clinical guidelines regarding this parameter. Although there are no specific data to support this recommendation, the chapter's authors suggest an empiric protocol of using 9 L (three 3-L bags) of fluid for Gustilo type III open fracture wounds, 6 L (two bags) for a type II wound, and 3 L for a type I wound. High-pressure irrigation has been shown to drive contamination into the tissue, damage bone, delay healing, and impair infection resistance in animal models and in vitro experiments.[8] Pulsatile delivery of fluid has no proven advantage.[9] Irrigation fluid additives have included antiseptics, antibiotics, and soaps. Antiseptics such as povidone-iodine or hydrogen peroxide are toxic to host immune cells and should not be used; antibiotics are of no proven value in open fracture wounds. Soap solutions help to remove dirt and bacteria through disruption of the hydrophobic and electrostatic forces that bind them to surfaces. In one prospective clinical study, soap solution was compared with antibiotic solution for open fracture wounds, and soap was found to have an advantage.[10]

Traditional teaching dictates that open fracture wounds should not be closed; however, low-energy wounds that have been adequately débrided and cleaned can be closed safely, if closure can be done without tension. If these conditions cannot be met, the fracture wound should be covered, within 1 week, by delayed primary closure, skin grafting, rotational flaps, or free tissue transfer. During the time before definitive coverage, the wound tissues should be protected from desiccation with appropriate dressing techniques. Two methods in use are the antibiotic bead-pouch technique and the Vacuum Assisted Closure device (wound VAC; KCI, San Antonio, TX). The antibiotic bead-pouch technique is a simple method in which handmade polymethylmethacrylate beads are placed on a strand of heavy suture or 18-gauge surgical wire and placed into the wound; the wound is covered with an occlusive adhesive barrier such as OPSITE Post-Op (Smith and Nephew, Memphis, TN) or Ioban (3M, St. Paul, MN).

Stabilizing open fractures promotes healing and infection resistance. The choice and timing of a fixation strategy depends on the characteristics of the patient, the injury, the surgeon, and the operating room resources. In general, immediate plate fixation of open fractures of the lower extremity should be avoided because of an increased risk of infection, although immediate plate fixation of upper extremity open fractures can often be done safely. Acute intramedullary nail fixation of open fractures of the lower extremity can be acceptable, provided that a clean wound with viable bone and soft tissues is achieved with irrigation and débridement. Temporary external fixation, often spanning injured joints, is a useful strategy to protect soft tissues, allow adequate time for planning, and avoid performing complex procedures in the middle of the night. When done for a severely multiply injured patient with unresolved physiologic issues, this strategy is known as damage control orthopaedics.[11]

Antibiotic treatment is one of the most important aspects of open fracture care. Traditionally, cephalosporin antibiotics were used for 3 days. For type III open fractures, aminoglycosides were added and treatment was extended to 5 days. It has been suggested that penicillin be added to the regimen for agricultural injuries with soil contamination because of the risk of clostridial infection; however, these recommendations are based on poorly designed studies done more than 20 years ago.[12,13] More recent data support a shorter duration (24 to 48 hours) of first-generation cephalosporin antibiotics and no additional drugs for coverage of gram-negative or clostridial organisms.[14,15]

Compartment Syndrome

Acute compartment syndrome can complicate any extremity injury, but it is most common in patients with a tibial fracture, especially in men younger than 35 years.[16] Patients with a forearm fracture are the second most common group. Although acute compartment syndrome occurs as a result of the initial injury, it is important to remember that acute surgical stabilization can increase the risk of the syndrome.[17,18] The diagnosis can be difficult, and it should be considered for all patients with an extremity injury. Acute compartment syndrome is a surgical emergency because a delay in treatment may be associated with substantial short- and long-term morbidity related to the degree of muscle necrosis that occurs. In the early phase, morbidity is related to potential renal impairment from rhabdomyolysis, whereas long-term disability is related to the degree of functional impairment caused by muscle fibrosis and neural dysfunction. Not surprisingly, delayed diagnosis of acute compartment syndrome is a common reason for litigation against physicians.[19,20]

Clinical Diagnosis of Compartment Syndrome

Acute compartment syndrome is typically diagnosed based on clinical factors. The classic symptoms of acute compartment syndrome are known as the "five P's"—pain, pallor, pulselessness, paresthesia, and paralysis—but these are late findings. Escalating pain, pain with passive stretching of the involved muscle, and numbness are the clinical clues of an acute compartment syndrome. These criteria are subjective and may be attributed to the associated fracture. This diminishes their diagnostic value. Avoiding regional anesthetic blockade and patient-controlled analgesia, which can completely mask the pain that occurs with acute compartment syndrome, is recommended.[21] Peripheral nerves are sensitive to ischemia; therefore, hypoesthesia in the distribution innervated by a peripheral nerve located within the involved compartment is an important early finding in acute compartment syndrome.[22,23] However, neurologic deficits may be caused by the initial trauma and are therefore not specific.

The variability in the clinical signs and symptoms of acute compartment syndrome makes the accuracy of clinical diagnosis poor, and the sensitivity and positive predictive value of clinical findings are low.[24] In contrast, the specificity and negative predictive value of clinical signs are high, meaning that the absence of clinical findings associated with compartment syndrome of the leg is more useful for excluding the diagnosis than the presence of findings is for confirming the diagnosis.[24] Given the uncertainty in the clinical diagnosis of acute compartment syndrome, a high index of suspicion must be maintained when caring for patients at risk.

Measurement of Intramuscular Pressure

By definition, intramuscular pressure is elevated in cases of acute compartment syndrome, but, because there is wide variation in intramuscular pressure among patients with tibial fractures and because many patients without compartment syndrome can have intramuscular pressures exceeding 30 mm Hg, the direct measurement of intramuscular pressure is not diagnostic.[25] Intramuscular pressure measurement is an adjunct to the clinical examination and is indicated for any patient with equivocal findings; no reliable diagnostic threshold has yet been described.[26-28] Intramuscular pressure measurement is the sole means of diagnosis for patients for whom a clinical examination is not possible, such as those who are intoxicated or have a head injury or those who are already intubated. Typically, intramuscular pressure is measured in the anterior, lateral, and deep posterior compartments of the leg with use of either a commercially available device such as the Stryker Intra-Compartmental Pressure Monitor System (Stryker, Kalamazoo, MI) or an arterial line manometer. Both techniques have acceptable accuracy.[29] Intramuscular pressures vary within each compartment, with measurable differences occurring at distances as close as 5 cm from the site at which the highest pressure was recorded.[30] Intramuscular pressures are also influenced by the position of the adjacent joints.[31]

The most well-supported threshold for fasciotomy appears to be a perfusion pressure of less than 30 mm Hg.[32-34] The perfusion pressure (delta P [ΔP]) is equal to the diastolic blood pressure minus the intramuscular pressure. When the perfusion pressure is 30 mm Hg or greater, it is safe to assume that the patient does not have an acute compartment syndrome. Conversely, when ΔP is less than 30 mm Hg for a sustained period of time, compartment syndrome may be present, and fasciotomy is recommended.

To improve the diagnosis of compartment syndrome and eliminate the need to perform multiple serial intramuscular pressure measurements, continuous intramuscular pressure monitoring has been advocated.[33,35] McQueen and associates[33] demonstrated that continuous pressure monitoring of the anterior compartment of the leg in a cohort of patients with a tibial fracture in whom a compartment syndrome developed led to a marked reduction in the sequelae of acute compartment syndrome, presumably because the diagnosis was made earlier. One important benefit of continuous monitoring is that the time trend of intramuscular pressure is an important variable that cannot be assessed on the basis of a single measurement. Prayson and associates[25] reported that 53% of the patients in their series had at least one intramuscular pressure measurement that was within 40 mm Hg of their mean arterial pressure (an alternative definition of a borderline perfusion pressure), yet none had signs of sequelae of compartment syndrome. Thus, a rising or sustained elevated pressure (or inadequate perfusion pressure) is a more important indication of an acute compartment syndrome and a better indicator of the need for fasciotomy than is a single pressure.

A method to accurately assess perfusion pressure in patients who are under anesthesia is not known. While a patient is under anesthesia, the blood pressure may be artificially low, leading to an inaccurately small perfusion pressure and to unneeded surgery if that pressure is used to decide whether a patient needs a fasciotomy. Kakar and associates[36] recorded blood pressures in a series of patients undergoing tibial nail fixation. Diastolic blood pressure during surgery was lower than that either before or after surgery, but the postoperative diastolic blood pressure was predicted by the preoperative blood pressure. Therefore, a more accurate measurement of an anesthetized patient's perfusion pressure should be based on the preoperative diastolic pressure rather than the intraoperative pressure. The only caveat to this is that, if the patient is to remain under anesthesia for some time, the intraoperative blood pressure should be used.

Surgical Treatment of Compartment Syndrome

Once identified, compartment syndrome must be treated with prompt fasciotomy. Early diagnosis of acute compartment syndrome and prompt fasciotomy have been shown to lead to more rapid union and improved function in patients with a tibial fracture.[32,33] In contrast, if fasciotomy is done too late, the procedure may have little benefit and may actually be harmful.[37] Fasciotomy that is performed after myonecrosis has occurred exposes the necrotic tissue and can lead to bacterial colonization and infection. Finkelstein and associates[37] reviewed the cases of five patients in whom fasciotomy had been performed more than 35 hours after the injury. Of these five patients, one died of multiple organ failure, and the others had amputation of the limb.

Technique of Fasciotomy

The fasciotomy is done by making a longitudinal skin and fascial incision over the entire compartment with release of all constricting tissues. An inadequate skin incision can contribute to persistent elevation of intramuscular pressure.[38] The precise incisions to be made and the structures that require release vary depending on the situation.

Two-Incision Fasciotomy of the Leg

Fasciotomy of the leg can be done safely and easily with two incisions: one lateral and one medial. The anterior and lateral compartments are released separately through the lateral incision. The superficial posterior compartment may be released through either incision. The deep posterior compartment is released through the medial incision. The intervening skin flap is at risk for necrosis if there has been damage to the anterior tibial artery. Therefore, when the anterior tibial artery is known to be or suspected of being injured, a single-incision four-compartment release from a lateral approach is recommended. To perform a two-incision fasciotomy, initially a lateral incision is made midway between the fibula and the anterior crest of the tibia. The skin is gently retracted anteriorly and posteriorly to expose the fascia of the anterior and lateral compartments, respectively. The lateral intermuscular septum that divides the anterior and lateral compartments and the superficial peroneal nerve are identified. The peroneal muscle fascia is usually released first. Finally, the anterior compartment fascia is completely released. Alternatively, the fascia overlying one compartment can be released, followed by division of the intermuscular septum to decompress the other compartment. However, iatrogenic injury to the superficial peroneal nerve may be more likely with this technique.[39] Next, the medial incision is made 1 cm posterior to the posteromedial border of the tibia. The saphenous vein and nerve should be identified. The fascia of the gastrocnemius-soleus complex should be completely released. Distally, the soleus bridge (representing the condensation of the anterior and posterior investing fibers of the soleus muscle) should be specifically released from the posterior aspect of the tibia to completely decompress the flexor digitorum longus and tibialis posterior muscles.

Single-Incision Fasciotomy of the Leg

To perform a single-incision fasciotomy, a single lateral incision, extending from the neck of the fibula to the lateral malleolus, is made. Fibulectomy is not necessary.[39] The anterior and lateral compartments are released in the manner described for the two-incision fasciotomy. The superficial posterior compartment (the gastrocnemius-soleus muscle complex) is released by elevating the skin posteriorly. Finally, a parafibular approach is used to decompress the deep posterior compartment. The peroneal muscles are retracted anteriorly, and the dissection is carried posteriorly to the fibula. With the lateral head of the gastrocnemius-soleus retracted posteriorly, the septum dividing the superficial and deep posterior compartments can be identified and released. If access to the deep posterior compartment is difficult, a medial incision can always be made as described above.

Upper Extremity Fasciotomy

The muscles of the entire upper extremity can be decompressed with an extended anterior incision extending from the shoulder to the wrist. In the upper arm, anterior release of the biceps and brachialis can be extended across the elbow and incorporated into a volar fasciotomy of the forearm. In turn, the volar forearm release can be extended into the palm of the hand to release the median (carpal tunnel) and ulnar nerves (Guyon canal). Beginning with the upper arm, an anterior incision is made along the medial edge of the biceps. The fascia of the biceps and underlying brachialis are released. The incision is extended across the flexion crease of the elbow in a zigzag fashion to avoid later contracture, and then it is continued distally along the volar aspect of the forearm as needed. Although rarely necessary, the triceps can be decompressed with a separate posterior incision. Adequate decompression of the forearm requires release of several potential sites of compression, including the lacertus fibrosus, all muscle fascia, and the flexor retinaculum. First, the incision is continued along the medial border of the mobile wad, consisting of the brachioradialis and radial wrist extensors, which are released. The fascia of the digital flexors, supinator, and pronator quadratus is released as needed. Rarely, a separate dorsal forearm fasciotomy is needed. Finally, a standard carpal tunnel release is performed at the wrist, with the incision again crossing the wrist flexion crease in a zigzag fashion to avoid contracture. Injury to the palmar cutaneous branch of the median nerve must be avoided. If the hand is also involved, release of the thenar, hypothenar, and interosseous muscles of the hand is performed separately with longitudinal dorsal incisions between the second and third metacarpals and between the fourth and fifth metacarpals.

Management of Fasciotomy Wounds

An advance in the management of fasciotomy wounds is the wound VAC device. When applied at the time of fasciotomy, the wound VAC device may allow earlier closure of the fasciotomy site and a decreased need for skin grafting.[40] Closure of the fasciotomy site before 5 days is not recommended and can be associated with recurrent compartment syndrome.[41] Skin grafting is associated with fewer complications than is either primary or delayed wound closure.[42]

Damage Control Orthopaedics

The understanding of the role of orthopaedic resuscitation in the overall management of multiply injured patients has changed dramatically in recent years. The potential benefits of optimal fracture care in this patient population include

(1) facilitating overall patient care, (2) controlling bleeding, (3) decreasing additional soft-tissue injury, (4) avoiding further activation of the systemic inflammatory response, (5) removal of devitalized tissue, (6) prevention of ischemia/reperfusion injury, and (7) pain relief.

Until recently, appropriate fracture care in a multiply injured patient was considered to be fixation of all fractures as soon as possible. This was believed to decrease the inflammatory load through stabilization of bone and soft tissue, and all long-bone fractures were definitively stabilized within 24 hours (or as soon as possible) so that the patient could be positioned upright for adequate pulmonary toilet. The paradigm at the time was "This patient is too sick not to be treated surgically." In a landmark study, Bone and associates[43] showed that this type of management resulted in fewer days of ventilator treatment, fewer days in the intensive care unit, and lower prevalences of multiple organ failure and mortality.

Approximately 15 years ago, published reports began to suggest that, in some cases, this aggressive initial management might be harmful.[44] The term damage control was originally coined by the United States Navy to describe the repair of damaged sea vessels in combat to allow continued use. An approach best described as damage control surgery was reported by Rotondo and associates[45] who used rapid but nondefinitive control of hemorrhage to avoid the lethal triad of acidosis, hypothermia, and coagulopathy in patients exsanguinating from penetrating abdominal trauma. In 1993, the report by Pape and associates[44] of increased pulmonary complications in multiply injured patients undergoing immediate femoral nailing ushered in the era of damage control orthopaedics and the new paradigm best described as "optimal surgery" rather than "maximal surgery."

In the past decade, substantial work has been done to define which group of patients can be safely treated with maximal fixation and which should have damage control surgery only. In general, the early death of a multiply injured patient is caused by primary brain injuries and major blood loss, whereas late death is caused by secondary brain injury and host defense failure.[46] The first "hit" (initial trauma) results in hypoxia, hypotension, organ and soft-tissue injuries, and fractures. The second and subsequent "hits" (surgical procedures and sepsis) lead to hypoperfusion, hypoxia/ischemia, reperfusion, blood loss caused by acute endothelial injury, and tissue damage causing local necrosis, inflammation, and acidosis. Any type of surgical procedure that induces substantial bleeding and/or soft-tissue damage can be sufficiently traumatic to the patient to represent a "second hit."

Damage control orthopaedics is defined as the provisional stabilization of musculoskeletal injuries to allow the patient's overall physiology to improve. The primary tactic of damage control orthopaedics is to use traction or external fixation as the means of provisional stabilization. The purpose of damage control orthopaedics is to avoid the worsening of physiologic parameters related to the second hit of a major orthopaedic procedure by delaying definitive fracture repair until the patient's physiology is optimized. In this approach, the focus is on controlling the bleeding, managing the injuries to the soft tissues, and achieving provisional fracture stability.

Pathophysiology of Trauma

Cytokines, leukocytes, the vascular endothelium, and endothelial-leukocyte interactions are the key determinants of the response to injury. Typical physiologic changes that occur after trauma are increased capillary permeability in the lung, gut, blood vessels, and muscle. The lung parenchyma is most affected in trauma patients. The largest capillary bed in the body is found in the lung, and pulmonary edema is a frequent sign of increased pulmonary permeability. As is the case in the lung, increased permeability of the blood vessels leads to movement of fluid into the third space. Increased tissue permeability also results in translocation of bacteria in the gut. In muscle, edema and bleeding can lead to compartment syndrome.

The inflammatory response to injury (first hit or second hit) includes the systemic inflammatory response syndrome, which is mediated by proinflammatory cytokines, arachidonic acid metabolites, proteins of the acute phase/coagulation systems, complement factors, and hormonal mediators. Systemic inflammatory response syndrome can lead to adult respiratory distress syndrome and/or multiple organ failure. Simultaneous with the onset of systemic inflammatory response syndrome is the counter regulatory anti-inflammatory response syndrome, which can cause immunosuppression and subsequent infection. The counter regulatory anti-inflammatory response syndrome is described as endothelial cell damage, accumulation of leukocytes, disseminated intravascular coagulopathy, and microcirculatory imbalances that lead to apoptosis and necrosis of parenchymal cells.

Measurement of specific markers can help to quantify the inflammatory responses. These markers include base deficit or serum lactate, soluble thrombomodulin, polymorphonuclear elastase, interleukin (IL)-6, IL-10, and human leukocyte antigen-DR (HLA-DR) (Table 1). Genetic influences have also been shown to play a role with IL-6, IL-10, tumor necrosis factor (TNF), and HLA-DR.[47] A base deficit or elevated serum lactate level is considered evidence of continued metabolic acidosis. A serum lactate level of more than 2.5 mmol/L can indicate occult hypoperfusion and can be used to judge a patient's suitability for surgery. Crowl and associates[48] showed that, when a nail is used to stabilize a femoral fracture within 24 hours after the injury, there is a twofold higher incidence of postoperative complications if the serum lactate level is more than 2.5 mmol/L. Four hours after femoral nailing (with or without reaming), markers associated with the systemic inflammatory response are elevated.[49] Waydhas and associates[50] demonstrated that patients with a high polymorphonuclear elastase level combined with a high C-reactive protein level and thrombocytopenia have a 79% incidence of lung, liver, or kidney failure. IL-6 concentration has also been shown to be a reliable index of the magnitude of injury (burden of trauma) and of the "second hit" produced by the surgical procedure.[49] If the initial IL-6 level is more than 500 pg/dL (> 5 μg/L), then definitive surgery should be delayed for at least 4 days after provisional stabilization surgery.[51] Patients with a high Injury Severity Score[52] have an elevated IL-6 level for more than 5 days. The potent anti-inflammatory cytokine IL-10 also inhibits TNF-α and IL-1 expression and negatively regulates HLA-DR expression. Giannoudis and associates[53] showed that elevated initial and persistently elevated IL-10 levels correlate with sepsis. HLA-DR is an indicator of resistance to infection and is expressed by circulating monocytes. It is required for antigen presentation and helper T-lymphocytes and thus plays a central role in the immune response to infection. Diminished HLA-DR expression is associated with sepsis and death.[54]

Table 1
Specific Markers and Mediators of Damage Control Surgery

Base deficit or serum lactate (hypovolemic shock)
Soluble thrombomodulin (endothelial injury)
Polymorphonuclear elastase (tissue injury)
Interleukin-6 (proinflammatory cytokine)
Interleukin-10 (anti-inflammatory cytokine)
Human leukocyte antigen-DR (resistance to infection)

Table 2
Parameters to Consider When Deciding to Implement Damage Control Orthopaedic Protocol

Polytrauma with Injury Severity Score of > 20 points and additional thoracic trauma (Abbreviated Injury Scale score[55] of > 2 points)
Polytrauma with abdominal and pelvic injuries and hemorrhagic shock (systolic blood pressure of < 90 mm Hg)
Injury Severity Score of ≥ 40 points without additional thoracic injury
Initial pulmonary artery pressure of > 24 mm Hg
Increased pulmonary artery pressure of > 6 mm Hg during intramedullary nailing
Difficult resuscitation
Platelet count < 90,000/μL (< 90 × 10^9/L)
Hypothermia (for example, temperature of < 35°C)
Transfusion of > 10 units of blood
Bilateral lung contusion on initial chest radiograph
Multiple long-bone fractures and truncal injury
Prolonged duration of anticipated surgery (> 90 min)

Timely analysis of specific markers and factors may not be possible in many facilities. In the absence of precise biomarker data, the orthopaedic surgeon may have to rely on physiologic and clinical parameters to guide decision making (Table 2).[55] The following injuries are usually best managed with the damage control orthopaedic protocol: femoral shaft fracture in a multiply injured patient, pelvic ring injuries with substantial hemorrhage, and polytrauma in a geriatric patient. Pape and associates[56] described the criteria for implementing the damage control orthopaedic protocol to include a serum lactate level of more than 2.5 mmol/L, a base excess of more than 8 mmol/L, a pH of less than 7.24, a temperature of less than 35°C, surgical time of more than 90 minutes, coagulopathy, and transfusion of more than 10 units of packed red blood cells. When damage control orthopaedic protocols are followed, initial stabilization of fractures is achieved with minimal blood loss, fluid shifts, hypothermia, or prolonged surgical time. Options for fracture stabilization in damage control orthopaedic protocols include skeletal traction, splints or casts, intramedullary nail fixation, conventional plates, minimally invasive plates, and external fixation. External fixation is the preferred method of initial stabilization because it can be done quickly with minimal blood loss. Nana and Kessinger[57] showed that the use of spanning external fixation for complex distal tibial fractures that are treated immediately improves skin perfusion.

After provisional stability has been obtained, definitive surgery is

Table 3
End Points for Damage Control Resuscitation

Giannoudis[58]
Stable hemodynamics
Stable oxygen saturation
Lactate level of < 2 mmol/L
No coagulopathy
Normal temperature
Urinary output of > 1 mL/kg/h
No inotropic support
Tscherne et al[59]
No increasing infiltrate on chest radiograph
Balanced or negative fluid balance
PaO_2/FiO_2 (arterial oxygen tension/fraction of inspired oxygen) of > 250
Pulmonary artery pressure of < 24 mm Hg
Maximal inspiratory airway pressure of < 35 cm H_2O
Platelet count of > 95,000/μL (> 95 × 10^9/L)
White blood cell count of < 12,000/μL (> 12 × 10^9/L)
Intracranial pressure of < 15 cm H_2O

considered only after the patient has been adequately resuscitated. End points for resuscitation with the use of damage control principles are outlined in Table 3.[58,59] A simplified guideline is to proceed with definitive surgery when fluid balance is negative.

Hemodynamic Instability in Patients With a Pelvic Ring Injury

Up to 40% of patients with an unstable pelvic ring injury die from their injuries, and hemodynamic instability is the main predictor of death. The initial management of patients with a pelvic ring injury, including the assessment and management of hemodynamic instability and acute (rather than definitive) stabilization of the pelvic injury, is critical. There are several key points to remember. (1) Pelvic ring injuries are markers of violent injury and are associated with life-threatening hemorrhage and injuries to other organs and sites, including the abdominal viscera and genitourinary system. It should not be assumed that the pelvis is the source of bleeding in an unstable patient. (2) Although the anatomic and mechanistic classifications of pelvic ring injuries are useful, they are not perfectly predictive of the risk of bleeding. (3) Pelvic ring compression with sheets is a simple and effective treatment of immediate management of bleeding in patients with an open-book injury. (4) The role of immediate angiography instead of surgical exploration remains controversial and probably varies depending on institutional resources and injury patterns. (5) The key to the correct initial assessment of a pelvic ring injury is careful evaluation of the radiographs for evidence of deformity and instability.

Assessment of Pelvic Ring Injury

The physical examination of patients with a pelvic ring injury is primarily aimed at defining the neurovascular status of the lower extremities. The motor function and the sensation in the lower extremities should be documented. The examiner should look for asymmetry and/or deformity of the iliac crest, limb-length inequality, and skin lesions (including any open wounds and areas of closed degloving). Every patient should have a rectal examination, the prostate should be examined in males, and the vagina should be examined in females, as lacerations in these locations may be the site of an open pelvic fracture.

Standard imaging of the pelvic ring includes both plain radiographs and CT scans. Radiographs should include AP, inlet, and outlet views. A cystogram should be done in all patients, and a retrograde urethrogram should be performed in male patients before passage of a Foley catheter. CT is done primarily to define the posterior part of the pelvic ring; axial views best demonstrate sacroiliac joint injuries and sacral fractures. Vertical displacement is underestimated on AP radiographs and cannot be measured on axial CT cuts. Vertical displacement can be determined on the inlet and outlet radiographs of the pelvis.

Deformity and instability should be established when radiographs of an injured pelvis are evaluated. Deformity is assessed on the basis of the relative degree of internal or external rotation of the iliac wing as well as anteroposterior and/or vertical displacement of the posterior aspect of the pelvis. A pelvic fracture is considered to be unstable when there is symphysis diastasis of more than 2.5 cm, more than 1 cm of displacement of the posterior part of the pelvis, complete widening of the posterior sacroiliac joint, and/or any neurologic injury.

Classification of Pelvic Ring Injuries

A fracture classification system should group together fractures that have a similar injury pattern, treatments, potential complications, and sequelae. With pelvic fractures, all of these are primarily related to the condition of the posterior aspect of the pelvic ring because stability, neurologic injury, pelvic asymmetry, limb-length inequality, and persistent lumbosacral pain are determined by the extent of injury to the posterior aspect of the pelvic ring.

Pennal and Associates Classification

Pennal and associates[60] classified injuries into three types. Type A injuries are stable with an intact posterior arch. Type B injuries are rotationally unstable, with incomplete disruption of the posterior arch. These are subdivided into open-book or external rotation injuries (type B1), lateral compression or internal rotation injuries (type B2), and bilateral injuries (type B3). Finally, type C injuries are both rotationally and vertically unstable, and they are subdivided into different types depending on the nature of the posterior injury.

Young-Burgess Classification

Young and Burgess proposed a mechanistic classification of pelvic ring injury, noting a correlation between the mechanism of injury and associated complications.[61] They proposed four types of injuries: anteroposterior compression (APC), lateral compression (LC), vertical shear (VS), and combined. Each of these major groups is further subtyped on the basis of the degree of displacement, deformity, and instability.

Hemodynamic Instability

Hemodynamic instability is defined by shock (low blood pressure), metabolic parameters (base deficit), and the need for blood products. The risk of bleeding is correlated with the fracture pattern, but hemodynamic instability can occur with any pelvic fracture.[62] APC pelvic injuries are more likely to be associated with posterior bleeding, whereas lateral compression injuries are more often associated with anterior vessel injury. Sarin and associates[63] reviewed the cases of 283 patients with a pelvic ring injury who were in shock (a systolic blood pressure of < 90 mm Hg) at the time of presentation. Thirteen percent required embolization because of persistent hypotension. In that series, the fracture pattern and orthopaedic management did not differ between the stable patients and those needing angiography. Advanced age was significantly correlated with an increased need for embolization in women only (the mean age of the women who needed embolization was 55 years compared with 40 years for women not needing embolization), whereas the Injury Severity Score correlated with the need for embolization in men but not in women.[63]

Treatment Options

Fluid replacement is the initial treatment of a patient with a pelvic ring injury who is hemodynamically unstable. Fluid replacement alone can increase bleeding in some instances and should be used judiciously. If the patient does not respond to fluid replacement, or initially responds but becomes hypotensive again, the source of bleeding should be found. Ultrasonographic examination of the abdomen and pelvis and CT angiography are the most common and expeditious means with which to evaluate bleeding. If there are no other sources of bleeding except the pelvic fracture, angiography, circumferential compression (by means of a sheet, pelvic binder, or external fixation), or an exploratory laparotomy with vascular repair and packing of the pelvis are three methods to control the bleeding. The most appropriate choice is institution and/or physician dependent, and the options have not been standardized.

Angiography has a limited role in the management of patients with pelvic ring injuries. Most bleeding after a pelvic ring injury is venous, and embolizable arterial lesions are uncommon. Large-vessel embolization also has been shown to cause extensive necrosis of the hip abductor muscles.[64] Balogh and associates[65] reported increased adherence to the key steps of the guidelines and better clinical outcomes after institution of evidence-based practice guidelines that included abdominal clearance with diagnostic peritoneal aspiration/lavage or ultrasound (Focused Assessment with Sonography in Trauma [FAST] examination), noninvasive pelvic binding within 15 minutes after presentation, pelvic angiography within 90 minutes after admission, and pelvic external fixation within 24 hours. In the period after the guidelines were instituted, the transfusion of packed red blood cells in the first 24 hours decreased from 16 ± 2 units to 11 ± 1 units, and the mortality rate decreased from 35% to 7% ($P < 0.05$).

Fangio and associates[66] used angiography in 32 patients with an average Injury Severity Score of 39 points who remained hypotensive despite controlled fluid resuscitation (500 mL of normal saline solution) and dopamine infusion and who did not have thoracic and abdominal bleeding, cardiac tamponade, or tension pneumothorax. Twenty-five patients had positive results on angiography and underwent embolization. There was no relationship between the presence of an arterial lesion and the pelvic fracture pattern; in fact, the only significant differences between those with and those without a lesion on angiography were the initial blood pressure (65 mm Hg compared with 78 mm Hg) and the amount of blood products received. Thirteen patients had a laparotomy because of expanding intra-abdominal fluid; three of six laparotomy procedures that were done before angiography revealed negative findings, whereas only one of seven done after angiography revealed negative findings. Twenty-five patients underwent embolization; pelvic arterial bleeding was stopped in 24 of them (96%) and was followed by hemodynamic improvement in 21 (84%).[66]

Cook and associates[67] reviewed 23 patients with a pelvic fracture who underwent angiography and found that the fracture morphology was not predictive of the location of the vascular injury. Six of 10 patients who died had angiography as the first therapeutic intervention. Five of the 10 patients had a fracture pattern that produced an increase in pelvic volume (APC or VS pattern), and two of those patients died during angiography. Cook and associates[67] believed that these patients would have been better treated with external fixation before the angiography. Shapiro and associates[68] demonstrated that repeat pelvic angiography might be necessary in patients with persistent hypotension after previous angiography, whether or not arterial bleeding was identified during the initial session.

Circumferential compression, external fixation, and pelvic packing to control pelvic stability are valuable methods to help control bleeding. They reduce bleeding, lessen pain, and allow the patient to be mobilized. Pelvic stability should be achieved as soon as possible after the injury and initial assessment. Simple wrapping of the pelvis with a sheet is now commonplace in the United States for any patient suspected of having a pelvic ring injury. It is cheap and simple, and it can be very effective.

Bottlang and associates[69] investigated stabilization of pelvic ring fractures with slings in cadavers. They demonstrated that circumferential compression with a noninvasive pelvic sling is an effective and safe method for reducing and stabilizing open-book pelvic fractures (Young-Burgess APC II, APC III, and LC II) at an emergency scene. Provisional pelvic external fixation as an initial method of controlling bleeding works but has a 21% rate of complications, which consist mostly of pin tract infections without sequelae.[70] Cothren and associates[71] reported a reduction in blood product requirements and no deaths caused by bleeding after instituting a protocol of preperitoneal pelvic packing and pelvic external fixation.

All patients identified with a pelvic ring injury during initial resuscitation should be treated with a pelvic binder and a Foley catheter (after a retrograde urethrogram and cystogram), and additional pelvic radiographs including inlet and outlet views and a pelvic CT scan should be obtained. Fluid resuscitation is given with continuous monitoring of urine output, the base deficit, hemoglobin levels, and coagulation function. Mechanical instability of the pelvis is determined and, in patients with persistent hypotension, subsequent management depends on the fracture pattern.

Rotationally Unstable Injuries

Patients with rotationally unstable fracture patterns may respond to wrapping of the pelvis with a sheet or application of a binder. If appropriate resources and expertise are available, anterior pelvic external fixation or symphyseal plate fixation can be done. Plate fixation is performed if the patient undergoes a laparotomy; otherwise, an external fixator is applied. Some apparent open-book injuries include vertically unstable posterior injuries for which posterior iliosacral fixation is also warranted. The challenge is to identify these.

Lateral Compression Injuries

Lateral compression injuries are more stable, and early pelvic fixation is not beneficial. If these patients remain hemodynamically unstable, angiography or laparotomy is indicated.

Rotationally and Vertically Unstable Injuries

Rarely, posterior pelvic clamping in the operating room is done after angiography if the patient is persistently hemodynamically unstable.

Upper Extremity Emergencies

The one absolute, nondeferrable, middle-of-the-night upper extremity surgical emergency procedure is the attempted replantation of an amputated finger or limb. Although a lengthy discussion of this subject is beyond the scope of this review, it is important to bear in mind that replantation is time sensitive. Restoration of arterial inflow and venous outflow is vital for the successful salvage of the amputated part and recovery of as much function as possible.

Infectious processes require early, if not immediate, intervention. Infection causes fibrosis, adhesions, edema, stiffness, and other detrimental effects that adversely affect the normal sliding and excursion of delicate hand and upper extremity structures. Immediate evacuation of pus and surgical control of infection are mandatory as soon as they are feasible. Suppurative tenosynovitis and septic arthritis caused by human bites, animal bites, or other penetrating injuries need immediate surgical treatment and antibiotic coverage with a third-generation cephalosporin. Ceftriaxone, or a similar antibiotic, should be used until specific culture and sensitivity results are available. An infectious disease consultation should be considered.

Deteriorating neurologic function is an indication for at least pro-

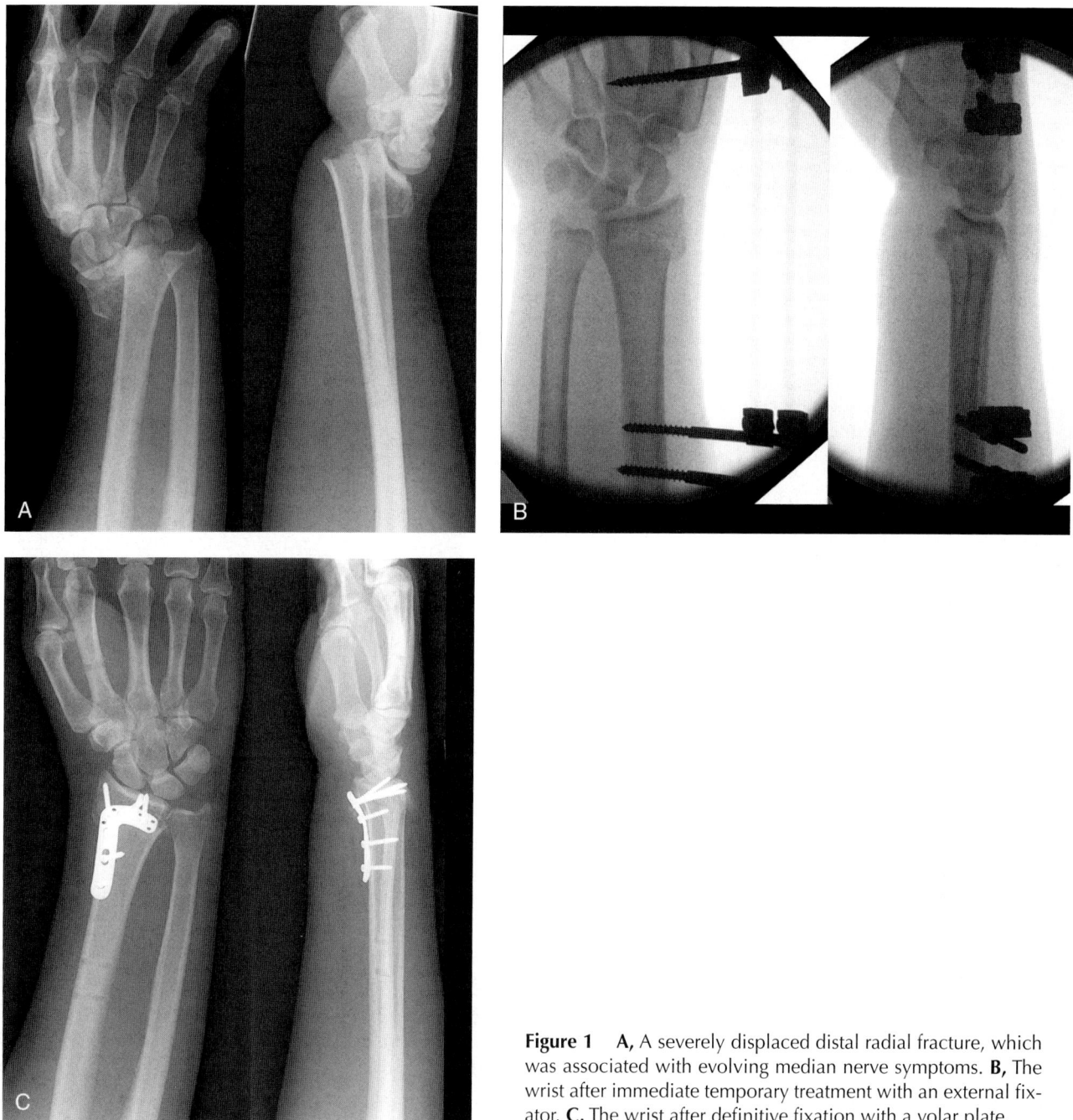

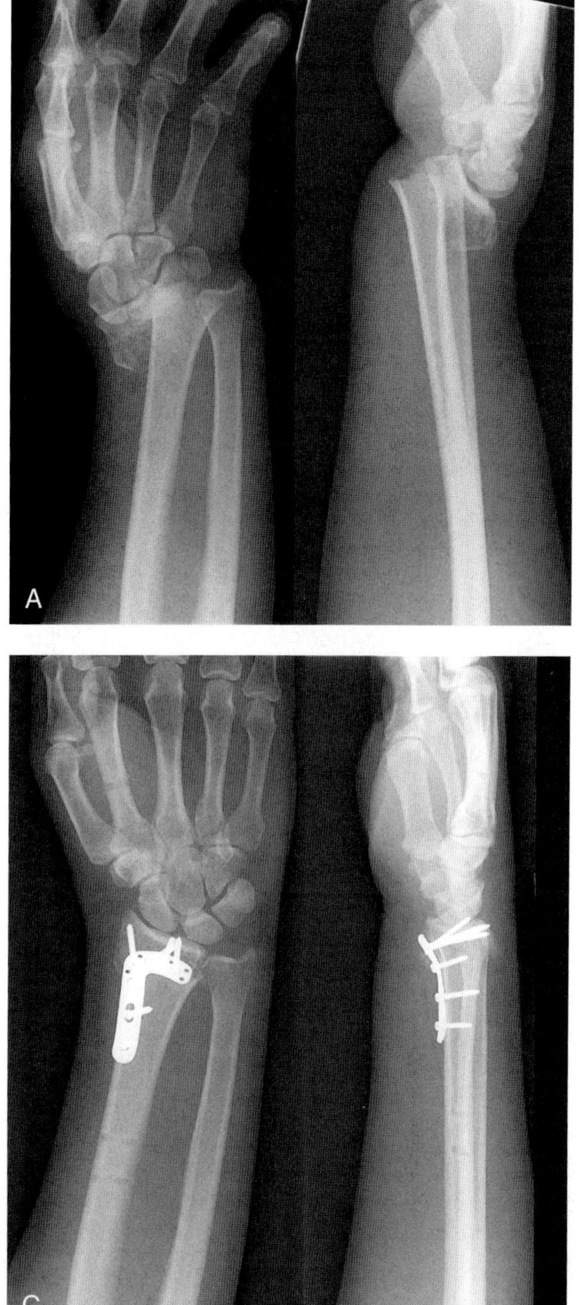

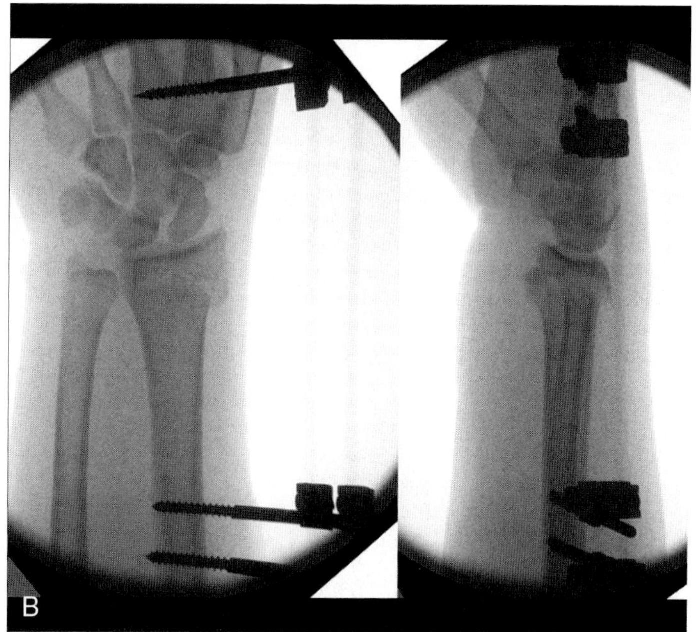

Figure 1 **A,** A severely displaced distal radial fracture, which was associated with evolving median nerve symptoms. **B,** The wrist after immediate temporary treatment with an external fixator. **C,** The wrist after definitive fixation with a volar plate.

visional, if not definitive, stabilization of an upper extremity fracture (Figure 1). A distal radial fracture caused by a high-energy injury is particularly noteworthy, if not notorious, in this regard, with respect to median nerve compromise. There are three possible situations that can arise after distal radial fracture that may lead to acute dysfunction of the median nerve. (1) The median nerve is found to be impaired or nonfunctional at the time of presentation. Under such circumstances, the nerve was probably injured at the time of impact, by stretch or laceration (uncommon), and immediate or early intervention will not change the natural history of the nerve's recovery. Emergent surgery is not warranted. (2) The neurologic function deteriorates during the process of examination, initial treatment, or early observation. This is

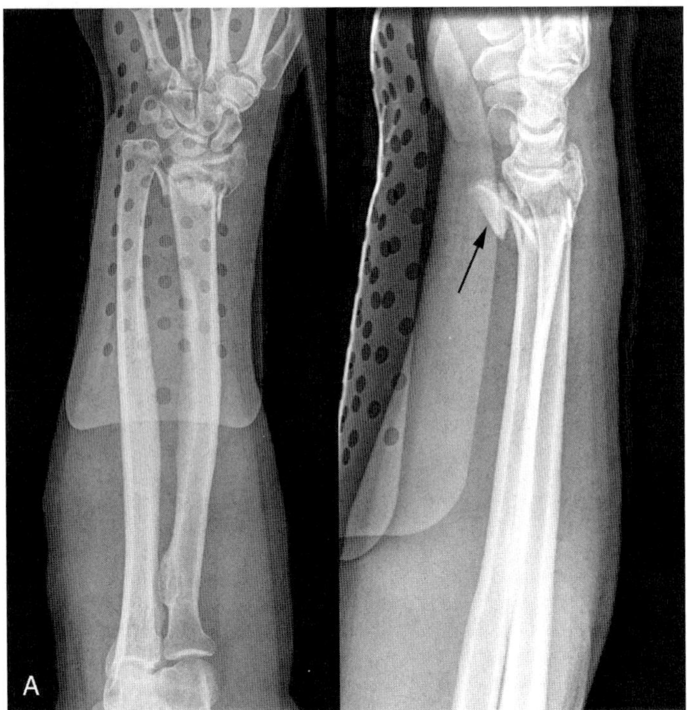

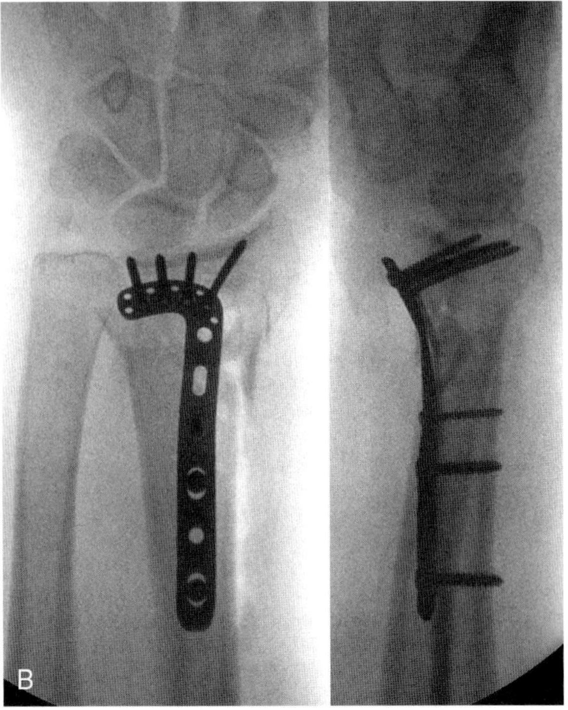

Figure 2 **A,** A high-energy distal radial fracture with acute carpal tunnel syndrome caused by a displaced volar fragment that was not reducible by closed means (*arrow*). **B,** Immediate open reduction and volar plate fixation with carpal tunnel release was performed.

essentially an impending compartment syndrome of the carpal tunnel and requires emergent carpal tunnel decompression (Figure 2). Fracture reduction alone can result in adequate decompression of the median nerve (in cases in which neurologic compromise is caused by pressure from a displaced bone fragment). (3) Nerve function changes over a period of several days or weeks. This most likely represents alteration in nerve physiology secondary to inflammation, hematoma organization, or accumulation of acute phase mediators. Nerve decompression and irrigation are indicated, but this should be done on an urgent, not an emergent, basis.

Lower Extremity Emergencies

Orthopaedic conditions in the lower extremity that are emergent problems include a hip dislocation, a displaced femoral neck fracture in any patient in whom femoral head salvage is desirable (most patients younger than 65 years), a knee dislocation, a talar neck fracture with displacement, and a subtalar dislocation.

Dislocation of the hip joint is usually a high-energy injury that can interrupt the blood supply to the femoral head and cause cartilage necrosis. Relocation should be done emergently to prevent irreversible damage to the joint, although reported time guidelines in the literature range from 6 to 24 hours. There are conflicting and strong opinions from various experts, but good data are lacking.[72] Theoretically, an associated acetabular fracture changes the urgency by decompressing both the soft-tissue tension and the hematoma. An expeditious relocation of the dislocated hip makes sense, if only from the point of view of reducing the patient's pain. Certainly, patients should not be transferred to other centers with a hip that is still dislocated.

A variety of reduction maneuvers have been described, including the Allis, Bigelow, Stimson, and East Baltimore lift maneuvers.[73] Adequate pain control, relaxation, and assistance are required. If one or two gentle and controlled attempts at reduction are unsuccessful, additional treatment should be performed in an operating room with the patient under general anesthesia and with the facilities available for open reduction. Repeated, forceful attempts are ill-advised. The inability to reduce a dislocation is often caused by interposed fragments from the femoral head or from the acetabulum, and such a dislocation should be treated in the operating room, where trochanteric osteotomy may be necessary to facilitate reduction.[74,75] If a patient has an unstable closed reduction or a dislocation with interposed fragments, skeletal traction should be used until definitive surgical treatment is accomplished.

A femoral neck fracture in a young patient requires emergent reduction and fixation to protect the blood supply to the femoral head; a controllable factor in outcome is the quality of the reduction. An anatomic reduction is recommended even if it must be performed in an open fashion. Fixation with three screws placed peripherally in an inverted triangle configuration provides good stability. The necessity for a capsulotomy to release the hemarthrosis is controversial. In a young patient with a nondisplaced or minimally displaced fracture, the capsule may be competent, and the formation of a tense hemarthrosis may compress the blood vessels supplying the femoral head. In that setting, an open or percutaneous capsulotomy may improve the blood flow to the head, although this remains unproven. However, there are risks to this procedure, including damage to those very same blood vessels.

Dislocation of the knee joint (that is, the femorotibial articulation, as opposed to the patellofemoral articulation) is a high-energy injury and can be limb-threatening because of associated vascular injury. If there is an abnormality of the pulses or of perfusion in the limb, emergent evaluation and treatment are indicated. If the pulses can be palpated and are clinically normal, and the ankle-brachial index is more than 0.9, arteriography is not necessary. If the limb is obviously not perfused, arteriography also is not necessary because the patient should be taken directly to the operating room for vascular exploration and repair. Delay of the vascular repair is an important risk factor for subsequent amputation.[76-78]

The knee should be gently reduced and stabilized with a splint or external fixation to allow close monitoring of the neurovascular status and compartment pressures. There is no advantage to emergent ligament repair. Rarely, the dislocation is irreducible by closed means. This is usually caused by the medial femoral condyle tearing through the capsule and becoming button-holed, with capsular-ligamentous tissue being caught in the intercondylar notch. If the patient is neurovascularly intact, this situation is not necessarily an emergency, but the patient should be monitored closely and taken on an urgent basis to the operating room for an open reduction.

Talar neck fracture is considered an emergency by some physicians because of the tenuous nature and retrograde flow of the blood supply to the talar dome, but emergent reduction and fixation have not been shown to improve outcomes.[79-81] However, if the displacement compromises the skin, as evidenced by tight blanched medial skin without capillary refill, the patient should be treated emergently to save the skin from dying. The same principle holds true for subtalar dislocation. If the skin is compromised, emergent reduction is warranted. Reduction can usually be accomplished in a closed fashion, but occasionally a surgical procedure is required if there is interposition of tendons.

Surgeon Performance and Fatigue

As with any orthopaedic emergency, the timing of the definitive procedure depends on multiple factors: availability of a suitable operating room, availability and operational integrity of appropriate equipment, availability of experienced assistants and scrub personnel, and other factors. Often overlooked, however, is the state of readiness of the surgeon. When deciding whether surgical treatment should be done in the middle of the night, surgeons are not always the most reliable judges of their own capabilities. Fatigue and sleeplessness have subtle but real negative influences on surgeons' performances.[82]

Because of the similar types of responsibilities and decision making involved with their jobs, surgeons are often compared with airline pilots with respect to performance accuracy and performance deterioration as fatigue comes into play. Sexton and associates[83] reported that more than 70% of surgeons refused to admit to fatigue-induced deterioration in performance as compared with only 23% of airline pilots. Like surgery, flying airplanes requires a coordinated and skilled team. More than 90% of pilots were able to relinquish some authority and responsibility when they were overly fatigued, as opposed to approximately 55% of surgeons. Others in the medical field do a much better job of recognizing fatigue; anesthesiologists are much better at preserving cohesiveness and team function when they are fatigued, doing almost twice as well as surgeons in these performance domains. Even residents and house officers far surpass surgeons.[83] Fischer and associates[84] studied petrochemical shift workers and found work performance and alertness were markedly impaired when they worked the nighttime shift. Not surprisingly, these parameters showed a marked

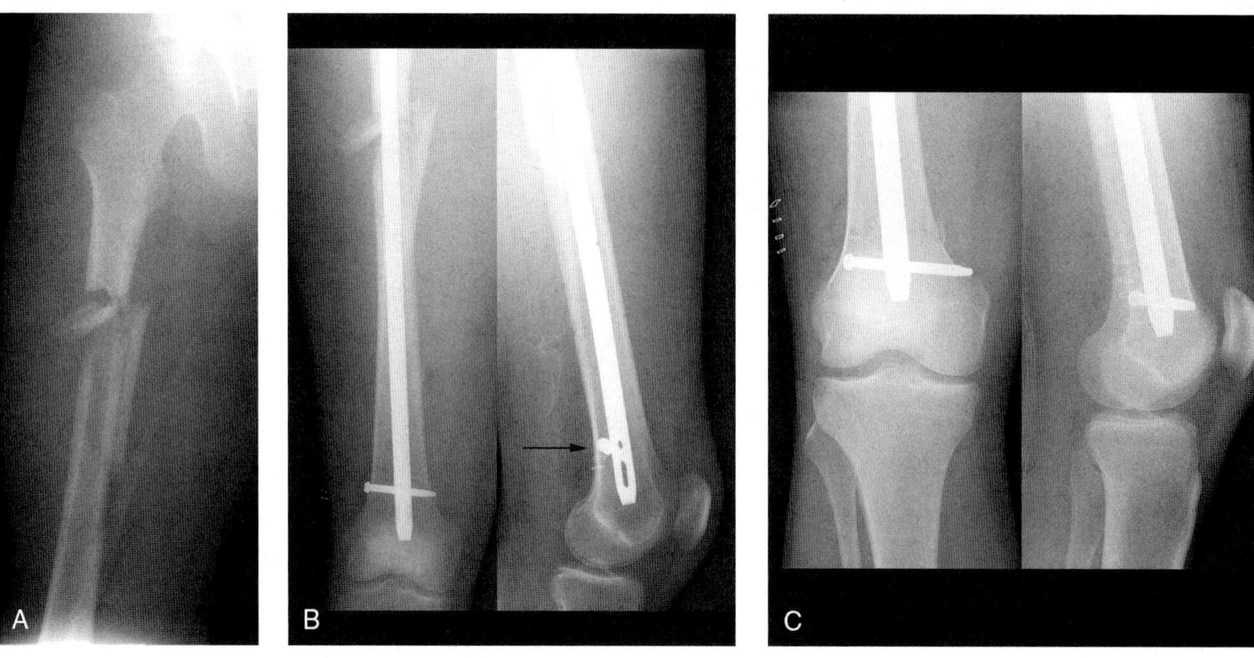

Figure 3 **A,** A comminuted femoral fracture presenting late in the evening. **B,** Immediate nailing was done during the middle of the night. Postoperative radiographs revealed a missed distal interlocking screw (*arrow*). **C,** Revision surgery was required to replace the distal interlocking screw.

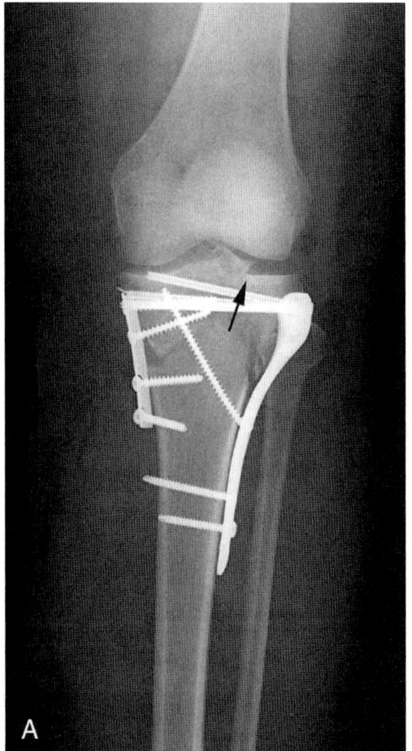

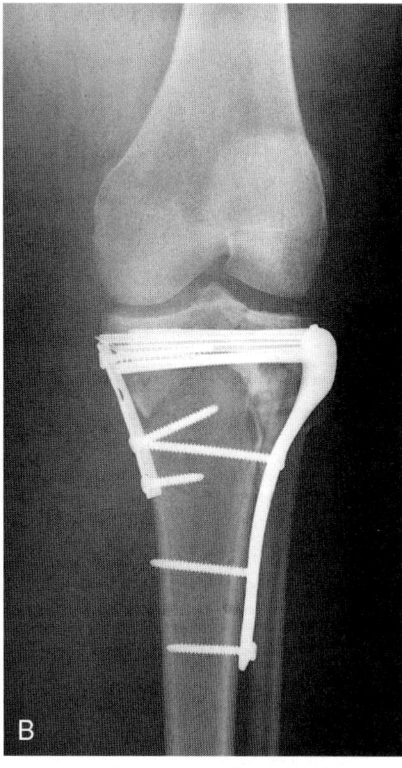

Figure 4 **A,** Postoperative AP radiograph of a malreduced bicondylar tibial plateau fracture, with unacceptable residual articular step-off (*arrow*). **B,** AP radiograph after revision fixation showing anatomic reduction of the articular surface.

tendency to worsen further as the nocturnal work shift passed. Bartel and associates[85] evaluated a cohort of anesthesiologists before and after a 24-hour period of call. The study group was tested for their ability to accurately complete a set of increasingly complex psychomotor tests. After a night on call, 30% of the doctors showed more than a 15% increase in simple-task reaction time and more than 50% showed similar increases in reaction times for more complex tasks. Surgeons are not the only ones affected by fatigue-induced deficits in accuracy and performance; however, they tend to be much less likely to recognize and acknowledge the fatigue effect.

Unfortunately, errors of commission probably take center stage more frequently than do most other errors when late-night or middle-of-the-night procedures are undertaken. Fatigue and accompanying decreases in decision-making accuracy and deterioration in motor skills can lead to imprecise reductions, inaccurate fixation, and incomplete treatment. Such circumstances often lead to poor outcomes and, worse, the need for revision surgery (Figures 3 and 4). Complex articular reconstructions are best deferred until the entire surgical team is well rested and ready to undertake these orthopaedic challenges.

References

1. Webb LX, Bosse MJ, Castillo RC, MacKenzie EJ; LEAP Study Group: Analysis of surgeon-controlled variables in the treatment of limb-threatening type-III open tibial diaphyseal fractures. *J Bone Joint Surg Am* 2007;89:923-928.
2. Charalambous CP, Siddique I, Zenios M, et al: Early versus delayed surgical treatment of open tibial fractures: Effect on the rates of infection and need of secondary surgical procedures to promote bone union. *Injury* 2005;36:656-661.
3. Khatod M, Botte MJ, Hoyt DB, Meyer RS, Smith JM, Akeson WH: Outcomes in open tibia fractures: Relationship between delay in treatment and infection. *J Trauma* 2003;55: 949-954.
4. Spencer J, Smith A, Woods D: The effect of time delay on infection in open long-bone fractures: A 5-year prospective audit from a district general hospital. *Ann R Coll Surg Engl* 2004; 86:108-112.
5. Crowley DJ, Kanakaris NK, Giannoudis PV: Debridement and wound closure of open fractures: The impact of the time factor on infection rates. *Injury* 2007;38:879-889.
6. Werner CM, Pierpont Y, Pollak AN: The urgency of surgical débridement in the management of open fractures. *J Am Acad Orthop Surg* 2008;16: 369-375.
7. Gainor BJ, Hockman DE, Anglen JO, Christensen G, Simpson WA: Benzalkonium chloride: A potential disinfecting irrigation solution. *J Orthop Trauma* 1997;11:121-125.
8. Bhandari M, Schemitsch EH, Adili A, Lachowski RJ, Shaughnessy SG: High and low pressure pulsatile lavage of contaminated tibial fractures: An in vitro study of bacterial adherence and bone damage. *J Orthop Trauma* 1999;13:526-533.
9. Owens BD, White DW, Wenke JC: Comparison of irrigation solutions and devices in a contaminated musculoskeletal wound survival model. *J Bone Joint Surg Am* 2009;91:92-98.
10. Anglen JO: Comparison of soap and antibiotic solutions for irrigation of lower-limb open fracture wounds: A prospective, randomized study. *J Bone Joint Surg Am* 2005;87:1415-1422.
11. Bose D, Tejwani NC: Evolving trends in the care of polytrauma patients. *Injury* 2006;37:20-28.
12. Patzakis MJ, Wilkins J, Moore TM: Use of antibiotics in open tibial fractures. *Clin Orthop Relat Res* 1983;178: 31-35.
13. Patzakis MJ, Wilkins J, Moore TM: Considerations in reducing the infection rate in open tibial fractures. *Clin Orthop Relat Res* 1983;178:36-41.
14. Hauser CJ, Adams CA Jr, Eachempati SR; Council of the Surgical Infection Society: Surgical Infection Society guideline: Prophylactic antibiotic use in open fractures. An evidence-based guideline. *Surg Infect (Larchmt)* 2006;7:379-405.
15. Gosselin RA, Roberts I, Gillespie WJ: Antibiotics for preventing infection in open limb fractures. *Cochrane Database Syst Rev* 2004;1:CD003764.
16. McQueen MM, Gaston P, Court-Brown CM: Acute compartment syndrome: Who is at risk? *J Bone Joint Surg Br* 2000;82:200-203.
17. Kenny C: Compartment pressures, limb length changes and the ideal spherical shape: A case report and in vitro study. *J Trauma* 2006;61: 909-912.
18. Nassif JM, Gorczyca JT, Cole JK, Pugh KJ, Pienkowski D: Effect of acute reamed versus unreamed intramedullary nailing on compartment pressure when treating closed tibial shaft fractures: A randomized prospective study. *J Orthop Trauma* 2000; 14:554-558.
19. Bhattacharyya T, Vrahas MS: The medical-legal aspects of compartment syndrome. *J Bone Joint Surg Am* 2004; 86-A:864-868.
20. Templeman D, Varecka T, Schmidt R: Economic costs of missed compartment syndromes. *60th Annual Meeting Proceedings*. Rosemont, IL, American Academy of Orthopaedic Surgeons, 1993.
21. Richards H, Langston A, Kulkarni R, Downes EM: Does patient controlled analgesia delay the diagnosis of compartment syndrome following intramedullary nailing of the tibia? *Injury* 2004;35:296-298.
22. Mubarak SJ, Hargens AR: Acute compartment syndromes. *Surg Clin North Am* 1983;63:539-565.
23. Rorabeck CH: The treatment of compartment syndromes of the leg. *J Bone Joint Surg Br* 1984;66:93-97.
24. Ulmer T: The clinical diagnosis of compartment syndrome of the lower leg: Are clinical findings predictive of the disorder? *J Orthop Trauma* 2002; 16:572-577.
25. Prayson MJ, Chen JL, Hampers D, Vogt M, Fenwick J, Meredick R: Baseline compartment pressure measurements in isolated lower extremity fractures without clinical compartment syndrome. *J Trauma* 2006;60: 1037-1040.
26. Janzing HM, Broos PL: Routine monitoring of compartment pressure in patients with tibial fractures: Beware of overtreatment! *Injury* 2001; 32:415-421.
27. Ovre S, Hvaal K, Holm I, Strømsøe K, Nordsletten L, Skjeldal S: Compartment pressure in nailed tibial fractures: A threshold of 30 mm Hg for decompression gives 29% fasciotomies. *Arch Orthop Trauma Surg* 1998;118:29-31.

28. Wall CJ, Richardson MD, Lowe AJ, Brand C, Lynch J, de Steiger RN: Survey of management of acute, traumatic compartment syndrome of the leg in Australia. *ANZ J Surg* 2007;77: 733-737.

29. Boody AR, Wongworawat MD: Accuracy in the measurement of compartment pressures: A comparison of three commonly used devices. *J Bone Joint Surg Am* 2005;87:2415-2422.

30. Heckman MM, Whitesides TE Jr, Grewe SR, Rooks MD: Compartment pressure in association with closed tibial fractures: The relationship between tissue pressure, compartment, and the distance from the site of the fracture. *J Bone Joint Surg Am* 1994;76:1285-1292.

31. Kumar P, Salil B, Bhaskara KG, Agrawal A: Compartment syndrome: Effect of limb position on pressure measurement. *Burns* 2003;29:626.

32. McQueen MM, Court-Brown CM: Compartment monitoring in tibial fractures: The pressure threshold for decompression. *J Bone Joint Surg Br* 1996;78:99-104.

33. McQueen MM, Christie J, Court-Brown CM: Acute compartment syndrome in tibial diaphyseal fractures. *J Bone Joint Surg Br* 1996;78: 95-98.

34. White TO, Howell GE, Will EM, Court-Brown CM, McQueen MM: Elevated intramuscular compartment pressures do not influence outcome after tibial fracture. *J Trauma* 2003;55: 1133-1138.

35. McQueen MM, Christie J, Court-Brown CM: Compartment pressures after intramedullary nailing of the tibia. *J Bone Joint Surg Br* 1990;72: 395-397.

36. Kakar S, Firoozabadi R, McKean J, Tornetta P III: Diastolic blood pressure in patients with tibia fractures under anaesthesia: Implications for the diagnosis of compartment syndrome. *J Orthop Trauma* 2007;21: 99-103.

37. Finkelstein JA, Hunter GA, Hu RW: Lower limb compartment syndrome: Course after delayed fasciotomy. *J Trauma* 1996;40:342-344.

38. Cohen MS, Garfin SR, Hargens AR, Mubarak SJ: Acute compartment syndrome: Effect of dermotomy on fascial decompression in the leg. *J Bone Joint Surg Br* 1991;73: 287-290.

39. Tornetta P III, Templeman D: Compartment syndrome associated with tibial fracture. *Instr Course Lect* 1997; 46:303-308.

40. Yang CC, Chang DS, Webb LX: Vacuum-assisted closure for fasciotomy wounds following compartment syndrome of the leg. *J Surg Orthop Adv* 2006;15:19-23.

41. Wiger P, Tkaczuk P, Styf J: Secondary wound closure following fasciotomy for acute compartment syndrome increases intramuscular pressure. *J Orthop Trauma* 1998;12:117-121.

42. Johnson SB, Weaver FA, Yellin AE, Kelly R, Bauer M: Clinical results of decompressive dermotomy-fasciotomy. *Am J Surg* 1992;164: 286-290.

43. Bone LB, Johnson KD, Weigelt J, Scheinberg R: Early versus delayed stabilization of femoral fractures: A prospective randomized study. *J Bone Joint Surg Am* 1989;71:336-340.

44. Pape HC, Auf'm'Kolk M, Paffrath T, Regel G, Sturm JA, Tscherne H: Primary intramedullary femur fixation in multiple trauma patients with associated lung contusion: A cause of posttraumatic ARDS? *J Trauma* 1993; 34:540-548.

45. Rotondo MF, Schwab CW, McGonigal MD, et al: "Damage control": An approach for improved survival in exsanguinating penetrating abdominal injury. *J Trauma* 1993;35:375-383.

46. Keel M, Trentz O: Pathophysiology of polytrauma. *Injury* 2005;36: 691-709.

47. Hildebrand F, Pape HC, van Griensven M, et al: Genetic predisposition for a compromised immune system after multiple trauma. *Shock* 2005;24: 518-522.

48. Crowl AC, Young JS, Kahler DM, Claridge JA, Chrzanowski DS, Pomphrey M: Occult hypoperfusion is associated with increased morbidity in patients undergoing early femur fracture fixation. *J Trauma* 2000;48: 260-267.

49. Giannoudis PV, Smith RM, Bellamy MC, Morrison JF, Dickson RA, Guillou PJ: Stimulation of the inflammatory system by reamed and unreamed nailing of femoral fractures: An analysis of the second hit. *J Bone Joint Surg Br* 1999;81:356-361.

50. Waydhas C, Nast-Kolb D, Trupka A, et al: Posttraumatic inflammatory response, secondary operations, and late multiple organ failure. *J Trauma* 1996; 40:624-631.

51. Pape HC, van Griensven M, Rice J, et al: Major secondary surgery in blunt trauma patients and perioperative cytokine liberation: Determination of the clinical relevance of biochemical markers. *J Trauma* 2001;50: 989-1000.

52. Baker SP, O'Neill B, Haddon W Jr, Long WB: The injury severity score: A method for describing patients with multiple injuries and evaluating emergency care. *J Trauma* 1974;14: 187-196.

53. Giannoudis PV, Smith RM, Perry SL, Windsor AJ, Dickson RA, Bellamy MC: Immediate IL-10 expression following major orthopaedic trauma: Relationship to anti-inflammatory response and subsequent development of sepsis. *Intensive Care Med* 2000;26:1076-1081.

54. Ditschkowski M, Kreuzfelder E, Rebmann V, et al: HLA-DR expression and soluble HLA-DR levels in septic patients after trauma. *Ann Surg* 1999; 229:246-254.

55. Committee on Injury Scaling: *The Abbreviated Injury Scale (AIS) 1990: Update 98*. Des Plaines, IL, Association for the Advancement of Automotive Medicine, 1998.

56. Pape HC, Giannoudis PV, Krettek C, Trentz O: Timing of fixation of major fractures in blunt polytrauma: Role of

conventional indicators in clinical decision making. *J Orthop Trauma* 2005; 19:551-562.

57. Nana A, Kessinger S: Improved soft-tissue perfusion following application of temporizing external fixation in complex distal tibia fractures. Annual Meeting of the Orthopaedic Trauma Association. Denver, CO, 2008. http://www.hwbf.org/ota/am/ota08/otapo/otp08099.htm. Accessed December 21, 2009.
58. Giannoudis PV: Surgical priorities in damage control in polytrauma. *J Bone Joint Surg Br* 2003;85:478-483.
59. Tscherne H, Regel G, Pape HC, Pohlemann T, Krettek C: Internal fixation of multiple fractures in patients with polytrauma. *Clin Orthop Relat Res* 1998;347:62-78.
60. Pennal GF, Tile M, Waddell JP, Garside H: Pelvic disruption: Assessment and classification. *Clin Orthop Relat Res* 1980;151:12-21.
61. Young JW, Burgess AR, Brumback RJ, Poka A: Pelvic fractures: Value of plain radiography in early assessment and management. *Radiology* 1986;160:445-451.
62. Metz CM, Hak DJ, Goulet JA, Williams D: Pelvic fracture patterns and their corresponding angiographic sources of hemorrhage. *Orthop Clin North Am* 2004;35:431-437.
63. Sarin EL, Moore JB, Moore EE, et al: Pelvic fracture pattern does not always predict the need for urgent embolization. *J Trauma* 2005;58:973-977.
64. Yasumura K, Ikegami K, Kamohara T, Nohara Y: High incidence of ischemic necrosis of the gluteal muscle after transcatheter angiographic embolization for severe pelvic fracture. *J Trauma* 2005;58:985-990.
65. Balogh Z, Caldwell E, Heetveld M, et al: Institutional practice guidelines on management of pelvic fracture-related hemodynamic instability: Do they make a difference? *J Trauma* 2005;58:778-782.
66. Fangio P, Asehnoune K, Edouard A, Smail N, Benhamou D: Early embolization and vasopressor administration for management of life-threatening hemorrhage from pelvic fracture. *J Trauma* 2005;58:978-984.
67. Cook RE, Keating JF, Gillespie I: The role of angiography in the management of haemorrhage from major fractures of the pelvis. *J Bone Joint Surg Br* 2002;84:178-182.
68. Shapiro M, McDonald AA, Knight D, Johannigman JA, Cuschieri J: The role of repeat angiography in the management of pelvic fractures. *J Trauma* 2005;58:227-231.
69. Bottlang M, Krieg JC, Mohr M, Simpson TS, Madey SM: Emergent management of pelvic ring fractures with use of circumferential compression. *J Bone Joint Surg Am* 2002; 84-A(suppl 2):43-47.
70. Mason WT, Khan SN, James CL, Chesser TJ, Ward AJ: Complications of temporary and definitive external fixation of pelvic ring injuries. *Injury* 2005;36:599-604.
71. Cothren CC, Osborn PM, Moore EE, Morgan SJ, Johnson JL, Smith WR: Preperitoneal pelvic packing for hemodynamically unstable pelvic fractures: A paradigm shift. *J Trauma* 2007;62:834-842.
72. Bhandari M, Matta J, Ferguson T, Matthys G: Predictors of clinical and radiological outcome in patients with fractures of the acetabulum and concomitant posterior dislocation of the hip. *J Bone Joint Surg Br* 2006;88:1618-1624.
73. Schafer SJ, Anglen JO: The East Baltimore Lift: A simple and effective method for reduction of posterior hip dislocations. *J Orthop Trauma* 1999; 13:56-57.
74. Anglen JO, Hughes M: Trochanteric osteotomy for incarcerated hip dislocation due to interposed posterior wall fragments. *Orthopedics* 2004;27: 213-216.
75. Moed BR, WillsonCarr SE, Watson JT: Results of operative treatment of fractures of the posterior wall of the acetabulum. *J Bone Joint Surg Am* 2002;84-A:752-758.
76. Hollis JD, Daley BJ: 10-year review of knee dislocations: Is arteriography always necessary? *J Trauma* 2005;59: 672-676.
77. Klineberg EO, Crites BM, Flinn WR, Archibald JD, Moorman CT III: The role of arteriography in assessing popliteal artery injury in knee dislocations. *J Trauma* 2004;56:786-790.
78. Mills WJ, Barei DP, McNair P: The value of the ankle-brachial index for diagnosing arterial injury after knee dislocation: A prospective study. *J Trauma* 2004;56:1261-1265.
79. Vallier HA, Nork SE, Barei DP, Benirschke SK, Sangeorzan BJ: Talar neck fractures: Results and outcomes. *J Bone Joint Surg Am* 2004;86-A:1616-1624.
80. Patel R, Van Bergeyk A, Pinney S: Are displaced talar neck fractures surgical emergencies? A survey of orthopaedic trauma experts. *Foot Ankle Int* 2005; 26:378-381.
81. Lindvall E, Haidukewych G, DiPasquale T, Herscovici D Jr, Sanders R: Open reduction and stable fixation of isolated, displaced talar neck and body fractures. *J Bone Joint Surg Am* 2004; 86-A:2229-2234.
82. Rothschild JM, Keohane CA, Rogers S, et al: Risks of complications by attending physicians after performing nighttime procedures. *JAMA* 2009; 302:1565-1572.
83. Sexton JB, Thomas EJ, Helmreich RL: Error, stress, and teamwork in medicine and aviation: Cross sectional surveys. *BMJ* 2000;320:745-749.
84. Fischer FM, de Moreno CR, Notarnicola da Silva Borges F, Louzada FM: Implementation of 12-hour shifts in a Brazilian petrochemical plant: Impact on sleep and alertness. *Chronobiol Int* 2000;17:521-537.
85. Bartel P, Offermeier W, Smith F, Becker P: Attention and working memory in resident anaesthetist after night duty: Group and individual effects. *Occup Environ Med* 2004;61: 167-170.

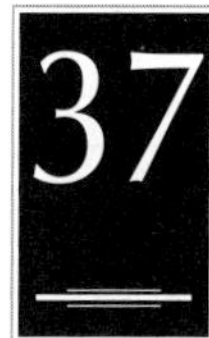

Pediatric Trauma: Getting Through the Night

Susan A. Scherl, MD
Andrew H. Schmidt, MD

Abstract

As is the case in adults, the timing and type of emergent treatment of fractures in children can be controversial. Some emergent conditions, such as compartment syndrome, pelvic fractures with hemodynamic instability, and open fractures, are managed similarly in adults and children. However, other types of fractures are unique to children or are managed differently in children and adults. To prevent complications, it is important to understand the appropriate treatment and timing of treatment of supracondylar humeral fractures and other specific elbow fractures, hip fractures and dislocations, and physeal fractures about the knee in pediatric patients.

Instr Course Lect 2010;59:455-463.

Although most orthopaedic surgeons do not specialize in pediatrics, almost all practicing orthopaedic surgeons, and certainly anyone on emergency trauma call, will be called on at some point to treat a child with a fracture. It is therefore imperative for practitioners to have some working knowledge of current pediatric fracture care. At a minimum, all orthopaedic surgeons should have an understanding of which pediatric fractures are emergencies and why, how to treat these fractures or at least temporize before definitive treatment, and how and why the treatment of children's fractures sometimes differs from that of adult fractures.

This chapter does not address emergent problems that present and are managed similarly in adults and children (for example, compartment syndrome, pelvic fractures with hemodynamic instability, and traumatic amputations and open fractures). Instead, it focuses on entities that are either unique to children or are managed differently in children and adults. Specifically, supracondylar humeral fractures and other specific elbow fractures, hip fractures and dislocations, and physeal fractures about the knee are discussed.

Supracondylar Humeral Fractures

Supracondylar humeral fractures are relatively common. They account for 30% of extremity fractures in children younger than 7 years and 60% of elbow fractures in that age group. They are most common in the first decade of life. Extension-type injuries account for 96% of supracondylar humeral fractures and result from a fall on an outstretched arm that forces the elbow into hyperextension. The much less common flexion-type injuries occur from a fall onto the point of the olecranon with the elbow flexed. According to the commonly used Gartland classification,[1] type I injuries are nondisplaced; type II injuries are angulated posteriorly, but

Dr. Scherl or an immediate family member is a board member, owner, officer, or committee member of the Orthopaedic Trauma Association and the Pediatric Orthopaedic Society of North America; has received research or institutional support from Arthrex, the National Institutes of Health, Tornier, and ESKA; and has received nonincome support (such as equipment or services), commercially derived honoraria, or other non–research-related funding (such as paid travel) from Lippincott Williams & Wilkins and UpTODATE. Dr. Schmidt or an immediate family member is a board member, owner, officer, or committee member of the Orthopaedic Trauma Association; has received royalties from Smith & Nephew; is a member of a speakers' bureau or has made paid presentations on behalf of Synthes; serves as a paid consultant for or is an employee of Smith & Nephew, Twin Star Medical, Medtronic, DigiMed, and AGA; serves as an unpaid consultant for Conventus Orthopedics and Anthem Orthopedics; has received research or institutional support from Synthes, Smith & Nephew, Twin Star Medical, and Medtronic; owns stock or stock options in Twin Star Medical, Conventus Orthopedics, and the International Spine and Orthopedic Institute; and has received nonincome support (such as equipment or services), commercially derived honoraria, or other non–research-related funding (such as paid travel) from Thieme.

the posterior cortex is intact; and type III injuries are completely displaced, usually with the distal part of the humerus and the elbow displaced posteromedially.

A patient with a supracondylar humeral fracture presents after a specific injury; has pain, swelling, and a decreased range of motion of the elbow; and usually has pain when motion of the arm is attempted. There is tenderness over the distal part of the humerus and, typically, an obvious deformity. There may be ecchymosis or buttonholing of the skin at the fracture site. The child holds the arm in extension and pronated at the forearm. A careful neurovascular examination is imperative. On initial presentation, the radial pulse may be absent secondary to draping of the artery over the spike of the proximal fracture fragment. Often, the pulse returns after fracture reduction. The function of the median, ulnar, radial, and anterior interosseous nerves must be documented and the forearm assessed for signs of ischemia or compartment syndrome.

AP and lateral radiographs of the elbow should be obtained. Comparison radiographs of the contralateral elbow can aid in interpreting the images. On the lateral radiograph, a line drawn along the anterior border of the humerus should pass through the center of the capitellum if there is no displacement. A posterior fat pad sign (a radiolucent area seen posterior to the distal part of the humerus, adjacent to the olecranon fossa, on a plain lateral radiograph) indicates a hemarthrosis and suggests an occult elbow fracture.[2]

Vascular injury occurs in approximately 1% of patients. Indications for vascular exploration are clinically obvious ischemia or loss of a pulse that had been previously palpable or apparent on Doppler examination after fracture reduction, because this may indicate that the vascular bundle has become entrapped in the fracture site. The use of arteriography in children is controversial, as is the management of the "pink, pulseless hand;" the usual recommendation is observation without vascular exploration in such situations.[3]

Neurologic injury occurs in about 7% of patients. Most nerve injuries are neurapraxias that resolve with time. The radial nerve is at the most risk of transection, which usually occurs with open fractures. The anterior interosseous nerve is the most frequently injured.[4] This nerve is injured when the posterolateral part of the distal fracture fragment compresses the nerve against the anterior structures in the forearm. Injury to the anterior interosseous nerve results in weak flexion of the interphalangeal joint of the thumb and the distal interphalangeal joint of the index finger. The radial nerve is more commonly injured in patients with a posteromedial fracture. The median nerve is more commonly injured in those with a posterolateral fracture, often in association with a brachial artery injury. A median nerve injury can mask a compartment syndrome because of the associated sensory loss in the forearm. Ulnar nerve injury is often iatrogenic, secondary to medial pin placement, but it also occurs in conjunction with a flexion-type supracondylar humeral fracture.

The treatment of supracondylar humeral fractures depends on the direction and degree of displacement. Gartland type I injuries may be treated, without reduction, in a long arm cast with the elbow flexed 90° to 110° for 3 to 4 weeks. Displaced Gartland type II and III injuries are treated with closed reduction and percutaneous pinning, with either two or three lateral pins or crossed medial and lateral pins. There is no substantial difference in the stability provided by the lateral and crossed-pin methods if proper technique and pin placement are used. The two lateral pins should be divergent, with one running up the lateral column and one crossing over to the medial column. The two pins should not cross at the fracture site; a third pin should be added when there is medial comminution or persistent instability with motion[5-8] (Figure 1 and Table 1).

The timing of surgery for a displaced supracondylar humeral fracture is controversial. A supracondylar humeral fracture is one of the classic pediatric orthopaedic emergencies, but the need to perform surgery in the middle of the night for these injuries has recently been challenged. Four retrospective studies showed no increase in complications in children for whom surgery had been delayed more than 12 hours.[9-12] Another study showed a possible increase in the prevalence of compartment syndrome in children with a delay of more than 22 hours before surgery.[13] In the opinion of the chapter's authors, if a delay of 12 to 24 hours is necessary or inevitable, the outcome should not be adversely affected. However, waiting is not a better option. Surgery should not be delayed unless the child has normal neurovascular function. Furthermore, surgery should not be delayed if there is excessive swelling or soft-tissue damage; the case must still be considered urgent, with the surgery being done at the earliest possible opportunity the following morning and not after the next day's elective surgery schedule, for example.

Vascular injury or interposition of the neurovascular bundle are the two most definitive indications for open reduction.[14] The antecubital approach is useful in both cases. Although vascular compromise usually can be managed without the need to operate on the artery, arterial repair may be needed and should be planned for. An inability to achieve an acceptable closed reduction because of lateral or medial soft-tissue or periosteal interposition is another indication for open reduction. An approach from the affected side allows removal of the offending soft tissue.

The pins are removed in the physician's office after periosteal new bone is visible radiographically, generally at 3 to 4 weeks. Additional protective immobilization is usually not necessary. Children generally regain range of motion within about 3 to 4 weeks without physical therapy, although the last few degrees of flexion may lag. Follow-up with radiographs and physical examination is recommended at 3, 6, and 12 months after injury.

Fortunately, complications are infrequent after supracondylar humeral fractures, and most are avoided by attention to detail during treatment.[15,16] Ulnar nerve injury—usually a neurapraxia that resolves in 3 to 6 months—is often the result of medial pin placement. Occupational therapy during resolution may be beneficial. Cubitus varus is caused by varus positioning of the fracture fragment as well as residual rotational deformity. Although cubitus varus is generally a cosmetic problem, ulnar nerve palsy can occur later; a distal humeral osteotomy is occasionally necessary. Loss of reduction is usually a result of

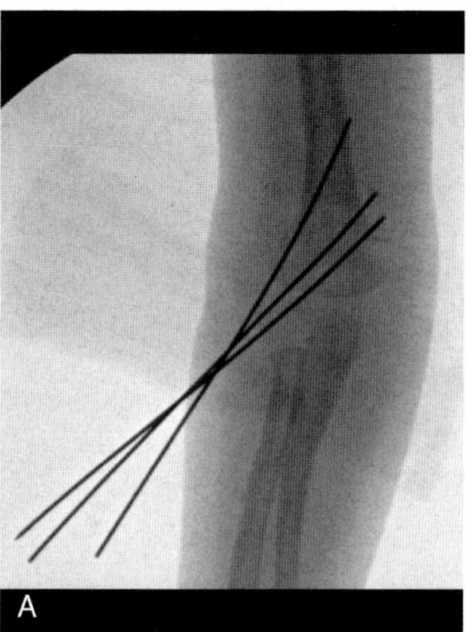

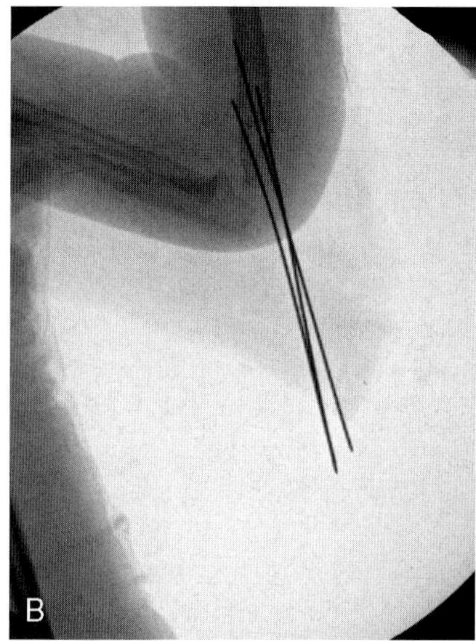

Figure 1 AP **(A)** and lateral **(B)** radiographs showing fixation of a Gartland type III supracondylar humeral fracture with a three-lateral-pin construct. Note the divergence of the pins, with one going up the lateral column and two traversing the olecranon fossa to the medial column.

Table 1
Pearls and Pitfalls for Closed Reduction and Percutaneous Pinning of Supracondylar Humeral Fractures

Place the patient supine.

Flip the C-arm, bring it perpendicular to the operating room bed, and use it as a table.

Reduction maneuver: straight traction, adjustment of the distal fragment medially or laterally, flexion of the elbow while pushing the distal fragment anteriorly, forearm pronation to "lock" the fragment in place

If no assistance is available, secure the arm in the reduced, flexed position with a roll of gauze.

Use 4-inch (10.2-cm) long, 0.062-inch (1.57-mm) diameter Kirschner wires.

Insert two pins from the lateral side.

If the fracture remains unstable, insert an additional pin: either a third lateral pin or a medial pin.

The medial pin can be inserted through a mini-open incision to ensure that the starting point is directly on the medial epicondyle and the ulnar nerve is out of the way.

Extend the arm to insert a medial pin; this drops the ulnar nerve posteriorly, further out of the way.

If the patient wakes up with an ulnar nerve palsy, first simply pull the medial pin.

Pay careful attention to rotational alignment; malrotation causes cubitus varus.

Splint with the elbow in 70° to 90° of flexion, in a posterior mold with side slabs.

Do not change the splint until it is time to pull the pin; doing so causes the child unnecessary discomfort and anxiety.

Leave the ends of the pins long enough to grab and pull out with your fingers; children do not like to be approached with pliers.

technical problems with pin placement.[16] Pin site infections are rare.

Transphyseal Elbow Fractures

The prevalence of transphyseal fractures of the distal part of the humerus is unknown, as these injuries are sometimes missed or misdiagnosed. They occur primarily in children younger than 4 years. They occur as a result of a fall on an outstretched arm but may be the result of abuse if the child is not yet walking; a high index of suspicion should be maintained in such cases. The fractures usually have a Salter-Harris type I or II pattern.[17] The diagnosis of transphyseal elbow fracture should be considered when a very young child presents with pain, swelling, and decreased use of the upper extremity. These injuries are frequently mistaken for elbow dislocations.

Because these fractures occur in very young children in whom much of the distal part of the humerus (often including the capitellum) is not yet ossified, radiographs may be difficult to interpret. When the elbow is dislocated, the normal radiocapitellar relationship is disrupted, but it is preserved with a transphyseal fracture. An arthrogram, a MRI scan, or a sonogram, all of which allow visualization of the nonossified capitellum, may aid in the diagnosis. A closed reduction, with or without percutaneous pinning, is needed. Often, these injuries present late, when there is already a periosteal reaction indicating healing. Reduction is not indicated in these cases.

The most common complication is malunion as a result of a late diagnosis. Luckily, there is substantial remodeling potential in young children. Rarely, osteonecrosis of the trochlea occurs.

Fractures of the Lateral Condyle

Seventeen percent of elbow fractures in children are fractures of the lateral condyle. The peak incidence is between 5 and 10 years of age. These injuries are caused by varus stress to an extended elbow with the forearm in supination. Children with a fracture of the lateral condyle present with lateral swelling and pain in the elbow. These fractures are much less likely to be associated with neurovascular injury than are supracondylar humeral fractures. AP and lateral radiographs of the elbow are essential. Sometimes, oblique radiographs help to visualize the fracture. Fractures of the lateral condyle are often mistaken for "chip" or "avulsion" fractures in very young children because most of the distal fracture fragment, including its articular surface, is not ossified. Although fractures of the lateral condyle may be classified with the Salter-Harris classification or the anatomically based Milch classification, many pediatric orthopaedic surgeons classify them simply on the basis of whether they are displaced because displacement dictates treatment.[17,18]

Nondisplaced fractures of the lateral condyle may be treated in a long arm cast with the elbow in 90° of flexion. Frequent follow-up and repeat imaging are necessary to watch for late displacement and the subsequent need for surgical treatment. Displaced fractures are best treated with an open reduction and pinning with two or three lateral pins. Direct visualization before pinning is necessary to ensure an anatomic reduction of the articular surface. An arthrogram can be made for minimally displaced fractures, and, if the articular surface of the humerus is congruent, the pins may be placed without opening the fracture. Because fractures of the lateral condyle are not likely to be associated with neurovascular injury, they are considered urgent but not in need of emergent surgical treatment.

Fractures of the lateral condyle are prone to late complications, including late displacement; malunion and nonunion, even after appropriate fixation; growth disturbance; late deformity; and loss of motion. Parents should be warned of these possibilities at the time of injury.

Monteggia Fracture-Dislocations

Monteggia fractures involve the proximal part of the ulna and are associated with a dislocation of the radial head. They are rare in children, accounting for about 0.4% of all forearm fractures. The peak incidence is between 4 and 10 years of age. The Bado classification is used to describe these injuries in children as well as in adults.[19] Bado type I injuries, which involve anterior angulation of the ulna and anterior dislocation of the radial head, are the most common variant in children, accounting for 70% of the fractures. Monteggia fractures in children are easy to miss. On all radiographic views, a line drawn through the center of the radial head should pass through the center of the capitellum. Any deviation from this is not normal and requires further evaluation. "Pure" radial head dislocations may not exist in children; therefore, it is advisable to look for plastic deformation of the ulna in children with a dislocated radial head.

Monteggia fractures can usually be treated with closed reduction (probably best performed with the patient under general anesthesia) and immobilization with the elbow in 90° to 110° of flexion and the forearm in full supination. Reduction is achieved by first correcting the ulnar deformity, then reducing the radial head, and finally relieving the deforming forces by positioning the elbow in flexion and the forearm in supination. Plastic deformation of the ulna is sometimes particularly difficult to reduce.

Associated neurovascular injuries are rare. A late diagnosis can be associated with so much fracture healing that an osteotomy of the ulna, open reduction of the radial head, and annular ligament reconstruction are necessary.

Table 2
Pearls and Pitfalls for Pediatric Hip Fractures

The goal of treatment is anatomic reduction of the proximal part of the femur.

An anterolateral (Watson-Jones) surgical approach is used for open reduction.

Consider internal fixation for nondisplaced fractures to avoid late displacement and the subsequent development of coxa vara.

Advise parents before treatment about the potential for serious late complications.

Do not compromise fracture stability/fixation to protect the physis; cross it with fixation pins if necessary.

The proximal femoral physis grows only 1/8 inch (3 mm) per year. If a limb-length discrepancy occurs, it can be readily managed.

Internal fixation options:
- 0 to 3 years of age: smooth pins (5/64 inch [2 mm] or 3/32 inch [2.4 mm]) or cannulated screws (3.5 or 4.0 mm)
- 4 to 8 years of age: cannulated screws (4.0 or 4.5 mm) or a pediatric hip-compression screw
- Older than 8 years: cannulated screws (6.5 or 7.3 mm) or a hip-compression screw

Pediatric bone is often denser than adult bone; consider predrilling and tapping.

Consider using a supplemental hip spica cast in children younger than 8 years.

Remove hardware in approximately 1 year.

Pathologic fractures may require additional treatment.

Osteonecrosis is probably predetermined by the fracture "personality." However, these fractures are still considered emergent; treatment should not be delayed unless medically necessary.

Consider hip joint aspiration when a fracture is treated closed.

Hip Fractures

Femoral neck and intertrochanteric femoral fractures are rare in children, accounting for less than 1% of all childhood fractures.[20] They are usually caused by high-energy trauma, and associated injuries, including other fractures, head injuries, and abdominal injuries, are common. Proximal femoral fractures in children are classified according to the scheme first reported in the French literature by Delbet in 1907 and popularized by Colonna in 1929.[21] In this classification, type I consists of transphyseal separation. This is an uncommon variant, accounting for 7% of these fractures. Fifty percent of type I fractures occur with a femoral head dislocation, there is an extremely high rate of osteonecrosis (up to 100%), and there is a high rate of growth arrest. Type II fractures are transcervical, and they are the most common, accounting for 50% of these fractures. Up to 80% of type II fractures are displaced, and there is a high rate of osteonecrosis (40% to 50%). Type III fractures are cervicotrochanteric, and account for 31% of these fractures. Fifty percent are displaced, and, although the risk of osteonecrosis is lower than the risk with type I and II fractures, it is still real. Type IV fractures are intertrochanteric. This is an uncommon variant, is associated with the fewest complications, and healing is rapid.

Transphyseal separations (type I) are treated with either closed or open reduction and transphyseal pinning[22-24] (Table 2). Femoral neck fractures (type II) are also treated with closed or open reduction and pin fixation of the femoral neck. Cervicotrochanteric fractures (type III) are treated similarly but also can be managed with a spica cast if the fracture is not displaced. Intertrochanteric fractures (type IV) can be treated with either a spica cast or internal fixation with a pediatric hip screw, depending on the size of the child and the degree of displacement.

Hip fractures in children are associated with an overall complication rate of 60%. Most complications are evident within 6 to 9 months after the injury. Necrosis of the femoral head is the most serious complication and is in large part a function of the initial fracture pattern. Coxa vara and coxa valga result from malunion, as does limb-length discrepancy. Nonunion is rare but can occur. Late arthritis can develop secondary to osteonecrosis and malunion.

Hip Dislocations

Hip dislocations are uncommon in children, but they are more common than hip fractures. They can occur with relatively minor trauma. Most (90%) are posterior, and 15% to 20% are associated with a hip fracture. Hip dislocations are usually easy to diagnose on the basis of the history, physical examination, an AP radiograph of the pelvis, and a cross-table lateral radiograph of the hip. Typically, with a posterior dislocation, the hip is flexed,

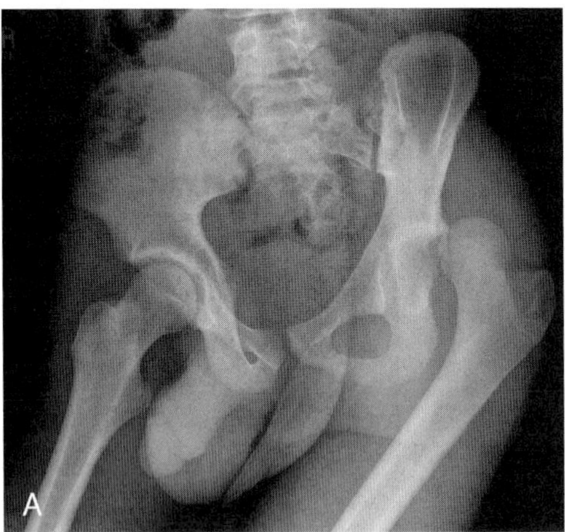

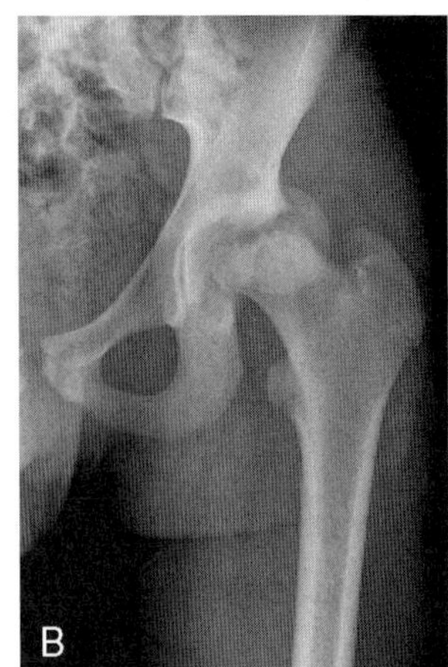

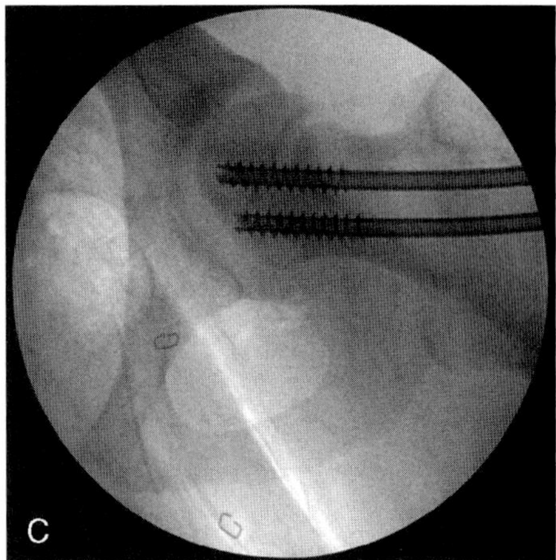

Figure 2 **A,** AP radiograph of the pelvis, showing a dislocation of the left hip sustained by a 13-year-old boy while playing football. **B,** AP radiograph of the left hip, made after an attempt at closed reduction in the emergency department with the patient under sedation. Note the resultant displaced transphyseal fracture of the femoral head. **C,** Lateral radiograph of the left hip, made immediately following open reduction and internal fixation of the fracture-dislocation.

adducted, and internally rotated. With an anterior dislocation, the hip is extended, abducted, and externally rotated.

A closed reduction should be performed with the patient under general anesthesia and with the use of muscle relaxation to minimize the risk of creating a transphyseal fracture when the femoral head contacts the acetabular rim (Figure 2). Preferably, the reduction should be performed within 6 hours after the injury, to reduce the chance of subsequent femoral head necrosis. The reduction maneuver for a posterior dislocation involves anterior traction with the hip and knee flexed. Longitudinal traction with the hip extended and the knee slightly flexed is used for an anterior dislocation. If it is irreducible, proceed to open reduction from the direction of the dislocation. After reduction, the stability and congruency of the joint should be assessed. If there is any doubt about the quality of the reduction, a CT scan should be performed to identify interposed soft tissue or intra-articular loose fragments. A spica cast or hip abduction brace is used for 6 weeks.

Femoral head necrosis develops after 10% to 16% of hip dislocations. Some patients experience a transient sciatic neurapraxia. Recurrent dislocation is rare in children.

Physeal Fractures About the Knee

Physeal fractures about the knee are relatively rare; they account for 1% to 6% of physeal injuries in children. The Salter-Harris system is used to classify these injuries.[17] Fractures through the growth plate should be anatomically reduced if the child has more than 2 years of growth remaining; restoration of the articular surface is critical to achieve a good outcome. Salter-Harris type I and II fractures can be treated with closed reduction and cast immobilization or with closed reduction and percutaneous pin or screw fixation. Salter-Harris type III and IV fractures are best treated with an open reduction and percutaneous or internal fixation, usually with screws that do not cross the physis.

Distal Femoral Physeal Fractures

These fractures are usually hyperextension injuries, but they can be caused by a hyperflexion force. They are a childhood analog of a knee dislocation, and injury to the neurovascular structures is a risk. Motor and sensory function and vascular supply to the distal part of the lower limb should be carefully examined. As is the case for a patient with a neurovascular injury after a supracondylar fracture, insufficiency of the vascular supply to the distal part of the lower limb requires emergent care.

Treatment of the fracture depends on the fracture pattern, the amount of displacement, and the nature of the physeal injury, as described according to the Salter-Harris classification[17] (Table 3). Salter-Harris type I fractures that are not displaced can be treated in a long leg cast, with or without a pelvic band, for 4 to 6 weeks. The prevalence of growth arrest is low after such injuries. Displaced Salter-Harris type I fractures should be reduced (usually with a closed reduction), and cross-pins should be placed to maintain the reduction. Reduction should be achieved, with the patient under general anesthesia, by applying traction in extension supplemented by slight flexion or extension of the distal fragment as needed. Cross-pin fixation is accomplished with smooth Steinmann pins that cross proximal to the fracture site. The pins are typically inserted retrograde, from distal to proximal, starting just posterior to the midpoint of the condyle and aiming 10° anteriorly. Alternatively, they may be inserted antegrade, from proximal to distal. This method is technically more demanding, but the advantage is that pins do not pass through the joint (Figure 3). The pins may be buried or be left outside the skin and can be removed in 4 weeks. The rate of growth arrest in association with displaced injuries is high (up to 40%).

Salter-Harris type II fractures are treated with closed reduction and percutaneous pin fixation. To treat these fractures, pins or screws should be placed in the metaphyseal (Thurston-Holland) fragment, if it is large enough, and parallel to the physis (Figure 4). Placing pins or screws across the physis should be avoided whenever possible.

Salter-Harris type III and IV fractures have intra-articular extensions, and should be reduced with an open procedure and internally fixed with pins or screws placed parallel to the physis. Crossing the physis with hardware should be avoided whenever possible. All patients with physeal injuries should be followed to determine if there is a growth disturbance, and the patient and parents should be advised of this risk at the initial assessment.

Proximal Tibial Fractures

Fractures through the growth plate of the proximal part of the tibia are uncommon but, like distal femoral physeal injuries, they are a childhood analog of a knee dislocation and can therefore be associated with neurovascular injury or compartment syndrome.

Table 3
Pearls and Pitfalls for Pediatric Distal Femoral Fractures

Salter-Harris fractures are more common than ligamentous injuries in children.

Nondisplaced Salter-Harris type I fractures may present with normal radiographs, and a high index of suspicion must be maintained if there is clinical evidence of the fracture (tenderness over the physis).

At a minimum, obtain orthogonal (AP and lateral) radiographs of the knee.

Obtain additional views, and contralateral comparisons, as needed.

The use of stress radiographs is controversial.

Never hesitate to treat a presumed Salter-Harris type I fracture on the basis of clinical findings.

The findings on physical examination are similar for all of these injuries. There is pain and knee effusion with or without an inability to bear weight, deformity, and point tenderness.

Distal femoral physeal fractures in particular are associated with a high rate of postinjury premature growth arrest.

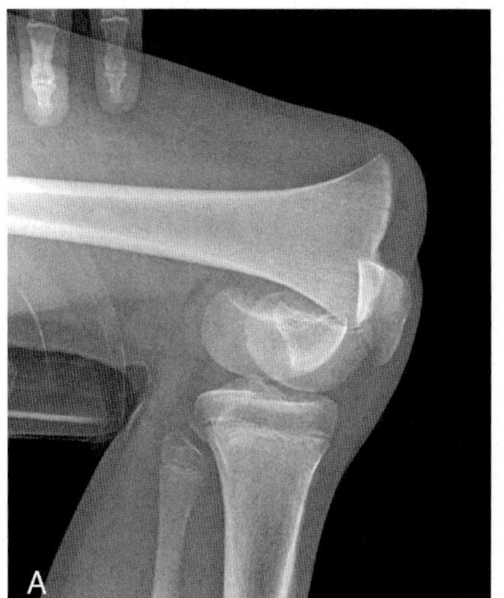

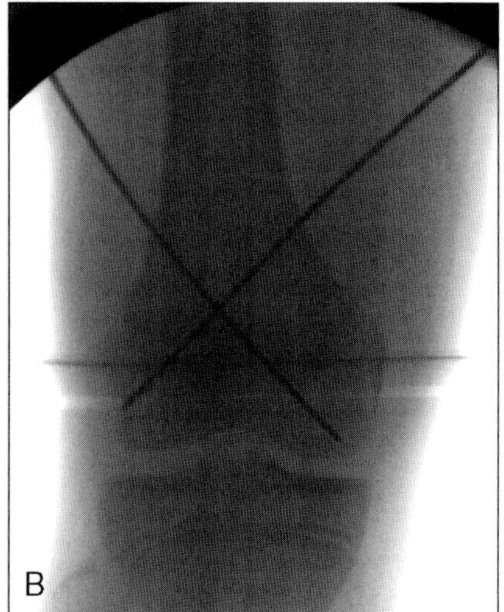

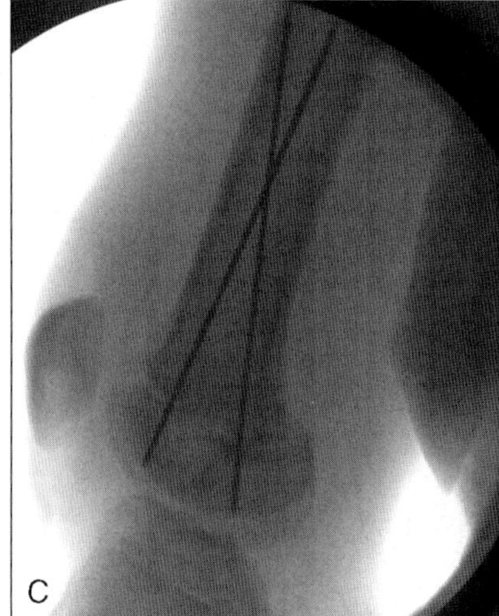

Figure 3 **A,** Lateral radiograph of a displaced Salter-Harris type I fracture of the distal part of the femur in a 12-year-old boy. AP **(B)** and lateral **(C)** radiographs of the knee, made after closed reduction and antegrade percutaneous pin fixation.

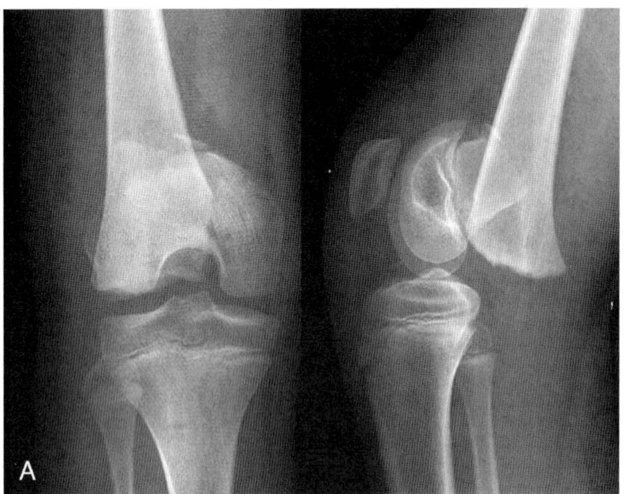

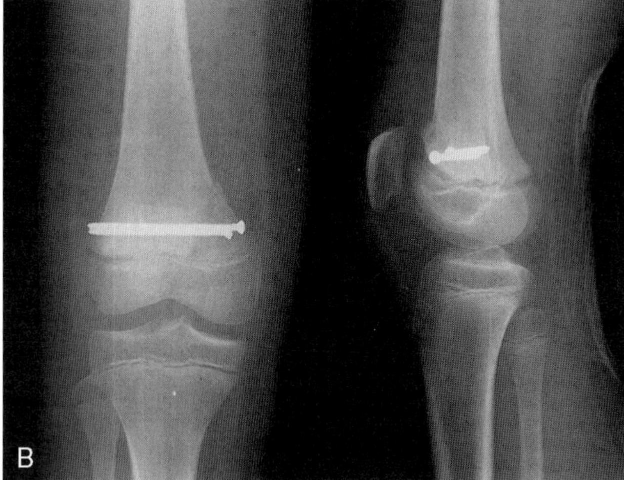

Figure 4 **A,** AP and lateral radiographs of a completely displaced Salter-Harris type II fracture of the distal part of the femur in an 11-year-old boy. **B,** Radiographs made immediately after open reduction and internal fixation with the use of two screws placed across the metaphyseal component of the fracture (the Thurston-Holland fragment).

Table 4
Pearls and Pitfalls for Pediatric Proximal Tibial Fractures

Physeal injuries about the knee are relatively uncommon.
Non–intra-articular (Salter-Harris type I and II) fractures can often be treated nonsurgically.
Most intra-articular (Salter-Harris type III and IV) fractures require surgical treatment.
One should not hesitate to open a Salter-Harris type I or II fracture if an adequate closed reduction cannot be achieved.
These fractures have a guarded prognosis. The prevalence of growth arrest is high. Parents must be informed of this at the time of injury.
Beware of neurovascular injury and compartment syndrome.

Most Salter-Harris type I and II injuries can be treated with closed reduction and cast immobilization or percutaneous pinning (Table 4). Salter-Harris type III and IV fractures require open reduction and internal fixation.

Summary

Pediatric fractures that require consideration for an emergent trip to the operating room include supracondylar humeral fractures, Monteggia fracture-dislocations, hip fractures and dislocations, and physeal fractures about the knee. These fractures are prone to neurovascular compromise and compartment syndrome, osteonecrosis, or growth arrest, which may be avoided by timely and accurate reduction and fixation.

References

1. Gartland JJ: Management of supracondylar fractures of the humerus in children. *Surg Gynecol Obstet* 1959; 109:145-154.
2. Skaggs DL, Mirzayan R: The posterior fat pad sign in association with occult fracture of the elbow in children. *J Bone Joint Surg Am* 1999;81: 1429-1433.
3. Sabharwal S, Tredwell SJ, Beauchamp RD, et al: Management of pulseless pink hand in pediatric supracondylar fractures of humerus. *J Pediatr Orthop* 1997;17:303-310.
4. Lyons ST, Quinn M, Stanitski CL: Neurovascular injuries in type III humeral supracondylar fractures in children. *Clin Orthop Relat Res* 2000;376: 62-67.
5. Davis RT, Gorczyca JT, Pugh K: Supracondylar humerus fractures in children: Comparison of operative treatment methods. *Clin Orthop Relat Res* 2000;376:49-55.
6. Skaggs DL, Cluck MW, Mostofi A, Flynn JM, Kay RM: Lateral-entry pin fixation in the management of supracondylar fractures in children. *J Bone Joint Surg Am* 2004;86-A:702-707.
7. Skaggs DL, Hale JM, Bassett J, Kaminsky C, Kay RM, Tolo VT: Operative treatment of supracondylar fractures of the humerus in children: The consequences of pin placement. *J Bone Joint Surg Am* 2001;83-A: 735-740.
8. Thomson JD, Stricker SJ, Williams MM: Fractures of the distal femoral epiphyseal plate. *J Pediatr Orthop* 1995;15:474-478.
9. Gupta N, Kay RM, Leitch K, Femino JD, Tolo VT, Skaggs DL: Ef-

fect of surgical delay on perioperative complications and need for open reduction in supracondylar humerus fractures in children. *J Pediatr Orthop* 2004;24:245-248.

10. Iyengar SR, Hoffinger SA, Townsend DR: Early versus delayed reduction and pinning of type III displaced supracondylar fractures of the humerus in children: A comparative study. *J Orthop Trauma* 1999;13: 51-55.
11. Leet AI, Frisancho J, Ebramzadeh E: Delayed treatment of type 3 supracondylar humerus fractures in children. *J Pediatr Orthop* 2002;22: 203-207.
12. Mehlman CT, Strub WM, Roy DR, Wall EJ, Crawford AH: The effect of surgical timing on the perioperative complications of treatment of supracondylar humeral fractures in children. *J Bone Joint Surg Am* 2001;83-A: 323-327.
13. Ramachandran M, Skaggs DL, Crawford HA, et al: Delaying treatment of supracondylar fractures in children: Has the pendulum swung too far? *J Bone Joint Surg Br* 2008;90:1228-1233.
14. Reitman RD, Waters P, Millis M: Open reduction and internal fixation for supracondylar humerus fractures in children. *J Pediatr Orthop* 2001;21: 157-161.
15. Mostafavi HR, Spero C: Crossed pin fixation of displaced supracondylar humerus fractures in children. *Clin Orthop Relat Res* 2000;376:56-61.
16. Sankar WN, Hebela NM, Skaggs DL, Flynn JM: Loss of pin fixation in displaced supracondylar humeral fractures in children: Causes and prevention. *J Bone Joint Surg Am* 2007;89: 713-717.
17. Salter RB, Harris WR: Injuries involving the epiphyseal plate. *J Bone Joint Surg Am* 1963;45:587-622.
18. Milch H: Fractures and fracture dislocations of the humeral condyles. *J Trauma* 1964;4:592-607.
19. Bado JL: The Monteggia lesion. *Clin Orthop Relat Res* 1967;50:71-86.
20. Canale ST: Fractures of the hip in children and adolescents. *Orthop Clin North Am* 1990;21:341-352.
21. Colonna PC: Fracture of the neck of the femur in children. *Am J Surg* 1929;6:793-797.
22. Cheng JC, Tang N: Decompression and stable internal fixation of femoral neck fractures in children can affect the outcome. *J Pediatr Orthop* 1999;19: 338-343.
23. Ng GP, Cole WG: Effect of early hip decompression on the frequency of avascular necrosis in children with fractures of the neck of the femur. *Injury* 1996;27:419-421.
24. Song KS, Kim YS, Sohn SW, Ogden JA: Arthrotomy and open reduction of the displaced fracture of the femoral neck in children. *J Pediatr Orthop B* 2001;10:205-210.

Joint and Long-Bone Gunshot Injuries

Paul J. Dougherty, MD
Rahul Vaidya, MD
Craig D. Silverton, DO
Craig S. Bartlett III, MD
Soheil Najibi, MD, PhD

Abstract

Gunshot wounds remain a major clinical problem, with the number of nonfatal gunshot wounds reported as 60,000 to 80,000 per year in the United States. Bone or joint injuries comprise a major portion of gunshot wound injuries. It is paramount for orthopaedic surgeons to be thorough in their treatment of patients with these injuries. Intra-articular injuries remain a source of significant clinical morbidity because of joint stiffness, arthritis, and the risk of infection. Treatment of long-bone fractures is a challenging clinical problem, and further studies are needed to investigate modern treatment methods. Lead toxicity is a potential risk for patients with gunshot injuries, particular for those with joint injuries. The clinician's recognition of the signs and symptoms of lead toxicity is important to achieve the best care for these patients.

Instr Course Lect 2010;59:465-479.

The care of patients with gunshot wounds can be clinically challenging as a result of the injury severity and systems-based factors, yet relatively few reports concerning the care of these patients have been written. To place the magnitude of the problem in perspective, it should be noted that there are 60,000 to 80,000 nonfatal gunshot wounds annually in the United States.[1] In comparison, in the 66 months from March 19, 2003, through October 4, 2008, only 30,072 individuals sustained battlefield wounds during Operation Iraqi Freedom.[2] Clearly, gunshot wounds are an enormous problem, and orthopaedic surgeons should be aware of these injuries and their treatment.

Prevalence

From 2001 to 2005, 1,059 patients with a total of 1,611 gunshot wounds were admitted to the authors' institution (Henry Ford Hospital, Detroit, MI); 988 (61.3%) of these gunshot wounds were to the extremities. Five hundred twenty-six wounds involved the lower extremity, and 462 involved the upper extremity. Ninety-eight injuries involved the spine, and an additional 525 did not involve the musculoskeletal system.

Similar to the situation in other urban trauma centers, 45.5% of patients who were admitted to the hospital had a fracture. Gunshot fractures are an important consideration for orthopaedic surgeons not only because of their frequency (Table 1) but also because of the amount of resources that must be provided to care for each patient. The patients require longer hospital stays and use more resources than patients without fractures.

Joint Injury

Injuries into or near the joint have been common according to the chapters authors' experience. The shoulder (intra-articular region, proximal part of the humerus, clavicle, and scapula) has been the most

Dr. Vaidya or an immediate family member has received research or institutional support from Synthes. Dr. Bartlett or an immediate family member has stock or stock options held in Merck Dow. None of the following authors or a member of their immediate families has received anything of value from or owns stock in a commercial company or institution related directly or indirectly to the subject of this chapter: Dr. Dougherty, Dr. Silverton, and Dr. Najibi.

Table 1
Gunshot Fractures Seen at Henry Ford Hospital, Detroit, Michigan, Between 2001 and 2005

	Number	%
Spine (cervical/thoracic/lumbar)	98	20.3
Clavicle	16	3.3
Scapula	12	2.5
Acetabulum	10	2.1
Hip	10	2.1
Pelvis	47	9.8
Humerus	42	8.7
Forearm	38	7.9
Hand	47	9.8
Femur	89	18.5
Patella	6	1.2
Tibia/fibula	50	10.4
Ankle	2	0.41
Foot	15	3.1
Total	482	100

Table 2
Periarticular Gunshot Wounds to Upper Extremity Joints Seen at Henry Ford Hospital, Detroit, Michigan, Between 2001 and 2005

Upper Extremity Joint	Number	%*
Shoulder	99	21.4
Elbow	47	10.2
Wrist	17	3.7

*Based on the total number of upper extremity gunshot wounds (462)

Table 3
Periarticular Gunshot Wounds to Lower Extremity Joints Seen at Henry Ford Hospital, Detroit, Michigan, Between 2001 and 2005

Lower Extremity Joint	Number	%*
Hip	20	3.8
Knee	50	9.5
Ankle	2	0.4

*Based on the total number of lower extremity gunshot wounds (526)

common upper extremity joint injured, with shoulder injuries accounting for 21.4% of all upper extremity gunshot wounds between 2001 and 2005. In contrast, the wrist, the least injured upper extremity joint, was involved 3.7% of the time (Table 2). A lower percentage of lower extremity injuries were intra-articular or near the joint; the knee was the most commonly injured joint (involved 9.5% of the time), whereas the ankle was the least commonly injured joint (involved 0.4% of the time; Table 3).

An intra-articular injury is not always obvious; therefore, a gunshot wound near a major joint should be suspected of penetrating that joint. Joint penetration is an indication for surgical exploration of the joint, with copious lavage to remove debris and contaminants and, if indicated, stabilization of the fracture. Clues of joint penetration include air in the joint, an intra-articular hematoma, and an intra-articular fracture. Aspiration of the joint may be beneficial, as is injection of saline solution or methylene blue dye, but these methods are not always diagnostic. Treatment should be on the side of caution when joint penetration is suspected; it is recommended that whenever there is doubt about joint penetration, the wound and joint be explored and débrided. There are two reasons to remove bullets and bullet fragments from the joint. First, a foreign body in the joint can cause mechanical trauma with subsequent arthritis and loss of function. Second, bullet lead in the joint is absorbed and can cause lead toxicity.[3-5]

Arthroscopy has been used to manage penetrating joint injuries of the shoulder, elbow, hip, and knee, but specific indications for this procedure have not been established and comparisons of arthroscopic and open exploration have not been done.[5-23] The advantages of arthroscopy are smaller incisions, potentially faster rehabilitation, and better visualization of the joint, whereas the disadvantages include prolonged time to set up, increased surgical time, and the risk of compartment syndrome. Fluid extravasation has been reported to lead to death after a hip arthroscopy.[24]

Shoulder

The experience of the authors of this chapter and the literature indicate that approximately 10% of all gunshot wounds of the extremities involve the shoulder. A minority (10%) of these shoulder injuries are intra-articular.[7,25-27] Penetrating injuries of the upper extremity are commonly associated with other injuries, with 15% being associated with a vascular injury. Although nerve injuries are less frequent, they are the most important determinant of long-term function of the limb.[6,25-28]

A multiteam approach should be used. Orthopaedic, vascular, microvascular, and plastic surgery may be needed for patients with severely injured limbs. Proximal humeral and glenoid fractures may be present. Muscle-tendon units, ligaments, articular cartilage and labrum, and capsule may be involved and can be repaired at the time of the initial surgery in patients with a low-velocity gunshot wound.

Although the authors of this chapter are not aware of any direct comparisons of open and arthroscopic techniques for the management of these injuries, case reports support the use of both techniques.[6,7,25,26] Fractures that are nondisplaced or easily reducible may be stabilized with arthroscopic techniques, whereas unstable fractures involving the articular surface require open reduction and internal fixation. Large osteochondral fragments can be stabilized with bioabsorbable pins, headless screws such as Herbert screws (Zimmer, Warsaw, IN), Acutrak screws (Acumed, Hillsboro, OR), or a combination of these devices (Figure 1). Small and nonviable fragments should be removed. The bullet and its fragments may be removed with arthroscopic or open techniques. In the presence of intra-articular fracture displacement, comminution, and/or metaphyseal-diaphyseal dissociation, an open technique through a deltopectoral approach is used to reconstruct the joint surface. Reconstruction of the humeral head is done with open reduction and internal fixation with the use of bioabsorbable pins and screws and headless screws. Fractures of the surgical neck and shaft are managed with internal fixation with a locked plate and screws. Hemiarthroplasty is an option when the humeral head cannot be reconstructed. Complications include stiffness, infection, nonunion, malunion, hardware failure, compartment syndrome, and neurovascular injury.

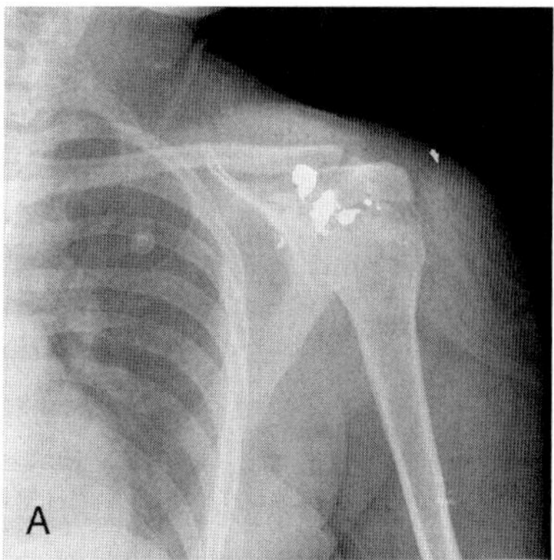

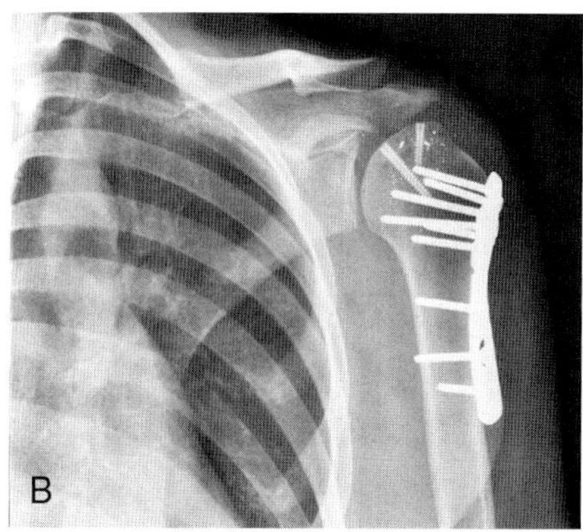

Figure 1 **A,** AP shoulder radiograph showing a proximal humeral and shoulder joint intra-articular fracture. **B,** Radiograph made after treatment with open reduction and internal fixation.

Elbow

The incidence of gunshot wounds to the elbow may be underestimated in the literature.[8,25,28-32] If the proximal part of the forearm (proximal part of the radius or proximal part of the ulna) and the distal part of the arm (distal part of the humerus) are included as part of the elbow, then the rate is higher than has been reported. On the basis of these criteria, gunshot wounds to the elbow account for 4.8% of all extremity gunshot wounds and 10.2% of upper extremity gunshot wounds. Associated injuries include nerve injuries and arterial and venous injuries.

Initial management includes vascular repair, irrigation and débridement, and stabilization with a bridging external fixator (Figure 2). Definitive treatment may involve a combination of various techniques, including internal and/or hinged external fixation (Figure 3).

Complications include stiffness, malunion, nonunion, infection, and nerve injury. A severely injured joint may be salvaged with a compression plate arthrodesis of the elbow or with arthroplasty.[31,32] Young, active patients are not good candidates for elbow arthroplasty. When such patients have an arthritic and painful elbow, an arthrodesis may be considered.[32] A loose bullet in the elbow joint is an indication for arthroscopic irrigation, débridement, and bullet removal.[8]

Wrist

In the authors' experience from 2001 through 2005, gunshot wounds to the wrist accounted for 1.7% of all extremity gunshot wounds and 3.7% of all upper extremity gunshot wounds. Associated injuries include fractures, neurovas-

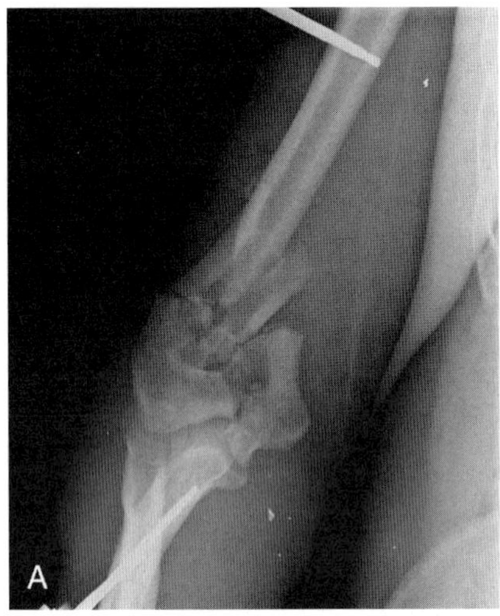

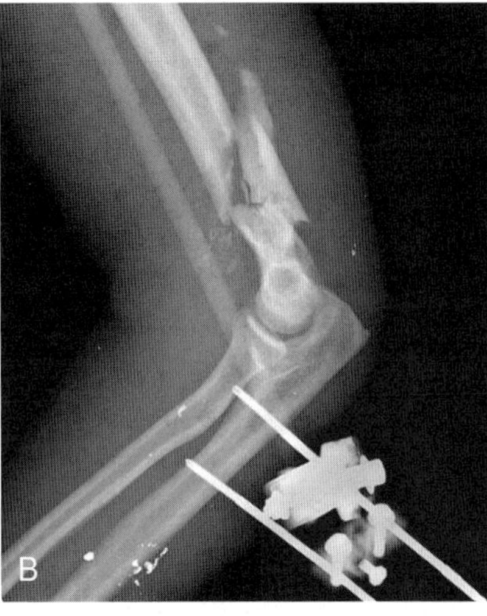

Figure 2 AP **(A)** and lateral **(B)** radiographs showing an intra-articular distal humeral fracture stabilized with a spanning external fixator of the elbow. This approach allowed staged reconstruction of the joint. A standard construct is to span the joint with two pins in the humerus and two pins in the ulna. This may be modified depending on the degree of fracture comminution and bone loss at the joint.

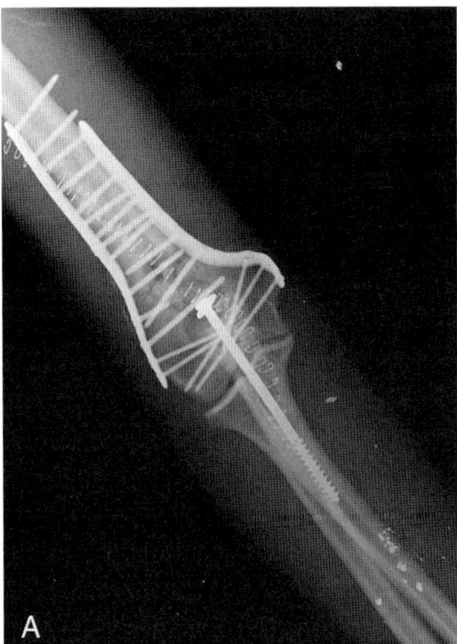

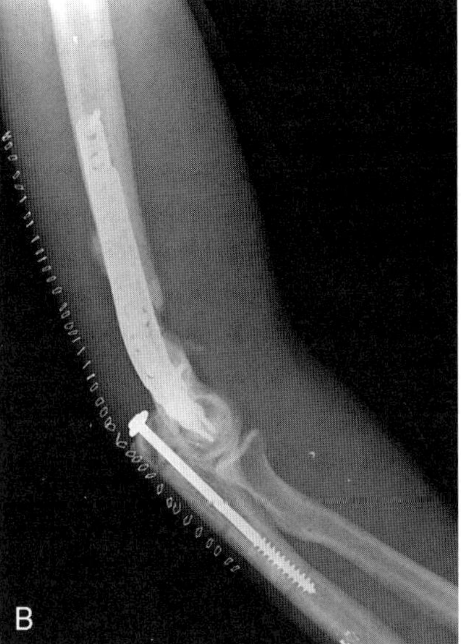

Figure 3 AP **(A)** and lateral **(B)** radiographs showing definitive open reduction and internal fixation, through a transolecranon approach, of the distal humeral fracture shown in Figures 2A and 2B.

cular injuries, and tendon ruptures. Fractures are very common in patients with a gunshot wound to the wrist and may involve the distal parts of the radius and ulna, the carpus, or both. Initial management includes irrigation and débridement, vascular repair if necessary, and spanning external fixation. A free flap or skin graft may be necessary to cover soft-tissue defects caused by high-energy gunshot wounds. Nerve repair, tendon repair, or reconstruction can be achieved after the initial irrigation and fracture stabilization. The role of arthroscopy in the treatment of gunshot wounds to the wrist is not clear, and because most of these injuries involve unstable fractures of the distal part of the radius and/or the carpus, open treatment is usually required.

Hip

The authors of this chapter have found that gunshot wounds to the hip joint account for 2% of all extremity gunshot wounds and 4% of lower extremity gunshot wounds. If nonarticular wounds to the hip region are included, these proportions increase to 9% and 17%, respectively.[9-16,24,25,33-38]

The recognition of an intra-articular injury is based on radiographic and CT findings (Figure 4). In the absence of a fracture, or when radiographs are inconclusive, a fluoroscopically assisted arthrogram is the most sensitive test to detect violation of the joint.[39]

When an associated injury to the femoral artery is suspected, an arteriogram is indicated. When a vascular injury is present, an emergent repair or bypass is necessary.

Transabdominal gunshot wounds to the hip pose a particularly difficult treatment challenge. The current recommendation for the treatment of hip joint violation with a transabdominal bullet is emergent irrigation and débridement and fracture stabilization in addition to antibiotic prophylaxis. Transpelvic bullets that traverse the urinary bladder require urologic assessment and primary bladder repair. Urinary diversion may be necessary to avoid infection or fistula formation.[36,39]

In a case study of 53 gunshot wounds to the hip, Long and associates[39] found the entry site to be the buttock in 32 patients, the anterior aspect of the thigh or inguinal area in 13, the lateral aspect of the hip in 6, and the lower part of the abdomen in 2. The authors of this study recommended antibiotic therapy (a 3-day course of cefazolin [Ancef; GlaxoSmithKline, Research Triangle Park, NC] and gentamicin) without an arthrotomy if the injury is caused by a low-energy gunshot, the injury is not transabdominal, the bullet is not in communication with synovial fluid, and there is a stable fracture that does not require internal fixation. Fifteen of the 53 patients met these criteria and were treated without an arthrotomy. Septic arthritis did not develop in any of these 15 patients. An arthrotomy was performed in hips with extensive comminution and/or transabdominal injury. An infection developed in 6 of the 53 hips, and 4 of the 6 patients with an infection had a transabdominal injury. One of the infections was associated with a missed bullet in the hip joint and one with a missed displaced femoral neck fracture.

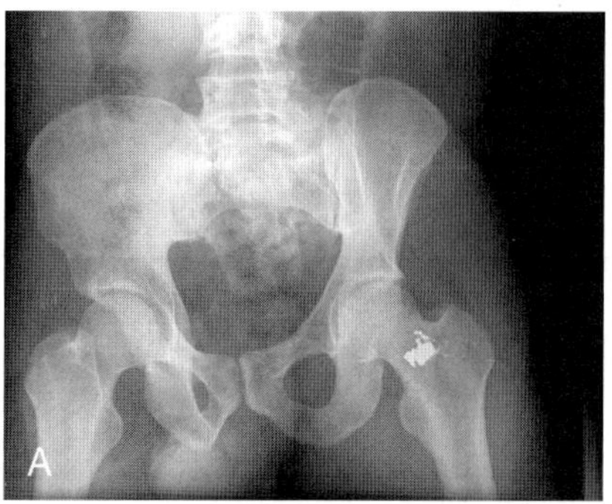

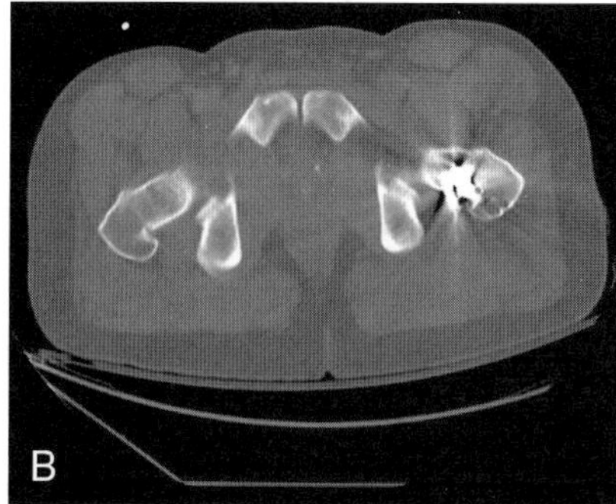

Figure 4 **A,** AP pelvic radiograph showing the intra-articular location of a bullet. **B,** Axial CT scan of the hips, showing the bullet embedded in the femoral neck.

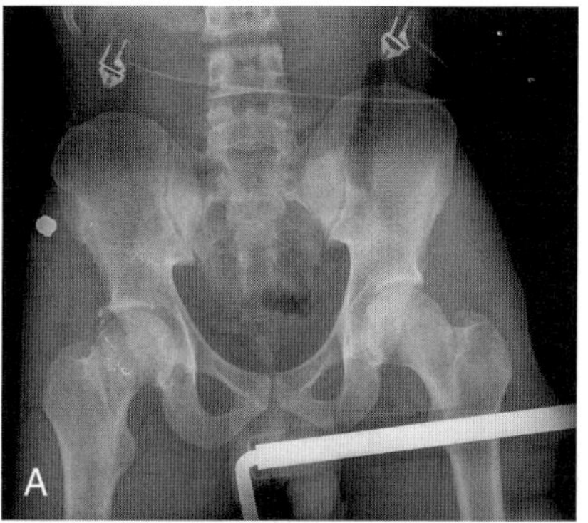

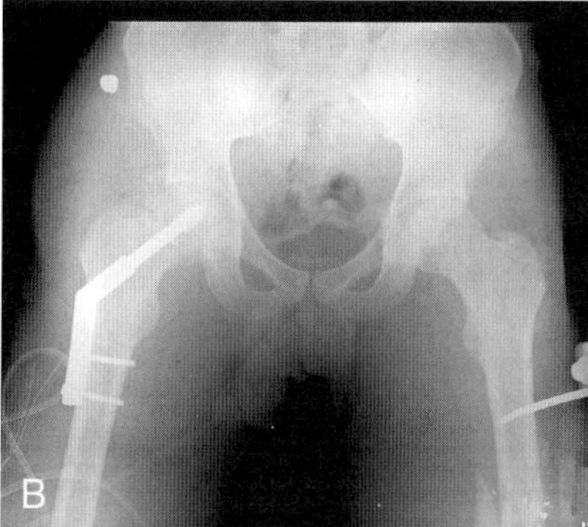

Figure 5 **A,** AP pelvic radiograph showing a gunshot femoral neck fracture. **B,** Radiograph made after treatment of the femoral neck fracture with a compression screw and side plate.

The recommended treatment of these fractures is open reduction and internal fixation (Figure 5). Hip arthroplasty or arthrodesis is not recommended in the acute setting. When there is severe comminution and adequate bone is not available for internal fixation, resection arthroplasty may be done.[39] Complications of gunshot wounds to the hip include arthrosis, infection, fistula formation, nonunion, malunion, and osteonecrosis.[39]

Bullets can be removed by means of arthrotomy or arthroscopy.[9,10,12-15,24,39] Hip arthroscopy requires special equipment, including a fracture table and fluoroscopy, as well as experience with the technique. Intra-abdominal fluid extravasation and abdominal compartment syndrome have been reported after hip arthroscopy for the treatment of a gunshot wound to the hip.[24] In the presence of an acetabular fracture, extreme care must be taken to measure the arthroscopy fluid inflow and outflow. If the inflow and outflow are not balanced, it is likely that fluid is extravasating into the pelvis and abdomen, and the procedure should be stopped.[24]

Knee

The chapter authors' experience has been that 5% of all extremity gunshot wounds and 9.5% of all lower extremity gunshot wounds involve the knee region (with or without an open joint injury and with or without a fracture). The literature suggests that 5% of all extremity gunshot wounds and 10% of lower extremity gunshot wounds involve the knee.[17,18,20,40]

Perry and associates[40] reported on 64 gunshot fractures of the knee. These included 37 intra-articular fractures and 27 extra-articular fractures. There were 29 femoral, 29 tibial, and 9 patellar fractures. Because a vascular injury was suspected, 23 patients had an arteriogram and 6 of these arteriograms were positive. All of the knees with a positive arteriogram were explored, and five of the six limbs required vascular repair. Of the five injuries that required vascular repair, one involved the common popliteal artery; one, a branch of the common femoral artery; two, both the peroneal and the posterior tibial arteries; and one, the superficial femoral artery. Only two patients had a nerve injury, which involved the peroneal nerve in both. Two infections were reported.

Spanning external fixation of the joint is recommended when there is a severely comminuted and unstable fracture about the knee. Multiple irrigation and débridement procedures and a delayed closure may be necessary for patients with extensive soft-tissue injury. Delayed reconstruction of the joint may be undertaken once the soft tissues have healed.

Acute reconstruction of knee ligaments is not recommended for patients with an unstable fracture or associated injuries. In these cases, a delayed reconstruction may be undertaken after fracture healing and rehabilitation. Meniscal tears and large osteochondral fragments may be fixed acutely.

Tornetta and Hui[18] reported on the role of arthroscopy in managing gunshot wounds of the knee. Of 33 patients who had an arthroscopic examination after sustaining a gunshot wound to the knee, 5 had a chondral injury, 14 had a meniscal injury, and 5 had intra-articular debris that had not been seen on radiographs. On the basis of these findings, the authors of this chapter recommend diagnostic arthroscopy, arthroscopic-assisted bullet removal, and irrigation and débridement for the treatment of gunshot wounds that involve the knee. In the presence of a meniscal tear or an osteochondral fragment, acute repair can be performed arthroscopically by an experienced arthroscopist. Complications with arthroscopy of the knee include fluid extravasation and compartment syndrome.

Ankle

In the chapter authors' experience, 0.4% of gunshot wounds to the lower extremity have involved the ankle. Treatment has varied from spanning external fixation or internal fixation for a low-velocity injury to arthrodesis or amputation for a high-velocity injury.[41,42] The role of arthroscopy is limited to bullet removal and irrigation and débridement of the joint, in the absence of an unstable fracture.

Lead Toxicity

Lead toxicity can occur with retained bullet fragments, most commonly when they are within the synovial fluid.[3-5,43-63] Lead becomes soluble in organic acids, such as synovial fluid, producing increased blood lead concentrations.[3] Another mechanism by which lead is introduced into the bloodstream is phagocytosis by macrophages. Although routine removal of bullets or their fragments is not recommended unless they are within a synovial fluid cavity, the possibility of lead toxicity from retained bullets anywhere should be considered.[3,4,44-47,51-57,61,64-66]

Approximately 90% to 95% of lead is stored in bone, taking the place of calcium in the calcium hydroxyapatite.[3,64] The half-life of lead in bone is 20 to 30 years.[4,51,57,61] Its blood half-life is approximately 30 days, and excretion is through the biliary and renal systems. Hypermetabolic states can mobilize bone stores and increase the blood lead concentration, causing a patient to become symptomatic. Hypermetabolic states can occur with fractures, surgery, alcohol use, diabetic ketoacidosis, pregnancy, infection, hyperthyroidism, Paget disease, neoplasia, and the use of medications or recreational drugs.

Surgeons should be aware of the symptoms of lead toxicity.[50] These symptoms are vague, and multiple organs can be affected. Because of this, the diagnosis of lead toxicity is often delayed. Patients with lead toxicity most often present with symptoms such as fatigue, malaise, abdominal complaints (pain, nausea, vomiting, and/or constipation), headache, or joint pain. Patients also can have difficulty with memory, attention span, and behavior. Signs of lead toxicity include microcytic hypochromic anemia, encephalopathy, peripheral nerve changes caused by demyelination of motor axons, and chronic renal failure. Later encephalopathic findings may be cerebral edema and seizures.

Lead toxicity should be suspected if the patient is found to have microcytic anemia or symptoms such as persistent abdominal pain. A whole blood lead concentration should be assessed to confirm the diagnosis.

Long-Bone Fractures

Humerus

Gunshot fractures to the humeral diaphysis occur less commonly than do those of the femur and tibia[67-70] (Table 1). Nerve injuries are relatively common in patients who sustain gunshot wounds of the humerus and are more common with distal injuries than with proximal injuries.[30,69,71-75]

The authors of this chapter are not aware of any prospective studies comparing the various methods of treatment of humeral fractures, and the management of these injuries is controversial.[28,30,68,72-76] A fracture brace or coaptation splint is recommended when there is minimal soft-tissue injury and the fracture can be held in alignment by these means. However, proximal or very distal fractures are often not amenable to this method of care.[68,69]

External fixation has been used for patients with more extensive injuries, such as battlefield wounds. Zinman and associates[74] reported on 26 Israeli war casualties who had external fixation of an open humeral fracture. A monolateral external fixator was used and resulted in union in 15 patients, whereas compression plate fixation was used in 5 patients and a cast was used for 6. Five of the six patients treated with a cast had a delayed union, and four were subsequently treated with plate fixation and bone grafting. Fifteen patients had a total of 20 nerve injuries. One of the injuries involved the radial nerve and was caused by distal, lateral pin placement. There were four brachial and two radial artery repairs. Twenty-three patients were followed for a mean of 6.5 years after the injury. The authors reported that the result was excellent in 14 patients, good in 4, fair in 3, and poor in 2. All fractures eventually healed. The authors of this study concluded that external fixation was the best treatment for patients with a severe open injury secondary to a war wound because it stabilized the fracture while allowing access for wound care. They recommended that an open method be used to place lateral pins in the distal part of the humerus and to avoid radial nerve injury; percutaneous placement should be reserved for posteriorly placed pins.

In 1995, Keller[73] reported a study of 37 refugees who had been treated for a gunshot fracture of the humerus at a Red Cross Hospital on the Sudanese border. The patients were seen at an average of 9.5 days after the injury, at which time 33 of the wounds were infected. Eight patients had nerve palsy. Twenty-three patients were treated with a plaster of Paris splint, 7 were treated with external fixation, and 7 were treated with skeletal traction. The average duration of the immobilization with the plaster of Paris splint was 35.8 days, and 21 of the 23 fractures so treated were adequately aligned. Four of the patients had an average of two surgeries. The seven patients treated with external fixation had the frame in place for an average of 46.3 days, and four of the fractures were adequately aligned. Five of the seven fractures did not unite and required a total of 11 surgeries. Of the seven patients treated with traction, which was maintained for an average of 27.7 days, five unions were obtained. There were six revisions in three of the seven patients. Although the patients treated with the splint had the best results, the groups were not comparable because those treated with external fixation or traction had more severe injuries.

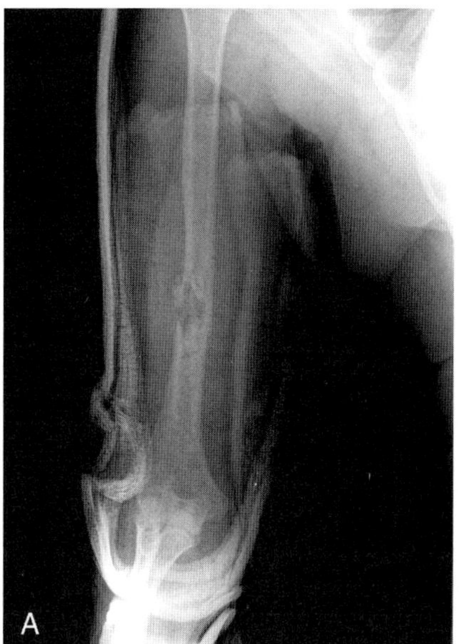

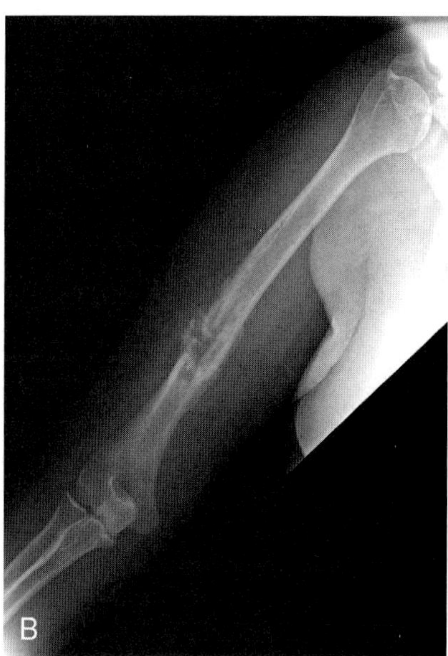

Figure 6 **A,** AP radiograph of a gunshot fracture of the humerus treated with a coaptation splint. **B,** The gunshot fracture after 4 months in a functional brace.

Hall and Pankovich[71] treated 89 humeral fractures with Ender nailing; 22 of these fractures were caused by gunshot wounds, and 4 of the 22 were caused by shotgun wounds. The authors of this study reported good results. As is the case with other traumatic indications, Ender nailing for the treatment of humeral fractures has been replaced with conventional intramedullary nailing. It remains to be seen whether intramedullary nailing or plate fixation is best for unstable or more extensive injuries.

The use of a functional brace, after a short time in a coaptation splint, for the treatment of simple fractures with minimal soft-tissue disruption yields acceptable results[68] (Figure 6). A spanning external fixator to provide initial stabilization for patients with more extensive injuries, such as those resulting from a short-range shotgun blast, is recommended[35] (Figure 7). The use of a small-pin external fixator for patients with extensive comminution and soft-

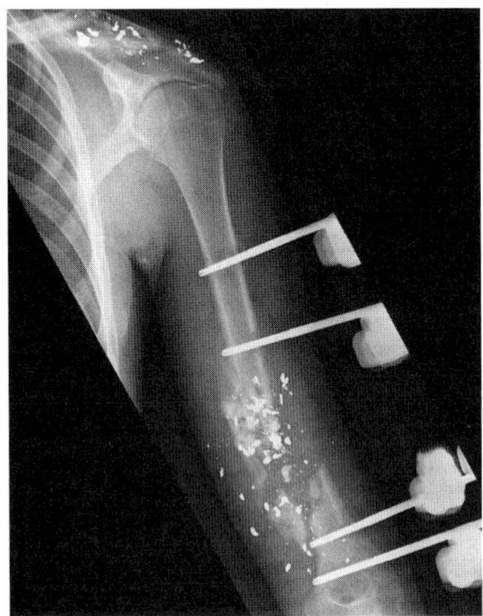

Figure 7 AP radiograph showing a gunshot fracture of the humerus treated with external fixation.

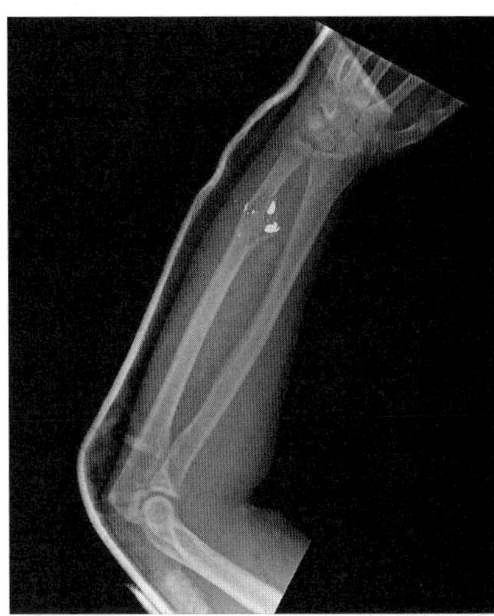

Figure 8 AP radiograph showing an ulnar shaft fracture treated with local wound care and a splint followed by a fracture brace. The fracture healed uneventfully.

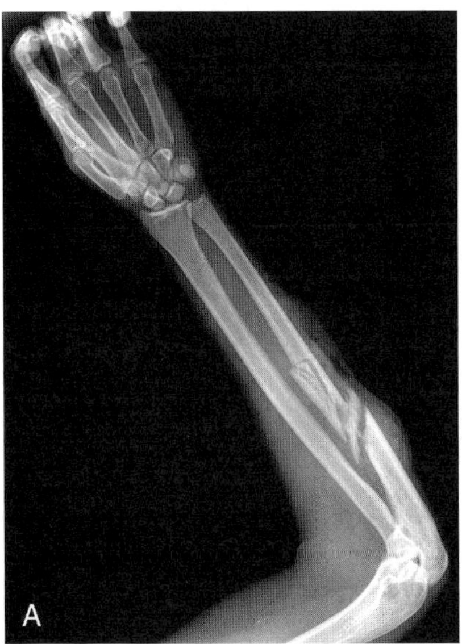

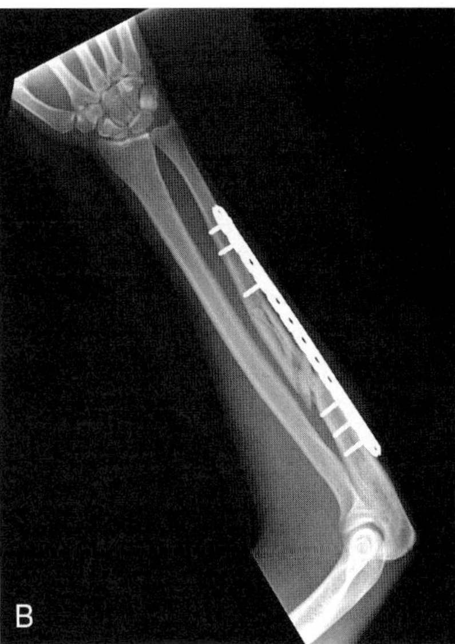

Figure 9 **A,** AP radiograph showing a comminuted ulnar shaft fracture. **B,** Radiograph made after treatment of the ulnar shaft fracture with open reduction and internal fixation.

tissue injury has been reported to have a good success rate.[28] When both the limb and the patient have become stable, planning for fracture stabilization and soft-tissue coverage can be done. The use of a cage with allograft or a fibular osteoseptocutaneous flap has been described for the treatment of skeletal defects.[77]

Forearm

There are relatively few reports describing the care of gunshot wounds to the forearm.[78-91] Nerve injury is commonly associated with gunshot wounds to the forearm, and there is a 10% prevalence of compartment syndrome.[84,86,88] The goals of fracture care are to restore forearm length and alignment as well as radial bow.

Elstrom and associates[92] treated 29 fractures of the radius and/or ulna in the 1970s. Fifteen patients were treated with a cast or with the pins-and-plaster technique. A nonunion developed in three of these patients, and a malunion developed in another three. Six displaced and comminuted fractures were treated with delayed open reduction and internal fixation, and none of them went on to malunion or nonunion. This suggests that open reduction and internal fixation may be safely used if the soft tissues are healthy.

External fixation is recommended for treating a displaced or comminuted forearm fracture that is unstable and associated with severe soft-tissue injury. Has and associates[93] reported a 10.3% infection rate following external fixation for treating upper extremity war injuries, primarily those resulting from explosive munitions.

Care for a diaphyseal forearm fracture depends on the severity of both the soft-tissue and the osseous injury, just as it does when the open forearm fracture is not caused by a firearm.[78] Patients with a relatively stable fracture of the ulna and minimal soft-tissue trauma may be treated with application of a cast after appropriate wound treatment (Figure 8). Displaced fractures should be treated with open reduction and internal fixation when the soft tissues permit (Figure 9).

Initial stabilization with external fixation should be used for patients with bone loss when both forearm bones are involved. If just the radius or the ulna is involved, splinting may be all that is required. A soft-tissue antibiotic-impregnated spacer may be used for initial care of the void.[79] A second-stage procedure to reconstruct bone defects should be done once the limb is stable. External fixation may also be used for patients with severe soft-tissue injury, such as those who have sustained a shotgun blast to the forearm. Initial stabilization with an external fixator allows staged bone and soft-tissue reconstruction. Autologous bone grafting to fill defects has been described;[79,80,84] however, the chapter authors are not aware of any reports on the use of allograft and bioactive substances, such as bone morphogenetic protein or demineralized bone matrix, for reconstruction of a forearm defect after a gunshot wound.

A salvage procedure may be performed by creating a "single-bone forearm" for the treatment of unreconstructible bone loss or osteomyelitis.[87] The proximal part of the ulna needs to be preserved to achieve a stable elbow, and the single bone based on the proximal part of the ulna does not allow pronation or supination.

Femur

Diaphyseal femoral fractures are the most common long-bone fractures associated with gunshot wounds[38,70,94-101] (Table 1). Prior to approximately 20 years ago, balanced skeletal traction was the mainstay of care for femoral fractures in war or peace.[102] Initial stabilization with traction is commonly used today as a temporary means of stabilization until more definitive care can be provided.[103]

External fixation has been used for open fractures on the battlefield. Reis and associates[70] reported on 19 femoral fractures that were initially treated with external fixation with the intention to use this method until bone union occurred. Six patients had conversion to a cast brace because of pin-tract infection, and five others had open reduction and internal fixation. Fourteen of the femora were treated with bone grafting. The authors of this study noted that no additional procedures were done until the limb was free of obvious infection. The average time to union was 19 weeks. External fixation is now more commonly used for patients who are physiologically unable to undergo more extensive surgery.[99,104] The use of temporary external fixation as a bridge from the injury to the definitive fracture stabilization has become a popular means of initially stabilizing the fracture.

Intramedullary Nailing

Use of intramedullary nailing to treat patients with a malunion, nonunion, or infection after a fracture secondary to a gunshot wound in the United States began after World War II.[105-107] Wiss and associates[101] retrospectively reviewed the cases of 77 patients who had sustained a gunshot femoral fracture; 56 of these patients had adequate records for follow-up. The patients were initially treated with skeletal traction for 10 to 14 days, and intramedullary nailing was performed when the wound tract had healed. No deep wound infections were reported. The average time to union was just over 5 months, and the average duration of follow-up was 16 months. Five patients had a limb-length discrepancy of more than 1 cm, one patient had angulation of 15°, and one had a clinically relevant rotational deformity. Five of the 56 patients required vascular repair in addition to the treatment of the femoral fracture. The authors of this study also reported an associated sciatic nerve injury in three patients, one of whom had a return of function, one of whom had partial return, and one of whom had no return of function. Two patients had a peroneal nerve palsy, and one of them had a return of function.

Hollmann and Horowitz[97] reported on 26 patients who had sustained a fracture as a result of a low-velocity gunshot wound and were treated with intramedullary nailing at an average of 9 days after the injury. Nineteen of the patients (2 treated with open nailing and 17 treated with closed nailing) were followed until union, which occurred at an average of 4.5 months after the injury.

Bergman and associates[95] reviewed the cases of 65 patients with a gunshot femoral fracture. The patients were treated with reamed intramedullary nailing at an average of 2 days (range, 0 to 14 days) after the injury, and they were followed for an average of 2 years (range, 9.5 months to 6 years). All fractures healed, at an average of just over 4 months (range, 13 to 31 weeks). Two patients had persistent drainage, which resolved within 3 weeks while they were being treated with antibiotics.

Tornetta and Tiburzi[100] reported on 55 patients with a gunshot femoral fracture. Thirty-eight were treated with intramedullary nailing and were followed for an average of 2 years (range, 14 to 36 months). The average time to union was 2 months (range, 5 to 22 weeks).

In a study by Nicholas and McCoy,[108] 12 patients with a total of 14 femoral fractures were treated with immediate intramedullary nailing (performed less than 8 hours after the injury). Three patients had vascular repair, and two patients had a sciatic nerve injury. The average time to union was 5.5 months (range, 3 to 8 months). None of the patients had an infection.

Retrograde nailing has become a popular technique for the treatment

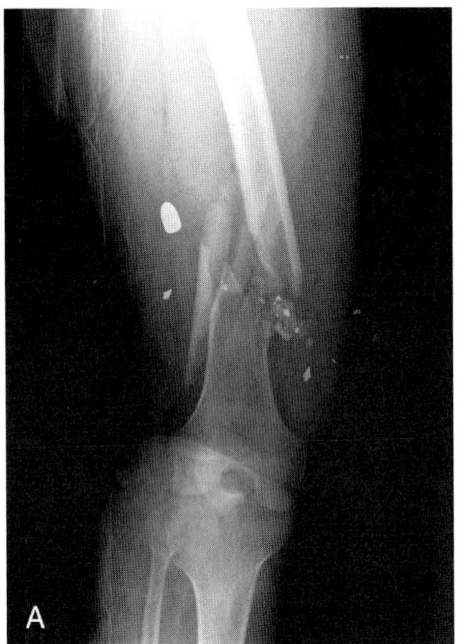

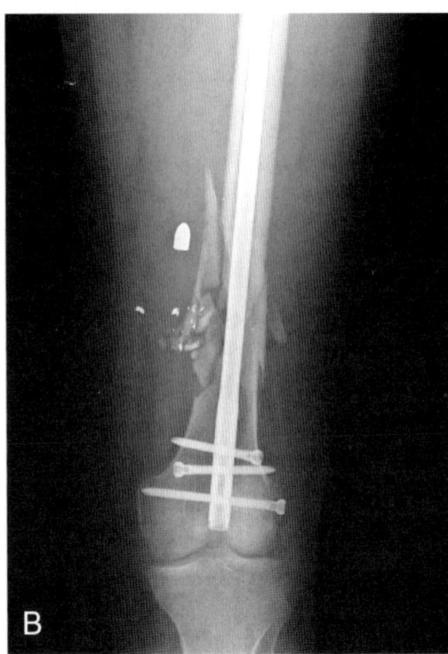

Figure 10 **A,** AP radiograph showing a diaphyseal femoral fracture, which was subsequently treated with immediate retrograde intramedullary nailing. **B,** Postoperative radiograph showing excellent fracture alignment.

of diaphyseal femoral fractures, particularly those near the knee. Initially, it was believed that this approach should not be used for an open fracture because of the risk of knee infection, but the chapter authors believe that two reports demonstrate that intramedullary nailing may be done safely, with a minimal risk of infection, in patients with a gunshot femoral fracture.[109,110] A recent study reported on a series of 196 gunshot femoral fractures, of which 56 were treated with retrograde nailing.[111] There was no increased rate of infection, at either the fracture site or the knee joint, associated with this method of treatment (Figure 10).

Compartment syndrome is an infrequent complication of femoral shaft fractures.[112,113] Three of 102 patients treated for a diaphyseal femoral gunshot wound between 2001 and 2006 at the Henry Ford Hospital were diagnosed with thigh compartment syndrome.

Tibia

Tibial fractures are the second most frequent long-bone fractures resulting from a gunshot wound (Table 1). A variety of methods have been reported for the treatment of these fractures, including the use of a cast or a fracture brace, external fixation, and intramedullary nailing.

Fracture bracing has been used in both war and peace since World War I. A walking brace was fashioned to treat fractures of the tibia during World War I.[114] Dehne and associates[114] popularized the use of nonsurgical ambulatory treatment of tibial fractures during the 1950s. This treatment was also developed by Sarmiento and associates[89] in the 1960s and has been a treatment method for a variety of both open and closed tibial fractures.

Witschi and Omer[115] reported the results of ambulatory treatment with a cast followed by fracture bracing in a series of 84 patients who had sustained a tibial fracture secondary to a missile injury. All of the fractures had some comminution. Despite this, the authors of this study reported less than 1 cm of shortening in 48 of 58 patients with an isolated injury and only 1 cm of shortening in the 10 additional patients. Osteomyelitis, which prolonged the time to union, developed in seven patients. Brown and Urban[116] reported on 60 patients with a total of 63 war-related tibial fractures that were treated with a fracture brace. The fractures healed in an average of 4.5 months. Shortening averaged 9 mm (range, 2 to 38 mm). Twenty-seven of the fractures had no shortening. Four of the 63 patients had persistent drainage. Sarmiento and associates[89] reported on 32 gunshot tibial fractures treated with a fracture brace. One fracture did not heal, but the average time to union of the others was 4 months.

Leffers and Chandler[117] reviewed the cases of 40 patients with a total of 41 tibial fractures caused by gunshot wounds. Thirty-five fractures were treated initially with a cast and then with a fracture brace. Because of their severity, five fractures were initially treated with external fixation, and then a functional brace was applied within the first 2 months. One patient was treated with pins and plaster. The fractures that were treated initially with a cast healed in an average of 3 months, whereas those that were initially treated with external fixation healed in an average of 5 months. Eight patients had persistent wound drainage, and two had a surgical procedure to care for the wound. It should be noted that these 40 patients accounted for fewer than one third of the patients with gunshot-associated tibial fractures who had been seen at the Henry Ford Hospital.

Ferraro and Zinar[118] reported on 90 of 133 patients with a tibial fracture caused by a gunshot wound who had been treated at Harbor/UCLA Medical Center. Fracture stabilization was achieved with a long leg cast in 58 patients, external fixation was used for 17, and unreamed intramedullary nailing was performed in 15. The authors of this study found that fractures classified as Winquist grade 0, I, or II healed within 3 months. In the group classified as Winquist grade III, IV, or V, those treated with intramedullary nailing healed at an average of 4 months, and those treated with external fixation healed at an average of 6.5 months.

Brien and associates[119] recommended a treatment algorithm based on both soft-tissue and bone injury. For stable fractures with minimal soft-tissue disruption, antibiotics and cast treatment were recommended. For "unstable" fractures, the recommended treatment was reamed intramedullary nailing, unreamed intramedullary nailing, or external fixation, depending on the degree of soft-tissue disruption. The authors of this study recommended the use of small-pin fixators for tibial metaphyseal fractures. It should be noted that the authors of this study did not precisely define "stable" or "unstable" fractures.[119]

Presently, the treatment of gunshot fractures of the tibial shaft depends on the amount of bone comminution and the degree of soft-tissue injury. Patients who have a tibial shaft fracture with minimal comminution, soft-tissue injury, displacement, or angulation may be treated successfully with local wound care in the emergency department and application of a cast, followed by a functional brace.

Although the chapter authors are not aware of any large clinical series in which the use of intramedullary nailing for the treatment of gunshot fractures was evaluated, it appears that more comminuted fractures are better managed with intramedullary nail fixation. If there is major soft-tissue injury requiring a soft-tissue transfer, consideration should be given to the use of external fixation until the soft tissues are reconstructed, at which point the fixator may be removed and an intramedullary nail can be inserted.

Summary

Gunshot injuries remain a major clinical problem for orthopaedic surgeons, particularly when the treatment of inner-city trauma is a major part of their practice. Additional research is needed to evaluate outcomes of gunshot fractures and joint injuries. The use of more modern fixation techniques developed since the 1980s has not been well documented for patients with humeral or tibial fractures. Likewise, prevention of arthritis, joint stiffness, infection, and lead toxicity are major concerns in the treatment of patients with gunshot joint injuries, and prevention of these complications should remain a focus of the treatment team.

References

1. Centers for Disease Control, National Center for Injury Prevention and Control: WISQUARS fatal injuries: Mortality reports. http://webappa.cdc.gov/sasweb/ncipc/mortrate.html. Accessed November 10, 2008.
2. DoD personnel and procurement statistics: Military casualty information. Operation Iraqi Freedom: Wounded in action. http://siadapp.dmdc.osd.mil/personnel/CASUALTY/castop.htm. Accessed November 10, 2008.
3. Leonard MH: The solution of lead by synovial fluid. *Clin Orthop Relat Res* 1969;64:255-261.
4. Linden MA, Manton WI, Stewart RM, Thal ER, Feit H: Lead poisoning from retained bullets: Pathogenesis, diagnosis, and management. *Ann Surg* 1982;195:305-313.
5. Ganocy K II, Lindsey RW: The management of civilian intra-articular gunshot wounds: Treatment considerations and proposal of a classification system. *Injury* 1998;29:SA1-SA6.
6. Otero F, Cuartas E: Arthroscopic removal of bullet fragments from the subacromial space of the shoulder. *Arthroscopy* 2004;20:754-756.
7. Tarkin IS, Hatzidakis A, Hoxie SC, Giangara CE, Knight RQ: Arthroscopic treatment of gunshot wounds to the shoulder. *Arthroscopy* 2003;19:85-89.
8. Jamdar S, Helm AT, Redfern DR: Arthroscopic removal of a shotgun pellet from the elbow joint. *Arthroscopy* 2001;17:E30.
9. Cory JW, Ruch DS: Arthroscopic removal of a .44 caliber bullet from the hip. *Arthroscopy* 1998;14:624-626.
10. Goldman A, Minkoff J, Price A, Krinick R: A posterior arthroscopic approach to bullet extraction from the hip. *J Trauma* 1987;27:1294-1300.
11. Lee GH, Virkus WW, Kapotas JS: Arthroscopically assisted minimally invasive intraarticular bullet extraction: Technique, indications, and results. *J Trauma* 2008;64:512-516.
12. Meyer NJ, Thiel B, Ninomiya JT: Retrieval of an intact, intraarticular bullet by hip arthroscopy using the lateral approach. *J Orthop Trauma* 2002;16:51-53.
13. Mineo RC, Gittins ME: Arthroscopic removal of a bullet embedded in the acetabulum. *Arthroscopy* 2003;19:E121-E124.
14. Singleton SB, Joshi A, Schwartz MA, Collinge CA: Arthroscopic bullet removal from the acetabulum. *Arthroscopy* 2005;21:360-364.

15. Teloken MA, Schmietd I, Tomlinson DP: Hip arthroscopy: A unique inferomedial approach to bullet removal. *Arthroscopy* 2002;18:E21.

16. Williams MS, Hutcheson RL, Miller AR: A new technique for removal of intraarticular bullet fragments from the femoral head. *Bull Hosp Jt Dis* 1997;56:107-110.

17. Petersen W, Beske C, Stein V, Laprell H: Arthroscopical removal of a projectile from the intra-articular cavity of the knee joint. *Arch Orthop Trauma Surg* 2002;122:235-236.

18. Tornetta P III, Hui RC: Intraarticular findings after gunshot wounds through the knee. *J Orthop Trauma* 1997;11:422-424.

19. White RR: Arthroscopic bullet retrieval. *J Trauma* 1987;27:455-456.

20. Nikolić D, Vulović R: Arthroscopy of the knee in war injuries. *Injury* 1996;27:175-176.

21. Hartford JM, Gorczyca JT: Late arthroscopic debridement of metal fragments and synovectomy after penetrating knee joint injury by low-velocity missile: A report of two cases. *J Orthop Trauma* 2001;15:222-224.

22. Oladipo JO, Creevy W, Remis R: Arthroscopic management of intra-articular low-velocity gunshot wounds of the knee. *Am J Knee Surg* 1999;12:229-232.

23. Ganocy TK II, Lindsey RW: Delayed diagnosis of an intra-articular gunshot injury of the knee: A case report. *J Trauma* 1999;47:158-160.

24. Bartlett CS, DiFelice GS, Buly RL, Quinn TJ, Green DS, Helfet DL: Cardiac arrest as a result of intraabdominal extravasation of fluid during arthroscopic removal of a loose body from the hip joint of a patient with an acetabular fracture. *J Orthop Trauma* 1998;12:294-299.

25. Davis GL: Management of open wounds of joints during the Vietnam War: A preliminary study. *Clin Orthop Relat Res* 1970;68:3-9.

26. Secer HI, Daneyemez M, Tehli O, Gonul E, Izci Y: The clinical, electrophysiologic, and surgical characteristics of peripheral nerve injuries caused by gunshot wounds in adults: A 40-year experience. *Surg Neurol* 2008;69:143-152.

27. Stewart MP, Birch R: Penetrating missile injuries of the brachial plexus. *J Bone Joint Surg Br* 2001;83:517-524.

28. Kömürcü M, Yanmiş I, Ateşalp AS, Gür E: Treatment results for open comminuted distal humerus intra-articular fractures with Ilizarov circular external fixator. *Mil Med* 2003;168: 694-697.

29. Brannon JK, Woods C, Chandran RE, Hansraj KK, Reyes CS: Gunshot wounds to the elbow. *Orthop Clin North Am* 1995;26:75-84.

30. Skaggs DL, Hale JM, Buggay S, Kay RM: Use of a hybrid external fixator for a severely comminuted juxta-articular fracture of the distal humerus. *J Orthop Trauma* 1998;12: 439-442.

31. Demiralp B, Komurcu M, Ozturk C, Tasatan E, Sehirlioglu A, Basbozkurt M: Total elbow arthroplasty in patients who have elbow fractures caused by gunshot injuries: 8- to 12-year follow-up study. *Arch Orthop Trauma Surg* 2008;128:17-24.

32. McAuliffe JA, Burkhalter WE, Ouellette EA, Carneiro RS: Compression plate arthrodesis of the elbow. *J Bone Joint Surg Br* 1992;74:300-304.

33. Becker VV Jr, Brien WW, Patzakis M, Wilkins J: Gunshot injuries to the hip and abdomen: The association of joint and intra-abdominal visceral injuries. *J Trauma* 1990;30:1324-1329.

34. Christie DB III, Bozeman AP, Stapleton TR, Ashley DW: Gunshot wound to the femoral neck: A unique case. *J Trauma* 2007;62:785.

35. Miric DM, Bumbasirevic MZ, Senohradski KK, Djordjevic ZP: Pelvifemoral external fixation for the treatment of open fractures of the proximal femur caused by firearms. *Acta Orthop Belg* 2002;68:37-41.

36. Morganstern S, Seery W, Borshuk S, Cole AT: Septic arthritis secondary to vesico-acetabular fistula: A case report. *J Urol* 1976;116:116-117.

37. Neviaser RJ, Clawson RS: Transabdominal gunshot wounds of the hip. *South Med J* 1976;69:757-763.

38. Nikolić D, Jovanović Z, Turković G, Vulović R, Mladenović M: Subtrochanteric missile fractures of the femur. *Injury* 1998;29:743-749.

39. Long WT, Brien EW, Boucree JB Jr, Filler B, Stark HH, Dorr LD: Management of civilian gunshot injuries to the hip. *Orthop Clin North Am* 1995;26:123-131.

40. Perry DJ, Sanders DP, Nyirenda CD, Lezine-Hanna JT: Gunshot wounds to the knee. *Orthop Clin North Am* 1995;26:155-163.

41. Bek D, Demiralp B, Kürklü M, Ateşalp AS, Başbozkurt M: Ankle arthrodesis using an Ilizarov external fixator in patients wounded by landmines and gunshots. *Foot Ankle Int* 2008;29:178-184.

42. Yildiz C, Ateşalp AS, Demiralp B, Gür E: High-velocity gunshot wounds of the tibial plafond managed with Ilizarov external fixation: A report of 13 cases. *J Orthop Trauma* 2003;17:421-429.

43. Bolanos AA, Demizio JP Jr, Vigorita VJ, Bryk E: Lead poisoning from an intra-articular shotgun pellet in the knee treated with arthroscopic extraction and chelation therapy: A case report. *J Bone Joint Surg Am* 1996;78: 422-426.

44. Coon T, Miller M, Shirazi F, Sullivan J: Lead toxicity in a 14-year-old female with retained bullet fragments. *Pediatrics* 2006;117:227-230.

45. de Madureira PR, De Capitani EM, Vieira RJ: Lead poisoning after gunshot wound. *Sao Paulo Med J* 2000; 118:78-80.

46. DeMartini J, Wilson A, Powell JS, Powell CS: Lead arthropathy and systemic lead poisoning from an intraarticular bullet. *AJR Am J Roentgenol* 2001;176:1144.

47. Dillman RO, Crumb CK, Lidsky MJ: Lead poisoning from a gunshot

wound: Report of a case and review of the literature. *Am J Med* 1979;66: 509-514.

48. Farber JM, Rafii M, Schwartz D: Lead arthropathy and elevated serum levels of lead after a gunshot wound of the shoulder. *AJR Am J Roentgenol* 1994; 162:385-386.
49. Gerhardsson L, Dahlin L, Knebel R, Schütz A: Blood lead concentration after a shotgun accident. *Environ Health Perspect* 2002;110:115-117.
50. Gracia RC, Snodgrass WR: Lead toxicity and chelation therapy. *Am J Health Syst Pharm* 2007;64:45-53.
51. Greenberg SR: The histopathology of tissue lead retention. *Histol Histopathol* 1990;5:451-456.
52. Grogan DP, Bucholz RW: Acute lead intoxication from a bullet in an intervertebral disc space: A case report. *J Bone Joint Surg Am* 1981;63:1180-1182.
53. Harding NR, Lipton JF, Vigorita VJ, Bryk E: Experimental lead arthropathy: An animal model. *J Trauma* 1999; 47:951-955.
54. Janzen DL, Tirman PF, Rabassa AE, Kumar S: Lead "bursogram" and focal synovitis secondary to a retained intraarticular bullet fragment. *Skeletal Radiol* 1995;24:142-144.
55. John BE, Boatright D: Lead toxicity from gunshot wound. *South Med J* 1999;92:223-224.
56. Khurana V, Bradley TP: Lead poisoning from a retained bullet: A case report and review. *J Assoc Acad Minor Phys* 1999;10:48-49.
57. Manton WI, Thal ER: Lead poisoning from retained missiles: An experimental study. *Ann Surg* 1986;204: 594-599.
58. Meggs WJ, Gerr F, Aly MH, et al: The treatment of lead poisoning from gunshot wounds with succimer (DMSA). *J Toxicol Clin Toxicol* 1994; 32:377-385.
59. Peh WC, Reinus WR: Lead arthropathy: A cause of delayed onset lead poisoning. *Skeletal Radiol* 1995;24: 357-360.
60. Rehman MA, Umer M, Sepah YJ, Wajid MA: Bullet-induced synovitis as a cause of secondary osteoarthritis of the hip joint: A case report and review of literature. *J Med Case Reports* 2007;1:171.
61. Slavin RE, Swedo J, Cartwright J Jr, Viegas S, Custer EM: Lead arthritis and lead poisoning following bullet wounds: A clinicopathologic, ultrastructural, and microanalytic study of two cases. *Hum Pathol* 1988;19: 223-235.
62. Sokolowski MJ, Sisson G Jr: Systemic lead poisoning due to an intraarticular bullet. *Orthopedics* 2005;28: 411-412.
63. Windler EC, Smith RB, Bryan WJ, Woods GW: Lead intoxication and traumatic arthritis of the hip secondary to retained bullet fragments: A case report. *J Bone Joint Surg Am* 1978; 60:254-255.
64. McQuirter JL, Rothenberg SJ, Dinkins GA, Kondrashov V, Manalo M, Todd AC: Change in blood lead concentration up to 1 year after a gunshot wound with a retained bullet. *Am J Epidemiol* 2004;159:683-692.
65. McQuirter JL, Rothenberg SJ, Dinkins GA, Manalo M, Kondrashov V, Todd AC: The effects of retained lead bullets on body lead burden. *J Trauma* 2001;50:892-899.
66. Reynolds SJ, Seem R, Fourtes LJ, et al: Prevalence of elevated blood leads and exposure to lead in construction trades in Iowa and Illinois. *Am J Ind Med* 1999;36:307-316.
67. Brown TD, Michas P, Williams RE, Dawson G, Whitecloud TS, Barrack RL: The impact of gunshot wounds on an orthopaedic surgical service in an urban trauma center. *J Orthop Trauma* 1997;11:149-153.
68. Balfour GW, Marrero CE: Fracture brace for the treatment of humerus shaft fractures caused by gunshot wounds. *Orthop Clin North Am* 1995; 26:55-63.
69. Sarmiento A, Kinman PB, Galvin EG, Schmitt RH, Phillips JG: Functional bracing of fractures of the shaft of the humerus. *J Bone Joint Surg Am* 1977; 59:596-601.
70. Reis ND, Zinman C, Besser MI, Shifrin LZ, Rosen H: A philosophy of limb salvage in war: Use of the fixateur externe. *Mil Med* 1991;156: 505-520.
71. Hall RF Jr, Pankovich AM: Ender nailing of acute fractures of the humerus: A study of closed fixation by intramedullary nails without reaming. *J Bone Joint Surg Am* 1987;69: 558-567.
72. Joshi A, Labbe M, Lindsey RW: Humeral fracture secondary to civilian gunshot injury. *Injury* 1998;29:SA13-SA17.
73. Keller A: The management of gunshot fractures of the humerus. *Injury* 1995;26:93-96.
74. Zinman C, Norman D, Hamoud K, Reis ND: External fixation for severe open fractures of the humerus caused by missiles. *J Orthop Trauma* 1997;11: 536-539.
75. Zagorski JB, Latta LL, Zych GA, Finnieston AR: Diaphyseal fractures of the humerus: Treatment with prefabricated braces. *J Bone Joint Surg Am* 1988;70:607-610.
76. Okçu G, Aktuğlu K: Management of shotgun induced open fractures of the humerus with Ilizarov external fixator. *Ulus Travma Acil Cerrahi Derg* 2005;11:23-28.
77. Attias N, Lehman RE, Bodell LS, Lindsey RW: Surgical management of a long segmental defect of the humerus using a cylindrical titanium mesh cage and plates: A case report. *J Orthop Trauma* 2005;19:211-216.
78. Fackler ML, Burkhalter WE: Hand and forearm injuries from penetrating projectiles. *J Hand Surg Am* 1992;17: 971-975.
79. Georgiadis GM, DeSilva SP: Reconstruction of skeletal defects in the forearm after trauma: Treatment with cement spacer and delayed cancellous bone grafting. *J Trauma* 1995;38: 910-914.

80. Hahn M, Strauss E, Yang EC: Gunshot wounds to the forearm. *Orthop Clin North Am* 1995;26:85-93.

81. Helber MU, Ulrich C: External fixation in forearm shaft fractures. *Injury* 2000;31:45-47.

82. Jabaley ME, Peterson HD: Early treatment of war wounds of the hand and forearm in Vietnam. *Ann Surg* 1973;177:167-173.

83. Kim DH, Kam AC, Chandika P, Tiel RL, Kline DG: Surgical management and outcome in patients with radial nerve lesions. *J Neurosurg* 2001; 95:573-583.

84. Lenihan MR, Brien WW, Gellman H, Itamura J, Kuschner SH: Fractures of the forearm resulting from low-velocity gunshot wounds. *J Orthop Trauma* 1992;6:32-35.

85. MacKinnon SE, Weiland AJ, Godina M: Immediate forearm reconstruction with a functional latissimus dorsi island pedicle myocutaneous flap. *Plast Reconstr Surg* 1983;71: 706-710.

86. Moed BR, Fakhouri AJ: Compartment syndrome after low-velocity gunshot wounds to the forearm. *J Orthop Trauma* 1991;5:134-137.

87. Reid RL, Baker GI: The single-bone forearm: A reconstructive technique. *Hand* 1973;5:214-219.

88. Rodrigues RL, Sammer DM, Chung KC: Treatment of complex below-the-elbow gunshot wounds. *Ann Plast Surg* 2006;56:122-127.

89. Sarmiento A, Sharpe FE, Ebramzadeh E, Normand P, Shankwiler J: Factors influencing the outcome of closed tibial fractures treated with functional bracing. *Clin Orthop Relat Res* 1995;315:8-24.

90. Wilson RH: Gunshots to the hand and upper extremity. *Clin Orthop Relat Res* 2003;408:133-144.

91. Wu CD: Low-velocity gunshot fractures of the radius and ulna: Case report and review of the literature. *J Trauma* 1995;39:1003-1005.

92. Elstrom JA, Pankovich AM, Egwele R: Extra-articular low-velocity gunshot fractures of the radius and ulna. *J Bone Joint Surg Am* 1978;60:335-341.

93. Has B, Jovanovic S, Wertheimer B, Mikolasević I, Grdic P: External fixation as a primary and definitive treatment of open limb fractures. *Injury* 1995;26:245-248.

94. Ateşalp AS, Kömürcü M, Demiralp B, Bek D, Oğuz E, Yanmiş I: Treatment of close-range, low-velocity gunshot fractures of tibia and femur diaphysis with consecutive compression-distraction technique: A report of 11 cases. *J Surg Orthop Adv* 2004;13: 112-118.

95. Bergman M, Tornetta P, Kerina M, et al: Femur fractures caused by gunshots: Treatment by immediate reamed intramedullary nailing. *J Trauma* 1993;34:783-785.

96. Grover J, Wiss DA: A prospective study of fractures of the femoral shaft treated with a static, intramedullary, interlocking nail comparing one versus two distal screws. *Orthop Clin North Am* 1995;26:139-146.

97. Hollmann MW, Horowitz M: Femoral fractures secondary to low velocity missiles: Treatment with delayed intramedullary fixation. *J Orthop Trauma* 1990;4:64-69.

98. Levy AS, Wetzler MJ, Guttman G, et al: Treating gunshot femoral shaft fractures with immediate reamed intramedullary nailing. *Orthop Rev* 1993;22:805-809.

99. Nowotarski P, Brumback RJ: Immediate interlocking nailing of fractures of the femur caused by low- to mid-velocity gunshots. *J Orthop Trauma* 1994;8:134-141.

100. Tornetta P III, Tiburzi D: Antegrade interlocked nailing of distal femoral fractures after gunshot wounds. *J Orthop Trauma* 1994;8:220-227.

101. Wiss DA, Brien WW, Becker V Jr : Interlocking nailing for the treatment of femoral fractures due to gunshot wounds. *J Bone Joint Surg Am* 1991;73: 598-606.

102. Harrison WE Jr, Chakales HH, Epright RH, DeBakey ME: Recent progress in the management of gunshot fractures of the femur. *J Trauma* 1963;3:52-62.

103. Urist MR, Quigley TB: Use of skeletal traction for mass treatment of compound fractures: A summary of experiences with 4,290 cases during World War II. *AMA Arch Surg* 1951; 63:834-844.

104. Scalea TM, Boswell SA, Scott JD, Mitchell KA, Kramer ME, Pollak AN: External fixation as a bridge to intramedullary nailing for patients with multiple injuries and with femur fractures: Damage control orthopedics. *J Trauma* 2000;48:613-623.

105. Dougherty PJ, Carter PR, Seligson D, Benson DR, Purvis JM: Orthopaedic surgery advances resulting from World War II. *J Bone Joint Surg Am* 2004;86:176-181.

106. Brav EA: A critical analysis of end results in fractures of the femoral shaft treated by intramedullary nailing. *Surgery* 1953;34:693-700.

107. Brav EA, Jeffress VH: Modified intramedullary nailing in recent gunshot fractures of the femoral shaft. *J Bone Joint Surg Am* 1953;35:141-152.

108. Nicholas RM, McCoy GF: Immediate intramedullary nailing of femoral shaft fractures due to gunshots. *Injury* 1995;26:257-259.

109. Moed BR, Watson JT: Retrograde nailing of the femoral shaft. *J Am Acad Orthop Surg* 1999;7:209-216.

110. Ostrum RF, DiCicco J, Lakatos R, Poka A: Retrograde intramedullary nailing of femoral diaphyseal fractures. *J Orthop Trauma* 1998;12: 464-468.

111. Hoegler J, Weir R, Dougherty P, Hurbanek J, Morandi M: Gunshot wounds of femoral shafts in urban populations: Is emergent retrograde intramedullary nailing appropriate? *Orthopaedic Trauma Association 22nd Annual Meeting Book*. Rosemont, IL, Orthopaedic Trauma Association, 2006, pp 315-316.

112. Newnham MS, Mitchell DI: Compartment syndrome of the thigh: A case report and review of the litera-

ture. *West Indian Med J* 2001;50: 239-242.

113. Foster RD, Albright JA: Acute compartment syndrome of the thigh: Case report. *J Trauma* 1990;30: 108-110.

114. Dehne E, Metz CW, Deffer PA, Hall RM: Nonoperative treatment of the fractured tibia by immediate weight bearing. *J Trauma* 1961;1: 514-535.

115. Witschi TH, Omer GE Jr: The treatment of open tibial shaft fractures from Vietnam War. *J Trauma* 1970;10: 105-111.

116. Brown PW, Urban JG: Early weight-bearing treatment of open fractures of the tibia: An end-result study of sixty-three cases. *J Bone Joint Surg Am* 1969; 51:59-75.

117. Leffers D, Chandler RW: Tibial fractures associated with civilian gunshot injuries. *J Trauma* 1985;25:1059-1064.

118. Ferraro SP Jr, Zinar DM: Management of gunshot fractures of the tibia. *Orthop Clin North Am* 1995;26: 181-189.

119. Brien EW, Long WT, Serocki JH: Management of gunshot wounds to the tibia. *Orthop Clin North Am* 1995;26:165-180.

The Surgical Treatment of Acetabular Fractures

Berton R. Moed, MD
Kyle F. Dickson, MD, MBA
Philip J. Kregor, MD
Mark C. Reilly, MD
Mark S. Vrahas, MD

Abstract

The goals of treating an acetabular fracture are to restore the congruity and stability of the hip joint. Some fracture types may not require surgery for a satisfactory outcome, but a displaced fracture in the weight-bearing area of the acetabulum generally should be treated with open reduction and internal fixation. The surgery is complex and demanding, and the fracture reduction must be anatomic to obtain the best result. There is no doubt, however, that an experienced surgeon can achieve an excellent result. Usually a poor result is related to residual fracture displacement or a perioperative complication. The evaluation and treatment protocols initially developed by Letournel and Judet continue to be important; in addition, the surgeon should be aware of the progress made during the past decade.

Instr Course Lect 2010;59:481-501.

An acetabular fracture routinely requires surgical intervention. The literature from the 1950s and 1960s offered conflicting recommendations for both nonsurgical and surgical treatment regimens.[1,2] It was agreed, however, that no matter the treatment, the result would be poor after a hip injury with residual joint instability or incongruity between the femoral head and the weight-bearing area of the acetabulum.[1-4] In 1964, Judet and associates[5] described the radiographic findings for acetabular fracture and outlined a plan of treatment. These authors refined several aspects of their seminal publication during the next three decades, but their basic principles did not change. These principles can be summarized as the need for the surgeon to understand the surgical anatomy of the innominate bone, define the injury through appropriate radiographic assessment, and use these findings to determine a suitable treatment plan. The results published by Letournel and Judet[6] in their definitive 1993 text still are considered optimal. Little new information appeared in the subsequent years,[7] however, during the past 5 to 10 years emerging trends have expanded the management of fractures of the acetabulum.

Imaging and Classification

Judet and associates[5] recognized that the plane of the ilium is approximately 90° to the plane of the obturator foramen and that both of these structures are oriented roughly 45° to the frontal plane. They proposed, therefore, that the AP view and two 45° oblique views of the pelvis be used to study the radiographic anatomy of the acetabulum, and they derived the

Dr. Moed or an immediate family member has received royalties from DePuy and has received research or institutional support from DePuy, Smith & Nephew, Stryker, and Synthes. Neither Dr. Dickson nor an immediate family member has received anything of value from or owns stock in a commercial company or institution related directly or indirectly to the subject of this article. Dr. Kregor or an immediate family member has received research or institutional support from the AO Foundation and Synthes. Dr. Reilly or an immediate family member serves as a board member, owner, officer, or committee member of the AO Foundation; is a member of a speakers' bureau or has made paid presentations on behalf of Synthes and Smith & Nephew; and has received research or institutional support from Biomet, EBI, the Musculoskeletal Transplant Foundation, Smith & Nephew, Stryker, Synthes, and Wright Medical Technology. Dr. Vrahas or an immediate family member has received research or institutional support from DePuy, Synthes, Zimmer, and AO and has stock or stock options held in Pioneer Medical.

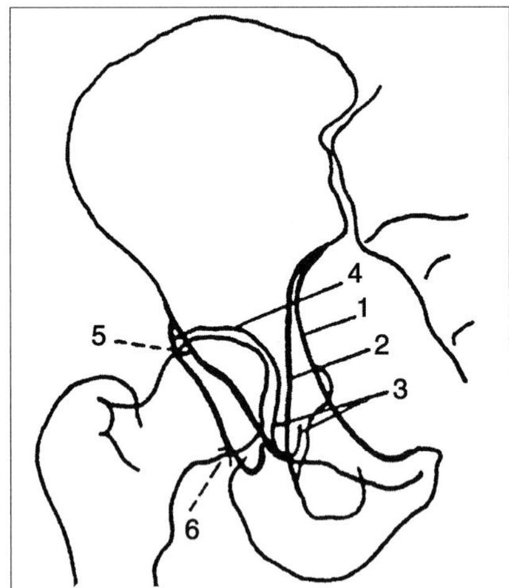

Figure 1 Schematic diagram showing the six acetabular landmarks seen on an AP radiograph: iliopectineal line (1), ilioischial line (2), U or teardrop (3), roof (4), anterior rim (5), and posterior rim (6). (Reproduced from Templeman D, Olson S, Moed BR, Duwelius P, Matta JM: Surgical treatment of acetabular fractures. *Instr Course Lect* 1999;48:481-496.)

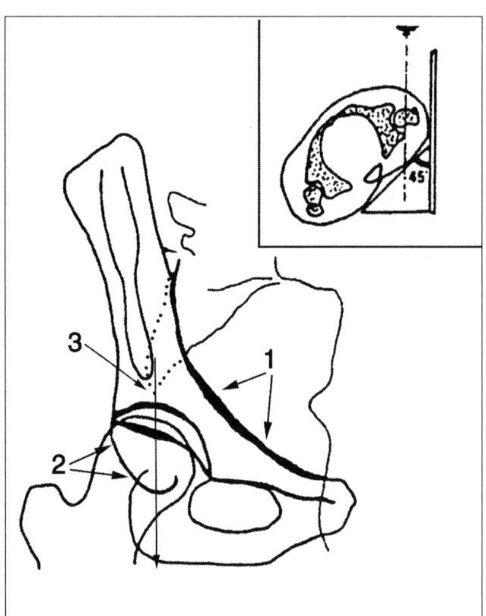

Figure 2 Schematic diagram showing the iliopectineal line (1) and posterior rim (2) as seen on an obturator oblique radiograph. The obturator ring is seen en face. The proper amount of rotation for the obturator oblique view (inset) is present when the tip of the coccyx lies just above the center of the ipsilateral femoral head (3). (Adapted from Templeman D, Olson S, Moed BR, Duwelius P, Matta JM: Surgical treatment of acetabular fractures. *Instr Course Lect* 1999;48: 481-496.)

first systematic classification of acetabular fractures based on the anatomic pattern of the fracture. This analysis was expanded to include preoperative two-dimensional CT.[6] Subsequent advances in CT technology have improved the information provided by the two-dimensional images and offer the promise of useful three-dimensional images. These newer imaging studies enhance but do not replace the use of the three plain radiographic projections. Accurate interpretation of the plain radiographs requires correlation of the normal anatomy of the innominate bone with the pertinent radiographic landmarks seen on each view of the pelvis.

AP Radiograph

The AP view shows six basic radiographic landmarks (Figure 1). The iliopectineal line is the major landmark of the anterior column.[6] The inferior three quarters of the iliopectineal line are directly correlated with the pelvic brim on the innominate bone. However, the superior one quarter of the iliopectineal line is formed by the x-ray beam tangent to the superior quadrilateral surface and the posterosuperior aspect of the greater sciatic notch. The ilioischial line, extending from the posterosuperior greater sciatic notch to the ischial tuberosity, generally is considered a radiographic landmark of the posterior column;[6] this radiographic landmark is formed by the x-ray beam tangent to the posterior portion of the quadrilateral surface of the innominate bone. The radiographic U, or teardrop, consists of a lateral and a medial limb;[6] the lateral limb represents the inferior aspect of the anterior wall of the acetabulum, and the medial limb is formed by the obturator canal and the anteroinferior portion of the quadrilateral surface. The teardrop and ilioischial lines always are superimposed on the AP view because these landmarks are from different parts of the quadrilateral plate;[6] therefore, dissociation of the teardrop from the ilioischial line suggests that the innominate bone is rotated or there has been displacement of the quadrilateral surface. The dense line of the superior articular surface of the acetabulum on the AP view is known as the roof; it results from the tangency of the x-ray beam to the subchondral bone in the superior acetabulum. The anterior and posterior rims of the acetabulum represent, respectively, the peripheral contours of the anterior and posterior walls of the acetabulum.

Obturator Oblique Radiograph

The obturator oblique radiograph is taken with the patient placed so that the injured hemipelvis is rotated 45° toward the x-ray beam (Figure 2). This view shows the obturator foramen in its largest dimension and profiles the anterior column. The iliopectineal line has the same relationship to the pelvic brim as on the AP radiograph. The posterior rim of the acetabulum is best seen in this view, as is a fracture involving the posterior wall. A comparison of the relationship between the femoral head and the posterior wall can reveal subtle posterior subluxation.

Iliac Oblique Radiograph

The iliac oblique radiograph is taken with the patient placed so that the injured hemipelvis is rotated 45° away from the x-ray beam (Figure 3). This view shows the iliac wing in its largest dimension and

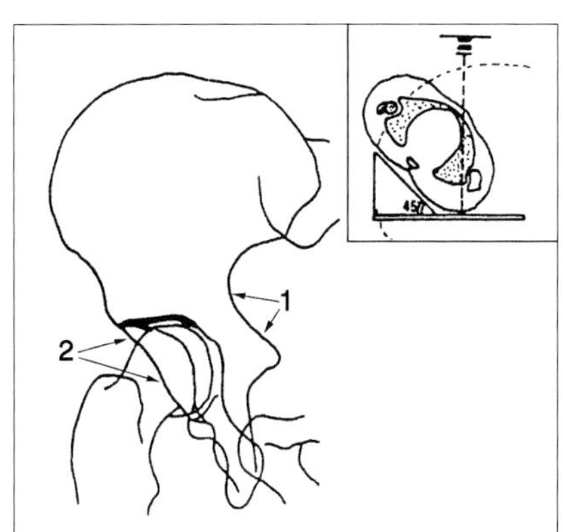

Figure 3 Schematic diagram showing the posterior border of the innominate bone (1) and anterior rim of the acetabulum (2) as seen on an iliac oblique radiograph. The iliac wing is seen en face. The anterior rim of the acetabulum can best be seen on this view. The proper amount of rotation for the iliac oblique view (inset) is present when the tip of the coccyx lies just above the center of the contralateral femoral head. (Adapted from Templeman D, Olson S, Moed BR, Duwelius P, Matta JM: Surgical treatment of acetabular fractures. *Instr Course Lect* 1999;48:481-496.)

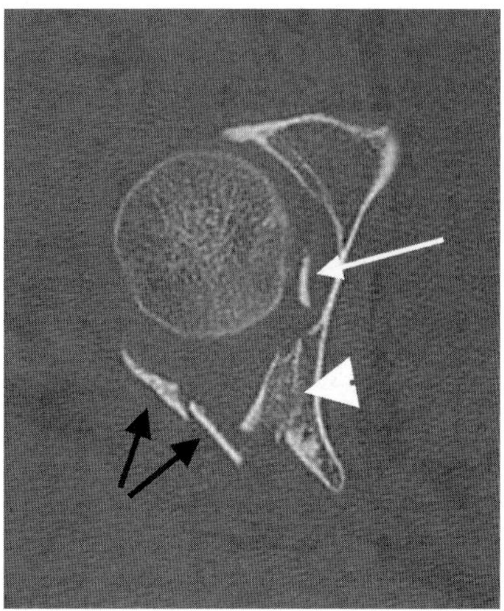

Figure 4 Axial CT scan showing a section through the acetabulum in which the posterior wall is fractured (*black arrows*) with marginal impaction (*white arrowhead*). An intra-articular loose body appears between the femoral head and acetabulum (*white arrow*). (Copyright Berton R. Moed, MD, St. Louis, MO.)

profiles the greater and lesser sciatic notches as well as the anterior rim of the acetabulum. Involvement of the posterior column often can best be seen on this view. Fractures of the anterior column traversing the iliac wing also can be detected.

Computed Tomography

CT is a helpful adjunct to the three plain radiographic projections to further define the fracture pattern and assess for associated injuries. The most reliable and useful information is obtained from contiguous CT sections of no more than 3 mm in thickness. After studying the plain radiographs, the surgeon should use CT scans to resolve specific unanswered questions about the fracture (Figure 4). Two-dimensional axial CT images are superior to plain radiographs in showing the extent and location of acetabular wall fractures, the presence of intra-articular free fragments or injury to the femoral head, the orientation of the fracture lines, the presence of any additional fracture lines (such as the vertical portion of a T-shaped fracture), the rotation of fracture fragments, and the status of the posterior pelvic ring. The orientation of one or more fracture lines can be helpful in distinguishing among fracture types.

CT also can help in identifying fractures of the quadrilateral plate that cannot be seen on the radiographs. Marginal impaction, which is defined as depression of the articular surface of the joint, is best seen using two-dimensional axial CT.[6] Two-dimensional CT was found to be superior to plain radiography for the detection of fracture step and fracture gap deformities.[8] However, displacements in the plane of CT imaging may be underappreciated or averaged out. Two-dimensional CT has proved unreliable for determining hip joint stability.[9]

Improvements in three-dimensional CT technology have made it a useful tool for further defining the fracture pattern and thereby assisting in preoperative planning. However, three-dimensional CT does not provide as much diagnostic detail as two-dimensional CT. Three-dimensional CT scans can help a surgeon who is inexperienced in interpreting plain radiographs to better understand the fracture pattern. The understanding of the fracture pattern can be further enhanced by drawing the fracture lines taken from the radiographic landmarks onto a plastic bone model or by making a line drawing of the pelvis as seen on each radiographic view. The fracture pattern can be fully appreciated only by understanding the location and orientation of each fracture line.

Fracture Classification

The AO[10] and Orthopaedic Trauma Association[11] comprehensive fracture classification systems use a basic alphanumeric coding of the acetabular fracture classification developed by Judet and Letournel.[5,6] and offer no clinical advantage. Therefore, the so-called Letournel acetabular fracture classification is preferred internationally by most surgeons treating these complex injuries. The classification is based on the anatomy of the fracture pattern and has 10 categories, including 5 elementary and 5 associated patterns (Figure 5). The five elementary fracture patterns are the anterior wall, anterior column, posterior wall, posterior column, and transverse. Each of the associated patterns is either a combination of elementary patterns or an elementary pattern with an additional fracture component. The five associated fracture patterns are the

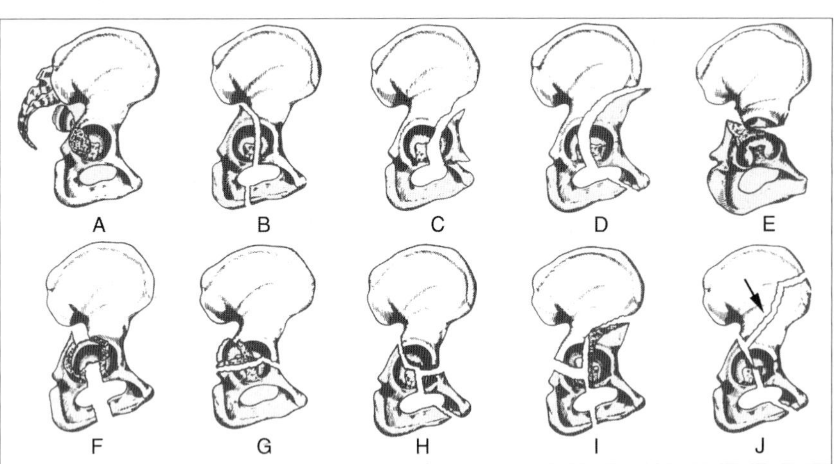

Figure 5 Schematic diagram showing the classification of acetabular fractures. **A,** Posterior wall fracture. **B,** Posterior column fracture. **C,** Anterior wall fracture. **D,** Anterior column fracture. **E,** Transverse fracture. **F,** Associated posterior column and posterior wall fracture. **G,** Associated transverse and posterior wall fracture. **H,** Associated T-shaped fracture. **I,** Associated anterior column and posterior hemitransverse fracture. **J,** Associated both-column fracture, with the supra-acetabular fracture line (*arrow*). (Adapted from Fitzgerald RH Jr, ed: Trauma: Pelvis and acetabulum, in *Orthopaedic Knowledge Update 2*. Park Ridge, IL, American Academy of Orthopaedic Surgeons, 1987, p 341-356.)

posterior column and posterior wall, anterior column (or wall) and posterior hemitransverse, transverse and posterior wall, T-shaped, and both-column. A variant pattern occasionally is seen, but usually it can easily be integrated into the system.

The Letournel system both describes the fracture and serves as a guide for subsequent surgical treatment. The fracture types are straightforward, with high rates of interobserver and intraobserver reliability.[12] However, those inexperienced with the system may be confused by the differentiation of the both-column type from the types with two-column fracture involvement (transverse, anterior column [or wall] and posterior hemitransverse, transverse and posterior wall, T-shaped). The both-column fracture is unique because it has both a displaced supra-acetabular fracture and a fracture line separating the anterior and posterior column components; no portion of the acetabular articular surface remains intact to the innominate bone (Figure 5, *J*).

Fracture Evaluation

Most fractures can be classified by using the information gleaned from high-quality plain radiographs. An organized approach must be used for examining the AP and oblique radiographs and the CT scan, so that each of the fracture types can be sequentially ruled in or ruled out. One useful method begins with a careful sequential analysis of each line on the AP radiograph (Figure 1). If the iliopectineal line is disrupted, the possible fracture types include the anterior wall, anterior column, transverse, transverse and posterior wall, T-shaped, anterior column and posterior hemitransverse, and both-column. If the ilioischial line is disrupted, the possible fracture types include the posterior column, transverse, transverse and posterior wall, T-shaped, anterior column and posterior hemitransverse, and both-column. If both lines are disrupted, the possible types are limited to the transverse, transverse and posterior wall, T-shaped, anterior column and posterior hemitransverse, and both-column. If the line along the posterior rim is disrupted, the possibility of a posterior wall fracture must be considered. Displacement of the ilioischial line from its normal relationship to the teardrop usually indicates that the two columns are separated from each other.

The obturator oblique radiograph is next examined to refine the diagnosis. A suspected posterior wall component will become obvious, as will a disruption involving the anterior wall or column. A fractured obturator ring suggests that the two columns are separated from each other. The presence of a supra-acetabular fracture line (the spur sign) is pathognomonic for a both-column fracture (Figure 6). The iliac oblique radiograph is examined to further define the injury to the posterior column and the possible presence and location of a fracture involving the iliac wing (anterior column, anterior column and posterior hemitransverse, or both-column).

Finally, the CT scan is studied for additional information (Figure 4). After this analysis, the plain radiographs are revisited to determine the fracture subtype, such as the level of a transverse fracture or the path of the stem of a T-shaped fracture. If the diagnosis still is unclear, three-dimensional CT can be helpful. However, three-dimensional CT has limitations (Figure 6, *B* and *C*).

Indications for Nonsurgical and Surgical Treatment

Nonsurgical Treatment

A stable, concentrically reduced acetabular fracture that does not in-

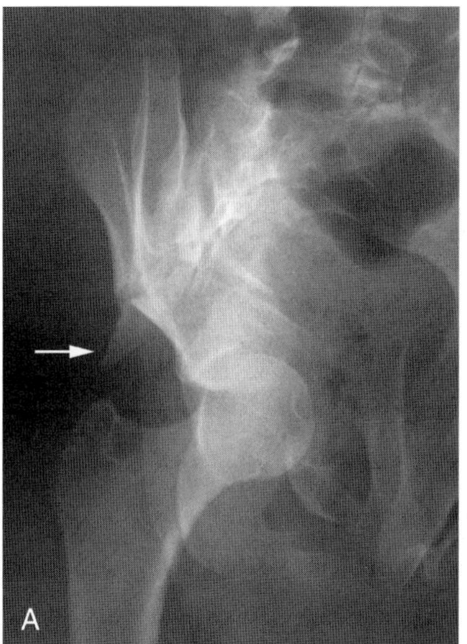

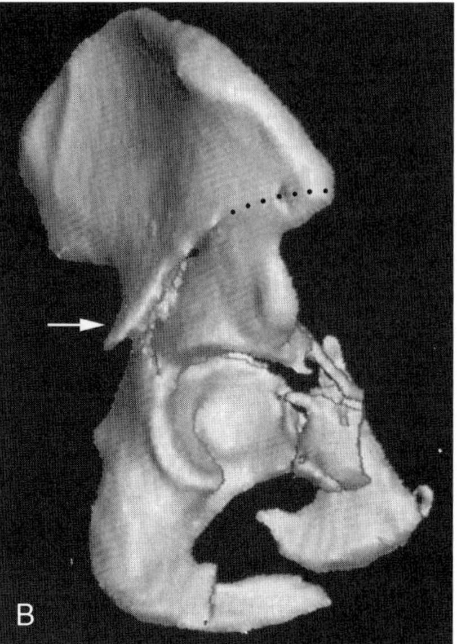

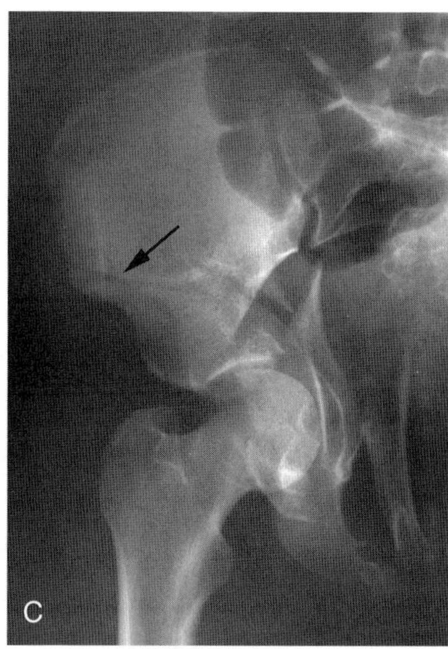

Figure 6 **A,** Obturator oblique radiograph showing a both-column fracture with the spur sign (arrow). **B,** Three-dimensional CT scan showing a supra-acetabular fracture (arrow), which creates the spur sign. The continuation of the anterior column fracture line (dotted line) cannot be seen on three-dimensional CT but was clearly visible (arrow) on a plain radiograph **(C)** and two-dimensional CT. (Copyright Berton R. Moed, MD, St. Louis, MO.)

volve the superior acetabular dome generally can be treated nonsurgically.[2,13-16] This group of fractures includes nondisplaced and minimally displaced fractures, fractures in which the intact part of the acetabulum is large enough to maintain stability and congruity, and both-column fractures in which the displaced articular fragments remain congruent with the femoral head without the application of skeletal traction (so-called secondary congruity[6]). Nonsurgical treatment also may be selected for a patient with severe osteoporosis or a severe comorbidity that precludes surgical intervention. There are relatively few such patients, most of whom are elderly.

Matta and associates[14] developed roof arc measurements to be used in deciding whether an acetabular fracture violates the weight-bearing dome. This measurement has been used to determine whether the remaining intact acetabulum is sufficient to maintain a stable and congruent relationship with the femoral head. Nonsurgical or surgical treatment can then be selected. The acetabular roof arc is measured on all three radiographic views with the leg out of traction. The AP view is used to measure the medial roof arc; the obturator oblique view, to measure the anterior roof arc; and the iliac oblique view, to measure the posterior roof arc. The measurements are obtained by drawing a vertical line through the center of the femoral head and a second line from the center of the femoral head to the fracture location at the articular surface (Figure 7, *A* through *C*). Initially, it was believed that roof arc values of greater than 45° on all three views indicated that the hip would remain stable and congruent.[17] However, these values have been revised.[18] Fractures with a medial roof arc angle greater than 45°, an anterior roof arc angle greater than 25°, and a posterior roof arc angle greater than 70° are currently believed to have sufficient intact acetabulum for nonsurgical treatment[18] (Figure 7, *D*). Therefore, displaced low anterior column, low transverse, and low T-shaped acetabular fractures are amenable to nonsurgical treatment, if, as expected, the fracture position is stable and the joint remains congruent.[2,6,15,19] These measurements are not applicable to both-column fractures or fractures involving the posterior wall.

Although it is generally recommended that all nondisplaced and minimally displaced acetabular fractures be considered for nonsurgical management, some authors believe that patients with such a fracture should be treated with percutaneous fracture fixation.[20-22] Their concern centers on the questionable stability of these fractures and the possibility that some of them later will become displaced. Early percutaneous fixation of these fractures with oc-

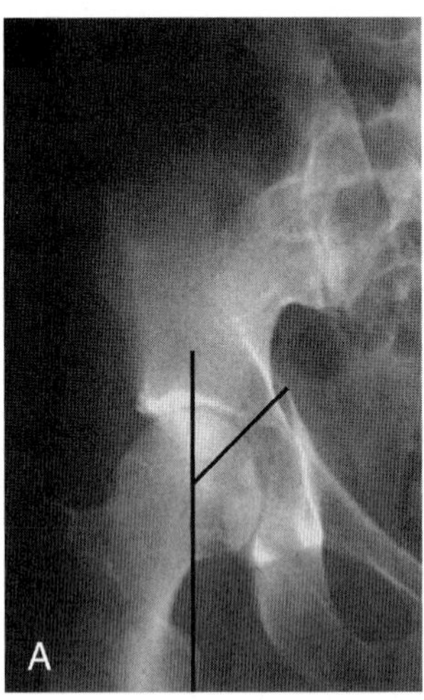

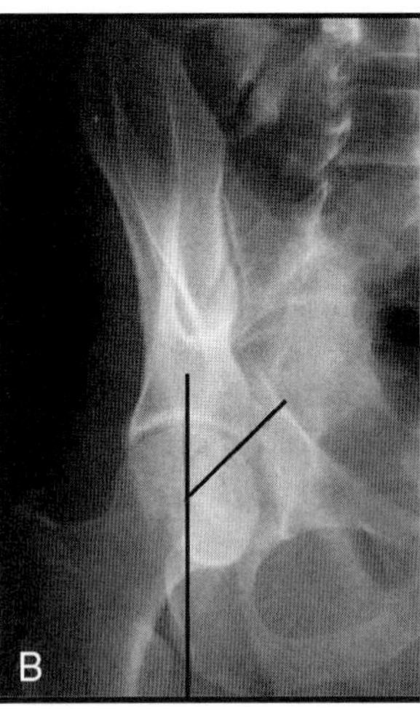

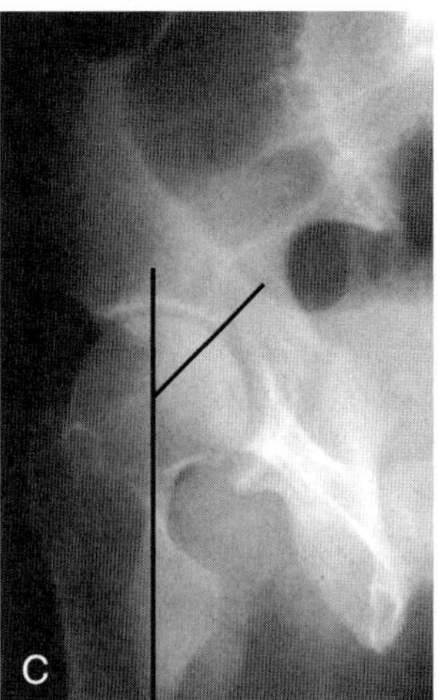

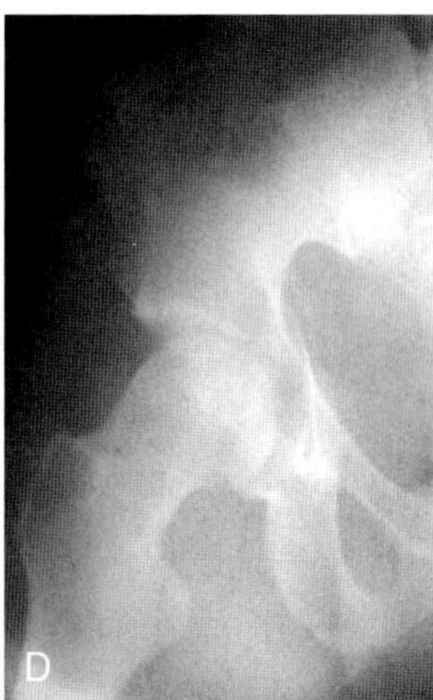

Figure 7 AP **(A)**, obturator oblique **(B)**, and iliac oblique **(C)** radiographs of the hip of a 35-year-old man treated approximately 15 years ago for a transverse fracture of the acetabulum. The lines in all views show roof arc measurements of approximately 50°, according to the initial recommendations of Matta and Merritt,[17] the hip joint is considered stable. **D,** AP radiograph taken 3 weeks later, showing gross medial subluxation of the hip, as could be predicted by using the criteria of Vrahas and associates.[18] (Copyright Berton R. Moed, MD, St. Louis, MO.)

cult instability may avoid a later, more extensive open procedure or prevent early traumatic arthritis (if the patient is not treated for the later displacement). However, fewer than 7% of nondisplaced or minimally displaced fractures have the potential to become significantly displaced without traction.[23] To avoid unnecessary surgical treatment of a large number of fractures in the interest of preventing displacement in a few, it is worthwhile to attempt to identify the fractures at risk for displacement. Dynamic fluoroscopic stress examination, done with the patient under general anesthesia, has been proposed for identifying these fractures at risk for displacement.[23] However, the exact technique for this examination is ill defined for fractures other than an isolated posterior wall fracture. Another method is close observation of every patient with a fracture suitable for nonsurgical treatment. Weekly radiographic follow-up is accompanied by readiness to shift immediately to percutaneous or open surgical treatment if joint instability or incongruity is detected.[13]

In summary, the prerequisites for nonsurgical treatment of an acetabular fracture include measurements indicating an intact roof arc and congruity of the femoral head to the intact acetabulum; both are evaluated on AP and oblique (also known as Judet) radiographs taken without traction applied to the leg. The patient's age, preinjury activity level, functional demands, and medical comorbidities also must be considered in deciding whether the patient is better served by surgical or nonsurgical treatment. Nonsurgical treatment may be appropriate for an elderly or infirm patient, particularly if the fracture displacement is minimal, with a plan for arthroplasty if symptomatic arthritis develops.[24-26]

Surgical Treatment

Surgical treatment is indicated for all acetabular fractures that result in hip joint instability or incongruity, regardless of how the fracture is classified or whether it is displaced or has occult instability. Fracture displacement of 2 mm or more in the weight-bearing dome results in joint incongruity, and it is one of the main indications for open reduction and internal fixation.[17,27] Posterior and anterior wall fractures with instability of the hip joint require surgical fixation. A fragment of bone or soft tissue incarcerated within the hip joint also can cause joint incongruity. Open reduction and removal of the loose body or obstructing tissue are indicated to prevent the early onset of traumatic arthritis. Recurrent dislocation, with disastrous consequences for the hip joint, is inevitable if stability is not restored.[28] Two-dimensional CT is unreliable for determining hip joint stability,[9] and therefore it should be assumed that all posterior wall fractures are unstable unless dynamic stress examination proves otherwise.[9] There is no need for dynamic stress examination of an obviously unstable hip. A both-column fracture may be significantly displaced but not require surgical treatment; however, surgi-

Table 1
Acetabular Fracture Patterns and Preferred Surgical Approaches

	Preferred Surgical Approach					
Fracture Pattern	**Kocher-Langenbeck**	**Ilioinguinal**	**Iliofemoral**	**Extended Iliofemoral**	**Modified Stoppa**	**Triradiate**
Posterior column	X					
Anterior column		X	X		X	
Posterior wall	X					
Anterior wall		X			X	
Transverse	X	X		X	X	X
T-shaped	X	X		X	X	X
Anterior column and posterior hemitransverse		X		X		X
Transverse and posterior wall	X			X		X
Posterior column and posterior wall	X					
Both-column		X		X		X

cal treatment is required if a loss of parallelism between the femoral head and acetabular articular surface is noted on any of the three radiographic views, indicating an incongruous hip joint.

Surgical Approaches

The main surgical approaches to the acetabulum, as described by Letournel and Judet,[6] are the Kocher-Langenbeck, ilioinguinal, iliofemoral, and extended iliofemoral approaches. The surgical approach usually is selected with the expectation that it will allow the entire fracture reduction and fixation[6,27,29] (Table 1). The Kocher-Langenbeck approach provides direct access only to the posterior column of the acetabulum, and the ilioinguinal and iliofemoral approaches provide direct access only to the anterior column. These three approaches rely on indirect manipulation for reduction of any fracture lines that traverse the opposite column. The extended iliofemoral approach allows almost complete direct access to all aspects of the acetabulum. This approach most often is used for an associated fracture that is surgically treated more than 21 days after injury or for a transverse, T-shaped or both-column fracture with a complicating feature that is not amenable to treatment by one of the more limited approaches.

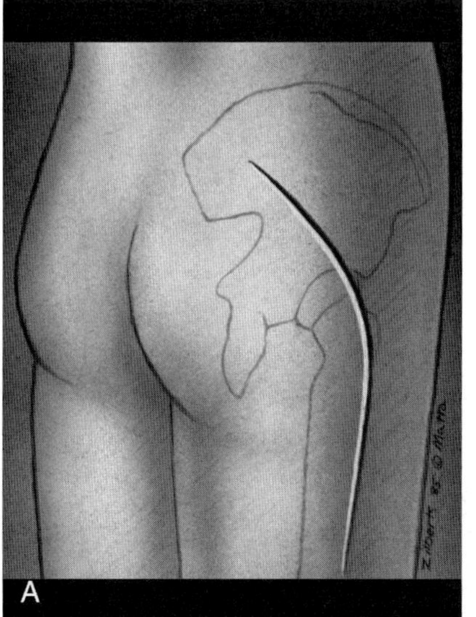

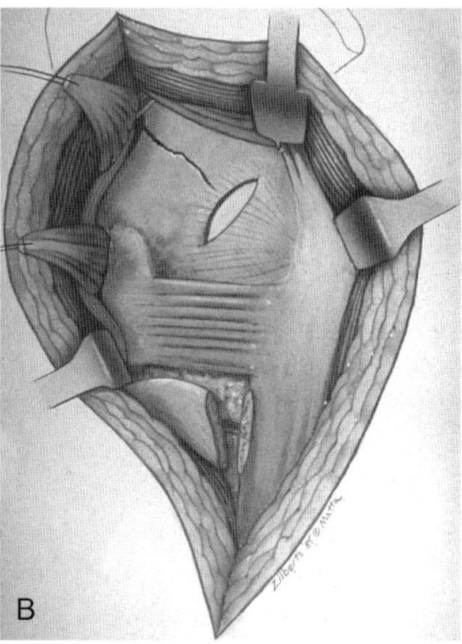

Figure 8 Schematic diagrams showing the Kocher-Langenbeck approach. **A,** Surgical incision. **B,** Final exposure of the retroacetabular surface. (Reproduced from Matta JM, Letournel E, Browner BD: Surgical management of acetabular fractures. *Instr Course Lect* 1986;35:382-397.)

Kocher-Langenbeck Approach

The Kocher-Langenbeck approach (Figure 8) is ideal for a posterior wall fracture or a posterior column fracture with or without an associated posterior wall fracture. A transverse or T-shaped fracture also is amena-

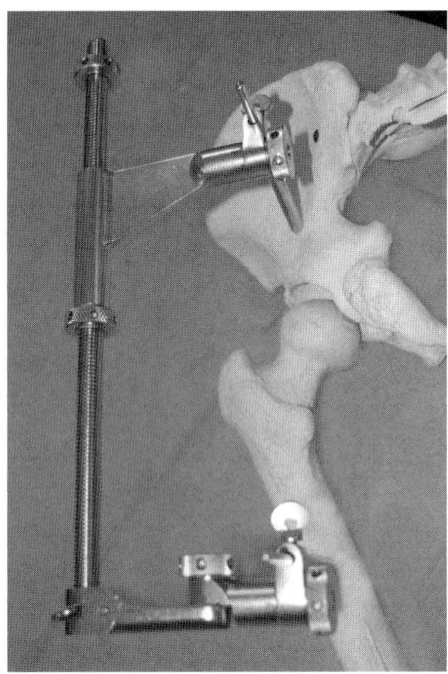

Figure 9 The application of a universal distractor, shown on a plastic bone model. (Copyright Berton R. Moed, MD, St. Louis, MO, and Mark S. Vrahas, MD, Boston, MA.)

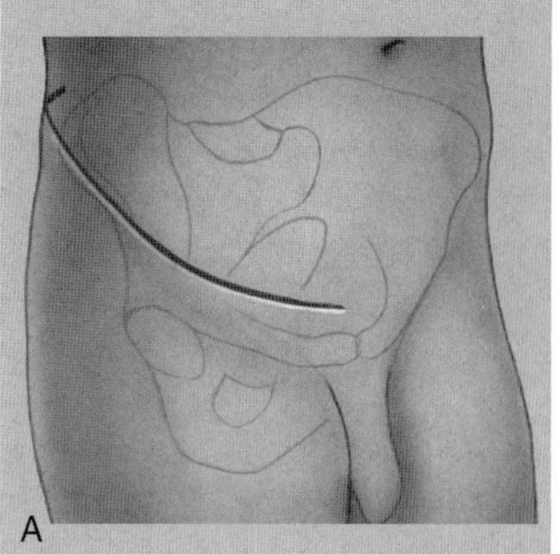

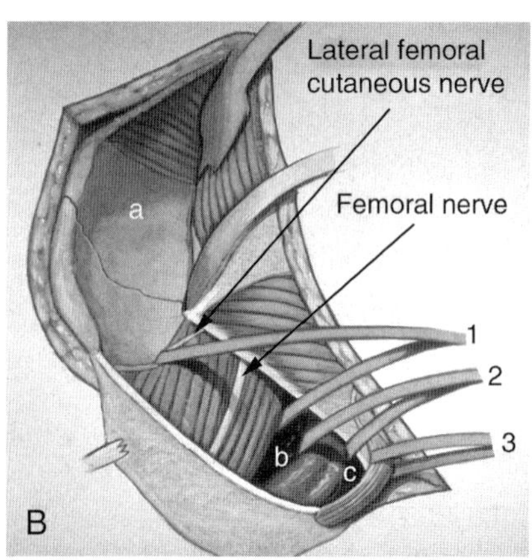

Figure 10 Schematic diagrams showing the ilioinguinal approach. **A,** Surgical incision. (Reproduced from Matta JM, Letournel E, Browner BD: Surgical management of acetabular fractures. *Instr Course Lect* 1986;35:382-397.) **B,** Final exposure, with isolation of the iliopsoas femoral and lateral femoral cutaneous nerves (1), external iliac vessels (2), and the spermatic cord in a male patient or round ligament in a female patient (3). Through the windows thus created, the surgeon gains access to the lateral (a), middle (b), and medial (c) innominate bone. (Adapted from Reilly MC, Olson SA: Treatment considerations for surgical and nonsurgical management of acetabular fractures, in Olson SA, Reilly MC, eds: *Acetabular and Pelvic Fractures*. Rosemont, IL, American Academy of Orthopaedic Surgeons, 2006, pp 43-66.)

ble to this surgical approach within 15 days of injury. In a T-shaped fracture, the major displacement should be posterior, with only minor anterior displacement at the pelvic brim. The patient can be in the lateral or prone position. Surgeons often choose to operate on posterior wall fractures with the patient lateral, allowing easier patient positioning, better visualization for the assistants, and a more familiar orientation. However, the patient should be positioned prone if the fracture involves the posterior column; in the lateral position, the weight of the leg displaces the femoral head medially and makes reduction of the column more difficult. The Kocher-Langenbeck approach is best used with a specialized fracture traction table. Such a table may not be available, however, and some means must be used to distract the femoral head from the acetabulum for fracture reduction. A universal distractor is a useful alternative to a specialized table (Figure 9).

Ilioinguinal Approach

The ilioinguinal approach (Figure 10) is indicated for anterior wall or anterior column fractures as well as most anterior column and posterior hemitransverse fractures. Transverse fractures in which the displacement is primarily anterior, with minimal posterior displacement, and both-column fractures having a noncomminuted posterior column fragment also can be treated using the ilioinguinal approach. Fractures of these complex types must have no displacement in the acetabular roof, and they must be treated within 15 days of injury. Both-column fractures that extend into the sacroiliac joint and have a fracture-dislocation component are not amenable to reduction through the ilioinguinal approach.

The ilioinguinal approach allows access to the internal aspect of the innominate bone from the sacroiliac joint to the symphysis pubis. The internal iliac fossa, pelvic brim, superior pubic ramus, and a portion of the quadrilateral surface can be directly visualized. Indirect access to the inferior portion of the quadrilateral surface is obtained using a palpating finger or special instruments. Limited access to the external aspect of the iliac wing is possible if the abductor origin is released. It is best to avoid dissection on the outer aspect of the pelvis. If this dissection is necessary, the sartorius origin always should be left intact to prevent overzealous exposure. Although the ilioinguinal approach offers extensive exposure, it is not convenient. The surgeon must work through small windows between major nerves and vessels to view the fracture (Figure 10, *B*). Many of the necessary reduction and fixation techniques are not intuitive when

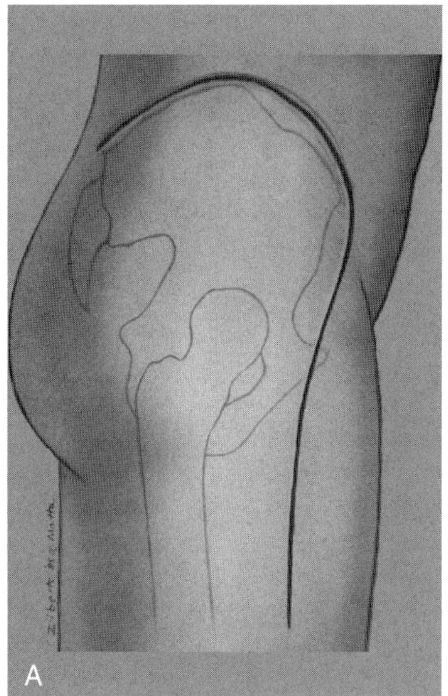

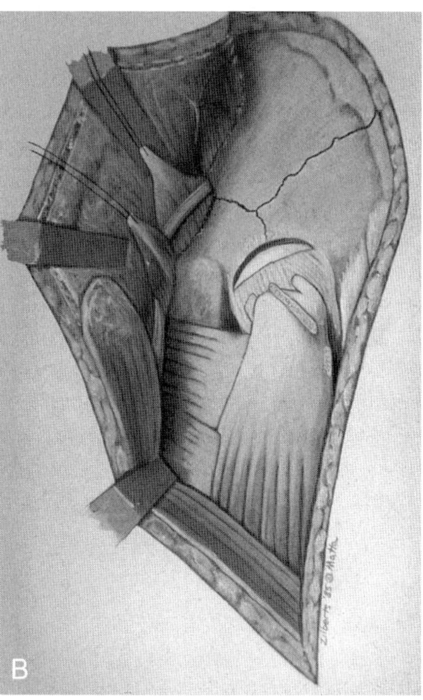

Figure 11 Schematic diagrams showing the extended iliofemoral approach. **A,** Surgical incision. **B,** Final exposure of the external aspect of the innominate bone. (Reproduced from Matta JM, Letournel E, Browner BD: Surgical management of acetabular fractures. *Instr Course Lect* 1986;35:382-397.)

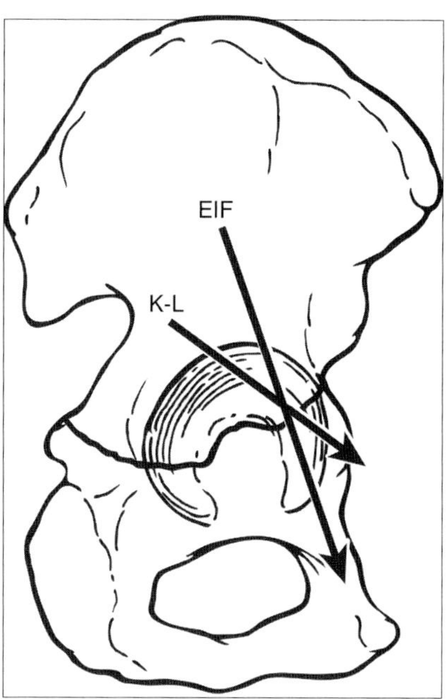

Figure 12 Schematic diagram showing the angles for insertion of an anterior column lag screw using the Kocher-Langenbeck (K-L) and extended iliofemoral (EIF) approaches. The angle shown for the extended iliofemoral approach also can be obtained with percutaneous techniques. (Copyright Berton R. Moed, MD, St. Louis, MO.)

the ilioinguinal approach is used; the work of an experienced pelvic surgeon should be closely observed before fracture fixation is attempted through this approach.

Iliofemoral Approach

The iliofemoral approach exposes the iliac fossa but does not allow access medial to the iliopectineal eminence. This approach has limited application. Although the ilioinguinal approach usually is preferable, the iliofemoral approach may be sufficient for a high anterior column fracture in which the main displacement is cephalad to the hip joint.

Extended Iliofemoral Approach

The extended iliofemoral approach (Figure 11) is used for selected complex acetabular fracture types and for surgery delayed more than 2 to 3 weeks following injury. These include transverse plus posterior wall fractures if the surgeon expects unusual difficulties with reduction.[6,27] Examples include a transtectal transverse component with an extended posterior wall fracture (those involving the posterior border of the bone), a T-shaped and posterior wall fracture, and fractures associated with dislocation of the symphysis pubis or fracture of the contralateral pubis ramus.[6,27] A suitable T-shaped fracture has a transtectal transverse component, a wide separation along the vertical stem of the T, or an association with dislocation of the symphysis pubis or fracture of the contralateral pubic ramus.[6,27] A suitable both-column fracture has a complex fracture of the posterior column, a displaced fracture line crossing the sacroiliac joint, or a wide separation of the anterior and posterior columns at the rim of the acetabulum.[27]

The extended iliofemoral approach provides maximal simultaneous access to both columns of the acetabulum. The entire lateral aspect of the iliac wing, the anterior column to the level of the iliopectineal eminence, the retroacetabular surface, and the interior of the hip joint are accessible. Unlike the Kocher-Langenbeck approach, the extended iliofemoral approach allows for a long screw to be placed down the anterior column under direct visualization (Figure 12). It is possible to expose the entire internal iliac fossa, however, this maneuver risks devascularizing the iliac wing.

Other Approaches

Modified Stoppa Intrapelvic Approach

The modified Stoppa intrapelvic approach has been advocated for treating anterior wall, anterior column, transverse, T-shaped, anterior column (or wall) and posterior hemitransverse, and both-column fractures.[30] Although this approach has not gained wide acceptance, it is especially useful for fractures that require buttress plating of the quadrilateral plate.[31] The pure modified Stoppa approach exposes only the true pelvis. Therefore, a second approach often is necessary for fracture reduction or hardware insertion. Combining these two approaches functions as the equivalent of using the lateral and medial windows of the ilioinguinal approach. As with the ilioinguinal approach, indirect reduction is required for posterior fracture lines. The advantage of the modified Stoppa approach over the ilioinguinal approach is that dissection of the iliac vessels is not required. However, this lack of access to the middle window of the ilioinguinal approach also is a disadvantage of the modified Stoppa approach.

Triradiate Approach

The triradiate approach described by Mears and Rubash[32] is used for many of the same fractures as the extended iliofemoral approach. However, the exposure is more limited, and the iliac crest cannot be completely seen. The skin incision is Y shaped, with a posterior limb nearly identical to that of the Kocher-Langenbeck incision. The anterior limb of the incision extends from the greater trochanter to the anterosuperior iliac spine. The skin incision is deepened through the fascia. The posterior portion of the triradiate approach is the same as that of the Kocher-Langenbeck approach. The triradiate approach is useful for transverse, transverse and posterior wall, and T-shaped fractures, especially for late fractures and those with substantial displacement of both the anterior and posterior columns. It is not ideal for fractures that exit high in the anterior column because only the anterior portion of the iliac crest is exposed.

The standard triradiate approach includes a trochanteric osteotomy, which provides more exposure than usually is necessary. Completing the anterior and posterior limbs of the approach without removing the trochanter allows visualization of the anterior and posterior columns and avoids extensive dissection of the abductors. The triradiate approach is similar to simultaneous anterior and posterior approaches, except that it allows both anterior and posterior column fractures to be treated from one side of the operating table.

Trochanteric Flip Osteotomy

The trochanteric flip osteotomy is used with the Kocher-Langenbeck approach to obtain greater anterosuperior exposure and facilitate intraoperative dislocation of the femoral head for inspection of the joint.[33,34] Although the patient is usually in the lateral position for this approach, the patient also can be placed in the prone position.[33] Indications for the use of this approach potentially include combined femoral head/posterior wall acetabular fractures, posterior wall fractures with anterosuperior extension, posterior wall and column fracture patterns, as well as certain transverse or T-shaped fractures.[34]

Simultaneous Anterior and Posterior Approaches

Many surgeons prefer to use an anterior (ilioinguinal or iliofemoral) and posterior (Kocher-Langenbeck) approach simultaneously as an alternative to the more extensive triradiate or extended iliofemoral approach or as the primary approach for transverse, T-shaped, and some both-column fractures. Although this combined approach is not generally considered the best method, excellent results have been obtained when two experienced surgical teams work together.[35]

Open Reduction and Internal Fixation of Specific Types of Fractures Grouped According to Common Features

The protocols developed by Letournel and Judet[6] call for strict adherence to patient positioning and the use of a fracture table. Fracture reduction is the most difficult and critical element of the surgical procedure. Before surgical intervention, the surgeon must use plain radiographs and two-dimensional CT to ascertain the pattern of displacement and fracture fragment malrotation. Drawing the fracture on paper or a plastic pelvic bone model is extremely helpful to establish a careful preoperative plan and determine the approximate clamp position required to achieve anatomic joint reduction. Intraoperative traction, which reduces the deforming force of the femoral head, permits a precise reduction of the fracture with the use of special clamps. Traction is best achieved by using a specialized fracture table, although alternative methods can be used (Figure 9). Obtaining an anatomic reduction is critical to consistently achieving a good clinical result.[27]

The fracture usually is fixed with 3.5-mm hardware; however, smaller screw sizes often are needed for fixation of a posterior wall or osteochondral fracture fragment.[36-38]

The standard fracture fixation constructs (Figure 13) often must be modified to accommodate the individual fracture morphology, as determined during preoperative planning. However, posterior wall fracture fixation always should include a buttress plate[37,38] (Figure 13, *A*). After fracture reduction and fixation are completed, the quality of the reduction and the hardware position should be assessed using intraoperative fluoroscopy through a 180° arc. Both the absence of a subchondral fracture gap or step-off and the congruity of the femoral head with the acetabular roof should be seen on the fluoroscopic images. Additional axial and tangential views can be used to ensure that all screws are extra-articular[39] (Figure 14). The acetabulum is a concave joint; therefore, only one projection showing extra-articular position of the entire screw is required. If this one projection cannot be found for a particular screw, then the screw should be removed.[39]

The three standard radiographs should be obtained postoperatively. Any concern generated from the review of these radiographs should be further evaluated with two-dimensional CT. Plain radiographs cannot adequately assess the posterior wall,[6,40] and therefore postoperative two-dimensional CT is required for fractures involving the posterior wall.

Posterior Wall, Posterior Column, and Posterior Column and Posterior Wall Fractures

Posterior Wall Fracture

Although a posterior wall fracture often is considered simple (Figure 5, *A*), an uncomplicated one-fragment posterior wall fracture rarely occurs.[6,37,40] Complicating factors in a posterior wall fracture include fragmentation of the wall, marginal impaction, the presence of intra-articular fragments, and femoral head damage.[27,37,40] Moed and associates[40] found that the quality of the reduction must be as anatomic as possible because imperfections are correlated with a poorer clinical outcome. The common mistakes in surgical treatment of a posterior wall fracture include an inadequate understanding of the complexity of the fracture, an inability to retrieve intra-articular fragments, difficulty in reducing and fixing small osteochondral fragments or marginal impaction, and poor reduction or fixation of the posterior wall fragment.

Appropriate fixation of a posterior wall fracture requires a well-executed Kocher-Langenbeck approach. The surgeon must minimize surgical devitalization of the abductors, preserve the vascular supply of the femoral head, maintain the capsular attachments to the posterior wall, and carefully débride the edges of the fracture and cancellous recipient bed of the posterior wall. Distraction of the hip joint is helpful for completely visualizing and débriding the hip joint. A specially designed fracture table that provides traction through a distal femoral pin allows flexion of the hip and approximately 1.5 cm of hip joint distraction, which enables removal of the torn ligamentum teres and any other small intra-articular fragments. Alternatively, a femoral distractor can be used across the hip joint, with one Schanz pin placed in the sciatic buttress region (1.5 cm lateral and 1.5 to 2 cm caudal to the sciatic notch) and another pin placed in the proximal femur (Figure 9).

After adequate débridement of the hip joint, the traction is released to allow the femoral head to assume its normal position against the intact articular surface of the acetabulum. The femoral head then can be used as a template for reducing the posterior wall. Often, there are multiple free osteochondral fragments that need to be reduced into position and held by mini-fragment screws.[36,37] Any marginal impaction should be reduced into position, possibly held with screws, and supported by bone graft placed into the void behind the elevated fragment. The key to the reduction is to elevate the marginal impaction as one fragment; this usually is best accomplished using a Freer elevator beneath the impacted fragment. A minifragment screw can be used to secure a fragment of adequate size that is unstable after being impacted into place.[36] After the osteochondral fragments and marginal impaction have been reduced into position, the posterior wall is reduced and fixed (Figure 13, *A*). The common errors in posterior wall fixation include overcontouring the plate so it does not adequately buttress the wall; failing to bring the plate sufficiently peripheral; and bringing the plate high above the greater sciatic notch, thereby placing the superior gluteal nerve at risk.

Posterior Column Fracture

The Kocher-Langenbeck approach is used for a posterior column fracture (Figure 5, *B*). The congruity of the hip joint is highly dependent on appropriate reduction of the posterior column, and obtaining a perfect reduction may be difficult. Therefore, placing the patient prone is preferred. The most common deformity is slight gapping superiorly and cephalad translation of the posterior column. Rotational mismatch of the posterior column is common and can best be assessed by palpation through the greater sciatic notch. Rotational control of the posterior

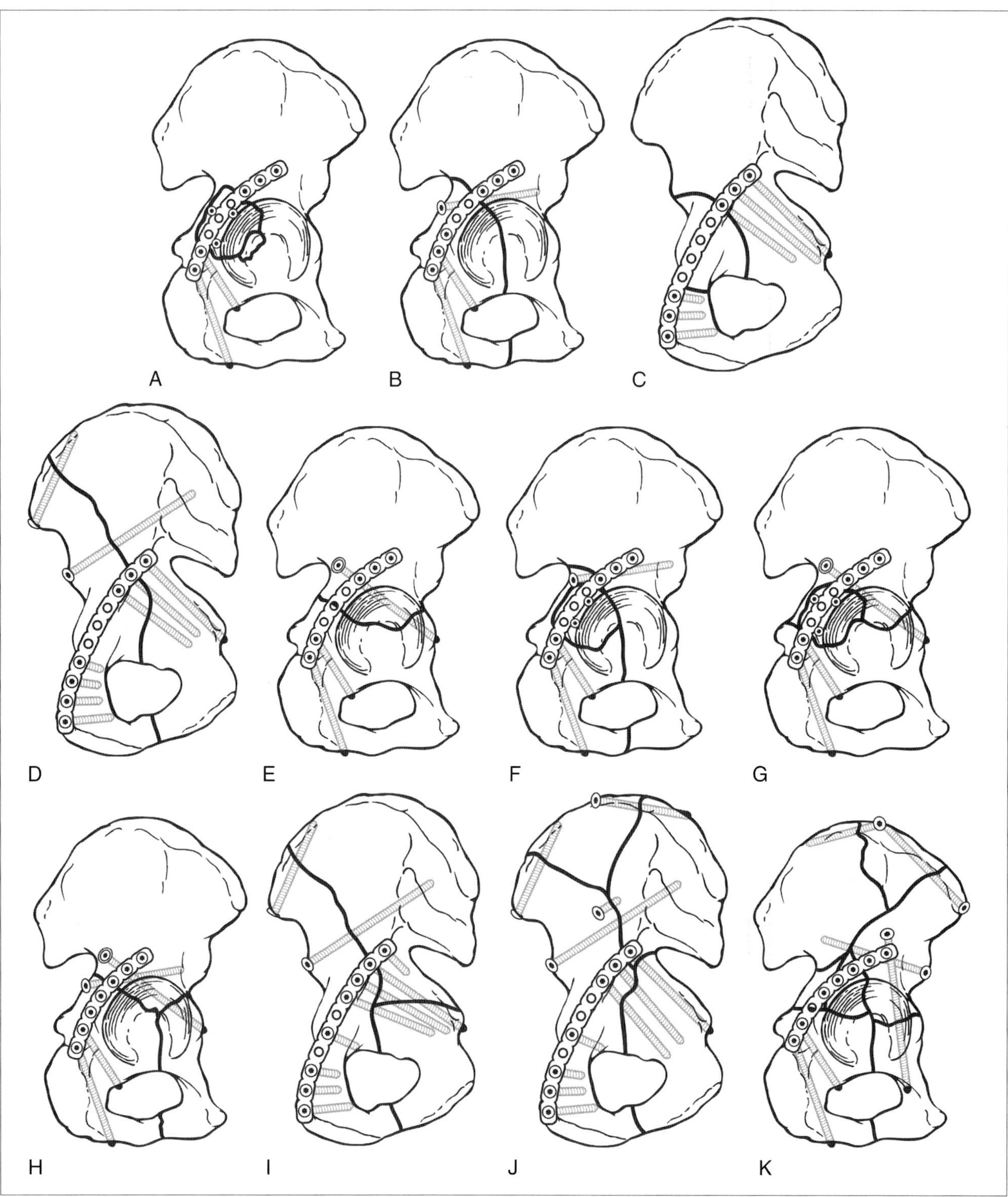

Figure 13 Schematic diagrams showing the 10 acetabular fracture types, with typical fixation constructs. (*A* through *E* show elementary types; *F* through *K* show associated types.) **A,** Multifragmented posterior wall fracture with intra-articular comminution. **B,** Posterior column fracture. **C,** Anterior wall fracture. **D,** High anterior column fracture. **E,** Juxtatectal transverse fracture. **F,** Posterior column and posterior wall fracture. **G,** Transverse and posterior wall fracture. **H,** T-shaped fracture. **I,** Anterior column and posterior hemitransverse fracture. **J,** Both-column fracture; the ilioinguinal approach was used. **K,** Both-column fracture with posterior column comminution; the extended iliofemoral approach was used. (Copyright Berton R. Moed, MD, St. Louis, MO.)

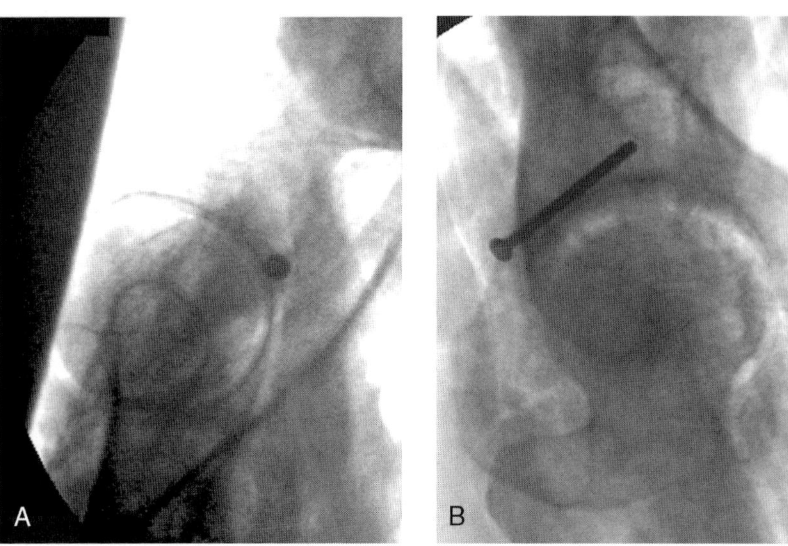

Figure 14 Axial **(A)** and tangential **(B)** fluoroscopic views of a cadaver specimen showing an extra-articular screw position. (Copyright Berton R. Moed, MD, St. Louis, MO.)

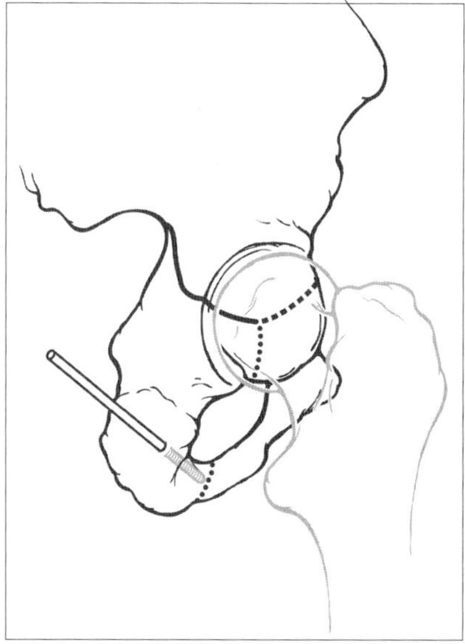

Figure 15 Schematic diagram of a hemipelvis with a Schanz screw in the ischium. A Schanz screw is used to control the rotational and translational displacement of the posterior column that occurs in several types of fractures. (Copyright Berton R. Moed, MD, St. Louis, MO.)

column can be obtained with a 6.0-mm Schanz screw driven into the ischium (Figure 15). The posterior column then is reduced through the greater sciatic notch using an angled-jaw bone forceps, a pointed reduction clamp, or a clamp applied to two temporary screws located on either side of the fracture. It may be helpful to use a ball spike pusher to push the posterior column from posterior to anterior. It is important that the surgeon not simply look at the posterior column reduction on the posterior aspect but also assess the rotation of the posterior column by palpation through the greater sciatic notch. After the posterior column is reduced, a lag screw from posterior to anterior is placed, keeping in mind the frontal plane nature of the fracture. A posterior column neutralization plate is then placed (Figure 13, *B*).

Posterior Column and Posterior Wall Fracture

The Kocher-Langenbeck approach is preferred for an associated posterior column and posterior wall fracture (Figure 5, *F*), with the patient in the prone position. The posterior column is reduced first. This reduction is facilitated by retracting the posterior wall fragment so that the joint can be inspected. After lag screw fixation of the posterior column fracture, the posterior wall is reduced and fixed. The fracture fixation construct is completed by the application of a buttress plate (Figure 13, *F*).

Anterior Wall and Anterior Column Fractures

Anterior Wall Fracture

The surgical treatment of an anterior wall fracture (Figure 5, *C*) usually requires all or part of the ilioinguinal surgical approach, with the patient in the supine position. A Pfannenstiel extension of the medial aspect of the ilioinguinal incision can be used to expose the entire quadrilateral surface to the sacroiliac joint; the exposure is similar to that obtained using a modified Stoppa approach.[30] Reduction of the anterior wall fracture starts with traction and internal rotation of the femur. Occasionally, intraoperative lateral traction with a Schanz pin placed in the greater trochanter aids reduction of the fractured anterior wall. The fracture usually can be reduced by direct posterior lateral force applied with a ball spike or a bone clamp positioned with one tine on the anterior wall fragment and the other lateral to the anteroinferior iliac spine. A curved buttress plate is placed along the pelvic brim, extending from the superior pubic ramus to the internal iliac fossa (Figure 13, *C*). This construct can be augmented by two lag screws inserted from the brim to the quadrilateral surface, with care to avoid penetrating the joint. Medial subluxation of the femoral head cannot occur if the anterior and posterior articular surfaces are intact or have been reconstructed, and any

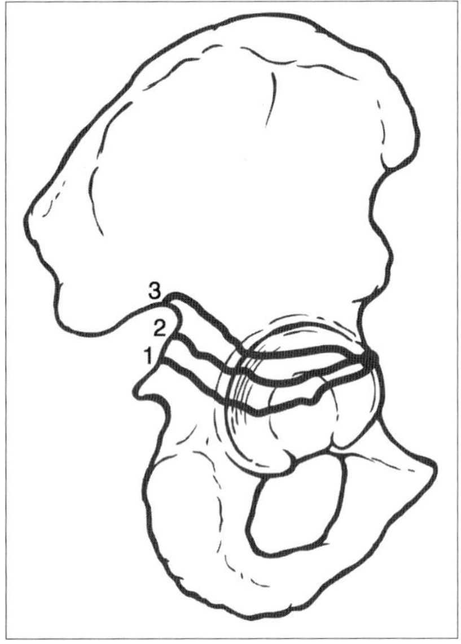

Figure 16 Schematic diagram of a hemipelvis showing the infratectal (1), juxtatectal (2), and transtectal (3) levels of the transverse fracture component and the component's exit at the iliopectineal eminence (dot). (Copyright Berton R. Moed, MD, St. Louis, MO, and Mark S. Vrahas, MD, Boston, MA.)

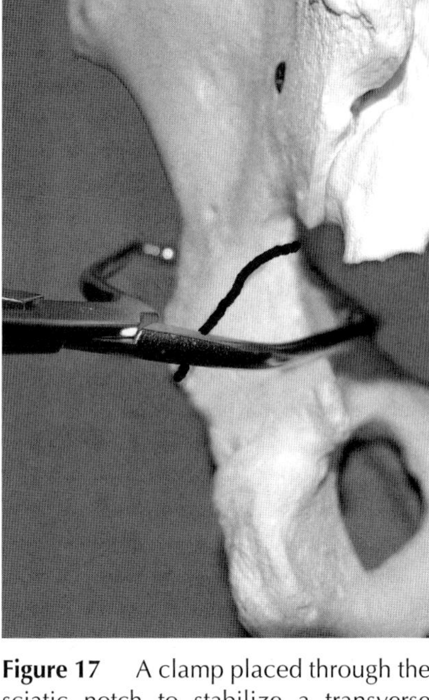

Figure 17 A clamp placed through the sciatic notch to stabilize a transverse fracture (line), shown on a plastic bone model. (Copyright Berton R. Moed, MD, St. Louis, MO, and Mark S. Vrahas, MD, Boston, MA.)

quadrilateral fracture fragments without articular involvement can be ignored.

Anterior Column Fracture

The treatment of an anterior column fracture (Figure 5, *D*) is similar to that of an anterior wall fracture. A complete or partial ilioinguinal approach is used, with the patient in the supine position. The anterior column fracture fragment usually is malrotated, and maximal displacement is observed at the pelvic brim. The reduction requires lateral traction on the femoral head and derotation of the anterior column. Traction and internal rotation places the femoral head on the intact posterior wall, often reducing the anterior column. Lateral traction through a Schanz pin placed from lateral to medial into the neck of the femur occasionally is helpful for reduction. In a high anterior column fracture (including the anterior border of the iliac wing), rotational control of the fracture can be obtained by gripping the anterior border of the bone with a clamp in the interspinous region. A second clamp can be placed across the fracture line at the iliac crest. The fracture usually is fixed with lag screws and a buttress plate (Figure 13, *D*).

Transverse, Transverse and Posterior Wall, and T-Shaped Fractures

In a transverse, transverse and posterior wall, or T-shaped fracture, the transverse fracture component commonly exits the anterior column at the iliopectineal eminence. The level at which it crosses the articular surface and exits the posterior column determines the effect on the joint (Figure 16). An infratectal fracture crosses below the acetabular roof and does not affect the weight-bearing surface, a juxtatectal fracture crosses just below the roof, and a transtectal fracture crosses the weight-bearing surface. Fracture reduction is most critical for a transtectal fracture; however, a juxtatectal fracture in many ways is the most difficult to reduce and stabilize.

Transverse Fracture

In a transverse fracture (Figure 5, *E*), the inferior (ischiopubic) segment is in one piece, and reduction requires the simultaneous control of the displacement and malrotation of the entire segment. The posterior column usually is the site of greatest fracture displacement, and therefore, the Kocher-Langenbeck approach is used. A reduction clamp is placed across the posterior column fracture to reduce the displacement, and a Schanz pin is secured near the ischial tuberosity to control the malrotation (Figure 15). Alternatively, a clamp can be placed across the fracture through the greater sciatic notch (Figure 17). The reduction is confirmed by palpation of the quadrilateral surface through the sciatic notch. A lag screw is directed from the retroacetabular surface across the fracture toward the anterior column. A neutralization plate is placed on the retroacetabular surface to complete the construct (Figure 13, *E*).

Transverse and Posterior Wall Fracture

The posterior wall component of an associated transverse and posterior wall fracture requires a posterior exposure (Figure 5, *G*). The choice of an extended iliofemoral or Kocher-Langenbeck approach is dictated by the configuration of the transverse component or the length of time from injury to surgical treatment. The transverse component is reduced first. Placing a reduction clamp across the posterior column fracture line with a posterior wall fracture present may be challenging; however, retraction of a posterior wall fracture improves visualization of the acetabular articular surface. After the transverse fracture component is fixed with a lag screw across the anterior column and plating or lag screw fixation across the posterior column, the posterior wall fracture is fixed (Figure 13, *G*).

T-Shaped Fracture

The Kocher-Langenbeck approach is used for most T-shaped fractures (Figure 5, *H*). Prone patient positioning on a fracture table is preferred. The anterior column fracture is exposed with longitudinal traction and retraction of the posterior column. As for a transverse fracture, the anterior column is reduced with a clamp (Figure 17) and fixed with a lag screw. The traction is released, the femoral head is repositioned, and the posterior column is reduced. The reduction is confirmed by palpation of the quadrilateral surface through the sciatic notch. A lag screw is inserted across the posterior column, and a plate is placed on the retroacetabular surface to complete the construct (Figure 13, *H*). If this strategy does not allow reduction of the anterior column, the posterior column is reduced and fixed, and the patient is repositioned for a second-stage anterior approach (usually the ilioinguinal approach). If a second-stage anterior approach is required, the posterior column fixation must not cross into the anterior column. Otherwise, independent manipulation of the anterior column fracture fragment will be impossible, and subsequent reduction maneuvers will be blocked.

Anterior Column and Posterior Hemitransverse and Both-Column Fractures

Anterior Column and Posterior Hemitransverse Fracture

In an associated anterior column and posterior hemitransverse fracture (Figure 5, *I*), the primary fracture line involves an anterior wall or column fracture. An associated transverse fracture component originates from the anterior fracture across the articular surface and extends to the posterior border of the innominate bone. The posterior hemitransverse fracture line is identical to the posterior half of a transverse fracture and usually is juxtatectal or infratectal. This fracture almost always is amenable to surgical treatment through the ilioinguinal approach. However, if there is segmental comminution or combined rotational and translational displacement of the posterior column fracture, the extended iliofemoral or staged combined approach is best used. The patient is positioned supine on the fracture table, with traction through a transcondylar femoral pin; or on the radiolucent table with the leg draped free. Sufficient flexion at the hip is necessary to relax the iliopsoas and allow dissection beneath the muscle.

The anterior column or wall is reduced and fixed first, as for an isolated anterior wall or column fracture. A plate is applied along the pelvic brim, leaving holes for subsequent lag screw fixation of the posterior column. The posterior column fracture is reduced using an angled clamp coursing around the iliopsoas; one tine is placed through the middle window onto the quadrilateral surface of the posterior column fragment, and the other tine is placed at the supra-acetabular ilium. An intrapelvic rotational reduction of the posterior column is achieved. The posterior column reduction to both the intact ilium and anterior column is assessed by visualization and fluoroscopic evaluation. However, the reduction of the articular surface can never be directly seen. The fixation construct is completed by screws placed from the internal iliac fossa and directed down the length of the posterior column to exit the ischium or lesser sciatic notch (Figure 13, *I*). In addition, a screw can be placed percutaneously from the outer cortex of the ilium to the quadrilateral surface to fix the posterior column. Screws often can be used alone for fixation of an anterior column and posterior hemitransverse fracture. However, buttress plates along the pelvic brim contribute additional stability, and they always should be used if there is any question about the stability of the screw-only construct, as in a comminuted fracture or a fracture in a patient with osteoporosis. An anterior wall fracture component may require additional buttress plate fixation.

Both-Column Fracture

The ilioinguinal approach is used for most associated both-column fractures (Figure 5, *J*), with the patient in the supine position. Frequently, the technique is similar to that of an anterior column and posterior hemitransverse fracture. The anterior column is first reduced and fixed with lag screws. A plate then is applied along the pelvic brim, with holes left for subsequent lag screw fixation of the posterior column. The posterior column fracture is reduced and fixed to complete the

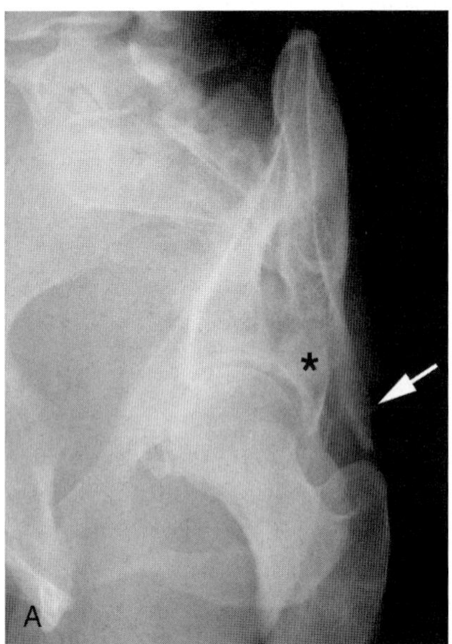

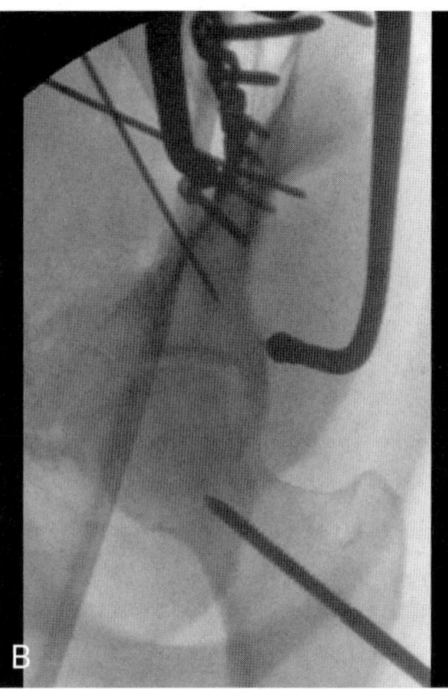

Figure 18 **A,** A preoperative obturator oblique radiograph showing the spur sign (arrow) and a large posterosuperior wall fracture fragment (asterisk). **B,** Intraoperative fluoroscopic view after reduction of the anterior column to the innominate bone; the spur sign is no longer evident, and the wall fracture has been reduced using a large clamp. (Copyright Berton R. Moed, MD, St. Louis, MO.)

construct (Figure 13, *J*). Like some anterior column and posterior hemitransverse fractures, many both-column fractures are amenable to lag screw fixation alone.

The extended iliofemoral approach commonly is used if there is a posterior wall fracture, comminution of the posterior column, or involvement of the sacroiliac joint (Figure 13, *K*). However, a posterior wall component of a both-column fracture differs from an isolated posterior wall fracture. The fragment is created at the junction of the anterior and posterior column fracture fragments, and frequently has a large cranial spike of cortical bone associated with it. Even in very comminuted both-column fractures, the acetabular labrum usually remains intact. Therefore, the fragment often can be manipulated by developing a small window of exposure through the interspinous region or over the iliac crest to the lateral surface of the ilium. A reduction clamp is used to reduce the posterior wall (Figure 18). The fracture then can be fixed by obliquely oriented screws inserted just lateral to the pelvic brim and directed posteriorly toward the superior iliac extension of the wall fragment. Buttress plate fixation of the fragment generally is not necessary because the intact capsule and labrum prevent posterior femoral head subluxation.

Acetabular Fracture Treatment With Associated Injuries

A fracture of the acetabulum usually is caused by high-energy blunt trauma. Surgery through a compromised soft-tissue envelope is ill advised because of the increased risk of infection. Therefore, the surrounding soft tissues should be carefully evaluated. Open wounds usually require débridement followed by delayed closure. Closed degloving soft-tissue injuries over the trochanteric region associated with underlying hematoma formation and fat necrosis (the Morel-Lavallé lesion) are associated with the presence of pathogenic bacteria.[41] Débridement followed by delayed wound closure and subsequent delayed fracture fixation often is required.[6,41] Recently, a percutaneous method has been reported, using a plastic brush to débride the injured fatty tissue.[42] A closed-suction drain is placed within the lesion and removed when drainage is less than 30 mL over 24 hours. Fracture fixation is deferred until at least 24 hours after drain removal.

An associated nonacetabular fracture can occur locally about the hip, distal to the hip at the location of the applied traumatic axial load, or at any location between these two points. Its initial treatment often affects later treatment of the acetabular fracture. A displaced fracture of the femoral head may be present, especially in association with a posterior fracture-dislocation, and usually is treated at the time of acetabular fracture fixation.[43] Treatment of a proximal femur fracture may compromise the optimal surgical approach to the acetabulum. This dilemma can be avoided if the proximal femur fracture is treated at the same time as acetabular fracture fixation or if a staged surgical procedure is planned so as not to interfere with optimal acetabular fracture care. A femoral neck fracture often requires immediate surgery, and it would be unusual to treat the acetabular fracture at the same time.[43] The acetabular fracture can be treated later, as required, through a separate, optimal approach. In contrast, an intertrochanteric or subtrochanteric femur fracture does not require urgent surgical treatment. Therefore, the treating physician can choose a staged procedure (proximal femur fracture fixation followed by acetabular fracture fixation) or an appropriately timed delayed fixation of both fractures during a single surgical procedure, using one or more separate incisions. Any treatment scheme should be planned to optimize the treatment of the acetabular fracture.

If both acetabular and femoral shaft fractures are present, the femur usually is stabilized first. Again, staged treatment should be planned for optimal acetabular fracture treatment. If an incision for antegrade nailing would compromise the surgical approach to the acetabulum, an alternative femoral shaft fracture treatment method, such as retrograde nailing, should be selected. When the femoral shaft and acetabular fracture surgeries are performed as sequential procedures during the same anesthesia, antegrade femoral nailing may not be the best choice. Compromised access to the proximal femur, which may occur with a severely displaced both-column fracture, or an irreducible dislocation of the femoral head that precludes satisfactory femoral shaft fracture reduction are two such situations. The alternatives to antegrade nailing include plating or retrograde nailing.

Prevention and Treatment of Postoperative Complications

The rate of infection is approximately 5% after surgical treatment of an acetabular fracture.[6,27,44] The adverse effects of a deep postoperative intra-articular wound infection cannot be minimized. Complete joint destruction occurs in approximately half of such infections.[27,44] The best preventive measures are perioperative antibiotic prophylaxis and meticulous surgical technique, including avoidance of operating through a compromised soft-tissue envelope. The treatment of infection in the acetabular region is similar to treatment in other anatomic regions. In an early infection, the hardware is preserved, if possible, until union to maintain the stability of the hip, and it is then removed. Late infection is treated with hardware removal. Long-term, culture-specific antibiotics are required for all infections, usually as an empiric course of 6 weeks.

Although the superior gluteal, inferior gluteal, obturator, and femoral nerves may be injured during acetabular surgery, these injuries appear to have a low prevalence. However, iatrogenic damage to the sciatic nerve is one of the most clinically important complications of acetabular fracture management, occurring in approximately 3% of cases.[27] These injuries usually are associated with the posterior and extended surgical approaches that involve direct exposure and retraction of the sciatic nerve.[6,45] Injury also can occur through an anterior surgical approach used for indirect reduction of posterior column displacement.[6,46,47] Although intraoperative nerve monitoring has been promoted, no data clearly indicate that nerve monitoring reduces the overall rate of iatrogenic sciatic nerve injury. There is no substitute for attention to detail in the operating room with respect to positioning the patient, maintaining the knee flexed to relax the sciatic nerve (for a posterior approach), placing retractors cautiously, and limiting traction on the nerve during fracture reduction.

Intra-articular placement of screws is a documented, destructive complication of acetabular fracture surgery. Letournel and Judet[6] originally proposed detecting intra-articular hardware by listening for crepitus as the hip is taken through the range of motion in the operating room, under conditions of complete silence. Anglen and DiPasquale[48] recommended using a sterile esophageal stethoscope for the same purpose. Other authors have recommended intraoperative and postoperative radiography to ensure that the hardware has been placed outside the joint.[49,50] Currently, intraoperative fluoroscopy appears to be the best method[39] (Figure 14). If hardware has been placed within the joint, removal of the implant is imperative.

Magnetic resonance venography identified proximal deep venous thrombosis in 34% of patients with an acetabular fracture.[51] Letournel and Judet[6] reported that 13 of 565 patients (2.3%) died after acetabular fracture surgery, and that 4 of these deaths were caused by massive pulmonary embolism. Some form of mechanical or chemical prophylaxis is recommended to decrease the risk of thromboembolic complications. The use of mechanical prophylaxis with a foot pump beginning at the time of hospital admission, with the addition of enoxaparin 5 days after all acute bleeding from the blunt trauma had resolved, was found to be successful for prophylaxis against venous thromboembolic disease after serious musculoskeletal injury.[52] The prevalence of large or occlusive deep venous thromboses among patients who had been managed with this protocol was significantly less than that among patients who had been managed with enoxaparin alone, initiated 24 to 48 hours after blunt trauma.[52] Enoxaparin was discontinued the night before surgery and resumed within 12 hours after surgery. Despite prophylactic treatment, the rate of posttraumatic and postoperative thromboembolism is approximately 11%.[52-54] Screening with Doppler ultrasonography or magnetic resonance venography remains controversial.[54] The placement of prophylactic vena cava filters is controversial, but it may be indicated for some high-risk patients.[54,55] The risk continues after discharge from the hospital, and it is prudent to continue postoperative prophylaxis until the patient is fully ambulatory.[6,56]

Severe heterotopic ossification of the hip is clinically defined as involving a loss of motion of at least 20%.[27] Using this criterion, Matta[27] reported its prevalence as 20% using the extended iliofemoral approach, 8% for the Kocher-Langenbeck, and 2% for the ilioinguinal. The most important risk factor for heterotopic ossification is the stripping of the gluteal muscles from the external surface of the ilium.[6,27,32,57,58] Although heterotopic ossification is an important postoperative complication, the risks associated with the available prophylactic treatments, their potential for failure, and the actual risk of occurrence must be weighed for each individual patient. A study of patients with acetabular fracture found that the use of indomethacin increases the risk of long-bone nonunion.[59] Induced malignant disease is a possible consequence of low-dose radiation therapy.[60] One study of a cohort of 2,067 women receiving 2.6 to 5.3 Gy of midline radiation for the benign condition metropathia hemorrhagica and followed for an average of 28 years found an increase in mortality from cancers of the irradiated pelvic sites.[60] However, for the radiation dosage and methods used for the prophylaxis of heterotopic ossification about the hip, the likelihood of induced malignancy is very low.[61] In deciding on prophylactic therapy, the clinician must keep in mind the actual rates of functionally important heterotopic ossification. Delayed excision of mature, functionally significant heterotopic ossification is a viable treatment option after unsuccessful prophylactic therapy and an alternative to prophylaxis. Functional improvement can be expected in patients with congruent joint surfaces, and Letournel and Judet[6] reported only one poor result in 14 patients. Delayed excision surgery is a relatively low risk procedure with good results, and a return to more than 80% of normal motion can be expected.[6,32,62]

Posttraumatic arthritis is the most common complication after an acetabular fracture. The quality of the fracture reduction appears to be the main determinant for clinical outcome and for the risk of late traumatic arthritis..[6,27,44] Damage to the femoral head at the time of initial injury is another important factor.[27] Osteonecrosis of the femoral head is known to result from acetabular fracture associated with hip dislocation and can also result in posttraumatic arthritis.[27,37] However, posttraumatic arthritis is more commonly caused by wear of the femoral head against a malreduced fracture.[6,27] Total hip arthroplasty or arthrodesis is indicated for patients who have disabling pain from posttraumatic arthritis.

Results of Surgical Treatment

The three largest studies of the outcome of acetabular fractures treated within 3 weeks of injury found a 75% to 81% rate of good or excellent results at long-term follow-up.[6,27,44] The most important objective of surgical treatment is to obtain an anatomic reduction of the articular surface, and the clinical outcome is strongly correlated with the adequacy of fracture reduction.[6,27] Letournel and Judet[6] studied 492 acetabular fractures followed for at least 1 year and found that anatomic reduction was achieved in 366 (74%), of which 316 (86%) had a good to excellent result. However, only 64% of those with an imperfect reduction (81 of 126 patients) had a good to excellent result. Among patients who had posttraumatic arthritis after a perfect articular reduction (10%), 50% had arthritis appearing 10 to 25 years after the injury. In contrast, among those who had posttraumatic arthritis after an imperfect reduction (36%), 80% had arthritis appearing within the first 10 years after injury.[6] Matta[27] found that achieving an anatomic reduction (defined 1 mm or less of residual displacement) is the most important determinant of the outcome of acetabular fracture surgery. Therefore, the surgeon must strive for a so-called inframillimetric reduction of every fracture to maximize the patient's quality of life after the injury.

The rate of anatomic reduction decreases with greater fracture complexity, patient age, and delay from injury to fixation.[27] The time from injury to fracture fixation has a dramatic effect on the outcome. Letournel and Judet[6] found that among 138 patients who were treated after a 3-week delay, the rate of good to excellent results was only 54%; Johnson and associates[63] found that 65% of 187 such patients had a good to excellent result. In a study of 237 patients, Madhu and associates[64] found that a fracture of an elementary type was more likely to be anatomically reduced and have a good to excellent clinical outcome if surgery was performed within 15 days; a fracture of an associated type was more likely to be anatomically reduced if the surgery was performed within 5 days and was more likely to have a good to excellent clinical outcome if the surgery was performed within 10 days.

Fractures of some types appear to have better outcomes after surgical treatment than fractures of other types. Both-column fractures are complex injuries and technically demanding; however, their outcome generally is better than that of many other fracture types despite a higher rate of nonanatomic reduction. Matta[27] obtained anatomic reduction in only 57% of these cases; nonetheless, 77% of patients had a good to excellent result. The treatment of posterior wall fractures is straightforward, with reported rates of anatomic reduction as high as 100%.[27] However, Matta[27] reported a 32% clinical failure rate in 22 treated fractures, despite having obtained anatomic reduction in every fracture. This rate was higher than that of any other fracture type. Aho and associates[65] and Chiu and associates[66] reported similar results. However, other researchers reported results of posterior wall fractures similar to those of other types of acetabular fractures (more than 80% good to excellent clinical outcomes).[6,36,37] Letournel and Judet[6] suggested and Moed and associates[40] later established that the disparity between apparent anatomic reduction, as determined by plain radiography, and clinical results is largely attributable to the inadequacy of radiographs for assessing the quality of the postoperative posterior wall reduction. Postoperative CT appears to be a more accurate means of documenting articular reduction after a posterior wall fracture.[40]

Summary

The goals of treating an acetabular fracture are to restore hip joint congruity and stability. Although some fracture types may not require surgery for a satisfactory outcome, in general a patient with a displaced fracture in the weight-bearing area of the acetabulum should be treated with open reduction and internal fixation. The surgery is complex and demanding, and fracture reduction must be anatomic to obtain the best results. However, there is no doubt that an experienced surgeon can obtain an excellent result. Poor results are related mainly to residual fracture displacement and perioperative complications. When treating an acetabular fracture, the surgeon must be cognizant of the importance of the evaluation and treatment protocols initially developed by Letournel and Judet, as well as the progress made during the past decade.

References

1. Knight RA, Smith H: Central fractures of the acetabulum. *J Bone Joint Surg Am* 1958;40:1-16.
2. Rowe CR, Lowell JD: Prognosis of fractures of the acetabulum. *J Bone Joint Surg Am* 1961;43A:30-59.
3. Stewart MJ: Discussion: Prognosis of fractures of the acetabulum. *J Bone Joint Surg Am* 1961;43A:59.
4. Stewart MJ, Milford LW: Fracture-dislocation of the hip: An end-result study. *J Bone Joint Surg Am* 1954;36:315-342.
5. Judet R, Judet J, Letournel E: Fractures of the acetabulum: Classification and surgical approaches for open reduction. Preliminary report. *J Bone Joint Surg Am* 1964;46:1615-1646.
6. Letournel E, Judet R: *Fractures of the Acetabulum*, ed 2. New York, NY, Springer-Verlag, 1993.
7. Templeman DC, Olson S, Moed BR, Duwelius P, Matta JM: Surgical treatment of acetabular fractures. *Instr Course Lect* 1999;48:481-496.
8. Borrelli J Jr, Goldfarb C, Catalano L, Evanoff BA: Assessment of articular fragment displacement in acetabular fractures: A comparison of computerized tomography and plain radiographs. *J Orthop Trauma* 2002;16:449-456.
9. Moed BR, Ajibade DA, Israel H: Computed tomography as a predictor of hip stability status in posterior wall fractures of the acetabulum. *J Orthop Trauma* 2009;23:7-15.
10. Helfet DL, Bartlett CS III: Acetabular fractures: Evaluation/classification/treatment concepts and approaches, in Ruedi TP, Murphy WM, eds: *AO Principles of Fracture Management*, New York, NY, Thieme, 2001, pp 419-442.
11. Marsh JL, Slongo TF, Agel J, et al: Fracture and dislocation classification compendium, 2007: Orthopaedic Trauma Association classification, database and outcomes committee. *J Orthop Trauma* 2007;21:S1-S133.
12. Beaulé PE, Dorey FJ, Matta JM: Letournel classification for acetabular fractures: Assessment of interobserver and intraobserver reliability. *J Bone Joint Surg Am* 2003;85:1704-1709.
13. Heeg M, Oostvogel HJ, Klasen HJ: Conservative treatment of acetabular fractures: The role of the weight-bearing dome and anatomic reduction in the ultimate results. *J Trauma* 1987;27:555-559.
14. Matta JM, Anderson LM, Epstein HC, Hendricks P: Fractures of the acetabulum: A retrospective analysis. *Clin Orthop Relat Res* 1986;205:230-240.
15. Olsen SA, Matta JM: The computerized tomography subchondral arc: A new method of assessing acetabular articular continuity after fracture. A preliminary report. *J Orthop Trauma* 1993;7:402-413.
16. Tile M, Helfet DL, Kellam JF: *Fractures of the Pelvis and Acetabulum*. Philadelphia, PA, Lippincott Williams and Wilkins, 2003.
17. Matta JM, Merritt PO: Displaced acetabular fractures. *Clin Orthop Relat Res* 1988;230:83-97.

18. Vrahas MS, Widding KK, Thomas KA: The effects of simulated transverse, anterior column, and posterior column fractures of the acetabulum on the stability of the hip joint. *J Bone Joint Surg Am* 1999;81:966-974.

19. Heeg M, Otter N, Klasen HJ: Anterior column fractures of the acetabulum. *J Bone Joint Surg Br* 1992;74: 554-557.

20. Crowl AC, Kahler DM: Closed reduction and percutaneous fixation of anterior column acetabular fractures. *Comput Aided Surg* 2002;7:169-178.

21. Kahler DM, DeGrange D, Wang G-J: Percutaneous fixation of selected acetabular fractures using computed tomographic guidance. *Orthop Trans* 1996;20:83.

22. Starr AJ, Reinert CM, Jones AL: Percutaneous fixation of columns of the acetabulum: A new technique. *J Orthop Trauma* 1998;12:51-58.

23. Tornetta P III: Non-operative management of acetabular fractures: The use of dynamic stress views. *J Bone Joint Surg Br* 1999;81:67-70.

24. Helfet DL, Borrelli J Jr, DiPasquale T, Sanders R: Stabilization of acetabular fractures in elderly patients. *J Bone Joint Surg Am* 1992;74: 753-765.

25. Sermon A, Broos P, Vanderschot P: Total hip replacement for acetabular fractures: Results in 121 patients operated between 1983 and 2003. *Injury* 2008;39:914-921.

26. Spencer RF: Acetabular fractures in older patients. *J Bone Joint Surg Br* 1989;71:774-776.

27. Matta J: Fractures of the acetabulum: Accuracy of reduction and clinical results in patients managed operatively within three weeks after the injury. *J Bone Joint Surg Am* 1996;78:1632-1645.

28. Dean DB, Moed BR: Late salvage of failed open reduction and internal fixation of posterior wall fractures of the acetabulum. *J Orthop Trauma* 2009;23:180-185.

29. Helfet DL, Schmeling GJ: Management of complex acetabular fractures through single nonextensile exposures. *Clin Orthop Relat Res* 1994;305: 58-68.

30. Cole JD, Bolhofner BR: Acetabular fracture fixation via a modified Stoppa limited intrapelvic approach: Description of operative technique and preliminary treatment results. *Clin Orthop Relat Res* 1994;305: 112-123.

31. Qureshi AA, Archdeacon MT, Jenkins MA, Infante A, DiPasquale T, Bolhofner BR: Infrapectineal plating for acetabular fractures: A technical adjunct to internal fixation. *J Orthop Trauma* 2004;18:175-178.

32. Mears DC, Rubash H: *Pelvic and Acetabular Fractures*. Thorofare, NJ, Slack, 1986.

33. Ellis TJ, Beck M: Trochanteric osteotomy for acetabular fractures and proximal femur fractures. *Orthop Clin North Am* 2004;35:457-461.

34. Siebenrock KA, Gautier E, Ziran BH, Ganz R: Trochanteric flip osteotomy for cranial extension and muscle protection in acetabular fracture fixation using the Kocher-Langenbeck approach. *J Orthop Trauma* 1998;12: 387-391.

35. Harris MA, Althausen P, Kellam JF, Bosse MJ: Simultaneous anterior and posterior approaches for complex acetabular fractures. *J Orthop Trauma* 2008;22:494-497.

36. Giannoudis PV, Tzioupis CC, Moed BR: Two-level reconstruction of comminuted posterior-wall fractures of the acetabulum. *J Bone Joint Surg Br* 2007;89:503-509.

37. Moed BR, WillsonCarr SE, Watson JT: Results of operative treatment of fractures of the posterior wall of the acetabulum. *J Bone Joint Surg Am* 2002;84:752-758.

38. Moed BR, McMichael JC: Outcomes of posterior wall fractures of the acetabulum: Surgical technique. *J Bone Joint Surg Am* 2008;90:87-107.

39. Carmack DB, Moed BR, McCarroll K, Freccero D: Accuracy of detecting screw penetration of the acetabulum with intraoperative fluoroscopy and computed tomography. *J Bone Joint Surg Am* 2001;83: 1370-1375.

40. Moed BR, Carr SE, Gruson KI, Watson JT, Craig JG: Computed tomography assessment of fractures of the posterior wall of the acetabulum after operative treatment. *J Bone Joint Surg Am* 2003;85:512-522.

41. Hak DJ, Olson SA, Matta JM: Diagnosis and management of closed internal degloving injuries associated with pelvic and acetabular fractures: The Morel-Lavallée lesion. *J Trauma* 1997;42:1046-1051.

42. Tseng S, Tornetta P III: Percutaneous management of Morel-Lavallee lesions. *J Bone Joint Surg Am* 2006;88: 92-96.

43. Kregor PJ, Templeman D: Associated injuries complicating the management of acetabular fractures: Review and case studies. *Orthop Clin North Am* 2002;33:73-95.

44. Mayo KA: Open reduction and internal fixation of fractures of the acetabulum: Results in 163 fractures. *Clin Orthop Relat Res* 1994;305:31-37.

45. Vrahas M, Gordon RG, Mears DC, Krieger D, Sclabassi RJ: Intraoperative somatosensory evoked potential monitoring of pelvic and acetabular fractures. *J Orthop Trauma* 1992;6: 50-58.

46. Dunbar RP Jr, Gardner MJ, Cunningham B, Routt ML Jr: Sciatic nerve entrapment in associated both-column acetabular fractures: A report of 2 cases and review of the literature. *J Orthop Trauma* 2009;23:80-83.

47. Helfet DL, Schmeling GJ: Somatosensory evoked potential monitoring in the surgical treatment of acute, displaced acetabular fractures: Results of a prospective study. *Clin Orthop Relat Res* 1994;301:213-220.

48. Anglen JO, DiPasquale T: The reliability of detecting screw penetration of the acetabulum by intraoperative auscultation. *J Orthop Trauma* 1994;8: 404-408.

49. Ebraheim NA, Savolaine ER, Hoeflinger MJ, Jackson WT: Radiological

diagnosis of screw penetration of the hip joint in acetabular fracture reconstruction. *J Orthop Trauma* 1989;3: 196-201.

50. Norris BL, Hahn DH, Bosse MJ, Kellam JF, Sims SH: Intraoperative fluoroscopy to evaluate fracture reduction and hardware placement during acetabular surgery. *J Orthop Trauma* 1999;13:414-417.

51. Montgomery KD, Potter HG, Helfet DL: The detection and management of proximal deep vein thrombosis in patients with acute acetabular fractures: A follow-up report. *J Orthop Trauma* 1997;11:330-336.

52. Stannard JP, Lopez-Ben RR, Volgas DA, et al: Prophylaxis against deep-vein thrombosis following trauma: A prospective, randomized comparison of mechanical and pharmacologic prophylaxis. *J Bone Joint Surg Am* 2006;88:261-266.

53. Stannard JP, Singhania AK, Lopez-Ben RR, et al: Deep-vein thrombosis in high-energy skeletal trauma despite thromboprophylaxis. *J Bone Joint Surg Br* 2005;87:965-968.

54. Borer DS, Starr AJ, Reinert CM, et al: The effect of screening for deep vein thrombosis on the prevalence of pulmonary embolism in patients with fractures of the pelvis or acetabulum: A review of 973 patients. *J Orthop Trauma* 2005;19:92-95.

55. Rogers FB, Shackford SR, Ricci MA, Huber BM, Atkins T: Prophylactic vena cava filter insertion in selected high-risk orthopaedic trauma patients. *J Orthop Trauma* 1997;11: 267-272.

56. Bjørnarå BT, Gudmundsen TE, Dahl OE: Frequency and timing of clinical venous thromboembolism after major joint surgery. *J Bone Joint Surg Br* 2006;88:386-391.

57. Bosse MJ, Poka A, Reinert CM, Ellwanger F, Slawson R, McDevitt ER: Heterotopic ossification as a complication of acetabular fracture: Prophylaxis with low-dose irradiation. *J Bone Joint Surg Am* 1988;70:1231-1237.

58. Moed BR, Maxey JW: The effect of indomethacin on heterotopic ossification following acetabular fracture surgery. *J Orthop Trauma* 1993;7:33-38.

59. Burd TA, Hughes MS, Anglen JO: Heterotopic ossification prophylaxis with indomethacin increases the risk of long-bone nonunion. *J Bone Joint Surg Br* 2003;85:700-705.

60. Darby SC, Reeves G, Key T, Doll R, Stovall M: Mortality in a cohort of women given x-ray therapy for metropathia haemorrhagica. *Int J Cancer* 1994;56:793-801.

61. Haas ML, Kennedy AS, Copeland CC, Ames JW, Scarboro M, Slawson RG: Utility of radiation in the prevention of heterotopic ossification following repair of traumatic acetabular fracture. *Int J Radiat Oncol Biol Phys* 1999;45: 461-468.

62. Webb LX, Bosse MJ, Mayo KA, Lange RH, Miller ME, Swiontkowski MF: Results in patients with craniocerebral trauma and an operatively managed acetabular fracture. *J Orthop Trauma* 1990;4:376-382.

63. Johnson EE, Matta JM, Mast JW, Letournel E: Delayed reconstruction of acetabular fractures 21-120 days following injury. *Clin Orthop Relat Res* 1994;305:20-30.

64. Madhu R, Kotnis R, Al-Mousawi A, et al: Outcome of surgery for reconstruction of fractures of the acetabulum: The time dependent effect of delay. *J Bone Joint Surg Br* 2006;88: 1197-1203.

65. Aho AJ, Isberg UK, Katevuo VK: Acetabular posterior wall fracture: 38 cases followed for 5 years. *Acta Orthop Scand* 1986;57:101-105.

66. Chiu FY, Lo WH, Chen TH, Chen CM, Huang CK, Ma HL: Fractures of posterior wall of acetabulum. *Arch Orthop Trauma Surg* 1996;115: 273-275.

Intertrochanteric Fractures: Ten Tips to Improve Results

George J. Haidukewych, MD

Abstract

Intertrochanteric hip fractures are among the most common types of fractures, and the numbers are increasing as the population ages. Most intertrochanteric fractures are treated surgically. It is therefore important that the treatment methods are effective and have a minimal risk of complications. The goals of treatment include a predictable union, unrestricted early weight bearing, and avoidance of fixation failure or excessive deformity of the proximal femur. Careful attention to the fracture pattern (obliquity or other hallmarks implying instability) can guide fixation device selection. Regardless of the device, accurate reduction and implant placement are important to a good outcome.

Instr Course Lect 2010;59:503-509.

Intertrochanteric hip fractures are becoming increasingly common as the population ages. These fractures typically occur in frail patients with multiple medical comorbidities and often result in loss of the patient's functional independence. The all-too-often problematic dispositions and prolonged hospital stays result in a tremendous cost to patients, their families, and society. Effective treatment strategies that result in high rates of union of these fractures and low rates of complications are important. Orthopaedic surgeons cannot control the quality of the bone, patient compliance, or comorbidities, but they should be able to minimize the morbidity associated with the fracture. Doing so requires choosing the appropriate fixation device for the fracture pattern, recognizing the problem fracture patterns, and performing accurate reductions with ideal implant placement while being conscious of implant costs. If these fractures are treated expeditiously, fixation failures minimized, and underlying osteoporosis is recognized and treated accordingly, patients outcomes will improve and the cost of treatment will decrease. The purpose of this review is to summarize 10 simple tips to help minimize failures and improve outcomes when treating intertrochanteric fractures.

Tip 1: Use the Tip-to-Apex Distance

The tip-to-apex distance has been described by Baumgaertner and associates[1,2] as a useful intraoperative indicator of deep and central placement of the lag screw in the femoral head, regardless of whether a nail or a plate is chosen to fix the fracture (Figure 1). This is perhaps the most important measurement of accurate hardware placement and has been shown in multiple studies to be predictive of success after the treatment of standard obliquity intertrochanteric fractures. Older theories about screw placement favored a low and occasionally a posterior position of the lag screw, thereby leaving more bone superior and anterior to the screw. This position effectively lengthens the tip-to-apex distance and should be avoided. The ideal position for a lag screw in both planes is deep and central in the femoral head within 10 mm of the subchondral bone[3,4] (Figure 2). A

Dr. Haidukewych or an immediate family member serves as a board member, owner, officer, or committee member of the Florida Orthopaedic Institute; has received royalties from DePuy and Zimmer; is a member of a speakers' bureau or has made paid presentations on behalf of DePuy; serves as a paid consultant to or is an employee of DePuy and Surmodics; has received research or institutional support from DePuy; and has stock or stock options held in Surmodics.

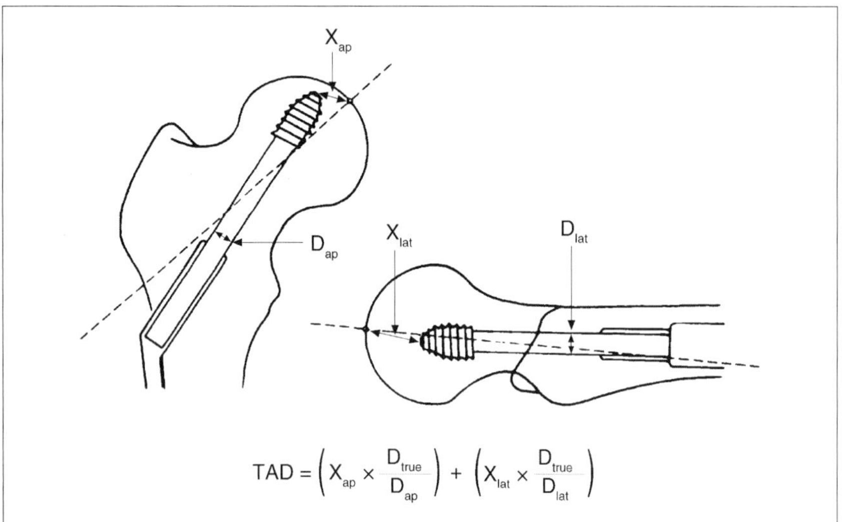

Figure 1 The technique for calculating the tip-to-apex distance (TAD). For clarity, a peripherally placed screw is depicted in the anteroposterior (ap) view, and a shallowly placed screw is depicted in the lateral (lat) view. D_{true} = known diameter of the lag screw. (Reproduced with permission from Baumgaertner MR, Curtin SL, Lindskog DM, Keggi JM: The value of the tip-apex distance in predicting failure of fixation of peritrochanteric fractures of the hip. *J Bone Joint Surg Am* 1995;77:1059.)

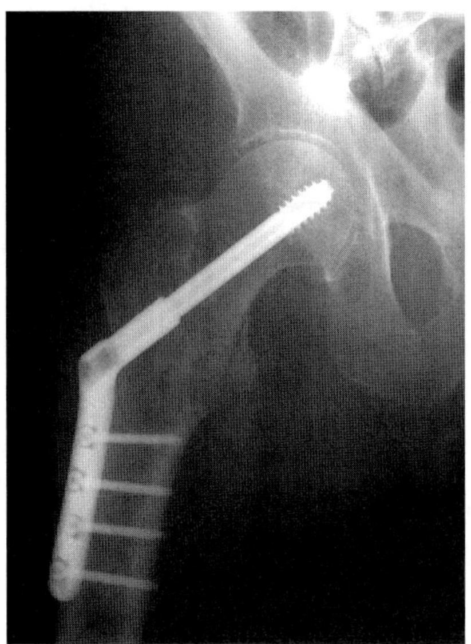

Figure 2 Radiograph showing excellent reduction and deep, central placement of the lag screw in the femoral head.

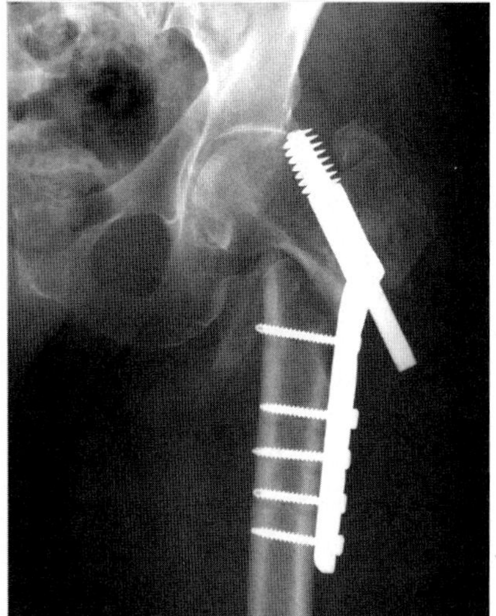

Figure 3 Radiograph showing failed fixation of a reverse obliquity fracture with lateralization of the proximal fragment and screw cutout.

tip-to-apex distance of less than 25 mm has been shown to be generally predictive of a successful result; however, most traumatologists aim for a tip-to-apex distance of less than 20 mm.

Tip 2: No Lateral Wall, No Hip Screw

Fractures that involve the lateral wall of the proximal part of the femur are, by definition, either reverse obliquity fractures or transtrochanteric fractures. These fractures do not have any lateral osseous buttress, and therefore, if a sliding hip screw is used, medial translation of the femoral shaft and lateralization of the proximal femoral fragment can occur. The result is deformity, nonunion, and screw cutout (Figure 3). Haidukewych and associates[5] found a 56% failure rate when a sliding hip screw had been used for reverse obliquity fractures of the proximal part of the femur. Although devices with a trochanteric stabilizing plate, those with a proximal trochanteric flare, and those that allow axial compression and locking of the sliding hip screw (such as the Medoff device) are reported to have reasonably good results, a hip screw should not be used if there is no lateral wall.[3-9] Locking plates and 95-degree condylar blade plates may function as prosthetic lateral cortices, but the results of using these devices for more problematic fractures of the proximal part of the femur are not available.[9-11] Intramedullary nails seem to be superior to dynamic condylar screws for reverse obliquity fractures, but comparative studies of intramedullary nails and proximal femoral locking plates are not available.

Tip 3: Know the Unstable Intertrochanteric Fracture Patterns and Nail Them

There are four classic intertrochanteric fracture patterns that signify instability. When internally fixed, the osseous fragments of these unstable fractures are not able to share the weight-bearing loads, and therefore the loads are predominantly borne by the internal fixation device. The unstable patterns include reverse obliquity fractures, transtrochanteric fractures, fractures with a large posteromedial fragment implying loss of the calcar buttress, and fractures with subtrochanteric extension[3-5,9,12-16] (Figures 4 through 7). These fractures, in general, should be treated with an intramedullary nail because of the more favorable biomechanical properties of an intramedullary nail compared with a sliding hip screw. An intramedullary nail is located closer to the center of gravity than is a sliding hip screw, and therefore the lever arm on the femoral fixation is shorter. Intramedullary nails can more reliably resist the relatively high forces across the medial calcar that are typically borne by the implant in an unstable fracture. The intramedullary position of the implant also prevents shaft medialization, which is a common complication associated with the transtrochanteric and reverse obliquity fracture patterns. Recognizing the unstable patterns preoperatively and choosing to use an intramedullary nail decrease the risk of fixation failure. A simple fracture of the lesser trochanter does not, in itself, automatically imply an unstable fracture, as many three-part and four-part fractures can include a small, relatively unimportant fracture of the lesser trochanter and yet have a primary fracture line that will tolerate compression well. It is not known how large the posteromedial fragment must be to be mechanically important. When there is doubt about the status of the calcar, however, an intramedullary nail is preferable to a sliding hip screw.

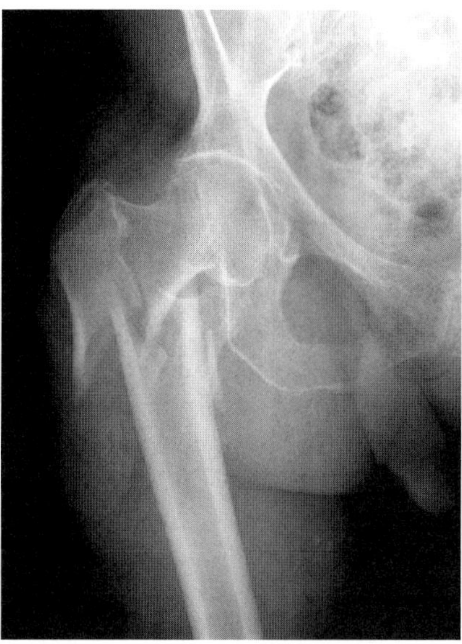
Figure 4 Radiograph showing a reverse obliquity fracture.

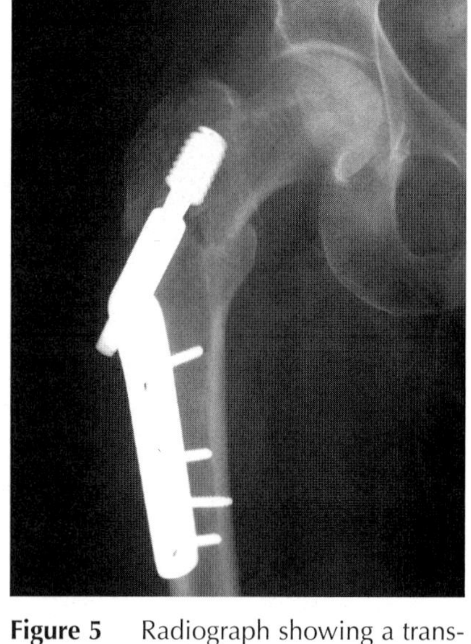
Figure 5 Radiograph showing a transtrochanteric fracture.

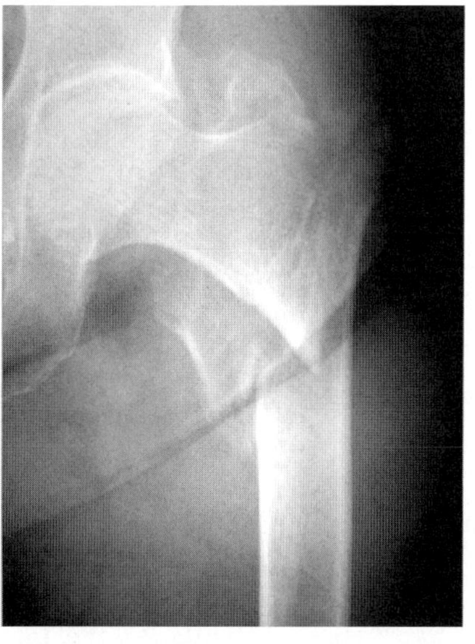
Figure 6 Radiograph showing a four-part fracture with a large posteromedial fragment.

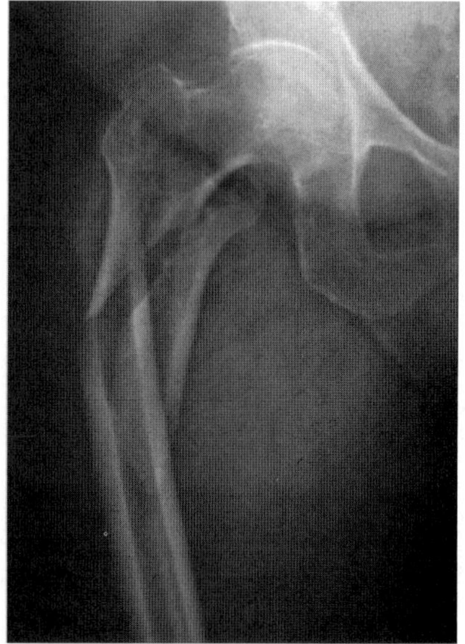
Figure 7 Radiograph showing a fracture with subtrochanteric extension.

Tip 4: Beware of the Anterior Bow of the Femoral Shaft

As a person ages, the femoral diaphysis enlarges, and the femoral bow increases.[17] Most commercial intramedullary nails have gradually evolved into a more bowed design, and many of them now have a radius of curvature of less than 2 m. The concern with using a straight intramedullary nail in a bowed osteopenic femur is that the nail can impinge on, and in some cases even perforate, the anterior femoral metaphyseal cortex distally (Figure 8). Additionally, when the nail hugs the anterior femoral cortex, any locking screws placed in the distal part of the femur may cause a stress riser in this area, which may lead to a fracture during the postoperative rehabilitation period. It is wise to know the radius of curvature of the particular device, which ideally should be no more than 2 m. Most commercially available in-

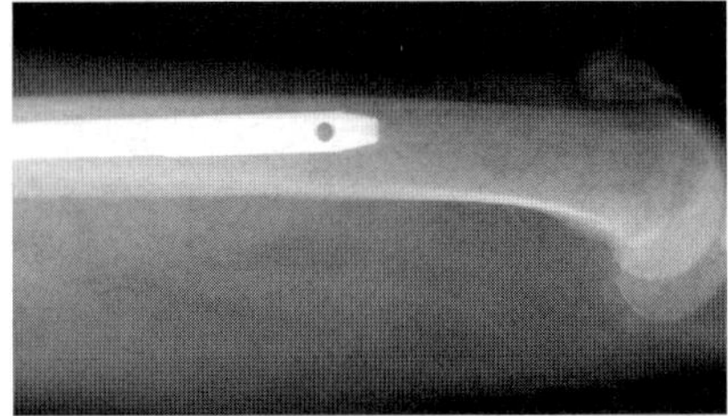

Figure 8 Radiograph showing a straight nail inserted into a bowed femur. Vigorous impaction or a bow mismatch may lead to perforation of the distal anterior femoral cortex.

tramedullary nails have a radius of curvature of between 1.5 and 2.2 m. It is also important to recognize that, if resistance is encountered during insertion of a long intramedullary nail for fixation of an intertrochanteric fracture, the surgeon should obtain a lateral radiograph of the distal part of the femur rather than trying to impact the device with a hammer. Hammering in a long intramedullary nail that is impinging on the anterior cortex can produce an iatrogenic fracture.

Tip 5: When Using a Trochanteric Entry Nail, Start Slightly Medial to the Exact Tip of the Greater Trochanter

The patient's soft-tissue mass, the surgical drapes, the trajectory of the reamer insertion and of the reaming, and the nail insertion can gradually enlarge the pilot hole in the greater trochanter laterally. This enlargement leads to more lateral placement of the intramedullary nail than intended. In turn, this can result in a varus reduction of the proximal fragment or a high lag-screw position in the femoral head, both of which are undesirable. A starting point slightly medial to the exact tip of the trochanter is recommended[18] (Figure 9). The starter reamer is used while it is observed with fluoroscopy, and subsequent reaming is performed very carefully. Use of the reamers should not be started until they are well contained in the proximal part of the femur. This avoids any gradual lateral enlargement of the pilot hole.

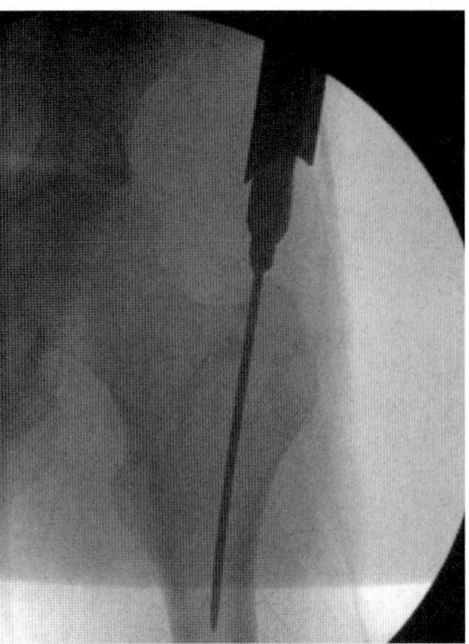

Figure 9 Fluoroscopic image showing the ideal starting point slightly medial to the exact tip of the greater trochanter. Note the good position of the guidewire distally.

Tip 6: Do Not Ream an Unreduced Fracture

In sharp contradistinction to diaphyseal fractures of the femur, which may be reamed in a position that is not necessarily well reduced because the interference fit in the diaphysis aligns the fracture as the intramedullary nail is passed, a misaligned intertrochanteric fracture cannot be reduced simply by passing the intramedullary nail across it. The intertrochanteric fracture should be reduced to an aligned position before reaming and passing of the intramedullary nail. One must remember that the way that these fractures look during reaming will not change after the nail has been inserted.

It is not possible to make a starting point in the proximal fragment and then manipulate this fragment with a reduction tool or even the intramedullary nail because the bone is too soft and the medullary canal is too large. Obtaining good muscle relaxation and then performing a gentle closed reduction with the patient on a fracture table while observing the fracture with fluoroscopy is recommended. If reduction cannot be obtained by closed means, then some form of percutaneous or miniopen reduction is recommended. A bone hook placed along the lesser trochanter, or even percutaneous joysticks or clamps, can be used to reduce the fragment without the need for substantial periosteal stripping or evacuation of the fracture hematoma (Figure 10). The fragment can then be reamed, and the intramedullary nail can be inserted.

Tip 7: Be Cautious About the Nail Insertion Trajectory and Do Not Use a Hammer to Seat the Nail

It is important to achieve a vertical trajectory with nail insertion. This can be difficult in obese patients. Even if care was taken with the starting point and the subsequent reaming, if the intramedullary nail is inserted at an oblique angle, the nail itself can impact the relatively soft bone of the lateral aspect of the greater trochanter and lead to a relatively oval entry point and a lateral position of the intramedullary nail in the proximal fragment. It is critical that the nail be inserted by hand with slight rotational motions. A hammer is not recommended because its use can lead to iatrogenic femoral fracture. It is safe to tap the jig with a mallet for the final seating; this is an easy way to fine-tune the final position of the intramedullary nail. The mallet should not be used if difficulty is encountered when inserting the intramedullary nail by hand. The variety of diameters at the distal end and valgus angles at the proximal end of modern intramedullary nail systems have decreased the frequency of iatrogenic femoral fractures.[19] It is still important to realize that, if a hammer is needed to advance the nail (as opposed to simply tapping it in a few final millimeters), there is a problem. The femoral shaft may need to be reamed further to prevent nail incarceration (this is not uncommon in younger patients), or there may be impingement on the anterior femoral cortex with a mismatch between the bows of the femur and the intramedullary nail. The cause of the difficulty should be identified and corrected because the intramedullary nail should be passed by hand. The suggested procedure is to ream the intramedullary canal to a diameter that is 1 mm larger than the diameter of the selected intramedullary nail and to ensure that the starter reamer has been inserted to the recommended depth. This prevents the funnel shape of the proximal nail from impinging on the endosteum proximally and preventing final seating.

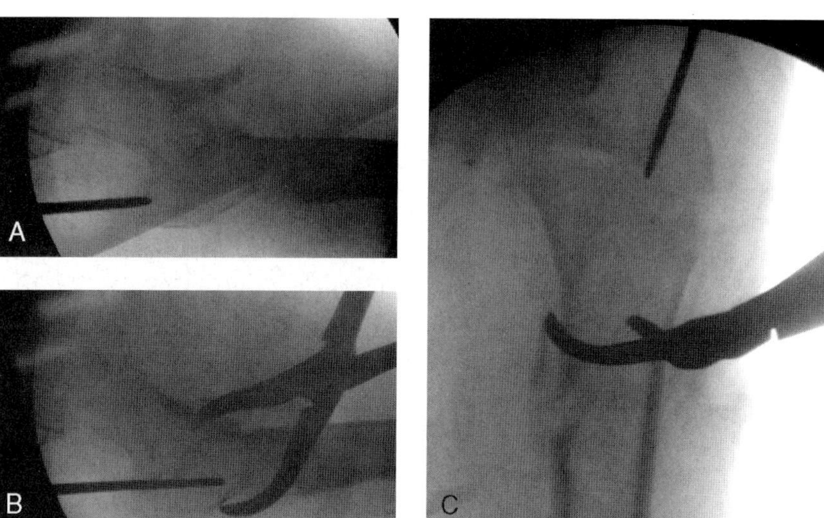

Figure 10 Fluoroscopic images of an unreduced fracture. **A,** An unreduced fracture cannot be reduced with nail passage because of the capacious metaphysis typically found in most patients with osteopenia. **B,** Reduction has been achieved with a clamp placed through a small lateral incision. **C,** A clamp is used to reduce a fracture with a subtrochanteric extension. Clamps can be inserted without evacuation of the fracture hematoma and with minimal soft-tissue disruption.

Tip 8: Avoid Varus Angulation of the Proximal Fragment—Use the Relationship Between the Tip of the Trochanter and the Center of the Femoral Head

Varus angulation of the proximal fragment increases the lever arm on the fixation because it makes the femoral neck more horizontal and therefore functionally longer when body weight is applied. This also results in the femoral head fixation being placed more superiorly in the head than is ideal and increases the risk of the device cutting out of the femoral head. It can be difficult to determine the appropriate femoral neck-shaft angle in a patient with an intertrochanteric fracture. When using an intramedullary nail for fixation of an intertrochanteric fracture, most surgeons choose a nail with a 130° neck-shaft configuration (Figure 11). It is important to know the neck-shaft angle of the device that is being used. One way to assess varus or valgus position during surgery is to look at the relationship between the tip of the greater trochanter and the center of the femoral head. These two points should be coplanar. If the center of the femoral head is distal to the tip of the greater trochanter, the reduction is in varus. If the center of the head is proximal to the greater trochanter, the reduction is in valgus. Preoperative plain radiographs of the uninjured hip can be used to assess the patient's normal neck-shaft angle because the two sides are normally symmetric. Varus and high lag screw placement are associated with an increased frequency of failure of fixation with an intramedullary nail and sliding hip screw.[20,21]

Tip 9: When Nailing, Lock the Nail Distally if the Fracture is Axially or Rotationally Unstable

Most unstable fractures of the proximal part of the femur require a long intramedullary nail. If there is any question about the stability of a fracture, then a long nail should be chosen and, in most instances, it should be locked distally.[15,22-24] Although short nails may be used for minimally displaced or nondisplaced fractures or very stable patterns, they can be associated with a subsequent fracture in the subtrochanteric area. Although most modern short nail designs have smaller diameter locking screws in this high-stress area to prevent the fractures that were en-

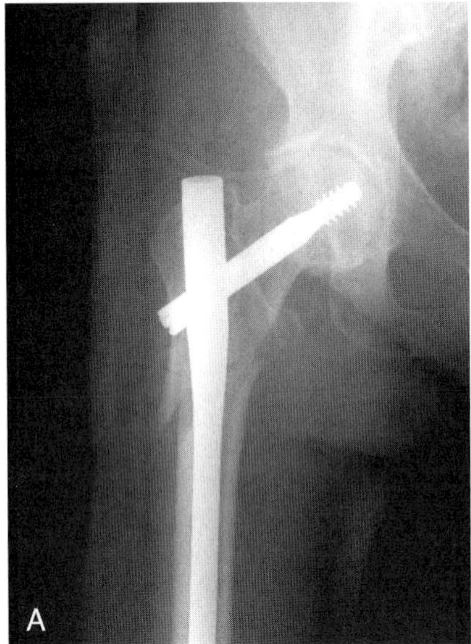

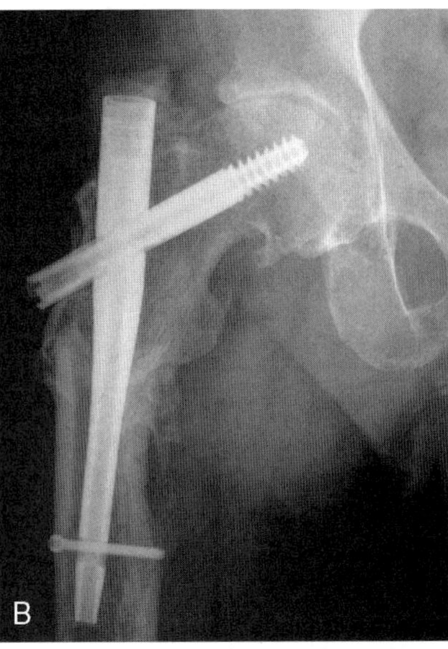

Figure 11 Radiographs of an intertrochanteric fracture. **A,** A well-aligned fracture. Note the central position of the lag screw in the femoral head. **B,** The relationship between the tip of the greater trochanter and the center of the femoral head is shown. Normally, this relationship is coplanar. Here, the proximal fragment is in varus, the starting point is lateral, and the screw is high in the head.

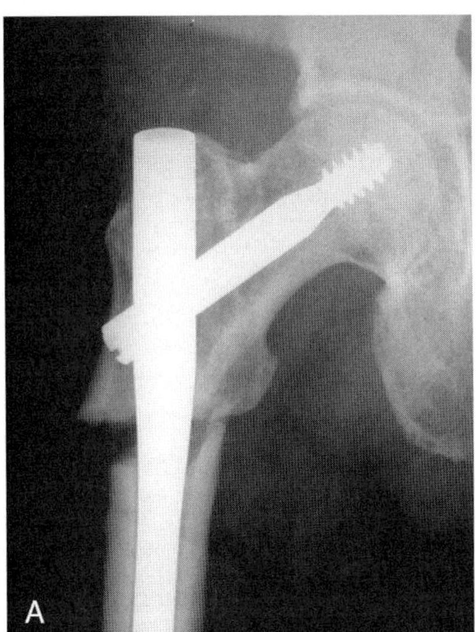

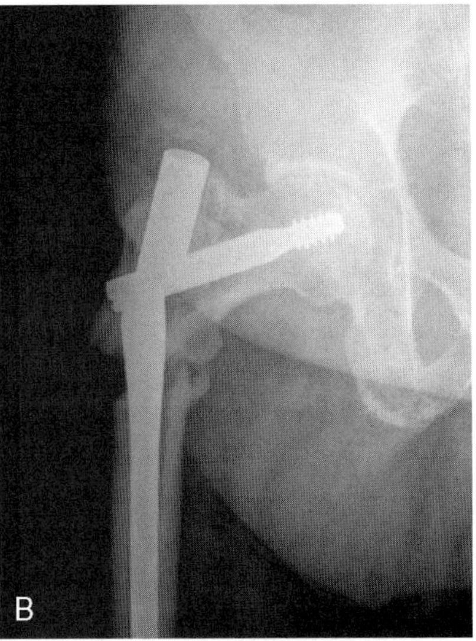

Figure 12 Radiographs showing a fracture locked in distraction. Note the typical lateral starting point and the high hip screw placement **(A)**. Distracted fracture in varus can result in high loads on the implant, causing nail fracture, typically through the aperture for the lag screw **(B)**.

countered with the older, large-diameter locking screw designs, it is probably wise to protect the length of the femur and choose a long nail. Using a long internal fixation device to protect the entire bone is a common principle for treating a pathologic fracture of bone caused by metastatic disease, and it is wise to consider most fragility fractures in elderly patients to be pathologic fractures. In addition, these patients have a propensity for falls, increasing their risk of subsequent fractures.

Tip 10: Avoid Fracture Distraction When Nailing

When nails are used for fractures with a transverse or reverse oblique configuration, it is not uncommon for the fracture to be either malrotated or distracted (Figure 12, *A*). If a fracture is locked in distraction, osseous contact that can accept some of the load with weight bearing does not occur, and the device must withstand all of the forces associated with the activities of daily living. Fractures that are internally fixed in distraction are at risk for nonunion and eventual hardware failure. The nail breaks through its weakest point, which is the large aperture in the nail for the lag screw (Figure 12, *B*). To eliminate distraction, the traction on the lower limb should be released during surgery before insertion of the distal locking screws, and fluoroscopy should be used to confirm that there is bone-on-bone contact.

Summary

Most intertrochanteric hip fractures are treated surgically. Intramedullary nail fixation has become more common, even for fractures that are stable or nondisplaced.[25] Intramedullary nails probably should not be used to treat these simpler types of fractures, and it is probably better to choose sliding hip screws for relatively simple patterns and basicervical patterns. Fixation of a stable or minimally displaced fracture with a sliding hip screw is acceptable, and the complication rate and costs are less. Meta-analyses have demonstrated that the rates of iatrogenic fracture with intramedullary nailing have improved over time, and the risk of femoral shaft fracture with nail insertion has decreased dramatically.[19] This is probably a reflection of the use of modern intramedullary nails with smaller diameters, smaller diameter locking screws, and less acute proximal valgus angles of the proximal nail, as well as the realization that aggressive impaction should be avoided in the nailing of these fractures.

References

1. Baumgaertner MR, Curtin SL, Lindskog DM, Keggi JM: The value of the tip-apex distance in predicting failure of fixation of peritrochanteric fractures of the hip. *J Bone Joint Surg Am* 1995;77:1058-1064.
2. Baumgaertner MR, Solberg BD: Awareness of tip-apex distance reduces failure of fixation of trochanteric fractures of the hip. *J Bone Joint Surg Br* 1997;79:969-971.
3. Kyle RF, Cabanela ME, Russell TA, et al: Fractures of the proximal part of the femur. *Instr Course Lect* 1995;44: 227-253.
4. Kyle RF, Gustilo RB, Premer RF: Analysis of six hundred and twenty-two intertrochanteric hip fractures. *J Bone Joint Surg Am* 1979;61:216-221.
5. Haidukewych GJ, Israel TA, Berry DJ: Reverse obliquity fractures of the intertrochanteric region of the femur. *J Bone Joint Surg Am* 2001;83:643-650.
6. Janzing HM, Houben BJ, Brandt SE, et al: The Gotfried PerCutaneous Compression Plate versus the Dynamic Hip Screw in the treatment of pertrochanteric hip fractures: Minimal invasive treatment reduces operative time and postoperative pain. *J Trauma* 2002;52:293-298.
7. Knight WM, DeLee JC: Nonunion of intertrochanteric fractures of the hip: A case study and review. *Orthop Trans* 1982;6:438.
8. Kosygan KP, Mohan R, Newman RJ: The Gotfried percutaneous compression plate compared with the conventional classic hip screw for the fixation of intertrochanteric fractures of the hip. *J Bone Joint Surg Br* 2002;84: 19-22.
9. Sadowski C, Lübbeke A, Saudan M, Riand N, Stern R, Hoffmeyer P: Treatment of reverse oblique and transverse intertrochanteric fractures with use of an intramedullary nail or a 95 degrees screw-plate: A prospective, randomized study. *J Bone Joint Surg Am* 2002;84:372-381.
10. Kinast C, Bolhofner BR, Mast JW, Ganz R: Subtrochanteric fractures of the femur: Results of treatment with the 95 degrees condylar blade-plate. *Clin Orthop Relat Res* 1989;238: 122-130.
11. Sanders R, Regazzoni P: Treatment of subtrochanteric femur fractures using the dynamic condylar screw. *J Orthop Trauma* 1989;3:206-213.
12. Haidukewych GJ, Berry DJ: Hip arthroplasty for salvage of failed treatment of intertrochanteric hip fractures. *J Bone Joint Surg Am* 2003;85: 899-904.
13. Haidukewych GJ, Berry DJ: Salvage of failed internal fixation of intertrochanteric hip fractures. *Clin Orthop Relat Res* 2003;412:184-188.
14. Koval KJ, Sala DA, Kummer FJ, Zuckerman JD: Postoperative weight-bearing after a fracture of the femoral neck or an intertrochanteric fracture. *J Bone Joint Surg Am* 1998;80: 352-356.
15. van Doorn R, Stapert JW: The long gamma nail in the treatment of 329 subtrochanteric fractures with major extension into the femoral shaft. *Eur J Surg* 2000;166:240-246.
16. Wu CC, Shih CH, Chen WJ, Tai CL: Treatment of cutout of a lag screw of a dynamic hip screw in an intertrochanteric fracture. *Arch Orthop Trauma Surg* 1998;117:193-196.
17. Ostrum RF, Levy MS: Penetration of the distal femoral anterior cortex during intramedullary nailing for subtrochanteric fractures: A report of three cases. *J Orthop Trauma* 2005;19: 656-660.
18. Ostrum RF, Marcantonio A, Marburger R: A critical analysis of the eccentric starting point for trochanteric intramedullary femoral nailing. *J Orthop Trauma* 2005;19:681-686.
19. Bhandari M, Schemitsch E, Jönsson A, Zlowodzki M, Haidukewych GJ: Gamma nails revisited: Gamma nails versus compression hip screws in the management of intertrochanteric fractures of the hip. A meta-analysis. *J Orthop Trauma* 2009;23:460-464.
20. Lindskog DM, Baumgaertner MR: Unstable intertrochanteric hip fractures in the elderly. *J Am Acad Orthop Surg* 2004;12:179-190.
21. Shukla S, Johnston P, Ahmad MA, Wynn-Jones H, Patel AD, Walton NP: Outcome of traumatic subtrochanteric femoral fractures fixed using cephalo-medullary nails. *Injury* 2007; 38:1286-1293.
22. Adams CI, Robinson CM, Court-Brown CM, McQueen MM: Prospective randomized controlled trial of an intramedullary nail versus dynamic screw and plate for intertrochanteric fractures of the femur. *J Orthop Trauma* 2001;15:394-400.
23. Barquet A, Francescoli L, Rienzi D, López L: Intertrochanteric-subtrochanteric fractures: Treatment with the long Gamma nail. *J Orthop Trauma* 2000;14:324-328.
24. Parker MJ, Pryor GA: Gamma versus DHS nailing for extracapsular femoral fractures: Meta-analysis of ten randomised trials. *Int Orthop* 1996;20: 163-168.
25. Anglen JO, Weinstein JN; American Board of Orthopaedic Surgery Research Committee: Nail or plate fixation of intertrochanteric hip fractures: Changing pattern of practice. A review of the American Board of Orthopaedic Surgery database. *J Bone Joint Surg Am* 2008;90:700-707.

Surgical Treatment of Osteoporotic Fractures About the Knee

Daniel S. Horwitz, MD
Erik N. Kubiak, MD

Abstract

The surgical treatment of fractures about the knee in elderly patients and/or those with osteoporosis remains a problematic and evolving challenge to many orthopaedic surgeons. The fundamental issues of poor bone quality, poor hosts, and associated medical comorbidities makes treating these fractures difficult both in terms of the decision-making process and the chosen surgical technique. It is important to review major treatment challenges and the potential solutions for minimizing complications.

Instr Course Lect 2010;59:511-523.

The treatment of osteoporotic fractures of the distal part of the femur and the tibial plateau continues to evolve. New developments with regard to implants and surgical technique now provide improved means of dealing with the numerous biologic and mechanical issues that directly affect patients with osteoporosis. These biologic and mechanical issues commonly include degenerative joint disease, multiple medical comorbidities, limited prefracture activity levels, multiple fracture planes with lower energy injuries, and difficulty with postoperative mobilization.

This patient population has, in general, lower physical demands and activity levels. Although there are some exceptions, most patients with osteoporosis are not running, skiing, or participating in heavy impact aerobic exercise. Further complicating treatment are the multiple medical comorbidities affecting not only the patient's final function but also the soft-tissue and osseous healing capabilities as well as the ability to recover from prolonged inactivity. Baseline weakness and dementia can dramatically affect an elderly patient's ability to protect the surgically treated extremity. This may lead to the use of additional internal fixation or protective spanning external fixation.

It is important to have a comprehensive understanding of a patient's functional level and comorbidities. Patients with osteoporotic bone are often elderly and may have functional, mental, and metabolic issues that affect the degree of correction necessary as well as their ability to withstand a surgical procedure. When a patient has internal fixation, there are additional issues related to the osteoporotic bone. The most common issue is subsidence of the articular surface during the postoperative period. This is the result of decreased bone quality, the inability of current implants to resist axial loads, and a patient's diminished ability to protect the injured lower extremity during mobilization. These problems make postoperative mobilization a challenge.

The complications inherent in the typical osteoporotic patient population are more challenging when there is preexisting degenerative arthritis of the knee. Degenerative arthritis makes precise anatomic restoration (< 2 mm of articular step-off) difficult, if not impossible. Additionally, a knee with degenerative arthritis is less tolerant of mechanical axis deviations;

Dr. Horwitz or an immediate family member has received royalties from DePuy; is a member of a speakers' bureau or has made paid presentations on behalf of DePuy; and serves as a paid consultant for or is an employee of DePuy. Neither Dr. Kubiak nor any immediate family members have received anything of value or own stock in a commercial company or institution related directly or indirectly to the subject of this chapter.

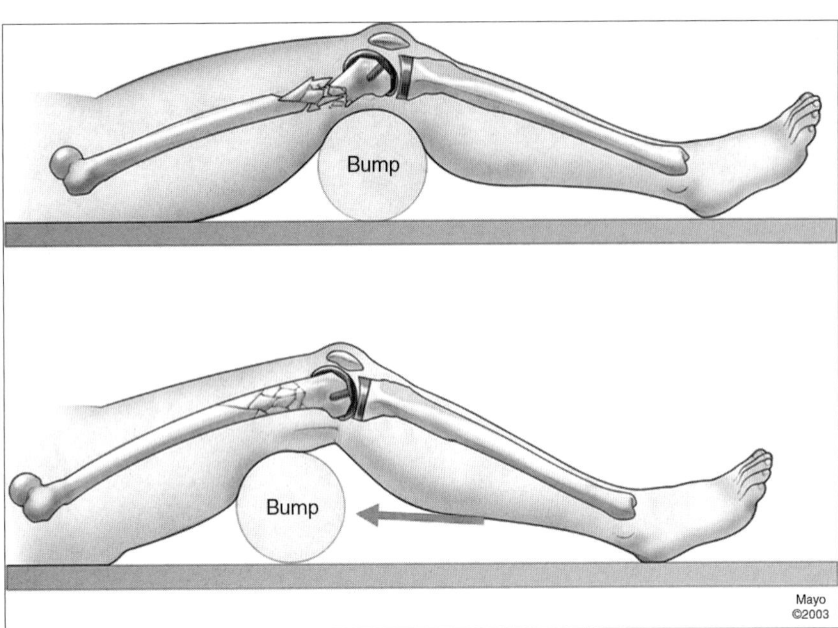

Figure 1 A small round bump is best suited for aiding reduction of the supracondylar fracture. Note that distal placement will result in an extension deformity that is corrected by moving the roll further proximally. (Reproduced with permission from the Mayo Foundation for Medical Education and Research, Rochester, MN.)

therefore, restoration of normal anatomic and mechanical alignment is critical.[1,2] Special instruments and recommendations are suggested to assist practitioners in the treatment of fractures in patients with osteoporosis, with or without degenerative arthritis, and to reduce the risks associated with this patient group.

Fracture Pattern

Osteoporotic bone often has a direct effect on the fracture pattern. Comminuted, multiplanar, intra-articular fractures around the knee seen in young patients are usually caused by high-energy injuries, whereas in patients with osteoporosis they are commonly caused by a low-energy fall. The soft-tissue injury is usually less severe with lower energy fractures, often allowing early or immediate fixation. The patient's comorbidities are more likely to be the factor most responsible for soft-tissue compromise.

Extra-articular Distal Femoral Fractures

A simple distal femoral shaft fracture can usually be treated with either retrograde or antegrade nail fixation; however, a supracondylar femoral fracture is different. When a fracture is distal to the metaphyseal flare, there is less bone available for fixation and there is a risk of malreduction. Treatment of a supracondylar fracture can be further complicated by the presence of a total knee replacement.

The surgical goal for a patient with a total knee replacement and a supracondylar fracture is, in general, restoration of the prefracture alignment. Restoration is necessary because correcting malaligned arthroplasty components results in either fracture gaps or a tilted joint line because the tibial component is not altered to match the new femoral position. When the femoral component is not well fixed, a revision total knee arthroplasty with a stemmed component is the preferred treatment option.

Evaluation and Planning

Evaluation and planning begin with obtaining the appropriate imaging studies. For femoral fractures, a complete set of plain radiographs that include the knee, the femoral shaft, and the hip should be obtained. In addition, if there is any suspicion that the fracture has entered the joint, a fine-cut CT scan with sagittal and coronal reconstructions should be obtained.

For fractures of the femur, it is particularly important to take into account the unique circumstances of patients with osteoporotic bone when choosing an implant. Poor bone quality and the possibility of metastatic bone disease are indications for selecting the longest implants available. Short retrograde nails and short locked plates should be avoided because they produce stress risers in the midpart of the diaphysis. Long implants improve the biomechanical strength of fracture fixation constructs and protect the entire length of the bone. Long locked plates provide axial stability in highly unstable fracture patterns and improved fixation in osteoporotic bone.[3-5]

Positioning and Approach

Malalignment can occur with any of the implants discussed here. To improve fracture reduction, the patient should be totally paralyzed. A roll should be used to correct flexion-extension deformity, with gentle traction applied to the leg, if necessary, to correct varus-valgus alignment (Figure 1). Several other important points with regard to determining the appropriate positioning and approach are specific to the implant that will be used.

Choice of Implants

Retrograde Nail

It is important to understand the most common complications associated with the use of a retrograde nail. These include malalignment caused by a poor starting point, flexion malalignment as a result of the knee flexion required for access to the joint during reaming and nail placement, and insufficient distal stability. Also, there are issues with regard to total knee replacements with fixed components and potentially uncontrollable malalignment.

Flexion of the knee so that the tibial plateau is not in the way is necessary to place a retrograde intramedullary nail. Even with the patient paralyzed, this maneuver generally flexes the distal fragment. It is tempting to move the starting point posteriorly to introduce more extension, but this produces anterior translation. The solution is to use provisional pin fixation from the medial and/or lateral condyle with the knee in extension along with limited roll support under the fracture site. The large intramedullary diameter of the distal part of the femur almost always allows room for both the pins and the reamers and nail. Provisional stabilization of the fracture makes it possible to flex the knee to gain access without producing a deformity at the fracture site.

The anatomy of the distal part of the femur allows good osseous contact of the retrograde nail in the subchondral region but no contact at the fracture site. As a result, the starting point for a retrograde nail determines flexion, extension, varus, valgus, and multidirectional translation. The ideal site for entry of a retrograde nail into the distal part of the femur has been well described, and, although absolute precision is not necessary, variance of more than several millimeters can be a problem.[6]

In almost all femora, the optimal entry site, in line with the long axis of the femur, is located 6 to 8 mm anterior to the posterior cruciate ligament insertion and slightly medial to the center of the intercondylar groove. The distal fracture fragment can be directly manipulated with the use of bone clamps or Steinmann pins, but the deforming forces caused by a misplaced starting hole often cannot be overcome. Starting too anterior or posterior results in flexion-extension deformity, and starting too medial or lateral results in translation of the distal fragment in the opposite direction unless varus or valgus deformity is accepted. Thus, the starting point for the retrograde nail is perhaps the most important and technically challenging part of the surgical procedure. Slight deformity at the fracture site can generally be manually corrected before placing distal interlocking screws, if close attention was paid to the initial entry site. For proper placement of the initial entry site, the starting guidewire should be inserted with fluoroscopic confirmation in two planes and to a depth of at least 8 to 10 cm so that actual alignment and orientation can be confirmed before drilling a larger entry hole.

In a patient with a periprosthetic supracondylar fracture in the femur, the approach may be limited by the previous surgery and the implant position. A femoral component that is medial or lateral in relation to the femoral shaft causes displacement of the distal fragment in the opposite direction when retrograde nail fixation is used. Similarly, if the femoral component is in excessive flexion or extension, the postfixation alignment will be opposite to this original deformity (Figure 2). An open-box total knee arthroplasty implant with metal extending posteriorly causes a similar deformity. In this circumstance, an extension deformity is produced by the retrograde intramedullary nail. There are situations in which a retrograde nail cannot be used because of the position or type of total knee replacement; in those instances a locked supracondylar plate is preferred.

Another limitation of retrograde nail fixation for these fractures that is beyond the control of the surgeon is the poor cancellous bone, even when multiple interlocking screws are used.[7] Many systems include an interference screw that can be placed in the most distal screw hole to convert the nail to a fixed-angle device. However, these systems still fail because the osteoporotic cancellous bone is inadequate, and it is not uncommon for these distal femoral fractures to drift into valgus at the site of the nail fixation.

Additional stability as well as some degree of angular correction can be achieved with blocking screws placed in the distal fracture fragment. The blocking screws must be in direct contact with the nail. To accomplish this, the drill used for the blocking screw should partially overlap the nail on the fluoroscopic image so that the nail deflects the drill as it passes from anterior to posterior. This technique ensures that the blocking screw will directly impinge against the nail, providing the desired stability.

Locked Supracondylar Plate

Several issues associated with retrograde nail fixation, the most important of which are distal fixation and stability, are addressed by using a locked supracondylar plate. The common issues related to the use of locked supracondylar plates for extra-articular distal femoral frac-

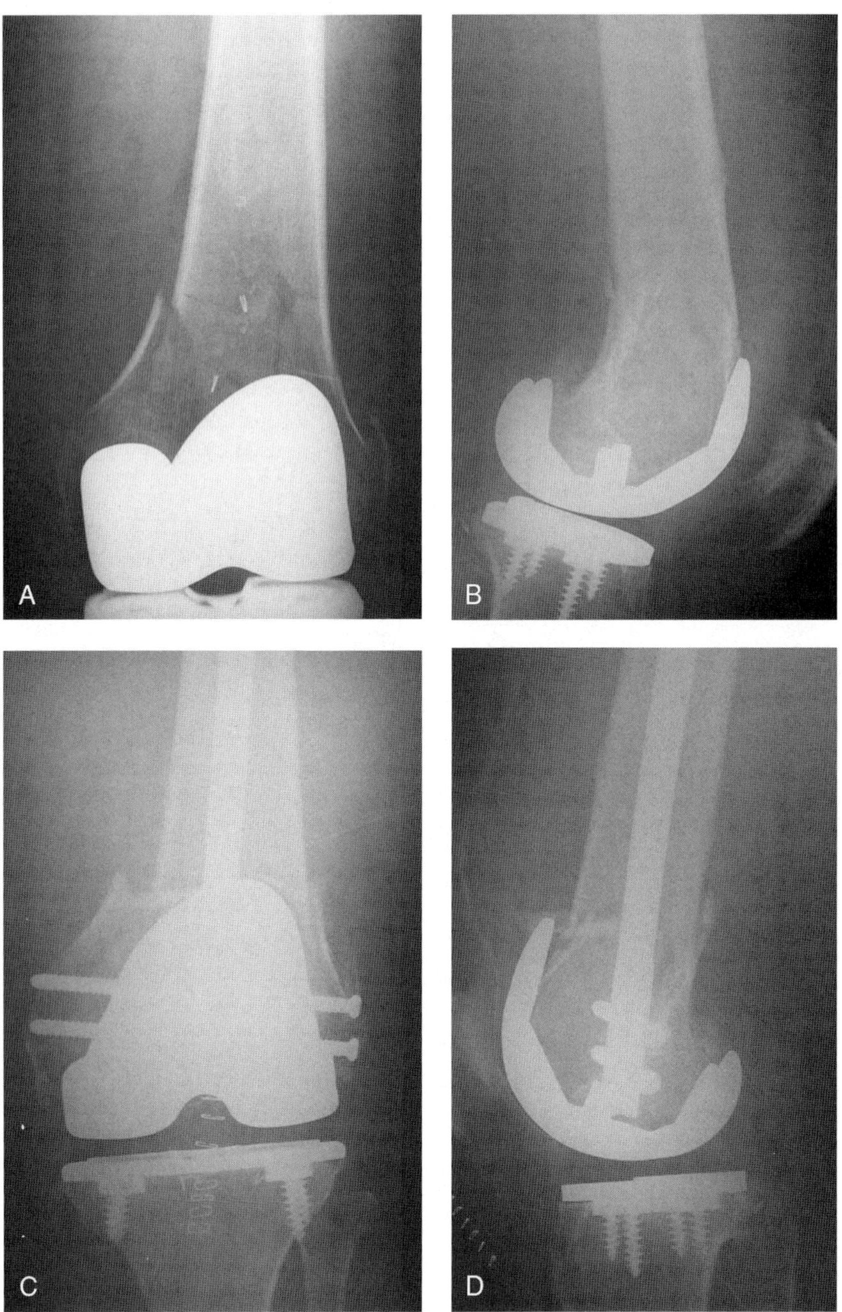

Figure 2 Preoperative (**A** and **B**) and postoperative (**C** and **D**) radiographs of a supracondylar periprosthetic fracture. Note the postoperative extension and medial displacement that are a direct result of the preoperative component position.

tures are appropriate plate length, malalignment, and interference with total knee arthroplasty pegs. Multiple locked screws in the distal part of the femur offer better overall stability and less motion after cyclic loading than do retrograde nails, and the success of these plates has been reported in clinical series.[3,8] Unfortunately, they bring their own new technical challenges.

Plate length is important in a patient with osteoporosis, both for fixation of the condylar fragment and to avoid creation of stress risers in the femoral shaft. Using a long plate, although leaving some screw holes without screws, provides better fixation with less chance of failure at the proximal part of the diaphysis caused by either pull-out of screws or a fracture at the tip of the plate.[9] There is no absolute rule for implant length, but it has been recommended that a lateral locked plate extend past the midpart of the diaphysis.

Medium-sized pins can be used for provisional fixation, and percutaneous techniques are recommended for placement of the long locking implant. In the absence of a prefracture deformity, the reference wire and subsequently used locked screw should be parallel to the joint surface. The chapter's authors prefer placing the reference wire with a distal clamp in place, clamping or lagging the diaphysis to the plate, and confirming alignment before placing any distal locked screws (Figure 3). When varus-valgus alignment is acceptable, any flexion-extension deformity can be corrected with the reference pin in place by manipulating the distal fragment either directly or by adjusting the roll under the lower limb. When the amount of comminution causes a large medial gap when the limb is brought to its proper length, it is better to accept shortening and achieve bone contact than to leave the gap. The same issues of prefracture implant position and risk of malalignment that were identified for intramedullary fixation in a patient with a fracture and a total knee replacement apply to the use of plate fixation in such a patient. The pegs in the femoral component can create problems. The reference wire and screw may pass them, although one or more of the

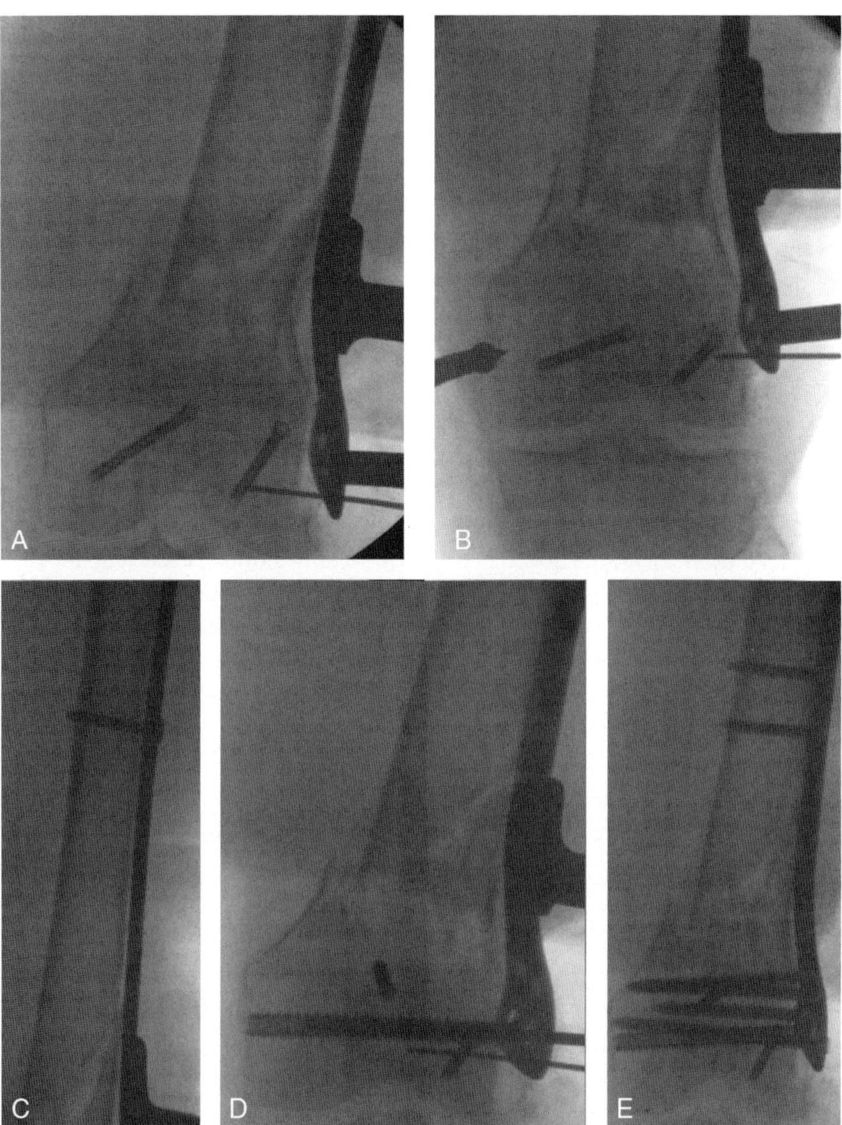

Figure 3 Intraoperative images show the sequence for plate application for a complex supracondylar fracture. Initially, the plate is clamped to the distal fragment (**A** and **B**). This is followed by proximal lag nonlocking fixation (**C**), then by placement of a distal reference wire and screw, and finally by complete proximal and distal screw fixation (**D** and **E**).

distal locked screws will impinge on or be blocked by them. Polyaxial locked screws are available and can be used in this situation. The stability and strength of polyaxial systems are adequate, and they allow the locked screws to be in direct contact with the prosthesis, which prevents osteopenic bone failure around the more rigid implant.[10]

Clamps on the distal fracture fragment can penetrate osteoporotic bone and reduce bone stock. Using the so-called lunar lander attachments on large periarticular clamps minimizes this risk. Large locked supracondylar femoral plates are difficult to revise, so one must be sure that the alignment is acceptable before most of the distal locked screws are placed. Intraoperative plain radiographs are recommended.

Intra-articular Distal Femoral Fractures

The challenges presented by intra-articular distal femoral fractures through osteoporotic bone are similar to those presented by such fractures through normal bone. The interventions for both injuries have the common goals of joint reduction, restoration of axial alignment, and early motion. Simple unicondylar fractures can be managed with direct exposure and buttress plate fixation. In contrast, locked supracondylar plates have made almost all other implants obsolete for the treatment of more complex bicondylar fractures. Complex comminuted fractures in osteoporotic bone are often caused by low-energy injuries, and, as a result, early definitive fixation is often possible. The issues specifically related to patients with osteoporotic bone are the need and/or desire for disimpaction of the articular surface, acceptance of shortening, and the potential need for bridging or protective external fixation.

When the distal articular surface of the femur is compressed or impacted, elevation is difficult, and restoration of the natural curved contour is almost impossible. This impaction pattern is more common in osteoporotic bone. Even when the articular surface can be elevated successfully, providing structural support beneath it becomes difficult. The choice is between accepting 1 to 2 mm of impaction in the weight-bearing surface or disimpacting the fragments and struggling to hold them in place. This decision is made on an individual basis, and it is important to recognize the inherent limitations and goals of the treatment of this injury.

Restoring anatomic length is less important than restoring overall axial alignment and achieving successful healing. After the articular surface has been restored to an acceptable degree, varus-valgus and flexion-extension alignment are obtained using the previously discussed techniques. The stability of the construct is determined after the joint has been reduced, alignment has been restored, and a long locked plate has been secured.

Fragmentation of the distal fracture fragment is the cause of early failure of the more complex intra-articular fractures in osteoporotic bone. Although interfragmentary screw fixation outside the plate helps to minimize this risk, additional protection may be needed. A bridging external fixator may be used because a brace or cast is insufficient. Applying an external fixator to the femur is difficult when there is a long plate; therefore, a shorter plate is often chosen when the possible use of a supplemental external fixator is anticipated. The fixator is placed in a neutral position so that the locked plate construct is protected rather than stressed by the fixator. In addition, neutral or slight distraction of the joint, not compression, should be the goal. The chapter's authors prefer to have the knee in full extension; the frame is removed after 6 to 8 weeks.

Tibial Plateau Fractures

Treatment goals for tibial plateau fractures in osteoporotic bone are the same as those for such fractures in normal bone. These goals are to restore articular congruity, limb length, anatomic rotation and alignment, and provide sufficient stability for union and function. However, the usual techniques require modifications in the presence of weak osteoporotic bone.

A patient's functional abilities are an important consideration, as those with limited function may not require the same degree of correction as those with greater function. Additionally, elderly patients may have several comorbidities that make it unlikely that they can tolerate a long surgical procedure. Midway through a dual approach to a bicondylar tibial plateau fracture is not the time to suspend the operation. Instead, a planned staged procedure may be more desirable for the patient and the surgical team.

Evaluation and Planning

A complete set of plain radiographs is essential. For tibial plateau fractures, this set should include four views of the knee and two views of the entire tibia. A fine-cut CT scan with coronal and sagittal reconstructions should be obtained for all fractures. If a fracture is axially unstable or associated with severe soft-tissue damage, joint-spanning external fixation should be placed before CT is performed.

The displacement of the unstable segment of the tibial plateau will be evident on inspection of the initial plain radiographs, and the direction of the displacement determines the position of the dominant segment. The CT scans and plain radiographs will clearly show the depressed articular fracture components. It is important to determine if the tibial tubercle is a free segment; if it is, it needs to be affixed to the distal part of the tibia. This may require additional implants to buttress the articular segments and fix the articular surface to the tibial shaft. Depressed articular segments are elevated regardless of whether they are medial or lateral. Most depressed articular fragments involve the lateral tibial plateau, but their position in the lateral condyle varies with the fracture pattern. Displaced metaphyseal-diaphyseal fragments are buttressed to the tibial shaft. The most common buttress plate positions are posteromedial and anterolateral, and not unexpectedly the most frequent surgical approaches are posteromedial and anterolateral.

Special Instruments

The surgical treatment of osteoporotic bicondylar fractures requires the same special instruments used for bicondylar fractures in normal bone. Key instruments are a complete set of bone tamps, including the curved tamps; a set of curved and straight osteotomes; and a large femoral distractor.

Patient Positioning

The patient is positioned supine on a radiolucent flat-top operating table with the ipsilateral arm across the chest. As a first step, the external rotation of the hip must be evaluated. If the patient has normal external rotation and an isolated tibial plateau fracture, no further positioning of the trunk is necessary. If the patient has an isolated tibial plateau fracture and restricted external rotation of the ipsilateral hip, a 6-inch (15.2-cm) diameter bump extending from under the ilium to the scapula positions the patient so that the patella points toward the ceiling. Additional bumps or a wedge may be necessary to support a rigid thoracic kyphosis, an ankylosed lumbar spine, or a rigid arthritic cervical spine. To allow easy access to the medial and lateral sides of the plateau and unobstructed imaging with the image intensifier, the leg that is to be operated is elevated on additional bumps. The patient's thorax and contralateral leg are then secured to the operating table. A well-padded tourniquet is applied to the proximal part of the thigh.

The image intensifier should be brought in from the contralateral side in most cases, but when the medial side is the most involved, the intensifier is brought in from the ipsilateral side. The image intensifier is used while the depressed fracture fragments are elevated with the bone tamp, the osteotome is positioned, and the amount of joint elevation and reduction is determined.

Choice of Approach

Careful attention to the soft tissue is important, particularly in elderly patients. In general, the tourniquet is not inflated unless it is necessary to improve visualization when the articular cartilage surface is being reduced. The use of self-retaining retractors should be avoided; instead, handheld Sofield or Langenbeck retractors should be used to minimize tension on the skin. Electrocautery is used sparingly during the initial dissection to minimize thermal injury to the dermis and subcutaneous tissues. Anterolateral flaps are elevated along with the deep fascia of the anterior compartment; the maximal safe medial extension of the lateral dissection is the lateral aspect of the tibial tubercle. The diaphyseal components of long periarticular plates are placed submuscularly and extraperiosteally.

There are key points specific to the lateral approach. The chapter's authors use a lazy-S incision to the lateral plateau because it does not compromise the iliotibial band and can be easily extended proximally and distally, but an L-shaped approach is useful, particularly if the primary aim of the lateral approach is joint elevation. The extensile medial approach is essential for the treatment of medial joint depression and fracture displacement. This approach is used for treating Schatzker type IV tibial plateau fractures[11] (Figure 4) and certain bicondylar tibial plateau fractures. The posteromedial fragment of the medial plateau can be properly buttressed only through the medial approach. When there is associated medial depression of the medial plateau, it can be elevated under direct visualization by using a submeniscal approach between the superficial and deep medial collateral ligaments. Release of the insertion of the semimembranosus from the proximal part of the tibia and the lateral aspect of the gastrocnemius from the femur allows maximal exposure, when necessary.

Methods of Joint Elevation and Grafting

Articular impaction typically occurs on the lateral side. Unlike the focal depressed segments observed in normal bone, the depressed segments in osteoporotic bone often are diffuse and multifragmentary and involve most of the tibial plateau. Often, the depressed segment is a thin section of corticocancellous subchondral bone lying above a cavitated metaphyseal-diaphyseal segment (Figure 5). This affects the choice of the bone graft, the method of fixation, and the approach. The meniscus in an elderly patient is typically firm and friable. Despite this, it is important to repair the meniscus to protect the articular surface. A submeniscal arthrotomy is performed to visualize the articular surface and facilitate the meniscal repair. Prior to the arthrotomy, a lateral femoral distractor is placed; one 5-mm Schanz pin is inserted in the distal part of the femur, and one 5-mm pin is placed in the lateral part of the tibia, distal to where the lateral plate is to be applied. The submeniscal arthrotomy leaves the coronary ligament inferior to the meniscus, which often appears bluish as a result of hemarthrosis, attached to the tibial plateau. A linear incision is first made parallel to the tibial plateau to ensure that the exposure is submeniscal. Once it is established that the incision is submeniscal, it is extended anteriorly and posteriorly. If the femoral condyle is visible, the meniscus is torn. If the meniscus is not visible, it is either trapped in the articular depression or flipped into the intercondylar notch. The meniscus often remains attached at its anterior and posterior horns. Varus stress to the joint with the femoral distractor permits visualization of the joint, and a Freer elevator can be used to free the meniscus and restore it to its native position. Temporary sutures placed in the periphery of the meniscus are used to aid in its retrieval. Size 1 or 0 sutures are placed perpendicular to the meniscus sequentially, from posterior to anterior through the periphery, and individually held with hemostats.

Critical to the treatment of tibial plateau fractures with joint depression is elevation of the depressed segment; this is particularly true for patients with poor bone quality. Elevation of the articular surface is performed under direct visualization. All attempts are made not to window open the lateral plateau fragments so that the periosteal ring of the proximal plateau is maintained. This prevents loss of containment of the multiple fragments of the tibial plateau. If the lateral split opens inadvertently during the approach, it can be gently opened fully for en bloc elevation of the articular sur-

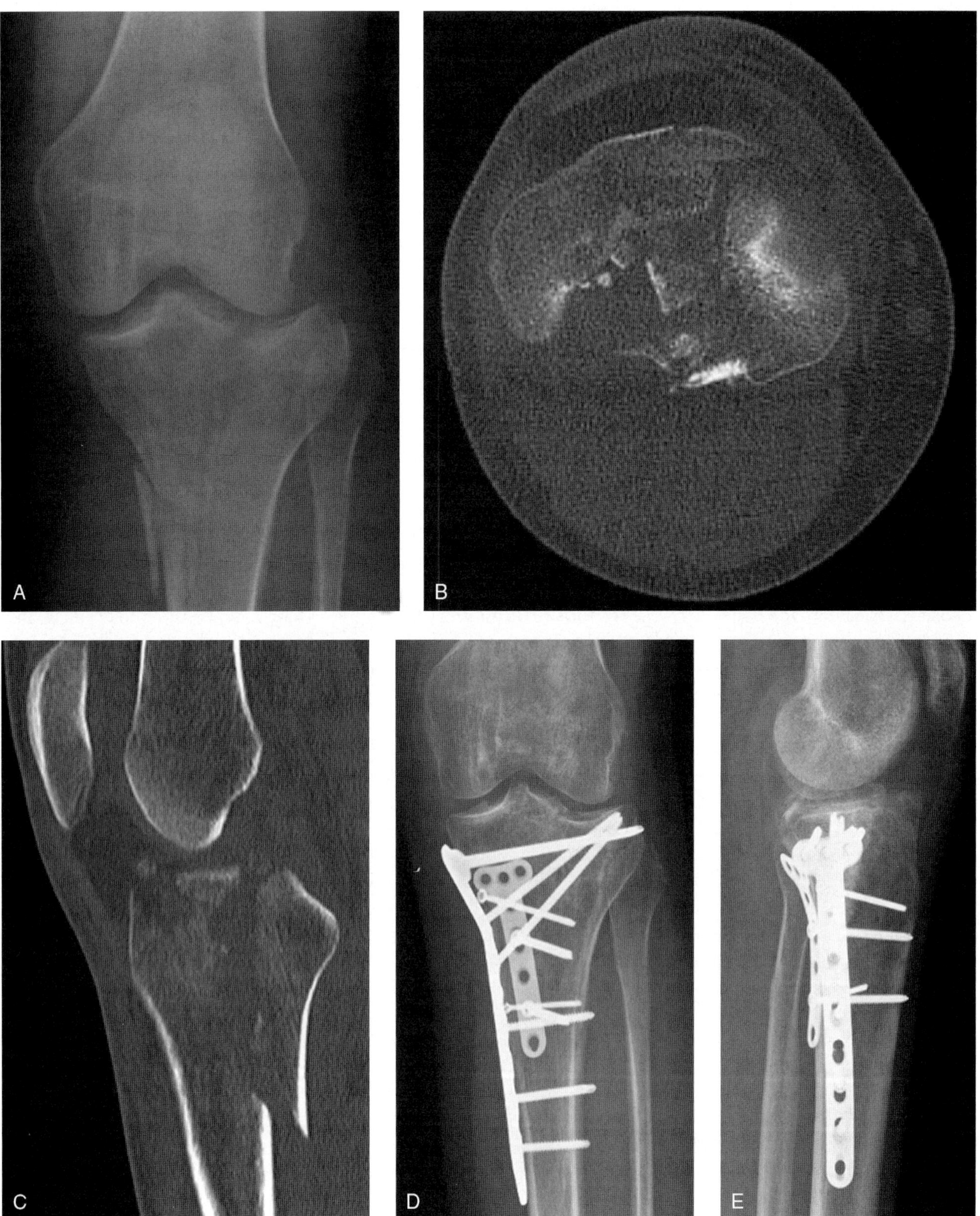

Figure 4 **A,** Radiograph of the knee of a 60-year-old woman who fell off her bicycle and sustained a Schatzker type IV tibial plateau fracture. **B,** The diffuse fragmentation of the tibial plateau is characteristic of osteopenic bone. **C,** The large posteromedial fragment will be difficult to reduce, fix, or buttress from the lateral side of the tibial plateau. **D** and **E,** The reduction and fixation were best achieved using a medial approach.

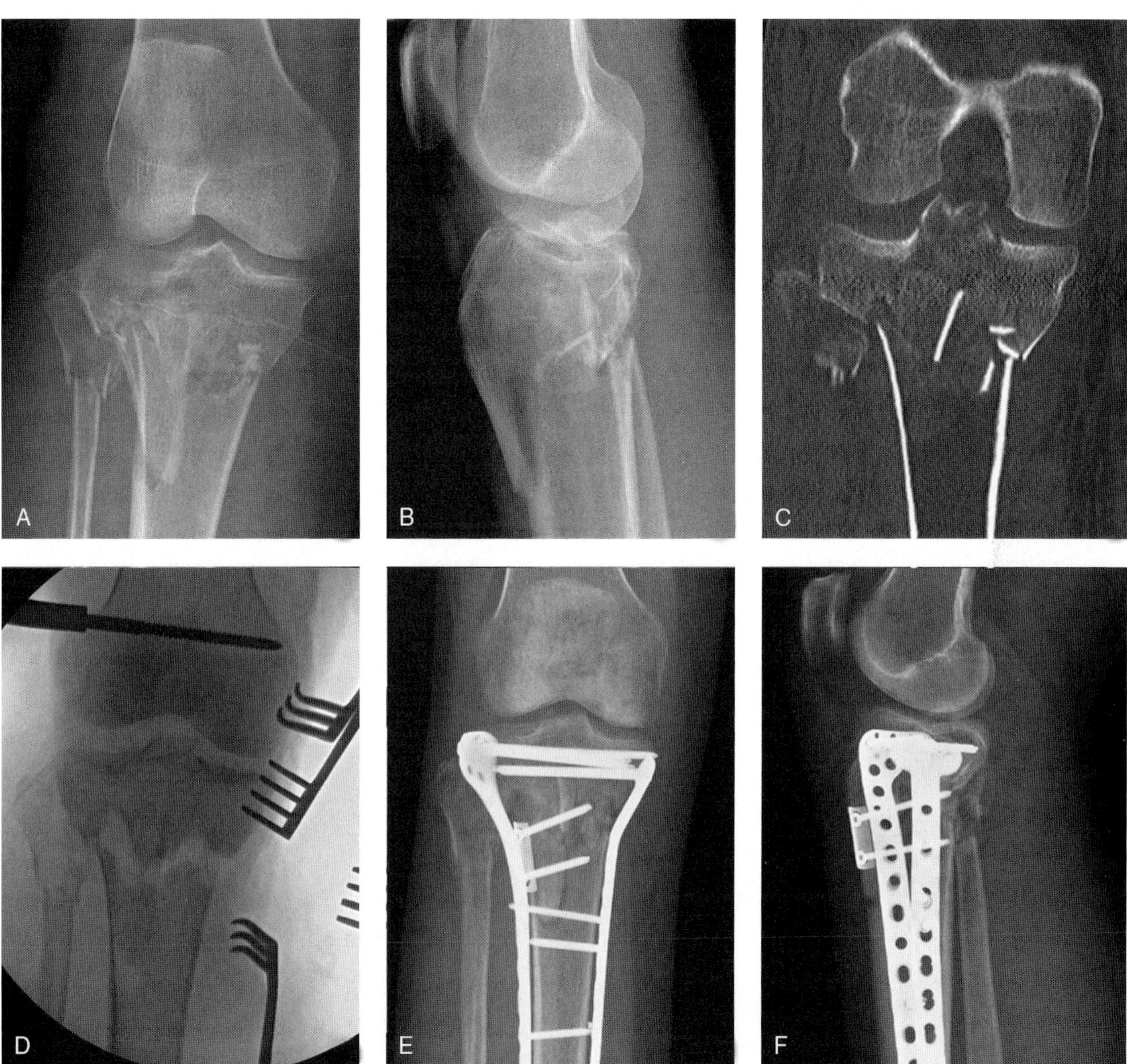

Figure 5 **A** and **B**, Radiographs of the knee of an 86-year-old woman who sustained a bicondylar tibial plateau fracture after falling 6 ft (1.8 m). **C**, The CT scan shows bicondylar metaphyseal-diaphyseal impaction. **D**, After reestablishment of limb length, transmetaphyseal-diaphyseal bone loss from impaction of osteopenic bone is readily apparent. **E** and **F**, Bilateral locked plates with supplemental tibial tubercle fixation reestablished limb length, rotation, and alignment of the proximal part of the tibia.

face. If the rim opens, the articular surface is elevated remotely (1 to 1.5 cm distal to the articular surface) with a wide osteotome acting as a skid. All impacted cancellous bone all of the way around the fragment should be freed before attempting to elevate the depressed fragment (Figure 6).

When the periphery of the plateau is intact, the depressed segment is elevated remotely on a "cloud" of bone. When the depressed articular segment is clearly visible through the arthrotomy site, the image intensifier is less necessary. A corticotomy of the anterolateral aspect of the tibia is created by drilling four holes with a 2.5-mm drill bit in a rectangular pattern in the anterolateral aspect of the cortex just inferior to the lateral flare of the plateau. Once created, the drill holes are connected with a 1-cm osteotome to create a cortical window. Bone graft is impacted with bone tamps through the remote corticotomy,

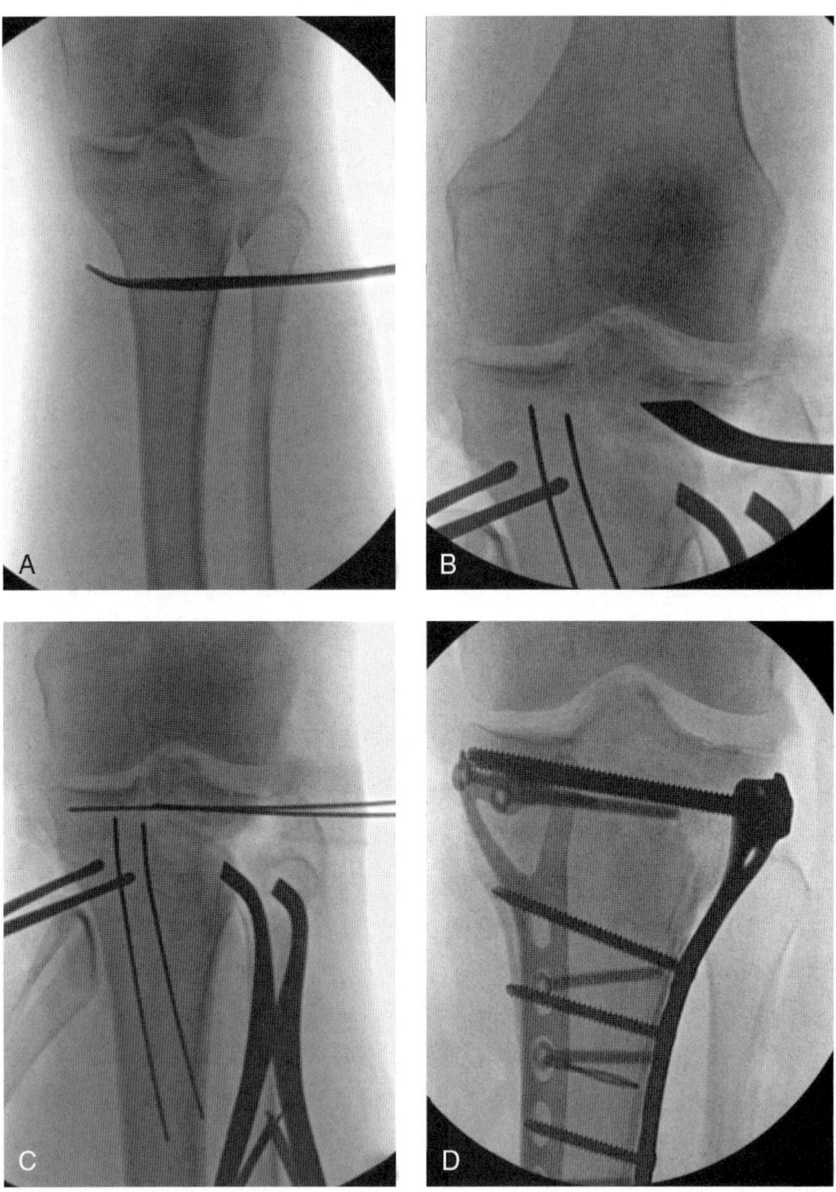

Figure 6 **A,** A bicondylar tibial plateau fracture with a lateral articular segment. **B,** The articular surface is elevated with an osteotome. **C,** Subchondral 0.062-inch (0.157-cm) Kirschner wires provisionally support the articular segment. **D,** A posteromedial buttress plate and a lateral periarticular plate have been used to stabilize the tibial plateau after elevation and bone grafting.

with or without the aid of an image intensifier. The impacted bone graft will elevate the articular surface (Figure 7). Use of gentle taps with a mallet to impact and elevate is a more controlled technique than gross movements of the hand. It is necessary to beware of inadvertent chondral perforation with the osteotome or bone tamps. Once the articular surface is elevated, provisional subchondral 0.062-inch (0.157-cm) Kirschner wires support the articular surface. These may be retained or removed after so-called raft screws have been placed through a periarticular plate or rim plate. Raft (or rafter) screws are a series of parallel or slightly divergent screws placed in a single plane just below the elevated articular surface. Their purpose is to act like the rafters in a roof and support the newly elevated articular surface.

Once elevated, the depressed articular segment is supported with bone graft or bone graft substitute. Allograft is ideally suited in these cases because it is available in almost unlimited quantities, is inexpensive, readily osteointegrates, can be impacted very densely, can be fine-tuned to a size that is ideal for elevation and support, and is more reliably directed than injectable cements. Both allograft and autograft, however, may be more likely to subside than biologic cements.[12] Allograft may also be less than ideal in very osteoporotic patients if it is harder than the native bone because it creates a risk of fragmentation of the subchondral surface during elevation.

There is increasing evidence supporting the use of biologic cements, despite their increased cost compared with allograft and autograft. The osteointegration of biologic cements and the durability of subchondral support vary with the composition of the cement, and the surgeon must evaluate each cement to ensure its appropriateness. Clinical and basic science data support the use of biologic cements to facilitate early weight bearing, which may be advantageous for an elderly patient.

The bone cements cannot be used to elevate the articular surface; this must be done manually by the surgeon. The elevated articular surface must be sealed to prevent extravasation of the cement into the knee joint, and the field must be as dry as possible before the cement is

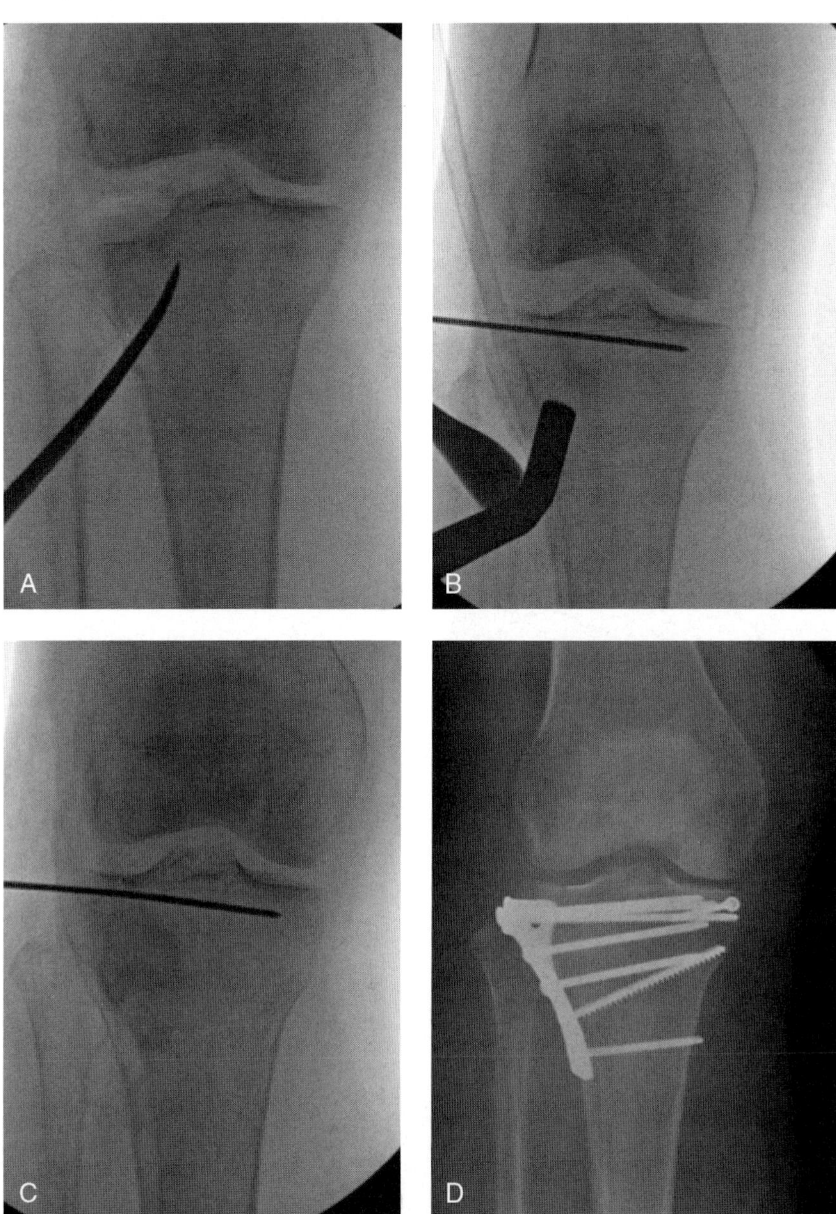

Figure 7 **A,** Through a lateral corticotomy, the narrow osteotome creates subarticular space for a bone graft "cloud." **B,** Bone graft elevates the articular surface when impacted with a bone tamp. **C,** Kirschner wires maintain articular elevation temporarily. **D,** Lateral fixation of the plateau, with bone graft in place.

placed. Placing the biologic cement in a warmer before use speeds up the setting process, thereby avoiding "wash away" by blood. Additionally, these fillers are not intended to be drilled, and instruments cannot be inserted into them. Thus, the cement must be used after the hardware is placed, or it must be injected into places where hardware is not intended to go. The authors of this chapter use biologic cements to fill large metaphyseal voids after joint elevation has been achieved (with or without allografting) and often after the instrumentation has been placed. In this setting, the cements prevent joint subsidence and protect the fixation construct during the initial phases of weight bearing.[13,14]

Choice of Implants

The implants used depend on the fracture type. As a general rule, multiple small articular raft (or rafter) screws provide better subchondral support than do a few large raft screws.[15,16] Depressed and minimally displaced split depressed unicondylar fractures are fixed with raft screws and nonlocked periarticular plates. When the contralateral condyle is osteoporotic, a periarticular locked plate is used so that the articular raft is fixed to the plate and not completely dependent on medial cortical support. Bicondylar fractures with a large minimally displaced medial fragment are treated with a lateral locked plate. If there is medial metaphyseal-diaphyseal comminution, a simple medial percutaneous plate can be added to prevent varus deformity (Figure 8). A medial locked plate is recommended in addition to the posteromedial buttress plate to fix fractures with metaphyseal-diaphyseal comminution (Figure 6) because the currently available locked plates do not adequately address the posteromedial fragment.[4,17] The medial plate is initially fixed to the shaft, and medial raft screws are not placed completely across the tibial plateau until the lateral plateau has been elevated and the width of the tibial plateau has been corrected. The correction of plateau width occurs after the lateral plateau has been elevated and the lateral buttress plate or lateral locked plate is in its provisional position and provisionally fixed with Kirschner wires to the tibia.

As discussed previously, there are occasions when bone quality is so poor that stability is inadequate despite multiple approaches and the

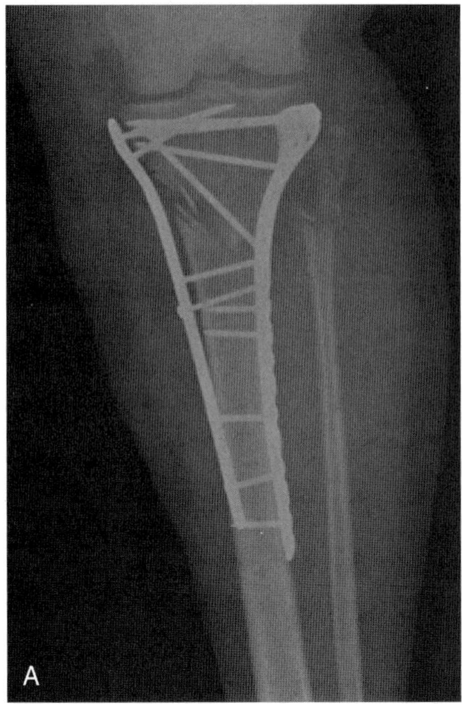

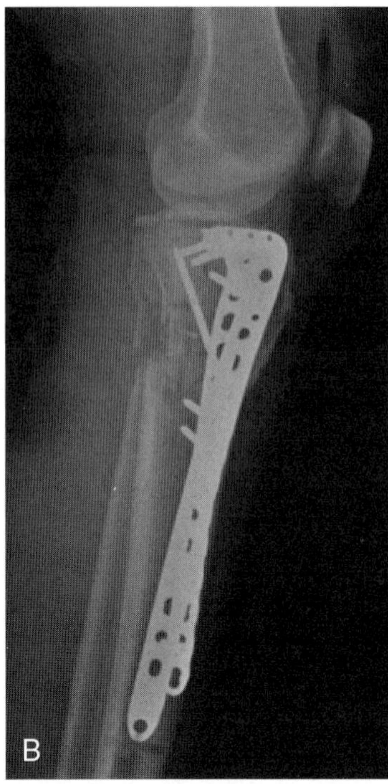

Figure 8 **A** and **B,** The dominant lateral fixation has been augmented by a percutaneously placed medial plate to prevent varus collapse.

aggressive use of locked plates. In these situations, bridging external fixation should be used to protect the reconstructed joint. As is the case with distal femoral fractures, the pins should be placed at least several centimeters away from any deep hardware, the knee should be kept in full extension, and the frame should be in a neutral position so that it does not load the restored joint in any way. The frame is left in place for 6 to 8 weeks, and passive, active, and active-assisted range-of-motion exercises are begun immediately after removal. However, weight bearing is delayed until 12 weeks after surgery.

Closure

The wounds should be closed in layers, with Hemovac drains (if necessary) placed in the deepest layer against the bone. It is very important to have a secure fascial layer over the lateral plate, and, if necessary, a fascial release is performed posteriorly in the lateral compartment to achieve this coverage. The subcutaneous and fascial layers are closed with 2.0 absorbable sutures. The skin is closed with 3.0 nylon sutures placed in a Donati-Allgower fashion or with an alternate retention suture technique.

Postoperative Care

Postoperative management of an elderly patient with osteoporotic bone is complicated by a loss of upper extremity muscle mass and decreased core strength, which make not bearing weight on the injured extremity extremely difficult. The use of crutches or a walker to protect a lower extremity of an elderly person is difficult and may result in partial weight bearing. The use of a wheelchair is preferred if the patient is unable to protect the extremity. Elderly patients often need to adhere to a non–weight-bearing protocol for 12 weeks, especially after internal fixation of a complex axially unstable fracture. At 3 to 4 weeks after surgery, mobilizing patients in a pool with water at the level of the shoulders is considered to be safe and beneficial. A knee immobilizer is also used for the first 2 weeks to protect the wound, with supervised gentle range-of-motion exercises usually started as soon as the wound can tolerate motion. A team approach with the aid of a geriatric provider or hospitalist may improve the patient's care.

References

1. Stevens DG, Beharry R, McKee MD, Waddell JP, Schemitsch EH: The long-term functional outcome of operatively treated tibial plateau fractures. *J Orthop Trauma* 2001;15:312-320.
2. Weigel DP, Marsh JL: High-energy fractures of the tibial plateau: Knee function after longer follow-up. *J Bone Joint Surg Am* 2002;84-A:1541-1551.
3. Zlowodzki M, Williamson S, Cole PA, Zardiackas LD, Kregor PJ: Biomechanical evaluation of the less invasive stabilization system, angled blade plate, and retrograde intramedullary nail for the internal fixation of distal femur fractures. *J Orthop Trauma* 2004;18:494-502.
4. Higgins TF, Klatt J, Bachus KN: Biomechanical analysis of bicondylar tibial plateau fixation: How does lateral locking plate fixation compare to dual plate fixation? *J Orthop Trauma* 2007;21:301-306.
5. Koval KJ, Hoehl JJ, Kummer FJ, Simon JA: Distal femoral fixation: A biomechanical comparison of the standard condylar buttress plate, a locked buttress plate, and the 95-degree blade plate. *J Orthop Trauma* 1997;11:521-524.

6. Krupp RJ, Malkani AL, Goodin RA, Voor MJ: Optimal entry point for retrograde femoral nailing. *J Orthop Trauma* 2003;17:100-105.
7. Janzing HM, Stockman B, Van Damme G, Rommens P, Broos PL: The retrograde intramedullary supracondylar nail: An alternative in the treatment of distal femoral fractures in the elderly? *Arch Orthop Trauma Surg* 1998;118:92-95.
8. Large TM, Kellam JF, Bosse MJ, Sims SH, Althausen P, Masonis JL: Locked plating of supracondylar periprosthetic femur fractures. *J Arthroplasty* 2008;23(6, suppl 1):115-120.
9. Sanders R, Haidukewych GJ, Milne T, Dennis J, Latta LL: Minimal versus maximal plate fixation techniques of the ulna: The biomechanical effect of number of screws and plate length. *J Orthop Trauma* 2002;16: 166-171.
10. Haidukewych G, Sems SA, Huebner D, Horwitz D, Levy B: Results of polyaxial locked-plate fixation of periarticular fractures of the knee: Surgical technique. *J Bone Joint Surg Am* 2008;90(suppl 2 pt 1):117-134.
11. Schatzker J, McBroom R, Bruce D: The tibial plateau fracture: The Toronto experience, 1968-1975. *Clin Orthop Relat Res* 1979;138:94-104.
12. Bajammal SS, Zlowodzki M, Lelwica A, et al: The use of calcium phosphate bone cement in fracture treatment: A meta-analysis of randomized trials. *J Bone Joint Surg Am* 2008;90:1186-1196.
13. Lobenhoffer P, Gerich T, Witte F, Tscherne H: Use of an injectable calcium phosphate bone cement in the treatment of tibial plateau fractures: A prospective study of twenty-six cases with twenty-month mean follow-up. *J Orthop Trauma* 2002;16:143-149.
14. Russell TA, Leighton RK; Alpha-BSM Tibial Plateau Fracture Study Group: Comparison of autogenous bone graft and endothermic calcium phosphate cement for defect augmentation in tibial plateau fractures: A multicenter, prospective, randomized study. *J Bone Joint Surg Am* 2008; 90:2057-2061.
15. Cooper HJ, Kummer FJ, Egol KA, Koval KJ: The effect of screw type on the fixation of depressed fragments in tibial plateau fractures. *Bull Hosp Jt Dis* 2002;60:72-75.
16. Patil S, Mahon A, Green S, McMurtry I, Port A: A biomechanical study comparing a raft of 3.5 mm cortical screws with 6.5 mm cancellous screws in depressed tibial plateau fractures. *Knee* 2006;13:231-235.
17. Barei DP, O'Mara TJ, Taitsman LA, Dunbar RP, Nork SE: Frequency and fracture morphology of the posteromedial fragment in bicondylar tibial plateau fracture patterns. *J Orthop Trauma* 2008;22:176-182.

Acute Trauma to the Upper Extremity: What to Do and When to Do It

Jennifer Moriatis Wolf, MD
George S. Athwal, MD, FRCS(C)
Alexander Y. Shin, MD
David G. Dennison, MD

Abstract

The management of acute trauma to the upper extremity includes the urgent treatment of injuries and the timing and choice of surgical stabilization and reconstruction. To evaluate and treat severe upper extremity trauma, the orthopaedic surgeon should understand the principles of emergency department and operating theater management of commonly seen traumatic injuries to the distal humerus, elbow, forearm, wrist, and hand. A review of the principles for treating these complex injuries, including principles of soft-tissue coverage, will aid surgeons in achieving the goal of providing optimal treatment for their patients.

Instr Course Lect 2010;59:525-538.

The management of any trauma patient begins with the standard trauma survey (ABCDE: airway, breathing, and circulation, followed by evaluation of disability [assessed with the Glasgow Coma Scale] and exposure for adequate examination while prevention of hypothermia is maintained). The purpose of the primary survey is the control and stabilization of life-threatening injury.[1] The secondary trauma survey, consisting of a detailed examination of each body region for possible injury, is then performed. Standard recommendations for identification of orthopaedic injuries include plain radiographs of the injured region and the joints proximal and distal to it.

Débridement coupled with intravenous antibiotics and administration of tetanus toxoid is the most important initial treatment of severe open injuries. Débridement includes copious irrigation and removal of skin, subcutaneous tissue, muscle, fascia, and bone. It should be completed with careful inspection of the entire wound and the medullary canals and an evaluation of muscle viability. In severe situations, such as forearm and wrist amputations, skeletal shortening may facilitate revascularization or replantation.

Acute Trauma to the Humerus and Elbow

Humeral Shaft Fractures

Fractures of the humeral shaft account for 1% to 3% of all fractures.[2] Indications for surgical treatment of such fractures include polytrauma, vascular injuries requiring surgery, open or segmental fractures, bilateral humeral fractures, floating elbow injuries, and most pathologic fractures. Methods of fixation include plate osteosynthesis, intramedullary nailing, and external fixation. The management of open fractures of the humeral shaft is similar to that of open fractures of other long bones. Prompt surgical débridement, irrigation, intravenous

Dr. Wolf or an immediate family member serves as a board member, owner, officer, or committee member of the Rocky Mountain Hand Surgery Society. Dr. Athwal or an immediate family member has received research or institutional support from Wright Medical Technology and Tornier. Dr. Shin or an immediate family member has received research or institutional support from the Mayo Foundation and Stryker. Dr. Dennison or an immediate family member has received research or institutional support from Aircast–DJ Orthopedics and DePuy.

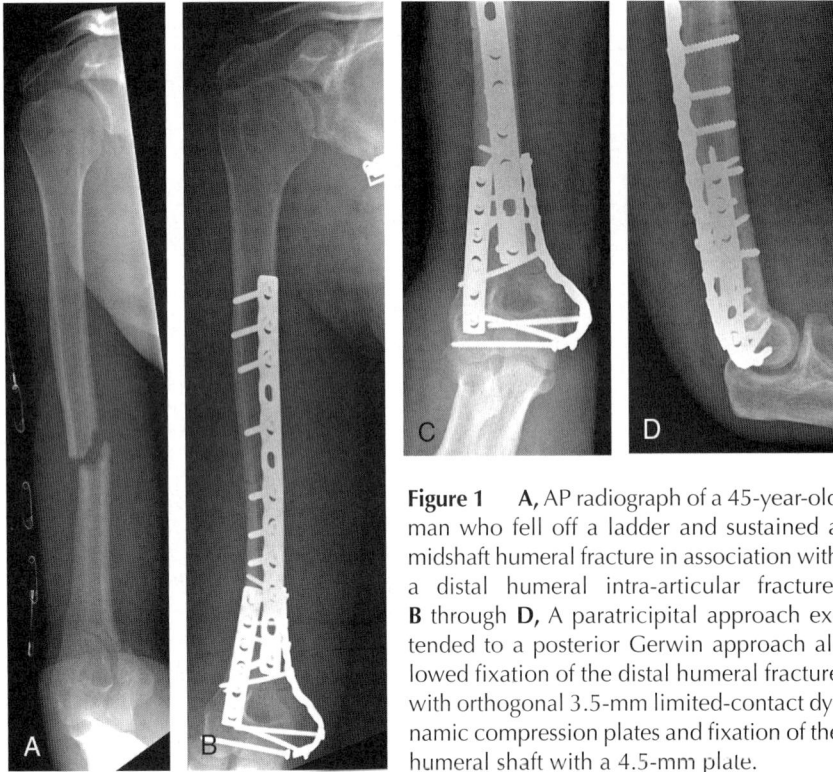

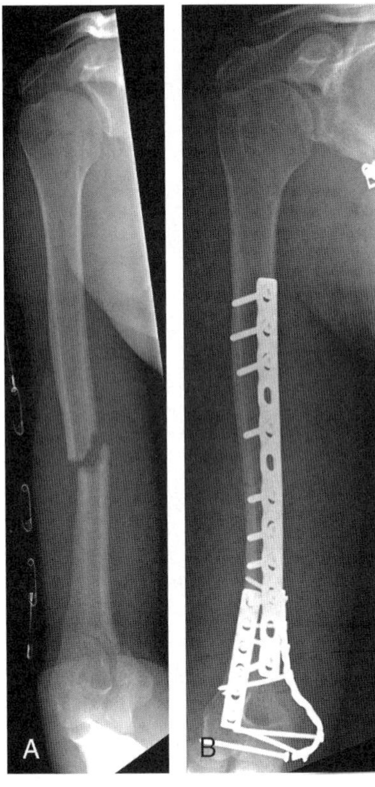

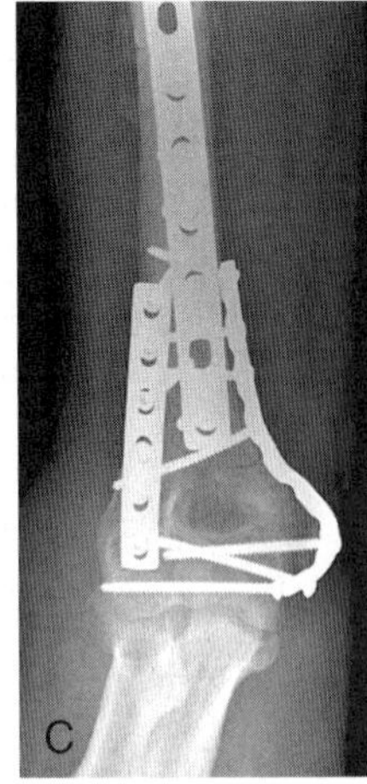

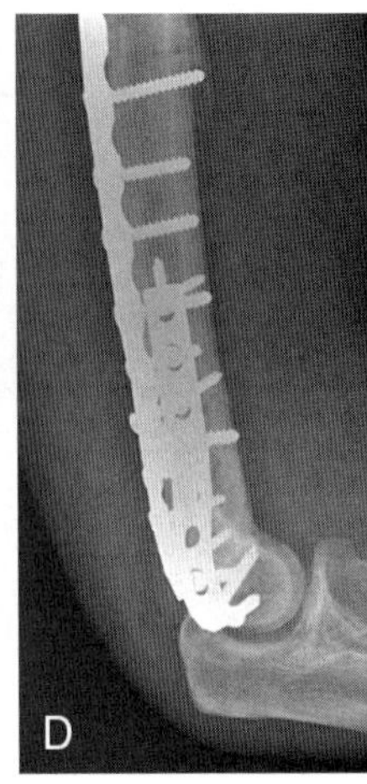

Figure 1 **A,** AP radiograph of a 45-year-old man who fell off a ladder and sustained a midshaft humeral fracture in association with a distal humeral intra-articular fracture. **B** through **D,** A paratricipital approach extended to a posterior Gerwin approach allowed fixation of the distal humeral fracture with orthogonal 3.5-mm limited-contact dynamic compression plates and fixation of the humeral shaft with a 4.5-mm plate.

antibiotics, and stabilization are the mainstay. There is controversy about the ideal form of fixation, with advocates of plate fixation and advocates of intramedullary nailing.[3-6]

Open reduction and internal fixation is the most acceptable form of surgical treatment. The surgical approach can be anterior, posterior, lateral, or medial. The anterior approach to the humerus is useful for the treatment of fractures of the proximal third of the humeral shaft as well as for polytraumatized patients because it is extensile and allows supine patient positioning for concurrent procedures, with good access to the airway. Disadvantages of the anterior approach include limited access to the radial nerve if microscopic repair is required and difficult access to the distal part of the humerus. The posterior approach described by Gerwin and associates[7] allows good access to the middle and distal parts of the humerus with nearly full exposure of the radial nerve (Figure 1). Limitations include the need for the lateral decubitus position and limited access to the humeral head and neck. Generally, open reduction and internal fixation should be done with a broad 4.5-mm dynamic compression plate with engagement of a minimum of six cortices, and ideally eight cortices, both proximal and distal to the fracture site.

Intramedullary nail fixation is also a viable option for treating acute humeral shaft fractures. The nail can be inserted antegrade through the proximal part of the humerus or retrograde through the apex of the olecranon fossa. Indications include burns, soft-tissue compromise, highly comminuted fractures, obesity, and pathologic fractures. The complication rate associated with intramedullary nails is slightly higher than that associated with plate osteosynthesis. These complications include nonunion, shoulder pain (after antegrade insertion), radial nerve injury, elbow stiffness (after retrograde insertion), and heterotopic ossification.

External fixation is not generally recommended as definitive treatment and is usually reserved for severely contaminated wounds or wounds with excessive soft-tissue loss.[8,9] External fixation may be used to stabilize a humeral fracture rapidly if that is required for vascular repair. The insertion of distal half-pins should be done through a mini-open approach to protect the radial nerve against injury.

Concurrent injury to the radial nerve is frequently associated with humeral shaft fractures. The reported prevalence ranges between 2% and 17%, and management is controversial.[2,10-14] In general, when there is no indication for surgical intervention, the patient can be observed, with an expectation that more than 70% of radial nerve injuries will resolve. When there is an indication for surgical fixation of the humeral fracture, nerve exploration should be conducted in association with open reduction and internal fixation. When a patient can tolerate a lateral decubitus position, the posterior approach to the humerus and radial nerve, as described by Gerwin and associates,[7] should be used. When there is a high risk of a nerve transection, such as in a patient with penetrating injuries or severe soft-tissue loss, early nerve exploration is recommended. If the nerve is transected, a primary microscopic repair should be done. When there is loss of a nerve segment, the humerus can be shortened for primary nerve repair. If the nerve is deemed unreparable, the ends should be tagged so that they can be found if nerve grafting is done later.

Distal Humeral Fractures

Distal humeral fractures remain some of the most challenging injuries to manage because they are commonly multifragmented, occur in osteopenic bone, and have a complex anatomy with limited options for internal fixation. In younger adults, these fractures are usually caused by higher-energy mechanisms. Although standard radiographs of the elbow are usually sufficient for diagnosis, CT with three-dimensional reconstructions improves the identification and visualization of fracture fragments.

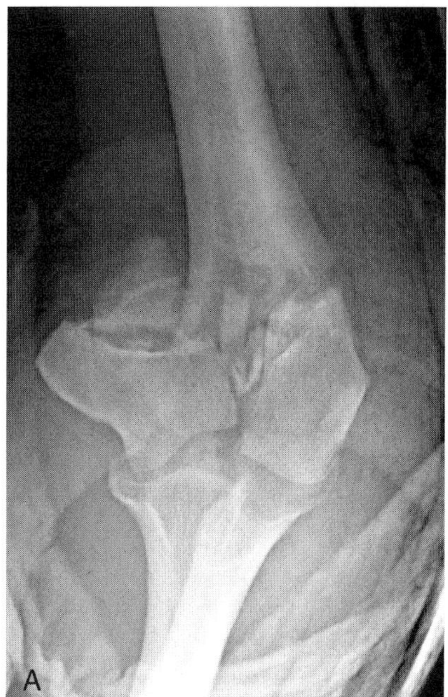

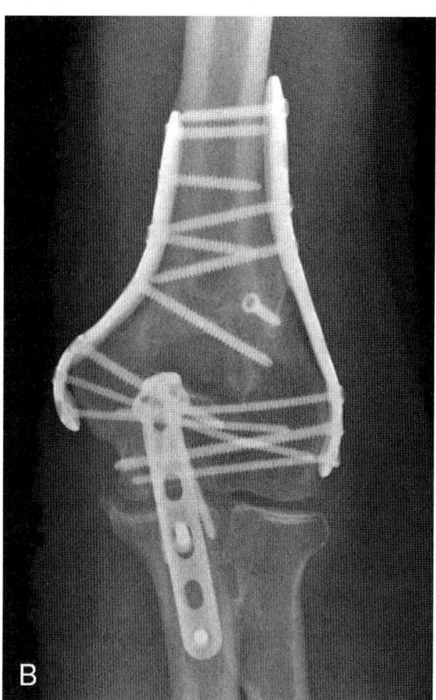

Figure 2 Parallel plate fixation of an intra-articular distal humeral fracture through an olecranon osteotomy. Preoperative **(A)** and postoperative **(B)** radiographs.

Several surgical approaches have been described for exposure and fixation of distal humeral fractures. The available types of posterior approaches include olecranon osteotomy[15-17] as well as paratricipital (triceps-on), triceps-splitting, triceps-reflecting, and triceps-dividing approaches.[18-23] The selection of the approach depends on how much articular visualization is required, the bone quality, the demand level of the patient, associated injuries such as triceps laceration, and whether the intraoperative decision is to proceed with arthroplasty as opposed to fixation.

Anatomic reduction and rigid internal fixation of displaced intra-articular distal humeral fractures provides stability for early range of motion. Patients who are medically fit and whose soft tissues are healthy may have surgery within 48 to 72 hours after the injury.[24] A closed distal humeral fracture in a multiply injured patient is splinted and treated after primary stabilization. Most surgeons prefer to perform definitive fixation within 2 or 3 weeks, but there are no data supporting this recommendation. When open reduction and internal fixation cannot be performed for several weeks, external fixation is recommended to stabilize the extremity to improve pain control and facilitate transfers, hygiene, and wound care. External fixator pins should be placed as far as possible from the planned internal fixation site to decrease the likelihood of infection.

Rigid fixation is obtained with orthogonal, parallel, or triple plates[25-28] (Figure 2). Generally, devascularized bone is débrided, but large segments that include articular cartilage are not necessarily removed. The risk of infection associated with retention of the fragments must be weighed against the risk of posttraumatic arthritis, and all attempts should be made to preserve articular cartilage.

Rigid fixation of the distal humeral fracture may not be possible in elderly patients with osteopenia, comminution, and/or articular fragmentation or in patients with a preexisting elbow disorder such as rheumatoid arthritis. In these situations, total elbow arthroplasty is a viable treatment option.[29-33]

Fracture-Dislocations of the Elbow

Fracture-dislocations of the elbow remain some of the most difficult and technically complex injuries to manage. These are loosely classified into three broad categories: terrible triad, Monteggia, and varus posteromedial injuries. The primary goal in managing these injuries is to stabilize the elbow to allow early motion. Failure to recognize complex elbow instability or to adequately stabilize the elbow leads to chronic instability, accelerated posttraumatic arthritis, or stiffness.[34-41]

The ulnohumeral joint, the anterior bundle of the medial collateral ligament, and the lateral ulnar collateral ligament are the primary stabilizers of the elbow. The secondary stabilizers include the radial head, the joint capsule, and the common flexor and extensor origins. Imaging should include AP and lateral radiographs with CT to better identify fracture patterns, comminution, and displacement. The initial management of an elbow fracture-dislocation is closed reduction. This reduces pain and soft-tissue swelling and allows more accurate radiographic interpretation. After the reduction, a repeat neurologic and vascular examination is documented. The management of open elbow fracture-dislocations is similar to that of open distal humeral fractures. The definitive surgical management of terrible triad, Monteggia, and varus posteromedial injuries varies. Most elbow fracture-dislocations require surgical management. When a patient has multiple traumatic injuries that include a closed elbow fracture-dislocation, the elbow fracture-dislocation should be reduced provisionally, be followed serially to ensure continued alignment, and then be treated after the patient's condition has stabilized. When definitive stabilization will be delayed for several weeks, static external fixation is recommended if the elbow displays instability.

Surgical management of an elbow dislocation with associated fractures of the radial head and coronoid, the so-called terrible triad, requires fixation of the osseous structures and repair of the ligaments. Fractures of the radial head should be internally fixed or the head should be replaced, depending on the specific characteristics of the fragments. All coronoid fractures, other than small tip fragments, require open reduction and internal fixation, or suture fixation if they are comminuted. After osseous stability is achieved, the lateral ulnar collateral ligament is repaired, and the elbow is examined for stability. If the elbow remains unstable, the anterior bundle of the medial collateral ligament is repaired. In the exceedingly rare circumstance that the elbow remains unstable after anatomic open reduction and internal fixation and ligament repair, a temporary dynamic or static external fixator may be used.

The ulnar fracture of the Monteggia injury is treated with rigid open reduction and internal fixation, which usually stabilizes the radiocapitellar joint. When there is a fracture of the radial head, it is treated with open reduction and internal fixation, radial head arthroplasty, or partial excision, depending on the characteristics of the fracture. If there is a coronoid fracture, anatomic and rigid fixation is required to re-create the anterior buttress of the ulnohumeral joint.

Varus posteromedial instability is caused by a coronoid fracture with an avulsion of the lateral collateral ligament. Repair of these injuries usually requires both a medial and a lateral approach to the elbow. A posterior skin incision can be used to achieve both medial and lateral exposure. The medial approach is used to repair a fracture that involves the anteromedial aspect of the coronoid, and the lateral approach is used to repair the lateral collateral ligament.

Acute Trauma to the Forearm, Distal Part of the Radius, and Distal Radioulnar Joint

Adult Forearm Fractures

Adult forearm fractures include a fracture of the radius or ulna alone or a fracture of both bones. The accepted treatment of fracture-dislocations such as a Monteggia fracture-dislocation (fracture of the ulna and dislocation of the radial head) and a Galeazzi fracture-dislocation (fracture of the radius and dislocation of the distal radioulnar joint) is open reduction and internal fixation.[42-46] Nonsurgical treatment is rare, but it can be used for a closed, minimally displaced (middle to distal) ulnar shaft fracture.[47,48]

As is the case for all fractures, treatment of forearm fractures includes management of the soft-tissue injury and restoration of skeletal alignment. If there is an open wound after débridement, open reduction and internal fixation of the radius and ulna is performed either through the traumatic wound or through a separate incision. A separate exposure for each bone is recommended to minimize the risk of radioulnar synostosis.[49,50] External fixation should be considered when the wound is contaminated or the soft-tissue injury is extensive (Figure 3). When there is an arterial injury with ischemia, stabilization (ideally definitive fixation) should be performed quickly, with temporary arterial shunting used to perfuse the distal part of the limb if necessary.

The radius is exposed through a volar Henry approach to expose its flat surface.[51] The dorsal Thompson approach allows exposure but is associated with a risk of injury to the posterior interosseous nerve.[52] The ulna is exposed through the interval between the extensor carpi ulnaris and the flexor carpi ulnaris. Attention to the radial length and radial bow (which should be approximately 12°) as well as the proximal ulnar varus bow (which should be

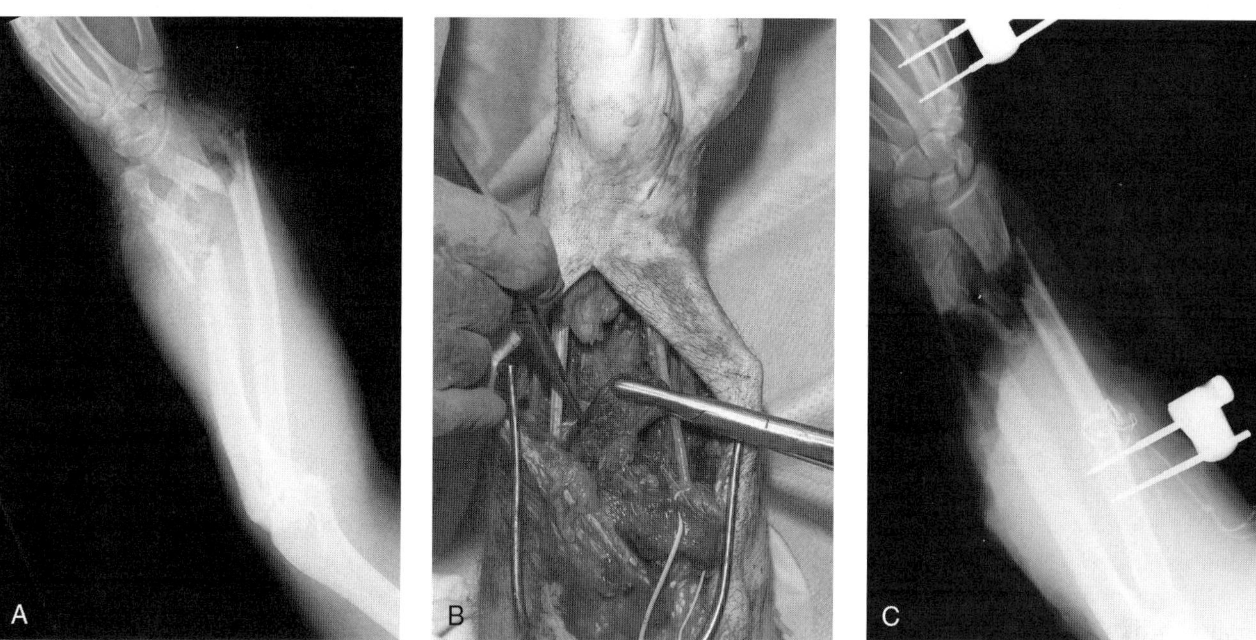

Figure 3 **A,** Radiograph of open radial and ulnar fractures with ischemia and severe soft-tissue injury. **B,** Débridement of the injury. **C,** Provisional external fixation to allow revascularization.

approximately 9°) and ulnar variance is key.[53] Rotational malalignment is avoided by reduction and provisional fixation, followed by examination of forearm rotation.[53-55] Open reduction and internal fixation with a 3.5-mm limited-contact dynamic compression plate provides balanced fixation with compression across the fracture with three bicortical screws on either side of the fracture. Locking plate fixation is recommended for osteoporotic bone, periarticular fractures, and fractures with segmental bone loss. Malleable reconstruction plates and partial tubular plates should not be used for diaphyseal forearm fractures because they routinely fail and break. The bone with the more easily reduced fracture should be reduced and fixed first. This makes the complex fracture easier to reduce. Radiographs of the contralateral extremity may provide a helpful "intact" template for reference when one is dealing with severely comminuted fractures.

When a patient has a distal radial or ulnar shaft fracture, stable fixation of the smaller, periarticular fragments may be obtained with the use of locking plates, nonlocked mini-fragment (2.7-mm) plates, or combination plates. Segmental fractures and comminution may be managed with bridge-plate or locking-plate techniques. Segmental fractures may be treated with two plates placed at 90° to one another, ideally with the plates overlapping by a minimum of two screw holes, with interdigitating screws.

When an incision is not prudent, particularly at the distal diaphyseal (or metaphyseal-diaphyseal) area of the ulna, percutaneous intramedullary fixation is considered to provide stability with minimal dissection of the soft tissues.[56] Finally, external fixation may be used temporarily, or definitively, when it is needed for a severely contaminated wound.[57,58]

Bone defects may be treated with cancellous or corticocancellous iliac crest bone graft alone if they are less than 6 cm in length and are located within a vascularized and clean wound.[17,59] Larger defects should be filled with autogenous or allogenic cancellous bone graft. When the soft tissues are compromised, as a result of either trauma, prior irradiation, or infection, a vascularized cortical graft is preferred.[60] Acute bone-grafting of simple or comminuted fractures remains controversial because it has not been shown to increase the rate of union.[44,61] Delayed grafting is preferable if the soft tissues are compromised. Space for a subsequent graft may be maintained by using antibiotic-impregnated bone cement.[62] Synostosis is a risk after bone graft is used, and the graft needs to be kept away from the interosseous membrane to reduce this risk.

When the injury is severe because of ischemia or crush, particularly with a segmental injury about the wrist, forearm, or elbow, amputation should be considered. Replantation or revascularization can often be done but may not be appropriate if there will be poor myotendinous function, joint contractures, or an insensate extremity. When a forearm-level amputation is necessary, every attempt should be made to preserve the elbow joint and sufficient forearm length and tissue to facilitate the use of a prosthesis.

Distal Radioulnar Joint

Stability of the distal radioulnar joint results from osseous, ligamentous (dorsal and volar radioulnar ligaments), and capsular constraints.[63-69] When the patient has a fracture with an associated distal radioulnar joint injury, the radius and/or ulna are stabilized first; then the distal radioulnar joint is evaluated.[46,70] When the distal radioulnar joint is reduced and stable, it is treated with a splint, with the forearm in either neutral rotation or supination. When the distal radioulnar joint is unstable, several types of treatment have been recommended.[46,71-73] These include fixation with two 0.062-inch (0.16-cm) Kirschner wires placed just proximal to the distal radioulnar joint across all four cortices (to facilitate removal if they break), external fixation cross-bridging the radius and ulna, or suture repair of the foveal insertion of the distal radioulnar ligaments.[74]

Ulnar styloid fixation and foveal repair may be completed at the same time through an ulnar incision by using a Kirschner wire and tension band, cannulated screws, or a simple suture technique. In general, ulnar styloid fractures do not require fixation unless the distal radioulnar joint is unstable.[75,76] When the distal radioulnar joint is unstable in the setting of an intra-articular distal radial fracture, the volar and dorsal lunate facet fragments must be reduced because they are attached to the radioulnar ligaments. The most common reason why the distal radioulnar joint cannot be reduced (provided that the radial fracture is reduced) is entrapment of the extensor carpi ulnaris, the triangular fibrocartilage complex, the extensor tendons, and the ulnar styloid.[77-81]

High-Energy Distal Radial Fractures

High-energy distal radial fractures include extra-articular and intra-articular fractures caused by impaction, shearing, or bending loads. While, in the past, shortening of up to 5 mm and articular displacement of up to 2 mm have been accepted in the alignment of distal radial fractures, Ruch[82] recommended a more anatomic goal for young, active adults, with articular step-off of less than 2 mm, radial shortening of less than 2 to 3 mm, and neutral tilt. CT imaging of intra-articular fractures provides a better understanding of fragment size and position to aid in treatment decisions.

There are several options for stabilizing these fractures, but there are insufficient data to indicate that one type of fixation is superior. Combined external fixation and percutaneous pin fixation has advantages, but its precise role is not clear. Associated complications include pin site infection, complex regional pain syndrome, stiffness, and malunion.[83-89] The best anatomic results are possible with open reduction and internal fixation, and an early return to function may follow.[90] The current trend of volar plate fixation (with distal locking screws or pegs) is supported by numerous reports of good outcomes, but most studies have not substantiated if overall long-term function is improved.[91-95] Complications include flexor and extensor tendon ruptures and subchondral screw penetration.[91,95] Dorsal plates are quite stable, but their use is associated with many complications.[96] Fragment-specific fixation with the use of separate pin-plate constructs for the volar, radial, and dorsal aspects of the fracture are powerful tools for reduction and stabilization. Finally, combinations of these techniques based on the fracture type and comminution may be required.

Volar plates take advantage of an anatomic recess at the pronator quadratus fossa for plate placement, minimizing the approach to the area of comminution dorsally.[92,93] During the reduction of these displaced fractures, the brachioradialis tendon may be released through the flexor carpi radialis approach,[94] which removes a deforming force and thus improves the reduction. Reduction of intra-articular fractures proceeds with reduction of the volar-ulnar cortex and then the dorsal lunate facet and the radial styloid. Subchondral Kirschner wires may be placed through Kirschner wire holes in the plate to maintain the reduction. They are later replaced with locking pegs to secure the articular reduction. Limitations of this approach include an inability to visualize interosseous ligament injuries and articular surfaces. Distal and ulnar fracture fragments are also difficult to stabilize because the plate-and-peg construct does not support or penetrate these small fragments. The volar-marginal fracture occurs at the volar-ulnar aspect of the distal part of the radius. It is important to identify and treat this intra-articular fracture because the radiocarpal ligaments are attached to the fragment, and the lunate will subluxate or dislocate volarly if the fracture is displaced.[97] Fragment-specific fixation works well for these relatively small fragments, as do Kirschner wire fixation and tension band techniques.[98,99] Severely comminuted fractures or those with volar and dorsal comminution may require adjunctive external fixation.

When an unstable distal ulnar fracture accompanies a distal radial fracture and remains unstable after fixation of the distal part of the radius, the ulnar fracture should be stabilized with a condylar bladeplate or a locking plate.[17,100] For severely comminuted and unstable distal radial fractures (especially those associated with multiple trauma), a 3.5-mm distraction plate may be used as an "internal external fixator" to stabilize the wrist with a temporary "wrist fusion"; this plate, spanning from the radius to the long-finger metacarpal, is used to distract the severely injured and comminuted metaphyseal-diaphyseal area of the radius.[101] The plate is removed after fracture healing, or at approximately 12 to 16 weeks.

Distal radial fractures and soft-tissue injuries may be so severe that acute salvage with a wrist arthrodesis or arthroplasty may be the best treatment.[102] Kafury and associates[103] as well as Richards and Roth[104] recommended that proximal row carpectomy, with provision of bone graft, decompression of the ulnocarpal joint, and shortening, be used to facilitate fusion in patients with severe injuries, such as those involving tendon, nerve, or arterial injury.

Acute Trauma to the Wrist and Hand

Perilunate Dislocations and Acute Carpal Tunnel Syndrome

Perilunate fracture-dislocations are generally caused by a high-energy injury.[105] However, there is a subset of these injuries that involves primarily ligamentous disruption, which is often missed without a high index of suspicion.[106] Perilunate dislocations usually involve a combination of osseous and soft-tissue injuries, with subtypes rated with the Mayfield classification.[107] Perilunate injury follows a predictable pattern, beginning on the radial side of the wrist with either the scaphoid or the scapholunate ligament, proceeding in an ulnar direction through either the carpal bones or the intercarpal ligaments, and culminating with Mayfield stage IV (complete volar dislocation of the lunate).

A perilunate fracture-dislocation requires urgent reduction, either open or closed, because of the risk of acute carpal tunnel syndrome. Reduction of the dislocation relieves pain and allows a more accurate radiographic assessment. Reduction is usually obtained in the emergency department with the use of finger traps, with 10 lb (4.5 kg) of traction applied for 10 to 15 minutes. The authors of this chapter recommend this type of reduction even for an open injury, unless the patient can be taken to the operating room urgently. The wrist is gently dorsiflexed while the physician's thumb maintains pressure on the lunate. Volar flexion should then allow the capitate to be reduced onto the lunate, and a palpable clunk should be felt with reduction. If the lunate is dislocated, it must first be reduced back onto the radius before the intercarpal reduction is performed.[107]

Acute carpal tunnel syndrome is a substantial risk, particularly in a patient with a volar dislocated-lunate type of perilunate injury, in whom carpal tunnel compression is caused by direct pressure on the nerve. Fractures of the distal part of the radius are the most common cause of acute carpal tunnel syndrome, and differentiating median nerve contusion from acute carpal tunnel syndrome is critical when deciding if acute carpal tunnel release in a patient with a traumatic injury to the wrist is necessary. A patient with a median nerve contusion generally has nonprogressive sensory changes immediately after the injury, whereas the sensory changes in a patient with acute carpal tunnel syndrome develop later and are associated with worsening pain.[108,109] Although Semmes-Weinstein monofilament tests and measurements of intracarpal canal pressure can be used to diagnose acute carpal tunnel syndrome, the diagnosis is usually based on the history. When an acute carpal tunnel syndrome is diagnosed, immediate surgical release of the transverse carpal ligament is indicated, with an extensile volar incision crossing the wrist crease, allowing full visualization of the nerve during decompression.[108]

If a perilunate fracture-dislocation is associated with acute carpal tunnel syndrome, decompression of the carpal canal is the first surgical priority and should be performed urgently. Definitive stabilization of the perilunate injury can be performed at the same time, or provisional pinning can be performed with surgery planned later (optimally within 3 to 5 days) for definitive stabilization. Definitive surgery for a perilunate injury includes fixation of the scaphoid and other carpal bones if necessary, fixation of the radial styloid if indicated, and ligament repair. Some advocate a single dorsal approach for definitive treatment, with repair of the scapholunate ligament, the lunotriquetral ligament, and the torn dorsal capsular ligaments.[110,111] Others recommend a combined dorsal and volar approach to directly repair the stout volar ligaments.[106,112-114] Perilunate injuries represent substantial trauma to the articular cartilage of the carpus and wrist, and sequelae of stiffness and subsequent arthritic changes are not uncommon.[112,115]

Radiocarpal Dislocation

Another type of high-energy injury is dislocation of the radiocarpal joint, which is mainly a ligamentous injury. Commonly, this is a dorsal dislocation, usually with avulsion of the cortical margin of the distal part of the radius.[116-118] Moneim and associates[119] classified these injuries on the basis of the presence or absence of intercarpal instability, whereas Dumontier and associates[117] subdivided radiocarpal dislocations on the basis of the size of the associated radial styloid fracture.

Initially, these injuries can be treated with closed reduction and splinting. Six of the 12 patients in the study by Mudgal and associates[118] had sensory impairment at presentation, and these resolved after reduction. Radiocarpal dislocations are often open and require acute stabilization, but even a closed injury should be stabilized within 7 days. The radial styloid fracture is reduced and fixed. Mudgal and associates[118] treated their patients with elevation of articular rim fragments, bone graft to fill any defect, buttress-plate fixation in some cases, repair of the ulnar styloid, suture repair of the palmar radiocarpal capsule, and scapholunate repair as needed.

High-Energy Axial Carpal, Carpometacarpal, and Metacarpophalangeal Joint Fracture-Dislocations

Severe traumatic injuries to the carpus and hand involve both soft tissue and bone. One of the most dramatic of these injuries is axial carpal dislocation, which is caused by a force of injury transmitted through the hand, splitting it into radial and ulnar columns.[120] Treatment of this type of "exploded hand" often requires several surgeries, with initial débridement of open wounds and provisional pinning of the carpus and metacarpals. An external fixator placed across the wrist can be used if needed to obtain stability. This is followed by repair of fractures; reconstruction of the intercarpal and intermetacarpal ligaments, with supportive pinning; and soft-tissue reconstruction.[121]

Injuries of the carpometacarpal joints are divided into two groups: those of the thumb carpometacarpal joint and those of the other carpometacarpal joints. An isolated thumb carpometacarpal joint dislocation without a fracture is rare and generally is caused by a high-energy injury or occurs in an individual with hyperlaxity. When this injury is acute, it can be reduced and then temporarily held in a splint, but it often requires the reconstruction of the anterior oblique ligament as described by Eaton and Littler to achieve definitive stability.[122,123] A Bennett-type fracture-dislocation of the thumb carpometacarpal joint is more common and can be treated either with closed methods, if it is minimally displaced; with percutaneous Kirschner wire pinning; or with miniscrews to fix the metacarpal shaft to the volar-ulnar fragment.[124]

Injuries to the other carpometacarpal joints of the hand are most common at the bases of the fourth and fifth metacarpals, as these joints are less intrinsically stable than are the second and third carpometacarpal joints. Dislocations are usually dorsal and are sometimes associated with fractures of the articular base of the metacarpal. These dislocations are easily missed on standard radiographs, especially when there is a small amount of subluxation. A pronated oblique radiograph of the hand should be obtained if an ulnar-sided hand injury is suspected. When acute, these injuries can be reduced and splinted and then treated within 7 to 10 days with percutaneous Kirschner wire fixation or application of small screws and plates as needed.[125,126]

Metacarpophalangeal joint dislocations are seen after high-energy injuries and often occur in the index finger. A single attempt at a closed reduction is recommended, but these injuries are often irreducible and generally require open reduction. Closed manipulation is performed with the wrist flexed to relax the flexor tendons. The metacarpophalangeal joint is then flexed, while the proximal phalanx is pushed dorsally. Metacarpophalangeal joint dislocations are frequently irreducible because of interposition of the volar plate between the proximal phalanx and the metacarpal head, and open reduction is performed through a dorsal incision, with incision of the extensor hood and capsule to expose the volar plate tented over the metacarpal head. The volar plate is released, and the joint is then reduced. Fractures are fixed as needed. Approximately 50% of these injuries are associated with an osteoarticular fracture fragment.[127]

Management of Soft-Tissue Injuries of the Upper Extremity

The spectrum of traumatic soft-tissue injuries of the upper extremity is vast, ranging from closed soft-tissue injuries (such as compartment syndrome) to composite soft-tissue and bone loss (amputations and segmental defects) to soft-tissue loss alone (degloving and avulsion-type injuries). Discussion of the management of every type of soft-tissue injury of the upper extremity is nearly impossible because of the tremendous variations in the types of injuries, the varying degrees of energy imparted to the injured arm, and the numerous mechanisms of injury. However, a key understanding of the principles of treatment of soft-tissue injuries can guide a surgeon in choosing the optimal treatment of such injuries of the upper extremity. An outline of the eight basic principles of soft-tissue reconstruction that can be applied to upper-extremity injuries follows.

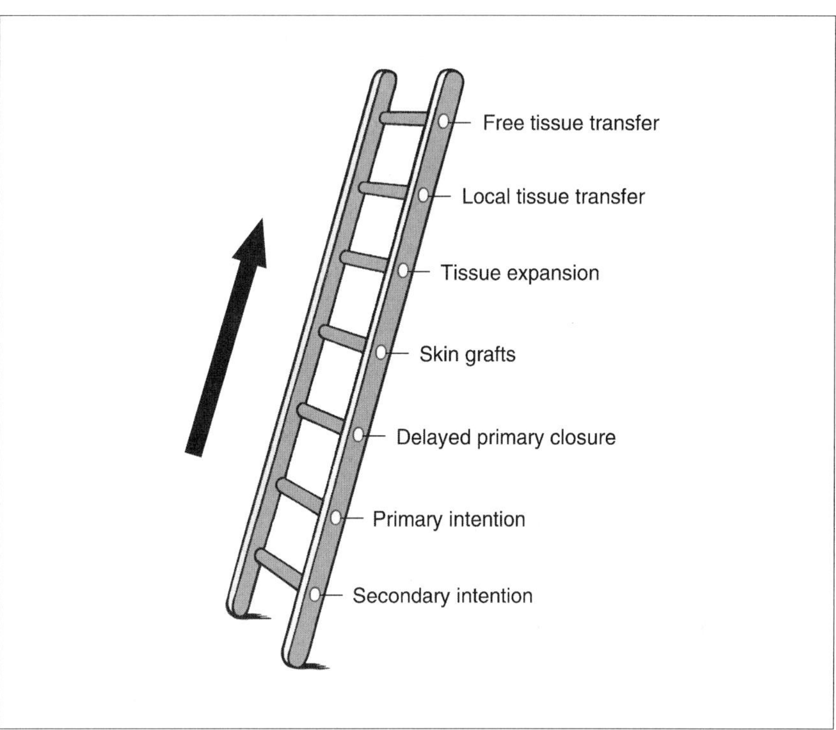

Figure 4 Illustration showing the reconstructive ladder.

Principle 1: Prevent Further Injury

Further injury to the upper extremity must be prevented. After determining the mechanism of injury, it is necessary to ascertain if compartment syndrome may be an issue or if a chemical burn must be neutralized.[128] Treating burns or frostbite injuries may be necessary.

Principle 2: Achieve Adequate Débridement

An aggressive tumorlike débridement of all necrotic and nonviable tissue, including bone, is essential.[129] This is often considered the most important single step in the management of soft-tissue injuries related to trauma. Appropriate cultures of contaminated tissue should be performed to guide antibiotic treatment. Reconstructive plans should not impede an adequate soft-tissue débridement. Repeat débridements should be performed every 24 to 48 hours as dictated by the wound and the patient's medical status.

Principle 3: Stabilize Bone

Once adequate débridement of soft tissue and bone has been accomplished, bone stability should be achieved. This can be done with external fixation or internal fixation, or both. External fixation is often preferred for highly contaminated wounds or wounds that have poor soft-tissue coverage. Internal fixation can be used for adequately débrided wounds that have good soft-tissue coverage of bone.

Principle 4: Achieve Soft-Tissue Coverage

When soft-tissue coverage is needed, acute coverage should be considered. Levin's reconstructive ladder identifies the simplest type of soft-tissue reconstruction procedure needed to cover a wound, with the procedures increasing in complexity as needed.[130,131] At the lowest level of the reconstructive ladder is healing by secondary intention, whereas free tissue transfer is at the highest level (Figure 4). When the wound is evaluated to determine possible options for coverage, it is imperative to consider patient factors; the genesis of the defect; the location, size, and depth of the defect; exposed structures; structures needing reconstruction; the degree of contamination; and the quality of surrounding tissues. All of these factors play a role in the decision.

Godina[129] popularized the concept of covering wounds within 72 hours. However, with advances in wound management with vacuum-assisted closure devices and antibiotic bead pouches, wound coverage can be performed more than 72 hours after the injury without untoward complications.[132]

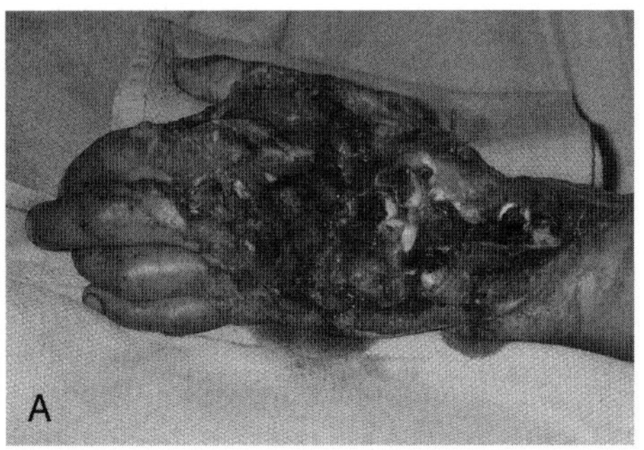

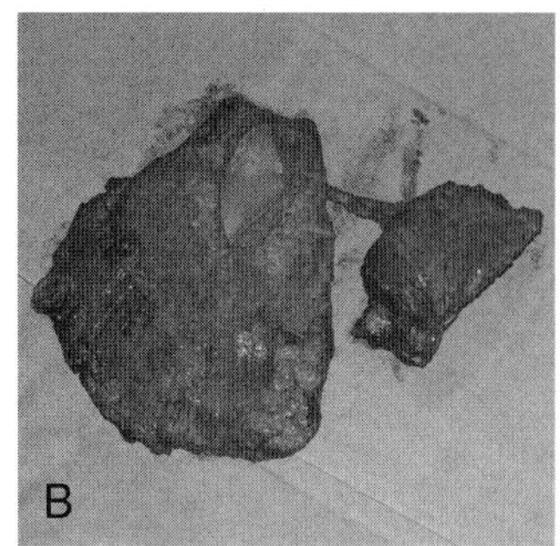

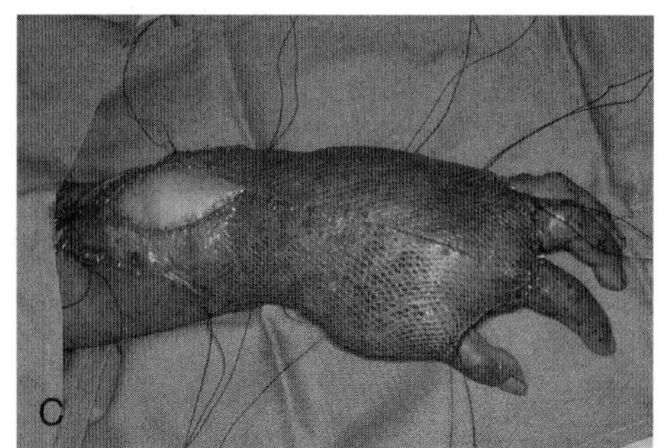

Figure 5 Composite flap reconstruction of the dorsal part of the hand with a combination of the latissimus dorsi, the serratus anterior, and two ribs on a combined thoracodorsal pedicle. **A,** The soft-tissue and bone defect. **B,** The free composite flap. **C,** Placement of the flap.

Principle 5: Determine Possible Secondary Reconstructive Procedures

It is necessary to determine what secondary reconstructions will be needed before the time of the soft-tissue coverage and the initial reconstructive procedure. If nerve grafts will be needed, the vascular pedicle of the free flap should be placed as far away from the nerve-graft sites as possible. If bone grafting (vascularized or conventional) or tendon procedures will be performed, it must be decided how these will be accomplished so that the pedicle is properly placed.

Principle 6: Consider Composite Soft-Tissue Reconstruction

Composite soft-tissue reconstruction should be considered when there is soft-tissue loss (Figure 5). A toe-to-thumb transfer is one such composite flap.

Principle 7: Evaluate Amputation Versus Limb Salvage

An amputation may be better than limb salvage. This is especially true in patients requiring a high amputation, in whom replantation is potentially associated with myoglobinuria, reperfusion injury, and systemic sequelae, all of which can place the patient at great risk. Although technically feasible, heroic efforts to reconstruct parts can lead to long recovery times with a prolonged loss of gainful employment and psychological problems.

Principle 8: Seek Advice

One should not hesitate to get assistance and advice. This is the most humbling of the principles but can be one of the most important. Collaboration with other surgeons may be extremely helpful in difficult cases.

Summary

The treatment of severe upper extremity injuries begins with standard trauma algorithms and débridement of devitalized soft tissue. The timing of osseous stabilization varies and is dependent on the quality and integrity of the soft-tissue envelope. A collaborative approach often represents the best care for the traumatized patient.

References

1. Thomson CB, Greaves I: Missed injury and the tertiary trauma survey. *Injury* 2008;39:107-114.
2. Ekholm R, Adami J, Tidermark J, Hansson K, Törnkvist H, Ponzer S: Fractures of the shaft of the humerus: An epidemiological study of 401 fractures. *J Bone Joint Surg Br* 2006;88: 1469-1473.
3. Bell MJ, Beauchamp CG, Kellam JK, McMurtry RY: The results of plating humeral shaft fractures in patients with multiple injuries: The Sunnybrook experience. *J Bone Joint Surg Br* 1985;67:293-296.
4. Heim D, Herkert F, Hess P, Regazzoni P: Surgical treatment of humeral shaft fractures: The Basel experience. *J Trauma* 1993;35:226-232.
5. Schoots IG, Simons MP, Nork SE, Chapman JR, Henley MB: Antegrade locked nailing of open humeral shaft fractures. *Orthopedics* 2007;30:49-54.
6. Vander Griend R, Tomasin J, Ward EF: Open reduction and internal fixation of humeral shaft fractures: Results using AO plating techniques. *J Bone Joint Surg Am* 1986;68:430-433.
7. Gerwin M, Griffith A, Weiland AJ, Hotchkiss RN, McCormack RR: Ligament reconstruction basal joint arthroplasty without tendon interposition. *Clin Orthop Relat Res* 1997; 342:42-45.
8. Marsh JL, Mahoney CR, Steinbronn D: External fixation of open humerus fractures. *Iowa Orthop J* 1999;19:35-42.
9. Mostafavi HR, Tornetta P III: Open fractures of the humerus treated with external fixation. *Clin Orthop Relat Res* 1997;337:187-197.

10. Amillo S, Barrios RH, Martinez-Peric R, Losada JI: Surgical treatment of the radial nerve lesions associated with fractures of the humerus. *J Orthop Trauma* 1993;7:211-215.

11. DeFranco MJ, Lawton JN: Radial nerve injuries associated with humeral fractures. *J Hand Surg Am* 2006; 31:655-663.

12. Holstein A, Lewis GM: Fractures of the humerus with radial-nerve paralysis. *J Bone Joint Surg Am* 1963;45: 1382-1388.

13. Pollock FH, Drake D, Bovill EG, Day L, Trafton PG: Treatment of radial neuropathy associated with fractures of the humerus. *J Bone Joint Surg Am* 1981;63:239-243.

14. Shao YC, Harwood P, Grotz MR, Limb D, Giannoudis PV: Radial nerve palsy associated with fractures of the shaft of the humerus: A systematic review. *J Bone Joint Surg Br* 2005;87:1647-1652.

15. Cassebaum WH: Open reduction of T & Y fractures of the lower end of the humerus. *J Trauma* 1969;9: 915-925.

16. Gainor BJ, Moussa F, Schott T: Healing rate of transverse osteotomies of the olecranon used in reconstruction of distal humerus fractures. *J South Orthop Assoc* 1995;4:263-268.

17. Hewins EA, Gofton WT, Dubberly J, MacDermid JC, Faber KJ, King GJ: Plate fixation of olecranon osteotomies. *J Orthop Trauma* 2007;21:58-62.

18. Alonso-Llames M: Bilaterotricipital approach to the elbow: Its application in the osteosynthesis of supracondylar fractures of the humerus in children. *Acta Orthop Scand* 1972;43:479-490.

19. Schildhauer TA, Nork SE, Mills WJ, Henley MB: Extensor mechanism-sparing paratricipital posterior approach to the distal humerus. *J Orthop Trauma* 2003;17:374-378.

20. Campbell WC: Incision for exposure of the elbow joint. *Am J Surg* 1932;15: 65-67.

21. Bryan RS, Morrey BF: Extensive posterior exposure of the elbow: A triceps-sparing approach. *Clin Orthop Relat Res* 1982;166:188-192.

22. O'Driscoll SW: Elbow dislocations, in Morrey BF, ed: *The Elbow and Its Disorders*, ed 3. Philadelphia, PA, Saunders, 2000, pp 409-420.

23. Van Gorder GW: Surgical approach in supracondylar "T" fractures of the humerus requiring open reduction. *J Bone Joint Surg Am* 1940;22:278-292.

24. Ilahi OA, Strausser DW, Gabel GT: Post-traumatic heterotopic ossification about the elbow. *Orthopedics* 1998;21:265-268.

25. Helfet DL, Schmeling GJ: Bicondylar intraarticular fractures of the distal humerus in adults. *Clin Orthop Relat Res* 1993;292:26-36.

26. Jupiter JB, Neff U, Holzach P, Allgöwer M: Intercondylar fractures of the humerus: An operative approach. *J Bone Joint Surg Am* 1985;67:226-239.

27. Self J, Viegas SF, Buford WL Jr, Patterson RM: A comparison of double-plate fixation methods for complex distal humerus fractures. *J Shoulder Elbow Surg* 1995;4:10-16.

28. Gofton WT, Macdermid JC, Patterson SD, Faber KJ, King GJ: Functional outcome of AO type C distal humeral fractures. *J Hand Surg Am* 2003;28:294-308.

29. Frankle MA, Herscovici D Jr, DiPasquale TG, Vasey MB, Sanders RW: A comparison of open reduction and internal fixation and primary total elbow arthroplasty in the treatment of intraarticular distal humerus fractures in women older than age 65. *J Orthop Trauma* 2003;17:473-480.

30. Kalogrianitis S, Sinopidis C, El Meligy M, Rawal A, Frostick SP: Unlinked elbow arthroplasty as primary treatment for fractures of the distal humerus. *J Shoulder Elbow Surg* 2008; 17:287-292.

31. Kamineni S, Morrey BF: Distal humeral fractures treated with noncustom total elbow replacement: Surgical technique. *J Bone Joint Surg Am* 2005; 87:41-50.

32. Morrey BF: Fractures of the distal humerus: Role of elbow replacement. *Orthop Clin North Am* 2000;31: 145-154.

33. Prasad N, Dent C: Outcome of total elbow replacement for distal humeral fractures in the elderly: A comparison of primary surgery and surgery after failed internal fixation or conservative treatment. *J Bone Joint Surg Br* 2008; 90:343-348.

34. Beingessner DM, Stacpoole RA, Dunning CE, Johnson JA, King GJ: The effect of suture fixation of type I coronoid fractures on the kinematics and stability of the elbow with and without medial collateral ligament repair. *J Shoulder Elbow Surg* 2007;16: 213-217.

35. Closkey RF, Goode JR, Kirschenbaum D, Cody RP: The role of the coronoid process in elbow stability: A biomechanical analysis of axial loading. *J Bone Joint Surg Am* 2000;82: 1749-1753.

36. McKee MD, Pugh DM, Wild LM, Schemitsch EH, King GJ: Standard surgical protocol to treat elbow dislocations with radial head and coronoid fractures: Surgical technique. *J Bone Joint Surg Am* 2005;87:22-32.

37. Pugh DM, Wild LM, Schemitsch EH, King GJ, McKee MD: Standard surgical protocol to treat elbow dislocations with radial head and coronoid fractures. *J Bone Joint Surg Am* 2004;86: 1122-1130.

38. Ring D: Fractures of the coronoid process of the ulna. *J Hand Surg Am* 2006;31:1679-1689.

39. Ring D, Doornberg JN: Fracture of the anteromedial facet of the coronoid process: Surgical technique. *J Bone Joint Surg Am* 2007;89: 267-283.

40. Ring D, Jupiter JB, Simpson NS: Monteggia fractures in adults. *J Bone Joint Surg Am* 1998;80:1733-1744.

41. Sotereanos DG, Darlis NA, Wright TW, Goitz RJ, King GJ: Unstable fracture-dislocations of the elbow. *Instr Course Lect* 2007;56: 369-376.

42. Sauter SL, Chapman LJ, Knutson SJ, Anderson HA: Case example of wrist

trauma in keyboard use. *Appl Ergon* 1987;18:183-186.

43. Wilson FC, Dirschl DR, Bynum DK: Fractures of the radius and ulna in adults: An analysis of factors affecting outcome. *Iowa Orthop J* 1997;17: 14-19.

44. Wright RR, Schmeling GJ, Schwab JP: The necessity of acute bone grafting in diaphyseal forearm fractures: A retrospective review. *J Orthop Trauma* 1997;11:288-294.

45. Moed BR, Kellam JF, Foster RJ, Tile M, Hansen ST Jr: Immediate internal fixation of open fractures of the diaphysis of the forearm. *J Bone Joint Surg Am* 1986;68:1008-1017.

46. Mikić Z: The blood supply of the human distal radioulnar joint and the microvasculature of its articular disk. *Clin Orthop Relat Res* 1992;275:19-28.

47. Szabo RM, Skinner M: Isolated ulnar shaft fractures: Retrospective study of 46 cases. *Acta Orthop Scand* 1990;61: 350-352.

48. Sarmiento A, Latta LL, Zych G, McKeever P, Zagorski JP: Isolated ulnar shaft fractures treated with functional braces. *J Orthop Trauma* 1998;12: 420-424.

49. Bauer G, Wörsdörfer O, Braun K: Radio-ulnar bridge callus following osteosynthesis of forearm fractures. *Aktuelle Traumatol* 1990;20:194-198.

50. Stern PJ, Drury WJ: Complications of plate fixation of forearm fractures. *Clin Orthop Relat Res* 1983;175:25-29.

51. Henry AK: *Extensile Exposure*, ed 2. Edinburgh, United Kingdom, Churchill Livingstone, 1973.

52. Spinner RJ, Berger RA, Carmichael SW, Dyck PJ, Nunley JA: Isolated paralysis of the extensor digitorum communis associated with the posterior (Thompson) approach to the proximal radius. *J Hand Surg Am* 1998;23:135-141.

53. Yasutomi T, Nakatsuchi Y, Koike H, Uchiyama S: Mechanism of limitation of pronation/supination of the forearm in geometric models of deformities of the forearm bones. *Clin Biomech (Bristol, Avon)* 2002;17: 456-463.

54. Dumont CE, Thalmann R, Macy JC: The effect of rotational malunion of the radius and the ulna on supination and pronation. *J Bone Joint Surg Br* 2002;84:1070-1074.

55. Tynan MC, Fornalski S, McMahon PJ, Utkan A, Green SA, Lee TQ: The effects of ulnar axial malalignment on supination and pronation. *J Bone Joint Surg Am* 2000;82: 1726-1731.

56. Walz M, Kolbow B, Möllenhoff G: Fracture of the distal ulna accompanying fractures of the distal radius: Minimally invasive treatment with elastic stable intramedullary nailing (ESIN). *Unfallchirurg* 2006;109:1058-1063.

57. Jackson RP, Jacobs RR, Neff JR: External skeletal fixation in severe limb trauma. *J Trauma* 1978;18:201-205.

58. Putnam MD, Walsh TM IV: External fixation for open fractures of the upper extremity. *Hand Clin* 1993;9: 613-623.

59. Barbieri PG, Colombini D, Occhipinti E, Vigasio A, Poli R: Epidemics of musculotendinous pathologies of the upper limbs (cumulative trauma disorders) in a group of assembly line workers. *Med Lav* 1993;84:487-500.

60. Ring D, Jupiter JB, Brennwald J, Büchler U, Hastings H II: Prospective multicenter trial of a plate for dorsal fixation of distal radius fractures. *J Hand Surg Am* 1997;22: 777-784.

61. Ring D, Rhim R, Carpenter C, Jupiter JB: Comminuted diaphyseal fractures of the radius and ulna: Does bone grafting affect nonunion rate? *J Trauma* 2005;59:438-442.

62. Georgiadis GM, DeSilva SP: Reconstruction of skeletal defects in the forearm after trauma: Treatment with cement spacer and delayed cancellous bone grafting. *J Trauma* 1995;38: 910-914.

63. Palmer AK, Werner FW: Biomechanics of the distal radioulnar joint. *Clin Orthop Relat Res* 1984;187:26-35.

64. Tay SC, Berger RA, Tomita K, Tan ET, Amrami KK, An KN: In vivo three-dimensional displacement of the distal radioulnar joint during resisted forearm rotation. *J Hand Surg Am* 2007;32:450-458.

65. Haugstvedt JR, Berger RA, Nakamura T, Neale P, Berglund L, An KN: Relative contributions of the ulnar attachments of the triangular fibrocartilage complex to the dynamic stability of the distal radioulnar joint. *J Hand Surg Am* 2006;31:445-451.

66. Watanabe H, Berger RA, An KN, Berglund LJ, Zobitz ME: Stability of the distal radioulnar joint contributed by the joint capsule. *J Hand Surg Am* 2004;29:1114-1120.

67. Stuart PR, Berger RA, Linscheid RL, An KN: The dorsopalmar stability of the distal radioulnar joint. *J Hand Surg Am* 2000;25:689-699.

68. Palmer AK: The distal radioulnar joint. *Orthop Clin North Am* 1984;15: 321-335.

69. Palmer AK: The distal radioulnar joint: Anatomy, biomechanics, and triangular fibrocartilage complex abnormalities. *Hand Clin* 1987;3:31-40.

70. Rettig ME, Raskin KB: Galeazzi fracture-dislocation: A new treatment-oriented classification. *J Hand Surg Am* 2001;26:228-235.

71. Nicolaidis SC, Hildreth DH, Lichtman DM: Acute injuries of the distal radioulnar joint. *Hand Clin* 2000;16: 449-459.

72. Cheng SL, Axelrod TS: Management of complex dislocations of the distal radioulnar joint. *Clin Orthop Relat Res* 1997;341:183-191.

73. Giannoulis FS, Sotereanos DG: Galeazzi fractures and dislocations. *Hand Clin* 2007;23:153-163.

74. Mestdagh H, Duquennoy A, Letendart J, Sensey JJ, Fontaine C: Long-term results in the treatment of fracture-dislocations of Galeazzi in adults: Report on twenty-nine cases. *Ann Chir Main* 1983;2:125-133.

75. Lindau T, Adlercreutz C, Aspenberg P: Peripheral tears of the triangu-

lar fibrocartilage complex cause distal radioulnar joint instability after distal radial fractures. *J Hand Surg Am* 2000; 25:464-468.

76. Nakamura R, Horii E, Imaeda T, Nakao E, Shionoya K, Kato H: Ulnar styloid malunion with dislocation of the distal radioulnar joint. *J Hand Surg Br* 1998;23:173-175.

77. Bruckner JD, Lichtman DM, Alexander AH: Complex dislocations of the distal radioulnar joint: Recognition and management. *Clin Orthop Relat Res* 1992;275:90-103.

78. Paley D, Rubenstein J, McMurtry RY: Irreducible dislocation of distal radial ulnar joint. *Orthop Rev* 1986; 15:228-231.

79. Kikuchi Y, Nakamura T: Irreducible Galeazzi fracture-dislocation due to an avulsion fracture of the fovea of the ulna. *J Hand Surg Br* 1999;24: 379-381.

80. Jenkins SA: Osteoarthritis of the pisiform-triquetral joint: Report of three cases. *J Bone Joint Surg Br* 1951; 33:532-534.

81. Alexander AH, Lichtman DM: Irreducible distal radioulnar joint occurring in a Galeazzi fracture: Case report. *J Hand Surg Am* 1981;6:258-261.

82. Ruch DS: Fractures of the distal radius and ulna, in Bucholz RW, Heckman JD, Court-Brown C, eds: *Rockwood and Green's Fractures in Adults*, ed 6. Philadelphia, PA, Lippincott Williams and Wilkins, 2006, pp 909-964.

83. Handoll HH, Huntley JS, Madhok R: External fixation versus conservative treatment for distal radial fractures in adults. *Cochrane Database Syst Rev* 2007;3:CD006194.

84. Handoll HH, Huntley JS, Madhok R: Different methods of external fixation for treating distal radial fractures in adults. *Cochrane Database Syst Rev* 2008;1:CD006522.

85. Handoll HH, Madhok R: Surgical interventions for treating distal radial fractures in adults. *Cochrane Database Syst Rev* 2003;3:CD003209.

86. Handoll HH, Vaghela MV, Madhok R: Percutaneous pinning for treating distal radial fractures in adults. *Cochrane Database Syst Rev* 2007;3:CD006080.

87. Chiou-Tan FY, Reno SB, Magee KN, Krouskop TA: Electromyographic localization of the palmaris brevis muscle. *Am J Phys Med Rehabil* 1998; 77:243-246.

88. Cooney WP: Distal radius fractures: External fixation proves best. *J Hand Surg Am* 1998;23:1119-1121.

89. Cooney WP, Dobyns JH, Linscheid RL: Fractures of the scaphoid: A rational approach to management. *Clin Orthop Relat Res* 1980;149:90-97.

90. Chung KC, Kotsis SV, Kim HM: Predictors of functional outcome after surgical treatment of distal radius fractures. *J Hand Surg Am* 2007;32: 76-83.

91. Arora R, Lutz M, Hennerbichler A, Krappinger D, Espen D, Gabl M: Complications following internal fixation of unstable distal radius fracture with a palmar locking-plate. *J Orthop Trauma* 2007;21:316-322.

92. Orbay JL: The treatment of unstable distal radius fractures with volar fixation. *Hand Surg* 2000;5:103-112.

93. Orbay JL, Fernandez DL: Volar fixation for dorsally displaced fractures of the distal radius: A preliminary report. *J Hand Surg Am* 2002;27: 205-215.

94. Orbay JL, Fernandez DL: Volar fixed-angle plate fixation for unstable distal radius fractures in the elderly patient. *J Hand Surg Am* 2004;29:96-102.

95. Rozental TD, Blazar PE: Functional outcome and complications after volar plating for dorsally displaced, unstable fractures of the distal radius. *J Hand Surg Am* 2006;31:359-365.

96. Kambouroglou GK, Axelrod TS: Complications of the AO/ASIF titanium distal radius plate system (pi plate) in internal fixation of the distal radius: A brief report. *J Hand Surg Am* 1998;23:737-741.

97. Jupiter JB, Fernandez DL, Toh CL, Fellman T, Ring D: Operative treatment of volar intra-articular fractures of the distal end of the radius. *J Bone Joint Surg Am* 1996;78:1817-1828.

98. Harness NG, Jupiter JB, Orbay JL, Raskin KB, Fernandez DL: Loss of fixation of the volar lunate facet fragment in fractures of the distal part of the radius. *J Bone Joint Surg Am* 2004; 86:1900-1908.

99. Bae DS, Koris MJ: Fragment-specific internal fixation of distal radius fractures. *Hand Clin* 2005;21:355-362.

100. Dennison DG: Open reduction and internal locked fixation of unstable distal ulna fractures with concomitant distal radius fracture. *J Hand Surg Am* 2007;32:801-805.

101. Shen J, Papadonikolakis A, Garrett JP, Davis SM, Ruch DS: Ulnar-positive variance as a predictor of distal radioulnar joint ligament disruption. *J Hand Surg Am* 2005;30:1172-1177.

102. Terral TG, Freeland AE: Early salvage reconstruction of severe distal radial fractures. *Clin Orthop Relat Res* 1996; 327:147-151.

103. Kafury AA, Freeland AE, Barbieri RA: Primary wrist arthrodesis in a severe intra-articular distal radial fracture. *Orthopedics* 1998;21:803-805.

104. Richards RS, Roth JH: Simultaneous proximal row carpectomy and radius to distal carpal row arthrodesis. *J Hand Surg Am* 1994;19:728-732.

105. Sauder DJ, Athwal GS, Faber KJ, Roth JH: Perilunate injuries. *Orthop Clin North Am* 2007;38:279-288.

106. Simic PM, Robison J, Gardner MJ, Gelberman RH, Weiland AJ, Boyer MI: Treatment of distal radius fractures with a low-profile dorsal plating system: An outcomes assessment. *J Hand Surg Am* 2006;31: 382-386.

107. Mayfield JK: Mechanism of carpal injuries. *Clin Orthop Relat Res* 1980;149: 45-54.

108. Szabo RM: Acute carpal tunnel syndrome. *Hand Clin* 1998;14:419-429.

109. Schnetzler KA: Acute carpal tunnel syndrome. *J Am Acad Orthop Surg* 2008;16:276-282.

110. Herzberg G, Comtet JJ, Linscheid RL, Amadio PC, Cooney WP, Stalder J: Perilunate dislocations and fracture-dislocations: A multicenter study. *J Hand Surg Am* 1993;18: 768-779.

111. Knoll VD, Allan C, Trumble TE: Trans-scaphoid perilunate fracture dislocations: Results of screw fixation of the scaphoid and lunotriquetral repair with a dorsal approach. *J Hand Surg Am* 2005;30:1145-1152.

112. Hildebrand KA, Ross DC, Patterson SD, Roth JH, MacDermid JC, King GJ: Dorsal perilunate dislocations and fracture-dislocations: Questionnaire, clinical, and radiographic evaluation. *J Hand Surg Am* 2000;25: 1069-1079.

113. Apergis E, Maris J, Theodoratos G, Pavlakis D, Antoniou N: Perilunate dislocations and fracture-dislocations: Closed and early open reduction compared in 28 cases. *Acta Orthop Scand Suppl* 1997;275:55-59.

114. Blazar PE, Murray P: Treatment of perilunate dislocations by combined dorsal and palmar approaches. *Tech Hand Up Extrem Surg* 2001;5:2-7.

115. Sotereanos DG, Mitsionis GJ, Giannakopoulos PN, Tomaino MM, Herndon JH: Perilunate dislocation and fracture dislocation: A critical analysis of the volar-dorsal approach. *J Hand Surg Am* 1997;22:49-56.

116. Arslan H, Tokmak M: Isolated ulnar radiocarpal dislocation. *Arch Orthop Trauma Surg* 2002;122:179-181.

117. Dumontier C, Meyer zu Reckendorf G, Sautet A, Lenoble E, Saffar P, Allieu Y: Radiocarpal dislocations: Classification and proposal for treatment. A review of twenty-seven cases. *J Bone Joint Surg Am* 2001;83:212-218.

118. Mudgal CS, Psenica J, Jupiter JB: Radiocarpal fracture-dislocation. *J Hand Surg Br* 1999;24:92-98.

119. Moneim MS, Bolger JT, Omer GE: Radiocarpal dislocation: Classification and rationale for management. *Clin Orthop Relat Res* 1985;192: 199-209.

120. Garcia-Elias M, Dobyns JH, Cooney WP III, Linscheid RL: Traumatic axial dislocations of the carpus. *J Hand Surg Am* 1989;14:446-457.

121. Graham TJ: The exploded hand syndrome: Logical evaluation and comprehensive treatment of the severely crushed hand. *J Hand Surg Am* 2006; 31:1012-1023.

122. Van Giffen N, Van Ransbeeck H, De Smet L: Stabilization of the prearthritic trapeziometacarpal joint using ligament reconstruction. *Chir Main* 2002;21:277-281.

123. Marcotte AL, Trzeciak MA: Nonoperative treatment for a double dislocation of the thumb metacarpal: A case report. *Arch Orthop Trauma Surg* 2008; 128:281-284.

124. Lutz M, Sailer R, Zimmermann R, Gabl M, Ulmer H, Pechlaner S: Closed reduction transarticular Kirschner wire fixation versus open reduction internal fixation in the treatment of Bennett's fracture dislocation. *J Hand Surg Br* 2003;28: 142-147.

125. Lawlis JF III, Gunther SF: Carpometacarpal dislocations: Long-term follow-up. *J Bone Joint Surg Am* 1991;73:52-59.

126. Stern PJ: Fractures of the metacarpals and phalanges, in Green DP, Hotchkiss RN, Pederson WC, Wolfe SW, eds: *Green's Operative Hand Surgery*, ed 5. Philadelphia, PA, Churchill Livingstone, 2005, pp 277-341.

127. Becton JL, Christian JD Jr, Goodwin HN, Jackson JG III: A simplified technique for treating the complex dislocation of the index metacarpophalangeal joint. *J Bone Joint Surg Am* 1975;57:698-700.

128. Friedrich JB, Shin AY: Management of forearm compartment syndrome. *Hand Clin* 2007;23:245-254.

129. Godina M: Early microsurgical reconstruction of complex trauma of the extremities. *Plast Reconstr Surg* 1986;78:285-292.

130. Levin LS: The reconstructive ladder: An orthoplastic approach. *Orthop Clin North Am* 1993;24:393-409.

131. Levin LS, Condit DP: Combined injuries: Soft tissue management. *Clin Orthop Relat Res* 1996;327:172-181.

132. Geiger S, McCormick F, Chou R, Wandel AG: War wounds: Lessons learned from Operation Iraqi Freedom. *Plast Reconstr Surg* 2008;122: 146-153.

Fixed-Angle Locking Plating of Displaced Proximal Humerus Fractures

Nata Parnes, MD
Jesse B. Jupiter, MD

Abstract

Proximal humerus fractures are common, especially among patients older than 60 years who have osteoporosis. Several techniques have been used within the past several decades to treat displaced proximal humerus fractures. Many different implants have been investigated and tested, all with inadequate results; debate continues as to the best method of fixation. Fixed-angle locking plates offer a relatively new treatment option for these complicated fractures, especially in patients with osteoporosis. The use of locking plates for treating comminuted proximal humerus fractures has biologic and biomechanical advantages over conventional fixation techniques. Complications including varus fracture collapse and screw penetration of the articular surface nonetheless remain problematic. Although the locking plate technique provides exceptional fixation stability, its use must be tailored to the individual patient, taking into account the extent of trauma, the fracture characteristics, and the patient's age and expectations; therefore, it must be carefully weighed against other forms of treatment. Prospective clinical trials and further study are necessary to generate data comparing locking plate fixation and alternative surgical treatments.

Instr Course Lect 2010;59:539-552.

Proximal humerus fractures are the third most common type of fracture among people older than 60 years, and they represent 5% of all fractures seen in emergency departments.[1-4] The risk factors for fracture of the proximal humerus include osteoporosis[5] and a pattern of frequent falls,[6,7] both of which are common in older adults. The incidence of these fractures increases sharply with age.[8] In people who are older than 60 years, a low-energy indirect injury to the shoulder is the cause of 97% of proximal humerus fractures.[9] In contrast, proximal humerus fractures in younger people usually result from high-energy trauma.

Between 80% and 85% of all proximal humerus fractures are nondisplaced or minimally displaced. These fractures can be treated nonsurgically, generally with a good outcome.[10] The remaining 15% to 20% of proximal humerus fractures are significantly displaced and may benefit from surgical treatment. No single surgical approach is considered the gold standard. Surgical stabilization of these fractures is challenging because of the relative deforming forces of the surrounding muscles, the blood supply pattern to the humeral head, and the poor bone quality common in older patients; it remains the subject of many clinical and experimental investigations.[11-13]

An understanding of the biomechanics and pathophysiology of the bones and soft tissues has guided the development of fixed-angle locking plates for treating displaced proximal humerus fractures.[14] Surgeons are advised to become familiar with

Neither Dr. Parnes nor an immediate family member has received anything of value from or owns stock in a commercial company or institution directly or indirectly related to the subject of this chapter. Dr. Jupiter or an immediate family member serves as an unpaid consultant to Synthes; has received research or institutional support from Aircast–DJ Orthopedics, Biomet, Hand Innovations, Linvatec, Mitek, SBI, Synthes, Wright Medical Technology, and Zimmer; and has received nonincome support (such as equipment or services), commercially derived honoraria, or other non–research-related funding (such as paid travel) from Elsevier-Saunders-Mosby and Wolters Kluwer–Lippincott Williams & Wilkins.

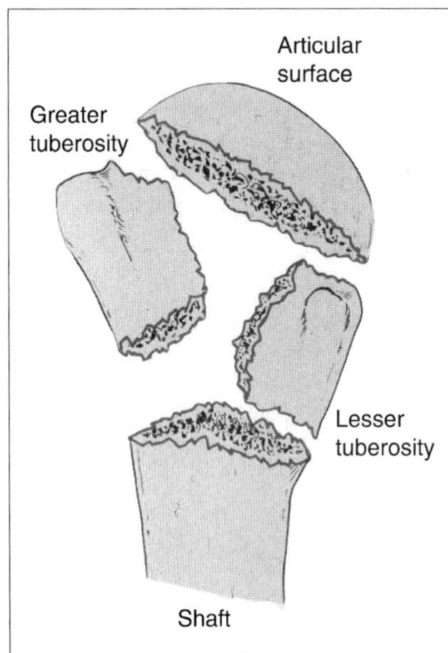

Figure 1 Schematic diagram showing the four bony segments of the proximal humerus: the humeral head, with a spherical articular surface; the greater tuberosity; the lesser tuberosity; and the humeral shaft. The proximal humerus usually fractures into these segments.

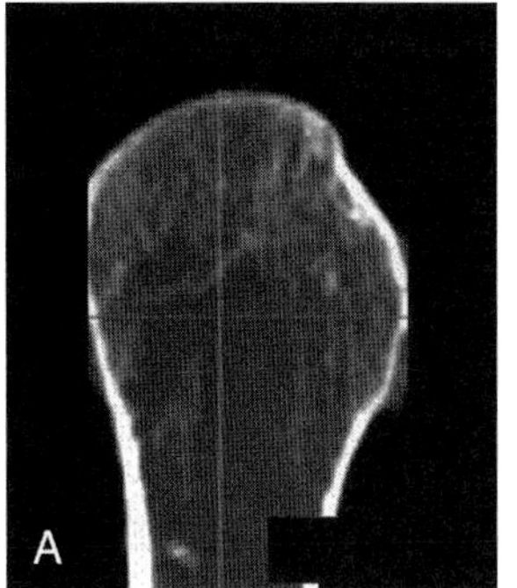

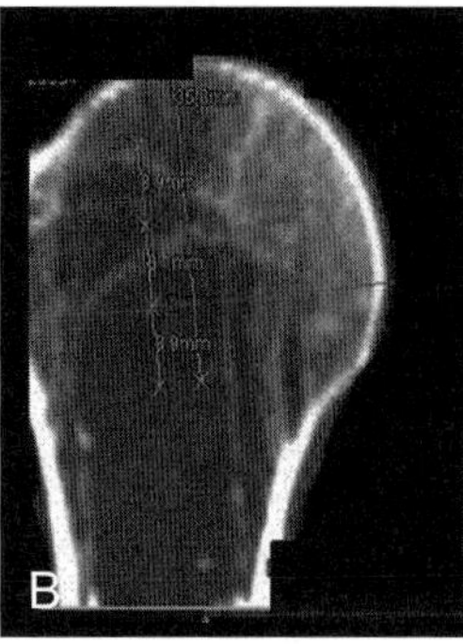

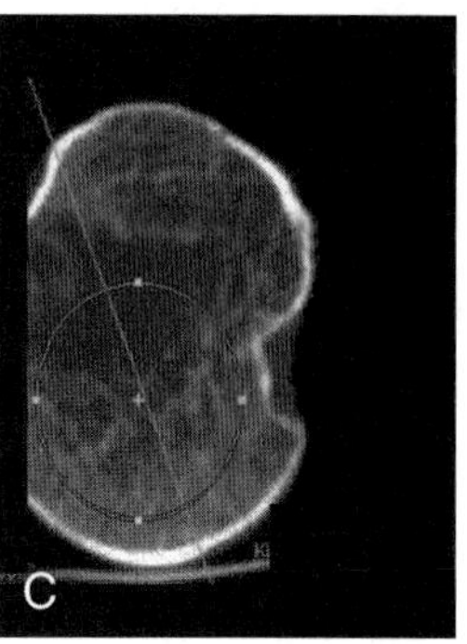

Figure 2 CT scans in the sagittal **(A)**, coronal **(B)**, and axillary **(C)** planes, showing an osteoporotic proximal humerus in which the central portion of the metaphysis is relatively devoid of bone.

locking plate technology for use when appropriate to facilitate humeral head preservation.

Anatomy

The unique anatomic characteristics of the proximal humerus must be considered when planning the treatment of a proximal humerus fracture. The proximal humerus is divided into four bony segments: the humeral head (with its spherical articular surface), the greater tuberosity, the lesser tuberosity, and the humeral shaft. The anatomic neck demarcates the junction between the humeral head and the metaphysis, the surgical neck demarcates the metaphyseal flares just distal to the tuberosities, and the bicipital groove separates the tuberosities. The proximal humerus fractures predictably through the anatomic junction lines into the bony segments (Figure 1). The fracture line between the tuberosities is an exception to this pattern, however; usually the fracture is located a few millimeters lateral to the bicipital groove rather than within the groove. Classifications of proximal humerus fractures based on these anatomic characteristics can be useful in determining treatment and have been shown to predict outcomes.[10]

The humeral articular segment is almost spherical, with a 46-mm average diameter of curvature (range, 37 to 57 mm). The average shaft-head angle is 130°; the humeral head center is offset from the humeral shaft axis by an average of 3 mm posteriorly and 7 mm medially.[15] There is an average 20° of humeral head retroversion; however, the variance among individuals is significant, ranging from 6.7° of anteversion to 47.5° of retroversion.[16]

The four rotator cuff tendons surround the humeral head and are attached to the tuberosities. By transmitting deforming muscular forces to the tuberosities, the rotator cuff tendons contribute to the typical pattern of fracture fragment displacement around the proximal humerus. The insertions of the supraspinatus, infraspinatus, and teres minor tendons onto the greater tuberosity contribute to the typical posterosuperior retraction of this fragment. The subscapularis tendon causes the lesser tuberosity fragment to retract medially. The head fragment rotates internally if the lesser tuberosity is still attached to the head fragment.

An osteoporotic proximal humerus can be thought of as resembling an eggshell because the central portion of the metaphysis is relatively devoid of bone[17](Figure 2). The best bone for securing the humeral head fracture fragments is in the subchondral bone.[18] Within the tuberosities, the bone at the tendinous insertion tends to be dense and strong. It is important to remember that the rotator cuff tendons usually are stronger than the bone that is the base for suture fixation of the tuberosities.[19]

It also is important to understand the blood flow dynamics of the proximal humerus because the humeral head is at risk of necrosis after the fracture and surgical intervention. The friction of a conventional plate and screws on the periosteum may cause the blood flow to be further reduced.[20,21] Studies of intact proximal humeri found that the major sources of blood perfusion to the humeral head are the anterior circumflex humeral artery and its interosseous branch (the arcuate artery)[20-22] (Figure 3). The anterior circumflex humeral artery is disrupted in most fracture patterns, and the implication is that perfusion from the posterior circumflex humeral artery often is sufficient for humeral head survival. Hertel and associates[23] found that the predictive factors for humeral head ischemia after a proximal humerus fracture are anatomic neck fracture, metaphyseal head extension of less than 8 mm (accuracy, 84%) and medial head disruption of more than 2 mm (accuracy, 79%) (Figure 4). The combination of these three factors had a positive predictive value of 97% for humeral head ischemia.

Classifications

In 1934, Codman[24] formulated a classification system based on the four segments of the proximal humerus. In 1970, Neer[10] modified and improved Codman's classification based on an analysis of 300 displaced proximal humerus fractures. Neer grouped the fractures by the number of fragments and their displacement from one another; the criteria for displacement were 45° of angulation or more than 1 cm of displacement. Neer's classification emphasizes the prognostic importance of fracture-dislocations and the

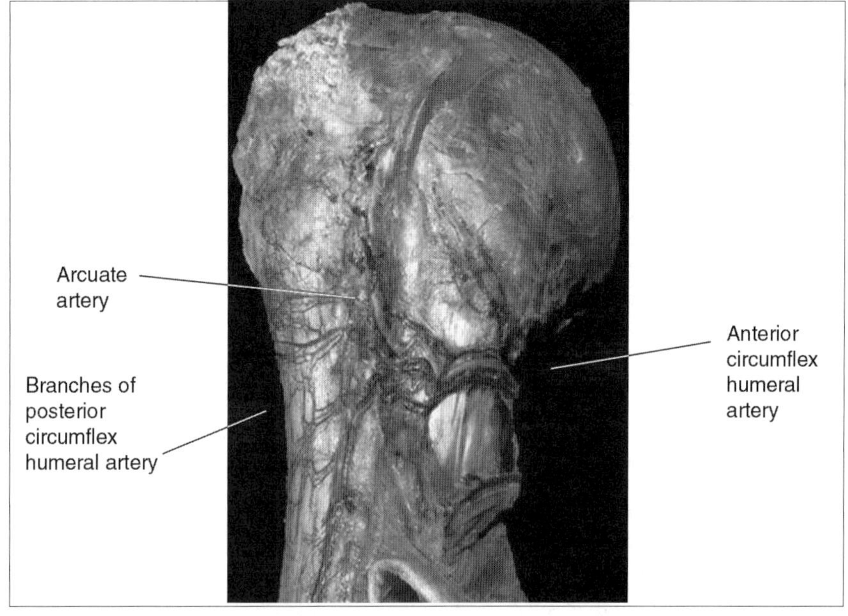

Figure 3 Photograph showing the anterior circumflex humeral artery and its interosseous branch, the arcuate artery, as well as the branches of the posterior circumflex humeral artery. The anterior circumflex and arcuate arteries are the most important sources of blood perfusion to the humeral head.

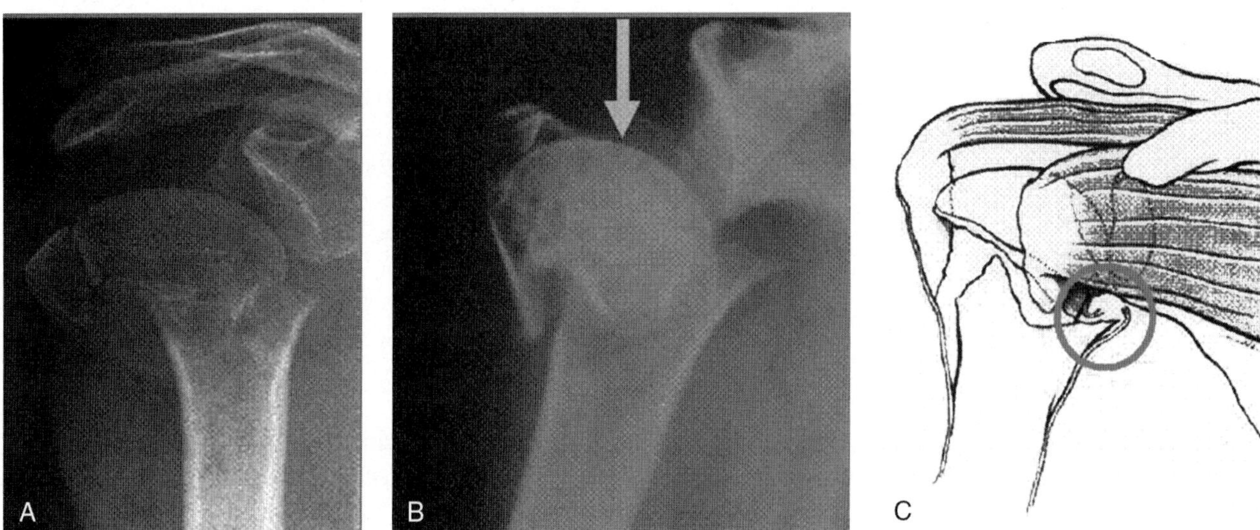

Figure 4 The three predictive factors for humeral head ischemia after a proximal humerus fracture. **A,** AP radiograph showing an anatomic neck fracture. **B,** AP radiograph showing metaphyseal head extension of less than 8 mm (*arrow*). **C,** Schematic diagram showing medial head disruption of more than 2 mm (circle).

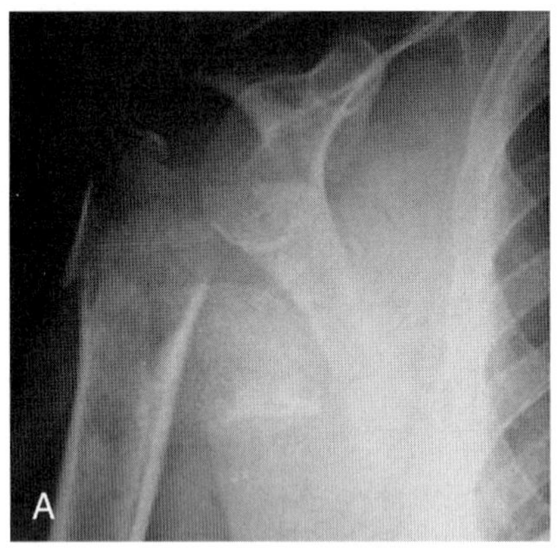

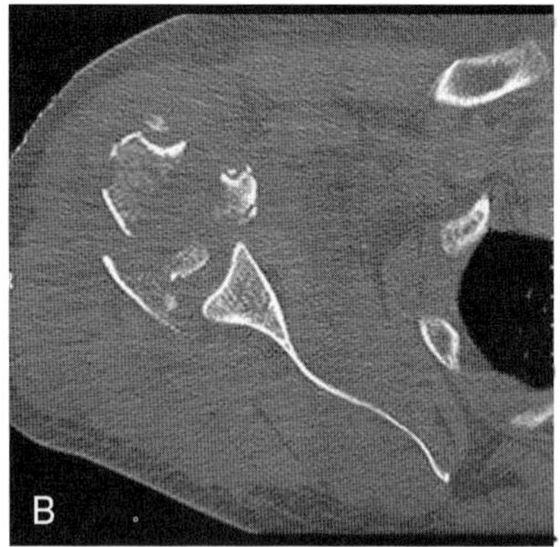

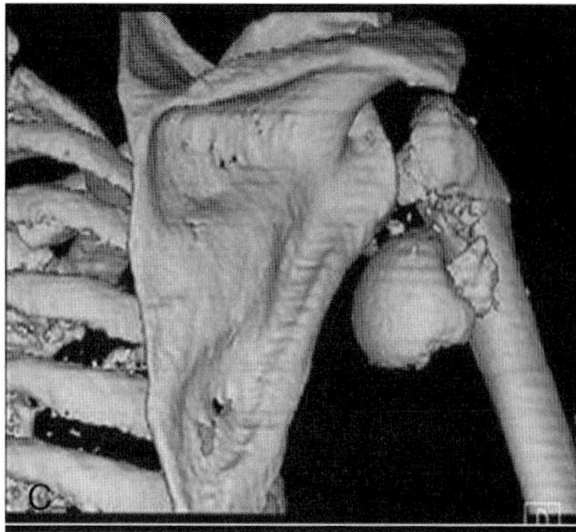

Figure 5 A comminuted, displaced proximal humerus fracture as seen on an AP radiograph **(A)**, an axillary CT scan **(B)**, and a three-dimensional CT reconstruction **(C)**.

significance of articular surface involvement for osteonecrosis of the humeral head.

Jakob and Ganz[25] studied 730 fractures and in 1982 proposed the AO-ASIF group classification, which was modified by the Orthopaedic Trauma Association. Proximal humerus fractures were divided into 27 subgroups based on the risk of osteonecrosis of the humeral head (as determined by the extent of articular involvement and likelihood of vascular injury).[26] Although this classification has not been widely used because of its complexity, it has a role in clinical research and cohort analysis.

No single classification of proximal humerus fractures is widely accepted. The Neer and AO-ASIF classifications[10,26] are the most widely used in evaluating proximal humerus fractures and determining their treatment. The fair to poor observer reliability and reproducibility of both classification systems cause difficulty in comparing the numerous clinical studies.[27,28] Most classification systems rely on the use of conventional radiographs in one to three planes, which is the standard diagnostic procedure for proximal humerus fractures. CT is especially useful for a fracture that cannot be fully assessed with conventional radiographs; in particular, a head split fracture is not adequately described by the classification systems[29] (Figure 5).

Principles of Treatment

The goals of treating a proximal humerus fracture are to maximize shoulder function and minimize shoulder pain. Both nonsurgical and surgical treatment may be considered. Neer's guidelines for deciding whether to use nonsurgical or surgical treatment for proximal humerus fractures cannot be considered the gold standard, according to the criteria of evidence-based medicine.[10,28-31] Both nonsurgical and surgical treatments have advantages and disadvantages, and each can lead to an excellent or poor outcome. The choice of treatment is still a controversial topic.[32,33]

A thorough history and physical examination are required, with particular attention to concomitant injuries and a thorough evaluation of neurovascular status. The radiographs should include the true AP shoulder, scapular lateral, and axillary views. CT is used to assess comminution, displacement of tuberosities, posterior dislocation, or concomitant glenoid fracture. CT is recommended, with or without three-dimensional reconstruction, if it appears necessary to fully assess the extent and pattern of the fracture.

It is recommended that a nondisplaced or minimally displaced proximal humerus fracture be treated nonsurgically. The treatment of a displaced humeral head fracture should be guided by a careful assessment of the fracture pattern, bone quality, degree of comminution, rotator cuff status, vascular status, and risk of humeral head osteonecrosis, as well as patient factors such as age, preinjury health, level of activity, and expectations. Proper patient selection perhaps is the most important factor in achieving a good outcome.

Methods of Surgical Treatment

A systematic approach to surgical fixation of proximal humerus fractures was first described by Lambotte in Belgium and Lane in England.[34,35] Other surgeons subsequently described methods of surgi-

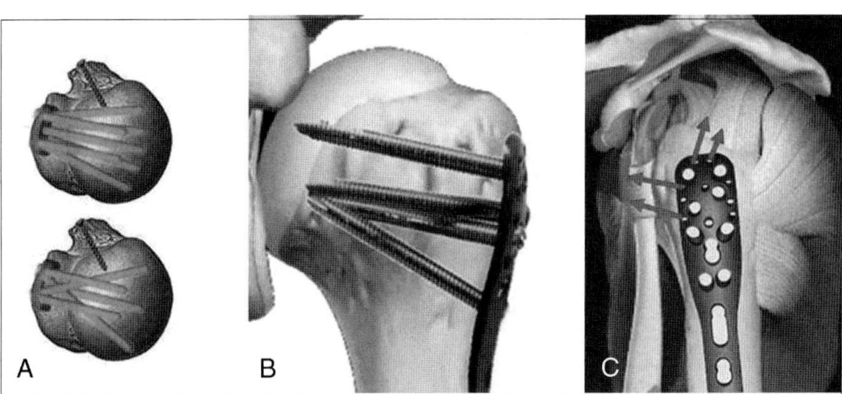

Figure 6 The locking screw plate design has multiple, diverging points of screw fixation in the humeral head **(A)**, a low profile **(B)**, and small holes for rotator cuff fixation **(C)**. The holes for supraspinatus and subscapularis fixation are shown in **C** (superior and anterior arrows, respectively).

Table 1
The Advantages of a Locking Plate System Over a Conventional Plate System for Fixation of a Proximal Humerus Fracture

Superior mechanical properties (stiffness, torsional resistance, load resistance)
Greater pullout strength
Better preservation of the blood supply to the bone
Decreased surgical time (because screw length is not measured)
Low profile
Greater suitability for osteoporotic bones (because the plate is less stiff)
Small holes for rotator cuff tendon fixation
Choice of plate fixation techniques in the shaft area

cal reduction and fixation of proximal humerus fractures using staples, percutaneous pins, intramedullary rods and pins, tension bands (with or without plates or rods), standard plates and screws, blade plate constructs, and hemiarthroplasty.[36-43] Many alternative surgical techniques evolved because standard plating initially had high failure rates. Several authors recommended hemiarthroplasty for the treatment of most three- and four-part proximal humerus fractures; however, the results of hemiarthroplasty for proximal humerus fractures were found to be inferior to those of hemiarthroplasty for glenohumeral arthritis or humeral head osteonecrosis, with higher rates of complications and revision surgery.[42] Locking plates were developed to provide a viable alternative to prosthetic replacement and to conserve the humeral head. Locking plates allow more secure fixation of proximal humerus fractures. The suture eyelets in locking plates enhance the fixation construct and resist deforming muscular forces to reduce the risk of failure.

The principle of conventional plate-and-screw fixation of fractures is to obtain the most stable fixation possible, after anatomic reduction, for the purpose of allowing early joint mobilization.[44] The use of conventional plates requires a surgical approach with a relatively large incision and complete bone exposure.[45] The plate is stabilized as a result of the friction between the undersurface of the plate and the bone; thus, surgeons are encouraged to tighten the screws forcefully to obtain a compression fit between the plate and the bone.[45] The construct is biomechanically stable, but healing can be delayed because of extensive soft-tissue dissection, bony devascularization, and damage to the periosteal blood supply at the contact area of the plate and the bone.[14] Another important disadvantage of this system is the dependence of the fixation on bone quality and the purchase of the two bone cortices by the screws. Screw engagement in the bone is compromised, and the failure rate is high in periarticular fractures with a short periarticular bony fragment, fractures in osteoporotic bone, and metaphyseal comminuted fractures.[14]

The Fixed-Angle Locking Plate Systems

The fixed-angle locking plate was developed to overcome these obstacles to fracture management. Biomechanical studies found improved periarticular fragment fixation when a fixed-angle device was used. The locking screw plate design has advantageous mechanical properties (Table 1). Locking plate fixation is superior in stiffness, torsional resistance, ultimate load, and displacement to buttress plate, blade plate, or T plate fixation of proximal humerus fractures.[46,47] The diverging screw insertion into the center of the humeral head increases the pullout strength of the locking plate[45] (Figure 6). The mechanical qualities of fixed-angle plate fixation allow functional physical therapy to start soon after surgery, without the risk of screw loosening or secondary loss of reduction. Loss of proximal humerus fracture fixation after the use of a fixed-angle plate was found to be 4%, compared with 22% after use of a conventional plate.[48] In a locking plate construct, threads on the screw head lock into corresponding

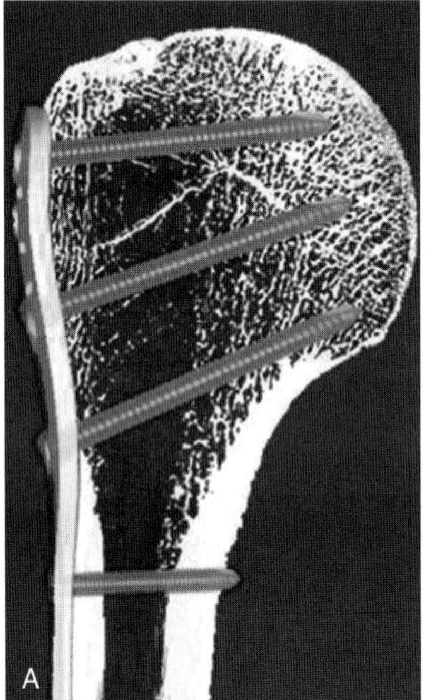

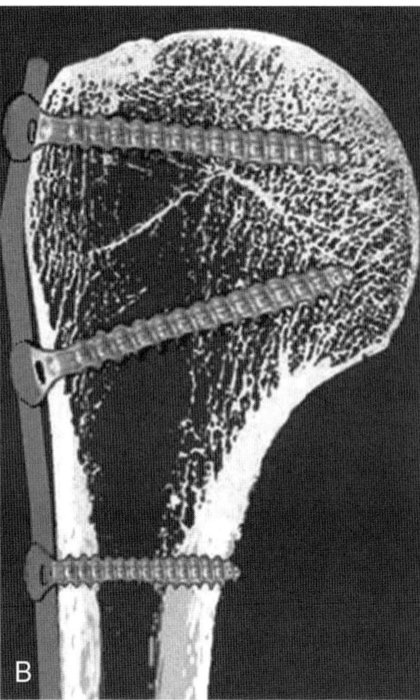

Figure 7 **A,** In a locking plate construct, the forces are transferred from the bone to the plate across the threaded connections between the screw and the plate, thus improving angular stability and preventing screw toggling. **B,** In a standard plate construct, there is no fixation between the screws and the plate, and the risk of screw toggling is greater.

Table 2
The Disadvantages of a Locking Plate System Over a Conventional Plate System for Fixation of a Proximal Humerus Fracture

Lack of tactile feedback during screw tightening

Inability to use the construct for obtaining or adjusting fracture reduction

Rigid fracture distraction (possibly causing delayed union or nonunion)

Inability to alter the angle of the screws in the plate holes

Inability to contour the plate to individual anatomy

More difficult hardware removal

Greater financial cost

threads on the screw hole of the plate. The forces are transferred from the bone to the plate across the threaded connection between the screw and the plate[49] (Figure 7). Bicortical purchase and compression of the plate to the underlying bone are not required to achieve construct stability, and the blood supply to the bone is better preserved. Eliminating the need for bicortical drilling allows surgical time to be minimized because there is no need for percutaneous screw length measurement, and the risk of refracture after plate removal is reduced.[49] A locking plate construct might be considered the ultimate internal-external fixator. The plate functions as a connecting bar placed extremely close to the mechanical axis of the bone; the ability to move the plate closer to the mechanical axis should markedly increase its stability in comparison with external fixators in which the bar is far from the limb axis and a large bending moment is created.

Locking plates have been developed for proximal humerus fracture fixation with particular attention to the specific anatomic characteristics of this region. Most of the plate designs are low profile to enable minimally invasive percutaneous insertion and proximal plate fixation and to avoid compromising the soft tissue (Figure 6). The risk of impingement decreases as range of motion improves during rehabilitation. These locking plates are less stiff than implants designed for lower extremity fractures, and thus they are better suited to osteoporotic bone and have a more positive effect on load capacity. Small holes in the humeral head area of all plate designs allow for rotator cuff fixation with sutures or cerclage wires, thus eliminating deforming forces on the fracture fragments. In the shaft area, different plate fixation techniques can be used because the plate has combination holes permitting insertion of locked screws or conventional small fragment screws (which can be introduced as compression screws, lag screws, or stationary holding screws).

The locking plate systems have several potential disadvantages, as listed in Table 2. The surgeon receives little tactile feedback while the screws are being tightened. All screws abruptly stop advancing when the threads are completely seated into the plate, regardless of bone quality. The locked screws cannot pull the plate down to the bone; locking plates can be used to maintain fracture reduction but not to obtain it. Full fracture reduction must be obtained before placement of any locked screw; after locked screws are placed above and below a fracture line, a reduction adjustment is possible only if the screws are completely removed. In addition, the rigidity of a locked screw construct means that any fracture distraction at the time of reduction or fracture resorption during healing is held rigidly and could result in delayed union or nonunion. With most currently used systems, the surgeon cannot alter the angle of the screw in the plate hole without destroying the ability of the screw to lock. The plate cannot be contoured because an attempt to contour the plate could distort the screw hole and adversely affect screw purchase. Hardware removal can be difficult if a locking plate was used, especially if the locked screws become cold welded to the plate. This difficulty is more common with titanium, rather than stainless steel, hardware. Cross-threaded screws also can cause difficulty in hardware removal. In some current systems, the use of torque-limiting screwdrivers may minimize the likelihood of this complication. A final disadvantage is that a locking plate system is more expensive than an equivalent nonlocking system.

Because of the disadvantages of locking plate systems, they should be used selectively for types of fractures that have a high failure rate when conventional plating is used. Locking plates are primarily indicated for patients who have a displaced three- or four-part fracture of the proximal humerus and for patients with severe osteoporosis who have an unstable fracture of the proximal humerus. (The radiographic width of the humeral cortices and the patient's medical history are used to determine the presence of severe osteoporosis.) A locking plate also can be used for a tilted and severely displaced two-part surgical neck fracture. A locking plate should not be used if the patient has an acute infection or is a child with open growth plates.

Surgical Treatment Using a Fixed-Angle Locking Plate

Operating Room Setup

A systematic approach to setup of the operating room is crucial for good intraoperative fluoroscopy. The patient is positioned on a beach chair operating table or a conventional operating table equipped with a long beanbag contoured medial to the scapula to ensure that the entire shoulder girdle is exposed for fluoroscopic imaging. After general anesthesia takes effect, the patient's buttocks are positioned at the break of the table, a wedge pillow is placed under the knees, and the back is elevated 30° into the modified beach chair position. All prominences are well padded.

After the bed is rotated 90° in relation to the anesthesiology equipment, a fluoroscopic C-arm is oriented parallel to the table so that it can be moved into position over or under the shoulder from a position at the head of the table. This C-arm positioning simplifies the use of fluoroscopy and allows an unobstructed intraoperative view of the shoulder with minimal repositioning. The image receiver is positioned near the foot of the table on the side opposite the C-arm so that it can be easily seen by the surgeon. AP and axillary radiographs are taken before the shoulder is prepared and draped, with the patient repositioned if necessary to obtain satisfactory images. The exact position and orientation of the C-arm are marked on the operating room floor so that it can be easily returned to the correct position after the shoulder and arm are prepared and draped. With an articulated arm holder, the extremity can be variably positioned throughout the procedure.

Approach, Reduction, and Fixation

A standard deltopectoral approach is used to expose the fracture site. The incision begins just superomedial to the coracoid process and travels distally to the middle of the humerus at the insertion of the deltoid. If a distal extension is needed, it can run straight down the anterolateral aspect of the arm. The cephalic vein is mobilized and retracted medially to prevent inadvertent injury during retraction and drilling. Numerous branches from the deltoid must be identified and cauterized. The subdeltoid interval is released, and the deltoid retracted. The leading edge of the coracoacromial ligament may be resected to improve visualization and mobilization of the fragments. The upper pectoralis major tendon may be released to facilitate the exposure and decrease the deforming force on the humeral shaft. The clavipectoral fascia is identified and released. The blood clot, incipient callus, and fibrous tissue, as well as the thick distended subacromial bursa, must be excised to obtain an adequate view of the fracture.

The fracture hematoma often obscures the normal landmarks. The biceps tendon, which can be palpated deep to the pectoralis major tendon, can be followed for orientation. The long biceps tendon may be interposed in the fracture fragments and require mobilization. Care should be taken to preserve the ascending branch of the anterior circumflex humeral artery, which is located laterally in the bicipital groove and is the primary blood supply to the head fragment. If further exposure is needed, the rotator cuff interval may be opened by following the course of the long biceps tendon to its attachment at the superior margin of the glenoid. An initial attempt

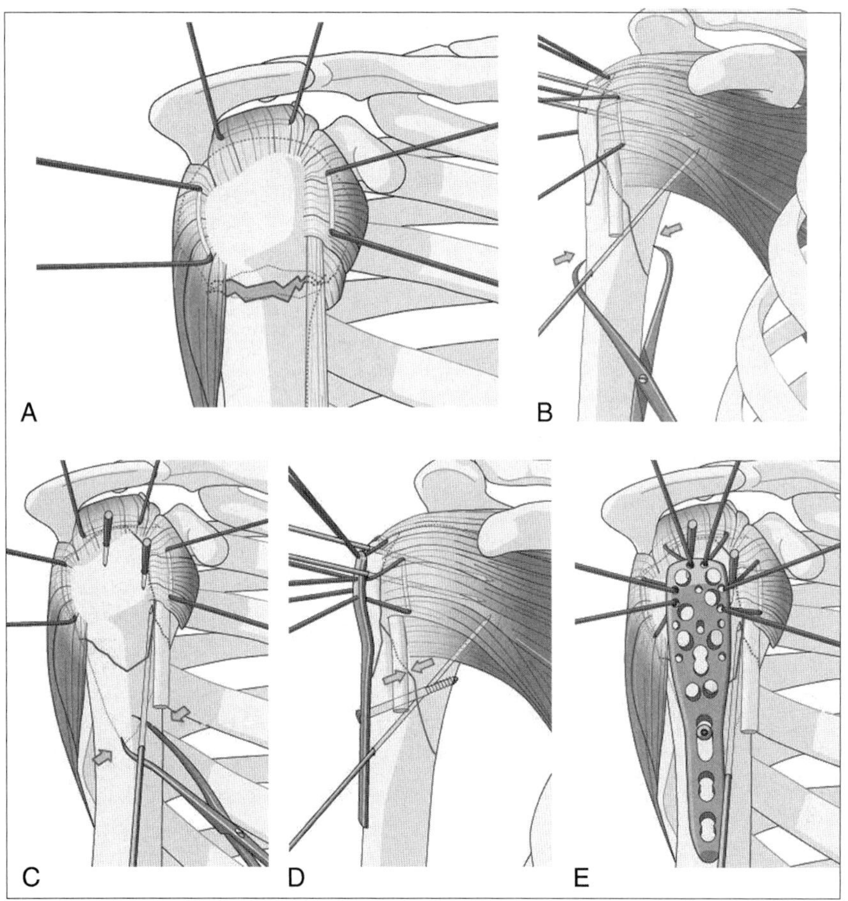

Figure 8 Drawings showing fixation of a proximal humerus fracture using a fixed-angle locking plate. **A,** Sutures are pulled through the insertions of the subscapularis, supraspinatus, and infraspinatus tendons to assist in fracture manipulation and reduction. The reduced fracture is provisionally secured with 2-mm Kirschner wires, as seen in AP **(B)** and lateral **(C)** views. The plate is fixed to the shaft through the slotted gliding hole to allow minor adjustments in plate height, as seen in AP **(D)** and lateral **(E)** views. To allow the plate to be compressed to the bone, the first shaft screw typically is not a locking screw; the screw also has compressed the fracture line in **D**. Arrows = reduction and compression of the fracture line. Solid and broken lines = bone margins.

should be made to preserve the tendon as a landmark for use in plate placement. However, it is usually advisable to perform a subpectoral biceps tenodesis after definitive fracture fixation to eliminate a potential source of pain and the risk of postoperative rupture. After the rotator cuff interval is opened, sutures are placed through the insertions of the subscapularis, supraspinatus, and infraspinatus tendons (Figure 8, *A*). These sutures are used for fracture manipulation and reduction; in particular, they can be pulled to bring the humeral head out of varus.

In an anterior fracture-dislocation, the humeral head usually is dislocated in the subcoracoid space. All releases should be performed first, and a gentle manipulation can be done using a Key or Cobb elevator to relocate the head fragment into the joint. Overzealous pulling on the fragment should be avoided to prevent neurovascular injury. It may be prudent for a vascular surgeon to be available during fracture relocation.

After adequate removal of fracture debris, the head is reduced into anatomic alignment with the assistance of a Key elevator. To help maintain the reduction, 2-mm Kirschner wires are placed through the head fragment and the shaft. Fluoroscopy is used to confirm proper head positioning until an acceptable reduction is established.

When the humeral head is correctly positioned in the joint, traction sutures are used at the rotator cuff tendon origins to reduce the tuberosities to the head. Finally, the shaft is reduced to the proximal segment, and the reduction is provisionally secured using 2-mm Kirschner wires (Figure 8, *B* and *C*). The reduction is confirmed using fluoroscopy.

If metaphyseal comminution is present, osteoconductive bone graft material or allograft is used to help buttress the head fragment and prevent a postoperative loss of reduction. The graft is placed in the canal of the proximal shaft, and the head is impacted onto the prominent allograft.

After the reduction is confirmed, an appropriately sized internal fixation plate is selected. The plate should be positioned just lateral to the bicipital groove, with the upper portion of the plate 8 mm distal to the top of the greater tuberosity (Figure 8, *D* and *E*). The implant height is confirmed under fluoroscopy. One or two screws are used to secure the plate to the shaft, and at least three more screws are used to secure the plate to the head fragment. The fixation is confirmed by manipulation of the construct under fluoroscopic imaging. When the plate placement is determined to be satisfactory, the screws are inserted, and the rotator cuff sutures are secured to the plate. Usually three or four screws are needed to secure the plate to the humeral head, and an additional three screws are needed to secure the plate to the humeral shaft. Fluoroscopic imaging is used to confirm adequate positioning and fixation (Figure 9). Orthogonal views must be taken to rule out head penetration by the fixation screws.

The rotator cuff interval is closed with size 2 Ethibond suture (Ethicon, Somerville, NJ), and the wound is carefully irrigated and closed in standard fashion.

A minimally invasive percutaneous approach can be chosen as an alternative to the standard approach. This technique involves two minimal skin incisions: a direct lateral longitudinal incision extending distally 4 cm from the lateral edge of the acromion and a 2-cm longitudinal distal shaft incision at the level of the most inferior holes of the plate (Figure 10). The lateral deltoid split approach is used, with careful identification and protection of the axillary nerve. The reduction can be supported by a blunt dissector, Kirschner wires, and traction sutures at the rotator cuff tendon origins.[50] The attachable insertion guide used to facilitate screw placement in the standard deltopectoral approach is too bulky to be safely used in this percutaneous approach, and the distal edge of the guide would impinge on the axillary nerve.[50] The locking plate can be safely fixed to the bone by using screws in the most proximal six holes of the plate and three or four screws in the shaft holes distal to the slot hole.[50,51]

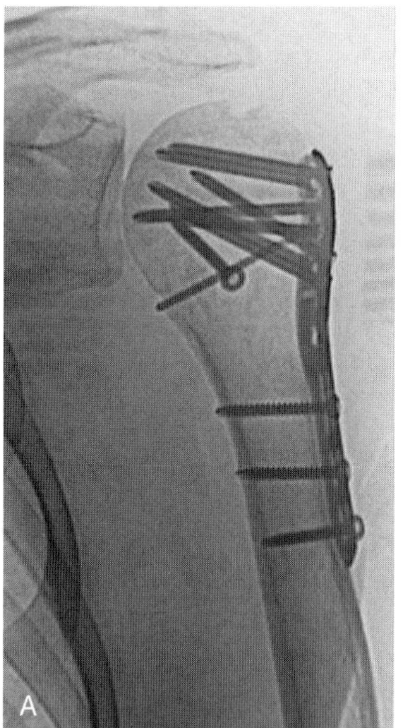

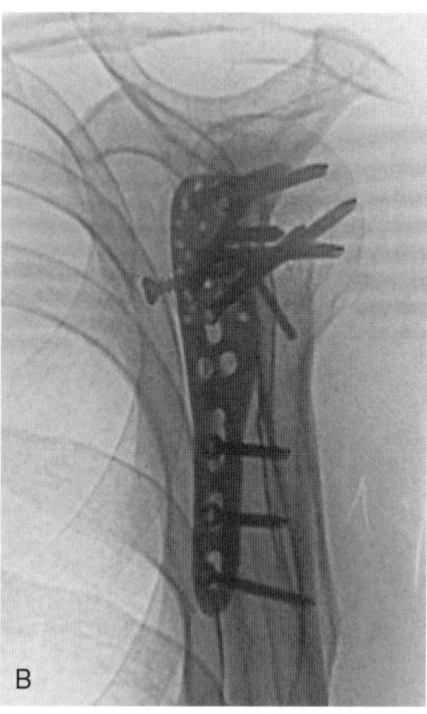

Figure 9 Final AP **(A)** and lateral Y scapular **(B)** fluoroscopic images used to confirm adequate positioning and fixation. Final imaging is done when the plate placement appears to be satisfactory, all screws are inserted, and the rotator cuff sutures are secured to the plate.

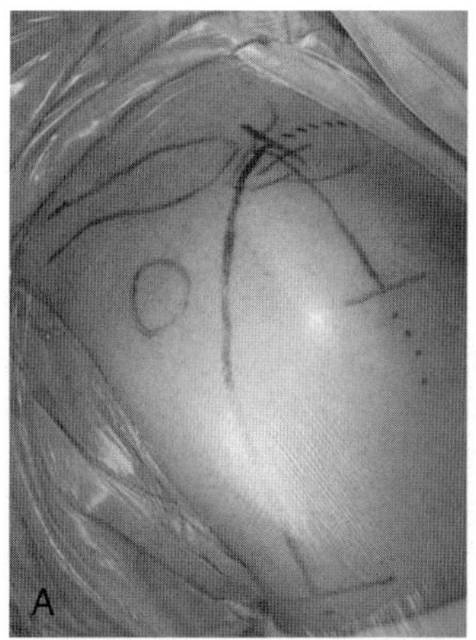

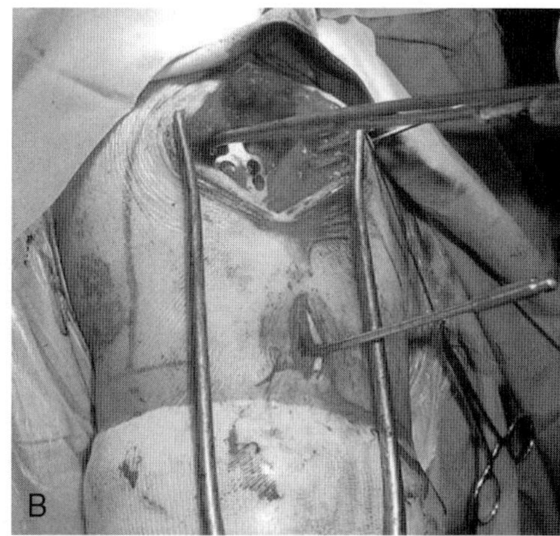

Figure 10 Photographs showing the minimally invasive percutaneous approach for fixation of a proximal humerus fracture. **A,** Incision-site skin marking. **B,** Plate placement.

Postoperative Management

A postoperative hospital stay of 1 or 2 days usually is required for pain control and administration of intravenous antibiotics. The patient's arm is placed in a sling on the operating table and is immobilized for approximately 1 month to allow early fracture healing. Simple pendulum exercises are allowed, and elbow, wrist, and finger movement is encouraged. After the first month,

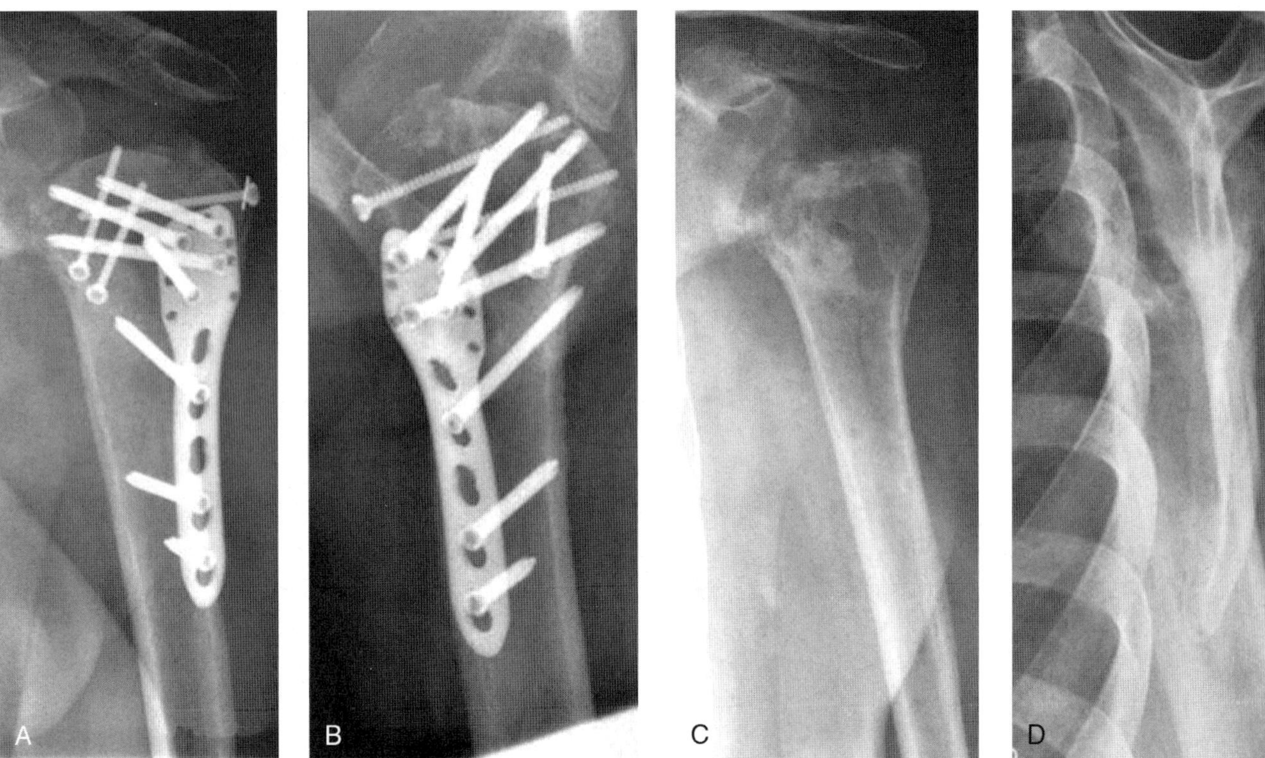

Figure 11 AP **(A)** and axillary **(B)** radiographs taken 6 months after fracture fixation with a proximal humerus locking plate, showing screw penetration of the humeral head. AP **(C)** and lateral Y scapular **(D)** radiographs taken 1 year after the fracture fixation, showing osteonecrosis of the humeral head.

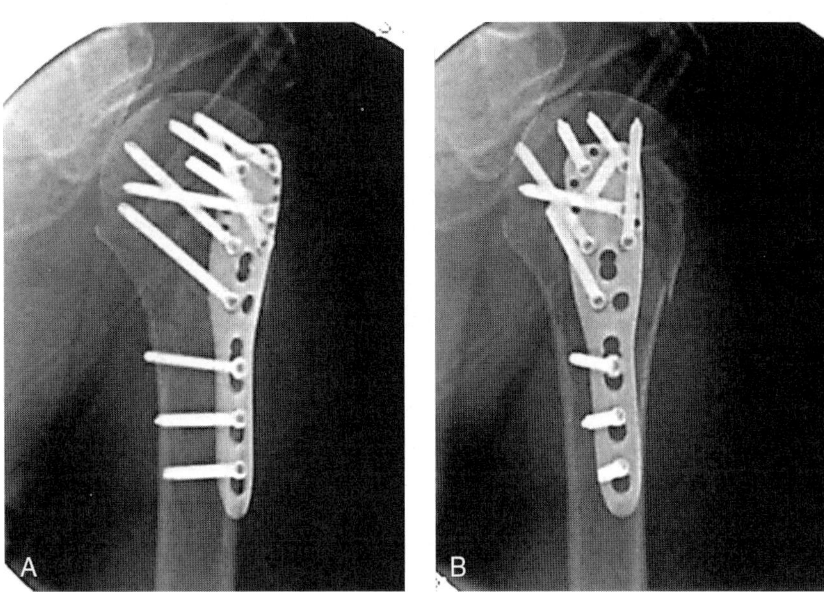

Figure 12 AP radiographs taken with the shoulder in internal **(A)** or external **(B)** rotation, showing humeral head screw penetration after proximal humerus fracture fixation with a locking plate.

the patient usually is ready to begin active assisted shoulder exercises using the other arm or a stick pushed by the other arm. Passive manipulation by a therapist is neither necessary nor helpful. Strengthening exercises (including isometric exercises) should be deferred until at least 3 months after surgery, when solid healing is well established.

Complications

Several clinical studies have described complications after the use of locking plates for the fixation of proximal humerus fractures. Although complications sometimes result from fracture characteristics or bone quality, more often the implant or the surgical technique is responsible. The reported incidence of complications is as high as 36%.[52]

The incidence of humeral head osteonecrosis reported in studies of proximal humerus locking plates ranges from 4% to 16%[53-57] (Figure 11). This relatively low rate of complications may be attributable to the surgical technique and the biomechanical advantages of locking plate designs. The incidence of humeral head screw penetration is 5% to 23%[52,57-59] (Figure 12). The exceptional fixation strength of the locking plate, the lack of mechanical support in the inferomedial region of the proximal humerus, and poor bone quality contribute to the incidence of this complication. Patients older than 60 years have a higher incidence of screw penetration, regardless of fracture type.[52,56,58] Other, less commonly reported complications of the proximal humerus locking plate include deep infection, plate buckling and breakage, screw loosening, varus malalignment (Figure 13), subacromial impingement, fracture malunion or nonunion, iatrogenic fracture comminution, nerve palsy, and deltoid paresthesia.[53-59]

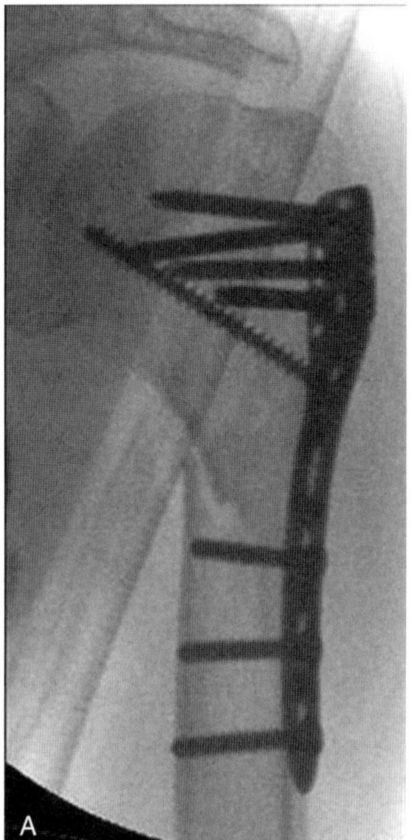

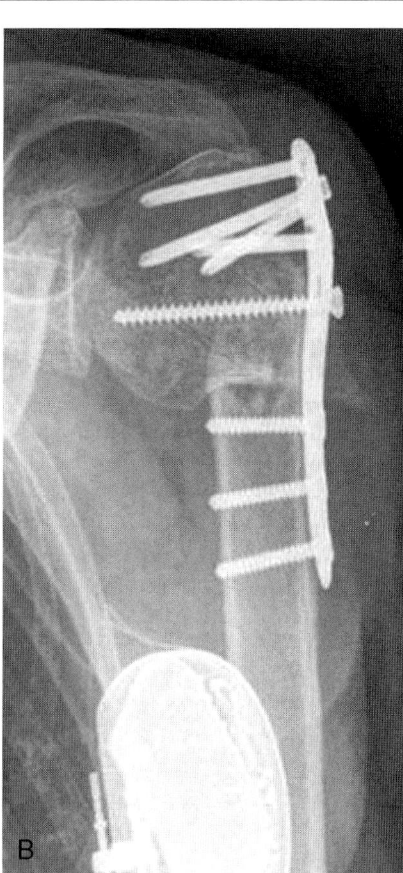

Figure 13 **A,** AP fluoroscopic image showing the final positioning and locking plate fixation of a proximal humerus fracture. **B,** AP radiograph showing varus displacement of the head fragment 6 months after surgery.

Research Results

The treatment of proximal humerus fractures with a fixed-angled locking plate requires caution because there is a lack of clinical data comparing this and other treatment methods. Several short-term studies have reported varying outcomes (Table 3). Plecko and Kraus[55] reviewed the outcomes of 36 patients at 31-month follow-up after locking plate fixation of an unstable displaced proximal humerus fracture. The mean Constant score was 63 points, and the mean age-related Constant score was 81%; the mean Disabilities of the Arm, Shoulder, and Hand Shoulder Disability Questionnaire score was 18 points, which was interpreted as a satisfactory result for 75% of the patients. Three patients had osteonecrosis, one had a deep infection, and one had a nonunion.

In a prospective cohort study of 29 proximal humerus fractures treated with a proximal humerus locking plate, Fankhauser and associates[56] reported an average Constant score of 75 at 1-year follow-up. One patient had plate breakage, four had loss of alignment, and one had a deep infection.

Laflamme and associates,[50] in a multicenter prospective clinical study of 34 patients who underwent percutaneous humeral plating of fractures of the proximal humerus, reported an average Constant score of 82 and a Disabilities of the Arm, Shoulder, and Hand Shoulder Disability Questionnaire score of 26 at 1-year follow-up. All fractures healed within the first 6 months after surgery. There was no axillary nerve injury or humeral head osteonecrosis. Two patients required revision surgery for removal of the plate or an intra-articular screw or because of acromial impingement.

Owsley and Gorczyca[52] recently reported on 53 patients treated with a locking plate for a proximal humerus fracture. At a minimum 1-year follow-up, 19 (36%) had radiographic signs of one or more

Table 3
Recent Studies of Locking Plate Fixation for Proximal Humerus Fractures

Study	Number of Shoulders	Fracture Patterns	Follow-Up (Months)	Final Constant Score	Complications
Egol et al[58]	51	Orthopaedic Trauma Association type A, 16; B, 12; C, 23	16	—	Screw penetration, 8 (16%); osteonecrosis, 2 (4%); implant failure, 2 (4%); deep infection, 1 (2%); nonunion, 1 (2%); heterotopic ossification, 1 (2%)
Owsley and Gorczyca[52]	53	Neer two-part fracture, 23; three-part, 28; four-part, 2	12	—	Screw penetration, 12 (23%); varus displacement, 13 (25%); osteonecrosis, 2 (4%)
Laflamme et al[50]	34	Neer displaced two-part surgical fracture or three-part severely impacted (> 160°) valgus fracture	12	82 (average)	Impingement, 1 (3%); screw penetration, 1 (3%)
Kettler et al[60]	176	—	9	81%	Malreduction, 25 (14%); screw penetration, 24 (14%); loss of reduction, 14 (8%); osteonecrosis, 5 (3%); infection, 2 (1%)
Plecko and Kraus[55]	36	AO-ASIF type A3, 8; B1, 1; B2, 5; B3, 3; C1, 1; C2, 16; C3, 2	31	81%	Osteonecrosis, 3 (8%); deep infection, 1 (3%); nonunion, 1 (3%)
Fankhauser et al[56]	29	AO-ASIF type A, 5; B, 15; C, 9	12	75 (average)	Redislocation, 4 (14%); varus malunion, 3 (10%); osteonecrosis, 2 (7%); plate breakage, 1 (3%); infection, 1 (3%)

complications, including 12 (23%) with intra-articular screw cutout, 13 (25%) with varus displacement, and 2 (4%) with osteonecrosis.

Egol and associates[58] recently reported that 47 of 51 patients (92%) who were treated with a proximal humerus locking plate had fracture healing within 3 months of the surgery. However, 12 (24%) had a complication, and 8 (16%) required further surgery.

Kettler and associates[60] studied 225 proximal humerus fractures treated with a locking plate. In the 176 patients available for review, the mean Constant score was 70 points, and the mean age-related Constant score was 81%. The complications included initial malreduction of the head and tuberosities in 25 (14%); screw perforation of the humeral head in 24 (14%); loss of reduction and secondary screw perforations in 14 (8%); complete or partial osteonecrosis of the humeral head in 5 (3%) or 9 (5%), respectively; and infection in 2 (1%) of the patients.

Summary

Proximal humerus fractures are common, especially among patients older than 60 years who have osteoporosis. Formerly, both nonsurgical therapy and hemiarthroplasty were considered to be a standard of care because plating was associated with a high complication rate and a poor outcome. The introduction of fixed-angle locking plates has provided a new treatment option for these complicated fractures, especially in patients with osteoporosis. Locking plates for treating comminuted proximal humerus fractures were found to have biologic and biomechanical advantages over conventional plates. Additional data are needed from prospective clinical studies to compare locking plate fixation with other surgical treatments.

References

1. Lind T, Kroner K, Jensen J: The epidemiology of fractures of the proximal humerus. *Arch Orthop Trauma Surg* 1989;180:285.
2. Horak J, Nilsson BE: Epidemiology of fractures of the upper end of the humerus. *Clin Orthop Relat Res* 1975; 112:250-253.
3. Green A, Norris T: Proximal humerus fractures and fracture dislocations, in Jupiter J, ed: *Skeletal Trauma*, ed 3. Philadelphia, PA, WB Saunders, 2003, pp 1532-1624.
4. Sporer SM, Weinstein JN, Koval KJ: The geographic incidence and treat-

ment variation of common fractures of elderly patients. *J Am Acad Orthop Surg* 2006;14:246-255.

5. Olsson C, Nordqvist A, Petersson CJ: Increased fragility in patients with fracture of the proximal humerus: A case control study. *Bone* 2004;34: 1072-1077.
6. Chu SP, Kelsey JL, Keegan TH, et al: Risk factors for proximal humerus fracture. *Am J Epidemiol* 2004;160: 360-367.
7. Schwartz AV, Nevitt MC, Brown BW Jr, Kelsey JL: Increased falling as a risk factor for fracture among older women: The study of osteoporotic fractures. *Am J Epidemiol* 2005;161:180-185.
8. Kannus P, Palvanen M, Niemi S, Parkkari J, Järvinen M Vuori I: Osteoporotic fractures of the proximal humerus in elderly Finnish persons: Sharp increase in 1970-1998 and alarming projections for the new millennium. *Acta Orthop Scand* 2000;71: 465-470.
9. Court-Brown CM, Garg A, McQueen MM: The epidemiology of proximal humerus fractures. *Acta Orthop Scand* 2001;72:365-371.
10. Neer CS II: Displaced proximal humeral fractures: I. Classification and evaluation. *J Bone Joint Surg Am* 1970; 52:1077-1089.
11. Sadowski C, Riand N, Stern R, Hoffmeyer P: Fixation of fractures of the proximal humerus with the PlantTan Humerus Fixator Plate: Early experience with a new implant. *J Shoulder Elbow Surg* 2003;12:148-151.
12. Astrand J, Thorngren KG, Tägil M: One fracture is enough! Experience with a prospective and consecutive osteoporosis screening program with 239 fracture patients. *Acta Orthop* 2006;77:3-8.
13. Mittlmeier TW, Stedtfeld HW, Ewert A, Beck M, Frosch B, Gradl G: Stabilization of proximal humeral fractures with an angular and sliding stable antegrade locking nail (Targon PH). *J Bone Joint Surg Am* 2003;85: 136-146.
14. Haidukewych GJ: Innovations in locking plate technology. *J Am Acad Orthop Surg* 2004;12:205-212.
15. Robertson DD, Yuan J, Bigliani LU, Flatow EL, Yamaguchi K: Three-dimensional analysis of the proximal part of the humerus: Relevance to arthroplasty. *J Bone Joint Surg Am* 2000; 82:1594-1602.
16. Boileau P, Walch G: The three-dimensional geometry of the proximal humerus: Implications for surgical technique and prosthetic design. *J Bone Joint Surg Br* 1997;79:857-865.
17. Hepp P, Lill H, Bail H, et al: Where should implants be anchored in the humeral head? *Clin Orthop Relat Res* 2003;415:139-147.
18. Tingart MJ, Apreleva M, Zurakowski D, Warner JJ: Pullout strength of suture anchors used in rotator cuff repair. *J Bone Joint Surg Am* 2003;85: 2190-2198.
19. Hawkins RJ, Bell RH, Gurr K: The three-part fracture of the proximal part of the humerus: Operative treatment. *J Bone Joint Surg Am* 1986;68: 1410-1414.
20. Gerber C, Schneeberger AG, Vinh TS: The arterial vascularization of the humeral head: An anatomical study. *J Bone Joint Surg Am* 1990;72: 1486-1494.
21. Duparc F, Muller JM, Fréger P: Arterial blood supply of the proximal humeral epiphysis. *Surg Radiol Anat* 2001;23:185-190.
22. Brooks CH, Revell WJ, Heatley FW: Vascularity of the humeral head after proximal humeral fractures: An anatomical cadaver study. *J Bone Joint Surg Br* 1993;75:132-136.
23. Hertel R, Hempfing A, Stiehler M, Leunig M: Predictors of humeral head ischemia after intracapsular fracture of the proximal humerus. *J Shoulder Elbow Surg* 2004;13: 427-433.
24. Codman EA: *The Shoulder: Rupture of the Supraspinatus Tendon and Other Lesions in or About the Subacromial Bursa.* Boston, MA, Thomas Todd, 1934.
25. Jakob RP, Ganz R: Proximal humerus fractures. *Helv Chir Acta* 1982;48: 595-610.
26. Müller ME:The comprehensive classification of fractures of long bones, in Müller ME, Allgower M, Schneider R, Willenegger H, eds: *Manual of Internal Fixation: Techniques Recommended by the AO-ASIF Group*. Berlin, Germany, Springer-Verlag, 1991, pp 118-125.
27. Kristiansen B, Andersen UL, Olsen CA, Varmarken JE: The Neer classification of fractures of the proximal humerus: An assessment of interobserver variation. *Skeletal Radiol* 1988;17:420-422.
28. Siebenrock KA, Gerber C: The reproducibility of classification of fractures of the proximal end of the humerus. *J Bone Joint Surg Am* 1993;75:1751-1755.
29. Brien H, Noftall F, MacMaster S, Cummings T, Landells C, Rockwood P: Neer's classification system: A critical appraisal. *J Trauma* 1995;38: 257-260.
30. Neer CS II: Displaced proximal humeral fractures: II. Treatment of three-part and four-part displacement. *J Bone Joint Surg Am* 1970;52: 1090-1103.
31. Tingart M, Bäthis H, Bouillon B, Tiling T: The displaced proximal humeral fracture: Is there evidence for therapeutic concepts? *Chirurg* 2001; 72:1284-1291.
32. Fjalestad T, Stromsøe K, Blücher J, Tennøe B: Fractures in the proximal humerus: Functional outcome and evaluation of 70 patients treated in hospital. *Arch Orthop Trauma Surg* 2005;125:310-316.
33. Olsson C, Nordquist A, Petersson CJ: Long-term outcome of a proximal humerus fracture predicted after 1 year: A 13-year prospective population-based follow-up study of 47 patients. *Acta Orthop* 2005;76: 397-402.
34. Colton CL: *The History of Fracture Treatment*. Philadelphia, PA, WB Saunders, 1992.

35. Van Der Ghinst M, Houssa P: Acrylic prosthesis in fractures of the proximal ends of the extremities. *Acta Chir Belg* 1951;50:31-40.

36. Lorenzo FT: Osteosynthesis with Blount's staples in fractures of the proximal end of the humerus: A preliminary report. *J Bone Joint Surg Am* 1955;37:45-48.

37. Jaberg H, Warner JJ, Jakob RP: Percutaneous stabilization of unstable fractures of the humerus. *J Bone Joint Surg Am* 1992;74:508-515.

38. Weseley MS, Barenfeld PA, Eisenstein AL: Rush pin intramedullary fixation for fractures of the proximal humerus. *J Trauma* 1977;17:29-37.

39. Darder A, Darder A Jr, Sanchis V, Gastaldi E, Gomar F: Four-part displaced proximal humeral fractures: Operative treatment using Kirschner wires and a tension band. *J Orthop Trauma* 1993;7:497-505.

40. Kristiansen B, Christensen SW: Plate fixation of proximal humeral fractures. *Acta Orthop Scand* 1986;57: 320-323.

41. Sehr JR, Szabo RM: Semitubular blade plate for fixation in the proximal humerus. *J Orthop Trauma* 1988; 2:327-332.

42. Boileau P, Krishnan SG, Tinsi L, Walch G, Coste JS, Molé D: Tuberosity malposition and migration: Reasons for poor outcomes after hemiarthroplasty for displaced fractures of the proximal humerus. *J Shoulder Elbow Surg* 2002;11:401-412.

43. Goldman RT, Koval KJ, Cuomo F, Gallagher MA, Zucherman JD: Functional outcome after humeral head replacement for acute three- and four-part proximal humeral fractures. *J Shoulder Elbow Surg* 1995;4:81-86.

44. Hintermann B, Trouillier HH, Schäfer D: Rigid internal fixation of fractures of the proximal humerus in older patients. *J Bone Joint Surg Br* 2000;82:1107-1112.

45. Wagner M: General principles for the clinical use of the LCP. *Injury* 2003; 34:B31-B42.

46. Weinstein DM, Bratton DR, Ciccone WJ II, Elias JJ: Locking plates improve torsional resistance in the stabilization of three-part proximal humeral fractures. *J Shoulder Elbow Surg* 2006;15:239-243.

47. Hessmann MH, Hansen WS, Krummenauer F, Pol TF, Rommens PM: Locked plate fixation and intramedullary nailing for proximal humerus fractures: A biomechanical evaluation. *J Trauma* 2005;58:1194-1201.

48. Lungershausen W, Bach O, Lorenz CO: Locking plate osteosynthesis for fractures of the proximal humerus. *Zentralbl Chir* 2003;128:28-33.

49. Frigg R: Locking Compression Plate (LCP): An osteosynthesis plate based on the Dynamic Compression Plate and the Point Contact Fixator (PC-Fix). *Injury* 2001;32:B63-B66.

50. Laflamme GY, Rouleau DM, Berry GK, Beaumont PH, Reindl R, Harvey EJ: Percutaneous humeral plating of fractures of the proximal humerus: Results of a prospective multicenter clinical trial. *J Orthop Trauma* 2008;22:153-158.

51. Smith J, Berry G, Laflamme Y, Blain-Pare E, Reindl R, Harvey E: Percutaneous insertion of a proximal humeral locking plate: An anatomic study. *Injury* 2007;38:206-211.

52. Owsley KC, Gorczyca JT: Fracture displacement and screw cutout after open reduction and locked plate fixation of proximal humeral fractures. *J Bone Joint Surg Am* 2008;90:233-240.

53. Björkenheim JM, Pajarinen J, Savolainen V: Internal fixation of proximal humeral fractures with a locking compression plate: A retrospective evaluation of 72 patients followed for a minimum of 1 year. *Acta Orthop Scand* 2004;75:741-745.

54. Strohm PC, Kostler W, Sudkamp NP: Locking plates fixation of proximal humerus fractures. *Tech Shoulder Elbow Surg* 2005;6:8-13.

55. Plecko M, Kraus A: Internal fixation of proximal humerus fractures using the locking proximal humerus plate. *Oper Orthop Traumatol* 2005;17:25-50.

56. Fankhauser F, Boldin C, Schippinger G, Haunschmid C, Szyszkowitz R: A new locking plate for unstable fractures of the proximal humerus. *Clin Orthop Relat Res* 2005; 430:176-181.

57. Koukakis A, Apostolou CD, Taneja T, Korres DS, Amini A: Fixation of proximal humerus fractures using the PHILOS plate: Early experience. *Clin Orthop Relat Res* 2006;442:115-120.

58. Egol KA, Ong CC, Walsh M, Jazrawi LM, Tejwani NC, Zukerman JD: Early complications in proximal humerus fractures (OTA Types 11) treated with locked plates. *J Orthop Trauma* 2008;22:159-164.

59. Lill H, Hepp P, Rose T, König K, Josten C: The angle stable locking-proximal-humerus-plate (LPHP) for proximal humeral fractures using a small anterior-lateral-deltoid-splitting-approach: Technique and first results. *Zentralbl Chir* 2004;129:43-48.

60. Kettler M, Biberthaler P, Braunstein V, Zeiler C, Kroetz M, Mutschler W: Treatment of proximal humeral fractures with the PHILOS angular stable plate: Presentation of 225 cases of dislocated fractures. *Unfallchirurg* 2006;109:1032-1040.

Technical Tips for Fixation of Proximal Humeral Fractures in Elderly Patients

Michael E. Torchia, MD

Abstract

Despite the application of modern locking plate technology, complications remain common after fixation of proximal humeral fractures in elderly patients. Varus deformity and intra-articular hardware are most often responsible; fortunately, both of these complications can be avoided. Recent advances in imaging, reduction techniques, fixation methods, and postoperative care have made surgical outcomes more reliable. Particular attention should be directed to obtaining high-quality fluoroscopic images, avoiding varus reductions, supporting the osteoporotic humeral head, using appropriate screw length, using tension band sutures liberally, and protecting the construct postoperatively. With these methods, many proximal humeral fractures in patients older than 75 years can be reliably fixed.

Instr Course Lect 2010;59:553-561.

Interest in the fixation of proximal humeral fractures has grown worldwide during the past several years. This change in practice has been fueled by recognition that humeral head replacement after an acute fracture has an unpredictable outcome;[1] an understanding that posttraumatic osteonecrosis of the humeral head is not a clinical disaster;[2] more accurate preoperative imaging using three-dimensional CT scans; improvements in intraoperative imaging using fluoroscopy; refined reduction maneuvers;[3-5] and improved implants, in the form of contoured locking plates. Despite these advances, clinical results continue to be inconsistent, and the reported rates of surgical complications remain far too high.[6-10] Most reported revision procedures are necessitated by varus reduction[11] or screw penetration beyond the subchondral bone of the humeral head,[7] both of which can be avoided with good surgical techniques.

Indications

Neer's guidelines, published almost 40 years ago, remain useful.[12,13] Minimally displaced one-part fractures are treated nonsurgically. Most displaced fractures typically are treated with surgery. However, if the anticipated demands on the extremity are very low, it is reasonable to allow a displaced fracture to malunite and accept the motion loss caused by tuberosity impingement. Most two- and three-part fractures can be reliably fixed using modern methods, even in patients with poor bone quality. Some four-part fractures also can be treated with open reduction and internal fixation (ORIF).[10,14,15] It was recently suggested that the outcome of a properly done osteosynthesis may be better than that of humeral head replacement.[10]

Preoperative Planning

Good surgical results begin with a sound preoperative plan. A comparison radiograph of the opposite shoulder is valuable for intraoperative assessment of the quality of the reduction (Figure 1), especially to avoid varus malreduction (one of the most common complications after ORIF).[4,7,10,11,16]

Three-dimensional CT scans can also be useful for understanding the geometry of more complex fractures

Neither Dr. Torchia nor an immediate family member has received anything of value from or owns stock in a commercial company or institution related directly or indirectly to the subject of this chapter.

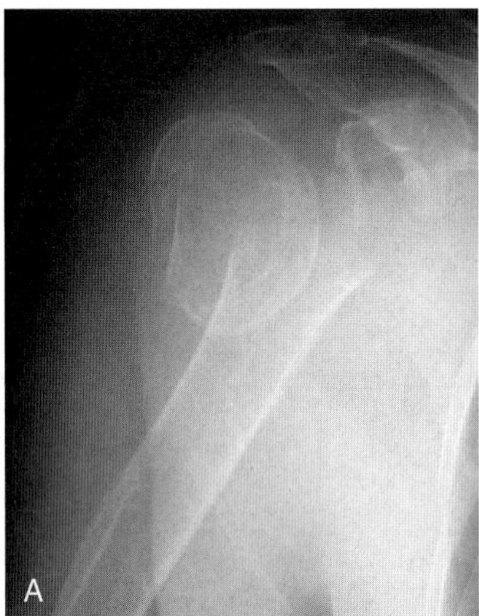

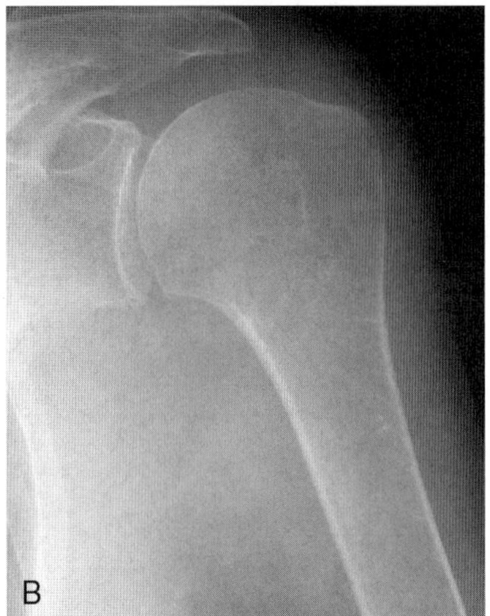

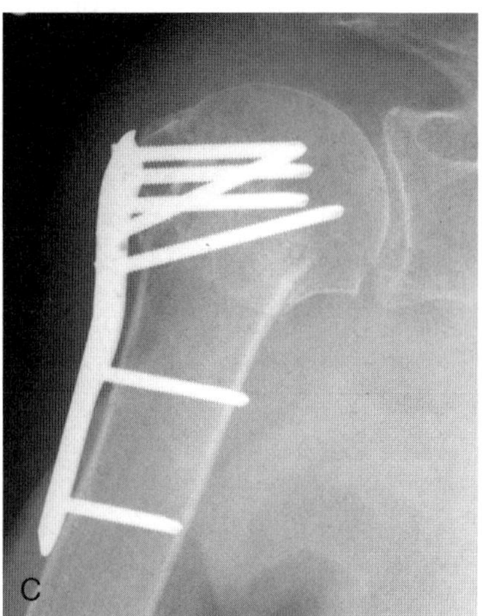

Figure 1 A two-part proximal humeral fracture in a 95-year-old woman. **A,** Preoperative AP radiograph. **B,** AP radiograph of the contralateral shoulder with the arm in external rotation. This comparison view serves as a template for reduction. **C,** AP external rotation radiograph taken at follow-up. Despite shortening to gain stability, the neck-shaft angle and the position of the greater tuberosity were restored.

and fracture-dislocations. Subtraction views show bony Bankart lesions and articular fractures of the humeral head that may be difficult to detect on some two-dimensional images. For a three- or four-part fracture, three-dimensional CT also reveals what, if any, part of the greater or lesser tuberosity is attached to the head segment. Any area of continuity between the tuberosities and head segment may serve as a "handle" to indirectly reduce the head segment with traction sutures placed at the bone-tendon junction of the rotator cuff (the so-called string puppet reduction technique). The use of three-dimensional CT has made it possible to plan the surgical exposure, reduction maneuvers, and hardware positioning and to anticipate the need for bone grafting (Figure 2).

Surgical Technique

Operating Room Setup for Fluoroscopic Imaging

The optimal operating room setup allows unrestricted access to the shoulder for fluoroscopic imaging. Most surgeons prefer using a standard operating table and some variation of the familiar beach chair patient position. The table is turned 90° after induction of anesthesia, so that the injured shoulder is opposite the anesthesia team and the equipment. This position allows the C-arm to enter and exit the field from the head of the operating table. Regardless of the setup and patient positioning, it is wise to verify that a minimum of two high-quality fluoroscopic views can be obtained prior to draping (Figure 3). This step is critical for the prevention of intraoperative screw penetration.

Exposure

The extended deltopectoral approach is preferred because of the options for extensile exposure to address almost any proximal humeral fracture pattern, including fracture-dislocations. The interval from the clavicle to the deltoid insertion is developed, while preserving the muscle origin and releasing a portion of the insertion as needed. The subdeltoid space is mobilized with care to avoid the terminal branches of the axillary nerve. A Brown deltoid retractor is placed. Abduction of the arm relaxes the deltoid and allows access to the entire greater tuberosity and rotator cuff.[17] During the exposure and placement of hardware, every attempt is made to respect the primary blood supply to the humeral head by avoiding the anterior circumflex vessels as they course along the subscapularis and the arcuate artery as it courses along the bicipital groove.

Extensile Maneuvers

Fractures of the proximal humerus occasionally extend into the diaphysis. For this pattern, the exposure is carried distally (the Henry approach), and a long plate is applied to the lateral aspect of the humerus. In this situation, the deltoid insertion is released, but doing so does not appear to have any clinical sequelae, in the absence of a brachial plexopathy.[18] Conversely, dissection can be extended proximally and medially to enter the glenohumeral joint so that a humeral head articular fracture or glenoid rim fracture can be treated. In patients with neurovascular injury, the brachial plexus and axillary artery can be explored through the deltopectoral interval.

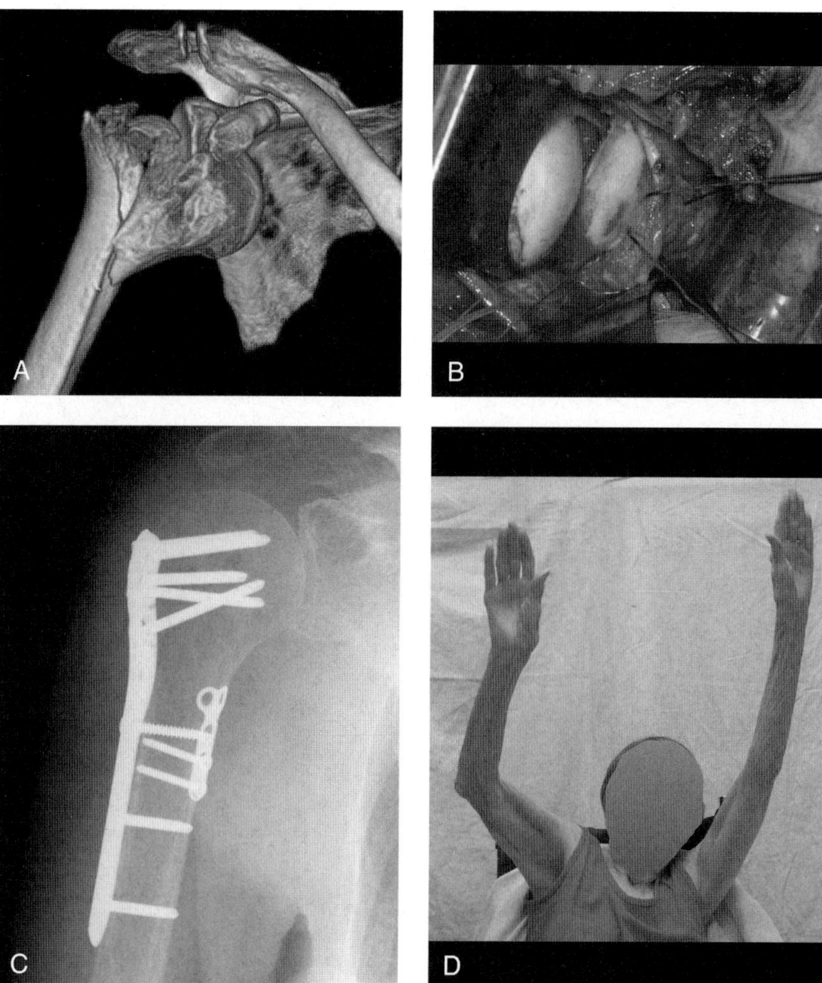

Figure 2 **A,** Three-dimensional CT scan showing a fracture-dislocation of the proximal humerus in an 87-year-old woman. The CT scan was used in planning the surgical exposure and positioning the implants. **B,** Intraoperative photograph showing an anterior arthrotomy for access to the glenoid rim fracture and placement of transosseous sutures. **C,** Postoperative AP radiograph showing placement of a minifragment antiglide plate along the medial aspect of the humerus; the pectoralis major tendon was divided and later repaired after the medial plate application. **D,** Clinical photograph of the patient (taken at 3-month follow-up) showing overhead elevation of the arm.

Reduction Maneuvers

Reduction maneuvers are determined by the fracture pattern. Impacted fractures are elevated using the method described by Jakob and associates[5] (Figure 4). Unimpacted fractures are compressed using the "parachute technique" described by Banco and associates[3] (Figure 5). A valgus impaction osteotomy allows balanced compression of the head segment on the shaft. This technique relies on tension band sutures and is ideally suited for reducing two-part surgical neck fractures. The method also can be used to reduce three-part fractures if the anterior portion of the greater tuberosity is connected to the head segment.

Although the principles of the parachute technique can be applied to most proximal humeral fractures, contraindications do exist. The reduction method is dependent on an intact rotator cuff and cannot be used in fractures in which the tuberosities are detached from the head segment, impacted fracture patterns, and fractures with severe metaphyseal comminution. In fractures with metaphyseal comminution, the parachute technique can result in excessive humeral shortening and inferior instability. In these cases, humeral length can be restored with bone grafting. Options for bone graft material include autograft, allograft, or a synthetic substitute.[4] Restoration of humeral length is also important in treating complex anterior fracture-dislocations in which the proximal humerus and glenoid are fractured (Figure 2). If humeral length is not restored, it can be difficult to keep the humeral head concentrically reduced in the postoperative period. This situation is particularly problematic in patients with an associated axillary nerve injury.

Humeral Head Support

The concept of humeral head support has been emphasized by several authors.[3,6,19] Most often, the head segment is supported by the shaft of the humerus. If there is moderate or severe traumatic bone loss, bone graft or a bone graft substitute is used. A soft humeral head supported only by rigid hardware tends to settle onto the metal. The result is

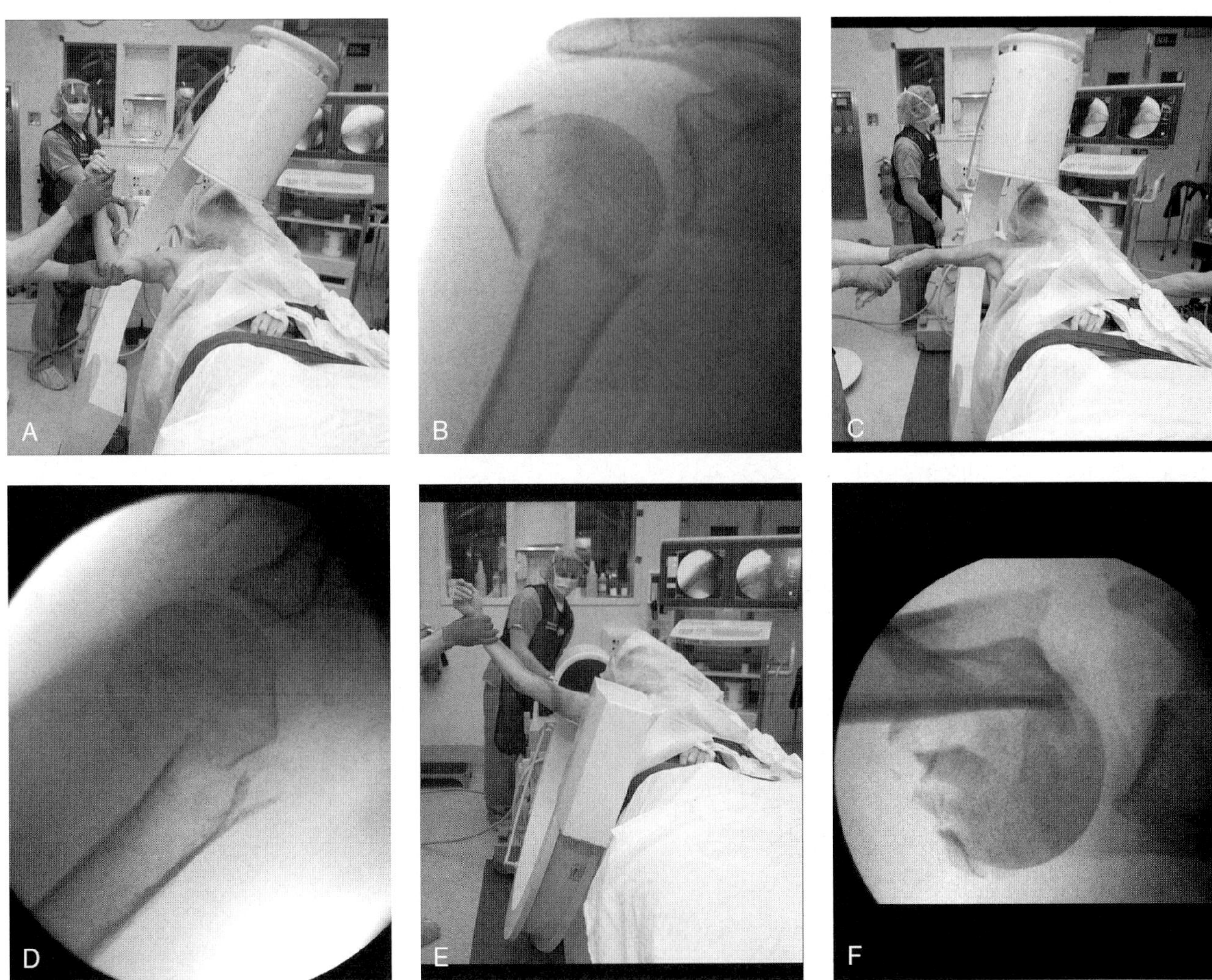

Figure 3 Fluoroscopic images are obtained in the operating room. **A,** Photograph showing positioning of the device to direct the fluoroscopic beam perpendicular to the scapula, with the patient's arm held in external rotation. **B,** An example of a preoperative AP external rotation fluoroscopic view. The relationship between the humeral shaft, the humeral head, and the greater tuberosity can be seen. **C,** Operating room photograph of patient positioning for the Velpeau axillary view taken with the arm held in internal rotation and slight longitudinal traction. Gentle traction lateralizes the scapula away from the operating room table and the patient's head. This allows unobstructed imaging of the proximal humerus and glenoid. **D,** An example of a preoperative Velpeau axillary internal rotation fluoroscopic view. Note the typical apex anterior angulation between the shaft and head segment. **E,** Operating room photograph showing patient positioning for the standard axillary view taken with the arm held in neutral rotation and longitudinal traction. **F,** An example of a preoperative fluoroscopic axillary view. This view shows the position of the lesser tuberosity and the relationship of the humeral head to the glenoid.

secondary screw cutout, which is a frequently reported reason for revision surgery.[7-10]

Provisional Fixation

After the initial reduction, provisional fixation is achieved with a Steinmann pin or pins placed just posterior to the long head of the biceps tendon. This location avoids interference with the plate that will later occupy the lateral surface of the proximal humerus. The traction sutures are tensioned and tied to the pin (Figure 6). This form of robust temporary tension band fixation allows the arm to be rotated so that the reduction can be fluoroscopically assessed in multiple planes.

Assessment of Reduction

The position of the shaft, head, and tuberosities is assessed with high-quality fluoroscopic imaging. On the AP external rotation fluoroscopic view (Figure 7), the shaft of the humerus should be under the humeral head, the greater tuberosity should be approximately 5 to 10 mm below the top of the head, and the articular surface should point toward the upper portion of the glenoid (RH Cofield, MD, Rochester MN, personal communication, 1998). Additional precision can be gained by referencing the image of the opposite shoulder. A reasonable attempt should be made to match the tuberosity height and neck-shaft angle of the opposite shoulder. Additional fluoroscopic views are used as necessary to assess translation and angulation of the humeral shaft relative to the head, the position of the lesser tuberosity, and the position of the head segment relative to the glenoid. The course of the long head of the biceps tendon is checked to confirm the rotational accuracy of the reduction. The provisional reduction should be scrutinized, and final adjustments should be made before the hardware is placed. The most common pitfall is the persistent varus position of the head segment. In most instances, this problem is easily resolved by slightly backing out the provisional Steinmann pin and adding additional provisional

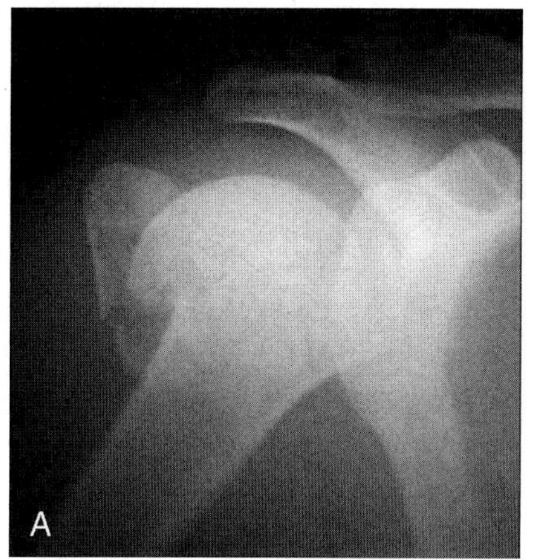

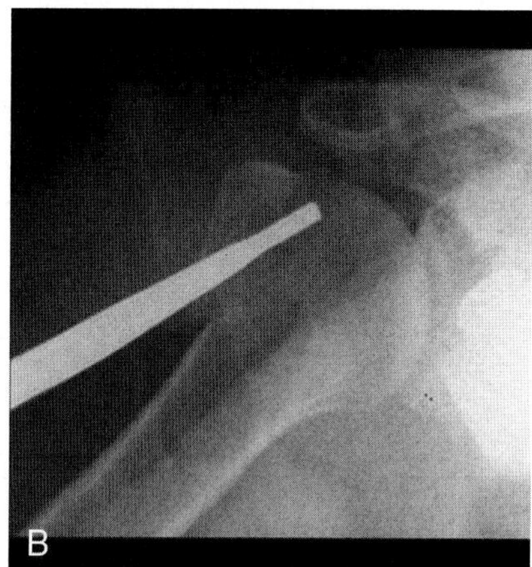

Figure 4 **A,** AP radiograph showing a valgus-impacted four-part fracture. **B,** Intraoperative fluoroscopic image showing elevation of the humeral head using a square-tipped impactor placed through a coronal split in the greater tuberosity.

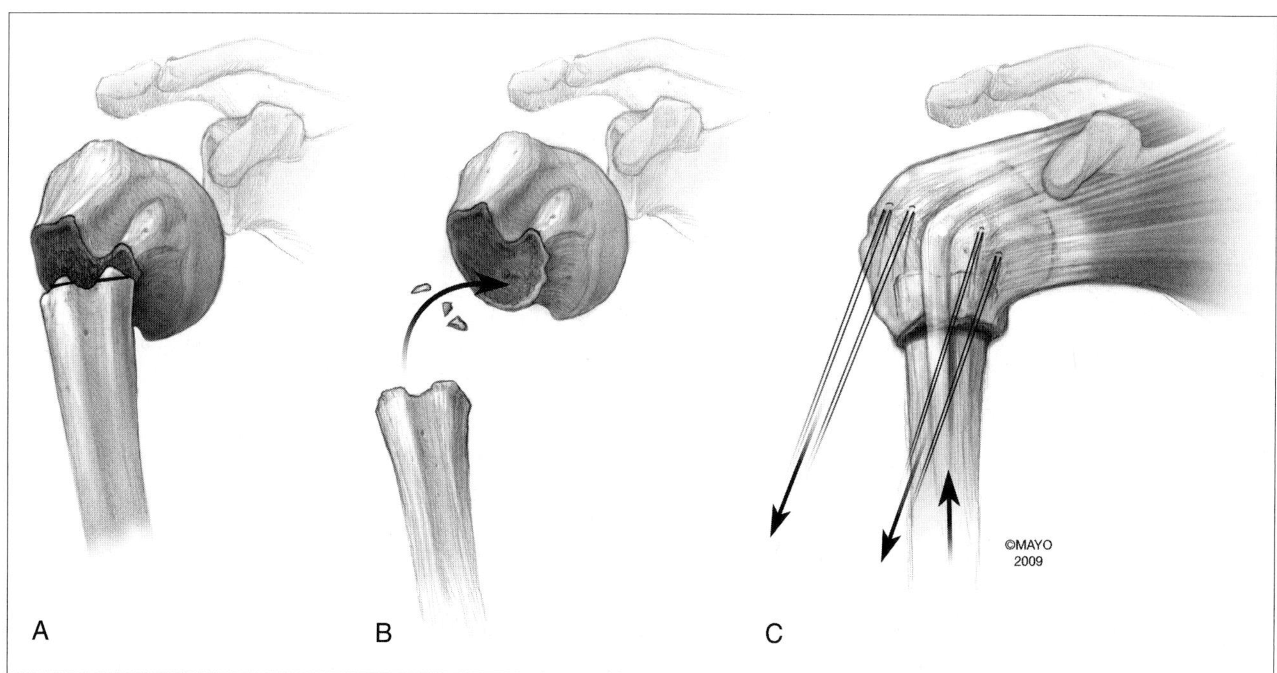

Figure 5 Schematic drawings showing a modification of the valgus impaction osteotomy. **A,** The transverse line delineates the intended level of the osteotomy. Prominent edges of the shaft anteriorly and laterally are trimmed with a rongeur to create a relatively flat surface that will allow balanced compression of the head segment. **B,** The "trimmings" are placed into the head segment and function as local bone graft. **C,** The head segment is supported by upward impaction of the shaft. The position of the head segment is adjusted with traction sutures placed at the bone-tendon junction of the subscapularis and supraspinatus tendons. (Reproduced with permission from the Mayo Foundation of Medical Education and Research, Rochester, MN.)

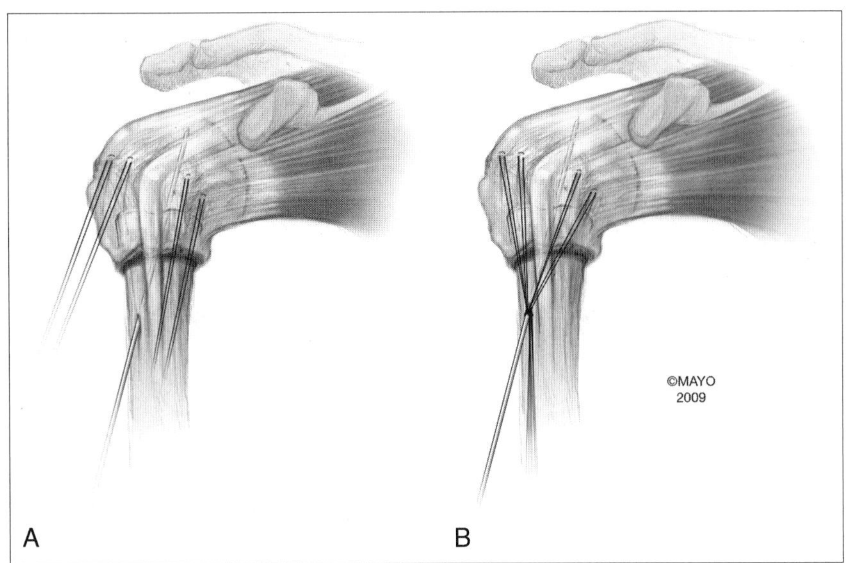

Figure 6 Schematic drawings showing a method of provisional fixation of proximal humeral fractures using pin and tension band suture fixation. This form of robust provisional fixation allows rotation of the arm for high-quality fluoroscopic imaging to assess the reduction in multiple planes. **A,** A long Steinmann pin is placed from the shaft into the head segment. **B,** Traction sutures are tensioned and tied to the pin. Tensioning the sutures pulls the head segment out of varus. (Reproduced with permission from the Mayo Foundation of Medical Education and Research, Rochester, MN.)

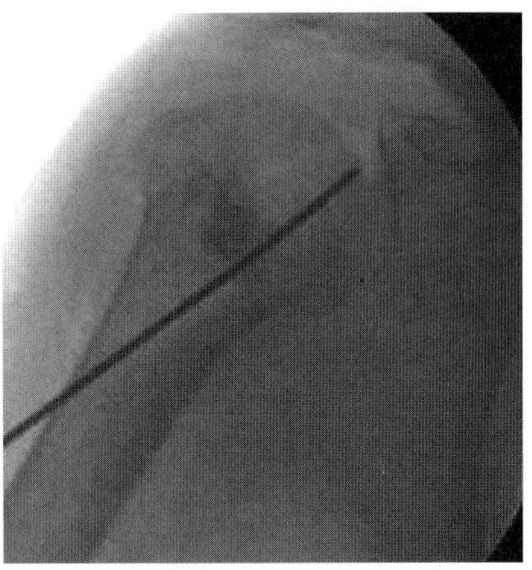

Figure 7 AP external rotation fluoroscopic image showing a provisional reduction of a three-part humeral fracture with a Steinmann pin and tension band sutures. A small amount of bone graft substitute was used to help support the humeral head.

tension band sutures extending from the bone-tendon junction of the supraspinatus to the provisional pin.

Definitive Fixation

A precontoured locking plate is applied laterally (Figure 8) and held with a push-pull reduction device (the so-called whirlybird). It is important to note that the plate is applied to the fracture after it is reduced and compressed. Hardware position is primarily assessed from the external rotation view (Figure 9). If the plate is positioned too high, it will cause impingement; if it is too low, the screw trajectory may be suboptimal. Gaps between the plate and the bone in the metadiaphysis are acceptable, and no attempt is made to contour the plate. This technique is quite different from the use of the plate as a reduction tool. Pulling the bone to the plate with screws or sutures tends to leave the head unsupported and at risk for varus drift or secondary screw penetration.[7,11] When the plate position is optimal, screws are placed into the osteoporotic humeral head (Figure 10). Because bone quality is often poor in this elderly patient population, only the outer cortex is drilled. The depth gauge is then inserted and gently advanced to the desired depth under fluoroscopic control. It is important to understand that if the head is supported and tension band sutures are used, the subchondral bone of the head need not be engaged. Placing shorter screws lowers the risk of screw penetration.[7] Following plate application, the provisional pin and suture fixation is removed. Next, definitive tension band sutures are placed, using any open holes in the plate as anchor points (Figure 11). It is preferable to use smooth holes to minimize the risk of suture abrasion.

Postoperative Care

Experience with caring for very elderly patients suggests that cognitive impairment is common. Many patients older than 75 years have limited understanding of their condition and are unable to participate in the gentle, passive range-of-motion program used in younger patients with good bone quality. In elderly patients, aggressive range-of-motion and strengthening exercises done prior to union of the fracture may increase the risk of fixation failure. With these concerns in mind, a variation of Neer's limited goals rehabilitation program seems appropriate for this patient population.[1,17] The primary focus of the program is protection of the fixation construct. Motion and strength are restored gradually over months.

During the first 6 weeks after surgery, patients are directed to wear a sling full time. After 6 weeks, supine

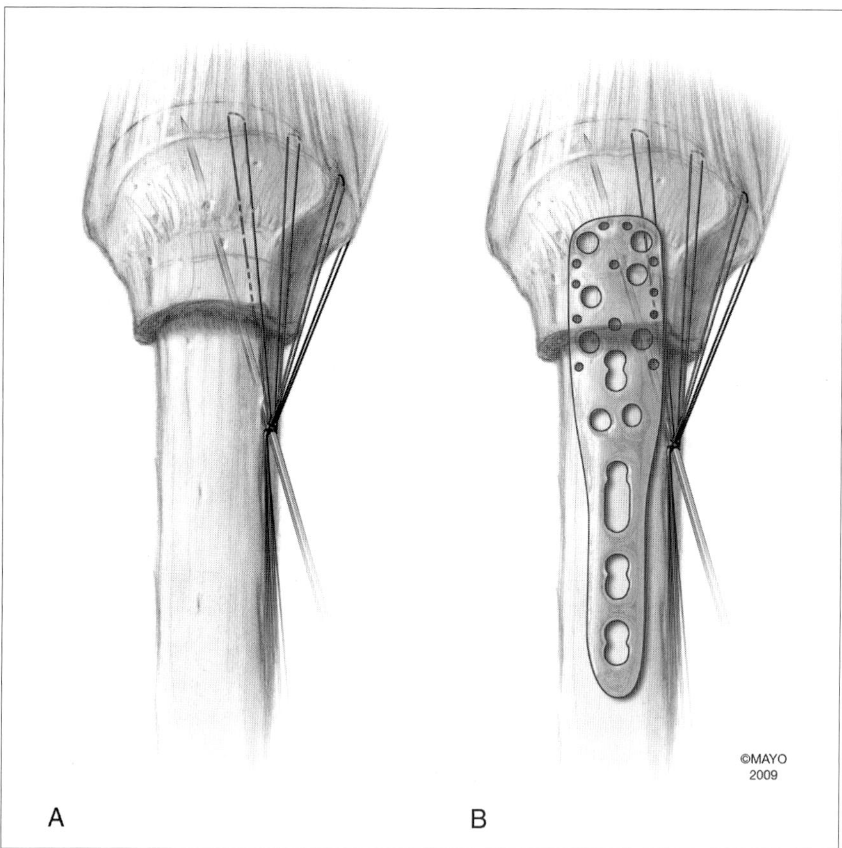

Figure 8 Schematic drawings showing a lateral view of the proximal humerus after provisional fixation. Note that the position of the pin and sutures **(A)** allow unobstructed access for definitive fixation with a precontoured locking plate **(B)**. (Reproduced with permission from the Mayo Foundation of Medical Education and Research, Rochester, MN.)

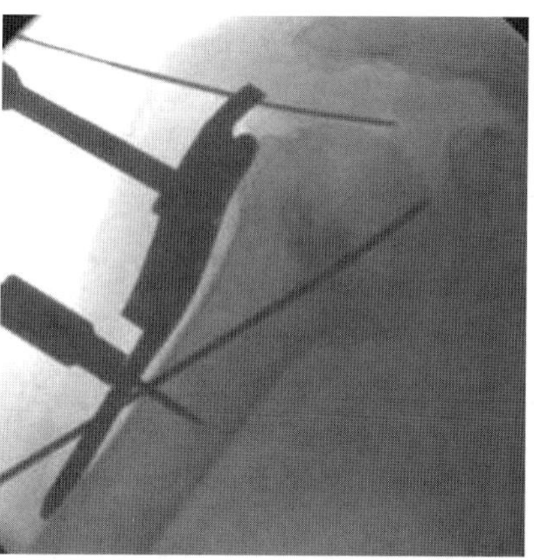

Figure 9 AP external rotation view fluoroscopic image showing plate positioning below the top of the humeral head.

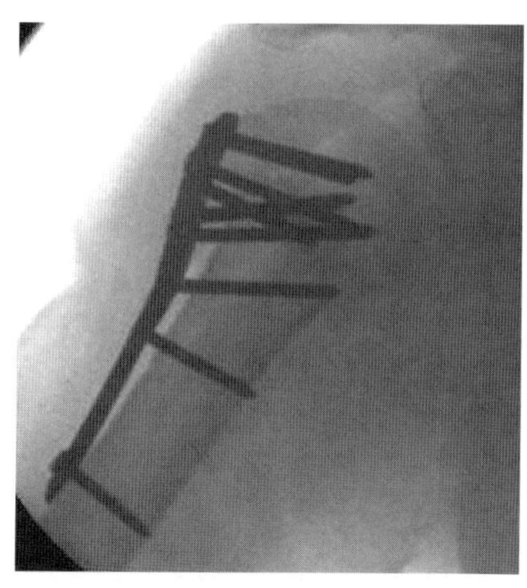

Figure 10 AP fluoroscopic image showing a method of screw placement that minimizes the risk of primary or secondary penetration. The arm is rotated under the fluoroscopy machine to check screw length in multiple planes.

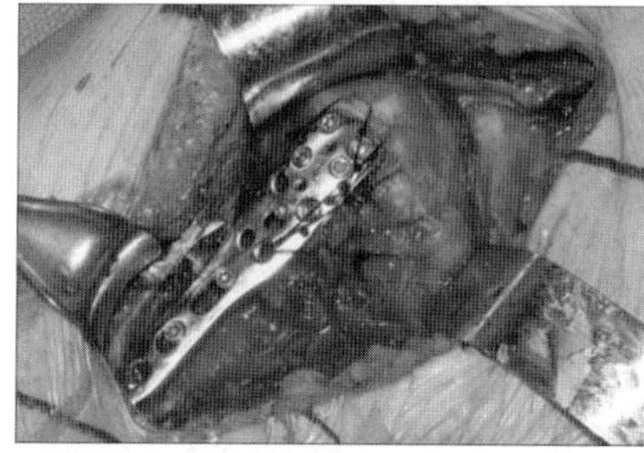

Figure 11 Intraoperative photograph showing the final construct. Heavy monofilament absorbable tension band sutures are applied liberally using empty holes in the plate as anchor points.

active assisted range-of-motion exercises are initiated. Radiographs taken 12 weeks after surgery usually show fracture consolidation (Figure 12). At this point, use of the sling is discontinued, and the patient is encouraged to use the arm for light daily activities, including driving and shopping. More forceful activities, such as yard work, tennis, and golf, are avoided for 6 months.

Results

General

There are few studies in the literature on the topic of proximal humeral fracture fixation in elderly patients.[3,7,10,16,20] Hintermann and associates[20] reported on 42 patients older than 50 years with three- and four-part humeral fractures who were treated with internal fixation with a blade plate. Although fracture healing was reliable, 11 secondary procedures were needed mainly to treat postoperative stiffness and prominent hardware. The authors advocated primary open reduction of all three- and four-part humeral fractures regardless of the patient's age.

Banco and associates[3] reviewed outcomes of a valgus impaction osteotomy for treating two-part fractures. Thirteen patients with a mean age of 68 years were treated with the

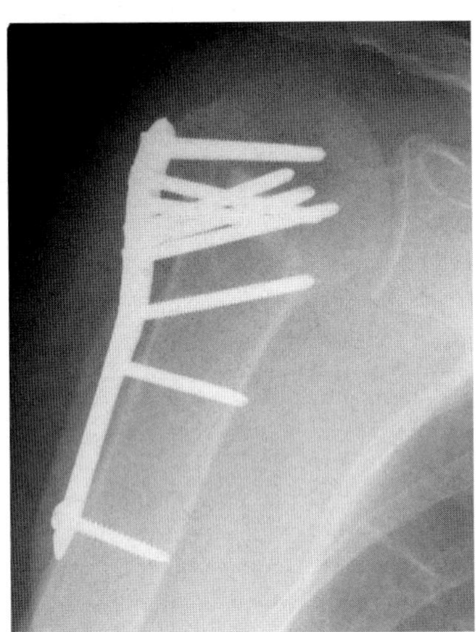

Figure 12 A typical 3-month follow-up AP external rotation radiograph of the proximal humerus showing consolidation of the fracture.

parachute technique using Dacron tapes as tension band sutures. All fractures healed after an average of 45 days. There were no reported complications or resurgeries. The authors concluded that using this technique to treat two-part fractures in elderly patients with osteopenic bone eliminates the morbidity of hardware implantation.

More recently, the results of locked plating for proximal humeral fractures in older patients have become available. Solberg and associates[10] reported on a group of 70 patients older than 55 years with three- and four-part humeral fractures. The patients were treated with a technique that involved placing screws within 5 mm of the subchondral bone of the humeral head. Active assisted range of motion was initiated postoperatively after 10 days. After 6 weeks, unrestricted motion and strengthening was allowed. Five patients had early return to the operating room for revision because of screw penetration of the humeral head seen on postoperative radiographs. By 18-month follow-up, an additional 29 patients required reoperation for complications such as secondary screw perforation, fixation failure, and osteonecrosis. The authors reported a particularly poor prognosis associated with varus reductions. Late subsidence developed in all fractures that had more than 5° of varus malreduction.

Two large multicenter studies from Europe also reported frequent complications with locked plating for proximal humeral fractures.[7,16] Brunner and associates[7] reported the results from eight centers in Switzerland where 158 fractures were treated by 53 surgeons between 2002 and 2005. The average age of the patients was 65 years, and 71% were women. At 1-year follow-up, 71 complications had been reported, and 25% of patients required reoperation. The most common cause for reoperation was screw perforation into the glenohumeral joint. Patients older than 60 years were more likely to have a complication than younger patients. The authors recommended using shorter screws, more accurate measurement of screw length, and more frequent use of tension band sutures to neutralize the deforming forces of the rotator cuff. In a similar study, Südkamp and associates[16] reported the results of 187 patients with proximal humeral fractures treated in nine German centers between 2002 and 2005. The fractures were treated with ORIF and a locking proximal humeral plate. The average patient age was 62.9 years, and 72% were women. The postoperative regimen involved early active range-of-motion exercises. Complications occurred in 34% of the patients, and 19% required reoperation. Again, many of the complications were related to primary screw penetration, varus reductions, and the placement of screws too close to the subchondral bone of the humeral head. The authors concluded that it was important for surgeons to use proper surgical techniques to avoid iatrogenic errors.

Mayo Clinic

The results of the Mayo Clinic's first 16 cases of locked plating for proximal humeral fractures were reported by Rose and associates[6] in 2007. Similar to other studies, a high rate of reoperation (19%) was reported. Surprisingly, older patients seemed to fare better than younger patients. This incidental finding prompted a critical analysis of the results. When the treatment of older patients was compared with the treatment of younger patients, four major differences were ascertained. (1) In most cases, elderly patients had been treated with a nonanatomic reduction using a valgus impaction osteotomy.[3] (2) In older patients, a greater emphasis was placed on supporting the humeral head with the proximal humeral shaft or bone graft.[3,4] (3) Tension band sutures were used liberally in all older patients to neutralize the forces of the rotator cuff. (4) In older patients with poor bone quality, the fixation was protected by delaying range-of-motion exercises for a period of 6 weeks.[1,17] This protocol has been called the hybrid technique because concepts from multiple sources were combined with modern locking plate technology. Results using the hybrid technique have been promising.

Hybrid Technique

During a 5-year period (2002 to 2007), the author used the hybrid protocol to treat 23 consecutive patients (mean age, 84 years; range, 75 to 97 years) with displaced proximal humeral fractures. The results were reviewed after a minimum of 1 year (range, 12 to 36 months; mean, 28 months). There were 10 Neer two-part fractures of the surgical neck, 10 Neer three-part fractures involving the surgical neck and greater tuberosity, and 3 severely impacted patterns as described by Jakob and associates.[5] At follow-up, all fractures healed, and all patients were able to perform daily activities independently. The mean elevation was 140°, and the mean external rotation was 42°. There were no cases of screw perforation, fixation failure, osteonecrosis, or infection. No reoperations were necessary in this group. The data suggest that advanced age is not a contraindication to ORIF, and a brief period of postoperative immobilization does not appear to cause disabling stiffness in elderly patients.

Summary

With a sound preoperative plan and attention directed to good surgical technique, many proximal humeral fractures in elderly patients can be reliably fixed. The key elements to successful treatment include high quality fluoroscopic imaging, an accurate reduction, support of the humeral head, locking plate fixation, generous tension band suturing, and postoperative protection of the construct.

References

1. Antuña SA, Sperling JW, Cofield RH: Shoulder hemiarthroplasty for acute fractures of the proximal humerus: A minimum five-year follow-up. *J Shoulder Elbow Surg* 2008;17: 202-209.
2. Gerber C, Hersche O, Berberat C: The clinical relevance of posttraumatic avascular necrosis of the humeral head. *J Shoulder Elbow Surg* 1998;7:586-590.
3. Banco SP, Andrisani D, Ramsey M, Frieman B, Fenlin JM Jr: The parachute technique: Valgus impaction osteotomy for two-part fractures of the surgical neck of the humerus. *J Bone Joint Surg Am* 2001;83:38-42.
4. Gardner MJ, Boraiah S, Helfet DL, Lorich DG: Indirect medial reduction and strut support of proximal humerus fractures using an endosteal implant. *J Orthop Trauma* 2008;22: 195-200.
5. Jakob RP, Miniaci A, Anson PS, Jaberg H, Osterwalder A, Ganz R: Four-part valgus impacted fractures of the proximal humerus. *J Bone Joint Surg Br* 1991;73:295-298.
6. Rose PS, Adams CR, Torchia ME, Jacofsky DJ, Haidukewych GG, Steinmann SP: Locking plate fixation for proximal humeral fractures: Initial results with a new implant. *J Shoulder Elbow Surg* 2007;16:202-207.
7. Brunner F, Sommer C, Bahrs C, et al: Open reduction and internal fixation of proximal humerus fractures using a proximal humeral locked plate: A prospective multicenter analysis. *J Orthop Trauma* 2009;23:163-172.
8. Egol KA, Ong CC, Walsh M, Jazrawi LM, Tejwani NC, Zuckerman JD: Early complications in proximal humerus fractures (OTA Types 11) treated with locked plates. *J Orthop Trauma* 2008;22:159-164.
9. Owsley KC, Gorczyca JT: Fracture displacement and screw cutout after open reduction and locked plate fixation of humeral fractures. *J Bone Joint Surg Am* 2008;90:233-240.
10. Solberg BD, Moon CN, Franco DP, Paiement GD: Locked plating of 3- and 4-part proximal humerus fractures in older patients: The effect of initial fracture pattern on outcome. *J Orthop Trauma* 2009;23:113-119.
11. Agudelo J, Schürmann M, Stahel P, et al: Analysis of efficacy and failure in proximal humerus fractures treated with locking plates. *J Orthop Trauma* 2007;21:676-681.
12. Neer CS II: Displaced proximal humeral fractures: I. Classification and evaluation. *J Bone Joint Surg Am* 1970; 52:1077-1089.
13. Neer CS II: Displaced proximal humeral fractures: II. Treatment of three-part and four-part displacement. *J Bone Joint Surg Am* 1970;52: 1090-1103.
14. Esser RD: Treatment of three- and four-part fractures of the proximal humerus with a modified cloverleaf plate. *J Orthop Trauma* 1994;8:15-22.
15. Robinson CM, Page RS: Severely impacted valgus proximal humerus fractures. *J Bone Joint Surg Am* 2004;86: 143-155.
16. Südkamp N, Bayer J, Hepp P, et al: Open reduction and internal fixation of proximal humeral fractures with use of the locking proximal plate: Results of a prospective, multicenter, observational study. *J Bone Joint Surg Am* 2009;91:1320-1328.
17. Neer CS: *Shoulder Reconstruction*. Philadelphia, PA, WB Saunders, 1990, pp 170-173.
18. Gill DR, Torchia ME: The spiral compression plate for proximal humeral shaft nonunion: A case report and description of a new technique. *J Orthop Trauma* 1999;13:141-144.
19. Gardner MJ, Weil Y, Barker JU, Kelly BT, Helfet DL, Lorich DG: The importance of medial support in locked plating of proximal humerus fractures. *J Orthop Trauma* 2007;21: 185-191.
20. Hintermann B, Trouillier HH, Schäfer D: Rigid internal fixation of fractures of the proximal humerus in older patients. *J Bone Joint Surg Br* 2000;82:1107-1112.

Periprosthetic Fractures of the Hip and Knee: A Problem on the Rise But Better Solutions

Craig J. Della Valle, MD
George J. Haidukewych, MD
John J. Callaghan, MD

Abstract

The absolute number of periprosthetic fractures seen by the orthopaedic surgeon is increasing. The basic principles of fracture management include preoperative patient optimization and determining the stability of the associated components. Loose components require revision, whereas fractures associated with well-fixed implants are generally treated with internal fixation. Although these fractures are challenging to manage, advances in surgical techniques, including the use of locking plates for internal fixation and improved revision systems and biomaterials (such as highly porous metals), offer the surgeon enhanced tools for treating these complex clinical disorders.

Instr Course Lect 2010;59:563-575.

The number of periprosthetic fractures associated with total hip arthroplasties (THAs) and total knee arthroplasties (TKAs) are increasing in number secondary to the increase in the total number of these procedures being performed annually; the concomitant increase in the number of implants in service, which may be affected by prosthetic loosening or osteolysis; the increase in the number of revision surgeries; and an aging population, which is at a higher risk for osteoporosis. Data from the Swedish hip registry suggest that since the year 2000, periprosthetic fractures of the femur are the third most common reason (following only aseptic loosening and recurrent instability) for revision surgery after THA. Periprosthetic fractures account for 6% of revision surgeries.[1] These fractures are the second leading cause of implant failure requiring revision surgery in patients 4 years or more after THA. It is estimated that the cumulative risk of a periprosthetic fracture occurring following THA within the first 10 years is 0.64% and up to 2.3% for patients in certain high risk categories, such as elderly patients, those with inflammatory arthritis or osteoporosis, and patients previously treated with prosthetic replacement for a hip fracture.[2,3]

The treatment of periprosthetic fractures following both THA and TKA is challenging and associated with a high rate of orthopaedic and systemic complications. Lindahl and associates[4] reported that 10-year implant survivorship without the need for surgery of the ipsilateral hip was 69.9%. The early failure rate (nearly 50% of all resurgeries occurred within 1 year) was particularly high,

Dr. Della Valle or an immediate family member is a member of a speakers' bureau or has made paid presentations on behalf of Angiotech; serves as a paid consultant to or is an employee of Zimmer; serves as an unpaid consultant to Biomet and Kinamed; has received research or institutional support from Zimmer; and has received nonincome support (such as equipment or services), commercially derived honoraria, or other non–research-related funding (such as paid travel) from Smith & Nephew and Stryker. Dr. Haidukewych or an immediate family member serves as a board member, owner, officer, or committee member of the Florida Orthopaedic Institute; has received royalties from DePuy and Zimmer; is a member of a speakers' bureau or has made paid presentations on behalf of DePuy; serves as a paid consultant to or is an employee of DePuy; has received research or institutional support from DePuy; and has stock or stock options held in Surmodics. Dr. Callaghan or an immediate family member has received royalties from DePuy; serves as an unpaid consultant to DePuy; has received research or institutional support from Arthrex and Smith & Nephew; and has received nonincome support (such as equipment or services), commercially derived honoraria, or other non–research-related funding (such as paid travel) from Wolters Kluwer Health–Lippincott Williams & Wilkins.

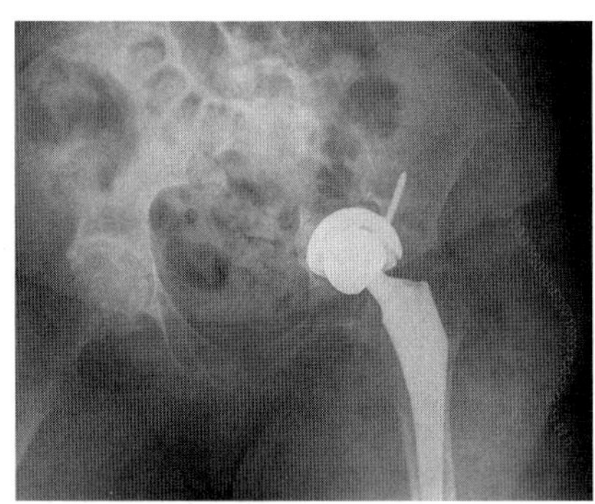

Figure 1 Radiograph showing an acute periprosthetic fracture of the pelvis following a primary THA with a fracture of the posterior column and a pelvic discontinuity treated with plating of the posterior column of the pelvis and staged revision of the acetabular component.

with most failures attributed to attempts at internal fixation as opposed to prosthetic revision in treating a loose femoral implant. Bhattacharyya and associates[5] reviewed the results of the treatment of 106 periprosthetic fractures of the femur associated with THA and found that 11% of the patients died within 1 year, which is similar to (albeit lower than) the mortality rate for patients with a fracture of the native proximal femur. Mortality increased among patients when surgery was delayed for more than 2 days. Patients treated with open reduction and internal fixation as opposed to femoral component revision also had a higher mortality rate (33% to 12%, respectively).

Risk Factors

The predominant risk factors for a periprosthetic fracture of the hip or knee are factors related to poor bone quality (female sex, older age, inflammatory arthritis) that increase the risks of fractures in general. Patients at high risk for falls, including those with poor vision and balance or neurologic disorders, have an increased risk for periprosthetic fractures. Most periprosthetic fractures are associated with low-energy trauma. Other factors that increase the risks include loose implants with associated bone loss and large osteolytic lesions. These risk factors highlight the need for radiographic surveillance of all patients treated with THA or TKA, even those who are asymptomatic.

Specific risk factors associated with a periprosthetic fracture of the femur following THA include a preoperative diagnosis of a proximal femoral fracture, certain implant types (those associated with high rates of osteolysis), and revision surgery compared with primary THA.[2] Intraoperative and early postoperative fractures are increasing in number secondary to the increased use of cementless rather than cemented implants in both primary and revision surgery.[6]

Periprosthetic Fractures of the Acetabulum

Acute Fractures in Primary THA

Periprosthetic fractures of the acetabulum are relatively rare and seem to be iatrogenic in nature, with a prevalence of less than 1%.[7] These fractures are a relatively recent phenomenon and are associated with the now common practice of underreaming the acetabulum and inserting a press-fit cementless acetabular component, particularly in an attempt to avoid the use of screws for adjunctive fixation. In a cadaver study, underreaming of the acetabulum by 2 mm was associated with a periprosthetic fracture in 26% of specimens, whereas underreaming by 4 mm was associated with a fracture in 93% of specimens.[8] The authors also reported that substantial impaction forces of 2,000 N were required to fully seat the components, and fractures were difficult to detect using plain radiographs only.

Clinical studies also have identified poor bone quality as an important risk factor in periprosthetic fractures of the acetabulum; this risk factor is common in older women and in patients with rheumatoid arthritis.[9] A more recent report identified more periprosthetic fractures of the acetabulum in elliptic compared with hemispheric acetabular components, with a particularly high rate in monoblock (as opposed to modular) elliptic shells.[7] If identified intraoperatively, the stability of the component should be carefully assessed. If the component is unstable, it should be removed and replaced with a component that can be fixed with multiple screws. Stable components have been associated with a high rate of osteointegration without the need for additional intervention, although bone graft from the acetabular reaming was placed in the fracture site in all patients in one study.[7] Rarely, an unstable intraoperative fracture may involve the acetabular columns and require plating of the posterior and, in some instances, the anterior column (Figure 1).

Stress Fractures of the Pelvis

Stress fractures of the pubic rami also occur following THA and can be an uncommon cause of groin pain after an otherwise successful THA.[10] These fractures typically occur in women with poor bone quality who were treated with THA using a cementless acetabular component. It is hypothesized that the patient's increased ambulatory capacity after successful THA is the cause of these fractures; they have been shown to heal reliably with nonsurgical treatment. Although early plain radiographs may be normal following the onset of pain, the fracture can be diagnosed with a bone scan or with serial radiographs over time. Stress fractures also may be associated with extensive retroacetabular osteolysis. If the component is stable, treatment should include exchange of the modular bearing surface and grafting of the osteolytic lesion.[11]

Pelvic Discontinuity

Pelvic discontinuity typically occurs in association with a loose acetabular component and can be considered a "chronic periprosthetic fracture of the acetabulum" in which the superior and inferior portions of the pelvis are separated by an area of bone loss.[12] Pelvic discontinuity is most commonly associated with female sex and a diagnosis of inflammatory arthritis.[13] Radiographic characteristics of a pelvic discontinuity include a transverse fracture line, medial translation of the inferior hemipelvis (with a break in the ilioischial line), and asymmetry of the obturator foramen. Vertical migration of the loose component of more than 3 cm is common[14] (Figure 2).

Traditional treatment includes extensive bone grafting, plating of the posterior column, and using a reconstruction cage that spans from the ilium to the ischium.[13] A recent report describes the successful use, at short-term follow-up, of trabecular metal acetabular components with augments.[15] The use of custom-made, porous-coated, triflanged components also has been described as a successful technique for reconstruction.[16]

Springer and associates[17] recently described a variant of a pelvic discontinuity associated with well-fixed components following revision THA, in which a trabecular metal acetabular component was used. All seven of the patients in the study were female and presented with groin pain. Five of the seven patients had a displaced fracture that was treated surgically; four required plating and bone grafting of the posterior column, and one was treated with a reconstruction cage to stabilize the pelvis.

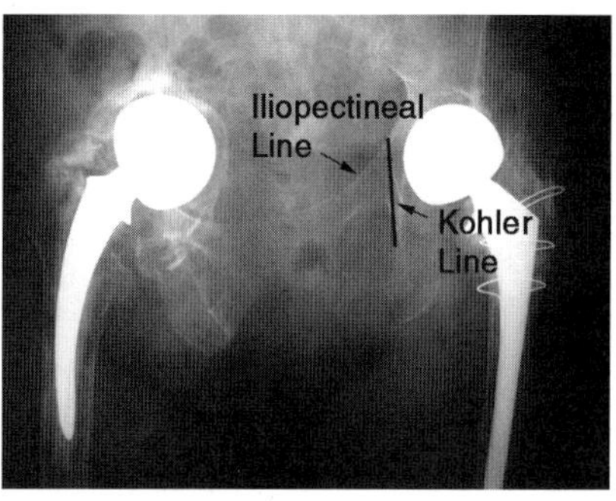

Figure 2 Pelvic discontinuity of the right hemipelvis. Note the break in the iliopectineal and ilioischial (Kohler) lines with significant superior and medial migration of the acetabulum, a transverse fracture line, and ischial lysis. Rotation of the inferior hemipelvis is seen as asymmetry of the obturator ring when compared with the contralateral side. Normal radiographic landmarks are shown on the left hemipelvis. (Reproduced from Della Valle CJ, Momberger NG, Paprosky WG: Periprosthetic fractures of the acetabulum associated with a total hip arthroplasty. *Instr Course Lect* 2003;52:281-290.)

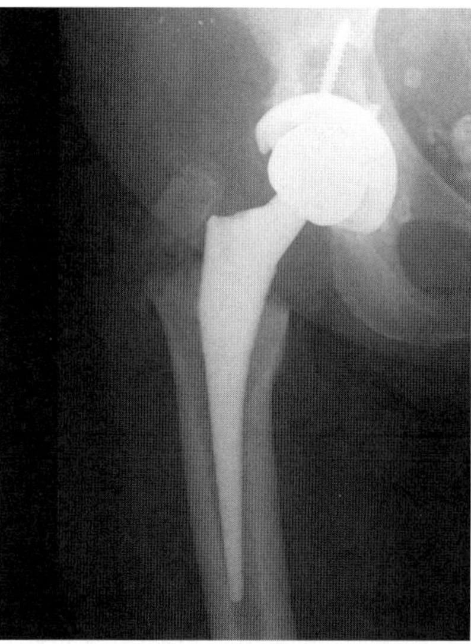

Figure 3 Radiograph showing a Vancouver type A periprosthetic fracture of the greater trochanter.

Periprosthetic Fractures of the Femur Associated With THA

Classification

The Vancouver classification system was developed for cemented prostheses and is clinically helpful in guiding treatment of periprosthetic femoral fractures. It is based on the location of the fracture, the fixation status of the femoral component, and the quality of the remaining bone stock. Vancouver type A fractures involve the greater or lesser trochanter and are almost always associated with osteolysis (Figure 3). Vancouver type B fractures occur around the stem and are the most common type of periprosthetic femoral fracture. Type B1 fractures occur around a well-fixed implant (Figure 4), type B2 fractures occur around a loose implant with good remaining bone stock (Figure 5), and type B3 fractures are associated with a loose implant and poor remaining proximal bone stock. Vancouver type C fractures occur well distal to the femoral component, and the component is almost always well fixed[18] (Figure 6).

Vancouver Type A Periprosthetic Fractures

The mainstay of managing Vancouver type A fractures is treating the associated osteolysis, typically with a modular polyethylene liner exchange. Osteolytic lesions can be grafted with cancellous allograft, and unstable greater trochanteric fractures should be stabilized; tension band techniques have been rec-

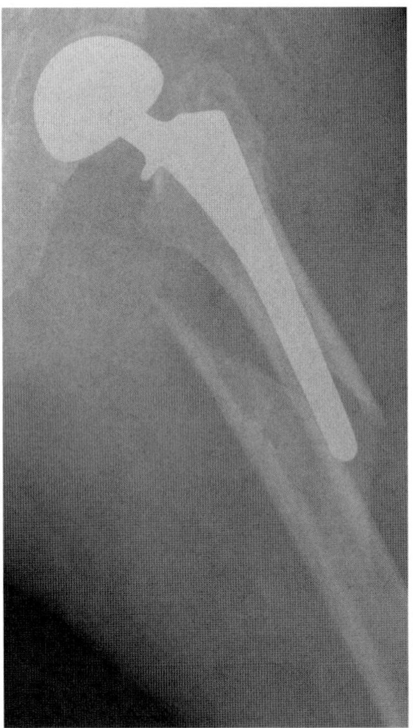

Figure 4 Radiograph showing a Vancouver type B1 fracture with a well-fixed femoral component.

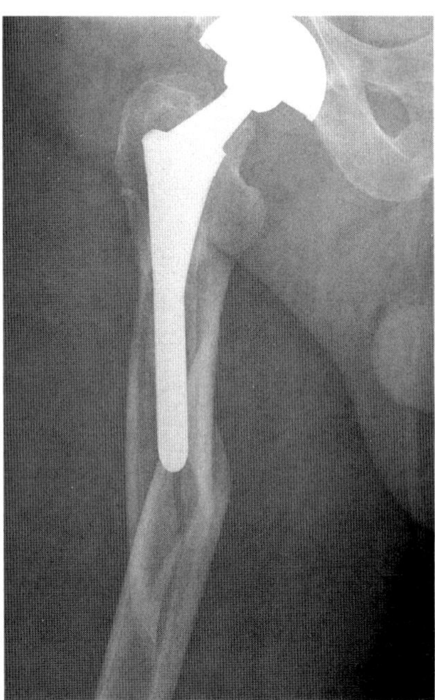

Figure 5 Radiograph showing a Vancouver type B2 periprosthetic fracture of the femur. A review of early postoperative radiographs showed clear subsidence of the femoral component, indicating loosening.

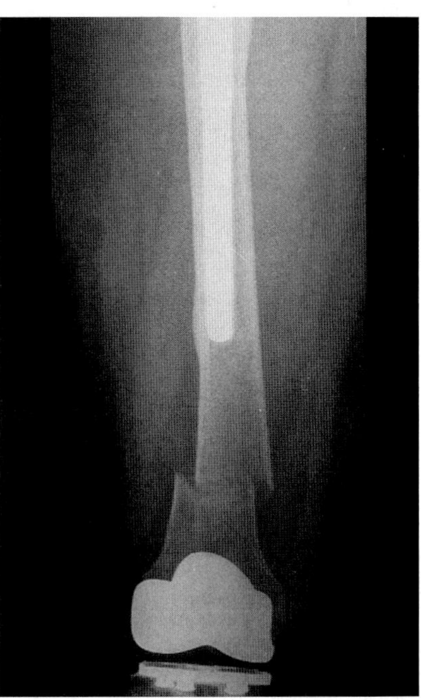

Figure 6 Radiograph showing a Vancouver type C periprosthetic fracture of the hip.

ommended using wire or heavy braided suture. It is important to understand that bone quality is typically poor because the trochanter has been "hollowed out" by the lytic process. If displaced and unstable, heavy suture fixation into the abductor tendon is recommended, which typically provides robust fixation. Internal fixation of the greater trochanter alone, without treating the wear problem with bearing exchange and bone grafting, will not resolve the underlying disorder and will likely lead to fixation failure. An abduction brace and protected weight bearing are recommended after trochanteric fixation.

Vancouver Type B1 Fractures

For type B1 fractures around a well-fixed implant, internal fixation with a plate with or without an allograft strut is recommended. It is critical to ensure that that stem is well fixed because treating a periprosthetic fracture of the femur with internal fixation when the femoral component is loose is a common cause of failure.

During internal fixation of type B1 fractures, obtaining stable proximal fixation is paramount. A lateral locked plate with a combination of unicortical locked screws and proximal cables generally provides adequate fixation. Proximal cable fixation alone is often inadequate because cables alone provide limited resistance to rotation. In general, three cables and three locked screws proximally and four bicortical screws distally (using a combination of locked and traditional screws) are used to achieve balanced internal fixation above and below the fracture (Figure 7). The authors of a cadaver study concluded that a combination of locked screws and cables is preferable.[19] The particular fracture geometry and length of the proximal segment will ultimately determine how many points of proximal fixation are possible. All proximal unicortical screws should be locked. It is important to preserve fracture biology and avoid medial dissection because most of the vascularity of the femur is medially based. The use of broad-based retractors and periosteal stripping is discouraged. It is important, however, to avoid fracture distraction when locked plating techniques are used. If possible, compression should be achieved to allow load sharing with the available bone; however, load sharing will vary with fracture geometry and the degree of comminution present. The use of hybrid plating techniques distally, using traditional nonlocked screws for compression and then locking the construct with bicortical locking screws, can facilitate obtaining a stable, compressed construct.

The use of supplementary allograft struts remains controversial. Struts were routinely used with good results before the advent of modern locked plating devices because some form of orthogonal bony support was necessary to minimize screw toggle and fixation failure. In the past, some authors have advocated "strut only" fixation constructs; however, in an era of modern locked plating devices, such constructs have generally fallen from favor. The need for strut augmentation is now typically based on bone quality. If a strut is used, it should be contoured with a high-speed burr to provide broad-based contact with the underlying host bone. Orthogonal placement of a locked plate (strut anterior on the femur) is generally preferred because medial dissection is avoided. Anterior placement can irritate the quadriceps and lead to knee stiffness, so careful attention is needed to prevent this potential postoperative complication, which can affect rehabilitation. The use of an allograft strut can be particularly problematic in thin patients of small stature in whom struts can add substantial bulk to the construct. Struts also add considerable expense and surgical time but carry a low risk of disease transmission. It is likely that as internal fixation implants and techniques evolve, the use of allograft struts for this indication will continue to decrease.

Vancouver Type B2 and B3 Fractures

Vancouver type B2 and B3 fractures are periprosthetic fractures of the femur associated with a loose implant. Treatment must include both revision of the femoral component and fracture fixation. A type B3 fracture is differentiated from type B2 by the presence of severe bone loss of the femur that further complicates treatment; however, a continuum of severity of femoral bone loss exists, and this differentiation is somewhat subjective.

For most type B2 fractures, the principal strategy for treatment includes the use of a cementless femoral component to achieve distal fixation beyond the fracture, effectively performing an intramedullary rodding of the femur. This treatment strategy is supported by the general success achieved with distally fixed, cementless femoral components, and reports suggest that the use of cemented femoral components for treating periprosthetic fractures is associated with a higher rate of failure.[20,21] Success with the use of impaction grafting has been reported.[22]

The first challenge in treating type B2 periprosthetic femoral fractures is removing the loose femoral component and the retained cement. Authors have described the successful use of an extended trochanteric osteotomy to facilitate cement removal, exposure, and implantation of the revision component.[23-25] The osteotomy is made distal to the tip of the fracture, the intact femoral diaphysis is prepared, the revision stem is implanted, and the proximal fragments are wrapped around the revision implant[23-25] (Figure 8). The amount of intact femoral diaphysis available for distal fixation and the diameter of the revision implant are important considerations in selecting an appropriate revision component. Cylindric, fully porous-coated stems have been shown to have higher rates of failure when less than 4 cm is available for distal fixation (in Paprosky type IIIB and type IV femoral defects). When the diameter of the implant is greater than 19 mm, a modular, titanium, fluted stem may be associated with a higher rate of success.[26,27]

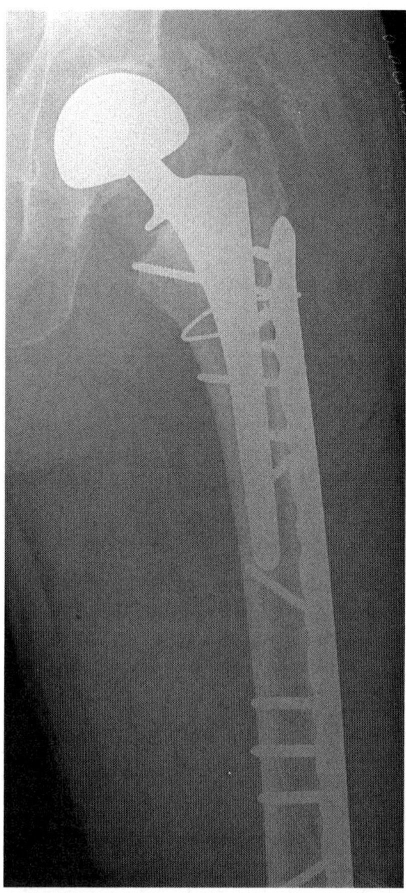

Figure 7 Postoperative radiograph of the fracture shown in Figure 4. Proximal fixation was achieved using a combination of unicortical and bicortical locking and unlocked screws as well as a cerclage cable.

Type B3 periprosthetic fractures of the femur have been successfully treated with the methods previously described for type B2 fractures, although other authors have advocated the use of proximal femoral replacement using an allograft-prosthetic composite or a tumor-type proximal femoral prosthesis.[28,29] If either of these treatment

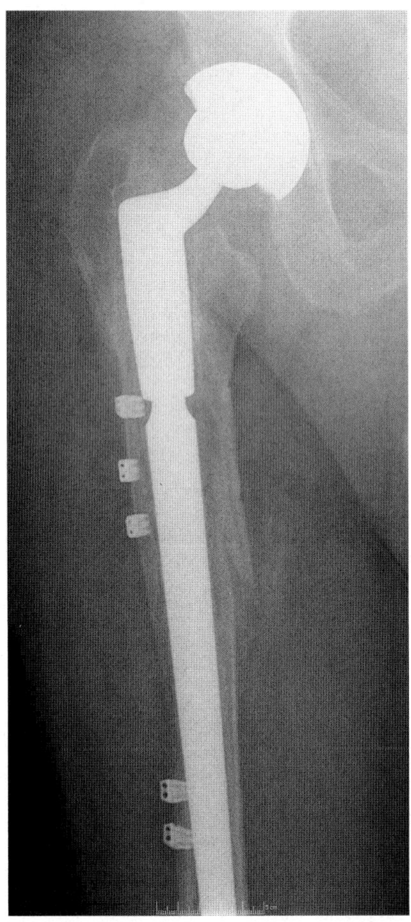

Figure 8 Postoperative radiograph of the fracture shown in Figure 5. An extended trochanteric osteotomy was used to remove the failed femoral component and facilitate implantation of the revision stem. The modular tapered revision femoral component was inserted first, achieving distal fixation, and the proximal fragments were wrapped around the revision femoral component.

options is considered, abductor deficiency can lead to instability, and a constrained acetabular liner should be considered.

Vancouver Type C Fractures

The principles of internal fixation of Vancouver type C injuries are similar to those of an osteopenic distal femoral fracture, with the added difficulty of proximally treating a potential stress riser from the existing

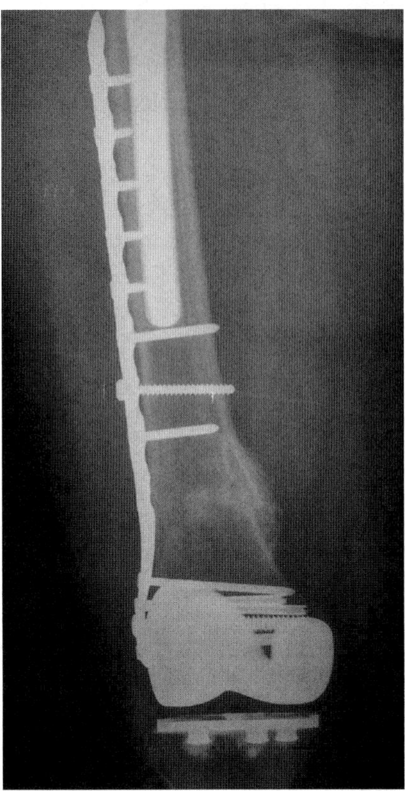

Figure 9 Postoperative radiograph of the fracture shown in Figure 6. A locked plate applied laterally was used to fix this Vancouver type C fracture.

femoral component. If a sufficient length of femoral diaphysis (at least 12 cm) is available between supracondylar fixation and the tip of the femoral stem, a short plate may be considered without bypassing the stem proximally. However, this situation is exceedingly rare and typically occurs only in tall patients with long femurs and very distal fractures. In most situations, it is preferable to bypass the femoral stem by two cortical diameters with the proximal part of the plate (Figure 9). Short retrograde nails are discouraged in this setting, and a long, locked plate that bypasses the tip of the ipsilateral femoral component is the treatment of choice.

The use of long, locked plates has been facilitated with modern jig-driven targeting of screws that avoids elevation of the vastus lateralis. This method theoretically preserves fracture vascularity and improves the rate of union. These concepts have generally been supported by the available trauma literature on distal femoral fractures.[30-33] With modern implants and biologically friendly implantation techniques, it is quite easy to insert a long plate that bypasses the femoral stem above without excessive soft-tissue dissection. An incision is made distally over the femoral condyles and another is made proximally below the greater trochanter. The plate is inserted submuscularly and extraperiosteally and is then stabilized with locked screw fixation proximally and distally, effectively bridging the fracture zone. Recent data have shown high union rates with such strategies without the need for the routine use of a femoral strut allograft.[34] After internal fixation, patients are mobilized postoperatively, and full weight bearing is typically delayed for at least 6 to 8 weeks until progressive radiographic healing is evident. Ambulatory aids are used for 12 weeks.

Periprosthetic Fractures of the Femur Associated With TKA

Important Considerations and Classification

The goals of treating periprosthetic femoral fractures after TKA include obtaining bony union; maintaining correct limb alignment, length, and rotation; and avoiding both local and systemic complications. Obstacles to achieving stable distal fixation include the often short, osteopenic distal bony fragments; fracture comminution; areas of osteolysis; and achieving fixation around the femoral component and associated stem, if present. Periprosthetic femoral fractures usually require an internal fixation device that provides coronal plane stability to avoid deformity (typically varus collapse) that can occur during the healing process. In general, nonsurgical treatment should be considered only for patients with nondisplaced or minimally displaced fractures that are associated with well-fixed implants, those at high risk of perioperative mortality, or patients who were nonambulatory before the fracture. The risks of both systemic (such as thromboembolic and other complications related to recumbency and immobilization) and local complications (such as a stiff knee joint and malunion of the fracture) must be carefully weighed against the risks of surgery. The Lewis and Rorabeck system is the most commonly used classification for periprosthetic fractures of the distal femur[35] (Table 1). As with other periprosthetic fractures, implants that are loose require revision for successful treatment.

Retrograde Nailing

Intramedullary nailing has been successfully used to manage complex periprosthetic distal femoral fractures. It limits soft-tissue disruption and provides excellent biomechanical stability.[36-41] Among the challenges to successful union with intramedullary techniques is that locking screws (even modern nail-locking screw clusters) provide marginal distal fixation of the typically comminuted, osteopenic distal bony fragments. Intramedullary nailing is not practical for use with implants that substitute for the posterior cruciate ligament because the femoral housing precludes access to the intramedullary canal. Intramedullary techniques are typically reserved for treating fractures located above cruciate-retaining femoral components with sufficient distal bone to allow purchase with a minimum of two distal locking screws. Recent biomechanical evidence suggests that in the presence of medial comminution, retrograde intramedullary nails may be mechanically more stable than laterally placed locking plates; however, this stability is based on achieving good distal fixation.[42] Occasionally, antegrade femoral nailing can be used for periprosthetic distal femur fractures if a sufficiently long distal fragment is present. The main challenges with antegrade techniques are obtaining appropriate alignment and stable distal fixation. With antegrade nailing techniques, an area of high stress concentration is created between the distal end of the nail and the femoral component. If a nailing strategy is chosen, a long retrograde nail may represent a more attractive option secondary to the benefits of distal locking bolts further from the fracture site.

Traditional Plate Fixation

In the past, devices such as the 95° blade plate and dynamic condylar screw have been used with mixed results.[36,38,39,43-47] Because of the extremely distal nature of these fractures, the blade of the blade plate or the lag screw of the dynamic condylar screw often must be inserted more proximally to avoid portions of the femoral component; thus, distal fixation is often suboptimal. Traditional condylar buttress plates offer more freedom of angulation of distal screws but no coronal plane stability. Unacceptable rates of varus collapse have been reported when this device is used for unstable fractures.[47,48] These implants have been largely abandoned in favor of static or polyaxial locked plates.

Table 1
Lewis and Rorabeck Classification of Periprosthetic Fractures of the Distal Femur

Type I	Prosthesis stable, fracture nondisplaced
Type II	Prosthesis stable, fracture displaced (most common)
Type III	Prosthesis loose

Locking Plate Fixation

Locking plate technology has been used for managing complex periarticular fractures about the knee for more than a decade.[30-33,49-55] Threads on the screw heads are threaded into corresponding threads in the plate holes, forming a fixed-angle construct and providing coronal plane stability.[56] These devices have been used with excellent results for managing complex periarticular injuries and provide reliable distal fixation. Such devices allow multiple locked screws to be placed around and between portions of the femoral component, improving distal fixation[51,57] (Figure 9). In a study of 38 periprosthetic fractures treated with the Less Invasive Stabilization System (LISS; Synthes, Paoli, PA), Kregor and associates[53] reported two failures (5%); one patient required revision knee arthroplasty and one required bone grafting to achieve a solid union. Ultimately, 37 of 38 fractures (97%) healed. Medical and orthopaedic complications were infrequent. To ensure predictable healing with this technique, the metaphyseal comminution should remain undisturbed to preserve the vascularity of the fragments.

In addition to providing excellent mechanical stability, several locked plating designs offer the theoretic biologic advantage of percutaneous insertion, which minimizes the need for additional large incisions

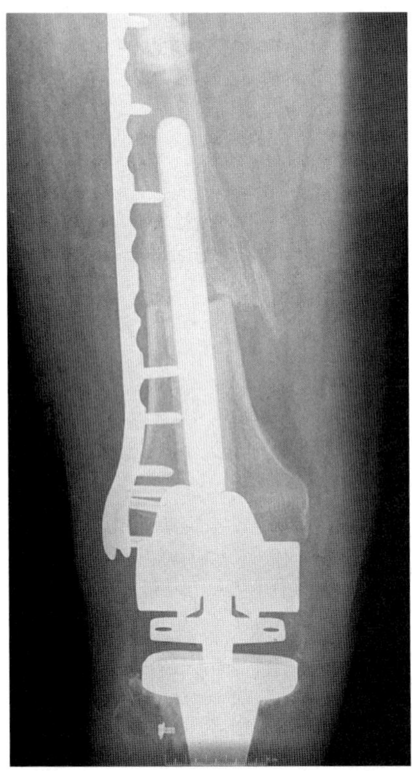

Figure 10 Radiograph showing nonunion of an allograft-prosthetic composite.

around the knee and potentially minimizes the soft-tissue complications and stiffness associated with traditional exposures used for open reduction and internal fixation.[30,51] When percutaneous techniques are used, vigilance is required to avoid malalignment, typically valgus positioning and hyperextension of the distal fragment.[51] Many commercially available locked plating designs offer the surgeon the option of either open or percutaneous insertion. When possible, percutaneous internal fixation takes advantage of the mechanical stability of a locking plate and the theoretic biologic advantages of percutaneous insertion.[58]

Prosthetic Revision

A periprosthetic fracture of the distal femur associated with a loose femoral component (type III) requires revision of the components and concomitant treatment of the fracture. Management of these injuries is particularly difficult because the remaining bone stock of the femur can be of particularly poor quality. Prosthetic revision can be performed with standard revision components that include a stem, the use of a distal femoral replacing hinged prosthesis, or an allograft-prosthetic composite.

If prosthetic revision with stemmed components is the selected treatment, the stem used should bypass the fracture by at least two cortical diameters.[35] Although a long, fully cemented stem can be considered, it may be difficult to prevent cement from entering the fracture site; this intrusion could lead to fracture nonunion. If a cementless stem is chosen, it must be of adequate length and diameter to provide both axial and rotational stability at the fracture site; augmentation with a plate or strut allograft can be considered if stability is not achieved intraoperatively.

Replacing the distal femur with a hinged, tumor-type prosthesis allows immediate weight bearing. Fracture healing is not required for successful treatment because the distal femur is removed. Although this strategy has been described as a successful treatment option, there is a substantial risk of complications, and it is probably best reserved for low-demand patients. This treatment option also has been described for patients with type II fractures (associated with a well-fixed prosthesis) when difficulties with distal fixation secondary to a small or osteopenic distal fragment are encountered.

The principles of using an allograft-prosthetic composite include cementing the allograft to the prosthesis and achieving union at the graft-host junction with a plate or strut allograft and typically a cementless stem that is placed into the retained more proximal aspect of the distal femur (Figure 10). Reattachment of the collateral ligaments to the allograft can be attempted; however, instability is a recognized complication of this approach, and the use of a constrained condylar insert or a resurfacing hinge-type implant should be strongly considered.

Periprosthetic Fractures of the Tibia

Periprosthetic fractures of the tibia are a relatively infrequent occurrence and are typically associated with loose components and/or extensive osteolysis. Because the components are either loose or the bone stock of the proximal tibia is compromised secondary to osteolysis, component revision is required. The primary goal of treatment is to bypass the fracture with a stemmed revision component if the component is loose. Because loss of proximal tibial bone stock is prevalent in this injury pattern, restoration of bone stock with impaction grafting has been described as a successful revision technique.[59] Although a fully cemented tibial stem can be used, interdigitation of cement at the fracture site may occur and inhibit bony healing. Consequently, a cementless, canal-filling stem is preferred, with cementation only in the metaphyseal region of the stem. Periprosthetic fractures of the tibia may be associated with well-fixed components in high-energy traumatic injuries or in elderly patients. In these scenarios, locked or standard plating techniques from the lateral side can be used (Figure 11).

Periprosthetic Fractures of the Patella

Periprosthetic fractures of the patella are relatively uncommon and occur in association with approximately 1% of TKAs.[60] Most of these fractures seem to occur without an identifiable traumatic event, and many are noted incidentally on routine follow-up radiographs without associated symptoms.[60] Surgical treatment of periprosthetic fractures of the patella have a high rate of complications (approximately 50% in most studies); therefore, surgical treatment is discouraged unless the extensor mechanism is disrupted or the patellar component is loose.[60-62] The most commonly reported complications include nonunion, recurrent extensor lag, painful hardware, and infection. The high rate of complications associated with surgical treatment is probably related to several factors, including damage to the blood supply of the patellar remnant secondary to a prior medially based arthrotomy (in some cases, a lateral retinacular release) and the potential difficulty of achieving rigid fixation in the thin patellar remnant. It also is difficult to balance the immobilization required for fracture healing against the stiffness that may result from extended periods of immobilization.

Risk Factors and Prevention

The primary patient-related factors associated with periprosthetic fractures of the patella include male sex, obesity, high activity levels, inflammatory arthritis, revision as opposed to primary procedures, and high range of motion. Several prosthetic design features, including the use of a metal-backed patella, cementless patellar components, and one large central peg as opposed to designs with three smaller pegs, have been associated with a higher prevalence of this complication.

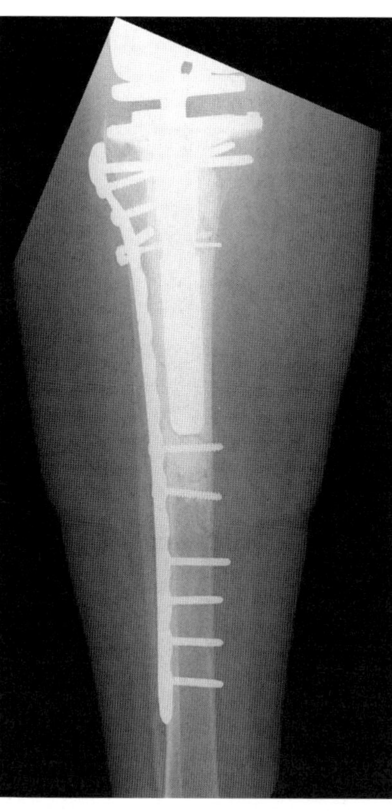

Figure 11 Radiograph showing a periprosthetic fracture of the tibia associated with a well-fixed component that was treated with a lateral locking plate.

Care in preparing both the patella itself and the tibiofemoral components are important in preventing periprosthetic fractures of the patella.[63] Appropriate external rotation and lateralization of the tibial and femoral components as well as medialization of the patellar component assist in patellar tracking and lower the risk of patellar complications. Patellae that are cut too thin (particularly less than 12 mm in thickness), remain too thick, or are cut asymmetrically seem to increase the risk of a periprosthetic fracture of the patella.[64] Lateral retinacular release, particularly with sacrifice of the superolateral geniculate artery, also has been associated with an increased risk of a periprosthetic fracture of the patella.[65]

Table 2
Classification of Periprosthetic Fractures of the Patella

Type I	Extensor mechanism intact, prosthesis stable (most common)
Type II	Extensor mechanism disrupted
Type III	Extensor mechanism intact, prosthesis loose
Type IIIA	"Reasonable" remaining bone stock (rare)
Type IIIB	Bone stock unsatisfactory for internal fixation and/or another resurfacing procedure

Classification

The most important considerations in treating a periprosthetic fracture of the patella include whether the extensor mechanism is intact or disrupted and if the patellar component itself is well fixed or loose. If the extensor mechanism is disrupted, surgery is required to restore active knee extension. The most commonly cited classification is that of Ortiguera and Berry[60] (Table 2).

Type I Fractures

In a type I periprosthetic fracture of the patella, the extensor mechanism is intact, and the patellar component is well fixed. These are often incidental radiographic findings that do not require specific treatment. If the patient is symptomatic, recommended treatment is a short course of immobilization followed by progressive, protected range of motion in a hinged knee brace. Surgical treatment is discouraged, regardless of the radiographic findings, because of the high rate of failure and complications. Nonsurgical treatment of type I fractures is associated with a high rate of success.[60]

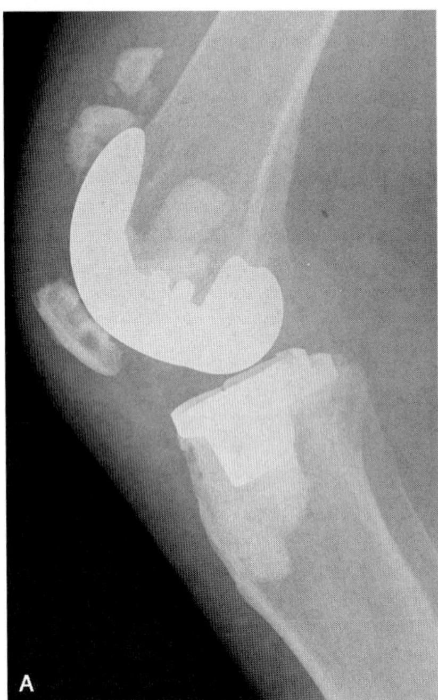

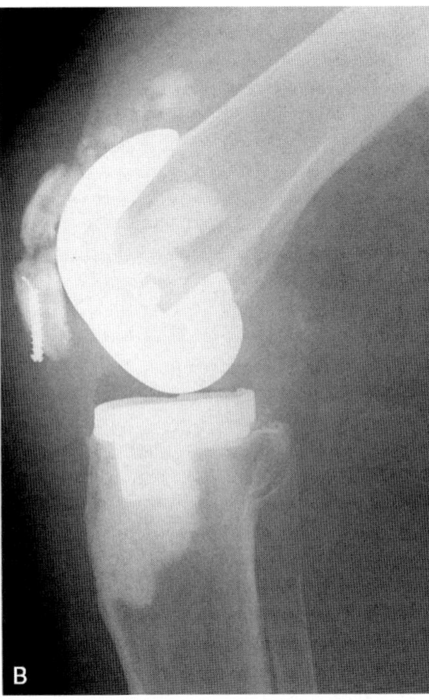

Figure 12 **A,** Radiograph of a type II periprosthetic fracture of the patella in a 57-year-old woman with rheumatoid arthritis. **B,** Despite fixation with cannulated lag screws, a tension band, and a cerclage wire, a nonunion developed.

Type II Fractures

If the extensor mechanism is not intact, surgical treatment is required to restore continuity and active knee extension. Patients who sustain this type of injury must be counseled preoperatively that the risk of complications is high but that surgical treatment is necessary to enable active knee extension and restore knee stability (Figure 12). Because there is a high risk of infection, it is critical to ensure that the skin overlying the knee is intact (and not abraded) before proceeding with surgery. Although the use of cannulated, partially threaded screws with a tension band running through them is the strongest construct biomechanically, it may be difficult to use this type of technique if the remaining patellar bone is thin; alternative methods, such as a standard tension band with a circumferential cerclage wire, may be required.[66] If the displaced fragment is small or otherwise unrepairable to the main body of the patella, excision of the fragment with primary soft-tissue repair of the extensor mechanism can be performed. Postoperative immobilization in a cast should be considered to allow bony union or soft-tissue healing. It must be recognized that concomitant tibiofemoral component revision may be required to correct rotational malalignment, which is a predisposing risk factor for the fracture; preoperative CT scans to objectively identify component rotation should be considered.[67]

Type III Fractures

In a type III fracture, the patellar component is loose, and the extensor mechanism is intact (fractures with a loose component and a disrupted extensor mechanism are classified as type II). Many of these fractures are associated with osteonecrosis of the patella. If the patellar component is loose and the patient can perform a straight leg raise, an initial course of nonsurgical treatment is recommended, particularly if the initial presentation was associated with a traumatic event. If the patient is persistently symptomatic, the component can be revised if there is adequate remaining bone stock. In most instances, however, the component is simply removed and the remaining bone contoured to optimize patellar tracking.

Management of Treatment Failures

If open reduction and internal fixation or attempts at primary extensor mechanism repair have failed, repeated attempts at repair are not recommended because of the high risk of infection and the low likelihood that repeated attempts at repair will result in restoration of extensor mechanism function. In these situations, a complete extensor mechanism allograft is recommended to restore active knee extension.[68]

Summary

Periprosthetic fractures are increasing common and are difficult clinical entities to treat. Challenges faced by the orthopaedic surgeon include gaining fracture fixation around a prosthesis that is implanted in bone that is often of poor quality or revising components in the setting of bone loss. These fractures also present biologic challenges because of prior damage to the endosteal blood supply. Postoperative treatment of some patients may be difficult because of medical comorbidities. A thorough understanding of the common pitfalls in treating and strategies for avoiding those pitfalls is paramount to achieving successful outcomes.

References

1. Lindahl H, Malchau H, Herberts P, Garellick G: Periprosthetic femoral fractures classification and demographics of 1049 periprosthetic femoral fractures from the Swedish National Hip Arthroplasty Register. *J Arthroplasty* 2005;20:857-865.
2. Lindahl H, Malchau H, Odén A, Garellick G: Risk factors for failure after treatment of a periprosthetic fracture of the femur. *J Bone Joint Surg Br* 2006;88:26-30.
3. Lowenhielm G, Hansson LI, Kärrholm J: Fracture of the lower extremity after total hip replacement. *Arch Orthop Trauma Surg* 1989;108:141-143.
4. Lindahl H, Oden A, Garellick G, Malchau H: The excess mortality due to periprosthetic femur fracture: A study from the Swedish national hip arthroplasty register. *Bone* 2007;40:1294-1298.
5. Bhattacharyya T, Chang D, Meigs JB, Estok DM II, Malchau H: Mortality after periprosthetic fracture of the femur. *J Bone Joint Surg Am* 2007;89:2658-2662.
6. Berry DJ: Epidemiology: Hip and knee. *Orthop Clin North Am* 1999;30:183-190.
7. Haidukewych GJ, Jacofsky DJ, Hanssen AD, Lewallen DG: Intraoperative fractures of the acetabulum during primary total hip arthroplasty. *J Bone Joint Surg Am* 2006;88:1952-1956.
8. Kim YS, Callaghan JJ, Ahn PB, Brown TD: Fracture of the acetabulum during insertion of an oversized hemispherical component. *J Bone Joint Surg Am* 1995;77:111-117.
9. Sharkey PF, Hozack WJ, Callaghan JJ, et al: Acetabular fracture associated with cementless acetabular component insertion: A report of 13 cases. *J Arthroplasty* 1999;14:426-431.
10. Christiansen CG, Kassim RA, Callaghan JJ, Marsh JL, Schmidt AH: Pubic ramus insufficiency fractures following total hip arthroplasty: A report of six cases. *J Bone Joint Surg Am* 2003;85:1819-1822.
11. Sánchez-Sotelo J, McGrory BJ, Berry DJ: Acute periprosthetic fracture of the acetabulum associated with osteolytic pelvic lesions: A report of 3 cases. *J Arthroplasty* 2000;15:126-130.
12. Della Valle CJ, Momberger NG, Paprosky WG: Periprosthetic fractures of the acetabulum associated with a total hip arthroplasty. *Instr Course Lect* 2003;52:281-290.
13. Berry DJ, Lewallen DG, Hanssen AD, Cabanela ME: Pelvic discontinuity in revision total hip arthroplasty. *J Bone Joint Surg Am* 1999;81:1692-1702.
14. Paprosky WG, Perona PG, Lawrence JM: Acetabular defect classification and surgical reconstruction in revision arthroplasty: A 6-year follow-up evaluation. *J Arthroplasty* 1994;9:33-44.
15. Sporer SM, Paprosky WG: Acetabular revision using a trabecular metal acetabular component for severe acetabular bone loss associated with a pelvic discontinuity. *J Arthroplasty* 2006;21:87-90.
16. DeBoer DK, Christie MJ, Brinson MF, Morrison JC: Revision total hip arthroplasty for pelvic discontinuity. *J Bone Joint Surg Am* 2007;89:835-840.
17. Springer BD, Berry DJ, Cabanela ME, Hanssen AD, Lewallen DG: Early postoperative transverse pelvic fracture: A new complication related to revision arthroplasty with an uncemented cup. *J Bone Joint Surg Am* 2005;87:2626-2631.
18. Brady OH, Garbuz DS, Masri BA, Duncan CP: Classification of the hip. *Orthop Clin North Am* 1999;30:215-220.
19. Dennis MG, Simon JA, Kummer FJ, Koval KJ, DiCesare PE: Fixation of periprosthetic femoral shaft fractures occurring at the tip of the stem: A biomechanical study of 5 techniques. *J Arthroplasty* 2000;15:523-528.
20. Maloney WJ, Herzwurm P, Paprosky W, Rubash HE, Engh CA: Treatment of pelvic osteolysis associated with a stable acetabular component inserted without cement as part of a total hip replacement. *J Bone Joint Surg Am* 1997;79:1628-1634.
21. Springer BD, Berry DJ, Lewallen DG: Treatment of periprosthetic femoral fractures following total hip arthroplasty with femoral component revision. *J Bone Joint Surg Am* 2003;85:2156-2162.
22. Tsiridis E, Narvani AA, Haddad FS, Timperley JA, Gie GA: Impaction femoral allografting and cemented revision for periprosthetic femoral fractures. *J Bone Joint Surg Br* 2004;86:1124-1132.
23. Levine BR, Della Valle CJ, Lewis P, Berger RA, Sporer SM, Paprosky W: Extended trochanteric osteotomy for the treatment of Vancouver B2/B3 periprosthetic fractures of the femur. *J Arthroplasty* 2008;23:527-533.
24. Stiehl JB: Extended osteotomy for periprosthetic femoral fractures in total hip arthroplasty. *Am J Orthop* 2006;35:20-23.
25. Ko PS, Lam JJ, Tio MK, Lee OB, Ip FK: Distal fixation with Wagner revision stem in treating Vancouver type B2 periprosthetic femur fractures in geriatric patients. *J Arthroplasty* 2003;18:446-452.
26. Della Valle CJ, Paprosky WG: Classification and an algorithmic approach to the reconstruction of femoral deficiency in revision total hip arthroplasty. *J Bone Joint Surg Am* 2003;85:1-6.
27. Sporer SM, Paprosky WG: Extensively coated cementless femoral components in revision total hip arthroplasty: An update. *Surg Technol Int* 2005;14:265-274.
28. Maury AC, Pressman A, Cayen B, Zalzal P, Backstein D, Gross A: Proximal femoral allograft treatment of Vancouver type-B3 periprosthetic femoral fractures after total hip arthroplasty. *J Bone Joint Surg Am* 2006;88:953-958.
29. Klein GR, Parvizi J, Rapuri V, et al: Proximal femoral replacement for the treatment of periprosthetic fractures.

J Bone Joint Surg Am 2005;87:1777-1781.

30. Kregor PJ: Distal femur fractures with complex articular involvement: Management by articular exposure and submuscular fixation. *Orthop Clin North Am* 2002;33:153-175.
31. Kregor PJ, Stannard J, Zlowodzki M, Cole PA, Alonso J: Distal femoral fracture fixation utilizing the Less Invasive Stabilization System (L.I.S.S.): The technique and early results. *Injury* 2001;32:SC32-SC47.
32. Schandelmaier P, Partenheimer A, Koenemann B, Grün OA, Krettek C: Distal femoral fractures and LISS stabilization. *Injury* 2001;32:SC55-SC63.
33. Schütz M, Müller M, Krettek C, et al: Minimally invasive fracture stabilization of distal femoral fractures with the LISS: A prospective multicenter study. Results of a clinical study with special emphasis on difficult cases. *Injury* 2001;32:SC48-SC54.
34. Ricci WM, Bolhofner BR, Loftus T, Cox C, Mitchell S, Borrelli J Jr: Indirect reduction and plate fixation, without grafting, for periprosthetic femoral shaft fractures about a stable intramedullary implant. *J Bone Joint Surg Am* 2005;87:2240-2245.
35. Rorabeck CH, Taylor JW: Periprosthetic fractures of the femur complicating total knee arthroplasty. *Orthop Clin North Am* 1999;30:265-277.
36. Ayers DC: Supracondylar fractures adjacent to total knee implants. *Instr Course Lect* 1997;46:197-203.
37. Engh GA, Ammeen DJ: Periprosthetic fractures adjacent to total knee implants: Treatment and clinical results. *Instr Course Lect* 1998;47:437-448.
38. Healy WL, Siliski JM, Incavo SJ: Operative treatment of distal femoral fractures proximal to total knee replacements. *J Bone Joint Surg Am* 1993;75:27-34.
39. Chen F, Mont MA, Bachner RS: Management of ipsilateral supracondylar femur fractures following total knee arthroplasty. *J Arthroplasty* 1994;9:521-526.
40. Henry SL, Busconi B, Gold S: Management of supracondylar femur fractures proximal to total knee prostheses with the GSH supracondylar intramedullary nail. *Orthop Trans* 1995;19:153.
41. Henry SL: Management of supracondylar fractures proximal to total knee arthroplasty with the GSH supracondylar nail. *Contemp Orthop* 1995;31:231-238.
42. Bong MR, Egol KA, Koval KJ, et al: Comparison of the LISS and a retrograde-inserted supracondylar intramedullary nail for fixation of a periprosthetic distal femur fracture proximal to a total knee arthroplasty. *J Arthroplasty* 2002;17:876-881.
43. Mulvey TJ, Thornhill TS, Kelly MA, Healy WL: Complications associated with total knee arthroplasty, in Pellici PM, Tria AJ Jr, Garvin KL, eds: *Orthopaedic Knowledge Update 2: Hip and Knee Reconstruction*. Rosemont, IL, American Academy of Orthopaedic Surgeons, 2000, pp 323-337.
44. Ayers DC, Dennis DA, Johanson NA, Pellegrini VD Jr: Common complications of total knee arthroplasty. *J Bone Joint Surg Am* 1997;79:278-311.
45. Sanders R, Regazzoni P, Ruedi TP: Treatment of supracondylar-intracondylar fractures of the femur using the dynamic condylar screw. *J Orthop Trauma* 1989;3:214-222.
46. Bolhofner BR, Carmen B, Clifford P: The results of open reduction and internal fixation of distal femur fractures using a biologic (indirect) reduction technique. *J Orthop Trauma* 1996;10:372-377.
47. Cordeiro EN, Costa RC, Carazzato JG, Silva Jdos S: Periprosthetic fractures in patients with total knee arthroplasties. *Clin Orthop Relat Res* 1990;252:182-189.
48. Davison BL: Varus collapse of comminuted distal femur fractures after open reduction and internal fixation with a lateral condylar buttress plate. *Am J Orthop* 2003;32:27-30.
49. Herrera DA, Kregor PJ, Cole PA, Levy BA, Jönsson A, Zlowodzki M: Treatment of acute distal femur fractures above a TKA: Systematic review of 415 cases (1981-2006). *Acta Orthop* 2008;79:22-27.
50. Cole PA, Zlowodzki M, Kregor PJ: Treatment of proximal tibia fractures using the less invasive stabilization system: Surgical experience and early clinical results in 77 fractures. *J Orthop Trauma* 2004;18:528-535.
51. Haidukewych GJ: Innovations in locking plate technology. *J Am Acad Orthop Surg* 2004;12:205-212.
52. Koval KJ, Hoehl JJ, Kummer FJ, Simon JA: Distal femoral fixation: A biomechanical comparison of the standard condylar buttress plate, a locked buttress plate, and the 95-degree blade plate. *J Orthop Trauma* 1997;11:521-524.
53. Kregor PJ, Hughes JL, Cole PA: Fixation of distal femoral fractures above total knee arthroplasty utilizing the Less Invasive Stabilization System (L.I.S.S.). *Injury* 2001;32:SC64-SC75.
54. Krettek C, Müller M, Miclau T: Evolution of minimally invasive plate osteosynthesis (MIPO) in the femur. *Injury* 2001;32:SC14-SC23.
55. Marti A, Fankhauser C, Frenk A, Cordey J, Gasser B: Biomechanical evaluation of the less invasive stabilization system for the internal fixation of distal femur fractures. *J Orthop Trauma* 2001;15:482-487.
56. Frigg R, Appenzeller A, Christensen R, Frenk A, Gilbert S, Schavan R: The development of the distal femur Less Invasive Stabilization System (LISS). *Injury* 2001;32:SC24-SC31.
57. Zlowodzki M, Williamson S, Zardiackas LD, Kregor PJ: Biomechanical evaluation of the less invasive stabilization system, angled blade plate, and retrograde intramedullary nail for the fixation of distal femur fractures. *J Orthop Trauma* 2004;18:494-502.
58. Farouk O, Krettek C, Miclau T, Schandelmaier P, Guy P, Tscherne H: Minimally invasive plate osteosynthesis: Does percutaneous plating disrupt femoral blood supply less than the traditional technique? *J Orthop Trauma* 1999;13:401-406.

59. Beharrie AW, Nelson CL: Impaction bone-grafting in the treatment of a periprosthetic fracture of the tibia: A case report. *J Bone Joint Surg Am* 2003; 85:703-707.

60. Ortiguera CJ, Berry DJ: Patellar fracture after total knee arthroplasty. *J Bone Joint Surg Am* 2002;84:532-540.

61. Keating EM, Haas G, Meding JB: Patella fracture after post total knee replacements. *Clin Orthop Relat Res* 2003;416:93-97.

62. Parvizi J, Kim KI, Oliashirazi A, Ong A, Sharkey PF: Periprosthetic patellar fractures. *Clin Orthop Relat Res* 2006;446:161-166.

63. Figgie HE III, Goldberg VM, Figgie MP, Inglis AE, Kelly M, Sobel M: The effect of alignment of the implant on fractures of the patella after condylar total knee arthroplasty. *J Bone Joint Surg Am* 1989;71:1031-1039.

64. Reuben JD, McDonald CL, Woodard PL, Hennington LJ: Effect of patella thickness on patella strain following total knee arthroplasty. *J Arthroplasty* 1991;6:251-258.

65. Tria AJ Jr, Harwood DA, Alicea JA, Cody RP: Patellar fractures in posterior stabilized knee arthroplasties. *Clin Orthop Relat Res* 1994;299: 131-138.

66. Carpenter JE, Kasman RA, Patel N, Lee ML, Goldstein SA: Biomechanical evaluation of current patella fracture fixation techniques. *J Orthop Trauma* 1997;11:351-356.

67. Berger RA, Crossett LS, Jacobs JJ, Rubash HE: Malrotation causing patellofemoral complications after total knee arthroplasty. *Clin Orthop Relat Res* 1998;356:144-153.

68. Burnett RS, Berger RA, Paprosky WG, Della Valle CJ, Jacobs JJ, Rosenberg AG: Extensor mechanism allograft reconstruction after total knee arthroplasty: A comparison of two techniques. *J Bone Joint Surg Am* 2004;86:2694-2699.

Orthopaedic Medicine

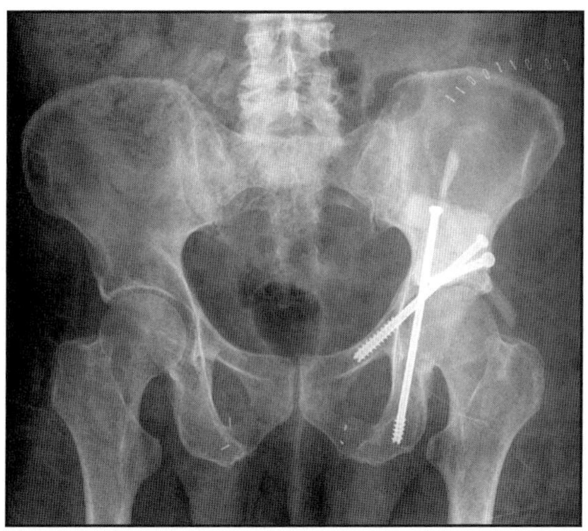

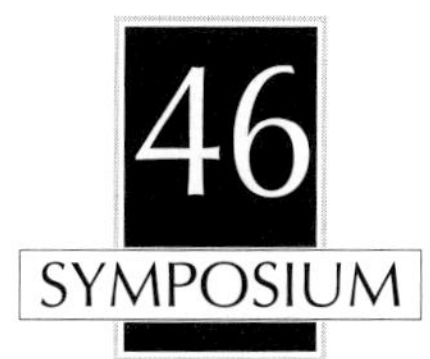

Tumors for the General Orthopedist: How to Save Your Patients and Practice

Kristy L. Weber, MD
Terrance Peabody, MD
Frank J. Frassica, MD
Michael P. Mott, MD
Theodore W. Parsons III, MD, FACS

Abstract

It is likely that most orthopaedic surgeons will see a patient with a benign or malignant musculoskeletal tumor sometime during their career. However, because of the rarity of these entities, many surgeons may benefit from a review of how to evaluate a patient with a bone lesion or soft-tissue mass. A logical approach is necessary in evaluating imaging studies as well as in the workup of children and adults with a possible tumor. It is important to have a good working relationship with a musculoskeletal radiologist to assist in interpreting the images. If the treatment algorithms lead to a conclusive diagnosis of a benign bone tumor, benign soft-tissue mass, or metastatic bone disease, the orthopaedic surgeon may choose to definitively treat the patient. If the workup indicates an indeterminate lesion, it may be prudent to discuss the situation with an orthopaedic oncologist or transfer the care of the patient to a physician with more specialized knowledge. A careful, logical workup is needed prior to surgery to limit risks to the patient and optimize the chances for a favorable outcome.

Instr Course Lect 2010;59:579-591.

Dr. Weber or an immediate family member serves as a board member, owner, officer, or committee member of the American Orthopaedic Association, the Ruth Jackson Orthopaedic Society, and the American Academy of Orthopaedic Surgeons Research Council. Dr. Peabody or an immediate family member serves as a board member, owner, officer, or committee member of the American Orthopaedic Association and the Musculoskeletal Tumor Society; and has received research or institutional support from Biomet. Dr. Frassica or an immediate family member is a member of a speakers' bureau or has made paid presentations on behalf of Stryker; serves as a paid consultant to or is an employee of Stryker; has received research or institutional support from Zimmer; has stock or stock options held in Zimmer and Stryker; and has received nonincome support (such as equipment or services), commercially derived honoraria, or other non–research-related funding (such as paid travel) from SLACK Orthopedics, Orthopedics Today, and Stryker. Dr. Mott or an immediate family member serves as a board member, owner, officer, or committee member of the Mid-America Orthopaedic Society and has stock or stock options held in Johnson & Johnson. Dr. Parsons or an immediate family member is a member of a speakers' bureau or has made paid presentations on behalf of Biomet and has received research or institutional support from Smith & Nephew, Tornier, Synthes, Zimmer, Medtronic, DePuy, and Biomet.

Practicing orthopaedic surgeons are likely to periodically encounter a patient with a benign or malignant musculoskeletal neoplasm during their careers. Approximately 12,000 new malignant musculoskeletal neoplasms are diagnosed each year in the United States, and it is important to categorize them correctly. Benign lesions are encountered much more often than malignant lesions.

Interpreting Imaging Studies of Musculoskeletal Tumors

Recognizing the imaging characteristics and anatomic details of musculoskeletal tumors from different imaging modalities provides the orthopaedic surgeon with a great deal of information and generally leads to an appropriate differential diagnosis.

Conventional Radiography

Good quality, biplanar radiographs remain the gold standard for evaluating bone lesions and providing useful information on soft-tissue lesions, such as the presence of mineralization, bone involvement, or

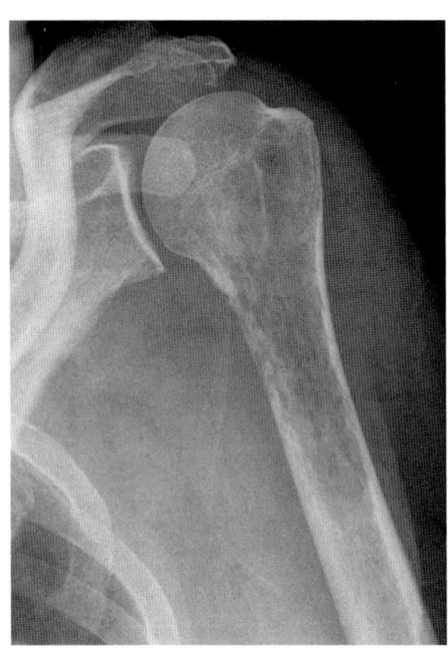

Figure 1 Radiograph showing a lymphoma in the humerus with the moth-eaten appearance typical of round cell tumors.

reactive changes. Plain radiographs should be obtained first.[1] Attention should be given to the zone of transition between the lesion and the bone. The Lodwick classification system helps determine the biologic activity of the lesion and response of the bone.[2] Type I lesions are geographic and have a sclerotic (type IA), well-defined (type IB), or poorly defined (type IC) margin. Type II lesions appear moth eaten (confluence of small lytic areas in bone) and suggest more aggressive processes (Figure 1). Type III lesions are permeative with diffuse destruction. Generally speaking, an increasing number in the Lodwick classification system corresponds to the increasing aggressiveness of the lesion.

The characteristics of the lesion help to differentiate aggressive from benign lesions. Larger lesions tend to be more aggressive. Cortical destruction, poor margination, and extension into the soft tissues are generally characteristics of a malignant tumor. Evaluating periosteal patterns, if present, also can be helpful. Benign or low-grade lesions generally demonstrate thick, wavy, and uniform changes on the bone surface, reflecting a slow response to the underlying condition. Lamellated (onion skin), spiculated (sunburst), or Codman triangle periosteal changes reflect aggressive lesions that are "blowing out" the bone.

The location of the lesion provides clues to an appropriate differential diagnosis (for example, chondroblastomas or giant cell tumors in the epiphyseal area; unicameral bone cysts in the proximal humerus or proximal femur). Patient age is similarly helpful in the diagnosis because many tumors manifest in specific age groups (for example, Ewing sarcoma in teenagers and multiple myeloma in older adults).[3]

Matrix mineralization is another feature that provides useful diagnostic clues. For example, the presence of stippled calcifications (rings and arcs) indicates a chondroid tumor. Amorphous ossification is common in osteosarcoma or osteoblastic metastasis. Fibrous dysplasia exhibits a "ground-glass" appearance; a central, swirling "smoke up the chimney" mineral pattern is consistent with a bone infarct.[4]

Bone Scintigraphy

Bone scintigraphy (bone scanning) is useful in determining whether a bone lesion is active (increased uptake) or indolent. The scan actually shows bone formation (in response to a stimulus) and blood flow. Slow growing or inactive lesions typically show minimal radiopharmaceutical uptake, whereas active bone-forming lesions, regardless of their biologic potential, typically show intense uptake. This test is generally sensitive in screening for distant metastatic bone disease, regional skip lesions within the bone, and radiographically occult disease. Transition from mild to intense radiopharmaceutical uptake in a known lesion is generally a poor prognostic sign. Multiple myeloma, renal cell carcinoma, thyroid cancer, and rapid infection with necrosis may show little uptake, giving a false-negative result.[5,6]

Computed Tomography

CT is particularly useful for identifying mineral densities in bone and soft-tissue lesions. This modality helps differentiate chondrogenic (calcification), osteogenic (cloud-like bone formation), and soft-tissue lesions that may have calcifications (hemangiomas, liposarcomas, and synovial sarcomas) in addition to myositis ossificans. CT also readily shows cortical thinning or breakthrough, the zone of transition (margination), and osteolytic and sclerotic changes in flat bones.[7] CT is helpful in evaluating axial skeletal (pelvis, spine) lesions where the anatomy is complex and in planning and performing needle biopsies and/or thermal ablation of lesions[8] (Figure 2). A contrast-enhanced CT scan of the chest, abdomen, and pelvis is one of the principal imaging tools used to detect the primary source of metastatic disease to bone.

Magnetic Resonance Imaging

MRI provides superior soft-tissue contrast and fine anatomic detail. This modality improves the physician's ability to appropriately stage musculoskeletal tumors and adequately plan limb-salvage surgery. Various sequences, which are influenced by relaxation and echo times between pulses, can be manipulated to maximize the visualization of dif-

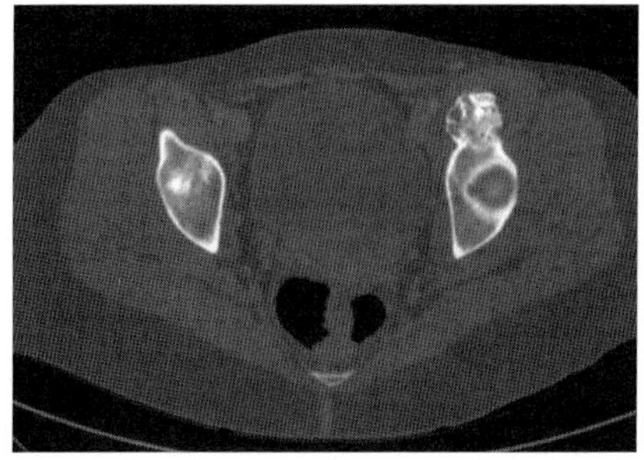

Figure 2 CT scan showing a benign osteochondroma arising from the anterior acetabular area. These lesions are poorly visualized with plain radiographs.

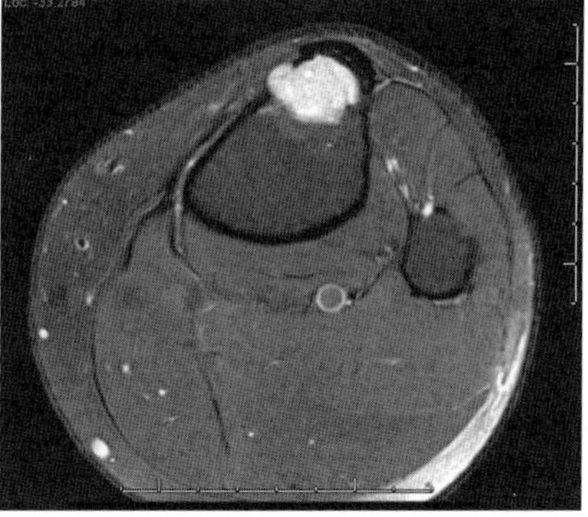

Figure 3 T2-weighted axial MRI scan of the tibia showing plasmacytoma with early cortical breakthrough of the soft-tissue mass.

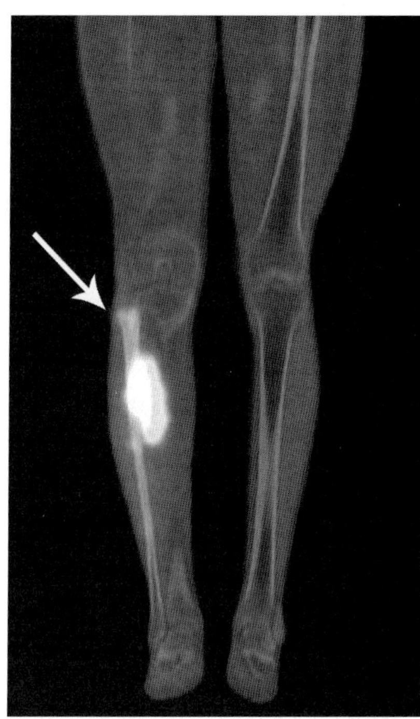

Figure 4 PET-CT fusion image of fibular Ewing sarcoma showing intense uptake.

ferent tissue types based on their signal characteristics. T1-weighted images (short echo and relaxation times) produce the greatest anatomic detail and tend to be the best method for evaluating bone marrow, which is largely composed of fat in an adult. Marrow replacement from a tumor or an infection tends to be at least as dark as adjacent muscle. Fat, methemoglobin (a blood product), gadolinium, proteinaceous fluid, melanin, and particulate calcium appear bright (white) on T1-weighted MRI scans.[9] Reduced venous flow, surgical packing, and hemostatic agents also may be bright on a postoperative T1-weighted MRI scan.[10] T2-weighted images (longer pulse sequences) are best for contrasting the difference between normal and abnormal tissues. Edema, cystic lesions, joint or synovial fluid, most tumors, and free water appear bright (white) on T2-weighted images (Figure 3). Fluid-fluid levels, the layering of different density materials (for example, blood and transudate or exudate) are common in lesions including an aneurysmal bone cyst, telangiectatic osteosarcoma, and synovial sarcoma. Other lesions, such as complex unicameral bone cysts, chondroblastoma, giant cell tumor, and fibrous dysplasia, may also exhibit fluid-fluid levels.

Gadolinium-contrasted T1-weighted images are used to further define tumor involvement and help distinguish between a tumor and postoperative scar tissue.[11] It should be noted that tumoral hyperemia associated with neoplasia revealed on gadolinium T1-weighted images can occasionally lead to an overestimation of the amount of tissue involvement by tumor. Gradient echo sequences (short relaxation, low angle) are useful in evaluating subtle calcifications or chronic blood products because of their sensitivity to signal loss from these tissues (bloom artifact). Certain conditions, such as pigmented villonodular synovitis, hemophilic hemorrhagic synovitis, and synovial chondromatosis, may be best shown with this sequence. Although MRI sensitivity is impaired by the presence of large metal implants, a prescanning consultation with a musculoskeletal radiologist often can produce a scan with useful information. Modified fast spin-echo and inversion recovery techniques can reduce the intravoxel dephasing and frequency misregistration adjacent to these implants.[12] Despite limitations associated with fine bony detail, subtle calcification, and implanted hardware, MRI is the modality of choice for evaluating many musculoskeletal tumors.

Positron Emission Tomography

Positron emission tomography (PET) is a functional imaging modality that is based on the presumption that neoplastic tissue has an increased metabolism compared with surrounding baseline tissue(s) and can be identified using radioactive glucose.[13] To increase its localization sensitivity, PET is often fused to a CT scan (PET-CT). To assess lesions, 18F-fluorodeoxyglucose (FDG) typically is used and is quite sensitive in identifying small and/or skip lesions. Increased FDG uptake is usually correlated with an increasing degree of tumor aggressiveness.[13] Typically, a standard uptake value greater than 2.0 or a tumor-to-background ratio greater than 3.0 is a cause for concern[14] (Figure 4). The wide overlap between normal and abnormal tissue leads to a relatively low specificity with a PET scan. PET is less useful in diagnosing inflammatory diseases such as osteomyelitis, Paget disease, fibrous dysplasia, and osteoblastic bone metastases. Sarcomas with extensive extracellular matrix can dilute the FDG signal, leading to an underestimation of the biologic aggressiveness of the lesion. In the future, PET may offer benefits in estimating tumor necrosis after neoadjuvant chemotherapy. A decreasing standard uptake value may be correlated with necrosis and theoretically will allow earlier or changing intervention for tumors that are responding poorly to treatment.[14,15]

Approach for the Older Patient With a Destructive Bone Lesion

In patients older than 40 years, destructive bone lesions will usually be diagnosed as metastatic carcinoma. Primary malignant bone tumors occur less commonly in this age group, and the surgical treatment is quite different for this subset of patients. A careful, stepwise approach to the evaluation of an older patient with a destructive bone lesion will minimize the chance of a misdiagnosis that could compromise the optimal outcome for the patient.[16,17]

Evaluation

Patient History

An appropriate patient evaluation begins with a thorough history.[16,17] Because destructive bone lesions are almost always painful, the nature of the pain, such as timing, duration, location, relation to weight bearing, exacerbating factors, and medications needed for pain relief, must be determined. Progressive pain that occurs at rest and at night is more suggestive of a malignant process. Constitutional symptoms, such as weight loss and lethargy, are important. Determining a personal or family history of cancer is critical. It is important to remember that cancers can metastasize more than 10 years after the primary site is treated. A history of radiation treatment or Paget disease may suggest the possibility of a secondary malignancy. Dates of screening mammograms, prostate examinations, and colonoscopies should be recorded. Cancer in any bodily site can metastasize to bone, but the most common primary sites of metastatic bone cancer include the breast, the lung, the prostate, the kidney, and the thyroid. Symptoms related to abnormal function of these organs should be documented.

Physical Examination

The physical examination should be complete and focus on the site of the painful lesion as well as the surrounding areas (for example, the entire affected extremity).[16,17] Potential primary sites of cancer (such as the breast, prostate, lung, or thyroid) should be evaluated. Any decreased joint range of motion, swelling, tenderness, neurologic deficits, gait abnormalities, and lymphadenopathy should be documented.

Laboratory Studies

A complete blood count with differential, basic metabolic panel, and urinalysis should be performed. Normal laboratory studies do not eliminate the possibility of malignancy or metastasis, but abnormal results sometimes are helpful in decision making. Anemia may suggest multiple myeloma, hypercalcemia occurs with hyperparathyroidism or widespread bone metastasis, and microscopic hematuria is associated with renal cell carcinoma. Alkaline phosphatase, phosphorus, and vitamin D levels may be helpful in identifying a particular metabolic bone disease. Other studies such as serum and urine electrophoresis, thyroid function tests, the prostate-specific antigen test, and other tumor markers can be ordered as necessary depending on radiographic findings and clinical suspicions.

Imaging

Plain radiographs of the destructive bone lesion often will provide clues to the eventual diagnosis.[16,17] Most bone metastases are osteolytic with the exception of prostate and some breast cancers, which create osteoblastic metastases. Multiple myeloma bone lesions are described as punched-out holes without visible matrix within the lesion. Lymphoma within the bone may not be visible on plain radiographs. Some bone tumors or metabolic abnormalities have unique characteristics (ossification in osteosarcoma, calcifications in chondrosarcoma, and coarsened trabeculae in Paget disease). The location of the bone lesion can be helpful. Most bone metastases occur in the thoracic spine. A lesser trochanteric avulsion implies an underlying pathologic process and impending hip fracture (Figure 5). Chordoma typically affects the sacrum. It is important to obtain orthogonal radiographic views and to image the entire bone.

Additional imaging is usually necessary for a definitive diagnosis. A total body technetium Tc 99m (^{99m}Tc) bone scan is a screening study for additional bone lesions and is often positive in metastatic disease. Because a bone scan documents osteoblastic response, it is usually falsely negative in patients with multiple myeloma.

A CT scan of the chest, abdomen,

and pelvis will usually identify a primary site of cancer in metastatic bone lesions.[16] A skeletal survey is suggested if the appearance of the bone lesion suggests multiple myeloma. Additional imaging, such as an FDG-PET scan, is not routinely used in the workup of a destructive bone lesion nor is it used for a staging workup for a high grade sarcoma; however, it is frequently used to stage and measure treatment response in patients with lymphoma. MRI is not necessary to define a destructive bone lesion unless it occurs in the spine, where it often cannot be clearly defined on plain radiographs. An MRI of the spine also can help differentiate between a vertebral compression fracture caused by osteoporosis and a fracture caused by metastatic disease.

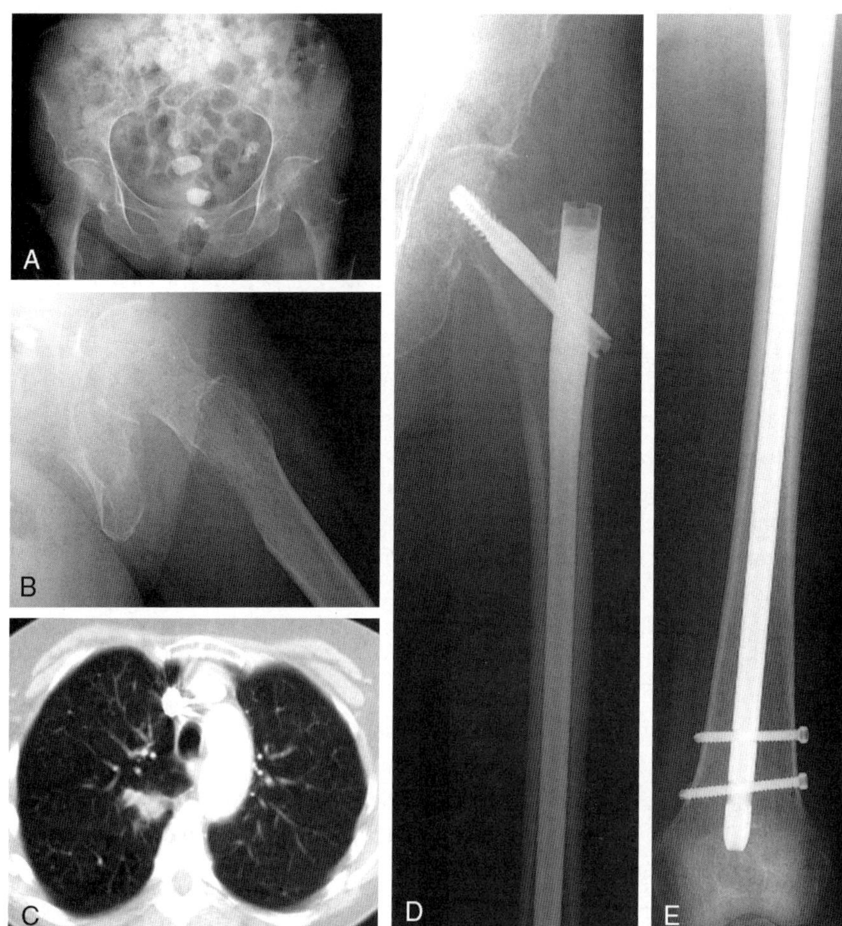

Figure 5 **A,** AP pelvic radiograph of a 67-year-old woman with left hip pain. Note the absence of the left lesser trochanter, signifying a destructive lesion. **B,** A lateral left hip radiograph better defines the osteolytic lesion, which places this patient at high risk for a pathologic fracture. A thorough history and physical examination revealed no history of cancer, a 30-pack per year history of cigarette use, pain on range of motion of the left hip, and an antalgic gait. **C,** A full radiographic staging workup was performed. This chest CT scan shows a probable primary lung cancer in the right upper lobe. Of note, the patient's abdominal CT scan showed multiple liver lesions and vertebral metastasis. A needle biopsy of the liver lesions showed metastatic lung cancer. AP radiographs of the proximal **(D)** and distal **(E)** left femur after placement of an intramedullary femoral reconstruction nail. A bone sample after reaming was sent to pathology to confirm the metastatic disease. This method of stabilization prevents a future femoral neck or diaphyseal fracture.

Biopsy

Sometimes, the previously described workup will lead to a definitive diagnosis (Figure 5); however, if there is any uncertainty, a biopsy must be performed. Bone lesions can be diagnosed by a needle biopsy under image guidance or by an incisional biopsy. If experienced radiologists and pathologists are available, a needle biopsy can be done expediently with minimal stress to the patient and a high rate of accuracy. With sophisticated immunohistochemical techniques, the primary site of a bone metastasis often can be identified, even if it was not apparent from the imaging workup.

If the workup and biopsy lead to a diagnosis of a primary malignant bone tumor, such as osteosarcoma, chondrosarcoma, chordoma, or malignant fibrous histiocytoma, referral to an orthopaedic surgeon with expertise in treating these conditions is warranted. If the lesion is a lymphoma, referral to a medical oncology team is suggested. Most destructive bone lesions caused by lymphoma are secondary to the systemic disease and will often heal with chemotherapy, thereby precluding surgical treatment. If the lesion is metastatic bone disease or multiple myeloma, surgical stabilization may be warranted. A proper understanding of the indications for fixation and the oncologic principles for treating metastatic bone disease is essential; much of this information can be found in the literature.

Associated Medical Disorders

Patients with metastatic bone disease should be treated with a multidisciplinary approach because their medical condition often requires expertise from physicians specialized in radiation oncology, medical oncology, interventional radiology, neurosurgery, and orthopaedic surgery. Depending on the extent of disease, patients may have physiologic disruptions related to the cancer.[17] Hypercalcemia is present in 10% to 15% of patients with bone metastasis, most commonly from lung and breast cancer. Early symptoms include polyuria and/or polydipsia, fatigue, weakness, and anorexia. Late symptoms include irritability, depression, nausea and/or vomiting, vision abnormalities, and coma. Hypercalcemia is a potentially life-threatening condition and requires hydration and possible intravenous bisphosphonate therapy. Other physiologic disruptions relate to the hematopoietic system (anemia), thromboembolic disease (hypercoagulability), and constipation (often related to the extensive medication required for adequate pain control).

Biomechanical Considerations and Indications for Stabilization

Patients with metastatic bone disease often present with a pathologic fracture. After stabilization with a brace or traction, the patient should be evaluated as previously described. If a patient presents with a destructive lesion, it is necessary to determine if the lesion puts the patient at risk for an impending fracture. A stress riser in the bone occurs whenever there is cortical destruction. When the length of an open section longitudinal bone defect exceeds 75% of the bone diameter, there is a 90% reduction in torsional strength. Cortical defects also reduce the bending strength of the bone. Indications for fixation of an impending fracture have been studied but remain somewhat imprecise because fractures are not entirely predictable and depend on other factors, including patient comorbidities and balance, histology of the tumor, and underlying general bone density.[18,19] Lesions are more likely to cause a fracture when they are osteolytic, located in the peritrochanteric region, affect more than two thirds of the cortex, and are painful. The decision to surgically treat extremity lesions is usually made based on plain radiographs; further local imaging is not necessarily required, although CT can better define the cortical integrity.

Noninvasive or minimally invasive alternative treatments that can be used alone or in combination with surgical treatment of metastatic bone disease include bisphosphonates, external beam radiation, CyberKnife (Accuray, Sunnyvale, CA) radiation, radiofrequency ablation, cryoablation, embolization, vertebroplasty, and kyphoplasty.

The complete technical details related to the stabilization of actual or impending fractures caused by metastatic bone disease or multiple myeloma are beyond the scope of this chapter;[20] however, a few technical pearls should be considered. (1) Methylmethacrylate can be used to supplement fixation when necessary. (2) Prosthetic replacement should be used for pathologic femoral neck fractures rather than in situ pinning or hip screw/side plate constructs. (3) The entire femur should be stabilized with a reconstruction type nail (Figure 5) regardless of where the femoral lesion or fracture is located. (4) Highly vascular lesions (such as renal cell carcinoma or thyroid cancer metastasis) should be embolized if a tourniquet cannot be used. (5) Postoperative external beam radiation can be used to supplement fixation after the skin heals to minimize the risk of disease progression and continued pain.

Approach for the Young Patient With a Destructive Bone Lesion

Three goals are necessary in treating a destructive bone lesion in a child. First, a diagnostic strategy is needed that leads to an effective and confident treatment plan. Second, an error that will result in the loss of the patient's life or limb must be avoided. Third, the treatment strategy should minimize unnecessary tests and interventions. It is important that the surgeon make sound recommendations to the child and the parents. These recommendations should provide a sense of competence and reassurance and should advise them of the need for the necessary tests and treatments that will achieve the best possible outcome.

Children differ from adults in many ways. They frequently have unrecognized infections and incidental trauma. As a result, most bone lesions are posttraumatic or inflammatory. Both children and adults may have metabolic bone disease but, with the exceptions of Paget disease, osteoporosis, and renal osteodystrophy, most metabolic bone diseases are diagnosed in patients younger than 20 years. Children frequently have developmental abnormalities or reactive, nonneoplastic lesions visible in bone. These nonneoplastic lesions often heal in children near the time of skeletal maturity. In contrast to adults, skeletal metastases are relatively rare in children, and primary malignant bone tumors in children are often high grade and associated with significant mortality.

Because there is a low incidence of primary malignant bone tumors in children (fewer than 2,000 cases per year in the United States), most surgeons have only a vague familiarity with the evaluation and treatment of these conditions. Similarly, radiologists involved in the interpretation of imaging studies may lack education and experience in reviewing primary malignant bone tumors in children and may provide opinions that are too generic to be helpful, are inaccurate, or lead to unnecessary tests and procedures.

Children and parents may not be able to provide an accurate patient history. Children often have vague symptoms that may not be reported to the parents. These may be interpreted, often correctly, as growing pains, muscle pulls, strains, and sprains. Once a bone abnormality is diagnosed, anxiety, guilt, and a need for a clear answer will be expressed by the parents. It is important to use a diagnostic rationale that will achieve the treatment goals and lessen anxiety for everyone who is involved. This scheme will involve a series of decision points with proposed action steps.

Findings Suggestive of a Primary Malignant Bone Tumor

If the child has a history of a focal lesion, increasing pain, physical findings of a soft-tissue mass and/or localized tenderness, and imaging findings consistent with a malignant tumor, a decision is needed on whether the orthopaedic surgeon will provide care or if the child will be referred to a trained orthopaedic oncologist (Figure 6). If the lesion is destructive, the child's ability to bear weight should be protected with an assistive device, and the family should be advised concerning the risk of a pathologic fracture. If the lesion is located in the upper extremity, a sling or splint is recommended.

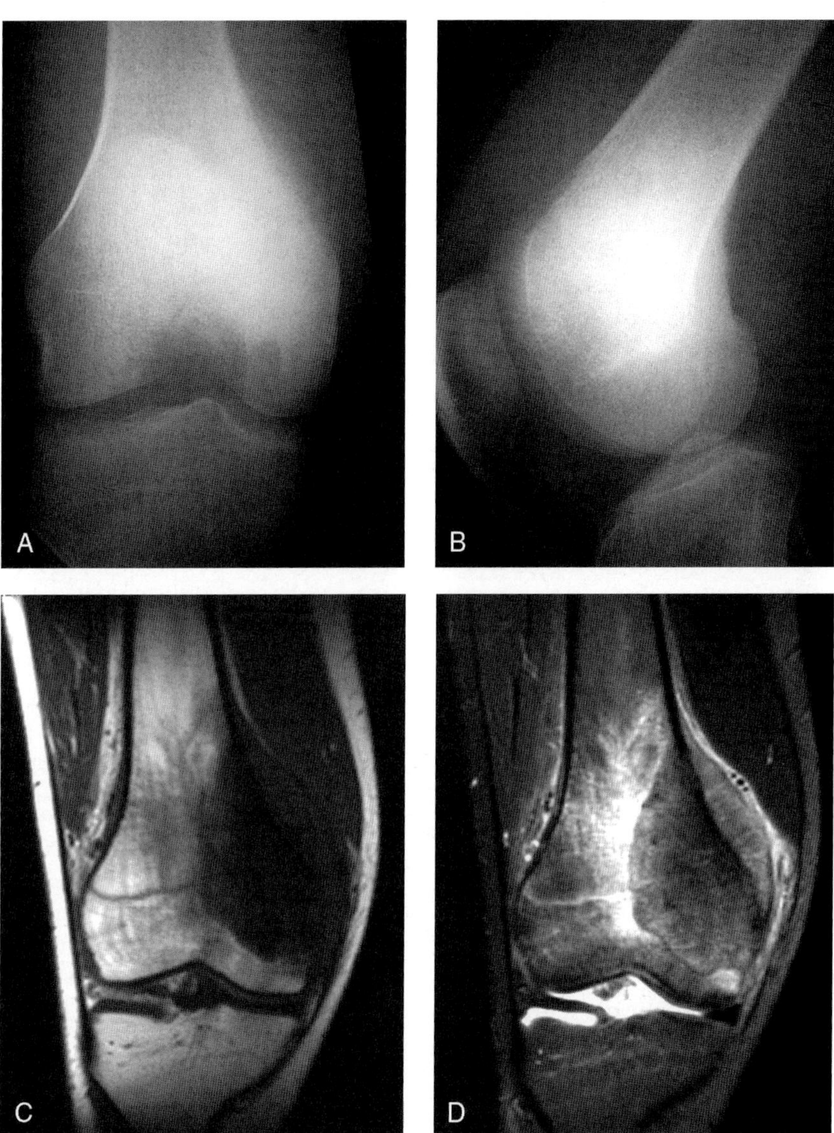

Figure 6 AP **(A)** and lateral **(B)** radiographs of a 17-year-old adolescent boy with right knee pain and swelling for 3 months. The radiographs show increased density in the medial femoral condyle with expansion of a mineralizing process into the adjacent soft tissues. The zone of transition is wide. These findings are most consistent with an osteosarcoma. **C,** The T1-weighted MRI scan shows decreased signal within the medial femoral condyle and a soft-tissue mass extending into the vastus medialis. **D,** The contrast-enhanced MRI scan shows extensive surrounding bone edema and a small effusion. The loss of the normal low signal cortex is particularly worrisome for a malignancy. A subsequent open biopsy confirmed a diagnosis of osteosarcoma.

Additional workup and a possible biopsy are indicated. If the surgeon is not familiar with the management of malignant bone tumors, including limb-salvage techniques, consultation with or referral to a colleague with such experience is necessary. Studies show improved outcomes for patients who are referred to physicians familiar with the treatment of bone sarcomas.[21]

The Incidental Bone Lesion

Incidental bone findings on plain radiographs are rarely worrisome but

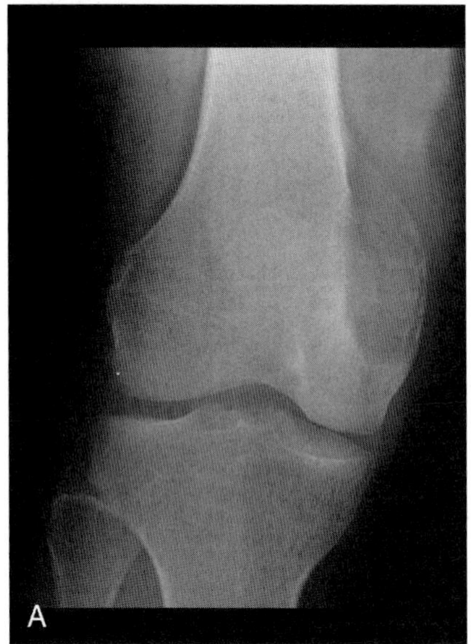

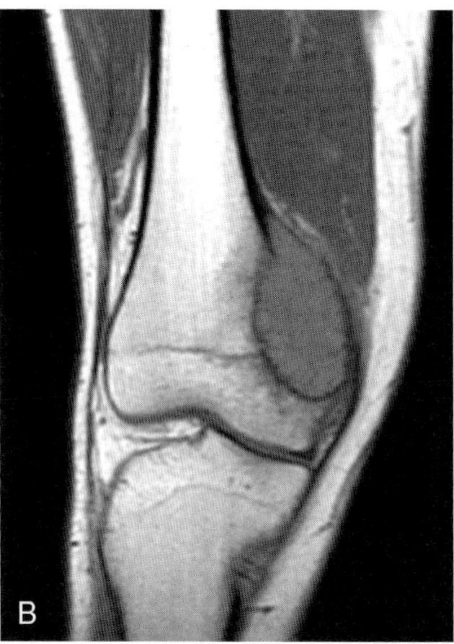

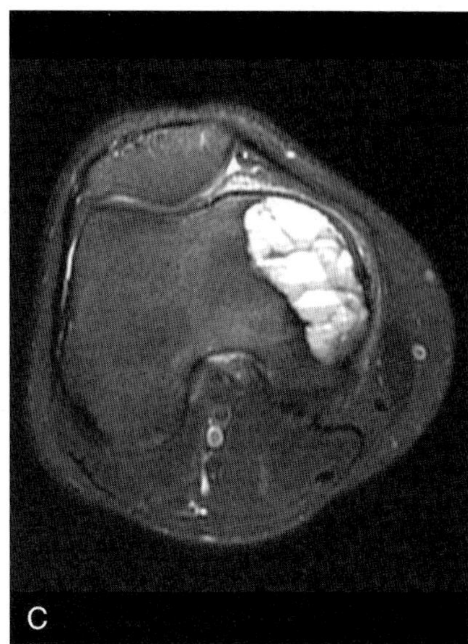

Figure 7 **A,** AP radiograph of a 15-year-old boy with 3 weeks of right knee pain. A lucency is seen in the medial femoral condyle with expansion of the cortex and periosteum. A fine line of peripheral ossification is present. Proximal periosteal elevation is apparent. There is no internal mineralization or calcification. The zone of transition is narrow. These are characteristics of an active lesion. **B,** The T1-weighted MRI scan shows a narrow zone of transition and a small rim of low signal bone about the lesion medially and is most consistent with a benign tumor. **C,** The T2-weighted axial MRI scan shows fluid-fluid levels consistent with an aneurysmal bone cyst. An open biopsy with frozen section confirmed the diagnosis, and definitive surgery with curettage and bone grafting was performed at the same setting.

merit observation. Occasionally, additional testing may be necessary, but treatment is usually not indicated. The absence of symptoms is most often associated with a latent bone lesion. In contrast, most active benign and malignant bone tumors are painful.

The presence of a fracture may add uncertainty to the diagnosis. The physician should be guided by imaging characteristics as previously described. If open treatment of the fracture is necessary, a biopsy to confirm the presence of a benign tumor is usually recommended.

In attempting to determine if a bone lesion is symptomatic, the physician should look for physical evidence of atrophy, deformity, tenderness, or a palpable mass. If the lesion is symptomatic, an active process may be involved. If there are no signs or symptoms associated with the radiographic findings, it is safe to observe most incidentally noted lesions with latent imaging characteristics. In general, follow-up examinations and radiographs at 3, 6, and 12 months are adequate to determine if there are any worrisome changes in the appearance of the lesion.

The Indeterminate Lesion

Indeterminate lesions require a diagnostic strategy involving additional imaging studies and possible biopsy.[22] After a careful history and physical examination, the physician should obtain laboratory tests including a complete blood count with differential, erythrocyte sedimentation rate, and C-reactive protein level, to look for infection. Rarely, the differential will indicate a hematologic malignancy. A chemistry panel including calcium, phosphate, and alkaline phosphatase is helpful if metabolic bone disease is suspected.

After the lesion is evaluated with plain radiographs, additional imaging may be required. A ^{99m}Tc bone scan can detect multifocal disease. CT can accurately assess cortical destruction or identify a nidus in an osteoid osteoma, but MRI with contrast is most helpful in determining the extent and nature of the lesion.[23] Marrow involvement may extend further than shown on plain radiographs. Soft-tissue involvement is worrisome, and MRI can define the relationship of the tumor to surrounding neurovascular structures. Fluid-filled lesions with only peripheral enhancement are often unicameral bone cysts. Fluid-fluid levels suggest an aneurysmal bone cyst (Figure 7).

The most common primary malignant bone tumors in children are osteosarcoma and Ewing sarcoma. Both diagnoses have radiographic findings that often include cortical destruction and a soft-tissue mass. If the eventual diagnosis proves to be eosinophilic granuloma, a skeletal survey is important in staging, but it is not as important in the initial workup.

Biopsy

When the diagnosis is not clear and the imaging findings suggest an active process, a biopsy is necessary. Biopsy is a simple technical procedure but requires significant planning.[24] The surgeon should be aware of nonconventional approaches and limb salvage options that allow the biopsy tract to be later resected with the tumor if it proves to be malignant. Complications may alter the ability to perform limb salvage surgery.

Biopsies can be open (incisional) or closed (core-needle or fine-needle aspiration). If a musculoskeletal radiologist performs the needle biopsy, it is recommended that the surgeon discuss the preferred site and route of needle entry. Many bone lesions that are suggestive of a particular lesion (such as chondroblastoma or an aneurysmal bone cyst) can be approached with an open biopsy because an accurate frozen section diagnosis may allow definitive treatment at the same surgical setting. It is recommended that prophylactic antibiotics be withheld until tissue cultures are obtained for bacteria, acid-fast bacilli, and fungus. Osteomyelitis often can be confused with an active bone tumor in a child.

Proper oncologic techniques involve selecting a direct approach to the tumor without exposing neurovascular structures. No flaps should be raised. The smallest necessary longitudinal incision should be used, and joint and tendon insertions should be avoided. A biopsy of the soft-tissue mass is preferable to creating a hole in the bone. If a bone biopsy is necessary, rounded edges should be made with a circular hole saw to minimize the chance of fracture. Meticulous hemostasis with polymethylmethacrylate or bone wax is important. A frozen section is important to ensure sufficient tissue for diagnosis and should be done before definitive surgery. Drains may be used but should be close to and in line with the incision.

Immediate Definitive Surgical Treatment

Definitive treatment should be performed in patients only when the preoperative evaluation suggests a benign tumor, which is confirmed by analyzing the frozen section. If findings are inconsistent, the surgeon should achieve hemostasis, close the incision, and await findings based on permanent sections. This approach requires the availability of an experienced musculoskeletal pathologist and is especially important when performing fracture fixation. Splinting or remote traction should be considered if there is any possibility that the underlying cause of the fracture is malignant. Plates and screws through a lateral approach will result in less contamination than intramedullary fixation, but neither technique is ideal.

Intralesional curettage is the definitive treatment for most benign bone lesions in children. A high-speed burr may be used to make a sufficiently large window in the bone to allow visualization and extend the curettage. Adjuvants such as polymethylmethacrylate, cryotherapy, phenol, or argon beams are often used. The approach, the extent of the resection, and the use of adjuvants and internal fixation must all be considered in the context of open growth plates in pediatric patients. Most surgeons use allograft or bone graft substitutes to reconstruct the defects. Children are followed postoperatively with serial radiographs at 3- to 4-month intervals for approximately 2 years to monitor for local relapse. A longer period of follow-up may be necessary to evaluate the development of a growth deformity in the child.

If the biopsy suggests a malignant process, such as an osteosarcoma or Ewing sarcoma, the patient should be treated by an orthopaedic surgeon experienced in limb-salvage techniques who has access to a multidisciplinary team. Malignant bone tumors in children generally require neoadjuvant and adjuvant chemotherapy.

A consistent and rational approach to treating a child with a destructive bone lesion will allow a confident evaluation of the significance of the lesion, preserve life and limb, and avoid unnecessary interventions and testing. Treatment may include observation, further testing, biopsy, or definitive surgery.

Soft-Tissue Masses

Soft-tissue masses are common. Primary care physicians and surgeons often must evaluate patients and decide whether a soft-tissue mass should be observed, biopsied, or removed.[25] Incorrect decisions may lead to a delay in the correct diagnosis or inappropriate excisional biopsy. In a 1982 study, Mankin and associates[26] reported a significant rate of biopsy errors that resulted in either a change in the management plan or even unnecessary amputation. In a second study by Mankin and associates[21] performed in 1992, there was no improvement in biopsy results for musculoskeletal malignancies in the 10-year interval between the two studies. Simply clas-

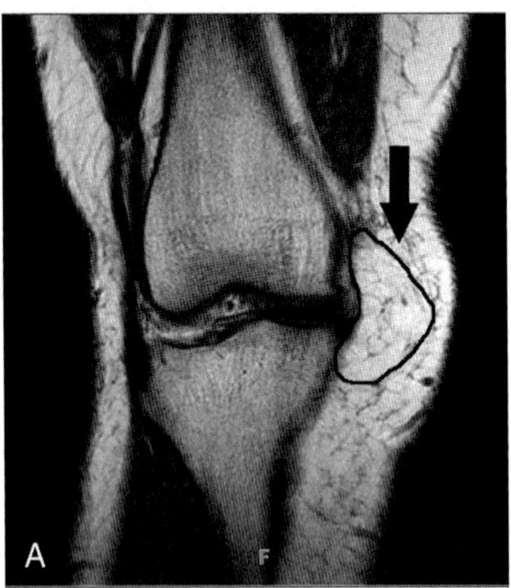

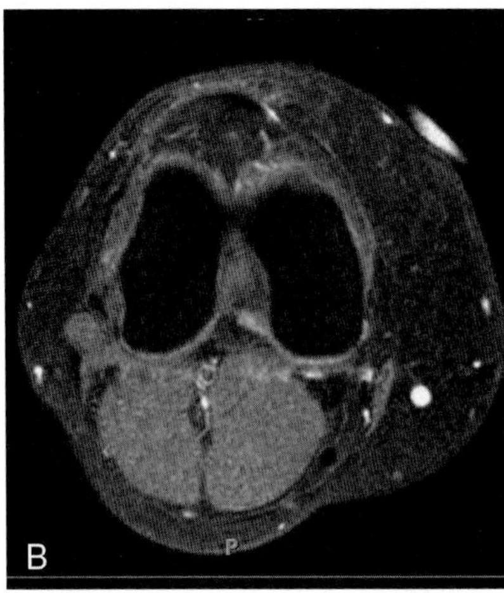

Figure 8 **A,** A T1-weighted coronal MRI scan shows a soft-tissue mass along the medial aspect of the knee (arrow; outlined area). It abuts the medial capsule and has high signal intensity (same signal as the subcutaneous fat). **B,** MRI scan with all of the medial soft tissues fat suppressed. The pattern shown in these images are diagnostic of a lipoma. This is a determinate mass, and treatment can be planned without a biopsy.

sifying the lesion as determinate or indeterminate can guide clinicians in making the correct decisions following the imaging evaluation of a soft-tissue tumor.[27]

Evaluation

If a patient presents with a soft-tissue mass on the extremities or the trunk, a thorough history and physical examination are necessary; however, these steps may provide only a few clues to the nature of the mass. Radiography and MRI are the two essential imaging studies necessary for making proper treatment decisions.

Radiographic Imaging

The first step in evaluating a soft-tissue mass is to obtain two orthogonal plain radiographs of the region. The radiographs are evaluated to ensure that the underlying osseous structures are normal. A fixed soft-tissue mass (one that does not move with palpation) may be the result of soft-tissue extension from an intramedullary or surface bone tumor (one arising from the cortex).

An MRI is the most definitive imaging technique for decision making and can be performed with or without contrast. A contrast-enhanced study should be performed if the clinician needs to differentiate a fluid-filled structure (cyst) from a solid tumor. The clinician should evaluate the MRI scan with an experienced musculoskeletal radiologist to classify the soft-tissue mass as determinate or indeterminate.[28]

Evaluation and Treatment of a Determinate Soft-Tissue Mass

Determinate soft-tissue masses are defined as masses for which the clinician and radiologist can establish a definitive diagnosis based on imaging studies.[27] If a definitive diagnosis can be established, the clinician can plan treatment without a biopsy. Common determinate masses include lipomas, synovial cysts, and soft-tissue hemangiomas.[29]

Lipomas

Lipomas show high signal intensity on T1-weighted images and low signal intensity on T2-weighted images (Figure 8). Fat suppression turns the entire lesion dark (low signal). To conclusively establish the diagnosis, the entire mass must be fat suppressed in a homogeneous fashion with no areas of high signal intensity. If there are areas of intermediate or high signal intensity within the lipomatous lesion, the mass may represent an atypical lipoma or dedifferentiated liposarcoma.

Synovial Cysts

Cysts are common, and patients may present with a soft-tissue mass as a manifestation of an articular disorder. Cysts are fluid-filled structures and have a uniform MRI appearance. On T1-weighted images, the cyst shows very low signal intensity, on T2-weighted images, the cyst shows high signal intensity. When a cyst arises from a joint in a characteristic location, contrast enhancement is not necessary to establish a diagnosis. For example, if the stalk (area of joint communication) of a popliteal (Baker) cyst can be identified arising between the semimembranosus and medial gastrocnemius muscles, contrast is not necessary to establish the diagnosis. However, if a soft-tissue mass is identified in an atypical location, contrast enhancement is necessary to establish the diagnosis.

Soft-Tissue Hemangiomas

Radiographs may show characteristic phleboliths, which allow a definitive diagnosis. On an MRI scan, the features of a soft-tissue hemangioma are round structures with low signal intensity interspersed within high signal areas on T1-weighted images. The low signal, round structures represent vascular channels, whereas the areas of high signal intensity represent adipose tissue. T2-

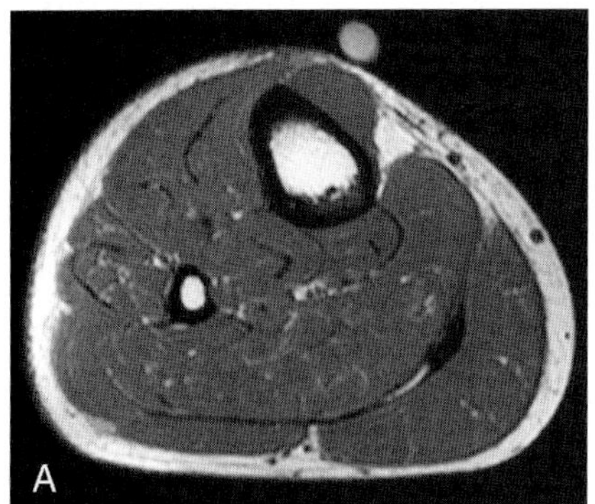

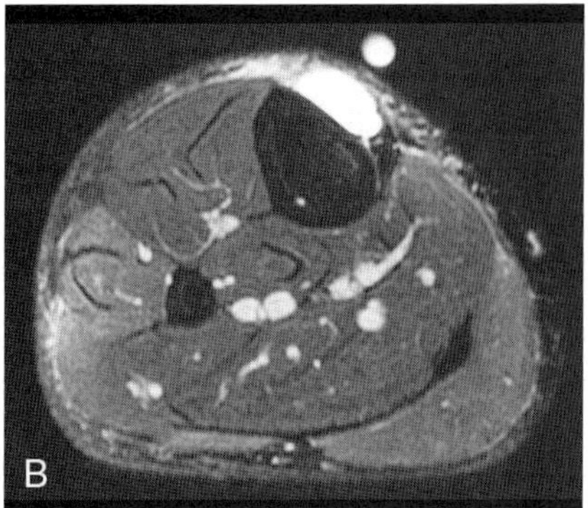

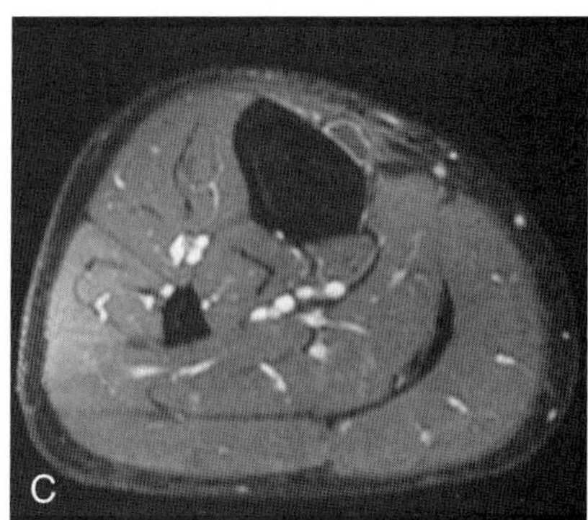

Figure 9 **A,** A T1-weighted axial MRI scan of a soft-tissue mass over the medial aspect of the tibia. On this scan, the mass has uniform low signal intensity characteristics. **B,** A T2-weighted axial MRI scan shows uniform high signal intensity within the lesion. **C,** A contrast-enhanced axial scan shows the rim enhancement (high signal intensity at the periphery of the mass). This lesion is a cyst. Because the cyst is over the tibial periosteum, this is a periosteal ganglion cyst. This patient is asymptomatic and can be managed with observation.

weighted images with fat suppression show round structures with very high signal intensity, with complete suppression for the prior high signal areas.

There are other determinate masses; however, the clinician and the radiologist must be able to identify the nature of the mass (Figure 9). Some teams of clinicians and radiologists may be able to identify only a few soft-tissue masses as determinate, whereas others may be capable of identifying many masses as determinate.

Treatment options for determinate masses include observation, excisional biopsy, or percutaneous treatment. The clinician and the radiologist must establish the exact diagnosis of a mass before recommending observation to the patient. Patients may choose observation as the method of treatment for an intramuscular lipoma or hemangioma if they are asymptomatic or only mildly symptomatic.

If the clinician is sure of the diagnosis, the patient may be advised to have the mass excised. If the mass is determinate, the clinician knows the diagnosis and can design the surgical procedure (or percutaneous treatment such as sclerotherapy for an intramuscular hemangioma) based on the biologic behavior of the process.

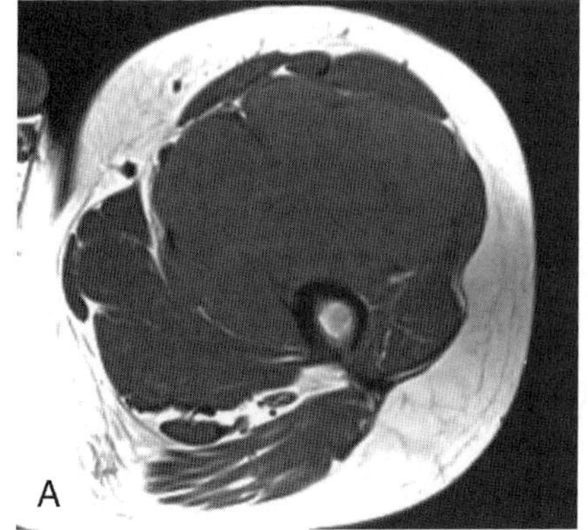

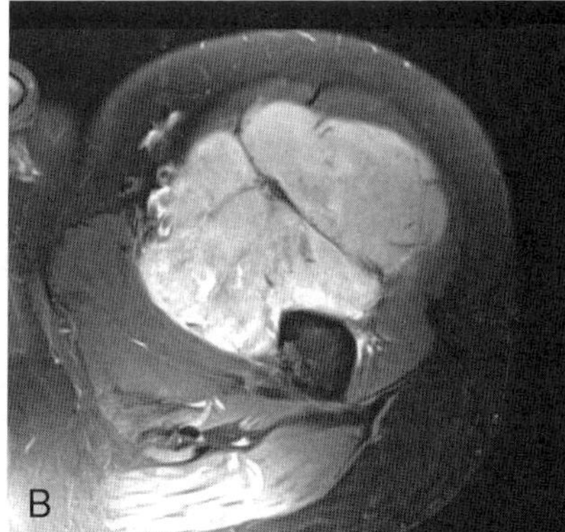

Figure 10 **A,** T1-weighted MRI scan showing a low signal intensity mass in the anterior compartment of the thigh. **B,** T2-weighted MRI scan showing a high signal mass in the anterior compartment that is an indeterminate lesion. A needle or incisional biopsy is necessary to establish the diagnosis.

Workup and Treatment of Indeterminate Soft-Tissue Masses

Soft-tissue masses that cannot be definitively identified by the clinician-radiologist team are classified as indeterminate. Examples include the entire spectrum of low- and high-grade soft-tissue sarcomas. There are no characteristic features of these sarcomas that enable accurate diagnosis based on the MRI scan (Figure 10). Many benign entities are also indeterminate.[30]

A needle or incisional biopsy must be performed to establish a diagnosis if the soft-tissue mass has been classified as indeterminate following an MRI evaluation. An indeterminate soft-tissue mass may be a malignant (low-, intermediate-, or high-grade sarcoma or other type of cancer) or a benign process. The surgeon cannot plan treatment without establishing a diagnosis through either needle or incisional biopsy.[31]

In two previously mentioned studies, Mankin and associates[21,26] documented a high error rate in diagnostic and technical factors following biopsy of bone and soft-tissue masses, with no reduction in management errors in the 10-year period between the studies. A possible explanation for a lack of improvement in management errors is that a method of decision making that would reduce errors was not developed. Removal (excisional biopsy) of sarcomas before a diagnosis had been established was one of the most frequently reported errors. Soft-tissue sarcomas may have a similar appearance to benign lesions, and both clinicians and radiologists often do not recognize that a patient has a malignant soft-tissue tumor.

Unplanned removal of soft-tissue sarcomas has several deleterious effects on the patient's outcome. Subsequent reexcision often requires a more extensive surgical procedure with removal of all areas possibly contaminated by the unplanned excision. Of even more concern is the potential for a higher local failure rate following reexcision.[32] Several studies have documented a compromised ability to obtain wide margins following an unplanned excision.[32,33]

A simple classification system that all clinicians and radiologists can use may help to reduce the number of errors in the decision-making process. The system of classifying lesions as determinate or indeterminate is simple and can be modified for all teams of clinicians and radiologists. These teams may have a small or large number of determinate masses in their armamentarium depending on their level of experience.

Summary

A logical evaluation of imaging studies and a stepwise, careful workup of a patient with a bone or soft-tissue lesion can help prevent mistakes in diagnosis and treatment. Patients frequently present to an orthopaedic oncologist after a soft-tissue sarcoma has been inadequately excised based on the false assumption that the mass was benign. Another scenario is the older patient with hip pain who is treated with a total hip arthroplasty for presumed osteoarthritis when the pain is actually emanating from an acetabular chondrosarcoma. Although benign bone lesions, benign soft-tissue lesions, and metastatic bone disease are much more common than primary malignant bone and soft-tissue tumors, the orthopaedic surgeon must remain vigilant and not make assumptions that are not substantiated by the patient history or findings from the examination and imaging studies. A biopsy is required if a conclusive diagnosis cannot be made. If the general orthopaedic surgeon lacks the training, experience, or team members needed to provide definitive care, the patient should be referred to an orthopaedic oncologist for treatment.

References

1. Parsons TW III, Filzen TW: Evaluation and staging of musculoskeletal neoplasia. *Hand Clin* 2004;20: 137-145.
2. Lodwick GS, Wilson AJ, Farrell C, Virtama P, Dittrich F: Determining growth rates of focal lesions of bone from radiographs. *Radiology* 1980;134: 577-583.
3. Peabody TD: Clinical presentation and recommended evaluation of a patient with a suspected bone tumor, in Fitzgerald RH, Kaufer H, Malkani AL, eds: *Orthopaedics*. St Louis, MO, Mosby, 2002, pp 1014-1027.
4. Sanders TG, Parsons TW: Radiographic imaging of musculoskeletal neoplasia. *Cancer Control* 2001;8: 221-231.
5. Parsons TW III, Frink SJ, Campbell SE: Musculoskeletal neoplasia: Helping the orthopaedic surgeon establish the diagnosis. *Semin Musculoskelet Radiol* 2007;11:3-15.
6. Bataille R, Chevalier J, Rossi M, Sany J: Bone scintigraphy in plasma-cell myeloma: A prospective study of 70 patients. *Radiology* 1982;145: 801-804.
7. Imhof H, Mang T: Advances in musculoskeletal radiology: Multidetector computed tomography. *Orthop Clin North Am* 2006;37:287-298.
8. Dupuy DE, Rosenberg AE, Punyaratabandhu T, Tan MH, Mankin HJ: Accuracy of CT-guided needle biopsy of musculoskeletal neoplasms. *AJR Am J Roentgenol* 1998;171: 759-762.
9. de Kerviler E, Cuenod CA, Clément O, Halimi P, Frija G, Frija J: What is bright on T1 MRI scans? *J Radiol* 1998;79:117-126.
10. Spiller M, Tenner MS, Couldwell WT: Effect of absorbable topical hemostatic agents on the relaxation time of blood: An in vitro study with implications for postoperative magnetic resonance imaging. *J Neurosurg* 2001;95:687-693.
11. May DA, Good RB, Smith DK, Parsons TW: MR imaging of musculoskeletal tumors and tumor mimickers with intravenous gadolinium: Experience with 242 patients. *Skeletal Radiol* 1997;26:2-15.
12. Kolind SH, MacKay AL, Munk PL, Xiang QS: Quantitative evaluation of metal artifact reduction techniques. *J Magn Reson Imaging* 2004;20: 487-495.
13. Toner GC, Hicks RJ: PET for sarcomas other than gastrointestinal stromal tumors. *Oncologist* 2008;13:22-26.

14. Bredella MA, Caputo GR, Steinbach LS: Value of FDG positron emission tomography in conjunction with MR imaging for evaluating therapy response in patients with musculoskeletal sarcomas. *AJR Am J Roentgenol* 2002;179:1145-1150.

15. Buck AK, Herrmann K, Büschenfelde CM, et al: Imaging bone and soft tissue tumors with the proliferation marker [18F] fluorodeoxythymidine. *Clin Cancer Res* 2008;14:2970-2977.

16. Rougraff BT: Evaluation of the patient with carcinoma of unknown primary origin metastatic to bone. *Clin Orthop Relat Res* 2003;415:S105-S109.

17. Weber KL, Lewis VO, Randall RL, Lee AK, Springfield D: An approach to the management of the patient with metastatic bone disease. *Instr Course Lect* 2004;53:663-676.

18. Mirels H: Metastatic disease in long bones: A proposed scoring system for diagnosing impending pathologic fractures. *Clin Orthop Relat Res* 1989; 249:256-264.

19. Damron TA, Morgan H, Prakash D, Grant W, Aronowitz J, Heiner J: Critical evaluation of Mirels' rating system for impending pathologic fractures. *Clin Orthop Relat Res* 2003; 415:S201-S207.

20. Weber KL, O'Connor MI: Operative treatment of long bone metastasis: Focus on the femur. *Clin Orthop Relat Res* 2003;415:S276-S178.

21. Mankin HJ, Mankin CJ, Simon MA: The hazards of the biopsy, revisited: Members of the Musculoskeletal Tumor Society. *J Bone Joint Surg Am* 1996;78:656-663.

22. Simon MA, Finn HA: Diagnostic strategy for bone and soft-tissue tumors. *J Bone Joint Surg Am* 1993;75: 622-631.

23. Letson GD, Greenfield GB, Heinrich SD: Evaluation of the child with a bone or soft-tissue neoplasm. *Orthop Clin North Am* 1996;27:431-451.

24. Peabody TD, Simon MA: Making the diagnosis: Keys to a successful biopsy in children with bone and soft-tissue tumors. *Orthop Clin North Am* 1996; 27:453-459.

25. Frassica FJ, McCarthy EF, Bluemke DA: Soft-tissue masses: When and how to biopsy. *Instr Course Lect* 2000;49:437-442.

26. Mankin HJ, Lange TA, Spanier SS: The hazards of biopsy in patients with malignant primary bone and soft-tissue tumors. *J Bone Joint Surg Am* 1982;4:1121-1127.

27. Frassica FJ, Khanna JA, McCarthy EF: The role of MR imaging in soft tissue tumor evaluation: Perspective of the orthopedic oncologist and musculoskeletal pathologist. *Magn Reson Imaging Clin N Am* 2000;8:915-927.

28. Frassica FJ, Thompson RC Jr: Evaluation, diagnosis, and classification of benign soft-tissue tumors. *Instr Course Lect* 1996;45:447-460.

29. Papp DF, Khanna AJ, McCarthy EF, Carrino JA, Farber AJ, Frassica FJ: Magnetic resonance imaging of soft-tissue tumors: Determinate and indeterminate lesions. *J Bone Joint Surg Am* 2007;89:103-115.

30. Ma LD, Frassica FJ, Scott WW Jr, Fishman EK, Zerbouni EA: Differentiation of benign and malignant musculoskeletal tumors: Potential pitfalls with MR imaging. *Radiographics* 1995; 15:349-366.

31. Sim FH, Frassica FJ, Frassica DA: Soft-tissue tumors: Diagnosis, evaluation, and management. *J Am Acad Orthop Surg* 1994;2:202-211.

32. Noria S, Davis A, Kandel R, et al: Residual disease following unplanned excision of soft-tissue sarcoma of an extremity. *J Bone Joint Surg Am* 1996; 78:650-655.

33. Goodlad JR, Fletcher CD, Smith MA: Surgical resection of primary soft-tissue sarcoma: Incidence of residual tumor in 95 patients needing re-excision after local resection. *J Bone Joint Surg Br* 1996;78:658-661.

Metastatic Bone Disease: Diagnosis, Evaluation, and Treatment

J. Sybil Biermann, MD
Ginger E. Holt, MD
Valerae O. Lewis, MD
Herbert S. Schwartz, MD
Michael J. Yaszemski, MD, PhD

Abstract

The management of bone metastases has changed considerably over the past decade, with the improved longevity of cancer patients, the advent of bisphosphonates, and the availability of other new treatment modalities. Of primary importance is the systematic establishment of the diagnosis of metastasis before treatment, which avoids improper management of primary bone malignancies and optimizes oncologic treatment. The decision to use surgical stabilization rests not only on structural concerns but also on the patient's anticipated longevity, activity goals, and preferences. Minimally invasive options are available to treat bone lesions in areas not amenable to surgical stabilization or in patients who are poor candidates for surgery. Selected patients with spinal metastases, especially those with cord compression, may benefit from decompression and/or stabilization.

Instr Course Lect 2010;59:593-606.

Metastatic bone disease is a major health care issue, affecting 4.9 million individuals in the United States. The cost of bone metastasis from cancer was estimated to be $13 billion per year in the United States in 2005, and the annual incident number of cancer cases in the United States is expected to double over the next 50 years.[1,2] With improved medical treatment of many cancers, patients are living longer, which places them at increased risk for the development of metastatic disease.[3,4] The skeleton is the third most common target of metastatic cancer and can be one of the earliest sites affected, especially in individuals with breast or prostate cancer. Ultimately, 60% to 84% of all cases of metastatic disease invade bone, and approximately 70% of patients with metastatic bone disease experience bone pain.[5] Patients with metastatic cancer involving bone are also at increased risk for fractures, spinal cord compression, hypercalcemia, and immobility resulting in substantial medical-associated morbidities.

Current treatment options for patients with bone metastases are primarily palliative. These options consist of local therapies, systemic treatment, and analgesics. Unfortunately, osseous metastases are generally refractory to systemic therapy. Local irradiation may be sufficient, but surgical treatment is necessary for patients with a pathologic fracture and often necessary for patients with an impending pathologic fracture.

Neither Dr. Biermann nor any immediate family members have received anything of value from or own stock in a commercial company or institution related directly or indirectly to the subject of this chapter. Dr. Holt or an immediate family member is a member of a speakers' bureau or has made paid presentations on behalf of Zimmer and serves as a paid consultant to or is an employee of Zimmer. Dr. Lewis or an immediate family member serves as a board member, owner, officer, or committee member of the Western Orthopaedic Association and the American Orthopaedic Association and has received research or institutional support from Stryker. Dr. Schwartz or an immediate family member serves as a board member, owner, officer, or committee member of the Musculoskeletal Tumor Society and the Musculoskeletal Transplant Foundation and has received research or institutional support from the Musculoskeletal Transplant Foundation, Stryker, Synthes, and Zimmer. Dr. Yaszemski or an immediate family member serves as a board member, owner, officer, or committee member of the Scoliosis Research Society and the Society of Military Orthopaedic Surgeons; serves as a paid consultant to or is an employee of the National Institutes of Health (NIAMS & NICHD), Osteotech, Wyeth, BonWRX, and K2M; and has received research or institutional support from Health and Human Services and the National Institutes of Health (NIAMS & NICHD).

Diagnosis

Orthopaedic surgeons are often the practitioners to whom a person with musculoskeletal pain is initially referred. If plain radiographs identify a bone lesion in the symptomatic area, the orthopaedic surgeon is then faced with a dilemma of how to proceed.

Plain radiographs yield more information about a bone tumor than any other diagnostic modality. Certain basic guidelines for interpretation of plain radiographs alert the clinician to pay particular attention to the anatomic site of the bone tumor, the zone of transition between the tumor and the host bone, and the presence of any internal characteristics that may determine the nature of the matrix that the tumor produces.

Aggressive features that can be identified on a plain radiograph include a tumor larger than 5 cm in diameter, interruption of the cortex, periosteal reaction, and pathologic fracture. Cortical interruption with concurrent symptoms can be considered evidence of a nondisplaced pathologic fracture.

Benign bone tumors are more common in young people, whereas malignant bone tumors, especially metastatic carcinomas, are much more common in individuals who are older than 40 years. The patient's medical history should be elicited to identify any personal or family history of malignant tumors, cancer risk factors, and systemic symptoms. The physical examination is important to identify the precise area of tenderness and the presence or absence of a soft-tissue mass. If a tumor originated in bone, the soft-tissue mass should not be mobile over the bone. Neurovascular compromise is uncommon, as is distal edema.

Laboratory tests offer some clues that may facilitate staging. The most important laboratory tests in the evaluation of an adult with a bone lesion are measurements of serum calcium, serum immunoglobulin, prostate-specific antigen level, and erythrocyte sedimentation rate. Hypercalcemia is not uncommon in patients with multiple myeloma or metastatic cancer, and it can be life threatening. A serum protein electrophoresis with a monoclonal protein spike is indicative of myeloma. An elevated level of serum prostate-specific antigen is unique to prostate carcinoma. The erythrocyte sedimentation rate is a nonspecific value that is often elevated in individuals with infection, immunologic disorders, or marrow cell neoplasms such as lymphoma, Ewing sarcoma, histiocytosis, or leukemia. A pregnancy test is warranted for a woman of child-bearing age to safely allow further radiographic imaging. Correlation among the history, findings on physical examination, and findings on plain radiographs is the key to the decision-making process, and the clinician bears the ultimate responsibility for correlating these important parameters. If a primary malignant tumor is considered a possibility, referral to an orthopaedic oncologist is justified at this stage. If the correlating clinical and radiographic data indicate that the tumor is benign, observation may be chosen. If it is more probable that the tumor is malignant, a sophisticated diagnostic and staging strategy should be used. Even the decision to perform a needle biopsy should be made judiciously by an experienced physician.

The orthopaedic surgeon should be aware that disorders other than bone tumors cause bone lesions. These include infection, stress fracture, myositis ossificans, metabolic bone disease, osteonecrosis, and synovial proliferative diseases.

Staging Studies

The chance that a solitary bone lesion is a metastatic carcinoma in an individual older than 40 years is approximately 500 times higher than the chance that the tumor is a primary bone sarcoma.

There are at least six good reasons to conduct a staging workup before biopsy:[6] (1) The tumor may be a sarcoma, and a staging workup could prevent an inappropriately placed biopsy site or needle trajectory; (2) there may be a site that is easier to biopsy or one that is associated with less morbidity; (3) preoperative embolization may be needed to prevent bleeding; (4) a biopsy can be avoided if the diagnosis can be made on the basis of the laboratory analysis, such as with multiple myeloma; (5) a working diagnosis or preoperative suspicion of a primary bone tumor on the basis of imaging studies can help the surgical pathologist make the diagnosis more accurately on frozen section analysis when surgery is contemplated at the time of biopsy; and (6) complete imaging combined with histopathologic analysis may make it more likely for the pathologist to accurately identify the primary site in metastatic lesions.

The most common steps in the workup for suspected bone metastasis of unknown origin consist of a medical history; physical examination; routine laboratory analysis; plain radiography of the involved bone and chest; whole-body bone scintigraphy (bone scanning); and CT of the chest, abdomen, and pelvis with oral and intravenous contrast media. Evaluation in this fashion will identify the primary site in 85% of patients with a metastatic bone tumor.[7] Local imaging, including MRI and CT of the involved site, needs to be performed only if a diagnosis of primary disease (sarcoma) is under consideration. Because breast carcinoma is common and rarely presents as a metastasis of unknown primary origin to bone, it may or may not be necessary to include a mammogram in the diagnostic strategy or workup.

Positron emission tomography is an emerging technology that has a high sensitivity for identifying malignant tumors, infections, and other physiologic processes in the skeleton and soft tissues throughout the body. Its specificity, however, is low. In several studies, positron emission tomography combined with CT identified the primary tumor in approximately 50% of individuals with a metastasis of previously unknown origin.[8-10] Use of positron emission tomography alone (without concomitant CT) decreases the specificity to 30%.

Once all of the data have been gathered, biopsy can be performed. It can be either percutaneous (needle) or open (incisional). Each of the two techniques has advantages and disadvantages. Nonetheless, it is imperative to make a pathologic diagnosis before proceeding with any further medical, surgical, or radiologic treatments. Unless the patient has a known history of histologically confirmed metastasis, radiographic findings are insufficient evidence on which to base treatment when cancer is suspected.

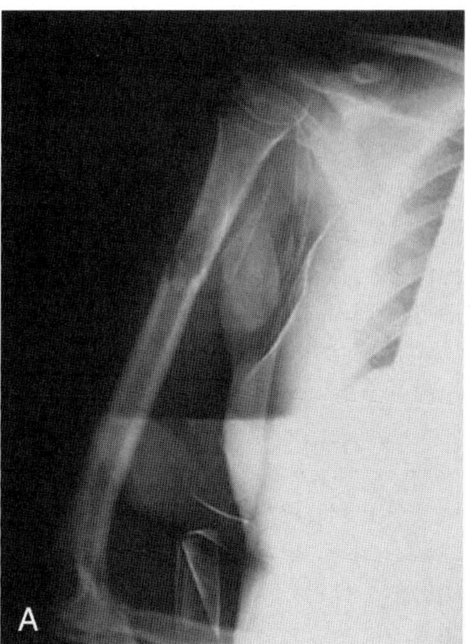

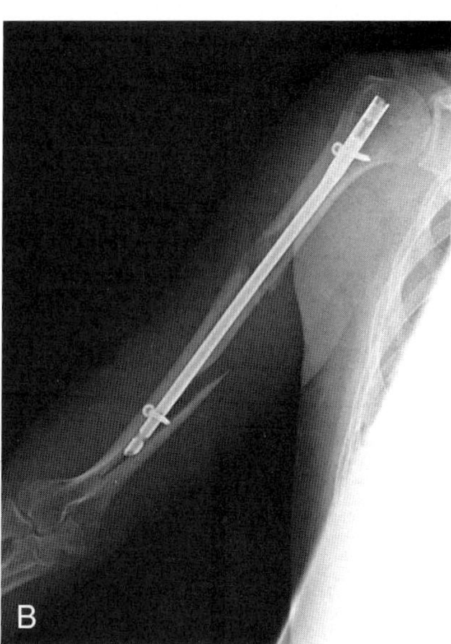

Figure 1 A rodded sarcoma. **A,** A pathologic fracture in the humerus with a radiographic diagnosis of metastatic carcinoma. **B,** An intramedullary nail was placed to treat a pathologic fracture in the humerus. One week later, it was discovered that the correct diagnosis was osteosarcoma.

Diagnostic Pitfalls and Premature Surgical Intervention

Perhaps the worst medical scenario for a patient who presents with an unknown bone lesion is the rodded sarcoma. A typical example is that of a 44-year-old man who sustained a pathologic fracture while swinging a hammer (Figure 1). A lytic lesion was detected in the humeral shaft. Statistical data and the radiologist's opinion suggested a metastatic malignant tumor of unknown origin. The surgeon assumed the radiographic diagnosis (metastatic carcinoma) to be correct and thus scheduled surgery for that evening. The postoperative radiograph showed an antegrade locked intramedullary nail in the humerus. Material obtained from reaming during the surgery was sent to the pathology department, and a week later the surgeon was notified that the diagnosis was osteosarcoma and not metastatic carcinoma. The treatment options now became incredibly complex, not to be outdone by the likely consequences with regard to the patient's survival and the medicolegal issues. The difficulty could have been entirely eliminated if the diagnosis had been made first. The lesson to be learned from this case is to proceed with the staging protocol described above. One should first perform a biopsy and frozen section analysis during the surgery and not proceed with additional surgery until the diagnosis is confidently made and the best management strategy is clear.

Considerations in Surgical Management

Goals of treatment of metastatic bone disease include pain relief, preservation of function, and provision of a long-lasting construct that can be used immediately. Accomplishing these goals in an environment of osteolysis and mechanical instability can be challenging. Common errors that lead to treatment failures include underestimating the life expectancy of the patient, underestimating the abnormal bone biology in pathologic defects, and undertreating current disease while not planning for future disease. Current strategies for treatment of metastatic disease have increased overall patient survival; therefore, careful consideration must be given not only to the immediate stability of the surgical construct but also to its durability. Despite some increases in survival, the shortened life span of this population makes a revision due to fixation failure especially undesirable.

Effect of Life Expectancy on Fixation Options

A clear understanding of the life expectancy of patients with metastatic bone disease can help to prevent many common fixation errors and failures. The life expectancy of patients with metastatic disease strongly influences the choice of the method of fixation of a pathologic fracture. Patients who are likely to survive for a longer duration are more likely to undergo some level of fracture healing and also to benefit from more extensive resections and reconstructions.[11,12] However, these patients are more likely to survive longer than the reconstruction was intended to last.[13] Surgical failures occur when local disease progresses or hardware failure occurs as a result of fracture nonunion.

Some general guidelines should be followed while it is kept in mind that treatment must be individualized. The 6-month survival rates associated with tumors that commonly metastasize to bone have been reported to be 98% for prostate cancer, 89% for breast cancer, 50% for lung cancer, and 51% for kidney tumors.[14] When the orthopaedic surgeon is not equipped to estimate life expectancy and weigh the risks and benefits of reconstruction against the anticipated life span, a medical oncologist or an orthopaedic oncologist should be consulted. Predicting the length of an individual patient's life is difficult and unreliable; therefore, it is better to assume that the patient will live longer than one anticipates.

Role of Patient Activity Level and Expectations in Choice of Fixation Method

A more active, mobile patient with a longer life expectancy should be considered for a more aggressive procedure that preserves a higher level of function as compared with what would be appropriate for an ill, immobile patient with a short life expectancy. A longer surgical procedure with greater risks can be justified for a patient who will obtain both short- and long-term benefits. It is important that the surgical goals be explained and reiterated so that the patients and families have realistic expectations. In particular, they should be reminded that care is palliative and not curative.

Need for Immediate Stability

The provision of immediate structural stability and the longevity of the construct must be considered when choosing the fixation technique. A mind-set toward treating normal bone that is fractured must be abandoned and replaced with an understanding of the implications of treating perpetually mechanically unstable bone with large, nonregenerating defects. Customary uses of polymethylmethacrylate, autogenous bone grafts, bone graft substitutes, and porous ingrowth implants must be reevaluated.[15] Constructs that would never be used to treat standard (nonpathologic) traumatic fractures are the mainstay of treatment of pathologic fractures secondary to metastatic disease.

Polymethylmethacrylate is a necessary adjunct that provides immediate structural stability and increased biomechanical rigidity when combined with the use of implants.[16] Its behavior is predictable, it does not degrade over time, it conforms to unusual tumor cavity geometry, and it allows evaluation of early construct failure caused by tumor recurrence. It has been proposed that its exothermic properties also result in some local tumor necrosis.[16] Polymethylmethacrylate should always be considered first for the filling of a large defect caused by metastatic tumor osteolysis.

In stark contrast, autogenous bone graft and bone graft substitutes should rarely be used. Autogenous bone graft causes donor site morbidity and pain, which is not justified in this patient population. Also, bone grafts and bone graft substitutes require osteointegration, which is unpredictable in the setting of tumor osteolysis. Equally important is the fact that, while integrating into the defect, the construct does not allow unrestricted weight bearing, which negates the important concept of immediate use.

Reasons to Avoid Planning for Bone Ingrowth

Another discordant concept is the use of bone ingrowth prostheses rather than cemented prostheses in this population.[17] Avoidance of weight bearing is commonly required for osteointegration of porous ingrowth implants. This may not be acceptable for a debilitated patient, who may also have upper extremity disease precluding weight bearing. In addition, the use of a porous ingrowth prosthesis at a site of microscopic residual disease is not recommended, as the residual tumor can cause rapid loosening. One must also consider the possibility that postoperative radiation therapy contributes to bone necrosis and may lead to peri-implant failure.[15]

Differences Between Pathologic and Conventional Traumatic Fractures

To treat metastatic bone disease, the surgeon must have a solid grasp of the biology of metastatic tumors and understand how it differs from that of normal bone that is fractured. Fracture healing rates in association with lesions that commonly metastasize to bone vary widely, with reported prevalences of 37% for breast cancer, 0% for lung cancer, 44% for kidney tumors, and 67% for myelomas.[18] A life expectancy of longer than 6 months is the most positive factor predicting fracture union.[11] A knowledge of fracture healing rates in particular settings may affect the choice of fixation device; for example, a distal femoral tumor with a pathologic fracture resulting from metastatic lung cancer may be better treated with a megaprosthesis, whereas a lesion from a myeloma may be amenable to open reduction and internal fixation with a plate and polymethylmethacrylate.

Understanding how aggressively a metastatic tumor needs to be treated helps in determining the appropriate degree of resection and reconstruction. The resections used to treat metastatic disease are most commonly intralesional. Intralesional resection leaves a large defect as well as microscopic (and sometimes macroscopic) disease that requires radiation therapy. The resection increases the size of the defect caused by the destructive tumor, and this defect requires a large, immediately structurally stable void filler as bone will not traverse a large defect, which consequently will not heal. Expecting a large defect to heal is a common mistake that leads to a high failure rate. Treatment of massive defects can require innovative and unconventional reconstruction solutions (for example, shortening of the bone with intercalary resection to achieve immediate bone apposition and stability or, more commonly, filling of the defect with polymethylmethacrylate).

Fixation that encompasses the entire bone, when possible, is a key element in treating metastatic disease and the large defects that it produces. Not only does it increase the mechanical stability of a construct that includes a large defect, it may also provide prophylaxis against future disease. The disease that presents in the future may arise from separate hematogenous deposits, or it may have been spread along the medullary canal when a nail was inserted through a site of macroscopic disease.

Role of Postoperative Radiation

Postoperative external beam radiation is necessary in most cases to obliterate residual microscopic disease and thus prevent disease progression and further osteolysis.[19] However, it also affects the bone's blood supply, which can lead to postradiation necrosis. Postoperative radiation should include the entire surgical field, which usually encompasses the entire bone.[20] Patients should be followed for the remainder of their lives to identify any postradiation necrosis at the tumor site as well as in the adjacent joints. Necrosis in these locations may require further treatment such as resection of necrotic bone and reconstruction with a prosthesis.

Fixation Specific to Tumor Location

Just as each patient requires individualized treatment, each osseous location requires special consideration with regard to the best type of fracture fixation. In general, pathologic fractures resulting from metastatic disease are treated by repairing or removing existing bone.[15] When there is enough remaining bone with structural integrity, it may be used to anchor a nail or a plate augmented with polymethylmethacrylate. When the host bone is mechanically incompetent, there is massive bone loss, or a joint surface is destroyed, bone is removed and replaced with a prosthesis.

Although there is agreement regarding the indications for most fixation methods, there is some controversy about the best treatment of metastatic bone disease. Controversial areas include the humeral diaphysis, the acetabulum, and the femoral neck. Some treatments are chosen solely on the basis of the surgeon's preference, whereas others are selected on the basis of experience combined with scientific principles. The principles described previously must be adhered to for treating any metastatic lesion optimally. In addition to predicting the patient's life expectancy and understanding tumor biology, one must be aware of the different biomechanical properties of the different areas of the same bone to achieve the best outcomes.

The humeral diaphysis may be fixed with an intramedullary nail or a combination of a plate and polymethylmethacrylate.[21] Although intramedullary nailing provides whole bone fixation, it does not allow tumor debulking unless the tumor is exposed through a separate incision.[22] It may be important to debulk a tumor that is not radiosensitive, such as a renal cell carcinoma. If debulking is planned, the tumor is usually exposed well enough for plate fixation, and open reduction and internal fixation may be a logical decision. Open reduction and internal fixation with a plate combined with use of polymethylmethacrylate allows additional biomechanical

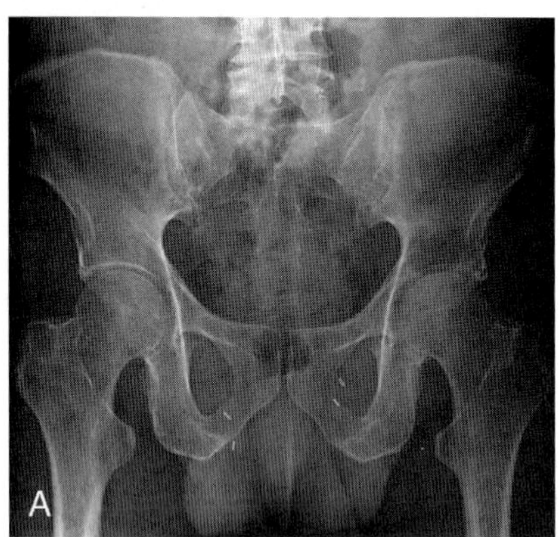

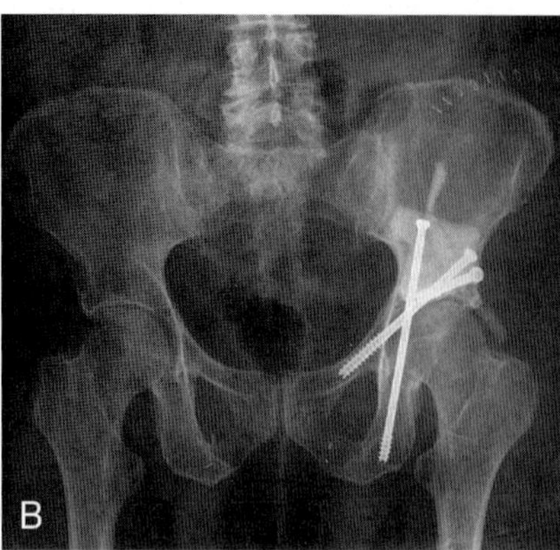

Figure 2 A 62-year-old man with a history of squamous cell carcinoma of the tongue presented with worsening pain in the proximal part of the left thigh and the left hip of 3 months' duration. **A,** The AP pelvic radiograph shows a lytic lesion in the left acetabular dome. An open biopsy confirmed metastatic squamous cell carcinoma. **B,** A postoperative AP radiograph shows a reconstruction with polymethylmethacrylate and cannulated screws that was performed through an extended iliofemoral approach.

fixation as well as reduction and control of less radiosensitive tumors. Biomechanically, a combination of plate and polymethylmethacrylate fixation is superior to intramedullary nail fixation.[23]

Reconstruction of periacetabular defects requires a stable construct that distributes weight from the lower extremity to the remaining pelvis and spine.[24] This may be accomplished with the use of a standard reconstruction cup, an antiprotrusio cage, polymethylmethacrylate, or polymethylmethacrylate with screw augmentation, as described by Harrington.[25] According to Harrington, the size of the construct that should be used to treat a periacetabular lesion increases as the size of the lytic defect increases.[25] Lesions that do not breach the joint may be treated with screws or pins and polymethylmethacrylate alone (Figure 2), whereas a larger defect is better treated with an antiprotrusio cage that bypasses the lytic zone and rests on solid host bone.

Common errors include underestimating the size of the lytic defect and underusing the surrounding ilium and ischium to anchor an implant or using standard arthroplasty implants because they are familiar to the surgeon.[26] If a hemispherical cup is chosen, it should be cemented into the acetabulum. A better construct is a cup-cement combination anchored to a large portion of the ilium with the Harrington technique.[27] However, this technique is demanding and is usually abandoned in favor of an antiprotrusio cage. Standard press-fit arthroplasty cups loosen,[22] especially when there is rapid tumor progression, and jumbo revision cups cannot appropriately fill large acetabular defects when fixation onto normal ilium (and ischium with discontinuity) is required. Antiprotrusio cages provide this necessary ilium-ischium fixation and, when augmented with polymethylmethacrylate, provide a construct that is immediately stable for full weight bearing.

Arthroplasty is the treatment method of choice for femoral neck lesions.[22,28] Reconstruction nails are commonly used in this setting, but they have a high failure rate because of the large biomechanical stresses on the femoral neck combined with lesions that progress instead of healing.[22] Arguments have been made in favor of intramedullary nail fixation of lesions that occur in the femoral neck and femoral shaft, but these lesions can be addressed with a long stem prosthesis. When a long stem prosthesis is used, the femoral neck lesion is removed, and the implant bypasses any additional femoral lesions. Polymethylmethacrylate should be used with care in this setting. Patients with extensive metastatic disease in the femur who undergo stabilization with an intramedullary rod or a long stem prosthesis combined with polymethylmethacrylate may have acute pulmonary compromise and hypotension intraoperatively. The anesthesiologist should be aware of this risk.

Once arthroplasty is chosen, the question of whether a cemented long stem or short stem should be used arises. A long stem prosthesis is technically more difficult to insert, but it fixes the entire bone, thereby providing prophylaxis against fractures through lesions that develop in the future. An argument against the use of a long stem is that it can be associated with intraoperative hypotension and postoperative sequelae secondary to fat emboli.[29] A secondary consideration is that a revision will be difficult should an infection or periprosthetic fracture occur.[22] Although a short stem is technically easier to insert, it does not protect the entire bone from fracture and thus requires close follow-up because periprosthetic metastases may occur. However, if such metastases do develop, the bone can be protected from fracture with a periprosthetic plate.

Avoiding Common Fixation Errors That Cause Construct Failures

Common fixation errors that may lead to construct failure can be avoided by understanding concepts that are paramount to the care of patients with metastatic bone disease.

The local biology that led to the lytic bone lesion and pathologic fracture also reduces the ability of the bone to heal. Not taking this into account when treating a pathologic fracture may lead to failure of fixation and additional difficulty for the patient. Relying on radiation or chemotherapy to overcome osteolytic damage resulting from a tumor is a recipe for failure. Periprosthetic fixation failure results from incomplete tumor debulking, inadequate bone fixation, failure to fix the entire length of bone, use of degradable substances instead of polymethylmethacrylate to fill the bone void, or use of familiar implants and techniques instead of ones that are more appropriate for fixation of pathologic fractures and may require greater exposure.

The surgeon must remember that pathologic fractures occur in perpetually mechanically unstable bone with large, nonregenerating defects. Fixation constructs that would never be considered in a standard trauma setting are the mainstay of treatment of pathologic fractures secondary to metastatic disease.

Minimally Invasive Treatment of Bone Metastases

Radiation therapy, usually external beam radiation, remains the standard of care for patients with localized bone pain but no impending risk of fracture. Recently, clinicians have begun to explore alternative strategies for the treatment of osseous metastases.

Minimally invasive procedures are excellent options for the treatment of skeletal metastases in patients who are otherwise poor surgical candidates because of their age, comorbidities, or the extent of their disease. In addition, patients in whom bone metastases are refractory to radiation therapy are excellent candidates for these minimally invasive procedures.

Radiofrequency Ablation

The aim of radiofrequency ablation is to ablate tumors as widely as possible but not beyond the outer margin of the tumor. To achieve this, an electrode, which is essentially an uninsulated length of wire that acts as a monopolar emitter of energy, is inserted directly into the tumor. Alternating electric current, emitted from the tip of the electrode, heats the tissue and causes cell death due to coagulative necrosis.[30] Thermal diffusion progressively raises the temperature of the tissue surrounding the probe until a steady state is reached. The surrounding blood flow cools the tissue and reduces the extent of thermal coagulation.

With the patient under local anesthesia or conscious sedation, a small skin incision is made and the probe is advanced up to the farthest part of the osteolytic lesion. Once the location of the probe is confirmed with use of CT or ultrasound, the electrode is advanced through the insulated needle tip. The temperature of the treated tissue as well as the skin is monitored constantly. The probe can be introduced into large lesions multiple times through additional routes, and the ablation is then extended. The use of multiple probes allows the clinician to treat larger lesions.

Radiofrequency ablation, which has been extensively studied for the treatment of tumors of the liver and kidney,[31-33] cardiac arrhythmias,[34,35] unresectable pulmonary tumors,[36-39] and osteoid osteomas,[40-43] appears to have been first reported for the treatment of bone metastases by Dupuy and associates[44] in 2000. Dupuy and associates[44] found a significant reduction in pain in a heterogeneous population of patients. Callstrom and associates[45] reported on the results of radiofrequency ablation in 12 patients with a metastatic bone lesion measuring between 1 and 11 cm, for whom radiation therapy or chemotherapy had failed to provide symptomatic relief. On average, the patients benefited from the treatment within 1 week. Four weeks after treatment, both the mean pain score and the mean score for pain interference with activities of daily living, as measured with the Brief Pain Inventory, had decreased significantly. Narcotic use was also significantly reduced.

Goetz and associates[46] performed a multicenter study of percutaneous image-guided radiofrequency ablation of painful bone metastases. They reported on 43 patients for whom the standard treatment of osseous metastases had failed or who were poor candidates for such treatment. The mean score for the worst pain before treatment, as recorded on the Brief Pain Inventory-Short Form, was 7.9 (range, 4 to 10) of a possible 10 points. Ninety-five percent of the patients experienced a significant initial decrease in pain, and the worst pain was decreased significantly at 4, 12, and 24 weeks.

More recently, Callstrom and associates[47] conducted a prospective clinical trial of the use of percutaneous radiofrequency ablation guided by CT and ultrasound in 14 patients who had one or two painful osseous metastases. Each patient had a score of at least 4 points (of a possible 10) for worst pain in a 24-hour period. The authors found that 4 weeks after treatment, the mean pain score decreased significantly, as did the mean score for pain interference with activities of daily living. All patients reported a reduction in narcotic use, and no serious complications were observed.

The mechanism by which radiofrequency ablation provides pain relief is likely multifold. It has been theorized that the intense heat that is generated may destroy local sensory nerves, thus effectively numbing the area.[46] Also, the decrease in tumor burden (cell death) may decrease the production of cytokines and tumor factors involved both in the sensitization of the nerve endings and in the stimulus of osteoclastic activity, or the radiofrequency ablation may prevent tumor progression and thus prevent development of additional painful microfractures of the bone.[46]

Radiofrequency ablation can provide effective palliation of localized and painful bone metastases. An additional benefit is that it can be performed on an outpatient basis. Furthermore, a biopsy, which is diagnostic in approximately 75% of cases, can be performed at the time of the procedure without decreasing or changing the structural integrity of the treated site. However, radiofrequency ablation is contraindicated when there is no safe needle access to the lesion, when there are important structures (especially nerves) within millimeters of the lesion, or when the lesions are immediately subcutaneous.

Percutaneous Cryoplasty

The use of freezing temperatures for the therapeutic destruction of tissue started in England in 1845 when James Arnott described the use of iced salt solutions to freeze certain cancerous tumors.[48,49] He reported a reduction in tumor size and amelioration of pain. Improved freezing techniques were possible early in the 1990s, when solidified carbon dioxide came into use and later when liquid nitrogen and nitrous oxide became available. Currently, with the development of an argon-based system and a smaller applicator diameter, use of this technique has become more feasible at other disease sites. Like radiofrequency ablation, percutaneous cryoplasty was initially used for nonosseous lesions such as hepatic and renal tumors.[50-54]

As a result of the size of the probe and the lack of proper insulation, the use of first-generation devices was limited to the intraoperative setting and open procedures. However, the development of sealed cryoprobes with small diameters (1.7 and 2.4 mm) and with insulation along the shaft not only allowed the use of these devices percutaneously but also afforded the user better control over the shape and size of the ablated area (with the use of multiple probes).

Cryoprobes are inserted percutaneously into the tissue with the patient under general anesthesia or conscious sedation. Argon gas is forced through a segmentally insulated probe. The rapid expansion of the gas results in rapid cooling, with the temperature reaching −100°C within a few seconds and the generation of an ice ball. Active thawing of the ice ball is achieved by the instillation of helium gas, instead of argon gas, into the cryoprobe. A single cryoprobe provides an ice ball of approximately 3.5 cm in diameter. The use of multiple cryoprobes allows the generation of large ice balls (more than 8 cm in diameter), and hence the management of large lesions, and also permits the clinician to contour the shape of the ice ball. The ablation zone can be shaped by varying the geometry of the probe placement. Up to eight cryoprobes can be used independently at a time, thus decreasing the procedure time for large lesions. In addition, synchronous ablation with several cryoprobes eliminates possible residual disease at the interface of overlapping zones.

Cell death from cryoablation is caused by two mechanisms: intracellular ice formation and cellular dehydration. The rapid freezing immediately adjacent to the probe results in intracellular ice formation and subsequent cell destruction; at a further distance from the probe, the gradual cooling causes osmotic differences across the cell membrane, resulting in secondary cellular dehydration and cell death.

Cryoablation treatments are more time consuming than radiofrequency ablation. Although complete radiofrequency ablation may require several overlapping procedures, the time for each procedure is short (5 to 10 minutes). However, each freeze-thaw-freeze cycle of cryoablation requires 25 to 30 minutes and an additional 10 minutes for warming before probe removal.[47] An advantage of cryoablation is that the edges of the ice ball can be seen with currently available imaging. The use of cryoablation for the treatment of primary and metastatic bone lesions was, to our knowledge, first reported by Sewell and associates.[55] In their study, 16 tumors in 14 patients underwent cryoablation under MRI guidance. They reported a reduction in pain in the postoperative period, and this reduction was apparently sustained.

Callstrom and associates[47] reported the results of a prospective study of 14 patients with osseous metastases that were treated with cryoablation. The lesions ranged from 1 to 11 cm in diameter. After treatment, the mean scores for the worst pain and pain interference with activities of daily living both decreased significantly. All patients who were taking narcotic pain medication reported a reduction in its use. No complications were reported. The authors concluded that percutaneous cryoablation is a safe and effective method for palliation of pain caused by osseous metastases. However, they did note that they did not treat patients who were at risk for pathologic fracture, and this may have slightly skewed the results.

Cementoplasty

Percutaneous injection of polymethylmethacrylate into metastatic vertebral body lesions has been used to palliate pain. Cementoplasty is an extension of the concept of vertebroplasty. It consists of the injection of opacified bone cement into an osseous cavity, and its goals are stabilization and pain relief. Like the procedures described earlier, cementoplasty provides pain relief, but it has the added potential benefit of restoring the mechanical stability of the bone.

To perform the cementoplasty, a needle is hammered into the osseous lesion percutaneously under three-dimensional imaging (CT or MRI). Injection of contrast can then be performed to evaluate the filling pattern and identify sites of leakage. Next, the polymethylmethacrylate is injected into the cavity under continuous fluoroscopic guidance. Although complete filling of the osteolytic defect with polymethylmethacrylate is preferred, complete filling may not be necessary to confer stability. Several authors have recommended radiation of the site after the procedure to ensure local tumor control.[47]

Serious complications include pulmonary embolus and fracture,[56,57] and imaging guidance is necessary during the procedure to prevent and/or assess the leakage of the polymethylmethacrylate into the soft tissues and, for acetabular lesions, into the hip joint.

Cotten and associates[56] reported the outcomes of acetabular cementoplasty for the treatment of 12 periacetabular lesions. All patients received postoperative radiation therapy at an average of 21 days after the procedure. Nine of the patients had pain relief, which was sustained in all but two of them. Improvement in mobility and walking was noted within 3 days.

More recently, Kelekis and associates[57] treated 23 lesions in 14 patients with cementoplasty. The lesions were located in the superior and inferior pubic rami and within the ischial tuberosity. All patients had pain that was refractory to radiation and narcotic therapy. The mean duration of follow-up was 9 months. The authors found that the procedure produced effective pain relief in 92% of the patients.

Cementoplasty and Radiofrequency Ablation

Although cementoplasty has been used to treat osteolytic lesions, several clinicians prefer to ablate a metastatic tumor before the cementoplasty.[47,58,59] This is especially true when a bone metastasis is bulky and extends outside the bone. In such cases, cementoplasty alone may be insufficient, and combination therapy can have a synergistic effect. The coagulation necrosis produced by the radiofrequency heat ablation makes homogeneous distribution of the polymethylmethacrylate in the lesion possible. The combination of the two modalities provides local tumor control, tumor necrosis, stabilization, and pain relief.

The procedure is a combination of the two techniques. Briefly, after the radiofrequency ablation is performed, a needle is introduced into the osteolytic lesion and positioned under CT guidance. The polymethylmethacrylate is then injected into the lesion under fluoroscopic guidance.

Toyota and associates[60] treated 23 bone metastases in 17 adult patients with radiofrequency ablation followed by cementoplasty. The mean tumor size was 5 cm (range, 2 to 12 cm). The technical success rate was 100%. The patients were followed for an average of 2 years. Initial pain relief was achieved in 100% of the patients, and the mean duration of pain relief was 7 months. Three patients had recurrence of the pain from 2 weeks to 3 months after the procedure.

Nakatsuka and associates[61] reported the outcomes of radiofrequency ablation and cementoplasty for the treatment of 23 metastatic bone lesions in 17 patients. The mean tumor size was 4.9 cm (range, 1.2 to 15 cm). The procedure was technically successful in 96% of the patients. Local therapeutic effects were evaluated with contrast-enhanced MRI, and tumor necrosis, indicated by a lack of tumor enhancement, was observed in 71% of the cases. Pain was relieved within 1 week in 100% of the patients, but it recurred in five patients at a mean of 4.9 months. The authors concluded that the combination of cementoplasty and radiofrequency ablation is a valuable treatment alternative.

Table 1
Treatment Algorithm for a Patient With Spinal Metastasis

I. Prognostic Factors Point Value	Primary Tumor	Visceral Metastasis*	Bone Metastasis†
1	Slow growth (eg, breast, thyroid)		Solitary or isolated
2	Moderate growth (eg, kidney, uterus)	Treatable	Multiple
4	Rapid growth (eg, lung, stomach)	Untreatable	

II. Treatment Prognostic Score	Treatment Goal	Surgical Strategy
2-3	Long-term local control	Wide or marginal excision
4-5	Middle-term local control	Marginal or intralesional excision
6-7	Short-term palliation	Palliative surgery
8-10	Terminal care	Supportive care

*No visceral metastasis = 0
†Including spinal metastasis
(Adapted with permission from Tomita K, Kawahara N, Kobayashi T, Yoshida A, Murakami H, Akamaru T: Surgical strategy for spinal metastases. *Spine* 2001;26:298-306.)

Spinal Metastases

The spine is the most common site for metastatic disease, and 40% to 80% of patients with cancer have spinal metastasis at the time of death. There are approximately 18,000 new cases of spinal metastasis per year in the United States. The ratio of skeletal metastases relative to that of primary bone tumors is 40:1, and skeletal metastasis must be considered in the differential diagnosis of a patient who presents with a spinal lesion.

Surgical treatment may be appropriate for spinal metastasis if there is a neurologic deficit resulting from compression by a surgically accessible lesion or if the patient has intractable pain. Surgical treatment may also be appropriate to establish a histologic diagnosis, obtain long-term local control, address impending or actual instability, or prevent or reduce deformity. Each of these indications is related to the goals of treatment of patients with spinal metastasis, which are to protect or improve neurologic function; to interfere as little as possible with systemic treatment; to be certain of the diagnosis of the spinal lesion before treating it; and to reduce unremitting pain so that the patient can return to his or her prior level of daily function, maximize mobility without using a brace if possible, and improve the quality of life in as little time as possible.[62-64] The need for a histologic diagnosis warrants additional discussion. Patients with a personal history of cancer do experience spinal conditions that are not metastases, such as infections and benign tumors, just as persons without cancer do. A special situation is a spinal lesion in a patient with cancer who has not yet had a metastasis from the cancer. It behooves the treating physician to verify that the lesion is cancer before initiating treatment of metastatic disease, so that a benign lesion or infection, should either be present, receives the appropriate treatment. Even if a patient has established metastases elsewhere, it is appropriate to perform a biopsy to obtain specimens for pathologic analysis and microbiologic culture before initiating treatment if the clinical situation, laboratory studies, and imaging studies lead to uncertainty regarding the spinal lesion in question.

The causes of pain from spinal metastases include tumor invasion of a vertebral body, pathologic vertebral fracture, spinal instability, and nerve root or spinal cord compression. Spinal instability is difficult to quantify, but there are several systems with which to classify it.[65,66] Once the decision has been made that a patient is an appropriate surgical candidate, it must be established that he or she does not have any contraindications to surgery, such as impaired nutritional status, anemia, coagulopathy, hypercalcemia, too short a life expectancy, or the inability to obtain skeletal fixation if reconstruction is part of the surgical plan. Life expectancy is particularly difficult to predict, but the surgeon and medical oncologist should try to make as good an estimate as possible. We have believed that an appropriate life expectancy before undergoing major spinal surgery is at least 3 months, but this is arbitrary and varies depending on the exact clinical setting.

There are several algorithms in the literature that can be used to guide decision making regarding patients with spinal metastatic disease. The approach described by Tomita and associates[67] is a revised version of the Tokuhashi score and includes consideration of the tumor's aggressiveness and the extent of skeletal and visceral metastases. Scores for these factors are combined to calculate a total score, which then links to

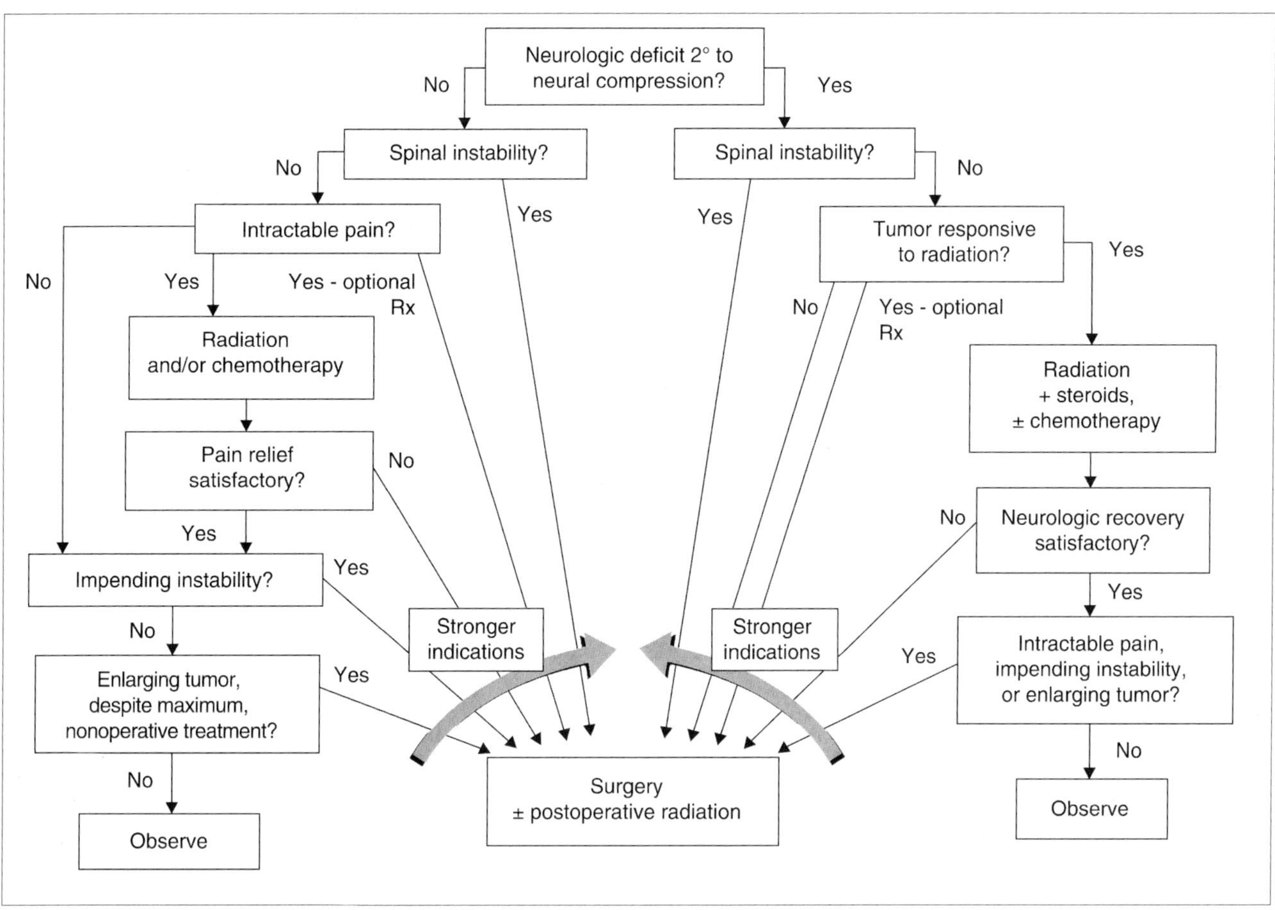

Figure 3 Treatment algorithm for a patient with spinal metastasis. (Adapted with permission from Walker MP, Yaszemski MJ, Kim CW, Talac R, Currier BL: Metastatic disease of the spine: Evaluation and treatment. *Clin Orthop Relat Res* 2003;415:S165-S175.)

treatments ranging from total en bloc tumor resection to palliative care. The system by Walker and associates[68] involves a sequence of questions about neurologic deficits, stability, pain, and the tumor's responsiveness to radiation. The answers to these questions lead to a decision regarding surgical or nonsurgical care. The strategies described by Tomita and associates[67] and by Walker and associates[68] are presented in Table 1 and Figure 3, respectively.

Between 1980 and 2000, there were several studies in which it was concluded that appropriate surgical decompression yielded useful improvement in neurologic function in about 80% of patients with spinal metastasis.[69,70] Klimo and associates[71] performed a meta-analysis of 28 articles on the treatment of spinal metastases that had been published between 1984 and 2002. The data were derived from 24 articles in which a total of 999 patients received surgical treatment and 4 articles in which a total of 543 patients received radiation treatment, and the studies mostly provided level III evidence. Eight hundred forty-three of the 999 patients in the surgically treated group were able to walk after the surgery, whereas only 357 of the 543 patients in the radiation-treated group were able to walk after the radiation. Of 384 patients who were unable to walk before surgical treatment, 228 regained the ability to walk after the surgery, but only 79 of 265 patients who could not walk before radiation were able to do so after it. Thus, the surgically treated patients were 1.3 times more likely to be able to walk after the surgery than the radiation-treated patients were likely to walk after the radiation, and they were twice as likely to regain ambulatory function after having been unable to walk at the time that treatment began. The overall success rates with regard to the ability to walk were 84% and 66% after surgery and radiation, respectively. The authors noted that the neurologic status, overall health, extent of the disease (spinal or extraspinal), and type of primary lesion all have an impact on the appropriate treatment selection.

Patchell and associates[72] reported the results of a prospective, randomized, multi-institutional nonblinded study of patients in whom a metastatic tumor resulting in spinal cord compression was treated either with surgery followed by radiation (50 patients) or with radiation alone (51 patients). The primary end point was the ability to walk, which was achieved for significantly more patients in the surgery group (43 of 50 [84%]) than in the radiation group (29 of 51 [57%]). In addition, of 16 patients who were unable to walk at the time that they received surgery, 10 regained the ability after the surgery, whereas only 3 of the 16 patients who could not walk before the radiation regained the ability after the radiation. This difference was significant. The patients in the radiation treatment arm of the study who lost their ability to walk and then had surgical decompression did not do as well as the nonambulatory patients who had surgery primarily. The patients treated with surgery retained the ability to walk significantly longer (122 days) than did those treated with radiation therapy alone (13 days). The rules for stopping a clinical trial were applied to this study because of the large difference in treatment effect between the two groups, and the conclusion was that direct decompressive surgery in addition to postoperative radiation therapy is superior to treatment with radiation therapy alone for patients with spinal cord compression caused by metastatic cancer.

The concept of performing surgical decompression first and then administering radiation was also supported by several other studies.[73,74] Wise and associates[74] addressed this issue from the perspective of complication rates in a retrospective study. They reported on 88 patients who had a spinal procedure for the treatment of metastatic disease; 44 had preoperative radiation and 43 did not. Six of the 45 patients with preoperative radiation had a major complication, and 10 of the 45 had a minor complication. In comparison, 4 of the 43 patients who had surgery first had a major complication, and 3 of the 43 had a minor complication. All of the deep wound infections in the entire series were in the patients who had had preoperative radiation.

Summary

Multiple factors must be carefully considered to arrive at a treatment plan for patients who have spinal metastatic disease. It should be remembered that spinal metastases are common and that primary spinal tumors are uncommon, and it is necessary to be certain of the diagnosis before initiating treatment. When metastatic disease is present, the treatment must address the tumor cells in addition to achieving neurologic decompression and spinal column stability. The treatment recommendations from medical and radiation oncology should be tailored to each particular patient's clinical situation.

References

1. Schulman KL, Kohles J: Economic burden of metastatic bone disease in the U.S. *Cancer* 2007;109:2334-2342.
2. American Cancer Society: Statistics for 2006. http://www.cancer.org/docroot/STT/stt_0_2006.asp?sitearea=STT&level=1. Accessed June 10, 2009.
3. Bagi CM: Targeting of therapeutic agents to bone to treat metastatic cancer. *Adv Drug Deliv Rev* 2005;57:995-1010.
4. Oien KA, Evans TR: Raising the profile of cancer of unknown primary. *J Clin Oncol* 2008;26:4373-4375.
5. Varadhachary GR, Abbruzzese JL, Lenzi R: Diagnostic strategies for unknown primary cancer. *Cancer* 2004;100:1776-1785.
6. Simon MA, Finn HA: Diagnostic strategy for bone and soft-tissue tumors. *J Bone Joint Surg Am* 1993;75:622-631.
7. Rougraff BT, Kneisl JS, Simon MA: Skeletal metastases of unknown origin: A prospective study of a diagnostic strategy. *J Bone Joint Surg Am* 1993;75:1276-1281.
8. Ambrosini V, Nanni C, Rubello D, et al: 18F-FDG PET/CT in the assessment of carcinoma of unknown primary origin. *Radiol Med* 2006;111:1146-1155.
9. Pelosi E, Pennone M, Deandreis D, Douroukas A, Mancini M, Bisi G: Role of whole body positron emission tomography/computed tomography scan with 18F-fluorodeoxyglucose in patients with biopsy proven tumor metastases from unknown primary site. *Q J Nucl Med Mol Imaging* 2006;50:15-22.
10. Scott CL, Kudaba I, Stewart JM, Hicks RJ, Rischin D: The utility of 2-deoxy-2-[F-18]fluoro-D-glucose positron emission tomography in the investigation of patients with disseminated carcinoma of unknown primary origin. *Mol Imaging Biol* 2005;7:236-243.
11. Nathan SS, Healey JH, Mellano D, et al: Survival in patients operated on for pathologic fracture: Implications for end-of-life orthopedic care. *J Clin Oncol* 2005;23:6072-6082.
12. Böhm P, Huber J: The surgical treatment of bony metastases of the spine and limbs. *J Bone Joint Surg Br* 2002;84:521-529.
13. Kelly CM, Wilkins RM, Eckardt JJ, Ward WG: Treatment of metastatic disease of the tibia. *Clin Orthop Relat Res* 2003;415:S219-S229.

14. Damron TA: Treatment principles and prediction of the impending pathologic fracture, in Schwartz HS, ed: *Orthopaedic Knowledge Update: Musculoskeletal Tumors 2*. Rosemont, IL, American Academy of Orthopaedic Surgeons, 2007, pp 369-374.

15. Ogilvie CM, Fox EJ, Lackman RD: Current surgical management of bone metastases in the extremities and pelvis. *Semin Oncol* 2008;35: 118-128.

16. Sim FH, Daugherty TW, Ivins JC: The adjunctive use of methylmethacrylate in fixation of pathological fractures. *J Bone Joint Surg Am* 1974;56:40-48.

17. Weber KL, Randall RL, Grossman S, Parvizi J: Management of lower-extremity bone metastasis. *J Bone Joint Surg Am* 2006;88:11-19.

18. Gainor BJ, Buchert P: Fracture healing in metastatic bone disease. *Clin Orthop Relat Res* 1983;178:297-302.

19. Frassica DA: General principles of external beam radiation therapy for skeletal metastases. *Clin Orthop Relat Res* 2003;415:S158-S164.

20. Townsend PW, Smalley SR, Cozad SC, Rosenthal HG, Hassanein RE: Role of postoperative radiation therapy after stabilization of fractures caused by metastatic disease. *Int J Radiat Oncol Biol Phys* 1995;31:43-49.

21. Frassica FJ, Frassica DA: Evaluation and treatment of metastases to the humerus. *Clin Orthop Relat Res* 2003; 415:S212-S218.

22. Damron TA, Rock MG, Choudhury SN, Grabowski JJ, An KN: Biomechanical analysis of prophylactic fixation for middle third humeral impending pathologic fractures. *Clin Orthop Relat Res* 1999;363:240-248.

23. Weber KL, Lewis VO, Randall RL, Lee AK, Springfield D: An approach to the management of the patient with metastatic bone disease. *Instr Course Lect* 2004;53:663-676.

24. Marco RA, Sheth DS, Boland PJ, Wunder JS, Siegel JA, Healey JH: Functional and oncological outcome of acetabular reconstruction for the treatment of metastatic disease. *J Bone Joint Surg Am* 2000;82:642-651.

25. Harrington KD: New trends in the management of lower extremity metastases. *Clin Orthop Relat Res* 1982; 169:53-61.

26. Wunder JS, Ferguson PC, Griffin AM, Pressman A, Bell RS: Acetabular metastases: Planning for reconstruction and review of results. *Clin Orthop Relat Res* 2003;415:S187-S197.

27. Harrington KD: The management of acetabular insufficiency secondary to metastatic malignant disease. *J Bone Joint Surg Am* 1981;63:653-664.

28. Camnasio F, Scotti C, Peretti GM, Fontana F, Fraschini G: Prosthetic joint replacement for long bone metastases: Analysis of 154 cases. *Arch Orthop Trauma Surg* 2008;128: 787-793.

29. Herrenbruck T, Erickson EW, Damron TA, Heiner J: Adverse clinical events during cemented long-stem femoral arthroplasty. *Clin Orthop Relat Res* 2002;395:154-163.

30. Simon CJ, Dupuy DE: Percutaneous minimally invasive therapies in the treatment of bone tumors: Thermal ablation. *Semin Musculoskelet Radiol* 2006;10:137-144.

31. de Baere T, Bessoud B, Dromain C, et al: Percutaneous radiofrequency ablation of hepatic tumors during temporary venous occlusion. *AJR Am J Roentgenol* 2002;178:53-59.

32. de Baere T, Kuoch V, Smayra T, et al: Radio frequency ablation of renal cell carcinoma: Preliminary clinical experience. *J Urol* 2002;167:1961-1964.

33. de Baère T, Risse O, Kuoch V, et al: Adverse events during radiofrequency treatment of 582 hepatic tumors. *AJR Am J Roentgenol* 2003;181: 695-700.

34. Belhassen B, Rogowski O, Glick A, et al: Radiofrequency ablation of accessory pathways: A 14 year experience at the Tel Aviv Medical Center in 508 patients. *Isr Med Assoc J* 2007;9: 265-270.

35. Topilski I, Rogowski O, Glick A, Viskin S, Eldar M, Belhassen B: Radiofrequency ablation of atrioventricular nodal reentry tachycardia: A 14 year experience with 901 patients at the Tel Aviv Sourasky Medical Center. *Isr Med Assoc J* 2006;8: 455-459.

36. Steinke K: Radiofrequency ablation of pulmonary tumours: Current status. *Cancer Imaging* 2008;8:27-35.

37. Steinke K, Sewell PE, Dupuy D, et al: Pulmonary radiofrequency ablation: An international study survey. *Anticancer Res* 2004;24:339-343.

38. Zhu JC, Yan TD, Morris DL: A systematic review of radiofrequency ablation for lung tumors. *Ann Surg Oncol* 2008;15:1765-1774.

39. Simon CJ, Dupuy DE, DiPetrillo TA, et al: Pulmonary radiofrequency ablation: Long-term safety and efficacy in 153 patients. *Radiology* 2007;243: 268-275.

40. Rosenthal DI: Radiofrequency treatment. *Orthop Clin North Am* 2006;37: 475-484.

41. Sans N, Galy-Fourcade D, Assoun J, et al: Osteoid osteoma: CT-guided percutaneous resection and follow-up in 38 patients. *Radiology* 1999;212: 687-692.

42. Woertler K, Vestring T, Boettner F, Winkelmann W, Heindel W, Lindner N: Osteoid osteoma: CT-guided percutaneous radiofrequency ablation and follow-up in 47 patients. *J Vasc Interv Radiol* 2001;12:717-722.

43. Rosenthal DI, Alexander A, Rosenberg AE, Springfield D: Ablation of osteoid osteomas with a percutaneously placed electrode: A new procedure. *Radiology* 1992;183:29-33.

44. Dupuy DE, Hong R, Oliver B, Goldberg SN: Radiofrequency ablation of spinal tumors: Temperature distribution in the spinal canal. *AJR Am J Roentgenol* 2000;175:1263-1266.

45. Callstrom MR, Charboneau JW, Goetz MP, et al: Painful metastases involving bone: Feasibility of percutaneous CT- and US-guided radiofrequency ablation. *Radiology* 2002; 224:87-97.

46. Goetz MP, Callstrom MR, Charboneau JW, et al: Percutaneous image-guided radiofrequency ablation of painful metastases involving bone: A multicenter study. *J Clin Oncol* 2004; 22:300-306.

47. Callstrom MR, Charboneau JW, Goetz MP, et al: Image-guided ablation of painful metastatic bone tumors: A new and effective approach to a difficult problem. *Skeletal Radiol* 2006;35:1-15.

48. Gage AA: History of cryosurgery. *Semin Surg Oncol* 1998;14:99-109.

49. Gage AA, Gonder MJ, Soanes WA, Emmings FG: Cancer cryotherapy. *Mil Med* 1967;132:550-556.

50. Sewell PE, Howard JC, Shingleton WB, Harrison RB: Interventional magnetic resonance image-guided percutaneous cryoablation of renal tumors. *South Med J* 2003;96:708-710.

51. Shingleton WB, Sewell PE Jr: Cryoablation of renal tumours in patients with solitary kidneys. *BJU Int* 2003; 92:237-239.

52. Zhou XD, Tang ZY: Cryotherapy for primary liver cancer. *Semin Surg Oncol* 1998;14:171-174.

53. Callstrom MR, Charboneau JW: Technologies for ablation of hepatocellular carcinoma. *Gastroenterology* 2008;134:1831-1835.

54. Desai MM, Gill IS: Current status of cryoablation and radiofrequency ablation in the management of renal tumors. *Curr Opin Urol* 2002;12: 387-393.

55. Sewell PE Jr, Jackson MS, Dhillon GS: Percutaneous MRI guided cryosurgery of bone tumors. *Radiology* 2002; 225(suppl):514.

56. Cotten A, Deprez X, Migaud H, Chabanne B, Duquesnoy B, Chastanet P: Malignant acetabular osteolyses: Percutaneous injection of acrylic bone cement. *Radiology* 1995;197:307-310.

57. Kelekis A, Lovblad KO, Mehdizade A, et al: Pelvic osteoplasty in osteolytic metastases: Technical approach under fluoroscopic guidance and early clinical results. *J Vasc Interv Radiol* 2005;16: 81-88.

58. Schaefer O, Lohrmann C, Herling M, Uhrmeister P, Langer M: Combined radiofrequency thermal ablation and percutaneous cementoplasty treatment of a pathologic fracture. *J Vasc Interv Radiol* 2002;13:1047-1050.

59. Marcy PY, Palussière J, Descamps B, et al: Percutaneous cementoplasty for pelvic bone metastasis. *Support Care Cancer* 2000;8:500-503.

60. Toyota N, Naito A, Kakizawa H, et al: Radiofrequency ablation therapy combined with cementoplasty for painful bone metastases: Initial experience. *Cardiovasc Intervent Radiol* 2005; 28:578-583.

61. Nakatsuka A, Yamakado K, Maeda M, et al: Radiofrequency ablation combined with bone cement injection for the treatment of bone malignancies. *J Vasc Interv Radiol* 2004;15:707-712.

62. Ecker RD, Endo T, Wetjen NM, Krauss WE: Diagnosis and treatment of vertebral column metastases. *Mayo Clin Proc* 2005;80:1177-1186.

63. Hosono N, Ueda T, Tamura D, Aoki Y, Yoshikawa H: Prognostic relevance of clinical symptoms in patients with spinal metastases. *Clin Orthop Relat Res* 2005;436:196-201.

64. North RB, LaRocca VR, Schwartz J, et al: Surgical management of spinal metastases: Analysis of prognostic factors during a 10-year experience. *J Neurosurg Spine* 2005;2:564-573.

65. Asdourian PL, Weidenbaum M, DeWald RL, Hammerberg KW, Ramsey RG: The pattern of vertebral involvement in metastatic vertebral breast cancer. *Clin Orthop Relat Res* 1990;250 :164-170.

66. Taneichi H, Kaneda K, Takeda N, Abumi K, Satoh S: Risk factors and probability of vertebral body collapse in metastases of the thoracic and lumbar spine. *Spine* 1997;22:239-245.

67. Tomita K, Kawahara N, Kobayashi T, Yoshida A, Murakami H, Akamaru T: Surgical strategy for spinal metastases. *Spine* 2001;26:298-306.

68. Walker MP, Yaszemski MJ, Kim CW, Talac R, Currier BL: Metastatic disease of the spine: Evaluation and treatment. *Clin Orthop Relat Res* 2003; 415:S165-S175.

69. Sundaresan N, Rothman A, Manhart K, Kelliher K: Surgery for solitary metastases of the spine: Rationale and results of treatment. *Spine* 2002; 27:1802-1806.

70. Wai EK, Finkelstein JA, Tangente RP, et al: Quality of life in surgical treatment of metastatic spine disease. *Spine* 2003;28:508-512.

71. Klimo P Jr, Thompson CJ, Kestle JR, Schmidt MH: A meta-analysis of surgery versus conventional radiotherapy for the treatment of metastatic spinal epidural disease. *Neuro Oncol* 2005;7: 64-76.

72. Patchell RA, Tibbs PA, Regine WF, et al: Direct decompressive surgical resection in the treatment of spinal cord compression caused by metastatic cancer: A randomised trial. *Lancet* 2005;366:643-648.

73. Ghogawala Z, Mansfield FL, Borges LF: Spinal radiation before surgical decompression adversely affects outcomes of surgery for symptomatic metastatic spinal cord compression. *Spine* 2001;26:818-824.

74. Wise JJ, Fischgrund JS, Herkowitz HN, Montgomery D, Kurz LT: Complication, survival rates, and risk factors of surgery for metastatic disease of the spine. *Spine* 1999;24: 1943-1951.

Nonsteroidal Anti-inflammatory Drugs in Orthopaedics

Omar Abdul-Hadi, MD
Javad Parvizi, MD, FRCS
Matthew S. Austin, MD
Eugene R. Viscusi, MD
Thomas A. Einhorn, MD

Abstract

It is important for orthopaedic surgeons to understand the role of prostaglandins in bone physiology and the mechanism of action of nonsteroidal anti-inflammatory drugs and their role in fracture healing, fusion, osteointegration, and aseptic loosening. Nonsteroidal anti-inflammatory drugs have benefits and risks in orthopaedic use, and their effects should be considered.

Instr Course Lect 2010;59:607-617.

Neither Dr. Abdul-Hadi nor an immediate family member has received anything of value from or own stock in a commercial company or institution related directly or indirectly to the subject of this article. Dr. Parvizi or an immediate family member serves as a board member, owner, officer, or committee member of the American Association of Hip and Knee Surgeons, the American Board of Orthopaedic Surgery, the British Orthopaedic Association, the Orthopaedic Research and Education Foundation, and SmartTech; serves as a paid consultant to or is an employee of Stryker; and has received research or institutional support from KCI, Medtronic, the Musculoskeletal Transplant Foundation, Smith & Nephew, and Stryker. Dr. Austin or an immediate family member serves as a board member, owner, officer, or committee member of the Jefferson Orthopaedic Society; is a member of a speakers' bureau or has made paid presentations on behalf of Stryker and DePuy; and has received research or institutional support from Stryker. Dr. Viscusi or an immediate family member serves as a paid consultant to or is an employee of Johnson & Johnson, Adolor, Anesiva, YM Biosciences, EKR Therapeutics, and Cadence and has received research or institutional support from Anesiva, Wyeth, Pacira, Johnson & Johnson, and Cadence. Dr. Einhorn or an immediate family member serves as a board member, owner, officer, or committee member of the Orthopaedic Research and Education Foundation; has received royalties from Stryker; is a member of a speakers' bureau or has made paid presentations on behalf of Stryker; serves as a paid consultant to or is an employee of Amgen, Eli Lilly, GlaxoSmithKline, the National Institutes of Health (NIAMS & NICHD), Novartis, Osteotech, Pfizer, Smith & Nephew, Stryker, Zelos, Biosurface Technologies, Procter and Gamble, and Anika; serves as an unpaid consultant to Harvest and ProgenStem; has received research or institutional support from Amgen, the National Institutes of Health (NIAMS & NICHD), Stryker, GlaxoSmithKline, and Zelos; has stock or stock options held in Osteogenix, Biomineral Holdings, and HealthpointCapital; and has received nonincome support (such as equipment or services), commercially derived honoraria, or other non–research-related funding (such as paid travel) from Elsevier.

Nonsteroidal anti-inflammatory drugs are widely used and prescribed in the United States. Between 35 and 70 million prescriptions for nonsteroidal anti-inflammatory drugs are written in the United States each year, and numerous agents are now available over the counter.[1] In particular, the prescription of cyclooxygenase-2 (COX-2) inhibitors has become widespread since they were approved by the US Food and Drug Administration in 1999, and in 2000 nearly 45 million prescriptions were written for celecoxib and rofecoxib.[2] More than 17 million Americans use various nonsteroidal anti-inflammatory drugs on a daily basis. Moreover, it has been estimated that 5% to 7% of all hospital admissions are related to adverse drug reactions, with nonsteroidal anti-inflammatory drugs being the culprit in 30% of these cases.[3] As a result of the aging of the population, there will be an increase in the use of nonsteroidal anti-inflammatory drugs parallel to the increase in the prevalence of painful degenerative musculoskeletal conditions. Despite the rising popularity of COX-2 inhibitors, their role in orthopaedic surgery remains controversial. Several studies have demonstrated the inhibitory effect of COX-2 inhibitors on bone healing, and the inhibitory effect of traditional nonsteroidal anti-inflammatory drugs is already well known.[4] The use of COX-2 inhibitors is growing in the elderly population, and there are multiple concerns regarding the adverse side effects and the theoretic basis of safety of COX-2 inhibitors in orthopaedic patients.

Role of Prostaglandins in Bone and Tendon Physiology

The skeleton is a metabolically active organ that undergoes continuous remodeling throughout life. Osteoblasts and osteoclasts, the most important contributors to bone remodeling, produce prostaglandins, which are shown to modulate the function of osteoblasts and osteoclasts in bone metabolism and healing.[5] Prostaglandins are multifunctional regulators with stimulatory and inhibitory effects on bone resorption and formation. They are autocrine and paracrine lipid mediators that act on a variety of cells, including platelets, as well as endothelial, uterine, and mast cells. Prostaglandins are found in virtually all tissues and organs. Skeletal tissue is also an abundant source of prostaglandin production, so it is likely that endogenous prostaglandins play important roles in skeletal physiology and pathophysiology.[6] Changes in prostaglandin synthesis and concentration have been shown to correlate with changes in the quantity of trabecular regeneration and with acceleration of bone healing.[7]

Prostaglandin E_2 is the most abundant prostaglandin produced by osteoblasts and was first shown to increase cyclic 3',5' adenosine monophosphate (cAMP) and stimulate bone resorption in cultured fetal rat long bones more than 30 years ago.[8] Its production by osteoblasts is regulated by several cytokines, including interleukin-1 (IL-1). The action of prostaglandin E_2 is mediated by rhodopsin-type receptors specific to prostaglandins. There are four subtypes of prostaglandin receptors, designated EP_1, EP_2, EP_3, and EP_4, which are encoded by different genes and expressed differently in each tissue. Intracellular signaling differs among the receptor subtypes; EP_1 is coupled to Ca^{2+} mobilization, EP_3 inhibits adenylate cyclase, and both EP_2 and EP_4 stimulate adenylate cyclase.[8]

Prostaglandin E_2 also has bone resorptive activity and is associated with an increased number of osteoclasts. Several studies have shown impaired osteoclast formation in cultures of cells from EP_4-deficient mice, and osteoclast formation is most potently induced by EP_4 agonist. Suzawa and associates[8] reported that bone resorption was markedly stimulated by EP_4 agonist and, to a lesser degree, by EP_2 agonist. The three regulatory steps are binding of prostaglandin E_2 to EP_4 and EP_2, an increase in cAMP, and induction of the osteoclast differentiation factor.

Mechanism of Action of Nonsteroidal Anti-inflammatory Drugs

Nonsteroidal anti-inflammatory drugs are structurally diverse compounds with common therapeutic and adverse effects. All nonsteroidal anti-inflammatory drugs, including the subclass of selective COX-2 inhibitors, are anti-inflammatory, analgesic, and antipyretic. The principal therapeutic effects of nonsteroidal anti-inflammatory drugs derive from the ability of the drugs to inhibit prostaglandin production.[9] The first enzyme in the prostaglandin synthetic pathway is prostaglandin G/H synthase, also known as cyclooxygenase or COX. This enzyme converts arachidonic acid to the unstable intermediates prostaglandin G_2 and H_2, leading to the production of thromboxane A_2 and a variety of prostaglandins.

Within the past decade, two cyclooxygenase isoforms have been identified and are referred to as COX-1 and COX-2.[10,11] COX-1 also is described as a "housekeeping enzyme" that regulates the normal cellular processes and is a primarily constitutive form found in most normal cells and tissues, including the stomach lining. In contrast, COX-2 is expressed at low levels unless it is induced by cytokines and inflammatory mediators and is responsible for the upregulation of the inflammatory system. COX-2 expression is inhibited by glucocorticoids, an important feature that led to the identification of the COX-2 enzyme.[10] Several studies suggest that COX-2 mediates increased prostaglandin production in bone in response to tumor necrosis factor-α (TNF-α), IL-1β, IL-6, IL-11, IL-17, and other osteotropic factors,[12-16] and many factors that either stimulate or inhibit bone resorption affect COX-2 expression in osteoblasts or stromal cells.[17,18] These studies suggest that COX-2 has a role distinct from that of COX-1 in bone resorption.[18] A splice variant derivative of the *COX-1* gene has been identified as COX-3, but the clinical relevance of this enzyme is unknown; whether it has cyclooxygenase activity remains controversial.[19,20]

Traditional nonsteroidal anti-inflammatory drugs inhibit both COX-1 and COX-2. The relatively high prevalence of gastrointestinal side effects (for example, gastric irritation) is attributed to COX-1 inhibition, whereas the desired effect is the subsidence of inflammation that results from COX-2 inhibition.

Effect of Nonsteroidal Anti-inflammatory Drugs on Fracture Healing

Prostaglandin E_2 induces substantial increases in bone formation, bone mass, and strength when administered systemically or locally to the skeleton.[21-23] Endogenous prostaglandin E_2 increases locally after fractures, and the inhibition of prostaglandin E_2 production interferes with bone healing.[24-27]

Li and associates[28] demonstrated osteopenic changes and impaired fracture healing in EP_4-receptor-deficient knockout mice (mice deficient with regard to one of the four receptor subtypes for prostaglandin E_2), confirming that the EP_4 receptor is a positive regulator in the maintenance of bone mass and fracture healing.

In theory, anti-inflammatory drugs that interfere with prostaglandin synthesis should delay fracture healing. Considerable evidence has accumulated that conventional nonspecific nonsteroidal anti-inflammatory drugs, such as ibuprofen, ketorolac, and indomethacin, have an inhibitory effect on fracture healing as well as on other forms of postoperative bone repair.[29-38] COX-2-selective nonsteroidal anti-inflammatory drugs also have been reported to impair and inhibit fracture healing in animal models, findings that are in agreement with observations of impaired fracture healing in mice lacking a functional *COX-2* gene.[39-41] Krischak and associates[42] showed that diclofenac, a nonselective nonsteroidal anti-inflammatory drug, impaired the appearance of osteoblasts in vivo during the early phase of bone healing, confirming the hypothesis that nonselective nonsteroidal anti-inflammatory drugs can inhibit osteoblasts in the early phase of bone healing.

Nonsteroidal anti-inflammatory drugs also impede cell proliferation by inhibiting angiogenesis. It has been proposed that a similar mechanism occurs in the initiation of nonsteroidal anti-inflammatory drug-induced nonunions. Murnaghan and associates[43] investigated this hypothesis in a randomized placebo-controlled trial of the nonsteroidal anti-inflammatory drug rofecoxib in a murine femoral fracture model. Their conclusion was that rofecoxib had a significant negative effect on blood flow across the fracture gap as well as an inhibiting effect on fracture repair.

COX-2 activity is necessary for normal endochondral ossification during fracture healing. The effects of COX-2-selective nonsteroidal anti-inflammatory drugs on fracture healing are caused by inhibition of COX-2 activity, not by a drug side effect. This was shown by Simon and associates,[39] who reported failure of fracture healing in the femora of mice homozygous for a null mutation in the *COX-2* gene. In that study, Simon and associates[39] also compared the effects of indomethacin, celecoxib, and rofecoxib on fracture healing in a rat femoral fracture model and found that treatment with COX-2-selective nonsteroidal anti-inflammatory drugs led to fracture nonunions and incomplete unions. The fracture was still clearly evident on the 8-week postfracture radiographs of the celecoxib- and rofecoxib-treated rats. No rofecoxib-treated rat was observed to have normal bridging callus radiographically, and nonunions, incomplete unions, and unions of the fractured femora were observed in the celecoxib-treated group. Torsional strength was found to be decreased in the group treated with rofecoxib. Rofecoxib was reported to have a drastic effect on the mechanical properties of the femora. In contrast, no significant differences in the mechanical properties were found between the healing fractured femora in the celecoxib-treated rats and those in the control group. Despite that finding, the fractured femora in that group failed as a result of either nonunion (complete failure of the femur along the original fracture site) or incomplete union (new bone bridging of the fracture site was evident, but the femur still failed primarily through the original fracture site). This was in contrast with the control group, in which most of the femora united (with failure caused by a spiral fracture through the diaphysis of the femur), an indication that the fracture sites in the celecoxib group were not bridged with bone. Indomethacin also initially reduced the mechanical properties of the fracture site; however, at 8 weeks, the mechanical properties were similar to those in the control group.

The histologic findings were consistent with delayed fracture bridging and remodeling in the celecoxib and rofecoxib groups. The fracture gap was still clearly evident at 8 weeks in these groups, and often it was filled with fibrous tissue. This study illustrates that, with the dose of celecoxib and the treatment regimen that were used, fracture healing was delayed and inhibited, but to a lesser extent than that found in the animals treated with the rofecoxib regimen. Indomethacin was also found to delay, but not prevent, fracture healing.

These findings were in contrast to the results reported by Brown and associates,[37] who compared the effects of indomethacin on fracture healing in rats with those of celecoxib. The drugs were administered starting on the first postoperative day, and the fractures were analyzed radiographically, histologically, and biomechanically at 4, 8, and 12 weeks. At 4 weeks, only the indomethacin group showed delayed healing. The fractures in the celecoxib group appeared to have more fibrous tissue than those in untreated rats at 4 and 8 weeks; however, radiographic signs of callus formation, mechanical strength, and stiffness did not differ significantly between the groups at 12 weeks. This indicated that COX-2-specific inhibitors caused less of a delay in fracture healing when compared with that associated with nonspecific nonsteroidal anti-inflammatory drugs.

COX-2-specific nonsteroidal anti-inflammatory drugs are only one third as effective as nonspecific nonsteroidal anti-inflammatory drugs in inhibiting prostaglandin E_2 levels within fracture calluses[38] and tissues from local sites of adjuvant-induced arthritis.[44] When the effects of a COX-2 inhibitor (valdecoxib) on experimental fracture healing were compared with those of a nonspecific nonsteroidal anti-inflammatory drug (ketorolac), ketorolac was found to lower prostaglandin E_2 levels two to three times more than valdecoxib.[38]

The effect of COX-2 inhibition on fracture healing is both dose and time dependent.[41] In a study of fractured rat femora, different doses of a COX-2-specific nonsteroidal anti-inflammatory drug (celecoxib) were given at different periods before and after the fracture. Celecoxib given within the first 2 weeks after the fracture reduced the mechanical properties of the fracture callus and caused significantly more nonunions. In contrast, celecoxib given before the fracture or 14 days after the fracture did not increase the proportion of nonunions significantly. The authors suggested that nonsteroidal anti-inflammatory drugs should be avoided by patients during fracture healing, especially during the immediate and early inflammatory phases.

The reversibility of the inhibitory effects of the COX-2 inhibitors on fracture healing were evaluated by Gerstenfeld and associates,[38] who found that withdrawal of either valdecoxib or ketorolac after 6 days of treatment led to a twofold rebound in the levels of prostaglandin E_2 at the fracture site by 14 days. Acetaminophen, an analgesic without anti-inflammatory activity, does not inhibit fracture healing.[45]

Although animal studies have demonstrated inhibitory effects of prostaglandins on bone metabolism, there have been few investigations of the effects in humans, and there remains considerable controversy regarding the effect of nonsteroidal anti-inflammatory drugs. Many factors have been found to correlate with clinical nonunions, including a history of smoking and the type of implant used for fixation. Several studies have demonstrated a higher risk of nonunion of fractures in association with the use of nonsteroidal anti-inflammatory drugs. Burd and associates[46] concluded that patients with an acetabular fracture and a concomitant fracture of a long bone who received indomethacin for prevention of heterotopic ossification were at greater risk for nonunion of the long-bone fracture than were those who did not receive indomethacin.

Giannoudis and associates[33] reported a correlation between clinical nonunions and the use of nonsteroidal anti-inflammatory drugs, especially when the drugs were taken for longer than 4 weeks.

In a study in the United Kingdom, Van Staa and associates[47] found no difference in the fracture risk between regular users of nonsteroidal anti-inflammatory drugs and incidental users. In a similar retrospective study, in Denmark, the effects of acetaminophen, nonsteroidal anti-inflammatory drugs, and acetylsalicylic acid (aspirin) were assessed in patients who had sustained a fracture.[48] A small increase in overall fracture risk was observed in association with acetaminophen, and no increase was seen with acetylsalicylic acid. Ibuprofen was associated with an increased overall fracture risk, whereas celecoxib was not.

In a randomized controlled trial involving 42 postmenopausal patients with a Colles fracture, Adolphson and associates[49] found no difference between a group treated with piroxicam (a nonsteroidal anti-inflammatory drug) and a control group with regard to either bone mineral density (as a measure of posttraumatic osteopenia) or the rate of functional recovery.

Bhattacharyya and associates[50] found no relationship between nonunion of humeral shaft fractures and the use of nonsteroidal anti-inflammatory drugs during the first 60 days after the fracture in older adults. The use of nonsteroidal anti-inflammatory drugs at 61 to 90 days after the humeral fracture was associated with nonunion, and this increased risk was also seen for patients exposed to opioid analgesics in the same period. This finding suggests that nonsteroidal anti-inflammatory drugs do not contribute to nonunion.

In summary, nonspecific nonsteroidal anti-inflammatory drugs inhibit osteoblasts in the early phases of bone healing. COX-2 activity is necessary for normal endochondral ossification during fracture healing. Although the newer COX-2 inhibitors are marketed as having a lower side-effect profile than traditional nonsteroidal anti-inflammatory drugs, particularly with regard to gastrointestinal effects, these drugs exert an inhibitory action on fracture repair in animal models. However, they have been found to cause less of a delay in fracture healing than is associated with nonspecific nonsteroidal anti-inflammatory drugs. It may be prudent for patients to avoid nonsteroidal anti-inflammatory drugs following osseous injury. This is more important for fractures that are associated with a delay in healing and that are often accompanied by a reduction in blood flow to the fracture site.

Effects of Nonsteroidal Anti-inflammatory Drugs on Spinal Fusion

Spinal fusion is a common procedure in the United States, with more than 185,000 operations performed each year.[51] In general, the results of spinal fusion are satisfactory, although a considerable number of patients do not obtain the desired outcome. Factors such as the composition of the bone graft, level of fusion, use of spinal instrumentation, electrical stimulation, and cigarette smoking have been shown to influence fusion rates.[32] The administration of nonsteroidal anti-inflammatory drugs is also reported to negatively influence the outcome.[2,32,52,53]

Physiologic doses of indomethacin were first reported to interfere with the healing of fractures of rat femora in 1976.[54] Early studies identified the pathophysiology as a net decrease in remodeling and woven bone formation, inhibition of endosteal bone-forming cells at the fracture site, inhibition of calcification of the bone matrix, and a decrease in the inflammatory response and blood flow at the fracture site.[52,55-57]

Dimar and associates[52] showed that indomethacin administered subcutaneously 1 week before posterior spinal fusion and 12 weeks after it resulted in an increased rate of nonunion in a rat model. Riew and associates[4] studied the time-dependent inhibitory effects of indomethacin on spinal fusion in a rabbit model and found that, when the indomethacin was begun at 2 weeks after the surgery, only 21% of the rabbits had fusion compared with 65% in the control group. Beginning indomethacin at 2 weeks also resulted in more than a twofold reduction in the fusion rate as compared with the rate when the drug was begun at 4 weeks. However, in another study, initiating indomethacin at 4 weeks after the surgery did not result in a significant difference in the fusion rate compared with that in the control group.[58] Deguchi and associates[59] tried to identify the risk factors for failure in a study of 83 consecutive adult patients with isthmic spondylolisthesis who had undergone identical decompressive surgery combined with posterolateral spine fusion. A history of smoking or postoperative use of nonsteroidal anti-inflammatory drugs had strong negative influences on the fusion and clinical success rates. Patients who continued to smoke after surgery had a substantially higher rate of pseudarthrosis. Patients who continued to take nonsteroidal anti-inflammatory drugs for more than 3 months after surgery showed substantially lower fusion and success rates. Similarly, Martin and associates[53] reported that administration of ketorolac for 7 days after a posterolateral intertransverse process arthrodesis was associated with a fivefold increase in the likelihood of pseudarthrosis developing.

Glassman and associates[32] reviewed the cases of 288 patients to determine the effect of postoperative administration of nonsteroidal anti-inflammatory drugs on spinal fusion. Nonunion was detected in 4% of the patients who received no nonsteroidal anti-inflammatory drugs, in contrast to 17% of the patients who received ketorolac.

Long and associates[60] investigated the effects of COX-2 inhibitors on spinal fusions in three groups of rabbits, which were randomly assigned to receive celecoxib, indomethacin, or saline solution daily for 8 weeks. The fusion rates, as determined with gross and histologic inspection and radiographic evaluation, were better in the control group and the celecoxib group than they were in the indomethacin group. The authors concluded that inhibitory effects on bone healing are likely mediated by the inhibition of COX-1, a finding that is in contrast with those of other studies.[39]

In conclusion, there is no consensus in the literature with regard to the effects of COX-2 inhibitors on spinal fusions and fracture healing. Nonspecific nonsteroidal anti-inflammatory drugs have a strong negative effect on spinal fusion rates. The inhibitory effects on bone healing are likely mediated by the inhibition of COX-1. There is a paucity of clinical studies evaluating the effects of COX-2 inhibitors on spinal fusions.

Effects of Nonsteroidal Anti-inflammatory Drugs on Osseointegration and Aseptic Loosening

Approximately 200,000 total hip arthroplasties are performed annually in the United States. Patients who have these operations require multimodal pain management, in which nonsteroidal anti-inflammatory drugs play a pivotal role. Also, nonsteroidal anti-inflammatory drugs have a role in the prevention of heterotopic bone formation after total hip arthroplasty. Therefore, the effect of these drugs on the outcome of total hip arthroplasty is an important issue that necessitates meticulous consideration.

Press-fit total hip arthroplasty implants, which are designed to achieve biologic fixation by means of bone ingrowth into a porous-coated surface, are being used with increasing frequency. There are two main issues with regard to the role of nonsteroidal anti-inflammatory drugs in the osseointegration of press-fit hip implants: (1) whether the drugs decrease bone ingrowth and thus affect the integration of bone into the prostheses and (2) whether they help to prevent aseptic loosening, a major cause of failure of total hip arthroplasty.

Bone Ingrowth

Trancik and associates[61] found a substantial decrease in bone growth into porous-coated cobalt-chromium implants in rabbits treated with indomethacin, ibuprofen, or high-dose aspirin when they were compared with controls. The inhibitory effects of indomethacin and aspirin were dose related, with higher doses having a greater inhibitory effect. Keller and associates[62] found a similar inhibitory effect with indomethacin. They reported that bone ingrowth into a porous cylindrical implant system did not increase between 2 and 8 weeks after implantation in rabbits treated with indomethacin; in contrast, a placebo control group exhibited a substantial increase in bone ingrowth in the same time period.

Cook and associates[63] reported that perioperative administration of indomethacin did not affect bone-implant-interface attachment strength of porous-coated implants except during the first 3 postoperative weeks. In an attempt to distinguish between the effects of COX-1 and COX-2, Goodman and associates[40] investigated the effects of naproxen and rofecoxib in vivo by using a harvest chamber. Both naproxen and rofecoxib were found to significantly decrease bone ingrowth. In addition, both decreased the number of CD51-positive osteoclast-like cells per section compared with that seen in the control group. Rofecoxib also decreased the area of osteoblasts per section area compared with that in the controls, although this difference did not reach significance. The conclusion was that bone formation was suppressed by oral administration of a nonsteroidal anti-inflammatory drug that contains a COX-2 inhibitor.

Aseptic Loosening

The potential role of nonsteroidal anti-inflammatory drugs in the prevention of aseptic loosening has been investigated in humans. The premise is that COX-2 expression contributes to activation of the macrophages responsible for the pseudomembrane surrounding loose implants and that inhibiting COX-2 activity can result in a decrease in the prevalence of aseptic loosening.

Hukkanen and associates[64] examined the bone-implant interface membranes of patients with aseptic loosening following total hip replacement in an attempt to determine whether there was an increase in inducible nitric oxide synthase (iNOS) and COX-2 expression in macrophages in these pseudomembranes, contributing to periprosthetic bone resorption. Prostaglandin E_2, an indicator of COX-2 activity, was measured with enzyme immunoassay, and COX-2 was evaluated with quantitative peroxidase immunocytochemistry. They found that iNOS and COX-2 proteins and the corresponding enzyme activities were present in the interface tissues surrounding loose implants. There was a colocalization of CD68+ macrophages with iNOS, nitrotyrosine, and COX-2, suggesting that both the iNOS and the COX-2 pathways may be directly involved in aseptic loosening.

Zhang and associates[18] provided further evidence of COX-2 involvement in osteolysis. To investigate the role of COX-2 in wear debris-induced osteolysis, titanium wear-debris particles were implanted in a calvarial model to induce an inflammatory response similar to osteolysis. In this study, celecoxib reduced inflammation and its associated bone resorption at doses that did not inhibit COX-1 activity. Furthermore, COX-2-lacking mice had substantially less bone resorption in response to the particles than did COX-1-lacking mice. This study also provided direct evidence of an important role of COX-2 that is distinct from that of COX-1 and suggested that selective COX-2 inhibition could have a therapeutic role for patients with inflammation-induced bone diseases.

More recently, Bukata and associates[65] investigated the importance of the COX-2 enzyme in vitro. Periprosthetic membranes from major osteolytic areas were obtained during revision surgeries. Histochemical analysis showed an abundance of COX-2 and minimal amounts of COX-1 along the membrane borders. Bukata and associates[65] also studied the relationship of prostaglandin E_2 production with COX-1 and COX-2 in a transgenic mouse model. The levels of prostaglandin E_2 produced in the COX-1-lacking fibroblasts were substantially increased in response to titanium particles. In contrast, prostaglandin E_2 levels in the COX-2-lacking cultures did not significantly increase above background levels under any conditions tested, indicating that a functional *COX-2* gene is required for prostaglandin E_2 production by fibroblasts and that particle-induced prostaglandin E_2 production is mediated by this enzyme. Consistent with the prostaglandin E_2 data, there were no increases in IL-6 production in any of the COX-2-lacking cultures, indicating a dependency of IL-6 production on prostaglandin E_2 levels. When exogenous prostaglandin E_2 was added to the COX-2-lacking cultures, there was a remarkable increase in the IL-6 levels compared with the levels in the cultures lacking exogenous prostaglandin E_2. This finding suggested that IL-6 production is dependent on prostaglandin E_2 levels at least in one pathway.

In conclusion, there is evidence that COX-2 inhibition causes suppression of bone ingrowth if the drug is administered in the early postoperative period. In cases of aseptic loosening, particle-induced prostaglandin E_2 production is mediated by the COX-2 enzyme. Therefore, COX-2 inhibition plays a role in decreasing the prevalence of aseptic loosening of cementless implants.

Soft-Tissue Healing

There is controversy regarding the effect of nonsteroidal anti-inflammatory drugs on soft-tissue healing.[66] These drugs are reported to not only reduce pain and swelling but also lead to earlier motion, which promotes early ligament healing. The use of COX-2 inhibitors may be beneficial when thickening of a healing tendon can cause problems (such as in the hand).[67] In cases of direct tissue trauma, tissue damage results from traumatically induced inflammatory reactions, with tissue hypoxia being the most likely trigger. In these cases, there is a transient upregulation of COX-2 expression. COX-2 has also been reported to be upregulated in surgery-associated paraspinal muscle injury, but levels were not found to reach their peak before 3 days.[68]

The effects of COX-2 inhibitors on soft-tissue healing have been investigated in several basic-science studies, with contradictory results. Several reports have illustrated the detrimental effects of COX-2 inhibitors on ligament healing,[69] whereas others have indicated a possible beneficial effect on ligament healing[70] and still others have revealed no relationship between ligament healing and the use of nonsteroidal anti-inflammatory drugs.[71,72]

Elder and associates[69] reported that the healed ligaments of rats that had received a COX-2 inhibitor had a 32% lower load to failure, measured 14 days after injury, than did a control group.

Bogatov and associates[71] found that treatment with a pure COX-1 inhibitor, SC-560, had no significant effect on the tensile strength of the site of healing of acute injuries of rat medial collateral ligaments. However, there was an increase in the strength of the uninjured collateral ligaments. This suggests that COX-1 inhibitors do not improve the strength of ligament-healing sites but do improve the strength of the contralateral uninjured ligament. Thus, a pure COX-1 inhibitor probably does not have a positive influence on ligament healing but might provide benefits in terms of prevention of ligament injury.

The lack of consensus in this area led Hanson and associates[70] to undertake a more comprehensive study to resolve the issue. They compared the effects of piroxicam, naproxen, rofecoxib, butorphanol, and acetaminophen on the healing of rat medial collateral ligaments with the findings in a control group. The only drug that improved ligament healing was piroxicam, which led to a 27% greater load to failure compared with that in the control group. This study showed that opioid analgesics, acetaminophen, and COX-2 inhibitors do not appear to categorically affect ligament healing and that piroxicam's effects cannot be attributed to all nonsteroidal anti-inflammatory drugs.

Ferry and associates[72] investigated the effects of ibuprofen, acetaminophen, naproxen, piroxicam, celecoxib, and valdecoxib on the healing of rat patellar tendons. The tendons in the acetaminophen and ibuprofen groups were significantly stronger than those in the celecoxib group; however, they were not significantly different from those in the control group. This study suggests that none of the tested nonsteroidal anti-inflammatory drugs, including piroxicam, had a beneficial effect on ligament healing.

The effects of nonsteroidal anti-inflammatory drugs in the setting of soft-tissue trauma and their role in angiogenesis were investigated by Gierer and associates.[73] Closed soft-tissue trauma to the hindlimb was induced in anesthetized rats, to which either parecoxib or an equal volume of saline solution was administered. Regardless of whether the parecoxib was administered before or after the injury, the microcirculatory flow was completely restored within the injured muscle. In contrast, skeletal muscle in the saline-solution-treated animals revealed persistent perfusion failure, with tissue hypoxia, and enhanced endothelial interaction of both leukocytes and platelets at 18 hours after the trauma. The authors concluded that treatment with parecoxib before as well as soon after a skeletal muscle soft-tissue injury may be effective in restoring disturbed microcirculation. Moreover, a reduced inflammatory cell response could help to prevent leukocyte or platelet-dependent secondary tissue injury.

Cohen and associates[74] studied the effect of nonsteroidal anti-inflammatory drugs on tendon healing to bone by administering celecoxib or indomethacin for 14 days to 180 rats that had undergone acute rotator cuff repair. Both the celecoxib and the indomethacin group had significantly lower failure loads compared with those in the control groups at 2, 4, and 8 weeks. The control groups demonstrated progressively increasing collagen organization during the course of the study, whereas the groups treated with the nonsteroidal anti-inflammatory drugs did not. There were no significant differences between these two drugs with regard to their negative effect on healing of the rotator cuff tendon, which implies that the inhibition of the healing process is linked to the COX-2 enzyme.

In summary, despite the common use of nonsteroidal anti-inflammatory drugs in the treatment of closed soft-tissue injuries, our understanding of the effect of these medications on soft-tissue healing is incomplete. COX-2-selective inhibitors exhibiting a low side-effect profile may be of superior therapeutic value in protecting the microcirculation and preserving skeletal muscle from secondary inflammatory tissue damage following closed soft-tissue injury. In addition, COX-2 inhibitors may play a role in postoperative management following ligament reconstructions and repairs by reducing pain and swelling and allowing an earlier return of motion.

Summary

Many orthopaedic surgeons rely on narcotic analgesia for pain control after fractures and surgical procedures in their patients because traditional nonsteroidal anti-inflammatory drugs have been shown to delay fracture healing and possibly impair tendon repair. This effect is thought to be smaller with COX-2-specific inhibitors.

The COX-2 enzyme plays an important role in bone and soft-tissue healing, and the inhibition of this enzyme can interfere with recovery. However, there is a considerable amount of evidence from several clinical studies that COX-2 inhibition is not detrimental to healing and recovery. It is believed that additional controlled clinical studies with appropriate randomization are essential to address concerns in this field and to discern the roles of COX-1 and COX-2 enzymes in the healing of musculoskeletal tissues.

References

1. Singh G, Ramey DR, Morfeld D, Fries JF: Comparative toxicity of nonsteroidal anti-inflammatory agents. *Pharmacol Ther* 1994;62:175-191.
2. Seidenberg AB, An YH: Is there an inhibitory effect of COX-2 inhibitors on bone healing? *Pharmacol Res* 2004; 50:151-156.
3. Pirmohamed M, James S, Meakin S, et al: Adverse drug reactions as cause of admission to hospital: Prospective analysis of 18,820 patients. *BMJ* 2004; 329:15-19.
4. Riew KD, Long J, Rhee J, et al: Time-dependent inhibitory effects of indomethacin on spinal fusion. *J Bone Joint Surg Am* 2003;85:632-634.
5. Sun JS, Tsuang YH, Lin FH, Liu HC, Tsai CZ, Chang WH: Bone defect healing enhanced by ultrasound stimulation: An in vitro tissue culture model. *J Biomed Mater Res* 1999;46: 253-261.
6. Radi ZA, Khan NK: Effects of cyclooxygenase inhibition on bone, tendon, and ligament healing. *Inflamm Res* 2005;54:358-366.
7. Sato Y, Tsuboi R, Lyons R, Moses H, Rifkin DB: Characterization of the activation of latent TGF-beta by cocultures of endothelial cells and pericytes or smooth muscle cells: A self-regulating system. *J Cell Biol* 1990; 111:757-763.
8. Suzawa T, Miyaura C, Inada M, et al: The role of prostaglandin E receptor subtypes (EP1, EP2, EP3, and EP4) in bone resorption: An analysis using specific agonists for the respective EPs. *Endocrinology* 2000;141:1554-1559.

9. Burke A, Smyth EM, FitzGerald GA: Analgesic-antipyretic and antiinflammatory agents: Pharmacotherapy of gout, in Brunton LL, Lazo JS, Parker KL, eds: *Goodman and Gilman's the Pharmacological Basis of Therapeutics*, ed 11. New York, NY, McGraw-Hill, 2005, pp 671-716.

10. Herschman HR, Fletcher BS, Kujubu DA: TIS10, a mitogen-inducible glucocorticoid-inhibited gene that encodes a second prostaglandin synthase/cyclooxygenase enzyme. *J Lipid Mediat* 1993;6:89-99.

11. Masferrer JL, Zweifel BS, Seibert K, Needleman P: Selective regulation of cellular cyclooxygenase by dexamethasone and endotoxin in mice. *J Clin Invest* 1990;86:1375-1379.

12. Min YK, Rao Y, Okada Y, Raisz LG, Pilbeam CC: Regulation of prostaglandin G/H synthase-2 expression by interleukin-1 in human osteoblast-like cells. *J Bone Miner Res* 1998;13: 1066-1075.

13. Tokushima T, Sato T, Morita I, Murota S: Involvement of prostaglandin endoperoxide H synthase-2 in osteoclast formation induced by parathyroid hormone. *Adv Exp Med Biol* 1997;433:307-309.

14. Tai H, Miyaura C, Pilbeam CC, et al: Transcriptional induction of cyclooxygenase-2 in osteoblasts is involved in interleukin-6-induced osteoclast formation. *Endocrinology* 1997; 138:2372-2379.

15. Kotake S, Udagawa N, Takahashi N, et al: IL-17 in synovial fluids from patients with rheumatoid arthritis is a potent stimulator of osteoclastogenesis. *J Clin Invest* 1999;103:1345-1352.

16. Morinaga Y, Fujita N, Ohishi K, Zhang Y, Tsuruo T: Suppression of interleukin-11-mediated bone resorption by cyclooxygenases inhibitors. *J Cell Physiol* 1998;175:247-254.

17. Kawaguchi H, Pilbeam CC, Harrison JR, Raisz LG: The role of prostaglandins in the regulation of bone metabolism. *Clin Orthop Relat Res* 1995;313:36-46.

18. Zhang X, Morham SG, Langenbach R, et al: Evidence for a direct role of cyclo-oxygenase 2 in implant wear debris-induced osteolysis. *J Bone Miner Res* 2001;16:660-670.

19. Botting R, Ayoub SS: COX-3 and the mechanism of action of paracetamol/acetaminophen. *Prostaglandins Leukot Essent Fatty Acids* 2005;72:85-87.

20. Snipes JA, Kis B, Shelness GS, Hewett JA, Busija DW: Cloning and characterization of cyclooxygenase-1b (putative cyclooxygenase-3) in rat. *J Pharmacol Exp Ther* 2005;313: 668-676.

21. Ke HZ, Shen VW, Qi H, et al: Prostaglandin E2 increases bone strength in intact rats and in ovariectomized rats with established osteopenia. *Bone* 1998;23:249-255.

22. Yang RS, Liu TK, Lin-Shiau SY: Increased bone growth by local prostaglandin E2 in rats. *Calcif Tissue Int* 1993;52:57-61.

23. Jee WS, Ma YF: The in vivo anabolic actions of prostaglandins in bone. *Bone* 1997;21:297-304.

24. Dekel S, Lenthall G, Francis MJ: Release of prostaglandins from bone and muscle after tibial fracture: An experimental study in rabbits. *J Bone Joint Surg Br* 1981;63:185-189.

25. Elves MW, Bayley I, Roylance PJ: The effect of indomethacin upon experimental fractures in the rat. *Acta Orthop Scand* 1982;53:35-41.

26. Keller J, Klamer A, Bak B, Suder P: Effect of local prostaglandin E2 on fracture callus in rabbits. *Acta Orthop Scand* 1993;64:59-63.

27. Sudmann E, Dregelid E, Bessesen A, Morland J: Inhibition of fracture healing by indomethacin in rats. *Eur J Clin Invest* 1979;9:333-339.

28. Li M Healy DR, Li Y, et al: Osteopenia and impaired fracture healing in aged EP4 receptor knockout mice. *Bone* 2005;37:46-54.

29. Allen HL, Wase A, Bear WT: Indomethacin and aspirin: Effect of nonsteroidal anti-inflammatory agents on the rate of fracture repair in the rat. *Acta Orthop Scand* 1980;51: 595-600.

30. Huo MH, Troiano NW, Pelker RR, Gundberg CM, Friedlaender GE: The influence of ibuprofen on fracture repair: Biomechanical, biochemical, histologic, and histomorphometric parameters in rats. *J Orthop Res* 1991;9:383-390.

31. Altman RD, Latta LL, Keer R, Renfree K, Hornicek FJ, Banovac K: Effect of nonsteroidal antiinflammatory drugs on fracture healing: A laboratory study in rats. *J Orthop Trauma* 1995;9:392-400.

32. Glassman SD, Rose SM, Dimar JR, Puno RM, Campbell MJ, Johnson JR: The effect of postoperative nonsteroidal anti-inflammatory drug administration on spinal fusion. *Spine (Phila Pa 1976)* 1998;23:834-838.

33. Giannoudis PV, Macdonald DA, Matthews SJ, Smith RM, Furlong AJ, De Boer P: Nonunion of the femoral diaphysis: The influence of reaming and non-steroidal anti-inflammatory drugs. *J Bone Joint Surg Br* 2000;82: 655-658.

34. Dumont AS, Verma S, Dumont RJ, Hurlbert RJ: Nonsteroidal anti-inflammatory drugs and bone metabolism in spinal fusion surgery: A pharmacological quandary. *J Pharmacol Toxicol Methods* 2000;43:31-39.

35. Gerstenfeld LC, Thiede M, Seibert K, et al: Differential inhibition of fracture healing by non-selective and cyclooxygenase-2 selective non-steroidal anti-inflammatory drugs. *J Orthop Res* 2003;21:670-675.

36. Goodman SB, Ma T, Genovese M, Lane SR: COX-2 selective inhibitors and bone. *Int J Immunopathol Pharmacol* 2003;16:201-205.

37. Brown KM, Saunders MM, Kirsch T, Donahue HJ, Reid JS: Effect of COX-2-specific inhibition on fracture-healing in the rat femur. *J Bone Joint Surg Am* 2004;86:116-123.

38. Gerstenfeld LC, Al-Ghawas M, Alkhiary YM, et al: Selective and non-selective cyclooxygenase-2 inhibitors and experimental fracture-healing:

Reversibility of effects after short-term treatment. *J Bone Joint Surg Am* 2007;89:114-125.

39. Simon AM, Manigrasso MB, O'Connor JP: Cyclo-oxygenase 2 function is essential for bone fracture healing. *J Bone Miner Res* 2002;17: 963-976.

40. Goodman S, Ma T, Trindade M, et al: COX-2 selective NSAID decreases bone ingrowth in vivo. *J Orthop Res* 2002;20:1164-1169.

41. Simon AM, O'Connor JP: Dose and time-dependent effects of cyclooxygenase-2 inhibition on fracture-healing. *J Bone Joint Surg Am* 2007;89:500-511.

42. Krischak GD, Augat P, Blakytny R, Claes L, Kinzl L, Beck A: The nonsteroidal anti-inflammatory drug diclofenac reduces appearance of osteoblasts in bone defect healing in rats. *Arch Orthop Trauma Surg* 2007;127: 453-458.

43. Murnaghan M, Li G, Marsh DR: Nonsteroidal anti-inflammatory drug-induced fracture nonunion: An inhibition of angiogenesis? *J Bone Joint Surg Am* 2006;88:140-147.

44. Anderson GD, Hauser SD, McGarity KL, Bremer ME, Isakson PC, Gregory SA: Selective inhibition of cyclooxygenase (COX)-2 reverses inflammation and expression of COX-2 and interleukin 6 in rat adjuvant arthritis. *J Clin Invest* 1996;97: 2672-2679.

45. Bergenstock M, Min W, Simon AM, Sabatino C, O'Connor JP: A comparison between the effects of acetaminophen and celecoxib on bone fracture healing in rats. *J Orthop Trauma* 2005;19:717-723.

46. Burd TA, Hughes MS, Anglen JO: Heterotopic ossification prophylaxis with indomethacin increases the risk of long-bone nonunion. *J Bone Joint Surg Br* 2003;85:700-705.

47. Van Staa TP, Leufkens HG, Cooper C: Use of nonsteroidal anti-inflammatory drugs and risk of fractures. *Bone* 2000;27:563-568.

48. Vestergaard P, Rejnmark L, Mosekilde L: Fracture risk associated with use of nonsteroidal anti-inflammatory drugs, acetylsalicylic acid, and acetaminophen and the effects of rheumatoid arthritis and osteoarthritis. *Calcif Tissue Int* 2006;79:84-94.

49. Adolphson P, Abbaszadegan H, Jonsson U, Dalen N, Sjöberg HE, Kalén S: No effects of piroxicam on osteopenia and recovery after Colles' fracture: A randomized, double-blind, placebo-controlled, prospective trial. *Arch Orthop Trauma Surg* 1993; 112:127-130.

50. Bhattacharyya T, Levin R, Vrahas MS, Solomon DH: Nonsteroidal antiinflammatory drugs and nonunion of humeral shaft fractures. *Arthritis Rheum* 2005;53:364-367.

51. Boden SD: Overview of the biology of lumbar spine fusion and principles for selecting a bone graft substitute. *Spine (Phila Pa 1976)* 2002;27: S26-S31.

52. Dimar JR II, Ante WA, Zhang YP, Glassman SD: The effects of nonsteroidal anti-inflammatory drugs on posterior spinal fusions in the rat. *Spine (Phila Pa 1976)* 1996;21:1870-1876.

53. Martin GJ Jr, Boden SD, Titus L: Recombinant human bone morphogenetic protein-2 overcomes the inhibitory effect of ketorolac, a nonsteroidal anti-inflammatory drug (NSAID), on posterolateral lumbar intertransverse process spine fusion. *Spine (Phila Pa 1976)* 1999;24:2188-2194.

54. Bo J, Sudmann E, Marton PF: Effect of indomethacin on fracture healing in rats. *Acta Orthop Scand* 1976;47: 588-599.

55. Keller J, Bünger C, Andreassen TT, Bak B, Lucht U: Bone repair inhibited by indomethacin: Effects on bone metabolism and strength of rabbit osteotomies. *Acta Orthop Scand* 1987;58:379-383.

56. Lindholm TS, Törnkvist H: Inhibitory effect on bone formation and calcification exerted by the anti-inflammatory drug ibuprofen: An experimental study on adult rat with fracture. *Scand J Rheumatol* 1981;10: 38-42.

57. Sudmann E, Bang G: Indomethacin-induced inhibition of haversian remodelling in rabbits. *Acta Orthop Scand* 1979;50:621-627.

58. Boden SD, Schimandle JH, Hutton WC: An experimental lumbar intertransverse process spinal fusion model: Radiographic, histologic, and biomechanical healing characteristics. *Spine (Phila Pa 1976)* 1995;20: 412-420.

59. Deguchi M, Rapoff AJ, Zdeblick TA: Posterolateral fusion for isthmic spondylolisthesis in adults: Analysis of fusion rate and clinical results. *J Spinal Disord* 1998;11:459-464.

60. Long J, Lewis S, Kuklo T, Zhu Y, Riew KD: The effect of cyclooxygenase-2 inhibitors on spinal fusion. *J Bone Joint Surg Am* 2002;84: 1763-1768.

61. Trancik T, Mills W, Vinson N: The effect of indomethacin, aspirin, and ibuprofen on bone ingrowth into a porous-coated implant. *Clin Orthop Relat Res* 1989;249:113-121.

62. Keller JC, Trancik TM, Young FA, St Mary E: Effects of indomethacin on bone ingrowth. *J Orthop Res* 1989; 7:28-34.

63. Cook SD, Barrack RL, Dalton JE, Thomas KA, Brown TD: Effects of indomethacin on biologic fixation of porous-coated titanium implants. *J Arthroplasty* 1995;10:351-358.

64. Hukkanen M, Corbett SA, Batten J, et al: Aseptic loosening of total hip replacement: Macrophage expression of inducible nitric oxide synthase and cyclo-oxygenase-2, together with peroxynitrite formation, as a possible mechanism for early prosthesis failure. *J Bone Joint Surg Br* 1997;79: 467-474.

65. Bukata SV, Gelinas J, Wei X, et al: PGE2 and IL-6 production by fibroblasts in response to titanium wear debris particles is mediated through a Cox-2 dependent pathway. *J Orthop Res* 2004;22:6-12.

66. Vogel HG: Mechanical and chemical properties of various connective tissue organs in rats as influenced by non-steroidal antirheumatic drugs. *Connect Tissue Res* 1977;5:91-95.

67. Forslund C, Bylander B, Aspenberg P: Indomethacin and celecoxib improve tendon healing in rats. *Acta Orthop Scand* 2003;74:465-469.

68. Lu K Liang CL, Chen HJ, et al: Nuclear factor-kappaB-regulated cyclooxygenase-2 expression in surgery-associated paraspinal muscle injury in rats. *J Neurosurg* 2003;98:181-187.

69. Elder CL, Dahners LE, Weinhold PS: A cyclooxygenase-2 inhibitor impairs ligament healing in the rat. *Am J Sports Med* 2001;29:801-805.

70. Hanson CA, Weinhold PS, Afshari HM, Dahners LE: The effect of analgesic agents on the healing rat medial collateral ligament. *Am J Sports Med* 2005;33:674-679.

71. Bogatov VB, Weinhold P, Dahners LE: The influence of a cyclooxygenase-1 inhibitor on injured and uninjured ligaments in the rat. *Am J Sports Med* 2003;31:574-576.

72. Ferry ST, Dahners LE, Afshari HM, Weinhold PS: The effects of common anti-inflammatory drugs on the healing rat patellar tendon. *Am J Sports Med* 2007;35:1326-1333.

73. Gierer P, Mittlmeier T, Bordel R, Schaser KD, Gradl G, Vollmar B: Selective cyclooxygenase-2 inhibition reverses microcirculatory and inflammatory sequelae of closed soft-tissue trauma in an animal model. *J Bone Joint Surg Am* 2005;87:153-160.

74. Cohen DB, Kawamura S, Ehteshami JR, Rodeo SA: Indomethacin and celecoxib impair rotator cuff tendon-to-bone healing. *Am J Sports Med* 2006;34:362-369.

Perioperative Strategies for Decreasing Infection: A Comprehensive Evidence-Based Approach

Joseph A. Bosco III, MD
James D. Slover, MD
Janet P. Haas, DNSc, RN, CIC

Abstract

Surgical site infections are a devastating complication of orthopaedic procedures and result in increased morbidity and mortality as well as higher costs. Universally, patients with surgical site infections have a worse outcome than uninfected patients. Payers of health care and regulatory organizations, such as the Centers for Medicare and Medicaid Services and the Joint Commission, are demanding both accountability and a reduction in the occurrence of surgical site infections. To effectively prevent such infections, the clinician must address preoperative, intraoperative, and postoperative factors, along with interventions. In the areas where evidence-based literature demonstrates a clear best practice, such as prophylactic antibiotic use and surgical scrub techniques, physicians and health care professionals will be held accountable for compliance with these standards. This accountability will be quantified and will be made available to the public. It is also evident that payers will reward and/or penalize physicians for failure to comply with established standards of care. For the health and safety of patients, surgeons are obligated to become familiar with the known best practices and standards of care with respect to the reduction of surgical site infections.

Instr Course Lect 2010;59:619-628.

Surgical site infections associated with orthopaedic surgical procedures are devastating complications. They increase morbidity, mortality, and cost and result in outcomes that are worse than those in uninfected patients.[1] Decreasing the incidence of surgical site infections is not only of interest to patients and surgeons, it is also a major focus of several groups of interested parties. These range from payers, including the Centers for Medicare and Medicaid Services (CMS), to institutions represented by the Surgical Care Improvement Project—a multiple-institution partnership between major public and private health care organizations, including the Joint Commission on Accreditation of Healthcare Organizations (Joint Commission). Decreasing the incidence of surgical site infections is, and will continue to be, a major focus in medicine.

To effectively prevent surgical site infections, the clinician must consider preoperative, intraoperative, and postoperative factors and interventions. Preoperative strategies for reducing infection rates include identification of high-risk patients, screening and decolonization of patients with methicillin-sensitive *Staphylococcus aureus* and methicillin-resistant *S aureus* colonization, preoperative preparation of the patient with chlorhexidine gluconate, use of proper hair removal techniques, and addressing preexisting dental and nutritional issues before surgery.

There are a variety of perioperative strategies that can and should be

Dr. Bosco or an immediate family member is a board member, owner, officer, or committee member of the American Orthopaedic Society for Sports Medicine and the New York State Society for Orthopaedic Surgeons; is a member of a speakers' bureau or has made paid presentations on behalf of Ortho McNeil Janssen; and has received research or institutional support from AO, Arthrex, DePuy, EBI, Exactech, Hand Innovations, Mitek, Small Bone Innovations, Smith & Nephew, Stryker, and Synthes. Dr. Slover or an immediate family member has received research or institutional support from Smith & Nephew and Stryker. Dr. Haas or an immediate family member serves as a paid consultant for or is an employee of Otsuka Pharmaceutical Co. Ltd.

used to decrease the risk of surgical site infections. Intraoperative interventions that have been shown to decrease surgical site infection rates include the proper selection, timing, and doses of prophylactic antibiotics and the use of best practices for hand hygiene and surgical site preparation. Maintaining a sterile operating room environment by decreasing operating room traffic, monitoring for breaks in sterile technique, and decreasing the use of flash sterilization is vital. Finally, postoperative strategies for reducing surgical site infection rates include the proper use and duration in situ of urinary catheters and surgical drains; standardization of wound care; the use of antibiotic-impregnated bandages; and, perhaps most importantly, maintenance of proper hand hygiene, isolation precautions, and room cleaning.

Preoperative Considerations

Although every precaution should be taken to prevent infection for all orthopaedic patients, the identification of high-risk patients enables clinicians to provide maximal prevention strategies for them. Furthermore, the identification of patients at high risk for infection allows appropriate preoperative counseling for shared decision making and establishes appropriate patient expectations regarding surgical risks.

Numerous high-risk patient populations and risk factors that place patients at high risk for infection after total joint arthroplasty or spine surgery have been described in the literature. Some of these factors can be modified, whereas others cannot. An explanation of the risk factors that cannot be modified should be included when patients are counseled about their increased risk of infection with the proposed surgical procedure. In this way, patients will more completely understand the risks and benefits when deciding on surgery. One factor that cannot be modified and that increases the risk of infection is a previous history of infection in the joint.[2] Some researchers have proposed that a history of intra-articular steroid injection may increase the risk of infection with total joint arthroplasty; however, some studies have not demonstrated this to be a risk factor.[3,4] Factors that cannot be modified that increase the risk of infection in patients undergoing spine surgery include trauma-related surgery, the use of instrumentation, and lumbar and posterior surgery.[5-7]

Other factors that increase the risk of infection are potentially modifiable and, therefore, provide the opportunity for patient optimization before elective orthopaedic procedures. For example, patients with inflammatory arthritis, sickle-cell disease, diabetes, renal failure, and human immunodeficiency virus (HIV) have increased infection rates with joint arthroplasty.[8-12] Although these risk factors cannot be eliminated, the risks can be minimized. For example, patients with inflammatory arthritis should have a preoperative consultation with their rheumatologist about reducing or discontinuing immunosuppressive medications perioperatively. Patients with sickle-cell disease should be screened for skin ulcerations or potential sources of osteomyelitis, which can cause seeding of the site of a prosthetic joint. Diabetic patients should have their hemoglobin A1C levels checked and normalized (to $< 6.9\%$, which reflects long-term glucose control) before surgery; consultation with an endocrinologist may be necessary. Patients with renal failure certainly should have their renal function optimized before surgery, and patients with HIV should be placed on regimens that achieve an undetectable viral load, if possible, before joint arthroplasty. Malnutrition is associated with an increased risk of infection; therefore, preoperative optimization, with the assistance of a nutritionist if necessary, is beneficial.[13]

Smoking and obesity increase the risk of infection with spine surgery.[14] Although these factors are often difficult to modify, patients should be counseled that a benefit of smoking cessation and weight reduction is a decreased risk of infection with spine surgery. Patients considering or planning surgical weight-loss treatments, such as gastric bypass surgery, probably should be advised to pursue these procedures first to reduce the risk of infection at the sites of hardware or prostheses as a benefit from weight loss. Working with patients and the appropriate consultants to optimize these factors before surgery may improve patient outcomes by lowering the risk of infection with high-risk joint replacement and spine procedures.

Another important preoperative consideration is preoperative bathing. Preoperative bathing has been used to reduce the bacterial load of the skin before surgery because skin preparation immediately before surgery does not completely sterilize the skin. In addition, direct contamination can occur at the time of surgery. A recent Cochrane review was performed to assess the information in the literature regarding preoperative bathing with antiseptics for the prevention of surgical site infection.[15] Chlorhexidine gluconate is the most commonly used antiseptic for preoperative bathing. The Cochrane review revealed evidence that the bacterial load of resident skin flora is reduced by the use of chlorhexidine gluconate preparations for preoperative bathing. Repeated, consecutive treatments reduce this load progressively over time. However, concerns about the development of resistant organisms and hypersensitivity remain. Therefore, the authors of the review concluded that there is no clear evidence that preoperative bathing with chlorhexidine gluconate is superior to preoperative bathing with other products, such as bar soap, for reducing the incidence of surgical site infection.

Hair removal has been used traditionally to keep hair from contaminating the wound. More recently, hair removal has allowed surgeons to apply occlusive dressings to the skin perioperatively to keep skin flora from directly contaminating the wound. Three methods used for hair removal include traditional razors, clippers, and hair removal creams or depilatories. Hairless surgical sites can make the surgery and application of dressings and protective draping easier, but the use of razors to shave the surgical site increases the risk of introducing primary infections through microscopic injuries to the skin. The Centers for Disease Control and Prevention (CDC) recommend that hair removal be minimized and that, when it is necessary, electric clippers or depilatories be used rather than razors.[16] A Cochrane review of the literature on hair removal before surgery supported the CDC recommendations and added that hair removal can be done on the day of the surgery.[17]

Dental care is another preoperative issue to be discussed with high-risk orthopaedic patients. All patients, but particularly those at high risk for infection, should be encouraged to maintain good dental health before and after surgery. Bacteremia from a dental infection can cause acute hematogenous infection at the site of a total joint arthroplasty. Evidence shows that the most critical period is the first 2 years after surgery.[18] Bacteremia also can occur after other invasive procedures. Given the potential for hematogenous seeding of a joint arthroplasty with bacteremia, the American Academy of Orthopaedic Surgeons (AAOS) has developed an information statement for clinicians regarding antibiotic prophylaxis for patients with total joint replacements prior to invasive procedures.[19] The antibiotics are given prior to the invasive procedure. The suggested regimens included in the AAOS information statement are shown in Table 1.

Antibiotics

Perioperative prophylactic antibiotics are effective in reducing the rate of surgical site infections in high-risk orthopaedic cases. In a 2002 meta-analysis of spine fusion surgery, Barker[20] reported that use of antibiotic therapy for such procedures is beneficial even when the infection rates without antibiotics are low. Similar studies have demonstrated the efficacy of preoperative antibiotics in general orthopaedic surgery and before total joint arthroplasty.[21,22]

The choice of antibiotic for patients with a low risk of methicillin-resistant *S aureus* colonization is either cefazolin (1 to 2 g administered intravenously) or cefuroxime (1.5 g administered intravenously). These doses must be adjusted for children. For patients with a β-lactam allergy, clindamycin (600 mg administered intravenously) or vancomycin (1.0 g administered intravenously) should be used in lieu of cephalosporins. Patients who are colonized with methicillin-resistant *S aureus* are at high risk for colonization (for example, nursing home residents) or have had a previous methicillin-resistant *S aureus* infection have an increased risk for the development of an infection with methicillin-resistant *S aureus*.[23,24] Prophylaxis with vancomycin (1.0 g administered intravenously) should be considered for these patients.[25]

The proper timing and duration of antibiotic prophylaxis are imperative for safety and effectiveness. In general, antibiotic therapy should be started within 1 hour before the surgical incision, and the drugs should be completely infused before tourniquet inflation. The exception to this recommendation is vancomycin, the administration of which may be started up to 2 hours before the surgical incision. This allows a slower infusion and decreases the likelihood of red man syndrome. Red man syndrome occurs when hypersensitivity to vancomycin causes degranulation of mast cells and a release of histamine. The histamine leads to hypotension and facial flushing. Red man syndrome is prevented by the slow administration of vancomycin over a period of 1 to 2 hours.

Antibiotic treatment should be stopped within 24 hours after wound closure. Administration of prophylactic antibiotics for longer than 24 hours has not been demonstrated to be effective and may actually lead to superinfection with drug-resistant organisms.[26] Repeat dosing with antibiotics is recommended during surgical procedures that last longer than 4 hours or when there is more than 1,500 mL of blood loss.[27]

The authors of this chapter recommend that, to ensure the proper

Table 1
AAOS Suggested Antibiotic Prophylaxis for Joint Replacement Patients Prior to Invasive Procedures

Procedure	Antimicrobial Agent	Dose	Timing	Duration
Dental	Cephalexin, cephradine, amoxicillin	2 gm PO	1 hour prior to procedure	Discontinued within 24 hours of the procedure. For most outpatient/office-based procedures a single preprocedure dose is sufficient.
Ophthalmic	Gentamicin, tobramycin, ciprofloxacin, gatifloxacin, levofloxacin, moxifloxacin ofloxacin, or meomycingramicidin -polymyxin B cefazolin	Multiple drops topically over 2 to 24 hours or 100 mg subconjunctivally	Consult ophthalmologist or pharmacist for dosing regimen	
Orthopaedic	Cefazolin Cefuroxime OR Vancomycin	1-2 g IV 1.5 g IV 1 g IV	Begin dose 60 minutes prior to procedure	
Vascular	Cefazolin OR Vancomycin	1-2 g IV 1 g IV	Begin dose 60 minutes prior to procedure	
Gastrointestinal				
Esophageal gastroduodenal	Cefazolin	1-2 g IV	Begin dose 60 minutes prior to procedure	
Biliary tract	Cefazolin	1-2 g IV		
Colorectal	Neomycin + erythromycin base (oral) OR metronidazole (oral)	1 g 1 g	Dependent on time of procedure; consult with GI physician or pharmacist	
Head and Neck	Clindamycin + gentamicin OR cefazolin	600-900 mg 1.5 mg/kg IV 1-2 g IV	Begin dose 60 minutes prior to procedure	
Obstetric and Gynecological	Cefoxitin, cefazolin Ampicillin/sulbactam	1-2 g IV 3 g IV	Begin dose 60 minutes prior to procedure	
Genitourinary	Ciprofloxacin	500 mg PO or 400 mg IV	1 hour prior to procedure Begin dose 60 minutes prior to procedure	

If a tourniquet is used, the entire dose of antibiotic must be infused prior to its inflation
PO = by mouth, IV = intravenously, GI = gastrointestinal

selection and timing of antibiotic prophylaxis, the choice of antibiotics and duration of administration be incorporated into the surgical "time-out." Rosenberg and associates[28] reported that compliance with the proper timing and selection of antibiotics increased from 65% to 99% when the protocol was incorporated into the time-out.

Surgical Hand Antisepsis

The objective of a preoperative hand scrub is to remove or kill as many bacteria as possible from the hands of the surgical team. Aqueous scrub solutions consisting of water-based solutions of either chlorhexidine gluconate or povidone-iodine have been traditionally used.

The authors of a recent Cochrane review[29] found alcohol-based rubs containing ethanol, isopropanol, or n-propanol to be as effective as aqueous solutions for preventing surgical site infections in patients.[30] Hajipour and associates[31] reported that alcohol rubs were more effective than either chlorhexidine gluconate or iodine-based scrubs for reducing bacterial colony-forming units on the hands of surgeons. Other investigators reported that the use of scrub brushes had no positive effect on asepsis and may actually increase the risk of infection as a result of skin damage.[32] On the basis of this evidence, the recommended procedure for preoperative surgical hand antisepsis is that, preceding the first scrub of the day or when the hands are grossly contaminated, the surgical team should wash with soap and water, use a nail pick to clean under the nails, and dry with paper towels. They should then use an alcohol-based rub for 3 minutes.[33] An alcohol-based rub should be used for each subsequent case. The use of scrub brushes is not recommended.

Surgical Site Preparation

Chlorhexidine gluconate–based solutions have supplanted alcohol and iodine-based solutions for surgical site preparation. Ostrander and associates[34] examined the residual amounts of bacteria on feet prepared with chlorhexidine gluconate, iodine/

isopropyl alcohol, or chloroxylenol scrub. They found that chlorhexidine gluconate was superior to the other two preparation solutions in reducing or eliminating bacteria from the feet before surgery. Chlorhexidine gluconate skin preparation was superior to either 70% alcohol or iodine in decreasing infection associated with the placement of central venous catheters and the drawing of blood for culture.[35,36] Thus, the current evidence-based recommendations and best-practice guidelines call for the use of chlorhexidine gluconate–based solutions for surgical site preparation and the placement of central venous catheters.

Decreasing the Risk of Surgical Site Infection Related to the Operating Room Environment

Although the arcane details of techniques used to sterilize surgical instruments are beyond the expected knowledge of most orthopaedic surgeons, many of a surgeon's actions can adversely affect sterilization and increase the risk of surgical site infections. Flash sterilization is a procedure used by operating room staff to sterilize instruments or implants with steam, on an as-needed basis. Flash sterilization is not equivalent to sterilization in central processing.[37,38] In central sterile processing, instruments are properly cleaned and all lumens are inspected; the instruments are then sterilized and allowed to dry completely, after which they are delivered in closed containers that ensure maintenance of sterility. Most importantly, the process is performed by trained, focused professionals. The entire process takes 3 to 4 hours. Flash sterilization should be used only for dropped instruments or in an emergency situation. Preventable reasons for flash sterilization include an insufficient quantity of instruments, loaner instruments and/or instruments not delivered in time for proper processing, and inaccurate or incomplete surgical booking requiring the emergency, unplanned use of instruments and/or implants.

Recommended changes to reduce the incidence of flash sterilization include an increase in physician awareness about the inadequacy of the technique; improvement in the accuracy of surgical booking; mandating cooperation from vendors to ensure timely delivery of equipment, including financial penalties for late delivery; purchase of more frequently flash-sterilized items; surgical scheduling to accommodate and mitigate equipment shortages; and, finally, generation of incident reports when a flash-sterilized implant is used in a patient. Adopting these policies and procedures leads to a decrease in the incidence of flash sterilization.[39]

Powderless Gloves

Traditionally, surgical gloves contained powder to aid in the manufacturing process and to make donning easier. The powder was either talc or lycopodium spores. Because of concerns about granuloma formation and adhesions associated with the use of these substances, cornstarch is now the powder of choice.[40] However, cornstarch is not benign. It causes foreign-body granuloma formation and delayed wound healing and can decrease the amount of bacteria required to cause a clinically apparent infection.[41] Cornstarch also leads to increased latex sensitivity in health care workers. Type I and type IV hypersensitivity reactions to latex protein in hospital staff led to increases in sick time and decreased job satisfaction.[42] Powderless gloves decrease staff absenteeism and eliminate the potential for foreign-body granuloma formation. These gloves cost 25% more than powdered gloves, but the added expense is mitigated by increased productivity of the operating room staff.[42]

Antiseptic-Coated Sutures

The use of antiseptic-coated sutures has generated increased interest. These sutures are typically coated with the antiseptic triclosan. Edmiston and associates[43] demonstrated the effectiveness of coated sutures in inhibiting bacterial growth and contamination in an in vitro model. In a randomized controlled trial, Rozzelle and associates[44] reported a significant reduction in surgical site infection rates following cerebral spinal fluid shunt surgery with the use of antiseptic-coated sutures compared with the rate following the same procedure without the use of such sutures. These sutures cost 7% to 10% more than their uncoated counterparts. The authors of this chapter do not believe that a cost-effectiveness analysis has been published; however, the use of these sutures in high-risk patients may be justified.

Operating Room Traffic

Maintaining a disciplined operating room culture can reduce the risk of surgical site infections. Unnecessary operating room traffic increases the rate of infections.[45] In a study of spine surgery, Olsen and associates[6] reported that two or more residents participating in the surgical procedure was an independent risk factor for surgical site infections, with an odds ratio of 2.2. Babkin and associates[46] found that the rate of surgical site infections associated with left knee replacements was 6.7 times higher than that associated with right knee replacements performed during the same time period and in the same operating rooms. When the door on the left side of the operating room was locked, preventing ingress or egress, the surgical site infection rate associated with the left knee replacements rapidly decreased to that associated with the right knee replacements, a finding that supports the importance of limiting operating room traffic.

Drains and Blood Transfusions

Whether to use drains at the end of orthopaedic surgical procedures is a decision that surgeons make on the basis of their training, opinions, and personal experience, in addition to research findings. A recent Cochrane review on this topic that included findings from 36 studies (5,464 patients) revealed that the use of closed drains reduced bruising and the need for reinforcement of dressings.[47] However, the use of closed drains was also associated with an increased need for transfusion. There was no difference in surgical site infection rates between drained and undrained wounds. The authors concluded that closed suction drains were of doubtful benefit.

In addition to the doubtful benefit of surgical drains in orthopaedic procedures, they are associated with a more frequent need for blood transfusion. Blood transfusion carries the general risk of infection with blood-borne pathogens, such as HIV or hepatitis, and with other bacteria or parasites. This risk is very small, although still present, in the United States and other developed countries that have rigorous testing procedures for donated blood.[48] The more immediate risk associated with transfusion is surgical site infection and an increased length of hospital stay.[49] Transfusion of blood induces immunomodulation that can lead to an increased risk of infection at the surgical site.[50] Talbot and associates[51] reported a 3.2-fold increase in the poststernotomy infection rate among patients who had a transfusion compared with the rate among those who had not. In a study of cardiac surgery, Bower and associates[52] reported that the rate of infection in patients who had a transfusion was almost twice as high as that in patients who had not. Weber and associates[49] found that patients who had a transfusion after hip arthroplasty had an increased length of hospital stay, even when the authors controlled for surgical site infection. Strategies to decrease the need for transfusion include preoperative assessment of hemoglobin levels and the hematocrit and prescription of drugs to improve these parameters, if indicated, as well as the use of an algorithm that depends on symptomatic anemia, rather than hemoglobin and hematocrit results alone, to determine transfusion need.

Postoperative Wound Management

The CDC recommends maintaining surgical dressings for 24 to 48 hours postoperatively.[53] Some surgeons use a 3-day rule, keeping the original surgical dressing in place for 72 hours. There is little evidence that keeping dressings on for an extra day or two decreases the infection risk; however, if the dressing is not clean and dry, it may become a source of microbes close to the incision.

Perhaps as important as the duration that the dressing is in place is ensuring the proper process for postoperative wound management. The surgeon should review policies and procedures to determine who changes dressings (for example, nurses or physicians only), under what circumstances they are changed, and if they are ever reinforced rather than changed. The basic concept of infection prevention is to keep the wound clean and dry. Soiled or blood-soaked dressings should be removed immediately rather than reinforced. If dressings do not stay intact, use of a different product may be warranted.

A multidisciplinary group should evaluate current practices and discuss ways to optimize postoperative wound care. Some basic issues are ensuring that an aseptic technique is used for dressing changes and having accurate descriptions of the amount and character of the wound drainage and of the wound itself in an accessible place. Restrictions on the use of products because of cost may hinder good wound care. For example, restricting the use of semipermeable occlusive dressings to the operating room leaves staff on the nursing units without an appropriate product with which to keep surgical dressings intact. When viewed with respect to the cost of surgical site infections, the cost of the occlusive dressing is very reasonable. Staff education is needed if long-standing policies and procedures are to be changed.

Antimicrobial dressings are available, and research indicates that they may be helpful in reducing infection risk. Silver-based dressings have been available for a long time, and they are effective in decreasing the risk of mediastinitis following cardiac surgery and following lumbar laminectomy and fusion.[54,55] They are not routinely used for surgical care, most likely because they are expensive and not always covered by insurance. Other compounds, such as polyhexamethylene biguanide (PHMB), have shown promise in small studies.[56,57] PHMB dressings look and feel similar to traditional gauze dressings and are much less expensive than silver-containing dressings. The cost of a PHMB-containing 4 × 4-inch sponge is roughly twice the cost of regular 4 × 4-inch gauze (the least expensive antimicrobial dressing). Gentian violet and methylene blue are combined for bacteriostatic effect in some dressings, but there is little evidence to support their use for clean surgical incisions.

Other Issues Concerning Infection Prevention

Hand Hygiene

Proper hand hygiene is the most important way to prevent infections in health care settings, yet compliance with hand-hygiene procedures is suboptimal. The authors of the 2002 CDC Guideline for Hand Hygiene in Health-Care Settings reported an average compliance rate of 40%.[58] Since that time, the Joint Commission has made decreasing rates of health care–associated infections one of its national patient-safety goals, and hospitals that are accredited by the Joint Commission are required to have a hand-hygiene monitoring and improvement program.[59] Studies have linked improved compliance with hand-hygiene protocols with decreased rates of marker organisms, such as methicillin-resistant *S aureus*.[60] Many studies have demonstrated that multipronged interventions that include strong administrative support are more successful over time than are traditional single interventions, such as education or feedback of hand-hygiene compliance data.[61] Another strategy that has helped increase hand-hygiene compliance is the use of alcohol-based hand sanitizers. These are recommended preferentially by the CDC for routine hand hygiene.[58] The rationale is that alcohol-based sanitizers can be more conveniently located than sinks and take less time to use than traditional hand washing. In addition, a counterintuitive finding is that alcohol hand sanitizers are less irritating to skin than hand washing with soap and water.[62,63]

Isolation Precautions

Contact isolation precautions are recommended by the CDC for patients with drug-resistant organisms, and this is now part of the national patient safety goals of the Joint Commission. Patients with drug-resistant organisms are placed in private rooms, if possible, or with other patients who harbor the same organism. Gowns and gloves are required for the care of these patients and should be donned on entry into the room. The decision about when to don gowns and gloves is no longer at the discretion of clinicians because that leads to substantial variability in adherence. The Joint Commission requires hospitals to monitor adherence to contact precautions and to have a program to improve compliance. Some issues regarding contact precautions are unclear. These include decisions about how to handle patients who have been decolonized for methicillin-resistant *S aureus*, a standardized definition of resistant gram-negative organisms, and how long to continue contact precautions for various organisms. More research is needed in these areas. Contact precautions are not without consequences. Recent study results indicate that patients subjected to contact isolation precautions are seen less frequently by attending physicians, are more likely to have skin breakdown or falls, and are more likely to complain about their care. Hospitals should include strategies to ameliorate these consequences when isolation precautions are indicated.[64]

Health Care–Associated Infections

The CMS is changing government payments for infections that arise as a result of hospital care. Successful interventions, such as the Institute for Healthcare Improvement's "100,000 Lives" campaign (currently, the "5 Million Lives" campaign) and the Keystone (Michigan Health and Hospital Association Keystone Center) initiative have shown that infections are not simply an unavoidable complication of health care and that, with attention to infection-prevention practices, many infections may be prevented. As a payer, the CMS has decided to reward institutions that use best practices and not pay extra for certain preventable complications that are referred to as "never events." As of October 2008, the CMS is not paying extra for infectious complications, including catheter-associated urinary tract infections; central venous catheter-associated bloodstream infections; surgical site infections following spine, neck, shoulder, or elbow procedures; or mediastinitis following cardiac surgery.[65]

Of these health care–associated events, urinary tract infections are the most numerous, so efforts at decreasing their occurrence are now a focus of hospitals around the country. Recent studies have shed light on the fact that many clinicians do not know which of their patients have urinary catheters and that there is a great opportunity to decrease the use of urinary catheterization. There are new guidelines and recommendations for the appropriate use of urinary catheters.[66] A daily assessment of the necessity for the device is among these recommendations and is probably the most straightforward approach to decreasing the use of urinary catheters and the associated infection risk.

Public Reporting of Health Care–Associated Infections

As a result of consumer and payer demands for more transparency about health care quality, many states now require some level of public reporting of health care–associated infections. The elements of required reporting and the methodology for reporting vary from state to state, but many are using the CDC National Healthcare Safety Network (NHSN) as the required system. The NHSN is a Web-based version of the CDC's hospital infection reporting system that has been in place since the 1970s. The standardized definitions of infection have been used for many years and have become the gold standard for surveillance definitions. In addition to its long track record, advantages of the NHSN system include the fact that it is a secure database and that it allows groups (such as states) to sign up together, allows a conferral of rights to see institutional data, provides some data analysis and data display capabilities, produces the national benchmarks for infection rates, and is free to use. NHSN modules can be accessed online.[67]

Infection prevention has become a focus of attention for patients, payers, and regulators. Physicians and hospitals must now incorporate infection-prevention practices into their care or risk losing payment and patients and having negative publicity when their rates become public. Fortunately, this gives surgeons the opportunity to collaborate with partners throughout the health care system to deliver the best care possible, paying attention to all processes of care for their patients.

Summary

Reduction of rates of surgical site infections promises to be an area of intense interest and activity in the foreseeable future. Health care payers and regulatory organizations such as CMS and the Joint Commission are demanding accountability and reductions in rates of surgical site infection. In the areas in which evidence-based literature has demonstrated a clear best practice, such as prophylactic use of antibiotics and surgical scrub techniques, physicians and hospitals will be held accountable for compliance with these standards. This accountability will be quantified, and the data will be made available to the public. It is also clear that payers will penalize those responsible for failure to comply with these standards of care. Thus, it is necessary for all to become familiar with the known best practices and standards of care for the reduction in the rates of surgical site infections.

References

1. Kirkland KB, Briggs JP, Trivette SL, Wilkinson WE, Sexton DJ: The impact of surgical-site infections in the 1990s: Attributable mortality, excess length of hospitalization, and extra costs. *Infect Control Hosp Epidemiol* 1999;20:725-730.
2. Jerry GJ Jr, Rand JA, Ilstrup D: Old sepsis prior to total knee arthroplasty. *Clin Orthop Relat Res* 1988;236:135-140.
3. Kaspar J, Kaspar S, Orme C, de Beer J de V: Intra-articular steroid hip injection for osteoarthritis: A survey of orthopedic surgeons in Ontario. *Can J Surg* 2005;48:461-469.
4. Joshy S, Thomas B, Gogi N, Modi A, Singh BK, et al: Effect of intra-articular steroids on deep infections following total knee arthroplasty. *Int Orthop* 2006;30:91-93.
5. Blam OG, Vaccaro AR, Vanichkachorn JS, et al: Risk factors for surgical site infection in the patient with spinal injury. *Spine (Phila Pa 1976)* 2003;28:1475-1480.
6. Sponseller PD, LaPorte DM, Hungerford MW, Eck K, Bridwell KH, Lenke LG: Deep wound infections after neuromuscular scoliosis surgery: A multicenter study of risk factors and treatment outcomes. *Spine (Phila Pa 1976)* 2000;25:2461-2466.
7. Olsen MA, Nepple JJ, Riew KD, et al: Risk factors for surgical site infection following orthopaedic spinal operations. *J Bone Joint Surg Am* 2008;90:62-69.
8. Sharma S, Nicol F, Hullin MG, McCreath SW: Long-term results of the uncemented low contact stress total knee replacement in patients with rheumatoid arthritis. *J Bone Joint Surg Br* 2005;87:1077-1080.
9. Hernigou P, Zilber S, Filippini P, Mathieu G, Poignard A, Galacteros F: Total THA in adult osteonecrosis related to sickle cell disease. *Clin Orthop Relat Res* 2008;466:300-308.
10. Yang K, Yeo SJ, Lee BP, Lo NN: Total knee arthroplasty in diabetic patients: A study of 109 consecutive cases. *J Arthroplasty* 2001;16:102-106.
11. Murzic WJ, McCollum DE: Hip arthroplasty for osteonecrosis after renal transplantation. *Clin Orthop Relat Res* 1994;299:212-219.
12. Parvizi J, Sullivan TA, Pagnano MW, Trousdale RT, Bolander ME: Total joint arthroplasty in human immunodeficiency virus-positive patients: An alarming rate of early failure. *J Arthroplasty* 2003;18:259-264.
13. Greene KA, Wilde AH, Stulberg BN: Preoperative nutritional status of total joint patients: Relationship to postoperative wound complications. *J Arthroplasty* 1991;6:321-325.

14. Capen DA, Calderone RR, Green A: Perioperative risk factors for wound infections after lower back fusions. *Orthop Clin North Am* 1996;27:83-86.

15. Webster J, Osborne S: Preoperative bathing or showering with skin antiseptics to prevent surgical site infection. *Cochrane Database Syst Rev* 2007; 2:CD004985.

16. Bratzler DW, Hunt DR: The surgical infection prevention and surgical care improvement projects: National initiatives to improve outcomes for patients having surgery. *Clin Infect Dis* 2006;43:322-330.

17. Tanner J, Woodings D, Moncaster K: Preoperative hair removal to reduce surgical site infection. *Cochrane Database Syst Rev* 2006;3:CD004122.

18. Hanssen AD, Osmon DR, Nelson CL: Prevention of deep periprosthetic joint infection. *Instr Course Lect* 1997;46:555-567.

19. American Academy of Orthopaedic Surgeons: Antibiotic prophylaxis for bacteremia in patients with joint replacements. http://www.aaos.org/about/papers/advistmt/1033.asp. Accessed November 4, 2009.

20. Barker FG II: Efficacy of prophylactic antibiotic therapy in spinal surgery: A meta-analysis. *Neurosurgery* 2002;51: 391-401.

21. Lidwell OM, Elson RA, Lowbury EJ, et al: Ultraclean air and antibiotics for prevention of postoperative infection: A multicenter study of 8,052 joint replacement operations. *Acta Orthop Scand* 1987;58:4-13.

22. Henley MB, Jones RE, Wyatt RW, Hofmann A, Cohen RL: Prophylaxis with cefamandole nafate in elective orthopedic surgery. *Clin Orthop Relat Res* 1986;209:249-254.

23. Kluytmans JA, Mouton JW, Vanden-Bergh MF, et al: Reduction of surgical-site infections in cardiothoracic surgery by elimination of nasal carriage of Staphylococcus aureus. *Infect Control Hosp Epidemiol* 1996;17: 780-785.

24. Kluytmans JA, Wertheim HF: Nasal carriage of Staphylococcus aureus and prevention of nosocomial infections. *Infection* 2005;33:3-8.

25. Prokuski L: Prophylactic antibiotics in orthopaedic surgery. *J Am Acad Orthop Surg* 2008;16:283-293.

26. Slobogean GP, Kennedy SA, Davidson D, O'Brien PJ: Single- versus multiple-dose antibiotic prophylaxis in the surgical treatment of closed fractures: A meta-analysis. *J Orthop Trauma* 2008;22:264-269.

27. Dehne MG, Mühling J, Sablotzki A, Nopens H, Hempelmann G: Pharmacokinetics of antibiotic prophylaxis in major orthopedic surgery and blood-saving techniques. *Orthopedics* 2001;24:665-669.

28. Rosenberg AD, Wambold D, Kraemer L, et al: Ensuring appropriate timing of antimicrobial prophylaxis. *J Bone Joint Surg Am* 2008;90:226-232.

29. Tanner J, Swarbrook S, Stuart J: Surgical hand antisepsis to reduce surgical site infection. *Cochrane Database Syst Rev* 2008;1:CD004288.

30. Parienti JJ, Thibon P, Heller R, et al: Hand-rubbing with an aqueous alcoholic solution vs traditional surgical hand-scrubbing and 30-day surgical site infection rates: A randomized equivalence study. *JAMA* 2002;288: 722-727.

31. Hajipour L, Longstaff L, Cleeve V, Brewster N, Bint D, Henman P: Hand washing rituals in trauma theatre: Clean or dirty? *Ann R Coll Surg Engl* 2006;88:13-15.

32. Furukawa K, Tajiri T, Suzuki H, Norose Y: Are sterile water and brushes necessary for hand washing before surgery in Japan? *J Nippon Med Sch* 2005;72:149-154.

33. Wheelock SM, Lookinland S: Effect of surgical hand scrub time on subsequent bacterial growth. *AORN J* 1997;65:1087-1098.

34. Ostrander RV, Botte MJ, Brage ME: Efficacy of surgical preparation solutions in foot and ankle surgery. *J Bone Joint Surg Am* 2005;87:980-985.

35. Adams D, Quayum M, Worthington T, Lambert P, Elliott T: Evaluation of a 2% chlorhexidine gluconate in 70% isopropyl alcohol skin disinfectant. *J Hosp Infect* 2005;61:287-290.

36. Barenfanger J, Drake C, Lawhorn J, Verhulst SJ: Comparison of chlorhexidine and tincture of iodine for skin antisepsis in preparation for blood sample collection. *J Clin Microbiol* 2004;42:2216-2217.

37. Carlo A: The new era of flash sterilization. *AORN J* 2007;86:58-72.

38. Leonard Y, Speroni KG, Atherton M, Corriher J: Evaluating use of flash sterilization in the OR with regard to postoperative infections. *AORN J* 2006;83:672-680.

39. Huggins KA, Mood R, Koch F: A process for improving flash sterilization. *AORN J* 2002;75:127-133.

40. Dave J, Wilcox MH, Kellett M: Glove powder: Implications for infection control. *J Hosp Infect* 1999;42:283-285.

41. Jaffray DC, Nade S: Does surgical glove powder decrease the inoculum of bacteria required to produce an abscess? *J R Coll Surg Edinb* 1983;28: 219-222.

42. Korniewicz DM, Chookaew N, El-Masri M, Mudd K, Bollinger ME: Conversion to low-protein, powder-free surgical gloves: Is it worth the cost? *AAOHN J* 2005;53:388-393.

43. Edmiston CE, Seabrook GR, Goheen MP, et al: Bacterial adherence to surgical sutures: Can antibacterial-coated sutures reduce the risk of microbial contamination? *J Am Coll Surg* 2006;203:481-489.

44. Rozzelle CJ, Leonardo J, Li V: Antimicrobial suture wound closure for cerebrospinal fluid shunt surgery: A prospective, double-blinded, randomized controlled trial. *J Neurosurg Pediatr* 2008;2:111-117.

45. Allo MD, Tedesco M: Operating room management: Operative suite considerations, infection control. *Surg Clin North Am* 2005;85:1291-1297.

46. Babkin Y, Raveh D, Lifschitz M, et al: Incidence and risk factors for surgical infection after total knee replacement. *Scand J Infect Dis* 2007;39:890-895.

47. Parker MJ, Livingstone V, Clifton R, McKee A: Closed suction surgical wound drainage after orthopaedic surgery. *Cochrane Database Syst Rev* 2007;3:CD001825.

48. Ceccherini-Nelli L, Filipponi F, Mosca F, Campa M: The risk of contracting an infectious disease from blood transfusion. *Transplant Proc* 2004;36:680-682.

49. Weber EW, Slappendel R, Prins MH, van der Schaaf DB, Durieux ME, Strümper D: Perioperative blood transfusions and delayed wound healing after hip replacement surgery: Effects on duration of hospitalization. *Anesth Analg* 2005;100:1416-1421.

50. Vamvakas EC, Blajchman MA: Transfusion-related immunomodulation (TRIM): An update. *Blood Rev* 2007;21:327-348.

51. Talbot TR, D'Agata EM, Brinsko V, Lee B, Speroff T, Schaffner W: Perioperative blood transfusion is predictive of poststernotomy surgical site infection: Marker for morbidity or true immunosuppressant? *Clin Infect Dis* 2004;38:1378-1382.

52. Bower WF, Cheung CS, Lai RW, Underwood MJ, van Hasselt CA: An audit of risk factors for wound infection in patients undergoing coronary artery bypass grafting or valve replacement. *Hong Kong Med J* 2008;14:371-378.

53. Mangram AJ, Horan TC, Pearson ML, Silver LC, Jarvis WR; Hospital Infection Control Practices Advisory Committee: Guideline for prevention of surgical site infection, 1999. *Infect Control Hosp Epidemiol* 1999;20:250-280.

54. Huckfeldt R, Redmond C, Mikkelson D, Finley PJ, Lowe C, Robertson J: A clinical trial to investigate the effect of silver nylon dressings on mediastinitis rates in postoperative cardiac sternotomy incisions. *Ostomy Wound Manage* 2008;54:36-41.

55. Epstein NE: Do silver-impregnated dressings limit infections after lumbar laminectomy with instrumented fusion? *Surg Neurol* 2007;68:483-485.

56. Mueller SW, Krebsbach LE: Impact of an antimicrobial-impregnated gauze dressing on surgical site infections including methicillin-resistant Staphylococcus aureus infections. *Am J Infect Control* 2008;36:651-655.

57. Lee WR, Tobias KM, Bemis DA, Rohrbach BW: In vitro efficacy of a polyhexamethylene biguanide-impregnated gauze dressing against bacteria found in veterinary patients. *Vet Surg* 2004;33:404-411.

58. Boyce JM, Pittet D; Healthcare Infection Control Practices Advisory Committee; HICPAC/SHEA/APIC/IDSA Hand Hygiene Task Force; Society for Healthcare Epidemiology of America/Association for Professionals in Infection Control/Infectious Diseases Society of America: Guideline for hand hygiene in health-care settings: Recommendations of the Healthcare Infection Control Practices Advisory Committee and the HICPAC/SHEA/APIC/IDSA Hand Hygiene Task Force. *MMWR Recomm Rep* 2002;51(RR-16):1-45.

59. Joint Commission on Accreditation of Healthcare Organizations: *Comprehensive Accreditation Manual for Hospitals: The Official Handbook*. Oakbrook Terrace, IL, Joint Commission Resources, 2008.

60. Pittet D: Compliance with hand disinfection and its impact on hospital-acquired infections. *J Hosp Infect* 2001; 48(suppl A):S40-S46.

61. Pittet D, Hugonnet S, Harbarth S, et al: Effectiveness of a hospital-wide programme to improve compliance with hand hygiene: Infection Control Programme. *Lancet* 2000;356:1307-1312.

62. Larson EL, Cimiotti J, Haas J, et al: Effect of antiseptic handwashing vs alcohol sanitizer on health care-associated infections in neonatal intensive care units. *Arch Pediatr Adolesc Med* 2005;159:377-383.

63. Boyce JM, Kelliher S, Vallande N: Skin irritation and dryness associated with two hand-hygiene regimens: Soap-and-water hand washing versus hand antisepsis with an alcoholic hand gel. *Infect Control Hosp Epidemiol* 2000;21:442-448.

64. Morgan DJ, Diekema DJ, Sepkowitz K, Perencevich EN: Adverse outcomes associated with contact precautions: A review of the literature. *Am J Infect Control* 2009;37:85-93.

65. Centers for Medicare and Medicaid Services Website: Hospital Acquired Conditions. http://www.cms.hhs.gov/HospitalAcqCond/06_Hospital-Acquired_Conditions.asp#TopOfPage. Accessed December 21, 2009.

66. Lo E, Lindsay N, Classen D, et al: Strategies to prevent catheter-associated urinary tract infection in acute care hospitals. *Infect Control Hosp Epidemiol* 2008;29:S41-S50.

67. Centers for Disease Control and Prevention Website: National Healthcare Safety Network. Device-associated module. http://www.cdc.gov/nhsn/psc_da.html. Accessed December 21, 2009.

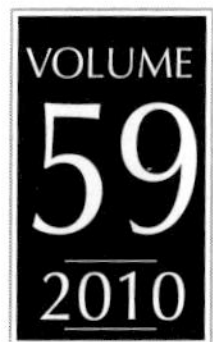

Index

Page numbers with *f* indicate figures
Page numbers with *t* indicate tables

A

B

C

D

M

P

Q

R

U